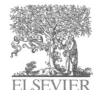
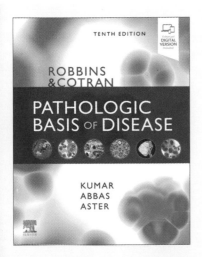
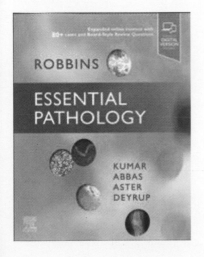

ROBBINS & KUMAR
BASIC PATHOLOGY

ELEVENTH EDITION

ROBBINS & KUMAR

BASIC PATHOLOGY

VINAY KUMAR, MBBS, MD, FRCPath
Lowell T. Coggeshall Distinguished Service
    Professor of Pathology
Biological Sciences Division and The Pritzker
    Medical School
University of Chicago
Chicago, Illinois

ABUL K. ABBAS, MBBS
Emeritus Professor
Department of Pathology
University of California San Francisco
San Francisco, California

JON C. ASTER, MD, PhD
Ramzi S. Cotran Professor of Pathology
Brigham and Women's Hospital and Harvard
    Medical School
Boston, Massachusetts

ANDREA T. DEYRUP, MD, PhD
Professor of Pathology
Duke University School of Medicine
Durham, North Carolina

ABHIJIT DAS, MD
Associate Professor of Pathology
Janakpuri Super Speciality Hospital
New Delhi, India

ELSEVIER

Elsevier
1600 John F. Kennedy Blvd.
Ste 1800
Philadelphia, PA 19103-2899

ROBBINS & KUMAR BASIC PATHOLOGY, ELEVENTH EDITION   ISBN: 978-0-323-79018-5
INTERNATIONAL EDITION   ISBN: 978-0-323-79019-2

Notice

Practitioners and researchers must always rely on their own experience and knowledge in evaluating and using any information, methods, compounds or experiments described herein. Because of rapid advances in the medical sciences, in particular, independent verification of diagnoses and drug dosages should be made. To the fullest extent of the law, no responsibility is assumed by Elsevier, authors, editors or contributors for any injury and/or damage to persons or property as a matter of products liability, negligence or otherwise, or from any use or operation of any methods, products, instructions, or ideas contained in the material herein.

Previous editions copyrighted 2018, 2013, 2007, 2003, 1997, 1992, 1987, 1981, 1976, and 1971.

Publisher: Jeremy Bowes
Director, Content Development: Rebecca Gruliow
Publishing Services Manager: Catherine Jackson
Senior Project Manager: Daniel Fitzgerald
Designer: Brian Salisbury

Printed in India

Last digit is the print number: 9 8 7 6 5 4 3 2

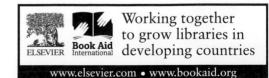

To our students who continue to challenge and inspire us.

PREFACE

Stanley Robbins conceived of *Basic Pathology* as a simple, clinically oriented textbook, published first in 1971. It had two authors: Robbins and Angell. Over the ensuing 50 years, driven by the goal of keeping the book up to date, most of the chapters were written by specialists. This has had the gradual (and inevitable) effect of making the book more complex. After careful thought, we decided a course correction was required. The eleventh edition reflects this in several ways:

- All chapters have been written and revised by the editors themselves.
- Over 150 new diagrams created by Dr. Abhijit Das (who joins us as an editor) have been added to illustrate complex disease mechanisms.
- To make *Basic Pathology* more useful for future physicians, tables listing commonly used laboratory tests with their pathophysiology and clinical relevance have been added to each chapter, an effort spearheaded by Dr. Andrea Deyrup, who has joined the editorial team.
- As an additional "tool" to help students focus on the fundamentals, we have created a Rapid Review section at the end of each chapter designed to provide key "take home" messages.
- Many new micrographs have been added to better illustrate disease processes. Additional figures, beyond those that appear in the text, have been added as eFigures that can be accessed in the online version of the textbook.
- Another major change has been to address the issue of health disparities and to reframe their relationship to socioeconomic factors and socially defined race. We engaged a consultant with expertise on the role of race in medicine, Dr. Joseph L. Graves, Jr., in this effort and have included a section on health disparities in

Chapter 7. Wherever possible, photographs of skin lesions in both lightly and more darkly pigmented skin have been included to reflect the range of clinical presentations, and illustrations that depict the human body have been made color neutral.

Although we have entered the "omics" era, the time-honored tools of gross and microscopic analysis remain central to understanding disease, and morphologic changes are highlighted for ready reference. The strong emphasis on clinicopathologic correlations is maintained, and, wherever understood, the impact of molecular pathology on the practice of medicine is emphasized. We are pleased that all of this was accomplished with a 10% "thinning" of the text.

We continue to firmly believe that clarity of writing and proper use of language enhance comprehension and facilitate the learning process. Those familiar with the previous editions will notice significant reorganization of the text in many chapters to improve the flow of information and make it more logical. We are in the digital age, so the text is available online along with 100 clinical cases with interactive features that are designed to be used as tutorials or self-study.

It is a privilege for us to edit this book, and we realize the considerable trust placed in us by students and teachers of pathology. We remain acutely conscious of this responsibility and hope that this edition will be worthy of and enhance the tradition of its forebears.

VK
AKA
JCA
ATD
AD

ACKNOWLEDGMENTS

Any large endeavor of this type cannot be completed without the help of many individuals. First and foremost, we thank the authors of various chapters in previous editions. Although the editors of this edition revised all chapters, the foundations were laid down by the previous contributors. They are acknowledged individually in the relevant chapters. We welcome two new editors—Andrea Deyrup and Abhijit Das—both of whom are seasoned educators. They have helped tremendously in our attempts to simplify the text and improve the illustrations.

We would like to recognize the Undergraduate Medical Educators Section of the Association of Pathology Chairs for their contributions to creating the laboratory test tables. In addition, we would like to express our gratitude to the Mayo Foundation for Medical Education and Research for allowing publication of reference values for the laboratory test tables from their website https://www.mayocliniclabs.com, accessed on 9/27/2022. Many additional colleagues have enhanced the text by carefully reviewing the laboratory tests to keep them at the levels appropriate for medical students. They are acknowledged individually with the relevant tables. Others have provided us with photographic gems from their personal collections; they are individually acknowledged in the credits for their contribution(s). Many new images have been taken from Dr. Edward Klatt's *Robbins and Cotran Atlas of Pathology* and Dr. Christopher Fletcher's *Histopathology of Tumors*. We are grateful to these authors for their generosity in allowing use of their pictures. In addition, we would like to thank the University of Michigan Department of Pathology for permission to use images from their virtual slide box (https://www.pathology.med.umich.edu/slides). We would like to thank Dr. Joseph Graves, Jr., for his recommendations about how race and ancestry should be addressed in the text. In addition, we are grateful to those who reviewed content of individual chapters. They include Dr. Julianne Elofson, the Dimmock Center of Roxbury, MA (addiction medicine); Dr. Sarah Wolfe, Duke University (dermatology); Dr. Susan Lester, Brigham and Women's Hospital (breast pathology); Dr. Thomas Cummings, Duke University (eye and brain pathology); Dr. Jessica Seidelman, Duke University (infectious disease); and Franca Alphin, Duke University (nutrition). For any unintended omissions, we offer our apologies.

Many at Elsevier deserve recognition for their roles in the production of this book. This text was fortunate to be in the hands of Rebecca Gruliow (Director, Content Development), who has been our partner for several editions. Others deserving of our thanks are Jim Merritt (Executive Content Strategist) and Jeremey Bowes (Publisher). We are especially grateful to the entire production team, in particular Dan Fitzgerald, Senior Project Manager, for tolerating our sometimes next to "impossible" demands and for putting up with our idiosyncrasies during the periods of extreme exhaustion that afflict all authors who undertake what seems like an endless task. We are thankful to the entire Elsevier team for sharing our passion for excellence, including Brian Salisbury (Senior Book Designer), Muthu Thangaraj (Senior Graphic Artist), Nijantha Priyadharshini (Graphics Coordinator), Narayanan Ramakrishnan (Graphics Coordinator), and Santhoshkumar Iaraju (Senior Producer, Digital Media). We also thank numerous students and teachers scattered across the globe for raising questions about the clarity of content and serving as the ultimate "copyeditors." Their efforts reassured us that the book is read seriously by them.

Ventures such as this exact a heavy toll from the families of the authors. We thank them for their tolerance of our absences, both physical and emotional. We are blessed and strengthened by their unconditional support and love and by their sharing with us the belief that our efforts are worthwhile and useful. We are especially grateful to our spouses Raminder Kumar, Ann Abbas, Erin Malone, Tony Williamson, and Kankana Roy who continue to provide steadfast support.

And, finally, we the editors salute each other; our partnership thrives because of a shared vision of excellence in teaching despite differences in opinions and individual styles.

VK
AKA
JCA
ATD
AD

ONLINE RESOURCES FOR INSTRUCTORS AND STUDENTS

RESOURCES FOR INSTRUCTORS

The following resources for instructors are available for use when teaching via Evolve. Contact your local sales representative for more information or go directly to the Evolve website to request access: https://evolve.elsevier.com. Note: *It may take 1–3 days for account access setup and verification upon initial account setup.*

Image Collection

To assist in the classroom, we have made the images available for instructors for teaching purposes. The images are provided in JPEG, PowerPoint®, and PDF versions with labels on/off and may be downloaded for use in lecture presentations.

Test Bank

Instructors can access a complete test bank of over 250 multiple-choice questions for use in teaching.

RESOURCES FOR STUDENTS

The following resources are available at eBooks.Health.Elsevier.com to students with purchase of *Robbins & Kumar Basic Pathology* (11th edition).

Textbook Online

The complete textbook is available online at eBooks.Health.Elsevier.com. The online version is fully searchable and provides all figures from the print book, with enhanced functionality for many, including clickable enlargements and slideshow views of multiple-part images.

Clinical Cases

Students can study over 100 clinical cases available online on eBooks.Health.Elsevier.com. The clinical cases are designed to enhance clinical pathologic correlations and pathophysiology.

Self-Assessment Questions

Students can test and score themselves with interactive multiple-choice questions linked to chapters online at eBooks.Health.Elsevier.com.

CONTENTS

CONTENTS

Cell Injury, Cell Death, and Adaptations

INTRODUCTION TO PATHOLOGY

The field of pathology is dedicated to understanding the causes of disease and the changes in cells, tissues, and organs that are associated with development of disease. Thus, **pathology provides the scientific foundation for the practice of medicine.** There are two important terms that students will encounter throughout their study of pathology and medicine:

- *Etiology* is the origin of a disease, including the underlying causes and modifying factors. Notably, many common diseases, such as hypertension, diabetes, and cancer, are caused by a combination of inherited genetic susceptibility and various environmental triggers. Elucidating the genetic and environmental factors underlying diseases is a major goal of modern medicine.
- *Pathogenesis* refers to the steps in the development of disease, from the initial etiologic trigger to the cellular and molecular changes that give rise to the specific functional and structural abnormalities which characterize any particular disease. Thus, etiology refers to *why* a disease arises and pathogenesis describes *how* a disease develops (Fig. 1.1).

Defining the etiology and pathogenesis of disease is essential not only for understanding disease but is also the basis for developing rational treatments. It is now appreciated that even diseases that present with similar morphologic features (e.g., cancer of a particular organ) show important molecular differences (e.g., mutations, epigenetic modifications) from case to case. This realization has launched the field of *precision* (or *personalized*) *medicine*, in which therapies are designed for each individual's disease rather than the diseases as a whole.

To render diagnoses and guide therapy in clinical practice, pathologists identify changes in the gross or microscopic appearance (morphology) of cells and tissues and in their constituents (e.g., genes and proteins), as well as biochemical alterations in body fluids (such as blood and urine). Defining these alterations in diseased tissues aids in diagnosis as well as in predicting outcomes and optimal therapies.

OVERVIEW OF CELLULAR RESPONSES TO STRESS AND NOXIOUS STIMULI

Cells actively interact with their environment, constantly adjusting their structure and function to accommodate changing demands and extracellular stresses in order to maintain a steady state, a process called *homeostasis*. As cells encounter physiologic stresses or injurious stimuli, they can undergo *adaptation*, achieving a new steady state and preserving viability and function. If the adaptive capability is exceeded or if the external stress is inherently harmful, *cell injury* occurs (Fig. 1.2). Within certain limits, injury is *reversible*, and homeostasis is restored; however, if the stress is severe or persistent, it results in *irreversible injury* and death of the affected cells. *Cell death* is a crucial event in the development of many diseases.

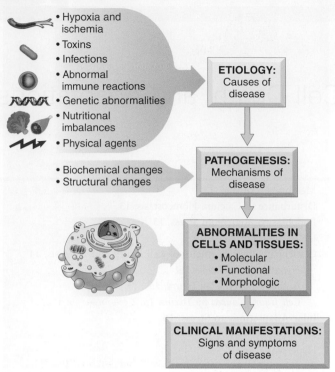

- Hypoxia and ischemia
- Toxins
- Infections
- Abnormal immune reactions
- Genetic abnormalities
- Nutritional imbalances
- Physical agents

ETIOLOGY: Causes of disease

- Biochemical changes
- Structural changes

PATHOGENESIS: Mechanisms of disease

ABNORMALITIES IN CELLS AND TISSUES:
- Molecular
- Functional
- Morphologic

CLINICAL MANIFESTATIONS: Signs and symptoms of disease

FIG. 1.1 Steps in the development of disease. Only some of the major etiologies are shown.

Cell injury is the basis of all disease, and in this chapter we discuss the causes, mechanisms, and consequences of reversible injury and cell death. We then consider cellular adaptations to stress and conclude with two other processes that affect cells and tissues, the deposition of abnormal substances and cell aging.

CAUSES OF CELL INJURY

The major causes of cell injury can be grouped into the following categories.

- *Hypoxia and ischemia.* Hypoxia refers to oxygen deficiency, and ischemia means reduced blood supply. These are among the most common causes of cell injury. Both deprive tissues of oxygen, the essential molecule for generating energy for cell function and survival, and ischemia also reduces the supply of nutrients. The most common cause of hypoxia is ischemia resulting from blockage of an artery, but it can also result from inadequate oxygenation of the blood, as in diseases of the lung, or from reduction in the oxygen-carrying capacity of the blood, as with anemia of any cause.
- *Toxins.* Potentially toxic agents are encountered daily in the environment; these include air pollutants, insecticides, carbon monoxide, asbestos, cigarette smoke, ethanol, and drugs. Many therapeutic drugs can cause cell or tissue injury in a susceptible patient or if used excessively or inappropriately (Chapter 7).
- *Infectious agents.* All types of infectious pathogens, such as viruses, bacteria, fungi, and parasites, can injure cells by diverse mechanisms, including liberation of toxins and eliciting harmful immune responses.
- *Immunologic reactions.* Although the immune system defends the body against pathogenic microbes, immune reactions can also result in cell and tissue injury. Examples are autoimmune reactions against one's own tissues, allergic reactions against environmental

substances, and excessive or chronic immune responses to microbes (Chapter 5). In all these situations, the immune responses elicit inflammatory reactions, and inflammation is often the cause of damage to cells and tissues.
- *Genetic abnormalities.* Some chromosomal abnormalities or mutations can result in pathologic changes as conspicuous as the congenital malformations associated with Down syndrome or as subtle as the single amino acid substitution in hemoglobin that gives rise to sickle cell anemia (Chapter 4). Mutations may cause cell injury as a consequence of a decrease (e.g., enzymes in inborn errors of metabolism) or an increase in the function of a protein, or through the accumulation of damaged DNA or misfolded proteins, which can trigger cell death. Mutations also have a central role in cancer development (Chapter 6).
- *Nutritional imbalances.* Protein-calorie insufficiency remains a major cause of cell injury, and specific vitamin deficiencies occur frequently even in countries with plentiful resources (Chapter 7). On the other hand, excessive dietary intake may result in obesity, which is an important underlying factor in many common diseases, such as type 2 diabetes and atherosclerosis.
- *Physical agents.* Trauma, extremes of temperature, radiation, electric shock, and sudden changes in atmospheric pressure all have damaging effects on cells (Chapter 7).

With this introduction, we proceed to a discussion of the process and morphologic manifestations of cell injury and then the biochemical mechanisms of injury caused by different noxious stimuli.

SEQUENCE OF EVENTS IN CELL INJURY AND CELL DEATH

Although injurious stimuli damage cells through diverse biochemical mechanisms, all tend to induce a stereotypic sequence of morphologic and structural alterations in most cell types.

Reversible Cell Injury

Reversible cell injury is defined as a derangement of function and morphology that cells can recover from if the damaging stimulus is removed (Fig. 1.3). In reversible injury, cells and intracellular

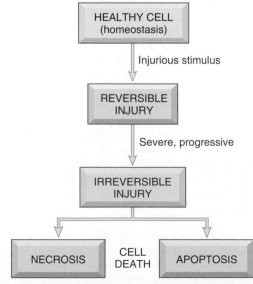

HEALTHY CELL (homeostasis)

Injurious stimulus

REVERSIBLE INJURY

Severe, progressive

IRREVERSIBLE INJURY

NECROSIS   CELL DEATH   **APOPTOSIS**

FIG. 1.2 Sequence of reversible cell injury and cell death.

organelles become swollen because they take in water as a result of the failure of energy-dependent ion pumps in the plasma membrane. In some forms of injury, degenerated organelles and lipids accumulate inside the injured cells.

MORPHOLOGY

The two most consistent morphologic correlates of reversible cell injury are cellular swelling and fatty change.

- **Cellular swelling** (Fig. 1.4B) is commonly seen when cells are injured by hypoxia, toxins, and other causes. It may be difficult to appreciate with the light microscope (since fluid from cells is extracted during tissue processing) but is often apparent grossly when the whole organ is examined. When many cells in an organ are affected, there can be pallor (due to compression of capillaries), increased turgor, and increased organ weight. Microscopic examination may reveal small, clear vacuoles within the cytoplasm; these represent distended and pinched-off segments of the endoplasmic reticulum (ER). This pattern of nonlethal injury is sometimes called **hydropic change** or **vacuolar degeneration.**
- **Fatty change** is manifested by the appearance of lipid vacuoles in the cytoplasm. It is principally encountered in organs that are involved in lipid metabolism, such as the liver, and hence it is discussed in Chapter 14.

The cytoplasm of injured cells also may become redder (eosinophilic, meaning stained red by the dye eosin—the *E* in the hematoxylin and eosin [H&E] stain)—a change that becomes more pronounced with progression to necrosis (described later). Other intracellular changes associated with cell injury, which are best seen by electron microscopy (eFig. 1.1), include: (1) plasma membrane alterations such as blebbing, blunting, or distortion of microvilli, and loosening of intercellular attachments; (2) mitochondrial changes such as swelling and the appearance of phospholipid-rich amorphous densities; (3) dilation of the ER with detachment of ribosomes and dissociation of polysomes; and (4) nuclear alterations, with clumping of chromatin. The cytoplasm may contain so-called **myelin figures,** collections of phospholipids resembling myelin sheaths that are derived from damaged cellular membranes.

In some situations, potentially injurious insults induce specific alterations in cellular organelles, like the endoplasmic reticulum (ER). The smooth ER is involved in the metabolism of various chemicals, including alcohol and drugs such as barbiturates (Chapter 7). Cells exposed to these chemicals show hypertrophy of the smooth ER as an adaptive response that may have important functional consequences. Cells adapted to one drug may have increased capacity to metabolize other compounds handled by the same system. Thus, if patients taking phenobarbital for epilepsy increase their alcohol intake, they may experience a drop in blood concentration of the antiseizure medication to subtherapeutic levels because of increased activity of the smooth ER in response to the alcohol.

Persistent or excessive injury causes injured cells to pass the nebulous "point of no return" and undergo cell death, typically by the process of necrosis. Although there are no definitive morphologic or biochemical correlates of irreversible injury, it is consistently characterized by three phenomena: the inability to restore mitochondrial function (oxidative phosphorylation and adenosine triphosphate [ATP] generation) even after resolution of the original injury; altered structure and loss of function of the plasma membrane and intracellular membranes; and the loss of structural integrity of DNA and chromatin. As discussed in more detail later,

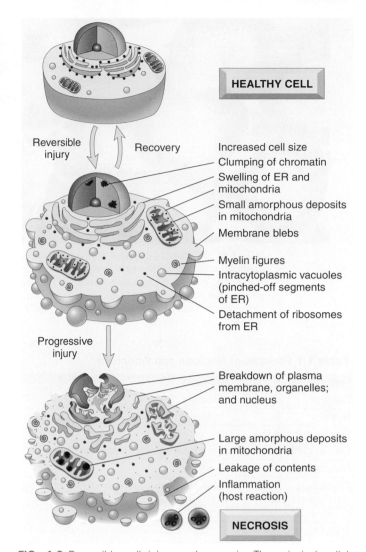

FIG. 1.3 Reversible cell injury and necrosis. The principal cellular alterations that characterize reversible cell injury and necrosis are illustrated. If an injurious stimulus is not removed, reversible injury culminates in necrosis.

Labels in figure:
HEALTHY CELL
Reversible injury — Recovery
Increased cell size
Clumping of chromatin
Swelling of ER and mitochondria
Small amorphous deposits in mitochondria
Membrane blebs
Myelin figures
Intracytoplasmic vacuoles (pinched-off segments of ER)
Detachment of ribosomes from ER
Progressive injury
Breakdown of plasma membrane, organelles; and nucleus
Large amorphous deposits in mitochondria
Leakage of contents
Inflammation (host reaction)
NECROSIS

injury to lysosomal membranes results in the enzymatic digestion of the injured cell, which is the culmination of necrosis.

Cell Death

When cells are injured, they die by different mechanisms, depending on the nature and severity of the insult (Table 1.1).

- *Necrosis.* Severe disturbances, such as loss of oxygen and nutrient supply and the actions of toxins, cause a rapid and uncontrollable form of death that has been called "accidental" cell death. The morphologic manifestation of accidental cell death is **necrosis** (Greek, *necros* = death). Necrosis is the major pathway of cell death in many commonly encountered injuries, such as those resulting from ischemia, exposure to toxins, various infections, and trauma. Necrosis is considered the inevitable end result of severe damage that is beyond salvage and is not thought to be regulated by specific signals or biochemical mechanisms; necrosis occurs because the injury goes beyond what a cell can repair or survive.

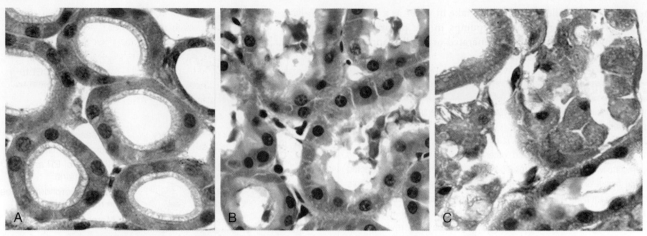

FIG. 1.4 Morphologic changes in reversible cell injury and necrosis. (A) Normal kidney tubules with viable epithelial cells. (B) Early (reversible) ischemic injury showing surface blebs, increased eosinophilia of cytoplasm, and swelling of occasional cells. (C) Necrosis (irreversible injury) of epithelial cells, with loss of nuclei and fragmentation of cells and leakage of contents. (Courtesy of Drs. Neal Pinckard and M.A. Venkatachalam, University of Texas Health Sciences Center, San Antonio, TX.)

Table 1.1 Features of Necrosis and Apoptosis

Feature	Necrosis	Apoptosis
Cell size	Enlarged (swelling)	Reduced (shrinkage)
Nucleus	Pyknosis → karyorrhexis → karyolysis	Fragmentation into nucleosome-sized fragments
Plasma membrane	Disrupted	Intact; altered structure, especially orientation of lipids
Cellular contents	Enzymatic digestion; may leak out of cell	Intact; may be released in apoptotic bodies
Adjacent inflammation	Frequent	Absent
Physiologic or pathologic role	Invariably pathologic (culmination of irreversible cell injury)	Often physiologic; means of eliminating unnecessary cells; may be pathologic after some forms of cell injury, especially DNA and protein damage

DNA, Deoxyribonucleic acid.

- *Apoptosis.* By contrast, when cells must be eliminated without eliciting a host reaction, a precise set of molecular pathways is activated in the cells that produce a form of cell death called **apoptosis** (see Table 1.1). Apoptosis relies on defined genes and biochemical pathways and must be tightly controlled because once it starts, it is irreversible; thus, it is referred to as "regulated" cell death. The discovery of regulated cell death was a revelation, since it showed that cell death can be an intentional, highly controlled process. Apoptosis serves to eliminate cells with a variety of intrinsic abnormalities and promotes clearance of the fragments of the dead cells without eliciting an inflammatory reaction. This "clean" form of cell suicide occurs in pathologic situations when a cell's DNA or proteins are damaged beyond repair or the cell is deprived of necessary survival signals. **But unlike necrosis, which is always an indication of a pathologic process, apoptosis also occurs in healthy tissues and is not necessarily associated with pathologic cell injury.** For example, it serves to eliminate unwanted cells during development and to maintain constant cell numbers. This type of physiologic cell death is also called *programmed cell death.*

It is important to recognize that **cellular function may be lost long before cell death occurs and that the morphologic changes of cell injury (or death) lag behind loss of function and viability** (Fig. 1.5). For example, myocardial cells become noncontractile after 1 to 2 minutes of ischemia but may not die until 20 to 30 minutes of ischemia have elapsed. Morphologic features indicative of the death of ischemic myocytes appear by electron microscopy within 2 to 3 hours after the death of the cells but are not evident by light microscopy until 6 to 12 hours later.

Necrosis

In necrosis, cellular membranes fall apart, cellular enzymes leak out and ultimately digest the cell, and there is an accompanying inflammatory reaction (see Fig. 1.3). The local host reaction, called *inflammation,* is induced by substances released from dead cells and serves to eliminate debris and start the subsequent repair process (Chapter 2). The enzymes responsible for digestion of the dead cells come from leukocytes that are recruited as part of the inflammatory reaction and from the disrupted lysosomes of the dying cells themselves.

The biochemical mechanisms of necrosis vary with different injurious stimuli and are described later.

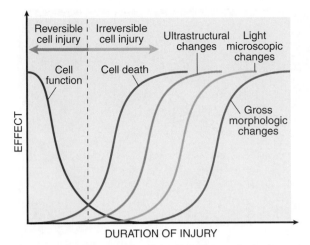

FIG. 1.5 The relationship of cellular function, cell death, and the morphologic changes of cell injury. Note that cells may rapidly become nonfunctional after the onset of injury yet still be viable, with potentially reversible damage; with a longer duration of injury, irreversible injury and cell death may result. Cell death typically precedes ultrastructural, light microscopic, and grossly visible morphologic changes.

MORPHOLOGY

Necrosis is characterized by changes in the cytoplasm and nuclei of the injured cells (see Figs. 1.3 and 1.4C).

- **Cytoplasmic changes.** Necrotic cells show increased eosinophilia, attributable in part to increased binding of eosin to denatured cytoplasmic proteins and in part to loss of basophilic ribonucleic acid (RNA) in the cytoplasm (basophilia stems from binding of the blue dye hematoxylin—the *H* in "H&E"). Compared with viable cells, necrotic cells may have a glassy, homogeneous appearance, mostly due to the loss of glycogen particles. When enzymes have digested cytoplasmic organelles, the cytoplasm becomes vacuolated and appears "motheaten." By electron microscopy, necrotic cells are characterized by discontinuities in plasma and organelle membranes, marked dilation of mitochondria associated with large amorphous intramitrochondrial densities, disruption of lysosomes, and intracytoplasmic myelin figures, which are more prominent in necrotic cells than in cells with reversible injury (eFig. 1.1).
- **Nuclear changes.** Nuclear changes assume one of three patterns, all caused by breakdown of DNA and chromatin. **Pyknosis** is characterized by nuclear shrinkage and increased basophilia; the DNA condenses into a dark, shrunken mass. The pyknotic nucleus can subsequently undergo fragmentation; this change is called **karyorrhexis**. At the same time, the nucleus may undergo **karyolysis**, in which the basophilia fades due to digestion of deoxyribonucleic acid (DNA) by DNase. In 1 to 2 days, the nucleus in a dead cell may undergo complete dissolution.
- **Fates of necrotic cells.** Necrotic cells may persist for some time or may be digested by enzymes and disappear. Dead cells may be replaced by myelin figures, which are either phagocytosed by other cells or further degraded into fatty acids. These fatty acids bind calcium salts, which may result in the dead cells ultimately becoming calcified (**dystrophic calcification**, see later).

Morphologic Patterns of Tissue Necrosis

Some severe injuries result in the death of many or all cells in a tissue or even an entire organ. This may happen in severe ischemia, infections, and inflammatory reactions. There are several morphologically distinct patterns of tissue necrosis, which may provide clues about the underlying cause. Although the terms that describe these patterns do not reflect underlying mechanisms, such terms are commonly used and their implications are understood by pathologists and clinicians. Most of the types of necrosis have distinctive gross appearances; fibrinoid necrosis is detected only by microscopic examination.

MORPHOLOGY

- In **coagulative necrosis,** the underlying tissue architecture is preserved for at least several days after the injury (Fig. 1.6). The affected tissues take on a firm texture. Presumably, the injury denatures not only structural proteins but also enzymes, limiting the proteolysis of the dead cells; as a result, eosinophilic, anucleate cells may persist for days or weeks. Ultimately, the dead cells are digested by the lysosomal enzymes of recruited leukocytes and the cellular debris is removed by phagocytosis. Coagulative necrosis is characteristic of infarcts (areas of necrosis caused by ischemia) in all solid organs except the brain.
- **Liquefactive necrosis** is seen at sites of bacterial or, occasionally, fungal infections, because microbes stimulate the accumulation of inflammatory cells and the enzymes of leukocytes digest ("liquefy") the tissue. For obscure reasons, hypoxic death of cells within the central nervous system often causes liquefactive necrosis (Fig. 1.7). In this form of necrosis, the dead cells are completely digested, transforming the tissue into a viscous liquid that is eventually removed by phagocytes. When the process is initiated by acute inflammation, as in a bacterial infection, the material is frequently creamy yellow and is called **pus**. A localized collection of pus is called an **abscess** (Chapter 2).
- Although **gangrenous necrosis** is not a distinctive pattern of cell death, the term is still commonly used in clinical practice. It usually refers to the condition of a limb (generally the lower leg) that has lost its blood supply and has undergone coagulative necrosis involving multiple tissue layers. When bacterial infection is superimposed, the morphologic appearance is often liquefactive because of destruction mediated by the contents of the bacteria and the attracted leukocytes (resulting in so-called **wet gangrene**).
- **Caseous necrosis** is encountered most often in foci of tuberculous infection. Caseous means "cheese-like," referring to the friable yellow-white appearance of the area of necrosis (Fig. 1.8). On microscopic examination, the necrotic focus appears as a collection of cellular debris with an amorphous granular pink appearance in H&E-stained tissue sections. Unlike coagulative necrosis, the tissue architecture is obliterated and cellular outlines cannot be discerned. Caseous necrosis is often surrounded by a collection of macrophages and other inflammatory cells; this appearance is characteristic of a nodular inflammatory lesion called a **granuloma** (Chapter 2).
- **Fat necrosis** refers to focal areas of fat destruction, which can be due to abdominal trauma or acute pancreatitis (Chapter 15), in which enzymes leak out of damaged pancreatic acinar cells and ducts and digest peritoneal fat cells and their contents, including stored triglycerides. The released fatty acids combine with calcium to produce grossly identifiable chalky white lesions (Fig. 1.9). On histologic examination, the foci of necrosis contain shadowy outlines of necrotic fat cells surrounded by granular basophilic calcium deposits and an inflammatory reaction.
- **Fibrinoid necrosis** is a special form of necrosis, visible by light microscopy. It may be seen in immune reactions in which complexes of antigens and antibodies are deposited in the walls of blood vessels, and in severe hypertension. Deposited immune complexes and plasma proteins that have leaked into the walls of injured vessels produce a bright pink, amorphous appearance on H&E preparations called fibrinoid (fibrin-like) by pathologists (Fig. 1.10). Fibrinoid necrosis is seen most often in certain forms of vasculitis (Chapter 3) and in transplanted organs undergoing rejection (Chapter 5).

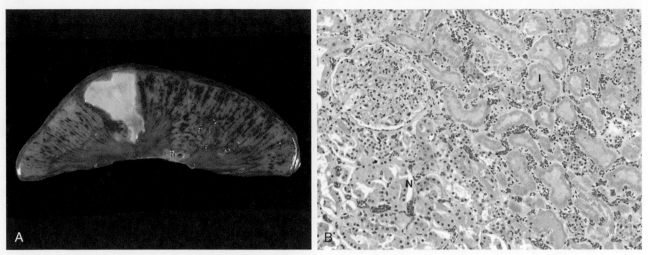

FIG. 1.6 Coagulative necrosis. (A) A wedge-shaped kidney infarct *(yellow)* with distinct margins. (B) Microscopic view of the edge of the infarct, with normal kidney *(N)* and necrotic cells in the infarct *(I)*. The necrotic cells show preserved outlines with loss of nuclei, and an inflammatory infiltrate is present (difficult to discern at this magnification).

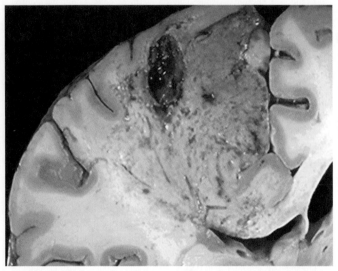

FIG. 1.7 Liquefactive necrosis. An infarct in the brain showing dissolution of the tissue.

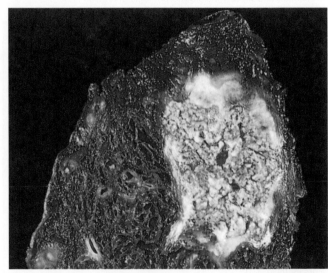

FIG. 1.8 Caseous necrosis. Tuberculosis of the lung, with a large area of caseous necrosis containing yellow-white (cheesy) debris.

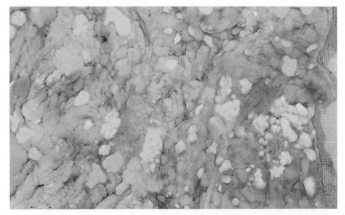

FIG. 1.9 Fat necrosis in acute pancreatitis. The areas of white chalky deposits represent foci of fat necrosis with calcium soap formation (saponification) at sites of lipid breakdown in the mesentery.

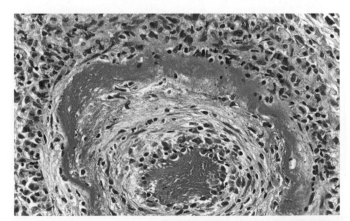

FIG. 1.10 Fibrinoid necrosis in an artery in a patient with polyarteritis nodosa, a form of vasculitis (Chapter 3). The wall of the artery shows a circumferential bright pink area of necrosis with protein deposition and inflammation.

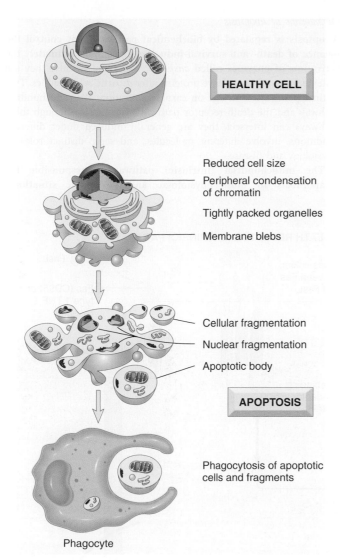

HEALTHY CELL

Reduced cell size

Peripheral condensation
of chromatin

Tightly packed organelles

Membrane blebs

Cellular fragmentation

Nuclear fragmentation

Apoptotic body

APOPTOSIS

Phagocytosis of apoptotic
cells and fragments

Phagocyte

FIG. 1.11 Apoptosis. The cellular alterations in apoptosis are illustrated. Contrast these with the changes that characterize necrotic cell death, shown in Fig. 1.3.

Leakage of intracellular proteins through the damaged cell membrane provides a means of detecting tissue-specific necrosis using blood or serum samples. Cardiac muscle, for example, contains a unique isoform of the contractile protein troponin, whereas hepatic bile duct epithelium contains a temperature-resistant isoform of the enzyme alkaline phosphatase, and hepatocytes contain transaminases. These proteins leak out of necrotic cells into the blood, where they serve as clinically useful markers of damage in the corresponding tissues.

Apoptosis

Apoptosis is a pathway of cell death in which cells activate enzymes that degrade the cells' own nuclear DNA and nuclear and cytoplasmic proteins (Fig. 1.11). Fragments of the apoptotic cells then break off, giving the appearance that is responsible for the name (*apoptosis*, "falling off"). The plasma membrane of the apoptotic cell remains intact, but the membrane is altered in such a way that the fragments, called apoptotic bodies, are recognized and rapidly phagocytosed by macrophages. In contrast to necrosis (see Table 1.1), the apoptotic cell and its fragments are cleared before cellular contents have leaked out, so apoptotic cell death does not elicit an inflammatory reaction in the host.

Causes of Apoptosis

Apoptosis occurs in many physiologic conditions and serves to eliminate potentially harmful cells and cells that have outlived their usefulness (Table 1.2). It also occurs as a pathologic event when cells are damaged beyond repair, especially when the damage affects the cells' DNA or proteins.

- *Physiologic apoptosis.* During the normal development of an organism, some cells die and are replaced by new ones. In mature organisms, highly proliferative and hormone-responsive tissues undergo cycles of proliferation and cell loss that are often determined by the levels of growth factors or survival signals. In these situations, the cell death is always by apoptosis, ensuring that unwanted cells are eliminated without eliciting potentially harmful inflammation. In the immune system, apoptosis removes excess leukocytes following immune

Table 1.2 Physiologic and Pathologic Conditions Associated With Apoptosis

Condition	Mechanism of Apoptosis
Physiologic	
During embryogenesis	Loss of growth factor signaling (presumed mechanism)
Turnover of proliferative tissues (e.g., intestinal epithelium, lymphocytes in lymph nodes and thymus)	Loss of growth factor signaling or survival signals (presumed mechanism)
Involution of hormone-dependent tissues (e.g., endometrium)	Decreased hormone levels lead to reduced survival signals
Decline of leukocyte numbers at the end of immune and inflammatory responses	Loss of survival signals as stimulus for leukocyte activation is eliminated
Elimination of potentially harmful self-reactive lymphocytes	Strong recognition of self antigens induces apoptosis by both the mitochondrial and death receptor pathways
Pathologic	
DNA damage	Activation of proapoptotic BH3-only proteins
Accumulation of misfolded proteins	Activation of proapoptotic BH3-only proteins, possibly direct activation of caspases
Infections, especially certain viral infections	Activation of proapoptotic proteins or caspases by viral proteins; killing of infected cells by cytotoxic T lymphocytes (CTLs), which activate caspases

responses, B lymphocytes in germinal centers that fail to produce high-affinity antibodies, and lymphocytes that recognize self antigens that could cause autoimmune diseases if they were to survive (Chapter 5).

- *Apoptosis in pathologic conditions.* Apoptosis eliminates cells with certain types of irreparable damage, such as severe DNA damage, e.g., after exposure to radiation and cytotoxic drugs. The accumulation of misfolded proteins also triggers apoptotic death; the underlying mechanisms of this cause of cell death and its significance in disease are discussed later, in the context of ER stress. Certain infectious agents, particularly some viruses, also induce apoptotic death of infected cells.

Mechanisms of Apoptosis

Apoptosis is regulated by biochemical pathways that control the balance of death- and survival-inducing signals and ultimately the activation of enzymes called *caspases*, so named because they are *cy*steine prote*ases* that cleave proteins after *asp*artic acid residues. Two distinct pathways converge on caspase activation: the mitochondrial pathway and the death receptor pathway (Fig. 1.12). Although these pathways can intersect, they are generally induced under different conditions, involve different molecules, and serve distinct roles in physiology and disease.

- **The mitochondrial (intrinsic) pathway is responsible for apoptosis in most physiologic and pathologic situations.**

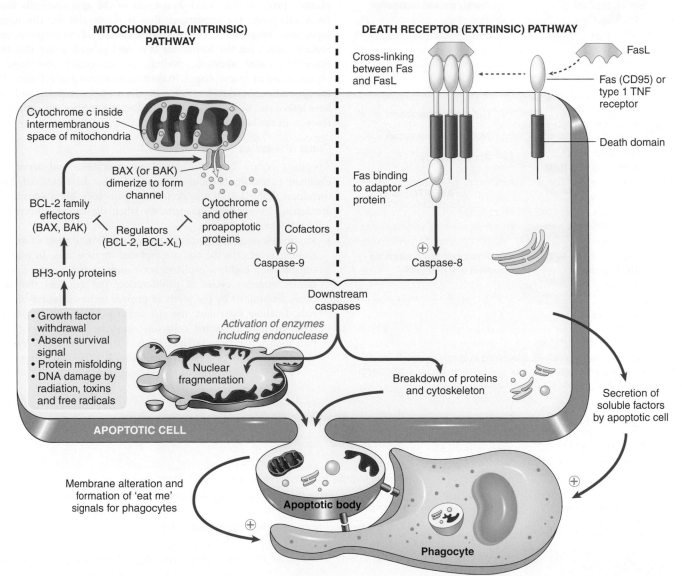

FIG. 1.12 Mechanisms of apoptosis. The two pathways of apoptosis differ in their induction and regulation, but both culminate in the activation of caspases. In the mitochondrial pathway, BH3-only proteins sense a lack of survival signals or DNA or protein damage and activate effector molecules that increase mitochondrial permeability. In concert with a deficiency of BCL-2 and other proteins that oppose mitochondrial permeability, the mitochondria become leaky and various substances, such as cytochrome c, enter the cytosol and activate caspases. Activated caspases induce the changes that culminate in cell death and fragmentation. In the death receptor pathway, signals from plasma membrane receptors lead to the assembly of adaptor proteins into a "death-inducing signaling complex," which activates caspases, and the end result is the same.

Mitochondria contain several proteins that are capable of inducing apoptosis, including cytochrome c. When mitochondrial membranes become permeable, cytochrome c leaks into the cytoplasm, triggering caspase activation and apoptotic death. The permeability of mitochondria is controlled by a family of more than 20 proteins, the prototype of which is BCL-2. In healthy cells, BCL-2 and the related protein BCL-X_L are produced in response to growth factors and other stimuli that keep cells viable. These antiapoptotic proteins maintain the integrity of mitochondrial membranes, in large part by holding two proapoptotic members of the family, BAX and BAK, in check. When cells are deprived of growth factors and survival signals, are exposed to agents that damage DNA, or accumulate unacceptable amounts of misfolded proteins, a number of sensors are activated. The most important of these sensors are called BH3-only proteins because they contain the third homology domain of the BCL-2 family. These sensors shift the balance in favor of BAK and BAX, which dimerize, insert into the mitochondrial membrane, and form channels through which cytochrome c and other mitochondrial proteins escape into the cytosol. At the same time, the deficiency of survival signals leads to decreased levels of BCL-2 and BCL-X_L, further compromising mitochondrial permeability. Once in the cytosol, cytochrome c interacts with certain cofactors and activates caspase-9, leading to the activation of a caspase cascade.

- **The death receptor (extrinsic) pathway of apoptosis.** Many cells express surface molecules, called death receptors, which trigger apoptosis. Most of these are members of the tumor necrosis factor (TNF) receptor family, which contain in their cytoplasmic regions a conserved "death domain," so named because it mediates interaction with other proteins involved in cell death. The prototypic death receptors are the type I TNF receptor and Fas (CD95). Fas ligand (FasL) is a membrane protein expressed mainly on activated T lymphocytes. When these T cells recognize Fas-expressing targets, Fas molecules are crosslinked by FasL and bind adaptor proteins via the death domain (see Fig. 1.12). These recruit and activate caspase-8, which in turn activates downstream caspases. The death receptor pathway is involved in elimination of self-reactive lymphocytes and in killing of target cells by some cytotoxic T lymphocytes that express FasL.
- **Terminal phase of apoptosis.** Activated caspase-8 and caspase-9 act through a final common series of reactions that first involve the activation of additional caspases, which through numerous substrates ultimately activate enzymes that degrade the cell's proteins and nucleus. The end result is the characteristic cellular fragmentation of apoptosis.
- **Clearance of apoptotic cells.** Apoptotic cells and their fragments entice phagocytes by producing a number of "eat-me" signals. For instance, in normal cells phosphatidylserine is present on the inner leaflet of the plasma membrane, but in apoptotic cells this phospholipid "flips" to the outer leaflet, where it is recognized by tissue macrophages. Cells that are dying by apoptosis also secrete soluble factors that recruit phagocytes. Numerous macrophage receptors are involved in the binding and engulfment of apoptotic cells. This process is so efficient that the dead cells disappear without leaving a trace, and there is no accompanying inflammation.

MORPHOLOGY

In H&E-stained tissue sections, the nuclei of apoptotic cells show various stages of chromatin condensation, aggregation, and, ultimately, karyorrhexis (Fig. 1.13). At the molecular level this is reflected in fragmentation of DNA into nucleosome-sized pieces. The cells rapidly shrink, form cytoplasmic buds, and fragment into apoptotic bodies that are composed of membrane-bound pieces of cytosol and organelles (eFig. 1.2; also see Fig. 1.11). Because these fragments are quickly shed and phagocytosed without eliciting an inflammatory response, even substantial apoptosis may be histologically undetectable.

Other pathways of cell death, in addition to necrosis and apoptosis, have been described. *Necroptosis* is a form of cell death caused by the cytokine tumor necrosis factor (TNF) that shows features of both necrosis and apoptosis, hence its name. *Pyroptosis* (*pyro*, fever) is induced by activation of inflammasomes (Chapter 5), which releases the cytokine interleukin-1 (IL-1), which cause inflammation and fever. *Ferroptosis* depends on levels of cellular iron. The roles of these mechanisms of cell death in normal physiology and pathologic states are not clearly established and remain topics of investigation.

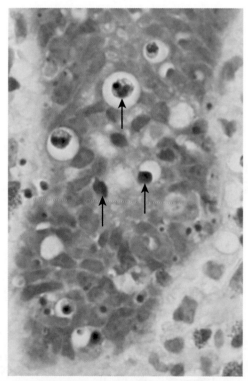

FIG. 1.13 Morphologic appearance of apoptotic cells. Apoptotic cells (some indicated by *arrows*) in a normal crypt in the colonic epithelium are shown. (The preparative regimen for colonoscopy frequently induces apoptosis in epithelial cells, which explains the abundance of dead cells in this normal tissue.) Note the fragmented nuclei with condensed chromatin and the shrunken cell bodies, some with pieces falling off. (Courtesy of Dr. Sanjay Kakar, Department of Pathology, University of California San Francisco, San Francisco, CA.)

Autophagy

Autophagy ("self-eating") refers to lysosomal digestion of the cell's own components. It is a survival mechanism in times of nutrient deprivation that enables the starved cell to live by eating its own contents and recycling these contents to provide nutrients and energy. In this process, intracellular organelles and portions of cytosol are first sequestered within an ER-derived double membrane (phagophore), which matures into an autophagic vacuole. The formation of this autophagosome is initiated by cytosolic proteins that sense nutrient deprivation (Fig. 1.14). The vacuole fuses with lysosomes to form an autophagolysosome, and lysosomal enzymes digest the cellular components. In some circumstances, autophagy may be associated with atrophy of tissues (discussed later) and represent an adaptation that helps cells survive lean times. If, however, the starved cell can no longer cope by devouring its contents, autophagy may also signal cell death by apoptosis.

Extensive autophagy is seen in ischemic injury and some types of myopathies. Autophagic vacuoles may also form around microbes in infected cells, leading to destruction of these infectious pathogens. Cancer cells acquire the ability to survive even in times of stress without autophagy (Chapter 6). Thus, a once little-appreciated survival pathway in cells may prove to have wide-ranging roles in human disease.

MECHANISMS OF CELL INJURY AND CELL DEATH

There are numerous and diverse extrinsic causes of cell injury and cell death, so it is not surprising that there are many intrinsic biochemical pathways that can initiate the sequence of events that lead to cell injury and culminate in cell death. Before discussing individual pathways of cell injury and their mechanisms, some general principles should be emphasized.

- **The cellular response to injurious stimuli depends on the type of injury and its duration and severity.** Thus, low doses of toxins or a brief duration of ischemia may lead to reversible cell injury, whereas larger toxin doses or longer ischemia times may result in irreversible injury and necrosis.
- **The consequences of an injurious stimulus also depend on the type of cell and its metabolic state, adaptability, and genetic makeup.** For instance, skeletal muscle in the leg can survive complete ischemia for 2 to 3 hours, whereas more metabolically active cardiac muscle dies after only 20 to 30 minutes. Genetically determined diversity in metabolic pathways can contribute to differences in responses to injurious stimuli. For instance, when exposed to the same dose of a toxin, individuals who inherit variants in genes encoding cytochrome P-450 may catabolize the toxin at different rates, leading to different outcomes.
- **Cell injury usually results from functional and biochemical abnormalities in one or more essential cellular components** (Fig. 1.15). Deprivation of oxygen and nutrients (as in hypoxia and ischemia) primarily impairs energy-dependent cellular functions, while damage to proteins and DNA triggers apoptosis. Because any one injurious insult may trigger multiple, overlapping biochemical pathways, it has proved difficult to prevent cell injury from any cause by targeting an individual pathway.

In the following sections, we discuss the mechanisms that lead to cell injury and death. While each of the mechanisms tends to cause cell death predominantly by necrosis or apoptosis, the two pathways may intersect. For instance, ischemia and the production of free radicals are typically associated with necrotic cell death, but they can also trigger apoptosis.

Mitochondrial Dysfunction and Damage

Mitochondria produce life-sustaining energy in the form of ATP. They may be damaged functionally or structurally by many types of injurious stimuli, including hypoxia, chemical toxins, and radiation. There are two major consequences of mitochondrial dysfunction.

- **Failure of oxidative phosphorylation, leading to decreased ATP generation and depletion of ATP in cells.** Since ATP is the energy source required for virtually all enzymatic and biosynthetic activities in cells, loss of ATP, which is often a consequence of ischemia (discussed later), has effects on many cellular systems.
  - *Reduced activity of plasma membrane ATP-dependent sodium pumps* results in intracellular accumulation of sodium and efflux of potassium. The net gain of solute is accompanied by osmotic gain of water, causing *cell swelling* and dilation of the ER.
  - The compensatory *increase in anaerobic glycolysis* leads to lactic acid accumulation, decreased intracellular pH, and decreased activity of many cellular enzymes.
  - Prolonged or worsening depletion of ATP causes *structural disruption of the protein synthetic apparatus*, manifested as detachment of ribosomes from the rough ER and dissociation of polysomes, with a consequent reduction in protein synthesis.
  - Ultimately, there is irreversible *damage to mitochondrial and lysosomal membranes*, and the cell undergoes necrosis.

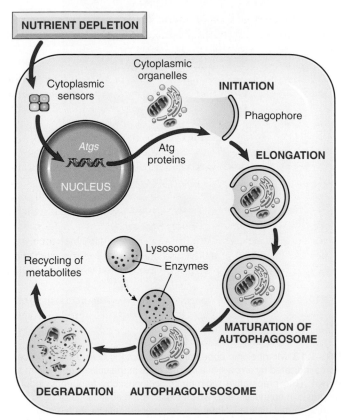

FIG. 1.14 Autophagy. Cellular stresses, such as nutrient deprivation, activate autophagy genes *(Atgs)*, whose products initiate the formation of membrane-bound vesicles in which cellular organelles are sequestered. These vesicles fuse with lysosomes, in which the organelles are digested, and the products are used to provide nutrients for the cell. The same process can trigger apoptosis by mechanisms that are not well defined.

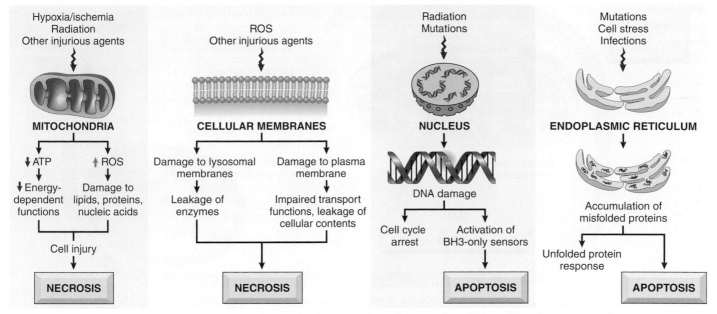

FIG. 1.15 The principal biochemical mechanisms and sites of damage in cell injury. Note that causes and mechanisms of cell death by necrosis and apoptosis are shown as being independent but there may be overlap; for instance, both may occur as a result of ischemia, oxidative stress, and radiation-induced cell death. *ATP,* Adenosine triphosphate; *ROS,* reactive oxygen species.

Although necrosis is the principal form of cell death caused by hypoxia, apoptosis by the mitochondrial pathway is also thought to contribute.

- Abnormal oxidative phosphorylation also leads to the formation of *reactive oxygen species*, described later.
- Damage to mitochondria is often associated with the formation of a high-conductance channel in the mitochondrial membrane, called the mitochondrial permeability transition pore. The opening of this channel leads to the loss of mitochondrial membrane potential and pH changes, further compromising oxidative phosphorylation.

As discussed earlier, mitochondria contain proteins such as cytochrome c that, when released into the cytoplasm, alert the cell to internal injury and activate apoptosis. The leakage of these proteins is regulated by other proteins and is a response to loss of survival signals and other proapoptotic triggers. Thus, mitochondria are life sustaining when healthy yet capable of activating numerous protective and pathologic reactions when damaged.

Oxidative Stress

Oxidative stress refers to cellular damage induced by the accumulation of reactive oxygen species (ROS), a form of free radical. Cell injury in many circumstances involves damage by free radicals; these situations include chemical and radiation injury, hypoxia, cellular aging, tissue injury caused by inflammatory cells, and ischemia-reperfusion injury (discussed later). Free radicals are chemical species with a single unpaired electron in an outer orbital. Such chemical species are extremely unstable and readily react with inorganic and organic compounds, such as nucleic acids, proteins, and lipids. During this reaction, the molecules that are "attacked" by free radicals are often themselves converted into other types of free radicals, thereby propagating the chain of damage.

Generation and Removal of Reactive Oxygen Species

The accumulation of ROS is determined by their rates of production and removal (Fig. 1.16). The properties and pathologic effects of the major ROS are summarized in Table 1.3.

ROS are normally produced by two major pathways.

- **ROS are produced in small amounts in all cells during the reduction-oxidation (redox) reactions that occur during energy generation.** In this process, molecular oxygen is reduced in mitochondria by the sequential addition of four electrons to produce water. This reaction is imperfect, however, and when oxygen is only partially reduced, small amounts of highly reactive, short-lived toxic intermediates are generated. These intermediates include superoxide ($O_2^{\cdot-}$), which is converted to hydrogen peroxide (H_2O_2) spontaneously and by the action of the enzyme superoxide dismutase (SOD). H_2O_2 is more stable than $O_2^{\cdot-}$ and can cross biologic membranes. In the presence of metals, such as Fe^{2+}, H_2O_2 is converted to the highly reactive hydroxyl radical •OH. Ionizing radiation and high doses of ultraviolet light can increase the production of ROS by hydrolyzing water into hydroxyl (•OH) and hydrogen (H•) free radicals.
- **ROS are produced in phagocytic leukocytes, mainly neutrophils,** as a weapon for destroying ingested microbes and other substances during inflammation (Chapter 2). ROS are generated in the phagolysosomes of leukocytes by a process that is similar to mitochondrial respiration and is called the *respiratory burst* (or oxidative burst). In this process, the enzyme phagocyte oxidase, located in the membranes of phagolysosomes, catalyzes the generation of superoxide, which is converted to H_2O_2. H_2O_2 is in turn converted to the highly reactive compound hypochlorite (the major component of household bleach) by the enzyme myeloperoxidase, which is abundant in leukocytes, especially neutrophils. ROS released from neutrophils may injure tissues.

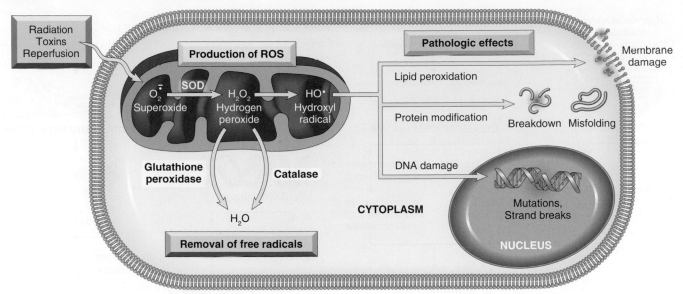

FIG. 1.16 The generation, removal, and role of reactive oxygen species (ROS) in cell injury. The production of ROS is increased by many injurious stimuli. These free radicals are removed by spontaneous decay and by specialized enzymatic systems. Excessive production or inadequate removal leads to accumulation of free radicals in cells, which may damage lipids (by peroxidation), proteins, and DNA, resulting in cell injury. *SOD,* Superoxide dismutase.

Table 1.3 Principal Free Radicals Involved in Cell Injury

Free Radical	Mechanisms of Production	Mechanisms of Removal	Pathologic Effects
Superoxide ($O_2^{\bar{\cdot}}$)	Incomplete reduction of O_2 during mitochondrial oxidative phosphorylation; by phagocyte oxidase in leukocytes	Conversion to H_2O_2 and O_2 by superoxide dismutase	Direct damaging effects on lipids (peroxidation), proteins, and DNA
Hydrogen peroxide (H_2O_2)	Mostly from superoxide by action of SOD	Conversion to H_2O and O_2 by catalase, glutathione peroxidase	Can be converted to •OH and ClO^-, which destroy microbes and cells
Hydroxyl radical (•OH)	Produced from H_2O, H_2O_2, and $O_2^{\bar{\cdot}}$ by various chemical reactions	Conversion to H_2O by glutathione peroxidase	Direct damaging effects on lipids, proteins, and DNA
Peroxynitrite ($ONOO^-$)	Interaction of $O_2^{\bar{\cdot}}$ and NO mediated by NO synthase	Conversion to nitrite by enzymes in mitochondria and cytosol	Direct damaging effects on lipids, proteins, and DNA

ClO⁻, Hypochlorite; *NO,* nitric oxide; *SOD,* superoxide dismutase.

Cells have evolved mechanisms that remove free radicals and thereby minimize their injurious effects. Free radicals are inherently unstable and decay spontaneously. There are also nonenzymatic and enzymatic systems, sometimes called free radical scavengers, that serve to inactivate free radicals (see Fig. 1.16):

- *Superoxide dismutases (SODs),* found in many cell types, convert superoxide into H_2O_2, which is degraded by catalase (see below).
- *Glutathione peroxidases* are a family of enzymes whose major function is to protect cells from oxidative damage. The most abundant member of this family, glutathione peroxidase 1, is found in the cytoplasm of all cells. It catalyzes the breakdown of H_2O_2 to H_2O.
- *Catalase,* present in peroxisomes, catalyzes the decomposition of hydrogen peroxide into O_2 and H_2O. It is highly efficient, being capable of degrading millions of molecules of H_2O_2 per second.

- *Endogenous or exogenous antioxidants* (e.g., vitamins E, A, and C and β-carotene) may either block the formation of free radicals or scavenge them once they have formed.

Cell Injury Caused by Reactive Oxygen Species

Reactive oxygen species cause cell injury by damaging multiple components of cells (see Fig. 1.16):

- *Peroxidation of membrane lipids.* ROS damage plasma membranes as well as mitochondrial and lysosomal membranes because the double bonds in membrane lipids are vulnerable to attack by free radicals. The lipid–radical interactions yield peroxides, which are themselves unstable and reactive, and an autocatalytic chain reaction ensues.
- *Crosslinking and other changes in proteins.* Free radicals promote sulfhydryl-mediated protein crosslinking, resulting in enhanced degradation or loss of functional activity. Free radical reactions

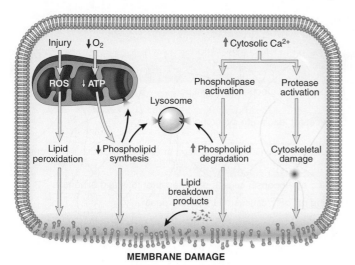

FIG. 1.17 Mechanisms of membrane damage. Decreased O_2 and increased cytosolic Ca^{2+} are typically seen in ischemia but may accompany other forms of cell injury. Reactive oxygen species, which are often produced on reperfusion of ischemic tissues, also cause membrane damage (not shown).

may also directly cause fragmentation of polypeptides. Damaged proteins may fail to fold properly, triggering the unfolded protein response, described later.

- *DNA damage.* Free radical reactions produce DNA damage of several types, notably mutations and DNA breaks. Such DNA damage has been implicated in apoptotic cell death, aging, and malignant transformation of cells.

In addition to their role in cell injury and killing of microbes, ROS at low concentrations may be involved in numerous signaling pathways in cells and thus in physiologic reactions.

Membrane Damage

Most forms of cell injury that culminate in necrosis are characterized by increased membrane permeability that ultimately leads to overt membrane damage. Cellular membranes may be damaged by ROS, decreased phospholipid biosynthesis (due to hypoxia and nutrient deprivation), increased degradation (e.g., following phosphatase activation due to increased intracellular calcium), and cytoskeletal abnormalities that disrupt the anchors for plasma membranes (Fig. 1.17). The most important sites of membrane damage are the following:

- *Mitochondrial membrane damage*, discussed earlier.
- *Plasma membrane damage*, which leads to loss of osmotic balance and influx of fluids and ions, as well as loss of cellular contents.
- *Injury to lysosomal membranes*, leading to leakage into the cytoplasm of lysosomal enzymes such as acid hydrolases, which are activated in the acidic intracellular pH of the injured (e.g., ischemic) cell. These enzymes digest numerous cellular components, producing irreversible damage and necrosis.

Disturbance in Calcium Homeostasis

Calcium ions normally serve as second messengers in several signaling pathways but if released into the cytoplasm of cells in excessive amounts are also an important source of cell injury. Cytosolic free Ca^{2+} is normally maintained at much lower concentrations (~ 0.1 μmol) than extracellular Ca^{2+} (1.3 mmol), and most intracellular Ca^{2+} is sequestered in mitochondria and the ER. Ischemia and certain toxins increase cytosolic Ca^{2+},

initially due to release from intracellular stores and later from increased influx across the dysfunctional plasma membrane. Excessive intracellular Ca^{2+} may cause cell injury by activating various enzymes, e.g., proteases and phospholipases, that damage cellular components.

Endoplasmic Reticulum Stress

The accumulation of misfolded proteins in a cell can stress compensatory pathways in the ER and lead to cell death by apoptosis. During protein synthesis, chaperones in the ER enhance the proper folding of newly synthesized proteins, but this process is imperfect, and some misfolded polypeptides are generated that are targeted for proteolysis by ubiquitination. When misfolded proteins accumulate in the ER, they induce a protective cellular response that is called the **unfolded protein response** (Fig. 1.18). This adaptive response activates signaling pathways that increase the production of chaperones and retard protein translation, thus reducing the levels of misfolded proteins in the cell. However, if the quantity of misfolded protein exceeds what can be handled by the adaptive response, additional signals are generated that activate proapoptotic sensors, leading to apoptosis mainly by the mitochondrial (intrinsic) pathway.

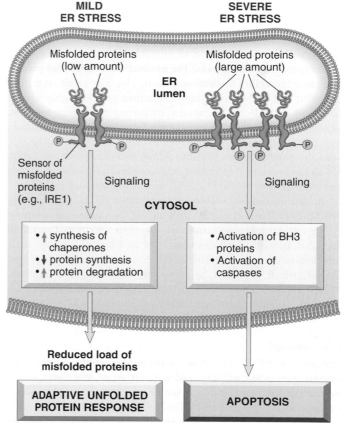

FIG. 1.18 The unfolded protein response and ER stress. The presence of misfolded proteins in the ER is detected by sensors in the ER membrane, such as the kinase IRE1, which form oligomers and are activated by phosphorylation (the extent of both being proportional to the amount of misfolded proteins). This triggers an adaptive unfolded protein response, which can protect the cell from the harmful consequences of the misfolded proteins. When the level of misfolded proteins is too great to be corrected, the mitochondrial pathway of apoptosis is induced and the irreparably damaged cell dies; this is also called the terminal unfolded protein response. *IRE1*, Inositol requiring enzyme-1.

Table 1.4 Diseases Caused by Misfolded Proteins

Disease	Affected Protein	Pathogenesis
Diseases Caused by Mutant Proteins That Are Degraded, Leading to Their Deficiency		
Cystic fibrosis[a]	Cystic fibrosis transmembrane conductance regulator (CFTR)	Loss of CFTR leads to defects in ion transport
Familial hypercholesterolemia[a]	LDL receptor	Loss of LDL receptor leading to hypercholesterolemia
Tay-Sachs disease[a]	Hexosaminidase α-subunit	Lack of the lysosomal enzyme leads to storage of GM_2 gangliosides in neurons
Diseases Caused by Misfolded Proteins That Result in ER Stress-Induced Cell Loss		
Retinitis pigmentosa[a]	Rhodopsin	Abnormal folding of rhodopsin causes photoreceptor loss and blindness
Creutzfeldt-Jakob disease	Prions	Abnormal folding of PrP^{sc} causes neuronal cell death
Diseases Caused by Misfolded Proteins That Result From Both ER Stress-Induced Cell Loss and Functional Deficiency of the Protein		
α-1-antitrypsin deficiency	α-1 antitrypsin	Storage of nonfunctional protein in hepatocytes causes apoptosis; absence of enzymatic activity in lungs causes destruction of elastic tissue, giving rise to emphysema

[a]Misfolding is responsible for protein dysfunction and cellular injury in a subset of molecular subtypes.

Shown are selected illustrative examples of diseases in which protein misfolding is a mechanism of functional derangement or cell or tissue injury.

CFTR, Cystic fibrosis transporter; *LDL,* low density lipoprotein; *PrP,* prion protein.

Intracellular accumulation of misfolded proteins may be caused by abnormalities that increase the production of misfolded proteins or reduce the ability to eliminate them. This may result from mutations that lead to the production of abnormal proteins; aging, which is associated with decreased capacity to correct misfolding; infections, especially viral infections, in which microbial proteins are synthesized in such large amounts that they overwhelm the quality control system that normally ensures proper protein folding; and changes in intracellular pH and redox state. Deprivation of glucose and oxygen, as in ischemia and hypoxia, may also increase the burden of misfolded proteins.

Protein misfolding within cells may cause diseases by creating a deficiency of an essential protein or by inducing apoptosis (Table 1.4). Misfolded proteins often lose their activity and are rapidly degraded, both of which can contribute to a loss of function. If this function is essential, cellular injury ensues. One example is cystic fibrosis, which is caused by inherited mutations in a membrane transport protein, some of which prevent its normal folding. Cell injury as a result of protein misfolding is recognized as a feature of a number of diseases (see Table 1.4).

DNA Damage

Exposure of cells to radiation or chemotherapeutic agents, intracellular generation of ROS, and acquisition of mutations may all induce DNA damage, which, if severe, may trigger apoptotic death. Damage to DNA is sensed by intracellular sentinel proteins, which transmit signals that lead to the accumulation of p53 protein. p53 first arrests the cell cycle (at the G1 phase) to allow the DNA to be repaired before it is replicated (Chapter 6). However, if the damage is too great to be repaired successfully, p53 triggers apoptosis, mainly by the mitochondrial pathway. When p53 is mutated or absent (as it is in certain cancers), cells with damaged DNA that would otherwise undergo apoptosis survive. In such cells, the DNA damage may result in various types of genomic alterations (e.g., chromosomal deletions) that lead to neoplastic transformation (Chapter 6).

Clinicopathologic Examples of Cell Injury and Necrosis

The mechanisms involved in some common causes of cell injury culminating in necrosis are summarized next.

Hypoxia and Ischemia

Oxygen deprivation is one of the most frequent causes of cell injury and necrotic cell death in clinical medicine. Oxygen is required for oxidative phosphorylation and the generation of ATP, the energy store of cells. Therefore, cells deprived of oxygen are at risk of suffering catastrophic failure of many essential functions. In contrast to hypoxia, in which blood flow is maintained and during which energy production by anaerobic glycolysis can continue, ischemia compromises the delivery of substrates for glycolysis. Thus, in ischemic tissues, not only does aerobic metabolism cease but anaerobic energy generation also fails after glycolytic substrates are exhausted or glycolysis is inhibited by the accumulation of metabolites, which otherwise would be washed out by flowing blood. For this reason, ischemia causes more rapid and severe cell and tissue injury than hypoxia.

Cells subjected to the stress of hypoxia that do not immediately die activate compensatory mechanisms that are induced by transcription factors of the hypoxia-inducible factor (HIF) family. HIF simulates the synthesis of several proteins that help the cell to survive in the face of low oxygen. Some of these proteins, such as vascular endothelial growth factor (VEGF), stimulate the growth of new vessels and thus increase blood flow and the supply of oxygen. Other proteins induced by HIF cause adaptive changes in cellular metabolism by stimulating the uptake of glucose and glycolysis. Anaerobic glycolysis can generate ATP in the absence of oxygen using glucose derived either from the circulation or from the hydrolysis of intracellular glycogen. Tissues with a greater glycolytic capacity due to the presence of glycogen (e.g., the liver and striated muscle) can survive loss of oxygen and decreased oxidative phosphorylation better than tissues with limited glycogen stores (e.g., the brain).

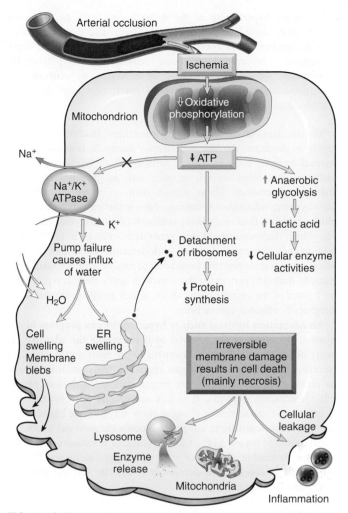

FIG. 1.19 The functional and morphologic consequences of hypoxia and ischemia. Only the lower left portion of the cell is shown as swollen but cell swelling is typically uniform throughout the injured cell.

Persistent or severe hypoxia and ischemia lead to depletion of ATP. Loss of this critical energy source results in failure of the plasma membrane sodium pump, decreased intracellular pH causing changes in the activities of many enzymes, increased generation of ROS, and defects in protein synthesis (Fig. 1.19). These alterations were described in the earlier discussion of mitochondrial damage.

Ischemia-Reperfusion Injury

Under certain circumstances, **the restoration of blood flow to ischemic but viable tissues results, paradoxically, in increased cell injury and necrosis.** This is the reverse of the expected outcome of restoration of blood flow, which should result in recovery of reversibly injured cells. This so-called *ischemia-reperfusion injury* is a clinically important process that may contribute significantly to tissue damage, especially after myocardial and cerebral ischemia.

Several mechanisms may account for the exacerbation of cell injury by reperfusion of ischemic tissues:

- *Increased ROS production* may occur during reoxygenation, exacerbating damage (described earlier). Some of the ROS may be generated by injured cells whose damaged mitochondria cannot carry out the complete reduction of oxygen, and cellular antioxidant defense mechanisms may be compromised by ischemia, worsening

the situation. ROS generated by infiltrating leukocytes may also contribute to the damage of vulnerable injured cells.
- *Influx of calcium* may cause injury by mechanisms described earlier.

The inflammation that is induced by ischemic injury increases with reperfusion because of increased influx and activation of leukocytes, the products of which cause additional tissue injury (Chapter 2). Activation of the complement system may also contribute to ischemia-reperfusion injury.

Cell Injury Caused by Toxins

Toxins, including environmental chemicals and substances produced by infectious pathogens, induce cell injury that culminates typically in necrosis. Different types of toxins cause cell injury by two general mechanisms:

- *Direct-acting toxins.* Some toxins act directly by combining with a critical molecular component or cellular organelle. For example, in mercuric chloride poisoning (as may occur from ingestion of contaminated seafood, Chapter 7), mercury binds to the sulfhydryl groups of various cell membrane proteins, inhibiting ATP-dependent transport and increasing membrane permeability. Many chemotherapeutic drugs used to treat cancers induce cell damage, often to DNA, by direct cytotoxic effects. Also included in this class are toxins made by infectious pathogens, which often cause damage by targeting host cell proteins that are needed for essential functions, such as protein synthesis and ion transport. For instance, diphtheria toxin produced by *Corynebacterium diphtheriae* inhibits protein synthesis, and different subunits of anthrax toxin produced by *Bacillus anthracis* promote water influx into cells and degrade critical enzymes such as MAP kinases that are involved in many cellular functions.
- *Latent toxins.* Other toxic chemicals are only active after they have been converted to reactive metabolites, which then act on target cells. This conversion is usually carried out by cytochrome P-450 in the smooth ER of the liver and other organs. Although the metabolites might cause membrane damage and cell injury by direct covalent binding to protein and lipids, the most important mechanism of cell injury involves the formation of free radicals. Two classic examples of this type of injury involve the solvent carbon tetrachloride and the drug acetaminophen.
  - *Carbon tetrachloride (CCl_4)* was once widely used in the dry-cleaning industry but is now banned. CCl_4 is converted to a toxic free radical $CCl_3\bullet$, principally in the liver, and this free radical is the cause of cell injury, mainly by membrane phospholipid peroxidation. In less than 30 minutes after exposure to CCl_4, there is sufficient damage to the ER membranes of hepatocytes to cause a decline in synthesis of enzymes and plasma proteins; within 2 hours, there is swelling of the smooth ER and dissociation of ribosomes from the rough ER. Because of reduced synthesis of transport proteins, there is also decreased triglyceride secretion, resulting in the fatty liver of CCl_4 poisoning. Mitochondrial injury and diminished ATP stores follow, resulting in defective ion transport and progressive cell swelling, and the plasma membranes are further damaged by lipid peroxidation. The end result can be cell death.
  - *Poisoning by acetaminophen*, a widely used analgesic and antipyretic, is the leading cause of acute liver failure in the United States (Chapter 14). Taken at recommended doses, metabolic pathways that convert acetaminophen to nontoxic products

dominate, but at high doses these pathways become saturated and the drug is metabolized in the liver by the P-450 system to a highly toxic intermediate capable of causing hepatocyte injury.

CELLULAR ADAPTATIONS TO STRESS

Adaptations are reversible changes in the number, size, phenotype, metabolic activity, or functions of cells in response to changes in their environment. *Physiologic adaptations* include the responses of cells to normal stimulation by hormones or endogenous chemical mediators (e.g., the hormone-induced enlargement of the breast and uterus during pregnancy) or to the demands of mechanical stress (in the case of bones and muscles). *Pathologic adaptations* are responses to stress that allow cells to modulate their structure and function and thus escape injury, but at the expense of normal function. Physiologic and pathologic adaptations can take several distinct forms, as described below.

Hypertrophy

Hypertrophy refers to an enlargement of cells that results in increase in the size of the organ. By contrast, hyperplasia (discussed next) is an increase in cell number. In pure hypertrophy, there are no new cells, just larger cells containing increased amounts of structural proteins and organelles. Pure hypertrophy is largely confined to cell types with a limited capacity to divide. In other tissues, hypertrophy and hyperplasia may occur together and combine to produce an enlarged (hypertrophic) organ.

Hypertrophy can be physiologic or pathologic and is caused either by increased functional demand or by growth factor or hormonal stimulation.

- *Physiologic enlargement of the uterus* during pregnancy occurs as a consequence of estrogen-stimulated smooth muscle hypertrophy and hyperplasia (Fig. 1.20). By contrast, in response to increased workload the striated muscle cells in both the skeletal muscle and the heart undergo only hypertrophy, as these cell types have a limited capacity to divide.

- *Pathologic hypertrophy of the heart* occurs with hypertension and other disorders that increase intracardiac pressures, such as narrowing of the aortic valve (stenosis) (Fig. 1.21). In these situations, myocardial cells are subjected to a persistently increased workload and adapt by enlarging to generate the required higher contractile force. Hypertrophy may also be a prelude to cell injury.

The mechanisms of hypertrophy have been studied most thoroughly in the heart. Cardiac hypertrophy occurs in response to mechanical triggers, such as stretch, with resultant release of soluble mediators that stimulate cell growth, such as growth factors and adrenergic hormones. These stimuli turn on signal transduction pathways that induce the expression of genes that encode a number of cellular proteins. One result is the synthesis of more myofilaments per cell, which increases the force generated with each contraction, enabling the cell to meet increased work demands. There may also be a switch of contractile proteins from adult to fetal or neonatal forms. For example, during hypertrophy, the α-myosin heavy chain is replaced by the β form of the myosin heavy chain, which produces slower, more energetically efficient contractions.

An adaptation to stress such as hypertrophy can progress to cell injury if the stress is not relieved or if it exceeds the adaptive capacity of the tissue. When this happens in the heart due to sustained hypertension, degenerative changes appear in the myocardial fibers, the most important of which are fragmentation and loss of myofibrillar contractile elements. It is not understood why hypertrophy progresses to these regressive changes; there may be finite limits on the ability of the vasculature to adequately supply the enlarged fibers, the mitochondria to supply ATP, or the biosynthetic machinery to provide sufficient contractile proteins or other cytoskeletal elements. The net result of these degenerative changes is ventricular dilation and ultimately cardiac failure.

Hyperplasia

Hyperplasia is an increase in the number of cells in an organ that stems from increased proliferation, either of differentiated cells or,

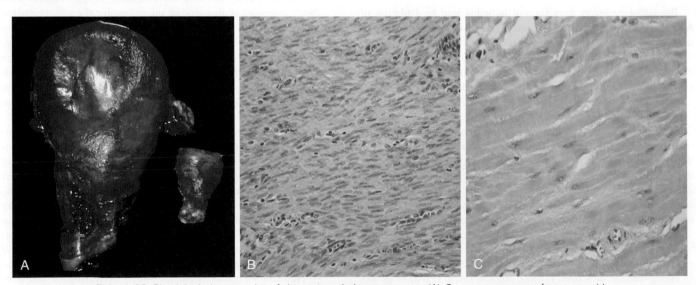

FIG. 1.20 Physiologic hypertrophy of the uterus during pregnancy. (A) Gross appearance of a nongravid uterus *(right)* and a gravid uterus *(left)* that was removed for postpartum bleeding. (B) Small spindle-shaped uterine smooth muscle cells from a nongravid uterus. (C) Large, plump hypertrophied smooth muscle cells from a gravid uterus; compare with B. (B and C, Same magnification.)

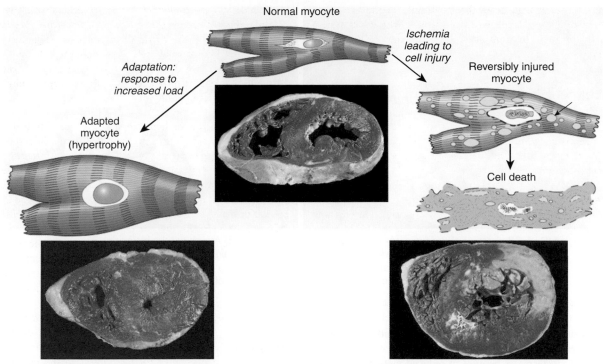

Normal myocyte

Ischemia leading to cell injury

Adaptation: response to increased load

Reversibly injured myocyte

Adapted myocyte (hypertrophy)

Cell death

FIG. 1.21 The relationship among normal, adapted, reversibly injured, and dead myocardial cells. The cellular adaptation depicted here is hypertrophy, the cause of reversible injury is ischemia, and the irreversible injury is ischemic coagulative necrosis. In the example of myocardial hypertrophy *(lower left)*, the left ventricular wall is thicker than 2 cm (normal, 1–1.5 cm). Reversibly injured myocardium *(upper right)* shows functional compromise without gross or light microscopic changes, or reversible changes like cellular swelling and fatty change *(arrow)*. In the specimen showing necrosis *(lower right)* the transmural light area in the posterolateral left ventricle represents an acute myocardial infarction. All three transverse sections of myocardium have been stained with triphenyltetrazolium chloride, an enzyme substrate that colors viable myocardium magenta. Failure to stain is due to enzyme loss after cell death.

in some instances, progenitor cells. As discussed earlier, hyperplasia happens if the tissue contains cell populations capable of replication; it may occur concurrently with hypertrophy and often in response to the same stimuli.

Hyperplasia can be physiologic or pathologic; in both situations, cellular proliferation is stimulated by hormones or growth factors.
- The two types of physiologic hyperplasia are (1) *hormonal hyperplasia*, exemplified by the proliferation of the glandular epithelium of the female breast at puberty and during pregnancy, and (2) *compensatory hyperplasia*, in which residual tissue grows after removal or loss of part of an organ. For example, when part of a liver is resected, mitotic activity in the remaining hepatocytes begins as early as 12 hours later, eventually restoring the liver to its normal weight. The stimuli for hyperplasia in this setting are polypeptide growth factors produced by uninjured hepatocytes as well as nonparenchymal cells in the liver (Chapter 2). After the liver returns to its normal size, cell proliferation is turned off by various growth inhibitors.
- *Hormonal imbalances can lead to pathologic hyperplasia.* For example, after a menstrual period there is a burst of uterine epithelial proliferation that is normally tightly regulated by the stimulatory effects of pituitary hormones and ovarian estrogen and the inhibitory effects of progesterone. A disturbance in this balance leading to increased estrogenic stimulation causes endometrial hyperplasia, a common cause of abnormal menstrual bleeding. Benign prostatic hyperplasia is another common example of pathologic

hyperplasia induced by responses to hormonal stimulation, in this case by androgens and estrogens.

An important point is that in all these situations, **the hyperplastic process remains controlled; if the signals that initiate it abate, the hyperplasia ceases.** It is this responsiveness to normal regulatory control mechanisms that distinguishes pathologic hyperplasia from cancer, in which growth control mechanisms become permanently dysregulated or ineffective (Chapter 6). Nevertheless, in many cases, pathologic hyperplasia constitutes a fertile soil in which cancers may eventually arise. For example, patients with hyperplasia of the endometrium are at increased risk of developing endometrial cancer (Chapter 17).

Atrophy

Atrophy is reduced size of an organ or tissue caused by reduction in the size and number of cells (Fig. 1.22). Causes of atrophy include a decreased workload (e.g., immobilization of a limb to permit healing of a fracture), loss of innervation, diminished blood supply, inadequate nutrition, loss of endocrine stimulation, and aging (senile atrophy). Although some of these causes are a physiologic part of life (e.g., the loss of hormone stimulation in menopause) and others are pathologic (e.g., denervation), the fundamental cellular changes are similar. Atrophy can be viewed as an adaptive retreat to a smaller cell size at which survival is still possible. Over time, however, as atrophy worsens, affected cells may pass a threshold and undergo apoptosis.

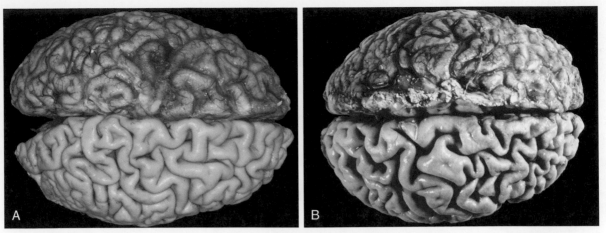

FIG. 1.22 Atrophy of the brain. (A) Normal brain of a young adult. (B) Atrophy of the brain in an 81-year-old man with atherosclerotic cerebrovascular disease. Atrophy of the brain is due to aging and reduced blood supply. Note that loss of brain substance narrows the gyri and widens the sulci. The meninges have been stripped from the bottom half of each specimen to reveal the surface of the brain.

Atrophy results from a combination of decreased protein synthesis and increased protein degradation.

- Protein synthesis decreases because of reduced metabolic activity.
- The degradation of cellular proteins occurs mainly by the ubiquitin-proteasome pathway. Nutrient deficiency and disuse may activate ubiquitin ligases, which attach multiple copies of the small peptide ubiquitin to cellular proteins and target them for degradation in the proteasome.
- In many situations, atrophy is also accompanied by increased autophagy, with resulting increases in the number of autophagic vacuoles. As discussed previously, autophagy is the process in which the starved cell eats its own organelles in an attempt to survive.

Metaplasia

Metaplasia is a change in which one adult cell type is replaced by another adult cell type. In this type of cellular adaptation, a cell type sensitive to a particular stress is replaced by another cell type better able to withstand the adverse environment. Metaplasia is thought to usually arise by reprogramming of stem cells to differentiate along a new pathway rather than a phenotypic change of differentiated cells (transdifferentiation).

Epithelial metaplasia is exemplified by the change in the respiratory epithelium that occurs with prolonged cigarette smoking. In this process, the normal, relatively delicate ciliated columnar epithelial cells of the trachea and bronchi are replaced by tough stratified squamous epithelial cells (Fig. 1.23), which are better suited to withstand the noxious chemicals in cigarette smoke. Although the metaplastic squamous epithelium has survival advantages, important protective mechanisms are lost, such as mucus secretion and ciliary clearance of particulate matter. Epithelial metaplasia is therefore a double-edged sword.

In other situations, e.g., in chronic gastric reflux, the normal stratified squamous epithelium of the lower esophagus may undergo metaplastic transformation to gastric or intestinal-type columnar epithelium. Metaplasia may also occur in mesenchymal cells, but in these situations it is generally a reaction to some pathologic alteration and not an adaptive response to stress. For example, bone is occasionally formed in soft tissues, particularly in foci of injury.

The influences that induce metaplastic change, if persistent, predispose to malignant transformation of the epithelium. Many

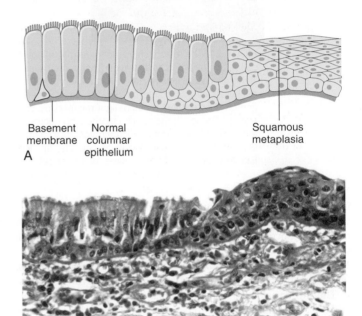

FIG. 1.23 Metaplasia of normal columnar (*left*) to squamous epithelium (*right*) in a bronchus, shown schematically (A) and histologically (B).

such examples exist. For example, the squamous metaplasia of the respiratory epithelium is a rich soil for the development of lung cancers composed of malignant squamous cells. Similarly, intestinal metaplasia of the stomach is associated with the development of gastric cancer.

INTRACELLULAR AND EXTRACELLULAR DEPOSITIONS

Under some circumstances cells or tissues accumulate abnormal amounts of various substances, which may be harmless or cause injury.

Intracellular Accumulations

The main mechanisms of abnormal intracellular accumulations are inadequate removal and degradation or excessive production of an endogenous substance, or deposition of an abnormal exogenous material (Fig. 1.24). Intracellular deposits may be located in the cytoplasm, within organelles (typically lysosomes), or in the nucleus. Examples of each are described.

Fatty Change (Steatosis). Fatty change refers to an abnormal accumulation of triglycerides within parenchymal cells. It is most often seen in the liver, since this is the major organ involved in fat metabolism, but it may also occur in the heart, skeletal muscle, kidney, and other organs. Steatosis may be caused by toxins, protein malnutrition, diabetes, obesity, or anoxia. Alcohol abuse and diabetes associated with obesity are the most common causes of fatty change in the liver (fatty liver) in higher-income nations. This process is discussed in more detail in Chapter 14.

Cholesterol and Cholesteryl Esters. Cellular cholesterol metabolism is tightly regulated to ensure normal synthesis of cell membranes (of which cholesterol is a key component) without significant intracellular accumulation. However, phagocytic cells may become overloaded with lipids (triglycerides, cholesterol, and cholesteryl esters) in several pathologic processes characterized by increased intake or decreased catabolism of lipids. Of these, atherosclerosis is the most important. The role of lipid and cholesterol deposition in the pathogenesis of atherosclerosis is discussed in Chapter 8.

Proteins. Morphologically visible protein accumulations are less common than lipid accumulations; they may occur because of increased uptake or increased synthesis. In the kidney, for example, trace amounts of albumin filtered through the glomerulus are normally reabsorbed by pinocytosis in the proximal convoluted tubules. However, in disorders with heavy protein leakage across the glomerular filter (e.g., nephrotic syndrome, Chapter 12), much more protein leaks into the urine. The excessive amounts of resorbed albumin accumulate in vesicles in the tubular epithelial cells, in which they are seen as pink, hyaline cytoplasmic droplets. This process is reversible: if the proteinuria abates, the protein is degraded and the hyaline droplets disappear. Another example is the marked accumulation of immunoglobulins that occurs in the rough ER of some plasma cells, forming rounded, eosinophilic Russell bodies. Other examples of protein aggregation are discussed elsewhere in this book, such as alcoholic hyaline in the liver (Chapter 14) and neurofibrillary tangles in neurons (Chapter 21).

Glycogen. Intracellular deposits of glycogen are associated with abnormalities in the metabolism of either glucose or glycogen. In poorly controlled diabetes, the prime example of abnormal glucose metabolism, glycogen accumulates in renal tubular epithelium, cardiac myocytes, and β cells of the islets of Langerhans. Glycogen also accumulates within cells in a group of genetic disorders collectively called glycogen storage diseases (Chapter 4).

Pigments. Pigments are colored substances that may be exogenous, coming from outside the body, or endogenous, synthesized within the body.

- *Carbon*, the most common exogenous pigment, is a ubiquitous urban air pollutant. When inhaled, it is phagocytosed by alveolar macrophages and transported through lymphatic channels to the regional tracheobronchial lymph nodes. Aggregates of the pigment blacken the draining lymph nodes and pulmonary parenchyma (*anthracosis*) (Chapter 11).
- *Lipofuscin*, or "wear-and-tear pigment," is an insoluble brownish-yellow granular intracellular material that accumulates in a variety

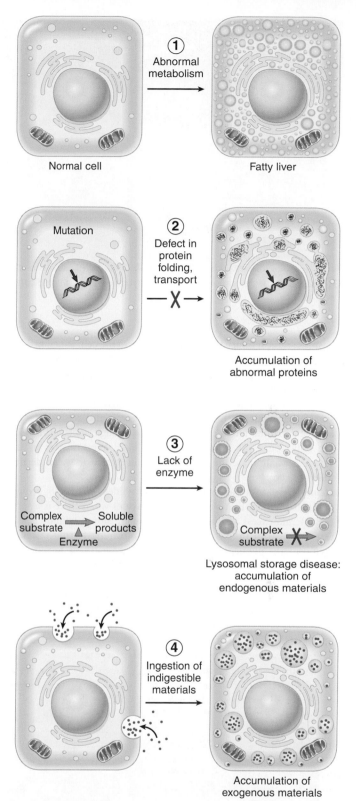

FIG. 1.24 Mechanisms of intracellular accumulations.

of tissues (particularly the heart, liver, and brain) as a function of age or atrophy. Lipofuscin represents complexes of lipid and protein produced by the free radical–catalyzed peroxidation of polyunsaturated lipids of intracellular membranes. It is a marker of

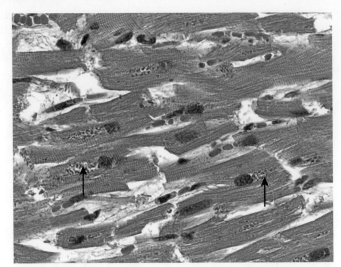

FIG. 1.25 Lipofuscin granules in cardiac myocytes (deposits indicated by *arrows*).

past free radical injury but is not injurious to the cell. When present in large amounts, the brown pigment (Fig. 1.25) imparts an appearance to the atrophic tissue, particularly the heart, that is called *brown atrophy*.

- *Melanin* is an endogenous, brown-black pigment that is synthesized by melanocytes located in the epidermis and acts as a screen against harmful ultraviolet radiation. Although melanocytes are the only source of melanin, adjacent basal keratinocytes in the skin can accumulate the pigment (e.g., in freckles), as can dermal macrophages.

- *Hemosiderin* is a hemoglobin-derived golden yellow to brown, granular pigment that accumulates in tissues when there is a local or systemic excess of iron. Iron is normally stored within cells in association with the protein apoferritin, forming ferritin micelles. Hemosiderin pigment represents large aggregates of ferritin micelles; these are readily visualized by light and electron microscopy, and the associated iron can be unambiguously identified by the Prussian blue histochemical reaction (Fig. 1.26). Although hemosiderin accumulation is usually pathologic, small amounts of this

pigment are normal in bone marrow, spleen, and liver mononuclear phagocytes, which phagocytose and degrade aging red cells and recycle their iron to support the production of new red cells (Chapter 10). Excessive deposition of hemosiderin, called hemosiderosis, and more extensive accumulations of iron seen in hereditary hemochromatosis, are described in Chapter 14.

Extracellular Deposits: Pathologic Calcification

Pathologic calcification, which is seen in a wide variety of disease states, is the result of abnormal deposition of calcium salts. It can occur in two ways.

- *Dystrophic calcification.* In this form, calcium metabolism is normal and the calcium deposits in injured or dead tissue, such as areas of necrosis of any type. It is virtually always seen in the arterial lesions of advanced atherosclerosis (Chapter 8). Although dystrophic calcification may be an incidental finding indicating insignificant past cell injury, it may also be a cause of organ dysfunction. For example, calcification can develop in aging or damaged heart valves, resulting in severely compromised valve motion (Chapter 9).

  Dystrophic calcification is initiated by the extracellular deposition of crystalline calcium phosphate in the form of membrane-bound vesicles, which may be derived from injured cells, or the intracellular deposition of calcium in the mitochondria of dying cells. It is thought that the extracellular calcium is concentrated in vesicles by its affinity for membrane phospholipids, while phosphates accumulate as a result of the action of membrane-bound phosphatases. The crystals are then propagated, forming larger deposits.

- *Metastatic calcification.* This form is associated with hypercalcemia and can occur in otherwise normal tissues. The major causes of hypercalcemia are (1) increased secretion of parathyroid hormone due to either primary parathyroid tumors or hyperplasia, or production of parathyroid hormone—related protein by malignant tumors; (2) destruction of bone due to the effects of accelerated turnover (e.g., Paget disease), immobilization, or tumors (increased bone catabolism associated with multiple myeloma, leukemia, or diffuse skeletal metastases); (3) vitamin D—related disorders including vitamin D intoxication and sarcoidosis (in which macrophages activate a vitamin D precursor); and (4) renal failure, in which phosphate retention leads to secondary hyperparathyroidism.

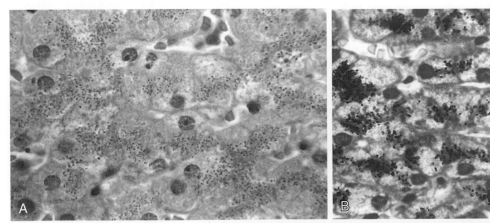

FIG. 1.26 Hemosiderin granules in liver cells. (A) Hematoxylin-eosin—stained section showing golden-brown, finely granular pigment. (B) Iron deposits revealed by a special staining process called the Prussian blue reaction.

Regardless of the site, calcium salts are seen on gross examination as fine white granules or clumps, often felt as gritty deposits. Dystrophic calcification is common in plaques of atherosclerosis, and in areas of caseous necrosis in tuberculosis. Sometimes a tuberculous lymph node is almost entirely converted to radiopaque stone. On histologic examination, calcification appears as basophilic deposits, which may be extracellular and intracellular. Over time, heterotopic bone may form in the focus of calcification.

Metastatic calcification can occur widely throughout the body but principally affects the interstitial tissues of the vasculature, kidneys, lungs, and gastric mucosa. The calcium deposits morphologically resemble those described in dystrophic calcification. Although they generally do not cause clinical dysfunction, extensive calcifications in the lungs may be evident on radiographs and may produce respiratory deficits, and massive deposits in the kidney (nephrocalcinosis) can lead to renal damage.

CELLULAR AGING

During early life in multicellular animals, natural selection strongly favors genetic variants that enhance reproduction, as these variants will be passed down to offspring and serve to maintain the population. By contrast, DNA repair mechanisms need not be perfect, as long as they are sufficient to allow survival through the reproductive years. As a result of imperfect DNA repair, with time mutations accumulate and those that are deleterious contribute to cellular aging. Aging is mediated by progressive decline of physiologic, cellular, and molecular homeostatic mechanisms after the reproductive years.

Aging has important health consequences, because age is one of the strongest independent risk factors for many chronic diseases including cancer, Alzheimer disease, and ischemic heart disease. Perhaps one of the most striking discoveries about the mechanisms of aging at the cellular level is that it is not simply an inevitable consequence of cells "running out of steam" because of the passage of time, but, in fact, is the consequence of alterations in genes and signaling pathways that are evolutionarily conserved from yeast to mammals. Indeed, experimental work has demonstrated that aging can be postponed; for instance, in animals, some manifestations of aging can be slowed by specific manipulations, such as calorie restriction and certain therapeutic drugs.

Cellular aging is the result of decreased replicative capacity and functional activity of cells. Several mechanisms contribute to cellular aging (Fig. 1.27):

- *DNA damage.* Nuclear and mitochondrial DNA frequently undergo mutations, which include base substitutions, copy number variations, and deletions or insertions. Many mutations are produced by the spontaneous deamination of cytosine residues, an event that (somewhat depressingly) occurs like clockwork over time. DNA damage is accelerated by endogenous stresses (e.g., ROS) and exogenous insults (e.g., exposure to UV radiation, chemotherapeutic agents). Although most DNA alterations are sensed by the cell and corrected by DNA repair enzymes, some are not, leading to mutations that accumulate as cells age. Predictably, several inherited syndromes characterized by premature aging are caused by mutations in genes that encode DNA repair proteins and thus maintain genomic stability. Damage of nuclear and mitochondrial DNA may contribute to aging through a number of deleterious effects:
  - Telomere dysfunction, described later
  - Epigenetic alterations that alter the expression of many genes
  - Synthesis of defective proteins that disturb protein homeostasis, also described later
  - Mitochondrial dysfunction, which may trigger cell death
  - Cellular senescence (proliferative arrest) and loss of stem cells
  - Effects on signaling pathways that regulate the aging process
- *Decreased cellular replication.* Normal cells (other than stem cells) have a limited capacity for replication and after a fixed number of divisions cells become arrested in a terminally nondividing state, known as *replicative senescence.* Aging is associated with progressive replicative senescence of cells. Cells from children have the capacity to undergo more rounds of replication than do cells from older people. By contrast, cells from patients with Werner syndrome, a rare disease that mimics aging, have substantially lower replicative potential.

Replicative senescence occurs in cells as they age because of progressive shortening of telomeres, which ultimately results in cell cycle arrest. *Telomeres* are short, repeated sequences of DNA present at the ends of chromosomes that are important for ensuring the complete replication of chromosome ends and for protecting the ends from fusion and degradation. When somatic cells replicate, a small section of the telomere is not duplicated, and telomeres become progressively shortened. Once the ends of

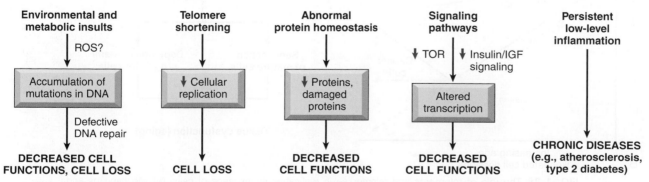

FIG. 1.27 Mechanisms of cellular aging. Multiple mechanisms contribute to cellular aging. Some environmental modifications, such as calorie restriction, counteract aging by activating various signaling pathways and transcription factors (not shown). *ROS,* Reactive oxygen species; *TOR,* target of rapamycin.

telomeres are completely eroded the ends of chromosomes are no longer protected and are sensed in cells as broken DNA, which signals cell cycle arrest. Telomere length is maintained by nucleotide addition mediated by an enzyme called *telomerase*. Telomerase is a specialized RNA-protein complex that uses its own RNA as a template for adding nucleotides to the ends of chromosomes. Telomerase is active in germ cells and present at low levels in stem cells but is absent in most somatic cells (Fig. 1.28). Therefore, as somatic cells age, their telomeres become shorter and they exit the cell cycle, resulting in an inability to generate new cells to replace damaged ones. Conversely, in immortalized cancer cells (Chapter 6), telomerase is usually reactivated and telomere length is stabilized, allowing the cells to proliferate indefinitely. However, the extent of the relationship between telomerase activity, telomere length, and aging has yet to be fully established. Inherited deficiencies in telomerase activities have been implicated in certain diseases, such as aplastic anemia (thought to be caused by a failure of hematopoietic stem cells) and pulmonary and liver fibrosis, as well as premature graying of hair and characteristic skin pigment and nail abnormalities. These disorders are sometimes considered "telomeropathies."

- *Altered protein homeostasis.* Over time, cells are unable to maintain normal protein homeostasis because of increased turnover and decreased synthesis of proteins and defective activity of chaperones (which promote normal protein folding) and proteasomes (which degrade misfolded proteins). The resultant abnormalities in protein production can have many deleterious effects on cell survival, replication, and functions, and the concomitant accumulation of misfolded proteins may trigger apoptosis.

- *Biochemical signaling pathways* may also play a role in regulating the aging process. Certain environmental stresses, such as calorie restriction, alter signaling pathways that influence aging. Biochemical alterations associated with calorie restriction may counteract aging and prolong lifespan. Specific agents that reduce aging in experimental models include inhibitors of insulin-like growth factor (IGF-1) and the molecular target of rapamycin (mTOR), both of which affect signaling pathways that regulate cellular metabolism. Partial inhibition of these pathways may switch cells from focusing on growth and proliferation to concentrating on repairing damage. These strategies have prolonged the lifespans of model organisms, but how relevant they are to humans remains uncertain.

- *Persistent inflammation.* As individuals age, the accumulation of damaged cells, lipids, and DNA may activate the inflammasome pathway (Chapter 5), resulting in low-level inflammation. Sustained inflammation in turn contributes to chronic diseases, such as atherosclerosis and type 2 diabetes. Cytokines produced during inflammatory reactions may themselves induce cellular alterations that exacerbate aging, and chronic metabolic disorders may further accelerate the process.

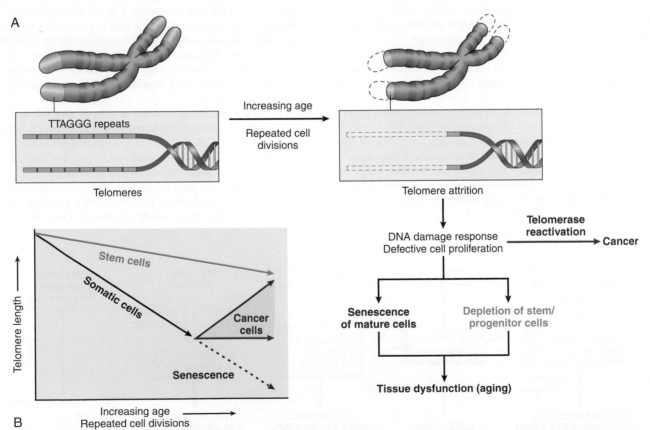

FIG. 1.28 The role of telomeres and telomerase in replicative senescence of cells. (A) Mechanisms and consequences of telomere attrition. Repeated cell division associated with aging leads to progressive shortening of telomeres, which triggers senescence and loss of stem cell pools. (B) Telomere attrition is characteristic of somatic cells. Stem cells maintain their telomeres and are, therefore, capable of unlimited replication. Cancer cells frequently activate telomerase and are thus able to maintain telomeres.

Clinical observations and epidemiologic studies have shown that physical activity and, as mentioned previously, calorie restriction slow aging, whereas many kinds of stress accelerate aging. The precise mechanisms underlying these effects remain to be defined, and for now we all remain vulnerable to the ravages of aging.

It should be apparent that the various forms of cellular derangements and adaptations described in this chapter cover a wide spectrum, ranging from reversible and irreversible forms of acute cell injury, to adaptations in cell size, growth, and function, to largely unavoidable consequences of aging. Reference is made to these alterations throughout this book, because all instances of organ injury and ultimately all clinical disease arise from derangements in cell structure and function.

■ RAPID REVIEW

Patterns of Cell Injury and Cell Death

- Causes of cell injury: ischemia, toxins, infections, immunologic reactions, genetic, nutritional imbalances, physical agents (e.g., trauma, burns), aging
- Reversible cell injury: cell swelling, fatty change, plasma membrane blebbing and loss of microvilli, mitochondrial swelling, dilation of the ER, eosinophilia (due to decreased cytoplasmic RNA), myelin figures
- Necrosis: eosinophilia; nuclear shrinkage, fragmentation, and dissolution; breakdown of plasma membrane and organellar membranes; leakage and enzymatic digestion of cellular contents; elicits inflammation
- Morphologic types of tissue necrosis: coagulative, liquefactive, gangrenous, caseous, fat, and fibrinoid.
- Apoptosis: regulated mechanism of cell death that eliminates unnecessary and irreparably damaged cells, without injurious host reaction; characterized by enzymatic degradation of proteins and DNA, initiated by caspases, and by recognition and removal of dead cells by phagocytes
- Two major pathways of apoptosis:
  - Mitochondrial (intrinsic) pathway is triggered by loss of survival signals, DNA damage, and accumulation of misfolded proteins (ER stress); associated with leakage of proapoptotic proteins from mitochondrial membrane into the cytoplasm, where they trigger caspase activation; inhibited by antiapoptotic members of the BCL family, which are induced by survival signals including growth factors.
  - Death receptor (extrinsic) pathway is responsible for elimination of self-reactive lymphocytes and damage by cytotoxic T lymphocytes; initiated by engagement of death receptors (members of the TNF receptor family) with ligands on adjacent cells.
- Autophagy is triggered by nutrient deprivation; characterized by degradation and recycling of cellular contents to provide energy during stress; can trigger apoptosis if the stress is not relieved.
- Other unusual pathways of cell death include necroptosis (features of both necrosis and apoptosis regulated by particular signaling pathways) and pyroptosis (cell death associated with the release of proinflammatory cytokines).

Mechanisms of Cell Injury

- Different initiating events cause cell injury and death by diverse mechanisms.

- Mitochondrial damage and increased permeability of cellular membranes are often late events in cell injury and necrosis from different causes.
- Oxidative stress refers to accumulation of ROS, which can damage cellular lipids, proteins, and DNA and is associated with numerous initiating causes.
- ER stress: Protein misfolding depletes essential proteins and, if the misfolded proteins accumulate within cells, triggers apoptosis.
- DNA damage, e.g., by radiation, can also induce apoptosis if it is not repaired.
- Hypoxia and ischemia lead to ATP depletion and failure of many energy-dependent functions, resulting first in reversible injury and, if not corrected, necrosis.
- In ischemia-reperfusion injury, restoration of blood flow to an ischemic tissue exacerbates damage by increasing production of ROS and by increasing inflammation.

Cellular Adaptations to Stress

- Hypertrophy: increased cell and organ size, often in response to increased workload; induced by growth factors produced in response to mechanical stress or other stimuli; occurs in tissues incapable of cell division
- Hyperplasia: increased cell numbers in response to hormones and other growth factors; occurs in tissues whose cells are able to divide or contain abundant tissue stem cells
- Atrophy: decreased cell and organ size, as a result of decreased nutrient supply or disuse; associated with decreased synthesis of cellular building blocks and increased breakdown of cellular organelles
- Metaplasia: change in phenotype of differentiated cells, often in response to chronic irritation, that makes cells better able to withstand the stress; usually induced by altered differentiation pathway of tissue stem cells; may result in reduced functions or increased propensity for malignant transformation

Abnormal Intracellular Depositions and Calcifications

- Abnormal deposits of materials in cells and tissues are the result of excessive intake or defective transport or catabolism.
  - Lipids
    - Fatty change: accumulation of free triglycerides in cells, resulting from excessive intake or defective transport (often because of defects in synthesis of transport proteins); manifestation of reversible cell injury
    - Cholesterol deposition: result of defective catabolism and excessive intake; in macrophages and smooth muscle cells of vessel walls in atherosclerosis
  - Proteins: reabsorbed proteins in kidney tubules; immunoglobulins in plasma cells
  - Glycogen: in macrophages of patients with defects in lysosomal enzymes that break down glycogen (glycogen storage diseases)
  - Pigments: typically indigestible pigments, such as carbon, lipofuscin (breakdown product of lipid peroxidation), or hemosiderin (usually due to iron overload)
- Pathologic calcifications
  - Dystrophic calcification: deposition of calcium at sites of cell injury and necrosis
  - Metastatic calcification: deposition of calcium in normal tissues, caused by hypercalcemia (usually a consequence of parathyroid hormone excess)

Cellular Aging

- Results from combination of multiple and progressive cellular alterations
- Accumulation of DNA damage and mutations
- Replicative senescence: reduced capacity of cells to divide secondary to progressive shortening of chromosomal ends (telomeres)
- Defective protein homeostasis: loss of normal proteins and accumulation of misfolded proteins
- Exacerbated by chronic diseases, especially those associated with prolonged inflammation, and by stress; slowed down by calorie restriction and exercise

Inflammation and Repair

Inflammation is a response of vascularized tissues to infections and tissue damage that brings cells and molecules of host defense from the circulation to the sites where they are needed, in order to eliminate the offending agents. Although in common medical and lay parlance inflammation suggests a harmful reaction, it is actually a protective response that is essential for survival. It serves to rid the host of both the initial cause of cell injury (e.g., microbes and toxins) and the consequences of such injury (e.g., necrotic cells and tissues) and initiates the repair of damaged tissues. The mediators of defense include phagocytic leukocytes, antibodies, and complement proteins (Fig. 2.1). Most of these normally circulate in the blood, where they are sequestered from tissues and unable to cause damage. Infections and dead cells are typically in the tissues, outside the vessels. The process of inflammation delivers leukocytes and proteins to foreign invaders, such as microbes, and to damaged or necrotic tissues and activates the recruited cells and molecules, which then remove the harmful or unwanted substances. Without inflammation, infections would go unchecked, wounds would never heal, and injured tissues might remain permanent festering sores.

We start with an overview of some of the important general features of inflammation, then discuss the major reactions of acute inflammation and the chemicals that mediate these reactions. We continue with a discussion of chronic inflammation and close with the process of tissue repair.

GENERAL FEATURES OF INFLAMMATION

Inflammation may be acute or chronic (Table 2.1). The initial, rapid response to infections and tissue damage is called *acute inflammation*. It develops within minutes to hours and lasts for several hours to a few days. Its main characteristics are the leakage of fluid and plasma proteins

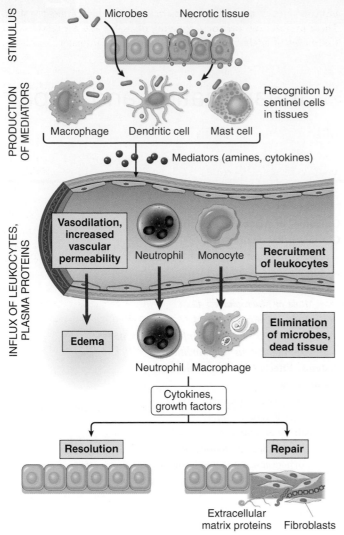

STIMULUS

PRODUCTION OF MEDIATORS

INFLUX OF LEUKOCYTES, PLASMA PROTEINS

Microbes　Necrotic tissue

Recognition by sentinel cells in tissues

Macrophage　Dendritic cell　Mast cell

Mediators (amines, cytokines)

Vasodilation, increased vascular permeability

Neutrophil　Monocyte

Recruitment of leukocytes

Edema

Elimination of microbes, dead tissue

Neutrophil　Macrophage

Cytokines, growth factors

Resolution

Repair

Extracellular matrix proteins　Fibroblasts

FIG. 2.1 Sequence of events in an inflammatory reaction. Macrophages and other cells in tissues recognize microbes and damaged cells and liberate mediators, which trigger the vascular and cellular reactions of inflammation. Influx of plasma proteins from the blood (not shown) accompanies edema.

(edema) and the accumulation of leukocytes, predominantly neutrophils (also called polymorphonuclear leukocytes). When acute inflammation achieves its desired goal of eliminating the offenders, the reaction quickly subsides, but if the response fails to clear the stimulus, it can progress to a protracted phase that is called *chronic inflammation*. Chronic inflammation is of longer duration and is associated with continuing tissue destruction and fibrosis (the deposition of connective tissue).

The external manifestations of inflammation, often called its cardinals signs, are heat (*calor* in Latin), redness (*rubor*), swelling (*tumor*), pain (*dolor*), and loss of function (*function laesa*). The first four of these were described more than 2000 years ago by a Roman encyclopedist named Celsus, who wrote the then-famous text *De Medicina*; the fifth was added in the late 19th century by Rudolf Virchow, known as the "father of modern pathology." These manifestations occur as consequences of the vascular changes and leukocyte recruitment and activation, as will be evident from the discussion that follows.

Inflammatory reactions develop in steps (which can be summarized as the five R's): (1) *recognition* of the offending agent; (2) *recruitment* of blood cells and proteins to the tissue site; (3) *removal* of the offending agent; (4) *regulation* of the reaction; and (5) *repair* of injured tissue. Each of these steps is described in detail in this chapter.

While normally protective, in some situations, the inflammatory reaction becomes the cause of disease, and the damage it produces is its dominant feature. Inflammatory reactions to infections are often accompanied by local tissue damage and pain. Typically, however, these harmful consequences resolve as the inflammation abates, leaving little or no permanent damage. By contrast, there are many diseases in which the inflammatory reaction is misdirected (e.g., against self tissues in autoimmune diseases), occurs against usually harmless environmental substances (e.g., in allergies), or is excessively prolonged (e.g., in infections by microbes that resist eradication such as *Mycobacterium tuberculosis*). These abnormal reactions underlie many common chronic diseases, such as rheumatoid arthritis, asthma and lung fibrosis (Table 2.2). Inflammation may also contribute to diseases that are thought to be primarily metabolic, degenerative, or genetic, such as atherosclerosis, type 2 diabetes, and Alzheimer disease. In recognition of the wide-ranging harmful consequences of inflammation, the lay press has rather melodramatically referred to it as "the silent killer."

Table 2.1 Features of Acute and Chronic Inflammation

Feature	Acute Inflammation	Chronic Inflammation
Onset	Fast: minutes to hours	Slow: days
Cellular infiltrate	Mainly neutrophils	Monocytes/macrophages and lymphocytes
Tissue injury	Usually mild and self-limited	May be significant
Fibrosis	None	May be severe and progressive
Local and systemic signs	Prominent	Variable, usually modest

Table 2.2 Disorders Caused by Inflammatory Reactions

Disorders	Cells and Molecules Involved in Injury
Acute	
Acute respiratory distress syndrome	Neutrophils
Glomerulonephritis, vasculitis	Antibodies and complement; neutrophils
Septic shock	Cytokines
Chronic	
Rheumatoid arthritis	Lymphocytes, macrophages; antibodies?
Asthma	Eosinophils; IgE antibodies
Pulmonary fibrosis	Macrophages; fibroblasts

Listed are selected examples of diseases in which the inflammatory response plays a significant role in tissue injury. Some, such as asthma, can present as a chronic illness with repeated bouts of acute exacerbation. These diseases and their pathogenesis are discussed in relevant chapters.

Inadequate inflammation is typically manifested by increased susceptibility to infections. Impairment of inflammation is caused by reduced production of leukocytes resulting from replacement of the bone marrow by cancers (e.g., leukemias), immunosuppressive agents used to treat graft rejection and autoimmune disorders, and many other conditions such as malnutrition. Inherited genetic disorders of leukocyte function are rare, but they provide valuable information about the mechanisms of leukocyte responses. These conditions are described in Chapter 5 in the context of immunodeficiency diseases.

Once inflammation has eliminated the offending agents, it subsides and also sets into motion the process of *tissue repair*. In this process, the injured tissue is replaced through *regeneration* of surviving cells and filling of residual defects with connective tissue *(scarring)*.

CAUSES OF INFLAMMATION

Of the myriad causes of inflammation, the following are the most frequent:

- *Infections,* in which the products of microbes are recognized by the host and elicit different types of inflammatory reactions.
- *Tissue necrosis,* which may be caused by *ischemia* (reduced blood flow, the cause of infarction in the heart, brain, and other tissues), *trauma,* and *physical and chemical injury* (e.g., thermal injury, irradiation, and exposure to toxins). Molecules released from necrotic cells trigger inflammation even in the absence of infection (so-called "sterile inflammation").
- *Foreign bodies,* such as sutures and tissue implants, also elicit sterile inflammation.
- *Immune reactions* (also called *hypersensitivity*) are reactions in which the normally protective immune system damages the individual's own tissues. As mentioned earlier, *autoimmune diseases* and *allergies* are diseases caused by immune responses; in both, inflammation is a major contributor to tissue injury (Chapter 5).

RECOGNITION OF MICROBES AND DAMAGED CELLS

The first step in inflammatory responses is the recognition of microbes and necrotic cells by cellular receptors and circulating proteins. All tissues contain resident cells whose primary function is to detect the presence of foreign invaders or dead cells, to ingest and destroy these potential causes of harm, and to elicit the inflammatory reaction that recruits cells and proteins from the blood to complete the elimination process. The most important of these sentinel cells are tissue-resident macrophages and dendritic cells. These cells express receptors for microbial products in multiple cell compartments: on their surface, where they recognize microbes in the extracellular space; in endosomes, into which microbes are ingested; and in the cytosol where certain microbes may survive. The best known of these receptors are the *Toll-like receptors (TLRs)* (Chapter 5). Activation of TLRs leads to the production of cytokines that trigger inflammation (discussed later). A different sensor system consists of cytosolic *NOD-like* receptors (NLRs) that, upon activation, recruit and activate a multiprotein complex (the *inflammasome,* Chapter 5) which generates the biologically active cytokine interleukin-1 (IL-1). NLRs recognize a wide range of stimuli, including microbial products and indicators of cell damage such as leaked DNA and decreased cytosolic potassium levels. The cytokine-induced inflammation then eliminates the stimulus that elicited the reaction (microbes and dead cell debris).

If microbes navigate the gauntlet of sentinels in tissues and enter the circulation, they are then recognized by a number of *plasma proteins,* such as antibodies and members of the complement system. These proteins can destroy circulating microbes and are recruited to tissue sites of infection, where they stimulate inflammatory reactions.

With this background, we proceed to a discussion of acute inflammation, its underlying mechanisms, and how it functions to eliminate microbes and dead cells.

ACUTE INFLAMMATION

Acute inflammation has three major components: (1) dilation of small vessels; (2) increased permeability of the microvasculature; and (3) emigration of the leukocytes from the microcirculation (see Fig. 2.1). Most of these changes happen in postcapillary venules at the site of infection or tissue injury. The walls of these vessels are capable of reacting to stimuli and are sufficiently thin to allow passage of fluid and proteins. Vasodilation slows down blood flow and sets the stage for the subsequent reactions, while increased vascular permeability enables plasma proteins to enter the tissue site. Transmigration moves leukocytes from their peaceful home inside the vessels into the maelstrom of infection or necrosis, where the cells perform their function of destroying noxious agents and cleaning up the damage. All these reactions are induced by cytokines and other molecules (collectively called *inflammatory mediators*) produced at the site of infection or necrosis (described later).

Vascular Reactions in Acute Inflammation

Vasodilation is one of the earliest reactions of acute inflammation and is responsible for the externally visible redness (*erythema*) and warmth that accompany most acute inflammatory reactions. The most important chemical mediator of vasodilation is histamine, discussed later.

Vasodilation is quickly followed by **increased permeability of the microvasculature** and the outpouring of protein-rich fluid into the extravascular tissues. The escape of fluid, proteins, and blood cells from the vascular system into the interstitial tissue or body cavities is known as *exudation* (Fig. 2.2). An *exudate* is an extravascular fluid that has a high protein concentration and contains cellular debris. Its presence implies that there is an increase in the permeability of small blood vessels, typically during an inflammatory reaction. By contrast, a *transudate* is a fluid with low protein content (most of which is albumin), little or no cellular material, and low specific gravity. A transudate is essentially an ultrafiltrate of blood plasma that is produced as a result of osmotic or hydrostatic imbalance across the vessel wall without an increase in vascular permeability and is usually not associated with inflammation (Chapter 3). *Edema* denotes an excess of fluid in the interstitial tissue or serous cavities; it can be either an exudate or a transudate. *Pus,* a *purulent* exudate, is an inflammatory exudate rich in leukocytes (mostly neutrophils), the debris of dead cells, and, in many cases, microbes.

The principal mechanism of increased vascular permeability is the contraction of endothelial cells, which creates interendothelial openings. It is elicited by histamine, bradykinin, leukotrienes, and other chemical mediators. It occurs rapidly after exposure to the mediator (within 15 to 30 minutes) and is usually short lived. In unusual cases (e.g., in burns), increased vascular permeability may result from direct endothelial injury. In these instances, leakage starts immediately after injury and is sustained for several hours until the damaged vessels become thrombosed or are repaired.

The loss of fluid and increased vessel diameter lead to slower blood flow and higher concentration of red cells in small vessels, raising the viscosity of the blood. Involved small vessels become engorged with

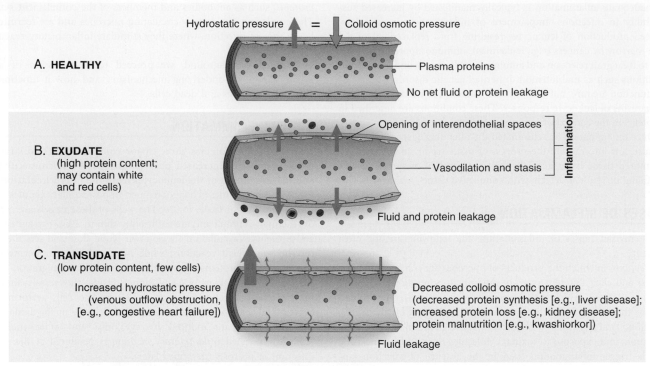

FIG. 2.2 Formation of exudates and transudates. (A) Normal hydrostatic pressure *(blue arrow)* is about 32 mm Hg at the arterial end of a capillary bed and 12 mm Hg at the venous end; the mean colloid osmotic pressure of tissues is approximately 25 mm Hg *(green arrow)*. Therefore, there is virtually no net flow of fluid across the vascular bed in the steady state. (B) An exudate is formed in inflammation because vascular permeability increases as a result of retraction of endothelial cells, creating spaces through which fluid and proteins can pass. (C) A transudate is formed when fluid leaks out because of increased hydrostatic pressure or decreased osmotic pressure.

red cells, a condition termed *stasis*, which is seen histologically as *vascular congestion* and externally as localized redness of the affected tissue.

In addition to the reactions of blood vessels, lymph flow is increased and helps drain edema fluid that accumulates because of increased vascular permeability. The lymphatics may become secondarily inflamed *(lymphangitis)*, appearing clinically as red streaks extending from an inflammatory focus along the course of lymphatic channels. Involvement of the draining lymph nodes may lead to enlargement (because of increased cellularity) and pain. The associated constellation of pathologic changes is termed *reactive* or *inflammatory lymphadenitis* (Chapter 10).

Leukocyte Recruitment to Sites of Inflammation

The journey of leukocytes from the vessel lumen to the tissue is a multistep process that is mediated and controlled by adhesion molecules and cytokines. Leukocytes normally transit rapidly through small vessels. In inflammation, they have to be stopped and then brought to the offending agent or the site of tissue damage, outside the vessels. This process can be divided into phases, consisting first of adhesion of leukocytes to endothelium at the site of inflammation, then transmigration of the leukocytes through the vessel wall, and finally, movement of the cells toward the offending agent (Fig. 2.3).

When blood flows from capillaries into postcapillary venules, under conditions of normal laminar flow, red cells are concentrated in the center of the vessel, displacing leukocytes toward the vessel wall. As the rate of flow slows early in inflammation (stasis), leukocytes, being larger than red cells, slow down more and assume a more peripheral position along the endothelial surface, a process called *margination*. By moving close to the vessel wall, leukocytes are able to detect and react to changes in the endothelium. When endothelial cells are activated by cytokines and other mediators produced locally, they express adhesion molecules to which the leukocytes attach loosely. These cells bind and detach and thus begin to tumble on the endothelial surface, a process called *rolling*. The cells finally come to rest at some point where they *adhere* firmly (resembling pebbles over which a stream runs without disturbing them).

The initial weak binding of leukocytes and their rolling on the endothelium are mediated by a family of proteins called *selectins* (Table 2.3). Selectins are receptors expressed on leukocytes and endothelium that have an extracellular domain that binds carbohydrates (hence the lectin part of the name). The ligands for selectins are sialic acid–containing oligosaccharides attached to glycoprotein backbones; some are expressed on leukocytes and others on endothelial cells. Endothelial cells express two selectins, E- and P-selectins, as well as the ligand for L-selectin, whereas leukocytes express L-selectin. E- and P-selectins are typically expressed at low levels or not at all on nonactivated endothelium but are upregulated after stimulation by cytokines and other mediators. Therefore, binding of leukocytes is largely restricted to endothelium at sites of infection or tissue injury (where the mediators are produced). For example, in nonactivated endothelial cells, P-selectin is found primarily in intracellular membrane-bound vesicles called Weibel-Palade bodies; however, within minutes of exposure to mediators such as histamine or thrombin, P-selectin traffics to the cell surface. Similarly, E-selectin and the ligand for L-selectin, which are not expressed on normal

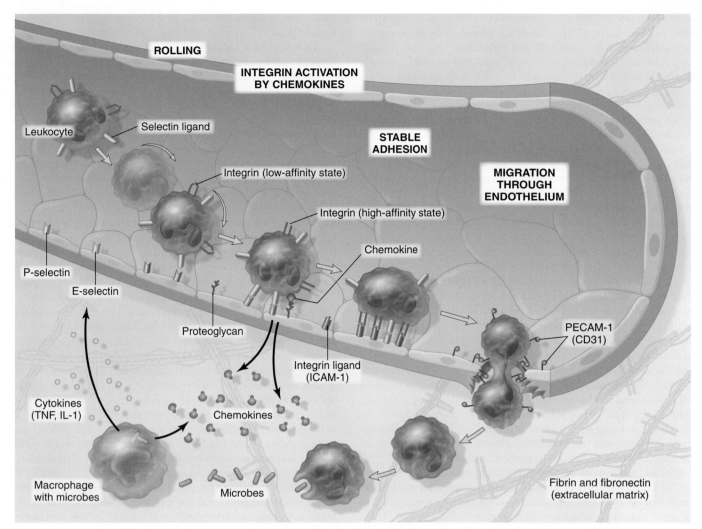

FIG. 2.3 The multistep process of leukocyte migration through blood vessels, shown here for neutrophils. The leukocytes first roll, then become activated and adhere to endothelium, then transmigrate across the endothelium, pierce the basement membrane, and move toward chemoattractants emanating from the source of injury. Different molecules play predominant roles at each step of this process: selectins in rolling; chemokines (displayed bound to proteoglycans) in activating the neutrophils to increase avidity of integrins; integrins in firm adhesion; and CD31 (PECAM-1) in transmigration. E- and P-selectins are expressed on endothelial cells; L-selectin is expressed on leukocytes (not shown). *ICAM-1,* Intercellular adhesion molecule-1; *IL-1,* interleukin-1; *PECAM-1 (CD31),* platelet endothelial cell adhesion molecule-1; *TNF,* tumor necrosis factor.

Table 2.3 Endothelial and Leukocyte Adhesion Molecules

Family	Adhesion Molecule	Major Cell Type	Principal Ligands
Selectin	L-selectin	Leukocytes	Sialyl-Lewis X on various glycoproteins expressed on endothelium
	E-selectin	Activated endothelium	Sialyl-Lewis X on glycoproteins expressed on neutrophils, monocytes, T lymphocytes
	P-selectin	Activated endothelium	Sialyl-Lewis X on glycoproteins expressed on neutrophils, monocytes, T lymphocytes
Integrin	LFA-1	T lymphocytes, other leukocytes	ICAM-1 expressed on activated endothelium
	MAC-1	Monocytes, other leukocytes	ICAM-1 expressed on activated endothelium
	VLA-4	T lymphocytes, other leukocytes	VCAM-1 expressed on activated endothelium
	α4β7	Lymphocytes, monocytes	MAdCAM-1 expressed on endothelium in gut and gut-associated lymphoid tissues

ICAM, Intercellular adhesion molecule; *LFA,* lymphocyte function-associated antigen; *MAC-1,* macrophage antigen 1; *MAdCAM-1,* mucosal addressin cell adhesion molecule-1; *VCAM,* vascular cell adhesion molecule; *VLA,* very late antigen.

endothelium, are induced after stimulation by the cytokines IL-1 and tumor necrosis factor (TNF), which are produced by tissue macrophages, dendritic cells, mast cells, and endothelial cells after encountering microbes or dead tissues. Selectin-mediated interactions have a low affinity with a fast off-rate, and they are easily disrupted by the flowing blood. As a result, the leukocytes bind, detach, and bind again to endothelium. These weak rolling interactions slow down the leukocytes sufficiently for them to recognize additional adhesion molecules on the endothelium.

Firm adhesion of leukocytes to endothelium is mediated by a family of leukocyte surface proteins called *integrins* (see Table 2.3). Integrins are transmembrane two-chain glycoproteins that mediate the adhesion of leukocytes to endothelium and of various cells to the extracellular matrix. They are normally expressed on leukocyte plasma membranes in a low-affinity form and do not adhere to their specific ligands until the leukocytes are activated by *chemokines*. Chemokines are chemoattractant cytokines that are secreted by many cells at sites of inflammation, bind to endothelial cell proteoglycans, and are displayed at high concentrations on the endothelial surface. When the rolling leukocytes encounter the displayed chemokines, the cells are activated and their integrins undergo conformational changes and cluster together, thereby converting to a high-affinity form. At the same time, other cytokines, notably TNF and IL-1 (also secreted at sites of infection and injury), activate endothelial cells to increase their expression of ligands for integrins. The combination of cytokine-induced expression of integrin ligands on the endothelium and increased affinity of integrins on the leukocytes results in firm integrin-mediated binding of the leukocytes to the endothelium at the site of inflammation. The leukocytes stop rolling, and engagement of integrins by their ligands delivers signals to the leukocytes that lead to cytoskeletal changes that arrest the leukocytes and firmly attach them to the endothelium.

A telling indication of the importance of leukocyte adhesion molecules is the existence of mutations affecting integrins and selectin ligands that result in recurrent bacterial infections as a consequence of impaired leukocyte adhesion and defective inflammation. These leukocyte adhesion deficiencies are described in Chapter 5. Antagonists of integrins are approved for the treatment of some chronic inflammatory diseases, such as multiple sclerosis and inflammatory bowel disease.

After arresting on the endothelial surface, leukocytes migrate through the vessel wall, primarily by squeezing between interendothelial junctions. This extravasation of leukocytes is called *transmigration* or *diapedesis*. Platelet endothelial cell adhesion molecule-1 (PECAM-1, also called CD31), a cellular adhesion molecule expressed on leukocytes and endothelial cells, mediates the binding events needed for leukocytes to traverse the endothelium. After crossing the endothelium, leukocytes pierce the basement membrane, probably by secreting collagenases, and enter the extravascular tissue. The directionality of leukocyte movement within tissues is controlled by locally produced chemokines, which create a diffusion gradient that the cells migrate along.

After exiting the circulation, leukocytes move in the tissues toward the site of injury by a process called *chemotaxis*, defined as locomotion along a chemical gradient. Among the many chemoattractants known, the most potent are bacterial products, particularly peptides with *N*-formylmethionine termini; cytokines, especially those of the chemokine family; components of the complement system, particularly C5a; and leukotrienes. These chemoattractants, which are described in more detail later, are produced in response to infections and tissue damage and during immunologic reactions. All of them bind to G protein–coupled receptors on the surface of leukocytes. Signals initiated from these receptors activate second messengers that induce the polymerization of actin at the leading edge of the cell and the localization of myosin filaments at the back. The leukocyte moves by extending filopodia that pull the back of the cell in the direction of extension, much as an automobile with front-wheel drive is pulled by the front wheels. The net result is that leukocytes migrate toward the inflammatory stimulus in the direction of the locally produced chemoattractants.

The nature of the leukocyte infiltrate varies with the age of the inflammatory response and the type of stimulus. In most forms of acute inflammation, neutrophils predominate in the inflammatory infiltrate during the first 6 to 24 hours and are replaced by monocytes in 24 to 48 hours (Fig. 2.4). There are several reasons for the early

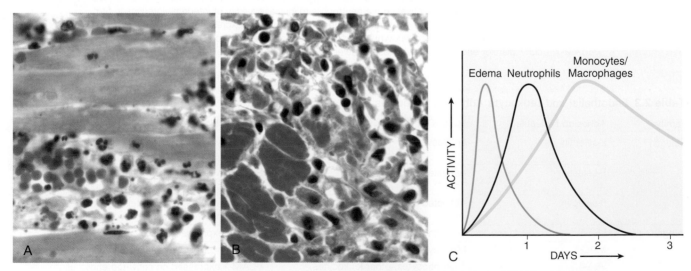

FIG. 2.4 Nature of leukocyte infiltrates in inflammatory reactions. The photomicrographs show an inflammatory reaction in the myocardium after ischemic necrosis (infarction). (A) Early neutrophilic infiltrates and congested blood vessels. (B) Later mononuclear cell infiltrates (mostly macrophages). (C) The approximate kinetics of edema and cellular infiltration. The kinetics and nature of the infiltrate may vary depending on the severity and cause of the reaction.

preponderance of neutrophils: they are more numerous in the blood than other leukocytes, they respond more rapidly to chemokines, and they may attach more firmly to adhesion molecules that are rapidly induced on endothelial cells, such as P- and E-selectins. After entering tissues, neutrophils are short lived; they undergo apoptosis and disappear within a few days. Monocytes develop into macrophages in tissues that not only survive longer but may also proliferate, and thus they become the dominant population in prolonged inflammatory reactions.

There are, however, exceptions to this stereotypic pattern of cellular infiltration. In certain infections—for example, those produced by *Pseudomonas* bacteria—the cellular infiltrate is dominated by continuously recruited neutrophils for several days; in viral infections, lymphocytes may be the first cells to arrive; some hypersensitivity reactions are dominated by activated lymphocytes, macrophages, and plasma cells (reflecting the immune response); and in allergic reactions and infections with certain parasites, eosinophils may be the main cell type.

The molecular understanding of leukocyte recruitment and migration has provided a large number of therapeutic targets for controlling harmful inflammation. As we discuss later, agents that block TNF, one of the major cytokines in leukocyte recruitment, are extremely useful therapeutics for chronic inflammatory diseases such as rheumatoid arthritis. Antibodies that block integrins were mentioned earlier.

Phagocytosis and Clearance of the Offending Agent

Neutrophils and monocytes that have been recruited to a site of infection or cell death are activated by products of microbes and necrotic cells and by locally produced cytokines. Activation induces several responses (eFig. 2.1), of which phagocytosis and intracellular killing are most important for destruction of microbes and clearance of dead tissues.

Phagocytosis

Phagocytosis is the ingestion of particulate material by cells. The body's most important phagocytes are *neutrophils* and *macrophages* (Table 2.4). Neutrophils are rapid responders but relatively short-lived. In inflammatory reactions, macrophages are derived from blood monocytes and can live for days or months. (As we will discuss later, some long-lived tissue-resident macrophages are derived from embryonic precursors that seed the tissues in early life and remain for years.) Macrophage responses tend to be slower but more long lasting.

Neutrophils and macrophages can ingest microbes following their recognition by phagocyte receptors, such as the mannose receptor (which recognizes terminal mannose residues found in microbial glycoproteins) and so-called "scavenger receptors." The efficiency of this process is greatly increased if the microbes are coated *(opsonized)* with molecules called *opsonins* for which the phagocytes also have specific receptors. Opsonins include antibodies, the C3b cleavage product of complement, and certain plasma lectins. Following binding to phagocyte receptors the particle is ingested into a membrane-bound vesicle called the *phagosome*, which then fuses with lysosomes, resulting in discharge of lysosomal contents into the *phagolysosome* (Fig. 2.5). During this process, neutrophils may also release granule contents into the extracellular space.

Intracellular Destruction of Microbes and Debris

Killing of microbes and destruction of ingested materials are accomplished by reactive oxygen species (ROS, also called *reactive oxygen intermediates*), reactive nitrogen species (mainly derived from nitric oxide [NO]), and lysosomal enzymes. All these substances are normally sequestered in lysosomes, to which phagocytosed materials are brought. Thus, potentially harmful substances are segregated from the cell's cytoplasm to avoid damage to the phagocyte while it is performing its normal function.

Table 2.4 Properties of Neutrophils and Macrophages

	Neutrophils	Macrophages
Origin	HSCs in bone marrow	HSCs in bone marrow (in inflammatory reactions) Stem cells in yolk sac or fetal liver (early in development, for some tissue-resident macrophages)
Life span in tissues	1–2 days	Inflammatory macrophages: days or weeks Tissue-resident macrophages: years
Responses to activating stimuli	Rapid, short-lived, mostly degranulation and enzymatic activity	More prolonged, slower, often dependent on new gene transcription
• Reactive oxygen species	Rapidly induced by assembly of phagocyte oxidase (respiratory burst)	Less prominent
• Nitric oxide	Low levels or none	Induced following transcriptional activation of iNOS
• Degranulation	Major response; induced by cytoskeletal rearrangement	Not prominent
• Cytokine production	Low levels or none	Major functional activity, requires transcriptional activation of cytokine genes
• NET formation	Rapidly induced, by extrusion of nuclear contents	Little or none
• Secretion of lysosomal enzymes	Prominent	Less

HSC, Hematopoietic stem cell; *iNOS*, inducible nitric oxide synthase; *NET*, neutrophil extracellular traps.

This table lists the major differences between neutrophils and macrophages. Note that the two cell types share many features, such as phagocytosis, ability to migrate through blood vessels into tissues, and chemotaxis.

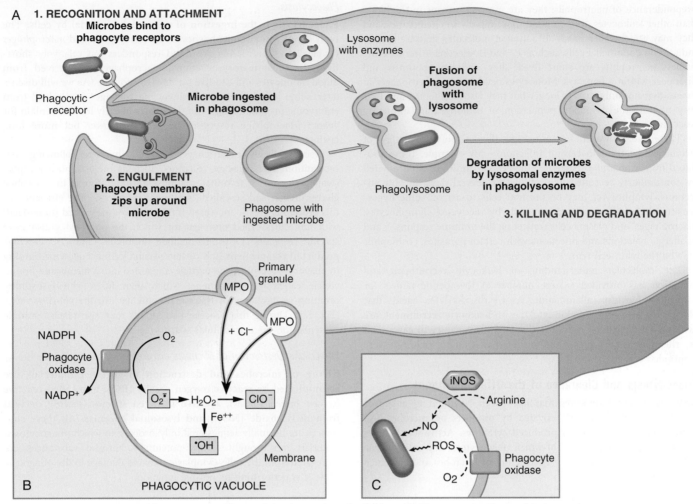

FIG. 2.5 Phagocytosis and intracellular destruction of microbes. (A) Phagocytosis of a particle (e.g., a bacterium) involves binding to receptors on the leukocyte membrane, engulfment, and fusion of the phagocytic vacuoles with lysosomes. This is followed by destruction of ingested particles within the phagolysosomes by lysosomal enzymes and by reactive oxygen and nitrogen species. (B) In activated phagocytes, cytoplasmic components of the phagocyte oxidase enzyme assemble in the membrane of the phagosome to form the active enzyme, which catalyzes the conversion of oxygen into superoxide $(O_2^{\cdot})$ and H_2O_2. Myeloperoxidase, present in the granules of neutrophils, converts H_2O_2 to hypochlorite. (C) Microbicidal reactive oxygen species (ROS) and nitric oxide (NO) kill ingested microbes. During phagocytosis, granule contents may be released into extracellular tissues (not shown). *iNOS,* Inducible NO synthase; *MPO,* myeloperoxidase; *ROS,* reactive oxygen species.

Reactive Oxygen Species. These free radicals are produced mainly in the phagolysosomes of neutrophils. Upon activation of neutrophils, a multicomponent enzyme called *phagocyte oxidase* (or NADPH oxidase) is rapidly assembled in the membrane of the phagolysosome (Fig. 2.5B). This enzyme oxidizes NADPH (reduced nicotinamide-adenine dinucleotide phosphate) and, in the process, reduces oxygen to superoxide anion $(O_2^{\cdot})$, which is then converted to H_2O_2. H_2O_2 is not able to efficiently kill microbes by itself. However, the azurophilic granules of neutrophils contain the enzyme *myeloperoxidase* (MPO), which, in the presence of a halide such as Cl^-, converts H_2O_2 to hypochlorite (ClO^-), a potent antimicrobial agent that destroys microbes by *halogenation* (in which the halide is bound covalently to cellular constituents) or by *oxidation* of proteins and lipids (lipid peroxidation). The H_2O_2-MPO-halide system is the most efficient bactericidal system of neutrophils. H_2O_2 is also converted to hydroxyl radical (•OH), another powerful destructive agent. As discussed in Chapter 1, these oxygen-derived free radicals bind to and modify cellular lipids, proteins, and nucleic acids and thus destroy cells such as microbes. The production of ROS coupled with oxygen consumption is called the *respiratory burst*. Genetic defects in the generation of ROS are the cause of an immunodeficiency disease called *chronic granulomatous disease*, described in Chapter 5.

Nitric Oxide. NO, a soluble gas produced from arginine by the action of nitric oxide synthase (NOS), also participates in microbial killing, especially in macrophages. Inducible NOS (iNOS) is upregulated in macrophages by transcriptional activation of the gene in response to microbial products and cytokines such as IFN-γ (Fig. 2.5C). NO reacts with superoxide $(O_2^{\cdot})$ generated by phagocyte oxidase to produce the highly reactive peroxynitrite ($ONOO^-$). These nitrogen-derived molecules, similar to ROS, attack and damage the lipids, proteins, and nucleic acids of microbes.

Leukocyte Granule Contents. Neutrophils have two main types of granules containing enzymes that degrade microbes and dead tissues and may contribute to tissue damage. The smaller *specific* (or secondary) granules contain lysozyme, collagenase, gelatinase, lactoferrin, plasminogen activator, histaminase, and alkaline phosphatase. The larger *azurophil* (or primary) granules contain myeloperoxidase, bactericidal factors (such as defensins), acid hydrolases, and a variety of neutral proteases (elastase, cathepsin G, nonspecific collagenases, proteinase 3). The contents of both types of granules are released when neutrophils are activated. Phagocytic vesicles containing engulfed material may fuse with these granules (and with lysosomes, as described earlier), allowing the ingested materials to be destroyed in the phagolysomes by the actions of the enzymes. Similarly, macrophages contain lysosomes filled with acid hydrolases, collagenase, elastase, and phospholipase, all of which can destroy ingested materials and cell debris.

In addition to granule contents, activated neutrophils liberate chromatin components, including histones, which form fibrillar networks called *neutrophil extracellular traps (NETs)* (eFig. 2.2). These networks bind and concentrate antimicrobial peptides and granule enzymes, forming extracellular sites for the destruction of microbes. In the process of NET formation, the nuclei of the neutrophils are lost, leading to death of the cells. NETs have also been detected in the blood during sepsis, as a consequence of widespread neutrophil activation.

Leukocyte-Mediated Tissue Injury

Leukocytes are important causes of injury to normal cells and tissues. This happens during normal defense reactions against microbes, especially if the microbes are resistant to eradication, such as mycobacteria. It is also the basis of tissue damage when the response is inappropriately directed against self antigens (as in autoimmune diseases) or against normally harmless environmental antigens (as in allergic diseases).

The mechanism of leukocyte-mediated tissue injury is release of the contents of granules and lysosomes. To some extent, this happens normally, when activated leukocytes try to eliminate microbes and other offenders. The process is exaggerated if phagocytes encounter materials that cannot be easily ingested, such as antibodies deposited on indigestible flat surfaces, or if phagocytosed substances, such as urate and silica crystals, damage the membrane of the phagolysosome. The harmful proteases released by leukocytes are normally controlled by a system of *antiproteases* in the blood and tissue fluids. Foremost among these is α_1-antitrypsin, which is the major inhibitor of neutrophil elastase. A deficiency of these inhibitors may lead to sustained protease activity, as is the case in patients with α_1-antitrypsin deficiency (Chapter 11).

While we have emphasized the role of neutrophils and macrophages in acute inflammation, other cell types also serve important roles. Some T cells, called *Th17 cells*, secrete cytokines such as IL-17 that recruit neutrophils and stimulate production of antimicrobial peptides that directly kill microbes. In the absence of effective Th17 responses, individuals are susceptible to fungal and bacterial infections. The skin abscesses that develop lack the classic features of acute inflammation, such as warmth and redness. Eosinophils are especially important in reactions to helminthic parasites and in some allergic disorders, and mast cells and basophils are critical cells of allergic reactions.

Once the acute inflammatory response has eliminated the offending stimulus, the reaction subsides because there is no further leukocyte recruitment, mediators are short lived and decline if they are no longer produced, and neutrophils have short life spans.

MEDIATORS OF INFLAMMATION

The inflammatory reaction is initiated and regulated by chemicals that are produced at the site of the reaction. The large number of mediators is daunting, but a basic understanding of the molecules is important because their identification has been the foundation for the development of many widely used and effective antiinflammatory drugs. We begin by summarizing the general properties of the mediators of inflammation and then discuss some of the more important molecules.

- **Mediators may be produced locally by cells at the site of inflammation or may be derived from circulating precursors that are activated at the site of inflammation.**
  - *Cell-derived mediators* are rapidly released from intracellular granules (e.g., amines) or are synthesized de novo (e.g., prostaglandins and leukotrienes, cytokines) in response to a stimulus. **The major cell types that produce mediators of acute inflammation are tissue macrophages, dendritic cells, and mast cells,** but platelets, neutrophils, endothelial cells, and most epithelia also elaborate some inflammatory mediators.
  - *Plasma-derived mediators* (e.g., complement proteins) are produced mainly in the liver and circulate as inactive precursors that enter and are activated at sites of inflammation, usually by a series of proteolytic cleavages.
- **Active mediators are produced only in response to various stimuli,** including microbial products and substances released from necrotic cells, which ensures that inflammation is triggered only when and where it is needed.
- **Most mediators are short lived.** They quickly decay or are inactivated by enzymes, or they are otherwise scavenged or inhibited. These built-in control mechanisms prevent excessive reactions.

The principal mediators of acute inflammation are summarized in Table 2.5 and discussed next.

Vasoactive Amines: Histamine and Serotonin

The major vasoactive amine is *histamine*, which is stored as a preformed molecule in the granules of mast cells, blood basophils, and platelets. It is rapidly released when these cells are activated, so it is among the first mediators to be produced during inflammation. The richest source of histamine is the mast cell, which is normally present in the connective tissue adjacent to blood vessels. Mast cell degranulation and histamine release occur in response to a variety of stimuli, including binding of IgE antibodies to mast cells, which underlies immediate hypersensitivity (allergic) reactions (Chapter 5); products of complement called *anaphylatoxins* (C3a and C5a), described later; and physical injury induced by trauma, cold, or heat, by unknown mechanisms. Antibodies and complement products bind to specific receptors on mast cells and trigger signaling pathways that induce rapid degranulation. Neuropeptides (e.g., substance P) and cytokines (IL-1, IL-8) may also trigger release of histamine.

Histamine causes dilation of arterioles and increases the permeability of venules. Its effects on blood vessels are mediated mainly via binding to histamine receptors called H_1 receptors on microvascular endothelial cells. Common antihistamine drugs that treat inflammatory reactions, such as allergies, bind to and block the H_1 receptor. Histamine also causes contraction of some smooth muscles, but leukotrienes, described later, are much more potent and relevant for causing spasms of bronchial smooth muscle, such as in asthma.

Serotonin (5-hydroxytryptamine) is a preformed vasoactive mediator present in platelets and certain neuroendocrine cells, for example,

Table 2.5 Principal Mediators of Inflammation

Mediators	Sources	Actions
Histamine	Mast cells, basophils, platelets	Vasodilation, increased vascular permeability, endothelial activation
Prostaglandins	Mast cells, leukocytes	Vasodilation, pain, fever
Leukotrienes	Mast cells, leukocytes	Increased vascular permeability, chemotaxis, leukocyte adhesion, and activation
Cytokines (e.g., TNF, IL-1, IL-6)	Macrophages, endothelial cells, mast cells	Local: endothelial activation (expression of adhesion molecules) Systemic: fever, metabolic abnormalities, hypotension (shock)
Chemokines	Leukocytes, activated macrophages	Chemotaxis, leukocyte activation
Platelet-activating factor	Leukocytes, mast cells	Vasodilation, increased vascular permeability, leukocyte adhesion, chemotaxis, degranulation, oxidative burst
Complement	Plasma (produced in liver)	Leukocyte chemotaxis and activation, direct target killing (membrane attack complex), vasodilation (mast cell stimulation)
Kinins	Plasma (produced in liver)	Increased vascular permeability, smooth muscle contraction, vasodilation, pain

IL, Interleukin; *TNF*, tumor necrosis factor.

in the gastrointestinal tract. It is a vasoconstrictor, but its importance in inflammation is unclear.

Arachidonic Acid Metabolites

Prostaglandins and *leukotrienes* **are lipid mediators produced from arachidonic acid (AA) present in membrane phospholipids that stimulate vascular and cellular reactions in acute inflammation.** AA is a 20-carbon polyunsaturated fatty acid that is released from membrane phospholipids through the action of cellular phospholipases, mainly phospholipase A_2, that are activated by inflammatory stimuli, including cytokines, complement products, and physical injury. AA-derived mediators, also called *eicosanoids* (from the Greek, *eicosa*, meaning 20, as they are derived from 20-carbon fatty acids), are synthesized by two major classes of enzymes, cyclooxygenases (which generate prostaglandins) and lipoxygenases (which produce leukotrienes and lipoxins) (Fig. 2.6). Eicosanoids bind to G protein–coupled receptors on many cell types and can mediate virtually every step of inflammation (Table 2.6).

Prostaglandins

Prostaglandins **(PGs) are produced by mast cells, macrophages, endothelial cells, and many other cell types and are involved in the vascular and systemic reactions of inflammation.** They are generated by the actions of two *cyclooxgenases*, called COX-1 and COX-2, which differ in where they are expressed. COX-1 is produced in response to inflammatory stimuli and is also constitutively expressed in most tissues, where it may have homeostatic functions (e.g., fluid and electrolyte balance in the kidneys, cytoprotection in the gastrointestinal tract). By contrast, COX-2 is induced by inflammatory stimuli and thus generates prostaglandins in inflammatory reactions but is low or absent in most healthy tissues.

Prostaglandins are named based on structural features coded by a letter, as in PGD, PGE, and others, and a subscript numeral (e.g., 1, 2), which indicates the number of double bonds in the compound. The most important prostaglandins in inflammation are PGE_2, PGD_2, PGF_{2a}, PGI_2 (prostacyclin), and TxA_2 (thromboxane A_2), each of which is derived by the action of a specific enzyme on an intermediate in the pathway. Some of these enzymes have restricted tissue distribution and functions.

- PGD_2 is the major prostaglandin made by mast cells; along with PGE_2 (which is more widely distributed), it causes vasodilation and increases the permeability of postcapillary venules, thus potentiating exudation and resultant edema. PGD_2 is also a chemoattractant for neutrophils.
- Platelets contain the enzyme thromboxane synthase, which produces TxA_2, the major eicosanoid in these cells. TxA_2 is a potent platelet-aggregating agent and vasoconstrictor.
- Vascular endothelium lacks thromboxane synthase and instead contains prostacyclin synthase, which is responsible for the formation of prostacyclin (PGI_2) and its stable end product PGF_{1a}. Prostacyclin is a vasodilator and a potent inhibitor of platelet aggregation and thus serves to prevent thrombus formation on normal endothelial cells. A thromboxane-prostacyclin imbalance has been implicated as an early event in thrombosis in coronary and cerebral arteries (Chapter 10).
- In addition to their local effects, prostaglandins are involved in the pathogenesis of *pain* and *fever*, two common systemic manifestations of inflammation (described later).

Leukotrienes

Leukotrienes **are produced by leukocytes and mast cells by the action of lipoxygenase and are involved in vascular and smooth muscle reactions and leukocyte recruitment.** The synthesis of leukotrienes involves multiple steps. The first generates leukotriene A_4 (LTA_4), which in turn gives rise to LTB_4 or LTC_4. LTB_4 is produced by neutrophils and some macrophages and is a potent chemotactic agent and activator of neutrophils. LTC_4 and its metabolites, LTD_4 and LTE_4, are produced mainly in mast cells and cause intense vasoconstriction, bronchospasm (important in asthma), and increased permeability of venules.

Other Arachidonic Acid–Derived Mediators

Lipoxins are also generated from AA by the lipoxygenase pathway, but unlike prostaglandins and leukotrienes, the lipoxins suppress inflammation by inhibiting neutrophil chemotaxis and adhesion to endothelium and hence the recruitment of leukocytes. Leukocytes, particularly neutrophils, produce intermediates in the lipoxin synthesis pathway that are converted to lipoxins by platelets interacting with the leukocytes.

Various other antiinflammatory AA-derived mediators have been described and given names such as resolvins because they resolve the active phase of acute inflammation. The role of these compounds in the inflammatory response is a topic of active study.

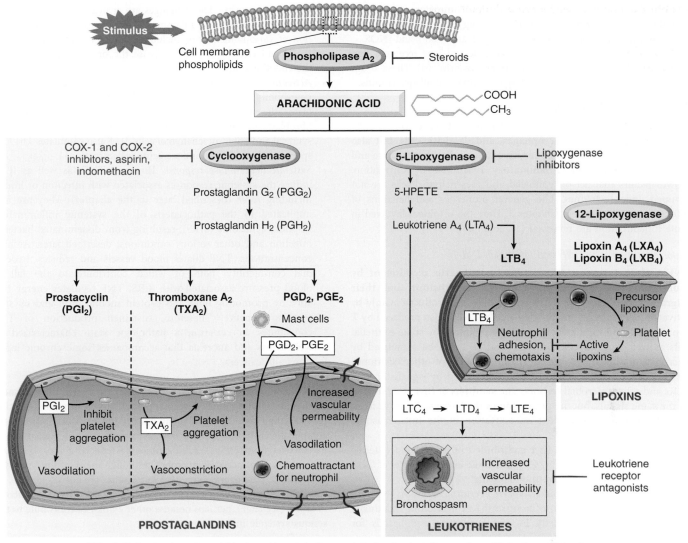

FIG. 2.6 Production of arachidonic acid metabolites and their roles in inflammation. Clinically useful antagonists of different enzymes and receptors are indicated in *red*. While leukotriene receptor antagonists inhibit all actions of leukotrienes, they are used in the clinic to treat asthma, as shown. *COX-1, COX-2,* Cyclooxygenase 1 and 2; *HPETE,* hydroperoxyeicosatetraenoic acid.

Table 2.6 Principal Actions of Arachidonic Acid Metabolites in Inflammation

Action	Eicosanoids
Vasodilation	Prostaglandins PGI_2 (prostacyclin), PGE_1, PGE_2, PGD_2
Vasoconstriction	Thromboxane A_2, leukotrienes C_4, D_4, E_4
Increased vascular permeability	Leukotrienes C_4, D_4, E_4
Chemotaxis, leukocyte adhesion	Leukotriene B_4

Pharmacologic Inhibitors of Prostaglandins and Leukotrienes

The importance of eicosanoids in inflammation has driven the development of antiinflammatory drugs, including the following:

- *Cyclooxygenase inhibitors* include aspirin and other nonsteroidal antiinflammatory drugs (NSAIDs), such as ibuprofen. They inhibit both COX-1 and COX-2 and thus inhibit prostaglandin synthesis (hence their efficacy in treating pain and fever); aspirin does this by irreversibly inactivating cyclooxygenases. Selective COX-2 inhibitors were developed to target prostaglandins involved solely in inflammatory reactions. However, COX-2 inhibitors may increase the risk of cardiovascular and cerebrovascular events, possibly by impairing endothelial cell production of prostacyclin (PGI_2), which is antithrombotic, while leaving intact the COX-1–mediated production by platelets of thromboxane A_2 (TxA_2), which promotes platelet aggregation. COX-2 inhibitors are now used mainly to treat arthritis and perioperative pain in patients who do not have cardiovascular risk factors.
- *Lipoxygenase inhibitors.* 5-lipoxygenase is not affected by NSAIDs. A pharmacologic agent that inhibits leukotriene production (zileuton) is useful in the treatment of asthma.

- *Corticosteroids* are broad-spectrum antiinflammatory agents that reduce the transcription of genes encoding COX-2, phospholipase A_2, proinflammatory cytokines (e.g., IL-1 and TNF), and iNOS.
- *Leukotriene receptor antagonists* block leukotriene receptors and prevent the actions of the leukotrienes (zafirlukast). These drugs are used in the treatment of allergic asthma and allergic rhinitis.

Cytokines and Chemokines

Cytokines **are proteins produced by many cell types (principally activated lymphocytes, macrophages, and dendritic cells, but also endothelial, epithelial, and connective tissue cells) that mediate and regulate immune and inflammatory reactions.** By convention, growth factors that act on epithelial and mesenchymal cells are not grouped under cytokines. The general properties and functions of cytokines are discussed in Chapter 5. Here the cytokines involved in acute inflammation are reviewed (Table 2.7).

Tumor Necrosis Factor (TNF) and Interleukin-1 (IL-1)

TNF and IL-1 serve critical roles in leukocyte recruitment by promoting adhesion of leukocytes to endothelium and their migration through vessels. These cytokines are produced mainly by activated macrophages and dendritic cells; TNF is also produced by T lymphocytes and mast cells, and IL-1 is produced by some epithelial cells as well. The secretion of TNF and IL-1 can be stimulated by microbial products, necrotic cells, and a variety of other inflammatory stimuli. The production of TNF is induced by signals through TLRs and other microbial sensors. The synthesis of IL-1 is stimulated by the same signals, but the generation of the biologically active form of this cytokine is dependent on activation of the inflammasome (Chapter 5).

The actions of TNF and IL-1 contribute to the local and systemic reactions of inflammation (Fig. 2.7). The most important roles of these cytokines in inflammation are the following.

- *Endothelial activation and leukocyte recruitment.* Both TNF and IL-1 act on endothelium to increase the expression of endothelial adhesion molecules, mostly E- and P-selectins and ligands for leukocyte integrins. These changes are critical for the recruitment of leukocytes to sites of inflammation. They also stimulate production of various mediators, including other cytokines and chemokines, and eicosanoids, and increase the procoagulant activity of the endothelium.
- *Activation of leukocytes and other cells.* TNF augments responses of neutrophils to other stimuli such as bacterial endotoxin and stimulates the microbicidal activity of macrophages. IL-1 activates fibroblasts to synthesize collagen and stimulates proliferation of synovial and other mesenchymal cells. IL-1 also stimulates Th17 responses, which in turn induce acute inflammation.
- *Systemic acute-phase response.* IL-1 and TNF (as well as IL-6) induce the systemic responses associated with infection or injury, including *fever* (described later in the chapter). They are also implicated in the pathogenesis of the systemic inflammatory response syndrome (SIRS), resulting from disseminated bacterial infection and other serious conditions, described later. At high concentrations, TNF dilates blood vessels and reduces myocardial contractility, both of which contribute to the fall in blood pressure associated with SIRS. TNF regulates energy balance by promoting lipid and protein mobilization and by suppressing appetite. Therefore, sustained production of TNF contributes to *cachexia*, a pathologic state characterized by weight loss and anorexia that accompanies some chronic infections and cancers.

TNF antagonists have been remarkably effective in the treatment of chronic inflammatory diseases, particularly rheumatoid arthritis, psoriasis, and some types of inflammatory bowel disease. One of the complications of this therapy is that patients become susceptible to mycobacterial infection, resulting from the reduced ability of macrophages to kill intracellular microbes. Although many of the actions of TNF and IL-1 are overlapping, IL-1 antagonists are not as effective, for obscure reasons. Blocking either cytokine does not affect the outcome of sepsis (see later), perhaps because other cytokines contribute to this serious systemic inflammatory reaction.

Table 2.7 Cytokines in Inflammation

Cytokine	Principal Sources	Principal Actions in Inflammation
In Acute Inflammation		
TNF	Macrophages, mast cells, T lymphocytes	Stimulates expression of endothelial adhesion molecules and secretion of other cytokines; systemic effects
IL-1	Macrophages, endothelial cells, some epithelial cells	Similar to TNF; greater role in fever
IL-6	Macrophages, other cells	Systemic effects (acute-phase response)
Chemokines	Macrophages, endothelial cells, T lymphocytes, mast cells, other cell types	Recruitment of leukocytes to sites of inflammation; migration of cells in healthy tissues
In Chronic Inflammation		
IL-12	Dendritic cells, macrophages	Increased production of IFN-γ
IFN-γ	T lymphocytes, NK cells	Activation of macrophages (increased ability to kill microbes and tumor cells)
IL-17	T lymphocytes	Recruitment of neutrophils and monocytes

IFN-γ, Interferon-γ; *IL,* interleukin; *NK cells,* natural killer cells; *TNF,* tumor necrosis factor.

Chemokines are divided into four groups based on the number of amino acids between two of the conserved cysteines in the protein. As indicated, the chemokines of these groups have somewhat different target cell specificities.

The most important cytokines involved in inflammatory reactions are listed. Many other cytokines may play roles in inflammation. There is also considerable overlap between the cytokines involved in acute and chronic inflammation. Specifically, all the cytokines listed under acute inflammation may also contribute to chronic inflammatory reactions.

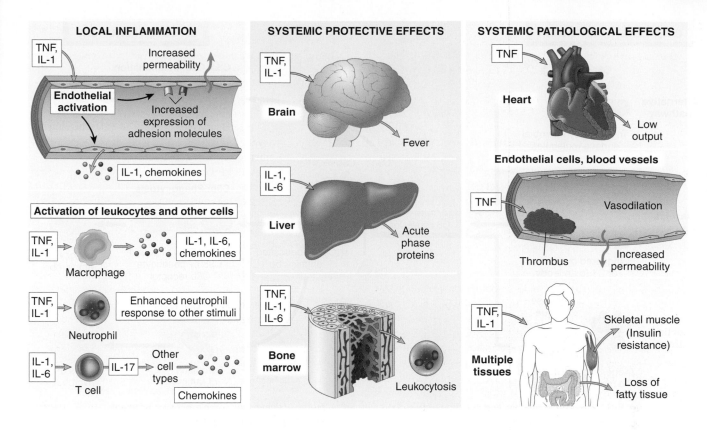

FIG. 2.7 Major roles of cytokines in acute inflammation.

Chemokines

Chemokines are a family of small (8 to 10 kD) proteins that act primarily as chemoattractants for specific types of leukocytes. About 40 different chemokines and 20 different receptors for chemokines have been identified. Different chemokines act on specific cell types according to their expression of various chemokine receptors (see Table 2.7). Chemokines bind to proteoglycans and are thus displayed at high concentrations on the surface of endothelial cells and in the extracellular matrix (see Fig. 2.3). They have two main functions:

- *In inflammation.* Production of *inflammatory chemokines* is induced by microbes and other stimuli. These chemokines bind to leukocyte receptors and stimulate both the integrin-dependent attachment of leukocytes to endothelium and the migration (chemotaxis) of leukocytes in tissues to sites of infection or tissue damage.
- *Maintenance of tissue architecture.* Some chemokines are produced constitutively by stromal cells in tissues (*homeostatic chemokines*) and promote the localization of various cell types to specific anatomic regions. Examples include the ability of certain chemokines to promote the localization of T and B lymphocytes to discrete areas of the spleen and lymph nodes (Chapter 5).

Although the role of chemokines in inflammation is well established, it has proved difficult to develop antagonists that block the activities of these proteins.

Other Cytokines in Acute Inflammation

The list of cytokines implicated in inflammation is huge and constantly growing. In addition to the ones described earlier, two that have received considerable recent interest are IL-6, which is made by macrophages and other cells and is involved in local and systemic reactions, and IL-17, which is produced mainly by T lymphocytes and promotes neutrophil recruitment. Antagonists against both have shown impressive efficacy in the treatment of inflammatory diseases. Type I interferons, whose normal function is to inhibit viral replication, contribute to some of the systemic manifestations of inflammation. Cytokines also play key roles in chronic inflammation (see later).

Complement System

The complement system is a collection of soluble proteins and their membrane receptors that function mainly in host defense against microbes and in pathologic inflammatory reactions. There are more than 20 complement proteins, some of which are numbered C1 through C9. The activation and functions of complement are outlined in Fig. 2.8.

Complement proteins are present as proforms that are activated during inflammatory reactions. They participate in a cascade of enzymatic reactions that is capable of tremendous amplification. **The critical step in complement activation is the proteolytic cleavage of the third (and most abundant) component, C3, which can occur by one of three pathways:**

- The *classical pathway*, which is triggered by fixation of C1 to antibody (IgM or IgG) that has combined with antigen
- The *alternative pathway*, which is triggered by microbial surface molecules (e.g., endotoxin, or lipopolysaccharide [LPS]), complex polysaccharides, and other substances, in the absence of antibody
- The *lectin pathway*, in which plasma mannose-binding lectin binds to carbohydrates on microbes and activates C1, also without a role for antibody

All three pathways of complement activation lead to the formation of an enzyme called the *C3 convertase*, which splits C3 into two functionally distinct fragments, C3a and C3b. C3a is released, and

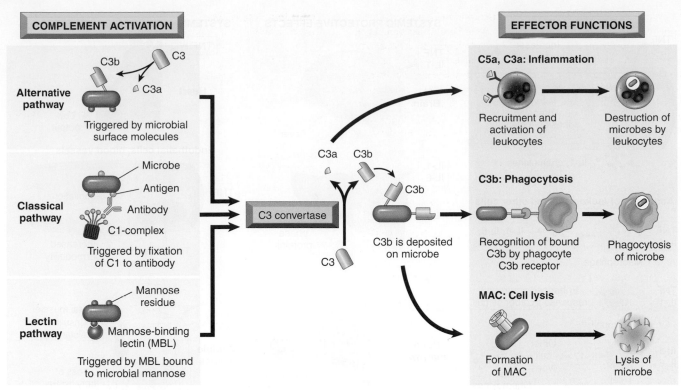

COMPLEMENT ACTIVATION

Alternative pathway
Triggered by microbial surface molecules

Classical pathway
Microbe
Antigen
Antibody
C1-complex
Triggered by fixation of C1 to antibody

Lectin pathway
Mannose residue
Mannose-binding lectin (MBL)
Triggered by MBL bound to microbial mannose

C3 convertase

C3a   C3b

C3

C3b is deposited on microbe

EFFECTOR FUNCTIONS

C5a, C3a: Inflammation
Recruitment and activation of leukocytes → Destruction of microbes by leukocytes

C3b: Phagocytosis
C3b
Recognition of bound C3b by phagocyte C3b receptor → Phagocytosis of microbe

MAC: Cell lysis
Formation of MAC → Lysis of microbe

FIG. 2.8 The activation and functions of the complement system. Activation of complement by different pathways leads to cleavage of C3. The functions of the complement system are mediated by breakdown products of C3 and other complement proteins and by the membrane attack complex (MAC).

C3b becomes covalently attached to the cell or molecule where complement is being activated. Additional C3b then binds to the previously generated fragments to form *C5 convertase*, which cleaves C5 to release C5a and leave C5b attached to the cell surface. C5b binds the late components (C6-C9), culminating in the formation of the membrane attack complex (MAC), composed of multiple C9 molecules.

The complement system has three main functions (see Fig. 2.8):
- *Inflammation. C5a*, and, to a lesser extent, *C4a* and *C3a*, are cleavage products of the corresponding complement components that stimulate recruitment of neutrophils and other leukocytes. They may also induce histamine release from mast cells and thereby increase vascular permeability and cause vasodilation. They are called *anaphylatoxins* because they have effects similar to those of mast cell mediators that are involved in the reaction called anaphylaxis (Chapter 5).
- *Opsonization and phagocytosis.* When fixed to a microbial wall, C3b and its cleavage product iC3b (inactive C3b) act as opsonins and promote phagocytosis by neutrophils and macrophages, which have cell surface receptors for these complement fragments.
- *Cell lysis.* The assembly of the MAC on cells creates holes in the cell membrane that allow intracellular water and ions to leak out, resulting in the death (lysis) of the cells, especially thin-walled microbes such as *Neisseria* bacteria. Notably, individuals with inherited deficiencies of the terminal components of complement or who are being treated with complement inhibitors are at high risk of disseminated infections with *Neisseria* species (meningococci and gonococci).

The activation of complement is tightly controlled by cell-associated and circulating regulatory proteins. The regulatory proteins inhibit the production of active complement fragments or remove fragments that deposit on cells. The regulators are expressed on normal host cells and thus prevent healthy tissues from being injured at sites of complement activation. These proteins can be overwhelmed when large amounts of complement are deposited on host cells and in tissues, as in autoimmune diseases in which individuals produce complement-fixing antibodies against their own cell and tissue antigens (Chapter 5). The most important of these regulatory proteins are the following:
- *C1 inhibitor (C1 INH)* blocks the activation of C1, the first protein of the classical complement pathway. Inherited deficiency of this inhibitor is the cause of *hereditary angioedema.*
- *Decay accelerating factor (DAF)* and *CD59* are two proteins that are linked to plasma membranes by a glycophosphatidylinositol (GPI) anchor. DAF prevents formation of C3 convertases and CD59 inhibits formation of the membrane attack complex. An acquired deficiency of the enzyme that creates GPI anchors leads to loss of these regulators and excessive complement activation and lysis of red cells (which are sensitive to complement-mediated cell lysis). This gives rise to a disease called *paroxysmal nocturnal hemoglobinuria (PNH)* (Chapter 10).
- Other complement regulatory proteins proteolytically cleave active complement components. For instance, *Factor H* is a plasma protein that promotes the inactivation of the C3 convertase; its deficiency results in excessive complement activation. Mutations in Factor H are associated with a kidney disease called the *hemolytic uremic syndrome* (Chapter 10) and *wet macular degeneration* of the eye (Chapter 21), characterized by increased permeability of retinal vessels.

The complement system contributes to disease in several ways. The activation of complement by antibodies or antigen-antibody complexes deposited on host cells and tissues is an important mechanism of cell and tissue injury (Chapter 5). Inherited deficiencies of complement proteins cause increased susceptibility to infections, and as mentioned previously, deficiencies of regulatory proteins cause a variety of disorders. Finally, through uncertain mechanisms, diseases of excessive complement activity such as hemolytic uremic syndrome and paroxysmal nocturnal hemoglobinuria are often marked by an increased risk of thrombosis. Antibodies that block complement activation have been developed to treat several of these disorders.

Other Mediators of Inflammation

- *Platelet-activating factor (PAF)* is a phospholipid-derived mediator that was discovered as a factor that caused platelet aggregation. A variety of cell types, including platelets, basophils, mast cells, neutrophils, macrophages, and endothelial cells, can elaborate PAF. In addition to platelet aggregation, PAF causes vasoconstriction and bronchoconstriction, and at low concentrations it induces vasodilation and increased venular permeability. Its role in acute inflammatory reactions remains unclear.
- Studies done more than 50 years ago suggested that inhibiting *coagulation factors* reduced the inflammatory reaction to some microbes, leading to the idea that coagulation and inflammation are linked processes. This concept was supported by the discovery of *protease-activated receptors (PARs)*, which are activated by thrombin and are expressed on platelets and leukocytes. It is, however, likely that the major role of the PARs is in platelet activation during clotting (Chapter 3). In fact, it is difficult to dissociate clotting and inflammation, since virtually all forms of tissue injury that lead to clotting also induce inflammation, and inflammation causes changes in endothelial cells that increase the likelihood of abnormal clotting (thrombosis, described in Chapter 3). Whether the products of coagulation, per se, have a significant role in stimulating inflammation is still not established.
- *Kinins* are vasoactive peptides derived from plasma proteins, called *kininogens*, by the action of specific proteases called *kallikreins*. Kallikrein cleaves a plasma glycoprotein precursor, high-molecular-weight kininogen, to produce *bradykinin*. **Bradykinin increases vascular permeability and causes contraction of smooth muscle, dilation of blood vessels, and pain when injected into the skin,** effects that are similar to those of histamine. The action of bradykinin is short lived because it is quickly inactivated by an enzyme called *kininase*. Bradykinin has been implicated as a mediator in some forms of allergic reaction, such as anaphylaxis (Chapter 5).
- *Neuropeptides* are secreted by sensory nerves and various leukocytes and may play a role in the initiation and regulation of inflammatory responses. These small peptides, such as substance P and neurokinin A, are produced in the central and peripheral nervous system. Substance P has many biologic functions, including the transmission of pain signals and increasing vascular permeability.

When Sir Thomas Lewis described the role of histamine in inflammation, one mediator was thought to be enough. Now, we are wallowing in them! Yet, from this large compendium, it is likely that a few mediators are most important for the reactions of acute inflammation in vivo, and these are summarized in Table 2.8. The redundancy of the mediators and their synergistic actions ensures that this protective response remains robust and is not readily subverted.

Table 2.8 Role of Mediators in Different Reactions of Inflammation

Reaction of Inflammation	Principal Mediators
Vasodilation	Histamine
Increased vascular permeability	Histamine C3a and C5a (by liberating vasoactive amines from mast cells, other cells) Leukotrienes C_4, D_4, E_4
Chemotaxis, leukocyte recruitment and activation	TNF, IL-1 Chemokines C3a, C5a Leukotriene B_4
Fever	IL-1, TNF Prostaglandins
Pain	Prostaglandins Bradykinin Neuropeptides
Tissue damage	Lysosomal enzymes of leukocytes Reactive oxygen species

IL, Interleukin; *TNF*, tumor necrosis factor.

MORPHOLOGIC PATTERNS OF ACUTE INFLAMMATION

The morphologic hallmarks of acute inflammatory reactions are dilation of small blood vessels and accumulation of leukocytes and fluid in the extravascular tissue. Although these general features are characteristic of most acute inflammatory reactions, morphologic patterns vary, depending on the severity of the reaction, the etiology, and the particular tissue and site involved. These distinct gross and microscopic patterns of inflammation often provide valuable clues about the underlying cause.

Serous Inflammation

Serous inflammation is marked by the accumulation of serumlike protein-rich exudates in body cavities lined by the peritoneum, pleura, or pericardium or spaces created by tissue injury. Typically, the fluid in serous inflammation is sterile and does not contain large numbers of leukocytes (which tend to produce purulent inflammation, described later). In body cavities the fluid may be derived from the plasma (as a result of increased vascular permeability) or from the secretions of mesothelial cells (due to local irritation); accumulation of fluid in a mesothelium-lined cavity is called an *effusion*. Skin blistering from a burn or viral infection represents accumulation of serous fluid within or immediately beneath the damaged epidermis (Fig. 2.9).

Fibrinous Inflammation

Fibrinous inflammation is characterized by the deposition of fibrin as a result of the local activation of coagulation. With large increases in vascular permeability, high-molecular-weight proteins such as fibrinogen accumulate within exudates, and if a procoagulant stimulus is present, fibrin forms. Fibrinous exudates are characteristic of inflammation of the lining of body cavities, such as the meninges, pericardium (Fig. 2.10A), and pleura. Histologically, fibrin appears as an eosinophilic meshwork of threads or sometimes as an amorphous coagulum (Fig. 2.10B). Fibrinous exudates may resolve through the

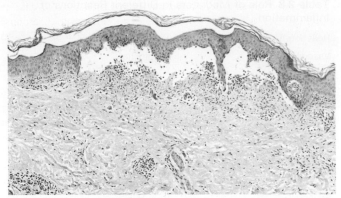

FIG. 2.9 Serous inflammation. Low-power view of a cross-section of a skin blister showing the epidermis separated from the dermis by a focal collection of serous effusion.

breakdown of fibrin (fibrinolysis) and clearance by macrophages or, if not resolved, may undergo *organization*, a process involving the ingrowth of fibroblasts and blood vessels that leads to scarring. This may have deleterious consequences. For example, conversion of a fibrinous exudate to scar tissue (organization) within the pericardial cavity, if extensive, may obliterate the pericardial space and result in a restrictive cardiomyopathy (Chapter 9).

Purulent (Suppurative) Inflammation, Abscess

Purulent inflammation is characterized by the production of pus, an exudate consisting of neutrophils, the liquefied debris of necrotic cells, and edema fluid. The most frequent cause of purulent (also called *suppurative*) inflammation is infection with bacteria that cause liquefactive tissue necrosis (e.g., staphylococci); these pathogens are referred to as *pyogenic* (pus-producing) bacteria. A common example of an acute suppurative inflammation is acute appendicitis. **Abscesses are localized collections of pus** caused by suppuration within a tissue, an organ, or confined space. They are produced by seeding of pyogenic bacteria into a tissue (Fig. 2.11). The central region of an abscess is a

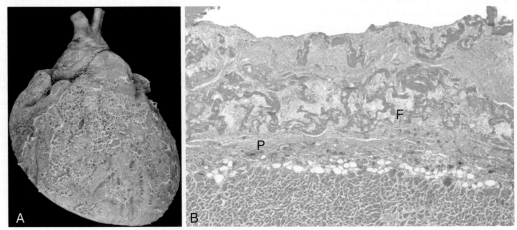

FIG. 2.10 Fibrinous pericarditis. (A) Deposits of fibrin on the pericardium. (B) A pink meshwork of fibrin exudate *(F)* overlies the pericardial surface *(P)*. (Courtesy of Dr. Joseph J. Maleszewski, Mayo Clinic, Rochester, MN USA.)

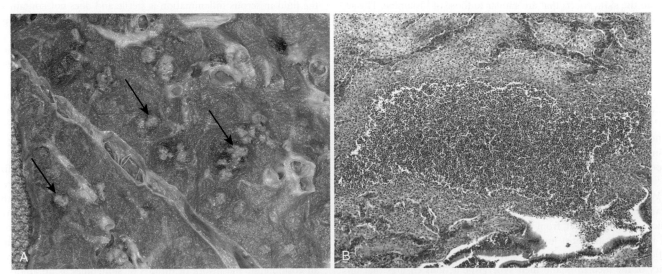

FIG. 2.11 Purulent inflammation. (A) Multiple bacterial abscesses *(arrows)* in the lung in a case of bronchopneumonia. (B) The abscess contains neutrophils and cellular debris and is surrounded by congested blood vessels.

mass of necrotic leukocytes and tissue cells. There is usually a rim of preserved neutrophils around the necrotic focus, and outside this region there may be vascular congestion and parenchymal and fibroblastic proliferation, indicating chronic inflammation and repair. In time the abscess may become walled off and replaced by connective tissue.

Ulcers

An ulcer is a local defect, or excavation, of the surface of an organ or tissue that is produced by the sloughing (shedding) of inflamed necrotic tissue (Fig. 2.12). Ulceration occurs only when tissue necrosis and resultant inflammation exist on or near a surface. It is most commonly encountered in the mucosa of the mouth, stomach, intestines, or genitourinary tract, and the skin and subcutaneous tissue of the lower extremities in individuals with circulatory disturbances that predispose to extensive ischemic necrosis (e.g., patients with peripheral vascular disease). Both acute and chronic inflammation may coexist. During the acute stage there is intense polymorphonuclear infiltration and vascular dilation in the margins of the defect. With time, the margins and base of the ulcer become scarred and chronic inflammatory cells (lymphocytes, plasma cells, and macrophages) accumulate.

OUTCOMES OF ACUTE INFLAMMATION

Although many variables may modify the basic process of inflammation, including the nature and intensity of the injury, the site and tissue affected, and the responsiveness of the host, **all acute inflammatory reactions typically have one of three outcomes** (Fig. 2.13):

- *Complete resolution.* In a perfect world, all inflammatory reactions, once they have eliminated the offending agent, should end and the tissue should return to normalcy. This is called *resolution* and is the usual outcome when the injury is limited or short lived or when there has been little tissue destruction and the damaged parenchymal cells can regenerate. Resolution involves removal of cellular debris and microbes by macrophages and resorption of edema fluid mainly through lymphatics.
- *Healing by connective tissue replacement (scarring, or fibrosis).* This occurs after substantial tissue destruction, when the inflammatory injury involves tissues that are incapable of regeneration, or when there is abundant fibrin exudation in tissue or in serous cavities (pleura, peritoneum) that cannot be fully cleared. In all these situations, connective tissue grows into the area of damage or exudate, converting it into a mass of fibrous tissue.

- *Progression to chronic inflammation* (discussed next). Acute to chronic transition occurs when the acute inflammatory response cannot be resolved because of either the persistence of the injurious agent or some interference with the normal process of healing.

CHRONIC INFLAMMATION

Chronic inflammation is a response of prolonged duration (weeks to months) in which inflammation, tissue injury, and attempts at repair coexist, in varying combinations. It may follow acute inflammation, as described earlier, or chronic inflammation may begin insidiously, as a smoldering, sometimes progressive, process without a preceding acute reaction. It may result in considerable tissue damage and scarring with relatively little inflammatory infiltrate, as seen in hepatic cirrhosis.

Causes of Chronic Inflammation

Chronic inflammation arises in the following settings:

- *Persistent infections* by microorganisms that are difficult to eradicate, such as mycobacteria and certain viruses, fungi, and parasites. In some infections, incompletely resolved acute inflammation may evolve into chronic inflammation, as in acute bacterial infection of the lung that progresses to a chronic lung abscess.
- *Hypersensitivity diseases.* Chronic inflammation plays an important role in a group of diseases that are caused by excessive and inappropriate activation of the immune system (Chapter 5). In *autoimmune diseases*, autoantigens evoke a self-perpetuating immune reaction that results in chronic tissue damage and inflammation; examples of such diseases are rheumatoid arthritis and multiple sclerosis. In *allergic diseases*, chronic inflammation is the result of excessive immune responses against common environmental substances, as in bronchial asthma. Such diseases may show morphologic patterns of mixed acute and chronic inflammation because they are characterized by repeated bouts of inflammation. Fibrosis may dominate the late stages.
- *Prolonged exposure to potentially toxic agents,* either exogenous or endogenous. An example of an exogenous agent is particulate silica, a nondegradable mineral that, when inhaled for prolonged periods, results in an inflammatory lung disease called *silicosis* (Chapter 11). *Atherosclerosis* (Chapter 9) is a chronic inflammatory process affecting the arterial wall that is induced, at least in part, by excessive production and tissue deposition of endogenous cholesterol and other lipids.

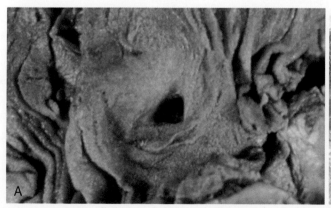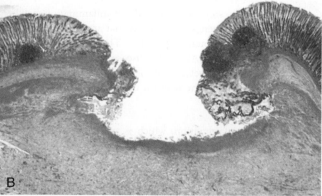

FIG. 2.12 Ulcer. (A) A chronic duodenal ulcer. (B) Low-power cross-section view of a duodenal ulcer crater with an inflammatory exudate in the base.

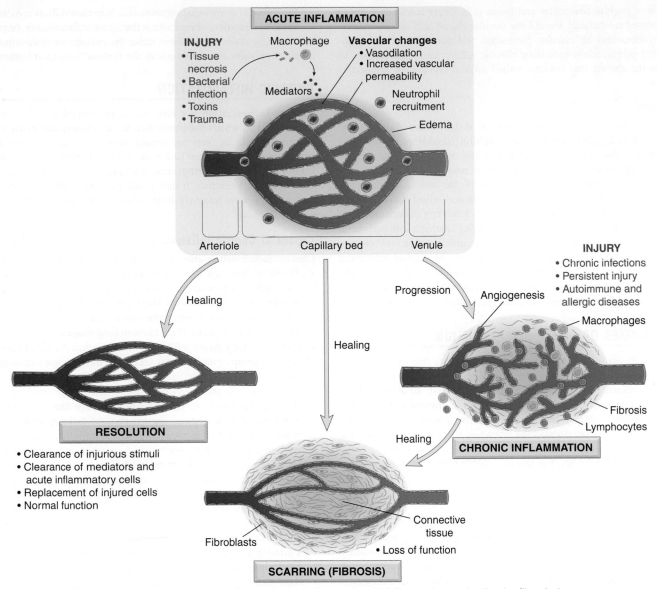

FIG. 2.13 Outcomes of acute inflammation: resolution, chronic inflammation, or healing by fibrosis (most often the outcome of chronic inflammation). The components of the various reactions and their functional outcomes are indicated.

- As mentioned earlier, some forms of chronic inflammation may be important in the pathogenesis of diseases that are not conventionally thought of as inflammatory disorders. These include neurodegenerative diseases such as Alzheimer disease, metabolic syndrome, and associated type 2 diabetes. The role of inflammation in these conditions is discussed in the relevant chapters.

Morphologic Features

In contrast to acute inflammation, which is manifested by vascular changes, edema, and predominantly neutrophilic infiltration, **chronic inflammation is characterized by the following:**

- *Infiltration by mononuclear cells,* which include macrophages, lymphocytes, and plasma cells (Fig. 2.14)
- *Tissue destruction,* induced by the persistent offending agent or by the inflammatory cells

- *Attempts at healing* by replacement of damaged tissue with connective tissue, accomplished by *angiogenesis* (proliferation of small blood vessels) and *fibrosis,* culminating in *scar* formation

Angiogenesis and fibrosis are discussed later, in the context of tissue repair.

Cells and Mediators of Chronic Inflammation

The combination of leukocyte infiltration, tissue damage, and fibrosis that characterize chronic inflammation is the result of the local activation of several cell types and the production of mediators.

Role of Macrophages

The dominant cells in most chronic inflammatory reactions are macrophages, which destroy foreign invaders and tissues, secrete

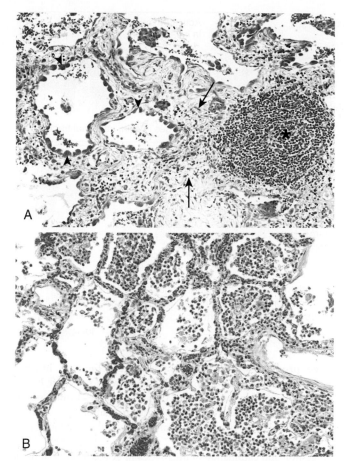

FIG. 2.14 Chronic inflammation. (A) Chronic inflammation in the lung, showing all three characteristic histologic features: (1) collection of chronic inflammatory cells *(*)*, (2) destruction of parenchyma (normal alveoli are replaced by spaces lined by cuboidal epithelium, *arrowheads*), and (3) replacement by connective tissue (fibrosis, *arrows*). (B) By contrast, in acute inflammation of the lung (acute bronchopneumonia), neutrophils fill the alveolar spaces and blood vessels are congested.

cytokines and growth factors, and activate other cells, notably T lymphocytes. Macrophages are professional phagocytes whose primary function is to ingest and destroy particulate matter, microbes, and dead cells. But, as we shall see shortly, they serve many other roles in host defense, inflammation, and repair. Macrophages are normally diffusely scattered in most connective tissues. Circulating cells of this lineage are known as *monocytes*. In addition, tissue-resident macrophages are found in specific locations in organs such

as the liver (Kupffer cells), spleen, and lymph nodes (sinus histiocytes), central nervous system (microglial cells), and lungs (alveolar macrophages). Together these cells make up the *mononuclear phagocyte system*. Blood monocytes are 10 to 15 μm in diameter and contain bean-shaped nuclei and finely granular cytoplasm (Fig. 2.15). Tissue macrophages have abundant cytoplasm containing phagocytic vacuoles, many filled with ingested material, as well as lysosomes and other organelles.

Macrophages in tissues are derived from hematopoietic stem cells in the bone marrow and from progenitors in the embryonic yolk sac and fetal liver during early development (Fig. 2.16). In inflammatory reactions, progenitors in the bone marrow give rise to monocytes, which enter the blood, migrate into various tissues, and differentiate into macrophages. Entry of blood monocytes into tissues is governed by the same factors that are involved in neutrophil emigration, such as adhesion molecules and chemokines. Because they have a longer life span in tissues than other leukocytes, macrophages often become the dominant cell population in inflammatory reactions within 48 hours of onset. Tissue-resident macrophages (e.g., microglia and Kupffer cells) arise from the yolk sac or fetal liver early in embryogenesis, populate the tissues, stay for long periods, and are replenished mainly by proliferation of resident cells.

There are two major pathways of macrophage activation, called classical and alternative (Fig. 2.17). The nature of the activating signals determines which of these two pathways is taken by a given macrophage.

- *Classical macrophage activation* may be induced by microbial products such as endotoxin, which engage TLRs and other sensors, and by T cell–derived mediators, especially the cytokine IFN-γ, in immune responses. Classically activated (also called M1) macrophages produce NO and ROS and upregulate lysosomal enzymes, all of which enhance their ability to kill ingested organisms, and they secrete cytokines that stimulate inflammation. These macrophages are important for eradicating infections and dominate many inflammatory reactions. As discussed earlier in the context of acute inflammation and leukocyte activation, activated macrophages are capable of injuring normal tissues.

- *Alternative macrophage activation* is induced by mediators other than IFN-γ, such as IL-4 and IL-13, produced by T lymphocytes and other cells. These alternatively activated (also called M2) macrophages are not actively microbicidal; instead, their principal function is tissue repair. They secrete growth factors that promote angiogenesis, activate fibroblasts, and stimulate collagen synthesis. They also inhibit inflammation. It seems plausible that in response to most injurious stimuli, the first activation pathway is the classical one, designed to destroy the offending agents, and this is followed by alternative activation, which terminates

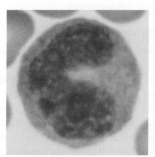
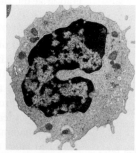
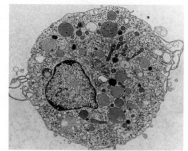

Monocyte   Activated macrophage

FIG. 2.15 The morphology of a monocyte and activated macrophage.

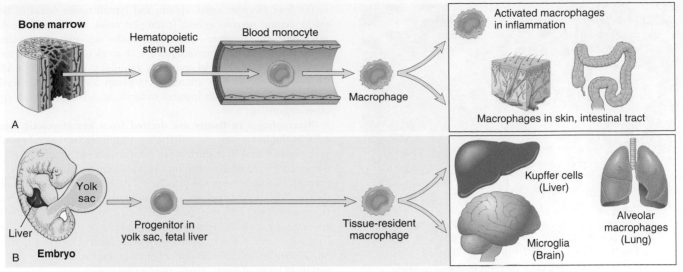

FIG. 2.16 Maturation of mononuclear phagocytes. (A) During inflammatory reactions, the majority of tissue macrophages are derived from hematopoietic precursors. (B) Some long-lived resident tissue macrophages are derived from embryonic precursors that populate the tissues early in development.

inflammation and initiates tissue repair. However, such a precise sequence is not well documented in most inflammatory reactions. Also, although these types of macrophages provide a useful conceptual framework, in reality many more subpopulations have been described that represent intermediates between the M1 and M2 phenotypes.

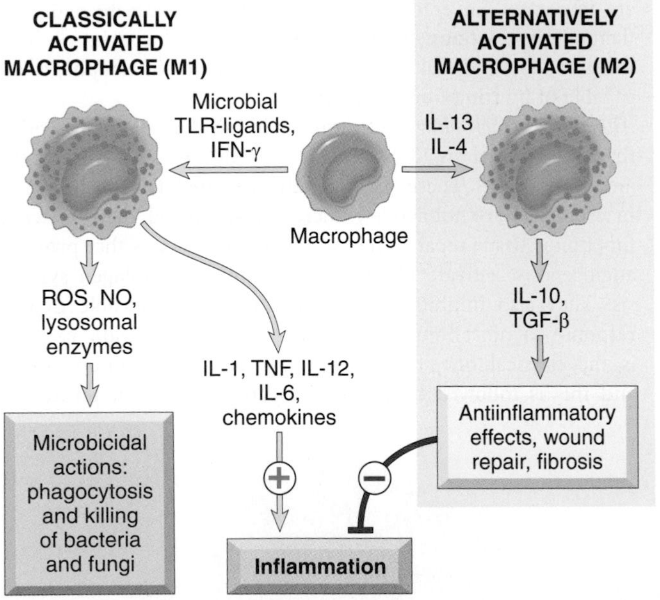

FIG. 2.17 Classical and alternative macrophage activation. Different stimuli activate tissue macrophages to develop into functionally distinct populations. Classically activated (M1) macrophages are induced by microbial products and cytokines, particularly IFN-γ. They phagocytose and destroy microbes and debris from dead tissues and can potentiate inflammatory reactions. Alternatively activated (M2) macrophages are induced by other cytokines and are important in tissue repair and the resolution of inflammation.

The products of activated macrophages eliminate injurious agents such as microbes and initiate the process of repair but are also responsible for much of the tissue injury in chronic inflammation. Several functions of macrophages are central to the development and persistence of chronic inflammation and the accompanying tissue injury. These include:

- Ingestion and elimination of microbes and debris from dead tissues
- Secretion of mediators of inflammation, such as cytokines (TNF, IL-1, chemokines, and others) and eicosanoids. Thus, macrophages are central to the initiation and propagation of inflammatory reactions
- Initiating the process of tissue repair and scar formation and fibrosis (discussed later)
- Displaying antigens to T lymphocytes and responding to signals from T cells, thus setting up a feedback loop that is essential for defense against many microbes by cell-mediated immune responses. These interactions are described further in the discussion of the role of lymphocytes in chronic inflammation in the next section and in more detail in Chapter 5, where cell-mediated immunity is considered.

Usually, once the irritant is eliminated, macrophages eventually disappear (either dying off or making their way via lymphatics into lymph nodes). However, at times, macrophage accumulation persists, due to continuous recruitment from the circulation and local proliferation at the site of inflammation.

Role of Lymphocytes

Microbes and other environmental antigens activate T and B lymphocytes, which amplify and propagate chronic inflammation. Although the principal role of lymphocytes is in adaptive immunity, which protects against infections (Chapter 5), these cells are often present in chronic inflammation. When they are activated, the inflammation tends to be persistent and severe. Some of the strongest chronic inflammatory reactions, such as granulomatous inflammation, described later, are dependent on interactions between lymphocytes and macrophages. In autoimmune and other hypersensitivity diseases, lymphocytes may be the dominant population.

CD4+ T lymphocytes secrete cytokines that promote inflammation and influence the nature of the inflammatory reaction. There are three subsets of CD4+ T cells that secrete different types of cytokines and elicit different types of inflammation.

- Th1 cells produce the cytokine IFN-γ, which activates macrophages by the classical pathway.
- Th2 cells secrete IL-4, IL-5, and IL-13, which recruit and activate eosinophils and are responsible for the alternative pathway of macrophage activation.
- Th17 cells secrete IL-17 and other cytokines, which induce the secretion of chemokines responsible for recruiting mainly neutrophils into the reaction.

Both Th1 and Th17 cells are involved in defense against many types of bacteria and viruses and in the chronic inflammation seen in many autoimmune diseases (e.g., rheumatoid arthritis, psoriasis, and inflammatory bowel disease). Th2 cells are important in defense against helminthic parasites and in allergic inflammation. These T cell subsets and their functions are described in more detail in Chapter 5.

Lymphocytes and macrophages interact in a bidirectional way, and these interactions play an important role in propagating chronic inflammation. Macrophages display antigens to T cells, express membrane molecules (called costimulators), and produce cytokines (IL-12 and others) that stimulate T-cell responses (Chapter 5). Activated T lymphocytes, in turn, produce cytokines that recruit and activate macrophages, promoting more antigen presentation and cytokine secretion. The result is a cycle of cellular reactions that fuel and sustain chronic inflammation.

Activated B lymphocytes and antibody-secreting plasma cells are often present at sites of chronic inflammation. The antibodies may be specific for persistent foreign or self antigens in the inflammatory site or against altered tissue components. However, the specificity and even the importance of antibodies in most chronic inflammatory disorders are unclear.

In some chronic inflammatory reactions, the accumulated lymphocytes, antigen-presenting cells, and plasma cells cluster together to form lymphoid structures resembling the follicles found in lymph nodes. These are called *tertiary lymphoid organs*; this type of lymphoid organogenesis is often seen in the synovium of patients with long-standing rheumatoid arthritis, in the thyroid in Hashimoto thyroiditis, and in the microenvironment of some cancers. The functional significance of these structures is not established.

Other Cells in Chronic Inflammation

Other cell types may be prominent in chronic inflammation induced by particular stimuli.

- *Eosinophils* are abundant in immune reactions mediated by IgE and in parasitic infections (Fig. 2.18). Their recruitment is driven by adhesion molecules similar to those used by neutrophils and by specific chemokines (e.g., eotaxin) derived from leukocytes and epithelial cells. Eosinophils have granules that contain *major basic protein*, a highly cationic protein that is toxic to parasites but also injures epithelial cells. This is why eosinophils are effective in controlling parasitic infections but also contribute to tissue damage in immune reactions such as allergies (Chapter 5).
- Although *neutrophils* are characteristic of acute inflammation, many forms of chronic inflammation continue to show large numbers of neutrophils, induced either by persistent microbes or by mediators produced by activated macrophages and T

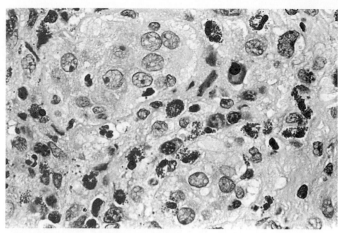

FIG. 2.18 A focus of inflammation containing numerous eosinophils.

lymphocytes. In chronic bacterial infection of bone (osteomyelitis), a neutrophilic exudate can persist for months (Chapter 19). Neutrophils are also important in the chronic damage induced in lungs by smoking and other irritant stimuli (Chapter 11).

Granulomatous Inflammation

Granulomatous inflammation is a form of chronic inflammation characterized by collections of activated macrophages, often with T lymphocytes, and sometimes associated with central necrosis. The name *granuloma* derives from the macroscopic granular appearance of these inflammatory nodules. Granulomatous inflammation is usually an attempt to contain offending agents that are difficult to eradicate and that induce strong T cell–mediated immune responses, such as persistent microbes. Granulomatous inflammation is also seen in response to indigestible foreign bodies, in the absence of T cell–mediated immune responses. These foreign bodies are not immunogenic but are too large to be phagocytosed by macrophages, resulting in persistent activation of the cells. Substances that induce foreign body granulomas include talc (associated with intravenous drug use) (Chapter 7), sutures, and other fibers. The foreign material can usually be identified in the center of the granuloma by microscopy, particularly if the material is refractile in polarized light.

MORPHOLOGY

In the usual hematoxylin and eosin preparations (Fig. 2.19), activated macrophages in granulomas have pink granular cytoplasm with indistinct cell boundaries and are called **epithelioid cells** because they resemble epithelia. The aggregates of epithelioid macrophages are often surrounded by a collar of lymphocytes. Older granulomas may have a rim of fibroblasts and connective tissue. Frequently, but not invariably, granulomas contain multinucleated **giant cells** 40 to 50 μm in diameter (Langhans giant cells) with abundant cytoplasm that are created by the fusion of numerous activated macrophages. In granulomas associated with certain infectious organisms (most classically *Mycobacterium tuberculosis*), a combination of hypoxia and free radical–mediated injury leads to a central zone of necrosis. Grossly, this has a granular, cheesy appearance and is therefore called **caseous necrosis.** Microscopically, this necrotic material appears as amorphous, structureless, eosinophilic, granular debris. The granulomas in Crohn disease, sarcoidosis, and foreign body reactions usually lack necrotic centers and are said to be *noncaseating*. Healing of granulomas is accompanied by fibrosis that may be extensive.

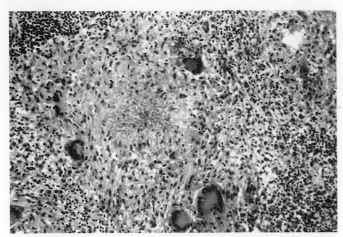

FIG. 2.19 Granulomatous inflammation. Typical tuberculous granuloma showing an area of central necrosis surrounded by multiple multinucleate giant cells, epithelioid cells, and lymphocytes.

Recognition of granulomas in an inflammatory reaction is important because only a limited number of conditions cause this type of inflammation (Table 2.9). **Tuberculosis is the prototype of a granulomatous disease caused by infection and should always be excluded as the cause when granulomas are identified.** Other infections, such as syphilis and some fungal infections, may also elicit granulomatous inflammation. Although the morphologic appearance of these diseases may be sufficiently different to allow reasonably accurate diagnosis (see Table 2.9), it is always necessary to identify the specific etiologic agent in the clinical laboratory using special stains (e.g., acid-fast stains for *M. tuberculosis*), microbial culture, molecular techniques, or serologic studies (e.g., in syphilis). Granulomas may also develop in some immune-mediated inflammatory diseases, notably Crohn disease (Chapter 13), a type of inflammatory bowel disease, and sarcoidosis (Chapter 11).

SYSTEMIC EFFECTS OF INFLAMMATION

Inflammation, even if it is localized, is associated with cytokine-induced systemic reactions. Anyone who has suffered through a severe bout of a viral illness (e.g., influenza) has experienced the systemic manifestations of inflammation. These changes are reactions to cytokines whose production is stimulated by bacterial products such as LPS and by other inflammatory stimuli. **The cytokines TNF, IL-1, and IL-6 are important mediators of the systemic response, and other cytokines, notably type I interferons, also contribute to the reaction.** The systemic reactions are typically more severe in acute than in chronic inflammation, reflecting the levels of cytokine production.

The systemic response to inflammation consists of several clinical and pathologic changes:

- *Fever*, characterized by an elevation of body temperature, usually by 1° to 4°C, is one of the most prominent manifestations of the systemic response, especially when inflammation is associated with infection. Substances that induce fever are called *pyrogens*. In infections, bacterial products such as LPS stimulate leukocytes to release the cytokines IL-1 and TNF, which upregulate the production of prostaglandins, particular PGE_2, in the vascular and perivascular cells of the hypothalamus. PGE_2 elevates the body's temperature by altering the firing of neurons in the preoptic nucleus of the hypothalamus. NSAIDs, including aspirin, reduce fever by inhibiting prostaglandin synthesis. Although fever has been postulated to have a protective role, the mechanism underlying this is unknown.

- *Leukocytosis* is a common feature of inflammatory reactions, especially those induced by bacterial infections. The leukocyte count usually climbs to 15,000 or 20,000 cells/μL, but sometimes it may reach extraordinarily high levels of 40,000 to 100,000 cells/μL. These extreme elevations are referred to as *leukemoid reactions*, because they are similar to the white cell counts observed in leukemia and have to be distinguished from this disease (Chapter 10). The leukocytosis occurs initially because of accelerated release of cells from the bone marrow postmitotic reserve pool (caused by cytokines, including TNF and IL-1) and is therefore associated with increased numbers of immature neutrophils in the blood ("band" cells), referred to as a *shift to the left* for historical reasons (based on how the cells were counted in the past). Prolonged infection also increases leukocyte production by stimulating the release of hematopoietic growth factors called colony stimulating factors (CSFs) from macrophages, stromal cells, endothelial cells, and T lymphocytes in the marrow. Most bacterial infections induce an increase in the blood neutrophil count, called *neutrophilia*. Viral infections, such as infectious mononucleosis, mumps, and German measles, cause an absolute increase in the number of lymphocytes

Table 2.9 Examples of Diseases With Granulomatous Inflammation

Disease	Cause	Tissue Reaction
Tuberculosis	*Mycobacterium tuberculosis* infection	Caseating granulomas (tubercles): foci of activated macrophages (epithelioid cells), rimmed by fibroblasts, lymphocytes; occasional Langhans giant cells; central necrosis with amorphous granular debris; acid-fast bacilli
Leprosy	*Mycobacterium leprae* infection	Acid-fast bacilli in macrophages; noncaseating granulomas
Syphilis	*Treponema pallidum* infection	Gumma: microscopic to grossly visible lesion; surrounding wall of macrophages; plasma cell infiltrate; central cells are necrotic without loss of cellular outline
Cat-scratch disease	*Bartonella henselae* (gram-negative bacillus) infection	Rounded or stellate granuloma containing central granular debris and recognizable neutrophils; giant cells uncommon
Sarcoidosis	Unknown etiology	Noncaseating granulomas with abundant activated macrophages
Crohn disease (inflammatory bowel disease)	Immune reaction against intestinal bacteria, possibly self antigens	Occasional noncaseating granulomas in the wall of the intestine, with dense chronic inflammatory infiltrate

(lymphocytosis). In some allergies and parasitic infestations, blood eosinophils increase *(eosinophilia)*. Certain infections (typhoid fever and infections caused by rickettsiae, and certain viruses and protozoa) are associated with a decreased number of circulating white cells *(leukopenia)*.

- The *acute-phase response* consists of the production of plasma proteins, called acute-phase proteins. They are mostly synthesized in the liver and their levels in the blood may increase up to several hundred-fold as part of the response to inflammatory stimuli. Three of the best known of these proteins are C-reactive protein (CRP), fibrinogen, and serum amyloid A (SAA) protein. Synthesis of these molecules in hepatocytes is stimulated by cytokines. Acute-phase proteins such as CRP and SAA bind to microbial cell walls and may have roles in host defense by acting as opsonins and by fixing complement. Fibrinogen neutralizes the negative surface charge of red cells, causing them to form stacks of cells (called *rouleaux*) that sediment more rapidly at unit gravity than do single red cells. This is the basis for measuring the *erythrocyte sedimentation rate* as a simple test for detecting inflammation. Acute-phase proteins have beneficial effects during acute inflammation, but prolonged production of these proteins (especially SAA) in states of chronic inflammation can cause *amyloidosis* (Chapter 5). Elevated serum levels of CRP have been proposed as a marker for increased risk of myocardial infarction in patients with coronary artery disease (Chapter 9). Inflammation is also associated with increased production of the iron-regulating peptide *hepcidin*, which reduces the availability of iron and is responsible for the *anemia* associated with chronic inflammation (Chapter 10).
- Other manifestations of the systemic response include increased heart rate and blood pressure; decreased sweating, mainly because of redirection of blood flow from cutaneous to deep vascular beds, to minimize heat loss through the skin; and rigors (shivering), chills, anorexia, somnolence, and malaise, probably because of the actions of cytokines on brain cells. In severe bacterial infections *(sepsis)*, the abundance of bacteria and their products in the blood stimulate the production of enormous quantities of several cytokines, notably TNF, IL-1, and IL-6. High blood levels of cytokines cause widespread abnormalities such as disseminated intravascular coagulation, hypotension, and metabolic disturbances (such as insulin resistance and hyperglycemia). This clinical triad is known as *septic shock* (Chapter 3). A syndrome similar to septic shock may occur as a complication of noninfectious disorders, such as severe burns, trauma, and pancreatitis. This is called the *systemic inflammatory response syndrome (SIRS)*.

TISSUE REPAIR

Repair, sometimes called healing, refers to the restoration of tissue architecture and function after an injury. The inflammatory response to microbes and injured tissues not only serves to eliminate these dangers but also sets into motion the process of repair.

Repair of damaged tissues occurs by two types of reactions, regeneration and scar formation (Fig. 2.20).

- *Regeneration.* Some tissues are able to replace the damaged components and essentially return to a normal state; this process is called *regeneration*. Regeneration occurs by proliferation of cells that survive the injury and retain the capacity to generate the mature cells of that tissue. The cells that are responsible for regeneration may be

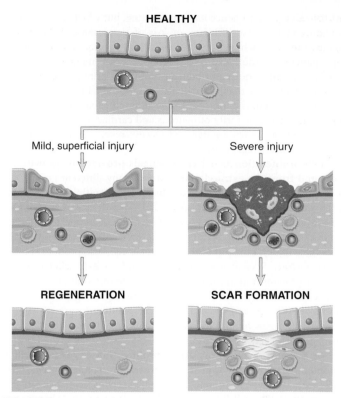

FIG. 2.20 Mechanisms of tissue repair: regeneration and scar formation. Following mild injury, which damages the epithelium but not the underlying tissue, resolution occurs by regeneration, but after more severe injury with damage to the connective tissue framework, repair is by scar formation.

mature differentiated cells or more commonly tissue stem cells (discussed later).

- *Scar formation.* When the injured tissues are incapable of complete restitution, or when the supporting structures of the tissue are damaged, repair occurs by the laying down of connective (fibrous) tissue, a process known as scarring. The fibrous scar provides enough structural stability that the injured tissue is usually able to function. When scarring, resulting from chronic inflammation, occurs in the lungs, liver, kidney, and other parenchymal organs it is referred to as fibrosis.

After many common types of injury, both regeneration and scar formation contribute in varying degrees to repair. We first discuss the mechanisms of cellular proliferation and regeneration and then healing by scar formation.

Cell and Tissue Regeneration

The ability of tissues to repair themselves is determined, in part, by their intrinsic proliferative capacity. In some tissues, cells are constantly being lost and must be continually replaced by new cells that are derived from tissue stem cells and from the remaining mature tissue cells. These types of tissues include hematopoietic cells in the bone marrow and many surface epithelia, such as the basal layers of the squamous epithelia of the skin and the columnar epithelium of the gastrointestinal tract. These tissues can readily regenerate after injury as long as the pool of stem cells is preserved. Other tissues are made up of cells that are normally in the G_0 stage of the cell cycle and hence not proliferating, but which are capable of dividing in response to injury or loss of tissue mass. These tissues include the parenchyma of most solid organs, such as liver, kidney, and pancreas. Endothelial cells, fibroblasts, and smooth muscle cells are also normally quiescent but can proliferate in response to growth factors, a reaction that is particularly important in wound healing. Some tissues consist of terminally differentiated nonproliferative cells, such as the majority of neurons and cardiac muscle cells. Injury to these tissues is irreversible and usually results in a scar, because the cells cannot regenerate.

Cell proliferation is driven by signals provided by growth factors and from the extracellular matrix. Many different growth factors have been described, some of which act on multiple cell types and others that are cell selective (Table 2.10). Growth factors are typically produced by cells near the site of damage. The most important sources of these growth factors are macrophages that are activated by the tissue injury, but epithelial and stromal cells also produce some of these factors. Several growth factors bind to extracellular matrix (ECM) proteins and are displayed at the site of tissue injury at high concentrations. All growth factors activate signaling pathways that stimulate cell division. In addition to responding to growth factors, cells use integrins to bind to ECM proteins; signals from integrins can also stimulate cell proliferation.

In the process of regeneration, proliferation of residual cells is supplemented by development of mature cells from stem cells. Stem cells were discovered in embryos as self-renewing cells that can give rise to all mature cell lineages (totipotent) and were called *embryonal stem cells (ES cells)*. Stem cells have subsequently been found in most adult tissues, where they are called *tissue stem cells*. Unlike ES cells, tissue stem cells have more limited self-renewal capacity, and they typically give rise to the tissue in which they reside. All stem cells have the important ability to undergo asymmetric cell division, defined as a mitosis in which one daughter cell remains a stem cell (accounting for self-renewal) and the other daughter cell begins to differentiate (accounting for the capacity of stem cells to generate mature cell types). Tissue stem cells live in specialized niches, and injury triggers signals that stimulate their proliferation and differentiation into mature cells that repopulate the injured tissue. Thus, they may contribute to regeneration of injured tissues, especially when the differentiated cells that survive the injury have limited or no intrinsic proliferative capacity.

The importance of regeneration in the replacement of injured tissues varies in different types of tissues and with the severity of injury.

- In epithelia of the intestinal tract and skin, provided the underlying basement membrane is intact, injured cells are rapidly replaced by proliferation of residual cells and differentiation of tissue stem cells.
- Tissue regeneration can occur in parenchymal organs whose mature cells are capable of proliferation, but with the exception of the liver, this is usually a limited process. The pancreas, adrenal, thyroid, and lung have some regenerative capacity. The surgical removal of a kidney elicits in the remaining kidney a compensatory response that consists of both hypertrophy and hyperplasia of proximal duct cells. The mechanisms underlying this response are not well defined. The extraordinary capacity of the liver to regenerate has made it a valuable model for studying this process, discussed below.

Restoration of normal tissue architecture can occur only if the residual tissue is structurally intact: for example, after partial surgical resection of the liver. By contrast, if the entire tissue, including the supporting framework, is damaged by infection or inflammation, regeneration is incomplete and is accompanied by scarring. For

Table 2.10 Growth Factors

Growth Factor	Sources	Functions
Epidermal growth factor (EGF)	Activated macrophages, salivary glands, keratinocytes, and many other cells	Mitogenic for keratinocytes and fibroblasts; stimulates keratinocyte migration; stimulates formation of granulation tissue
Transforming growth factor-α (TGF-α)	Activated macrophages, keratinocytes, many other cell types	Stimulates proliferation of hepatocytes and many other epithelial cells
Hepatocyte growth factor (HGF) (scatter factor)	Fibroblasts, stromal cells in the liver, endothelial cells	Enhances proliferation of hepatocytes and other epithelial cells; increases cell motility
Vascular endothelial growth factor (VEGF)	Mesenchymal cells	Stimulates proliferation of endothelial cells; increases vascular permeability
Platelet-derived growth factor (PDGF)	Platelets, macrophages, endothelial cells, smooth muscle cells, keratinocytes	Chemotactic for neutrophils, macrophages, fibroblasts, and smooth muscle cells; activates and stimulates proliferation of fibroblasts, endothelial, and other cells; stimulates ECM protein synthesis
Fibroblast growth factors (FGFs), including acidic (FGF-1) and basic (FGF-2)	Macrophages, mast cells, endothelial cells, many other cell types	Chemotactic and mitogenic for fibroblasts; stimulates angiogenesis and ECM protein synthesis
Transforming growth factor-β (TGF-β)	Platelets, T lymphocytes, macrophages, endothelial cells, keratinocytes, smooth muscle cells, fibroblasts	Chemotactic for leukocytes and fibroblasts; stimulates ECM protein synthesis; suppresses acute inflammation
Keratinocyte growth factor (KGF) (i.e., FGF-7)	Fibroblasts	Stimulates keratinocyte migration, proliferation, and differentiation

ECM, Extracellular matrix.

example, extensive destruction of the liver with collapse of the reticulin framework, as occurs in a liver abscess, leads to scar formation even though the remaining liver cells have the capacity to regenerate.

Liver Regeneration

The liver has a remarkable capacity to regenerate, as demonstrated by its growth after partial hepatectomy, which may be performed for tumor resection or for living-donor hepatic transplantation. The mythologic image of liver regeneration is found in the story of Prometheus, whose liver was eaten every day by an eagle sent by Zeus as punishment for stealing the secret of fire and grew back overnight. The reality, although less dramatic, is still quite impressive.

Regeneration of the liver occurs by the same two mechanisms described earlier: proliferation of remaining hepatocytes and repopulation from stem cells. Which mechanism plays the dominant role depends on the nature of the injury.

- *Proliferation of hepatocytes following partial hepatectomy.* In humans, up to 90% of the liver can be regenerated by the proliferation of the residual hepatocytes. Hepatocyte proliferation in the regenerating liver is triggered by the combined actions of cytokines and polypeptide growth factors. Initially, cytokines such as IL-6 produced mainly by Kupffer cells act on hepatocytes to make the parenchymal cells competent to receive and respond to growth factor signals. In the next phase, growth factors such as HGF and TGF-α, produced by many cell types (see Table 2.10), act on the primed hepatocytes to stimulate their proliferation.
- *Liver regeneration from stem cells.* In situations in which the proliferative capacity of hepatocytes is impaired, such as after chronic liver injury or inflammation, stem cells in the liver contribute to repopulation. Some of these stem cells reside in specialized niches called *canals of Hering,* where bile canaliculi connect with larger bile ducts.

Repair by Scarring

If repair cannot be accomplished by regeneration alone, there is replacement of the injured cells with connective tissue, leading to the formation of a scar. As discussed earlier, scarring may happen when the tissue injury is severe or chronic with damage to parenchymal cells

and epithelia as well as to the connective tissue framework, or when nondividing cells are injured. In contrast to regeneration, which involves the restitution of tissue components, scar formation is a response that "patches" rather than restores the tissue. The term *scar* is most often used in connection to wound healing in the skin but may also be used to describe the replacement of parenchymal cells in any tissue by collagen, as in the heart after myocardial infarction.

Steps in Scar Formation

Scar formation is best illustrated by healing of skin wounds. Within minutes after a traumatic injury, a hemostatic plug comprising platelets (Chapter 3) is formed, which stops bleeding and provides a scaffold for infiltrating inflammatory cells and the formation of a stable clot. The subsequent steps are summarized below (Fig. 2.21):

- *Inflammation.* Over the next 6 to 48 hours, neutrophils and then monocytes are recruited to the site to eliminate the offending agents and clear the debris. **Macrophages are the central cellular players in the repair process.** As discussed earlier, different macrophage populations clear microbes and necrotic tissue, promote inflammation, and produce growth factors that stimulate the proliferation of many cell types in the next stage of repair. As the injurious agents and necrotic cells are cleared, the inflammation resolves.
- *Cell proliferation.* In the next stage, which takes up to 10 days, several cell types, including epithelial cells, endothelial cells, and other vascular cells and fibroblasts, proliferate and migrate to close the now-clean wound. Each cell type serves unique functions:
  - *Epithelial cells* respond to locally produced growth factors and migrate to cover the wound.
  - *Endothelial and other vascular cells* proliferate to form new blood vessels, a process known as *angiogenesis,* described in more detail later.
  - *Fibroblasts* proliferate and migrate into the site of injury and lay down collagen fibers that form the scar.
  - The combination of proliferating fibroblasts, ECM, and new blood vessels forms a type of tissue unique to healing wounds that is called *granulation tissue.* This term derives from its pink, soft, granular gross appearance.

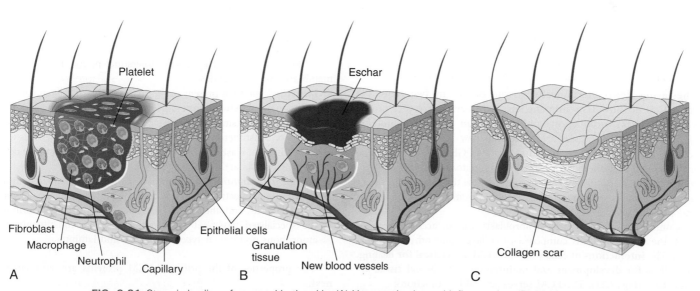

FIG. 2.21 Steps in healing of a wound in the skin. (A) Hemostatic clot and inflammation. (B) Proliferation of epithelial cells; formation of granulation tissue by vessel growth and proliferating fibroblasts. An eschar is the scab that forms over the damaged skin. (C) Remodeling to produce the fibrous scar. This is an example of healing by second intention.

- *Remodeling.* The connective tissue that has been deposited is reorganized to produce the stable fibrous *scar*. This process begins 2 to 3 weeks after injury and may continue for months or years.

Healing of skin wounds can be classified into *healing by first intention (primary union)*, referring to epithelial regeneration with minimal scarring, as in well apposed surgical incisions, and *healing by second intention (secondary union)*, referring to larger wounds that heal by a combination of regeneration and scarring. The key events involved in both types of wound healing are identical hence they are not described separately. We discuss next some of the major events in repair by healing.

Angiogenesis

Angiogenesis is the process by which new blood vessels form from existing vessels. It is critical in healing at sites of injury, in the development of collateral circulations at sites of ischemia, and in allowing tumors to grow. Much work has been done to understand the mechanisms of angiogenesis, and therapies to either augment the process (e.g., to improve blood flow to a heart ravaged by coronary atherosclerosis) or inhibit it (e.g., to frustrate tumor growth or block pathologic vessel growth, as in wet macular degeneration of the eye) have been developed.

Angiogenesis involves the sprouting of new vessels from existing ones. Although many angiogenic and antiangiogenic factors have been described that are involved in regulating vessel growth during tissue repair, the most important factor is *vascular endothelial growth factor (VEGF)*, which stimulates both the migration and proliferation of endothelial cells. In areas of injury, VEGF is produced by cells such as macrophages in response to hypoxia, which increases levels of hypoxia inducible factor (HIF), a transcription factor that is an important regulator of VEGF production. In response to VEGF, nearby intact vessels dilate and become permeable and the basement membrane is digested by matrix metalloproteases, allowing a sprout to form. Endothelial cells at the leading front (the "tip") of the sprout migrate toward the area of tissue injury, and the cells behind the tip proliferate and are remodeled into vascular tubes. In parallel, pericytes (in capillaries) or smooth muscle cells (in larger vessels) are recruited and remodeled, eventually producing a mature vessel. With time, there is progressive vascular regression, transforming the highly vascularized granulation tissue into a pale, largely avascular scar.

Activation of Fibroblasts and Deposition of Connective Tissue

The laying down of connective tissue occurs in two steps: (1) migration of fibroblasts into the site of injury, where they proliferate, and (2) production and deposition of ECM proteins (Fig. 2.22). These processes are orchestrated by locally produced cytokines and growth factors, including PDGF, FGF-2, and TGF-β. The major sources of these factors are inflammatory cells, particularly macrophages that infiltrate sites of injury. Since the major component of scar is connective tissue, we next briefly summarize its composition and properties.

Connective tissue consists of fibroblasts and an acellular component, the ECM, which is composed of collagen and other glycoproteins. **The interactions of cells with the ECM are critical for healing, as well as for development and maintenance of normal tissue architecture** (Fig. 2.23). The ECM serves several key functions:
- *Mechanical support* for cell anchorage and cell migration, and maintenance of cell polarity.

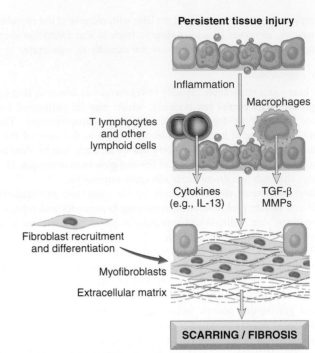

FIG. 2.22 Mechanisms of connective tissue deposition. Persistent tissue injury leads to chronic inflammation and loss of tissue architecture. Cytokines produced by macrophages and other leukocytes stimulate the migration and proliferation of fibroblasts and myofibroblasts and the deposition of collagen and other extracellular matrix proteins. The net result is replacement of normal tissue by connective tissue.

- *Control of cell proliferation*, by binding and displaying growth factors and by signaling through cellular receptors of the integrin family. The ECM provides a depot for a variety of latent growth factors that can be activated within a focus of injury or inflammation.
- *Scaffold for tissue renewal.* Because maintenance of normal tissue structure requires a basement membrane or stromal scaffold on which tissue cells can rest, the integrity of the basement membrane (in epithelia) or the stroma (in parenchymal organs) is critical for the regeneration of tissues.

ECM occurs in two basic forms, interstitial matrix and basement membrane (see Fig. 2.23).
- *Interstitial matrix* is present in the spaces between cells in connective tissue, and between the epithelium and the underlying supportive vascular and smooth muscle structures in parenchymal organs. Its major constituents are fibrillar and nonfibrillar collagens, as well as fibronectin, elastin, proteoglycans, hyaluronate, and other constituents (see later).
- *Basement membrane.* The seemingly random array of interstitial matrix in connective tissues becomes highly organized around epithelial cells, endothelial cells, and smooth muscle cells, forming the specialized basement membrane. Its major constituents are amorphous nonfibrillar type IV collagen and laminin.

The properties of the principal ECM proteins are summarized next.
- *Collagen.* This is the major ECM component of the interstitial matrix and scar tissue. There are over 30 different types of collagen, all

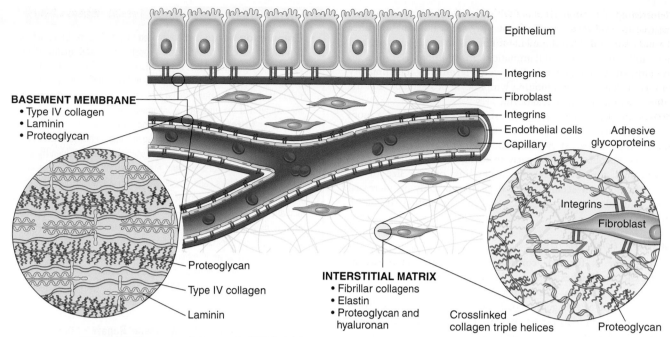

FIG. 2.23 The extracellular matrix (ECM). Main components of the ECM include collagens, proteoglycans, and adhesive glycoproteins. Both epithelial and mesenchymal cells (e.g., fibroblasts) interact with ECM via integrins. Basement membranes and interstitial ECM have different architecture and general composition, although certain components are present in both. Many ECM components (e.g., elastin, fibrillin, hyaluronan, and syndecan) are not shown.

consisting of three polypeptide chains braided into a triple helix. The fibrillar collagens (types I, II, III, and V) are the main types found in scar tissue, tendons, bones, and skin. Fibrillar collagens derive their tensile strength from lateral crosslinking of the triple helices by covalent bonds, a structural modification involving an enzymatic process that requires vitamin C (ascorbic acid) as a cofactor. This requirement explains why individuals with vitamin C deficiency (*scurvy*) show poor healing of wounds and bleed easily.

- *Elastin.* The ability of tissues to recoil and recover their shape after physical deformation is conferred by elastin. Elasticity is especially important in cardiac valves and large blood vessels, which must accommodate recurrent pulsatile flow, as well as in the uterus, skin, and ligaments.
- *Proteoglycans and hyaluronan.* Proteoglycans form highly hydrated gels that confer resistance to compressive forces; in joint cartilage, proteoglycans also provide a layer of lubrication between adjacent bony surfaces. Besides providing compressibility to tissues, proteoglycans also serve as reservoirs for secreted growth factors (e.g., FGF and HGF). Some proteoglycans are integral cell membrane proteins that have roles in cell proliferation, migration, and adhesion, for example, by binding and concentrating growth factors and chemokines.
- *Adhesive glycoproteins and adhesion receptors.* These are structurally diverse molecules involved in cell-cell, cell-ECM, and ECM-ECM interactions. Prototypical adhesive glycoproteins include fibronectin (a major component of the interstitial ECM) and laminin (a major constituent of the basement membrane).
  - *Fibronectin* occurs in tissue and plasma and is synthesized by a variety of cells, including fibroblasts, monocytes, and endothelium.

In healing wounds, fibronectin provides a scaffold for subsequent ECM deposition, angiogenesis, and reepithelialization.
  - *Laminin* is the most abundant glycoprotein in the basement membrane. Besides mediating attachment to the basement membrane, laminin can also modulate cell proliferation, differentiation, and motility.

The attachment of cells to ECM constituents such as laminin and fibronectin is mediated by integrins, which were discussed earlier in the context of leukocyte recruitment into tissues (see Table 2.3). Thus, integrins functionally and structurally link the intracellular cytoskeleton with the outside world. Integrins also mediate cell-cell adhesive interactions. In addition to providing focal attachment to underlying substrates, binding through integrins can also trigger signaling cascades that influence cell locomotion, proliferation, shape, and differentiation.

With this background of ECM structure and functions, we return to the deposition of connective tissue during scar formation (see Fig. 2.22). In response to cytokines and growth factors, fibroblasts enter the wound from the edges and migrate toward the center. Some of these cells may differentiate into cells called *myofibroblasts*, which contain smooth muscle actin and have increased contractile activity; they help close the wound by pulling its margins toward the center. When fibroblasts and myofibroblasts are activated, they increase their synthetic activity and produce connective tissue proteins, mainly collagen and also other ECM proteins.

Transforming growth factor-β (TGF-β) is the most important cytokine for the synthesis and deposition of connective tissue proteins. It is produced by most of the cells in granulation tissue, including activated macrophages. TGF-β stimulates fibroblast migration and proliferation, increased synthesis of collagen and fibronectin, and decreased degradation of ECM due to inhibition of metalloproteinases. TGF-β is involved not only in scar formation after injury but also in the development of fibrosis in the lung, liver, and kidneys following chronic inflammation. In addition, TGF-β is an antiinflammatory cytokine that limits and terminates inflammatory responses. It does this by inhibiting lymphocyte proliferation and the functional activity of other leukocytes.

As healing progresses, the fibroblasts progressively adopt a more synthetic phenotype, leading to increased ECM deposition. Collagen synthesis, in particular, strengthens the healing wound site. Collagen synthesis by fibroblasts begins early in wound healing (days 3 to 5) and continues for several weeks, depending on the size of the wound. Net collagen accumulation depends not only on increased synthesis but also on diminished collagen degradation (discussed later).

Remodeling of Connective Tissue

After the scar is formed, continued remodeling increases its strength and diminishes its size. Wound strength increases due to crosslinking of collagen and increased size of collagen fibers. In addition, the type of collagen deposited shifts from type III collagen early in repair to the more resilient type I collagen. In well-sutured skin wounds, strength may recover to 70% to 80% of normal skin by 3 months.

Over time, the scar shrinks due to the action of *matrix metalloproteinases (MMPs)*, so called because they are dependent on metal ions (e.g., zinc) for their activity. MMPs are produced by a variety of cell types (fibroblasts, macrophages, neutrophils, synovial cells, and some epithelial cells), and their synthesis and secretion are regulated by growth factors, cytokines, and other agents. They include interstitial collagenases, which cleave fibrillar collagen (MMP-1, -2, and -3); gelatinases (MMP-2 and -9), which degrade amorphous collagen and fibronectin; and stromelysins (MMP-3, -10, and -11), which degrade a variety of ECM constituents, including proteoglycans, laminin, fibronectin, and amorphous collagen. MMPs are inhibited by specific tissue inhibitors of metalloproteinases (TIMPs) that are produced by most mesenchymal cells, and the balance of MMP and TIMP activity regulates the ultimate size and makeup of the scar.

Factors That Interfere With Tissue Repair

Variables that prevent healing may be extrinsic (e.g., infection) or intrinsic to the injured tissue, and systemic or local:
- *Infection* is clinically one of the most important causes of delay in healing; it prolongs inflammation and may increase local tissue injury.
- *Diabetes* is a metabolic disease that compromises tissue repair for many reasons (Chapter 18) and is an important systemic cause of delayed wound healing.
- *Nutritional status* has profound effects on repair; protein and vitamin C deficiencies inhibit collagen synthesis and retard healing.
- *Glucocorticoids (steroids)* are antiinflammatory agents that inhibit production of TGF-β, already mentioned as a cytokine that promotes collagen deposition. Thus, in the postsurgical setting the administration of glucocorticoids may prevent adequate wound healing. On the other hand, glucocorticoids are sometimes

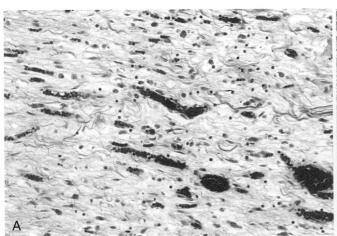
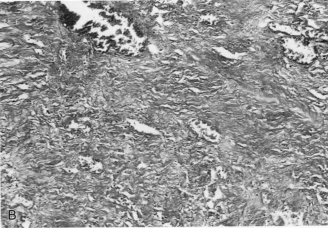

FIG. 2.24 Healing wound. (A) Granulation tissue showing numerous blood vessels, edema, and a loose extracellular matrix containing occasional inflammatory cells. Collagen is stained blue by the trichrome stain; minimal mature collagen can be seen at this point. (B) Mature scar, showing dense collagen (*blue*, trichrome stain) and scattered vascular channels.

prescribed (along with antibiotics) to patients with corneal infections to reduce the likelihood of collagen deposition and vision loss.

- *Mechanical factors* such as increased local pressure or torsion caused by mobility may cause wounds to pull apart.
- *Poor perfusion*, due either to arteriosclerosis and diabetes or to obstructed venous drainage (e.g., in varicose veins), also impairs healing.
- *Foreign bodies* such as fragments of steel, glass, or even bone impede healing.

Clinical Examples of Abnormal Wound Healing and Scarring

Complications in tissue repair can arise from abnormalities in any of the basic components of the process, including deficient scar formation, excessive deposition of the repair components, and the development of contractures.

Defects in Healing: Chronic Wounds

These are seen in numerous clinical situations, typically associated with local and systemic factors that interfere with healing. The following are some common examples.

- *Venous leg ulcers* (Fig. 2.25A) develop most often in elderly people as a result of chronic venous hypertension, which may be caused by severe varicose veins or congestive heart failure, resulting in poor delivery of oxygen.
- *Arterial ulcers* (Fig. 2.25B) develop in individuals with atherosclerosis of peripheral arteries, especially associated with diabetes. Ischemia resulting from the vascular compromise interferes with repair and may cause necrosis of the skin and underlying tissues, producing painful lesions.
- *Diabetic ulcers* (Fig. 2.25C) affect the lower extremities, particularly the feet. The necrosis and failure to heal are the result of small vessel disease causing ischemia and neuropathy, as well as secondary infections. Histologically, these lesions are characterized by epidermal ulceration (Fig. 2.25E) and extensive granulation tissue in the underlying dermis (Fig. 2.25F).
- *Pressure sores* (Fig. 2.25D) are areas of skin ulceration and necrosis of underlying tissues caused by prolonged compression of tissues against a bone, e.g., in bedridden individuals. The lesions are caused by mechanical pressure and local ischemia.

In some situations, failure of healing may lead to dehiscence or rupture of a wound. Although not common, this occurs most frequently after abdominal surgery and is due to vomiting, coughing, or ileus, which can generate mechanical stress on the abdominal wound, leading to its rupture.

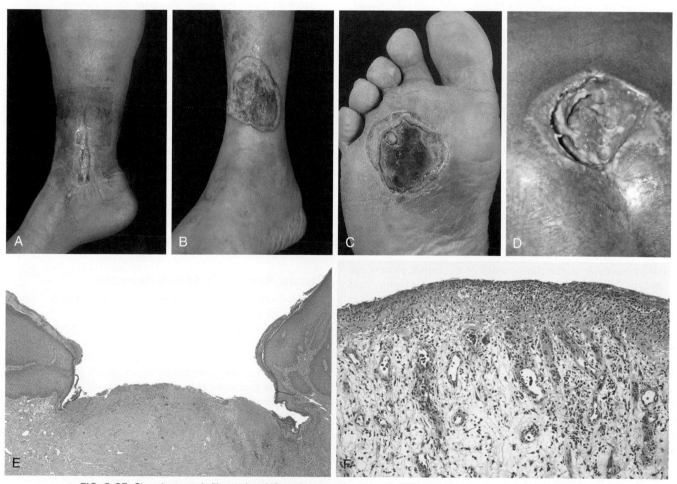

FIG. 2.25 Chronic wounds illustrating defects in wound healing. (A–D) External appearance of skin ulcers. (A) Venous leg ulcer; (B) arterial ulcer, with more extensive tissue necrosis; (C) diabetic ulcer; and (D) pressure sore. (E–F) Histologic appearance of a diabetic ulcer. (E) Ulcer crater; (F) chronic inflammation and granulation tissue. (From Eming SA, Martin P, Tomic-Canic M: Wound repair and regeneration: mechanisms, signaling, and translation. *Sci Transl Med* 6:265, 2014.)

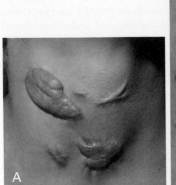

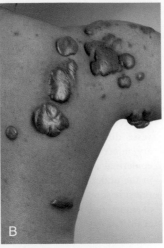

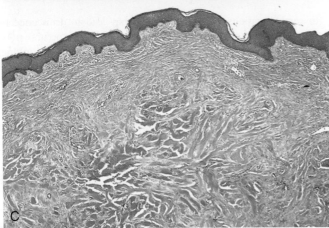

FIG. 2.26 Keloid. Keloids may appear erythematous in light skin tones (A) or hyperpigmented in darker skin (B). (C) Microscopic appearance of a keloid. Note the thick connective tissue deposited in the dermis. (A from Zitelli BJ, Davis HW: *Atlas of Pediatric Physical Diagnosis*, ed 5, Philadelphia, 2007, Mosby; B from Eming SA, Martin P, Tomic-Canic M: Wound repair and regeneration: mechanisms, signaling, and translation. *Sci Transl Med* 6:265, 2014.)

Excessive Scarring

Excessive formation of the components of the repair process can give rise to hypertrophic scars and keloids. Hypertrophic scars contain abundant myofibroblasts and often grow rapidly but tend to then regress over several months. Hypertrophic scars generally develop after thermal or traumatic injury that involves the deep layers of the dermis. When the scar tissue grows beyond the boundaries of the original wound and does not regress, it is called a *keloid* (Fig. 2.26). Keloid formation seems to be an individual predisposition.

Contraction in the size of a wound is an important part of the normal healing process. An exaggeration of this process gives rise to *contracture* and results in deformities of the wound and the surrounding tissues. Contractures are particularly prone to develop on the palms, the soles, and the anterior aspect of the thorax. Contractures are commonly seen after serious burns and can compromise the movement of joints.

Fibrosis in Parenchymal Organs

The term *fibrosis* is used to denote the excessive deposition of collagen and other ECM components in a tissue. The terms *scar* and *fibrosis* are often used interchangeably, but fibrosis usually refers to the abnormal deposition of collagen in internal organs in chronic diseases. The basic mechanisms of fibrosis are the same as those of scar formation in the skin during tissue repair. Fibrosis is induced by persistent injurious stimuli, such as chronic infections and immunologic reactions, and may be responsible for substantial organ dysfunction and even organ failure. As discussed earlier, the major cytokine involved in fibrosis is TGF-β, but cytokines such as IL-13 produced by T lymphocytes may also contribute (see Fig. 2.22).

Fibrotic disorders include diverse chronic and debilitating diseases such as liver cirrhosis, systemic sclerosis (scleroderma), fibrosing diseases of the lung (idiopathic pulmonary fibrosis, pneumoconioses, and drug- and radiation-induced pulmonary fibrosis), end-stage kidney disease, and constrictive pericarditis. These conditions are discussed in the relevant chapters in the book. Because of the tremendous functional impairment caused by fibrosis in these conditions, there is great interest in the development of antifibrotic drugs.

■ RAPID REVIEW

General Features and Causes of Inflammation

- Inflammation is a beneficial host response to foreign invaders and necrotic tissue, but it may also cause tissue damage.
- The main components of inflammation are a vascular reaction and a cellular response; both are activated by mediators that are derived from plasma proteins and various cells.
- The steps of the inflammatory response can be remembered as the five R's: (1) recognition of the injurious agent; (2) recruitment of leukocytes; (3) removal of the agent; (4) regulation (termination) of the response; and (5) repair.
- The causes of inflammation include infections, tissue necrosis, foreign bodies, trauma, and immune responses.
- Epithelial cells, tissue macrophages and dendritic cells, leukocytes, and other cell types express receptors that sense the presence of microbes and necrotic cells. Circulating proteins recognize microbes that have entered the blood.
- The outcome of acute inflammation is either elimination of the noxious stimulus followed by decline of the reaction and repair of the damaged tissue, or persistent injury resulting in chronic inflammation.

Vascular Reactions in Acute Inflammation

- Vasodilation is induced by chemical mediators and is the cause of erythema and stasis of blood flow.
- Increased vascular permeability is induced by histamine, kinins, and other mediators that produce gaps between endothelial cells, or by direct or leukocyte-induced endothelial injury.
- Increased vascular permeability allows plasma proteins and leukocytes, the mediators of host defense, to enter sites of infection or tissue damage. Fluid leak from blood vessels (exudation) results in edema.
- Lymphatic vessels and lymph nodes are also involved in inflammation and often show redness (the vessels) and swelling (lymph nodes).

Leukocyte Recruitment to Sites of Inflammation

- Leukocytes are recruited from the blood into the extravascular tissue where infectious pathogens or damaged tissues may be located and are activated to perform their defensive functions.

- Leukocyte recruitment is a multistep process consisting of loose attachment to and rolling on endothelium (mediated by selectins); firm attachment to endothelium (mediated by integrins); and migration through interendothelial spaces.
- Various cytokines promote expression of selectins and integrin ligands on endothelium (TNF, IL-1), increase the avidity of integrins for their ligands (chemokines), and promote directional migration of leukocytes (also chemokines). Many of these cytokines are produced by tissue macrophages and other cells responding to the pathogens or damaged tissues.
- Neutrophils predominate in the early inflammatory infiltrate and are later replaced by monocytes, which differentiate into macrophages in the tissues.

Leukocyte Activation and Removal of Offending Agents

- Leukocytes can eliminate microbes and dead cell debris by phagocytosis, followed by their destruction in phagolysosomes.
- Destruction is caused by free radicals (ROS, NO) generated in activated leukocytes and by granule enzymes.
- Neutrophils can extrude their nuclear contents to form extracellular nets that trap and destroy microbes.
- Enzymes and ROS may be released into the extracellular environment and cause tissue injury.
- The mechanisms that function to eliminate microbes and dead cell debris (the physiologic role of inflammation) are also capable of damaging normal tissues (the pathologic consequences of inflammation).

Mediators of Inflammation

- Vasoactive amines, mainly histamine: Vasodilation and increased vascular permeability
- Arachidonic acid metabolites (prostaglandins and leukotrienes): Several forms exist and are involved in vascular reactions, leukocyte chemotaxis, and other reactions of inflammation; antagonized by lipoxins.
- Cytokines: Proteins produced by many cell types; usually act at short range; mediate multiple effects, in inflammatory reactions mainly in leukocyte recruitment and migration; principal ones in acute inflammation are TNF, IL-1, and chemokines
- Complement proteins: Activation of the complement system by microbes or antibodies leads to the generation of multiple breakdown products, which are responsible for leukocyte chemotaxis, opsonization, and phagocytosis of microbes and other particles, and cell killing
- Kinins: Produced by proteolytic cleavage of precursors; mediate vascular reaction, pain

Morphologic Patterns of Inflammation

- Serous inflammation is accumulation of protein-rich exudate in body cavities and spaces created by tissue necrosis.
- Fibrinous inflammation is characterized by formation of fibrin, usually on the surfaces of organs such as the heart and lungs.
- Purulent inflammation is characterized by formation of pus, which consists of dead cells, neutrophils, and microbes, and is most often caused by bacterial infection. An abscess is localized purulent inflammation.
- An ulcer is a discontinuity in an epithelium, with underlying acute and chronic inflammation.

Chronic Inflammation

- Chronic inflammation is a prolonged host response to persistent stimuli.
- It is caused by microbes that resist elimination, immune responses against self and environmental antigens, and some toxic substances (e.g., silica); underlies many medically important diseases.
- It is characterized by coexisting inflammation, tissue injury, attempted repair by scarring, and immune response.
- The cellular infiltrate consists of macrophages, lymphocytes, plasma cells, and other leukocytes.
- It is mediated by cytokines produced by macrophages and lymphocytes (notably T lymphocytes); bidirectional interactions between these cells tend to amplify and prolong the inflammatory reaction.
- Granulomatous inflammation is a pattern of chronic inflammation induced by T cell and macrophage activation in response to an agent that is resistant to eradication. It is characterized by an aggregation of macrophages that acquire an epithelioid morphology; caused by tuberculosis, fungal infections, and syphilis.

Systemic Effects of Inflammation

- Fever: Cytokines (TNF, IL-1) stimulate production of prostaglandins in the hypothalamus.
- Leukocytosis: Caused by release of cells from the bone marrow; cytokines (colony-stimulating factors) stimulate production of leukocytes from precursors in the bone marrow
- Production of acute-phase proteins: C-reactive protein, others; synthesis stimulated by cytokines (IL-6, others) acting on liver cells
- In some severe infections, septic shock: Fall in blood pressure, disseminated intravascular coagulation, metabolic abnormalities; induced by high levels of TNF and other cytokines

Repair by Regeneration

- Different tissues consist of continuously dividing cells (epithelia, hematopoietic tissues), normally quiescent cells that are capable of proliferation (most parenchymal organs), and nondividing cells (neurons, skeletal and cardiac muscle). The regenerative capacity of a tissue depends on the proliferative potential of its constituent cells.
- Cell proliferation is stimulated by growth factors and interactions of cells with the extracellular matrix.
- Regeneration of the liver is a classic example of repair by regeneration; triggered by cytokines and growth factors produced in response to loss of liver mass and inflammation; in different situations, may occur by proliferation of surviving hepatocytes or differentiation of stem cells.

Repair by Scar Formation

- Repair occurs by replacement with connective tissue and scar formation if the injured tissue is not capable of proliferation or if the structural framework is damaged and cannot support regeneration.
- The main steps in repair by scarring are clot formation, inflammation, angiogenesis with formation of granulation tissue, migration and proliferation of fibroblasts, collagen synthesis, and connective tissue remodeling.
- Macrophages are critical for orchestrating the repair process, by eliminating offending agents and producing cytokines and growth

factors that stimulate the proliferation of the cell types involved in repair.

- TGF-β is a potent fibrogenic agent; ECM deposition depends on the balance between fibrogenic agents, matrix metalloproteinases (MMPs) that digest ECM, and tissue inhibitors of MMPs (TIMPs).

Clinicopathologic Aspects of Tissue Repair

- Cutaneous wounds can heal by primary union (healing by first intention) or secondary union (healing by secondary intention);

secondary healing involves more extensive scarring and wound contraction.
- Wound healing can be altered by many conditions, particularly infection and diabetes; the type, volume, and location of the injury are important factors that influence the healing process.
- Excessive production of collagen can cause keloids in the skin.
- Persistent stimulation of collagen synthesis in chronic inflammatory diseases leads to fibrosis of the tissue, often with extensive loss of the tissue and functional impairment.

■ Laboratory Tests

Test	Reference Value	Pathophysiology/Clinical Relevance
Blood cell counts		See Chapter 10
C-reactive protein (CRP), serum	≤8 mg/L	CRP is an acute-phase reactant that acts as an opsonin. In acute inflammation, IL-6 stimulates production of CRP from hepatocytes. CRP is a sensitive but nonspecific marker of inflammation. CRP is increased in a variety of acute illnesses and inflammatory conditions (e.g., bacterial infection, myocardial infarction). Higher baseline levels of plasma CRP are associated with increased risk of chronic heart disease and stroke, possibly through the inflammatory response associated with atherosclerosis.
Erythrocyte sedimentation rate (ESR); aka Sed rate, Westergren test	Male 0–22 mm/hr Female 0–29 mm/hr	In health, the negatively charged red cell membrane prevents red cell aggregation. In the setting of inflammation, positively charged immunoglobulins and acute-phase proteins (e.g., prothrombin, plasminogen, fibrinogen, C-reactive protein) bind to the cell membrane, neutralizing the negative charge and causing clumping into stacks (rouleaux). These large aggregates sediment more rapidly than individual red cells, increasing the ESR. ESR can be elevated in multiple conditions, including infections, chronic inflammation, pregnancy, malignancy, end-stage renal disease, and nephrotic syndrome.

References values from https://www.mayocliniclabs.com/ by permission of Mayo Foundation for Medical Education and Research. All rights reserved.

Adapted from Deyrup AT, D'Ambrosio D, Muir J, et al. Essential Laboratory Tests for Medical Education. *Acad Pathol.* 2022;9. doi: 10.1016/j.acpath.2022.100046.

Hemodynamic Disorders, Thromboembolism, and Shock

The health of cells and tissues depends on the circulation of blood, which delivers oxygen and nutrients and removes wastes generated by cellular metabolism. Under normal conditions, as blood passes through capillary beds, there is little net movement of water and electrolytes into the tissues (discussed later). This balance is often disturbed by pathologic conditions that alter endothelial function, increase vascular hydrostatic pressure, or decrease plasma protein content, all of which promote *edema*—the accumulation of fluid in tissues resulting from a net movement of water into extravascular spaces. Depending on its severity and location, edema may have minimal or profound effects. In the lower extremities, it may only make one's shoes feel snugger after a long, sedentary day; in the lungs, however, edema fluid can fill alveoli, causing life-threatening hypoxia.

The structural integrity of blood vessels is frequently compromised by trauma. *Hemostasis* is the process of blood clotting that follows blood vessel damage. Inadequate hemostasis results in *hemorrhage* (excessive bleeding), which may compromise tissue perfusion and, if massive and rapid, lead to hypotension, shock, and death. Conversely, inappropriate clotting *(thrombosis)* or migration of clots in the vasculature *(embolism)* may lead to blood vessel obstruction and ischemic cell death *(infarction)*. Importantly, thromboembolism underlies three major causes of morbidity and death: myocardial infarction, pulmonary embolism, and cerebrovascular accident (stroke).

With this as background, we begin our discussion of hemodynamic disorders with conditions that increase blood volumes, either locally or systemically.

HYPEREMIA AND CONGESTION

Hyperemia and congestion both refer to an increase in blood volume within a tissue but have different underlying mechanisms. *Hyperemia* is an active process resulting from arteriolar dilation and increased blood inflow; it occurs at sites of inflammation and in exercising skeletal muscle. Hyperemic tissues are redder than normal because they are engorged with oxygenated blood. *Congestion* is a passive process resulting from impaired outflow of venous blood from a tissue. Congestion occurs systemically in cardiac failure and locally as a consequence of venous obstruction. Congested tissues have an abnormal blue-red color *(cyanosis)* that stems from the accumulation of deoxygenated hemoglobin. In long-standing chronic congestion, inadequate tissue perfusion and persistent hypoxia may lead to parenchymal cell death and secondary tissue fibrosis, and the elevated intravascular pressures may cause edema or rupture capillaries, producing focal hemorrhages.

Cut surfaces of hyperemic or congested tissues feel wet and typically ooze blood. Microscopically, **acute pulmonary congestion** is marked by blood-engorged alveolar capillaries and variable alveolar septal edema and intraalveolar hemorrhage. In **chronic pulmonary congestion,** the septa become thickened and fibrotic and the alveolar spaces contain numerous macrophages laden with hemosiderin (**"heart failure cells,"** eFig. 3.1) derived from phagocytosed red cells. In **acute hepatic congestion,** the central vein and sinusoids are distended with blood and centrally located hepatocytes may undergo necrosis. Periportal hepatocytes, which experience less severe hypoxia because of their proximity to hepatic arterioles, may develop fatty change. In **chronic passive liver congestion,** the central regions of the hepatic lobules are congested, red-brown, and slightly depressed (owing to necrosis and cell loss) and are accentuated by surrounding zones of tan, sometimes fatty, periportal hepatocytes (**nutmeg liver**) (Fig. 3.1A, B).

EDEMA

Approximately 60% of lean body weight is water, two-thirds of which is intracellular. Most of the remaining water is found in tissues in the form of interstitial fluid; only 5% of the body's water is in blood plasma. As noted earlier, edema is an accumulation of interstitial fluid within tissues. Extravascular fluid can also collect in body cavities, where it is often referred to as an effusion. Examples include effusions in the pleural cavity *(hydrothorax)*, the pericardial cavity *(hydropericardium)*, and the peritoneal cavity (hydroperitoneum, or *ascites*). *Anasarca* is severe, generalized edema marked by profound swelling of subcutaneous tissues and accumulation of fluid in body cavities.

Table 3.1 lists the major causes of edema. In inflammation, edema is due to increased vascular permeability (Chapter 2); the noninflammatory causes are described in the following discussion.

Fluid movement between the vascular and interstitial spaces is governed mainly by two opposing forces: vascular hydrostatic pressure and colloid osmotic pressure produced by plasma proteins. Normally, the outflow of fluid produced by hydrostatic pressure at the arteriolar end of the microcirculation is nearly balanced by inflow at the venular end owing to osmotic pressure. The small net outflow of fluid into the interstitial space is drained by lymphatic vessels to the bloodstream by way of the thoracic duct, keeping the tissues "dry." Either increased hydrostatic pressure or diminished colloid osmotic pressure will result in increased movement of water into the interstitium (Fig. 3.2), and if the drainage capacity of the lymphatics is exceeded, edema results.

The edema fluid that accumulates due to high hydrostatic pressure or low colloid pressure typically is a protein-poor *transudate*; by contrast, because of increased vascular permeability, inflammatory

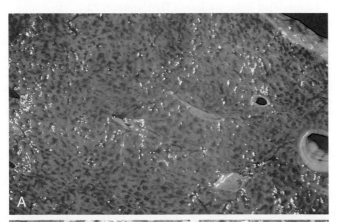
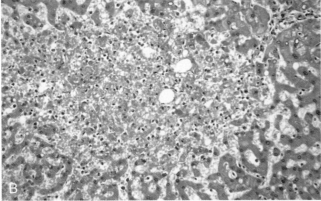

FIG. 3.1 Liver with chronic passive congestion and hemorrhagic necrosis. (A) In this autopsy specimen, centrilobular areas are red and slightly depressed compared with the surrounding tan viable parenchyma, creating "nutmeg liver" (so called because it resembles the cut surface of a nutmeg). (B) Microscopic preparation shows centrilobular hepatic necrosis with hemorrhage and scattered inflammatory cells. (Courtesy of Dr. James Crawford.)

Table 3.1 Causes of Edema

Increased Hydrostatic Pressure
Impaired Venous Return
Congestive heart failure
Constrictive pericarditis
Liver cirrhosis
Venous obstruction or compression
Thrombosis
External pressure (e.g., mass)
Lower extremity inactivity with prolonged dependency
Arteriolar Dilation
Heat
Neurohumoral dysregulation
Reduced Plasma Osmotic Pressure (Hypoproteinemia)
Protein-losing glomerulopathies (nephrotic syndrome)
Reduced protein synthesis (e.g., advanced liver disease)
Malnutrition
Protein-losing gastroenteropathy
Lymphatic Obstruction
Inflammatory
Neoplastic
Postsurgical
Postirradiation
Sodium Retention
Excessive salt intake with renal insufficiency
Decreased renal excretion of sodium
Renal hypoperfusion
Increased renin-angiotensin-aldosterone secretion
Inflammation
Acute inflammation
Chronic inflammation
Angiogenesis

Data from Leaf A, Cotran RS: *Renal Pathophysiology*, ed 3, New York, 1985, Oxford University Press, p 146.

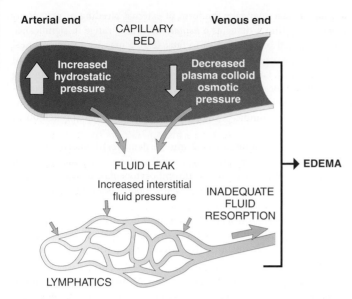

FIG. 3.2 Factors influencing fluid movement across capillary walls. Capillary hydrostatic and osmotic forces are normally balanced, so there is little net movement of fluid into the interstitium. If hydrostatic pressure rises or plasma osmotic pressure decreases, the flux of fluid into the interstitium increases. Tissue lymphatics drain much of the excess fluid back to the circulation by way of the thoracic duct; however, if the interstitial fluid accumulation exceeds the capacity for lymphatic drainage, tissue edema results.

edema fluid is a protein-rich *exudate*. Next we discuss the various causes of edema.

Increased Hydrostatic Pressure

Increases in hydrostatic pressure are mainly caused by disorders that impair venous return. For example, deep venous thrombosis in the lower extremity may cause edema restricted to the distal portion of the affected leg, whereas congestive heart failure (Chapter 11) leads to a systemic increase in venous pressure and, often, widespread edema. Fig. 3.3 illustrates the mechanisms underlying the generalized edema that may be seen in the context of cardiac, renal, or hepatic

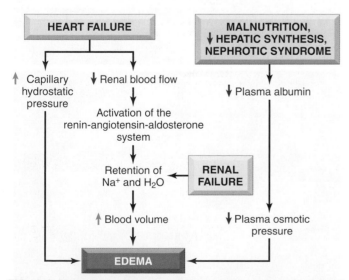

FIG. 3.3 Pathways leading to systemic edema resulting from heart failure, renal failure, or reduced plasma osmotic pressure, which has several causes including liver failure.

failure. Several factors increase venous hydrostatic pressure in patients with congestive heart failure. Reduced cardiac output leads to pooling of blood in the venous circulation and increased capillary hydrostatic pressure. The reduction in cardiac output also results in hypoperfusion of the kidneys, triggering the renin-angiotensin-aldosterone axis and inducing sodium and water retention (*secondary hyperaldosteronism*). In patients with normal heart function, this adaptation increases cardiac filling and cardiac output, resulting in improved renal perfusion. However, the failing heart often cannot increase its output in response to increases in cardiac filling, and a vicious cycle of fluid retention, increased venous hydrostatic pressures, and worsening edema ensues. Unless cardiac output is restored or renal water retention is reduced (e.g., by salt restriction or treatment with diuretics or aldosterone antagonists), this downward spiral continues. Secondary hyperaldosteronism is also a feature of noncardiac generalized edema, which may also benefit from treatment with salt restriction, diuretics, and aldosterone antagonists.

Reduced Plasma Osmotic Pressure

Reduced plasma albumin is a common feature of disorders in which edema is caused by decreases in colloid osmotic pressure. Normally, albumin accounts for almost half of the total plasma protein and is the biggest contributor to colloid osmotic pressure. Albumin levels fall if urinary loss increases or hepatic synthesis decreases.

- *Nephrotic syndrome* is the most important cause of albuminuria. In diseases associated with nephrotic syndrome (Chapter 12), damage to glomeruli allows albumin (and other plasma proteins) to pass into the urine.
- Reduced albumin synthesis is seen in the setting of severe liver disease (e.g., cirrhosis) (Chapter 14) and protein malnutrition (Chapter 7).

Regardless of cause, low albumin levels lead to edema, reduced intravascular volume, renal hypoperfusion, and secondary hyperaldosteronism. Unfortunately, increased salt and water retention by the kidney not only fails to correct the plasma volume deficit but also exacerbates the edema, because the primary defect—low serum protein—persists.

Lymphatic Obstruction

Edema may result from lymphatic obstruction that compromises resorption of fluid from interstitial spaces. Impaired lymphatic drainage and consequent lymphedema usually results from a localized obstruction caused by an inflammatory or neoplastic condition. For example, the parasitic infection *filariasis* can cause massive edema of the lower extremity and external genitalia (so-called "elephantiasis") secondary to fibrosis of the inguinal lymphatics and lymph nodes (eFig. 3.2). Infiltration and obstruction of superficial lymphatics by breast cancer may cause edema of the overlying skin; the characteristic finely pitted appearance of the skin of the affected breast is called *peau d'orange* (orange peel). Lymphedema may also occur as a complication of therapy, as in patients with breast cancer who undergo axillary lymph node resection and/or irradiation; both may disrupt and obstruct lymphatic drainage and cause severe lymphedema of the arm.

Sodium and Water Retention

Excessive retention of salt (and associated water) can lead to edema by increasing hydrostatic pressure (owing to expansion of the intravascular volume) and reducing plasma osmotic pressure (because of decreased plasma protein concentration). Excessive salt and water retention are seen in a wide variety of diseases that compromise renal function, including poststreptococcal glomerulonephritis and acute renal failure (Chapter 12).

Clinical Features. The effects of edema vary, ranging from merely annoying to rapidly fatal. Subcutaneous edema is important to recognize because it may often signal underlying cardiac or renal disease; if severe, it may also impair healing of cutaneous wounds and the clearance of skin infections. Pulmonary edema is a common clinical problem. It is seen most frequently with left ventricular failure but also may occur with renal failure, acute lung injury (Chapter 11), and inflammatory and infectious disorders of the lung. It may cause death by interfering with normal ventilatory function, and alveolar edema fluid also creates a favorable environment for superimposed infection. Brain edema is life threatening: if the swelling is severe, the brain may herniate (extrude) through the foramen magnum. With increased intracranial pressure, the brain stem vascular supply may be compromised, leading to death due to injury to the medullary centers that control respiration and other vital functions (Chapter 21).

HEMORRHAGE

Hemorrhage, defined as the extravasation of blood from vessels, results from damage to blood vessels and may be exacerbated by defects in blood clotting. As described earlier, capillary bleeding can occur in chronically congested tissues. Trauma, atherosclerosis, or inflammatory or neoplastic erosion of a vessel wall also may lead to hemorrhage, which may be massive if the affected vessel is a large vein or artery.

   The risk of hemorrhage (often after a seemingly insignificant injury) is increased in a wide variety of disorders collectively called *hemorrhagic diatheses.* These have diverse causes, including inherited or acquired defects in vessel walls, platelets, or coagulation factors, all of which must function properly to ensure hemostasis. These are discussed in the next section. Here we focus on clinical features of hemorrhages, regardless of the cause.

   Hemorrhage may be manifested by different appearances and consequences.

- Hemorrhage may take the form of external bleeding or may accumulate within a tissue as a *hematoma.* These range in significance from trivial (e.g., a bruise) to fatal (e.g., a massive retroperitoneal hematoma caused by rupture of a dissecting aortic aneurysm) (Chapter 8). Large bleeds into body cavities are described according to their location—*hemothorax, hemopericardium, hemoperitoneum,* or *hemarthrosis* (in joints). Large hemorrhages can occasionally result in jaundice as red cells and hemoglobin are broken down by macrophages.
- *Petechiae* are minute (1 to 2 mm in diameter) hemorrhages into skin, mucous membranes, or serosal surfaces (Fig. 3.4A). Causes include low platelet counts (thrombocytopenia), defective platelet function, and loss of vascular wall support, as in vitamin C deficiency (scurvy, Chapter 7).
- *Purpura* are slightly larger (3 to 5 mm) hemorrhages. Purpura can result from the same disorders that cause petechiae, as well as trauma, vascular inflammation (vasculitis), and increased vascular fragility.
- *Ecchymoses* are larger (1 to 2 cm) subcutaneous hematomas (colloquially called "bruises"). Extravasated red cells are phagocytosed and degraded by macrophages; the characteristic color changes of a bruise result from the enzymatic conversion of hemoglobin (red-blue color) to bilirubin (blue-green color) and eventually hemosiderin (golden-brown).

   The clinical impact of a hemorrhage depends on the volume of blood that is lost, the rate of bleeding, the location of the bleed, and the

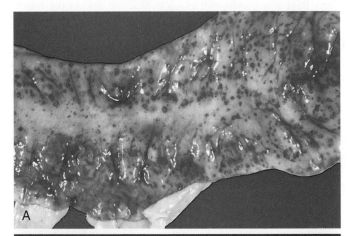

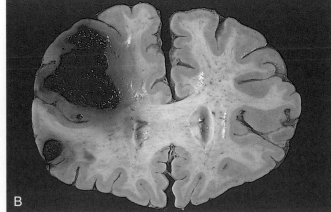

FIG. 3.4 (A) Punctate petechial hemorrhages of the colonic mucosa, a consequence of thrombocytopenia. (B) Fatal intracerebral hemorrhage.

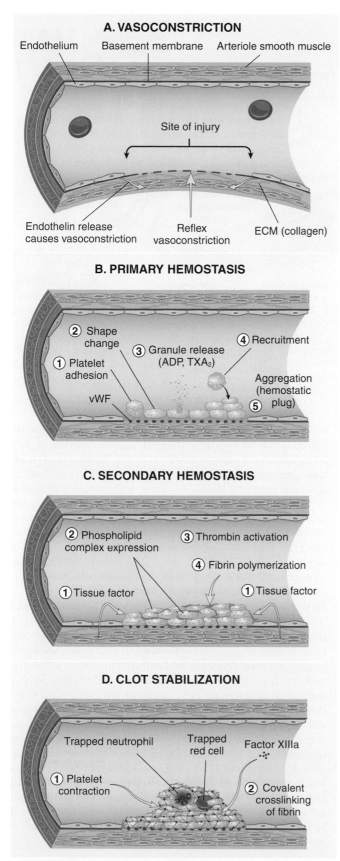

A. VASOCONSTRICTION

Endothelium   Basement membrane   Arteriole smooth muscle

Site of injury

Endothelin release causes vasoconstriction   Reflex vasoconstriction   ECM (collagen)

B. PRIMARY HEMOSTASIS

② Shape change
③ Granule release (ADP, TXA₂)
④ Recruitment
① Platelet adhesion
vWF
Aggregation (hemostatic plug) ⑤

C. SECONDARY HEMOSTASIS

② Phospholipid complex expression
③ Thrombin activation
④ Fibrin polymerization
① Tissue factor
① Tissue factor

D. CLOT STABILIZATION

Trapped neutrophil   Trapped red cell   Factor XIIIa
① Platelet contraction
② Covalent crosslinking of fibrin

FIG. 3.5 Normal hemostasis. (A) After vascular injury, local neurohumoral factors induce a transient vasoconstriction. (B) Exposure of von Willebrand factor (vWF) in the extracellular matrix (ECM) leads to binding of platelets, which adhere and become activated, undergoing a shape

health of the individual affected. Rapid loss of up to 20% of the blood volume may be well tolerated in healthy adults yet cause cardiovascular decompensation in individuals with underlying heart or lung disease. Greater losses may cause hemorrhagic (hypovolemic) shock (discussed later) even in those who are healthy. A bleed that is relatively trivial in the subcutaneous tissues may cause death if located in the brain (Fig. 3.4B). Finally, chronic or recurrent external blood loss (e.g., due to peptic ulcer or menstrual bleeding) frequently leads to iron deficiency anemia owing to loss of the iron in hemoglobin. By contrast, iron is efficiently recycled from phagocytosed red cells, so internal bleeding (e.g., a hematoma) does not lead to iron deficiency.

HEMOSTASIS AND THROMBOSIS

Hemostasis is a process initiated by a traumatic vascular injury that leads to the formation of a blood clot. The pathologic counterpart of hemostasis is thrombosis, the formation of a clot (a thrombus) within vessels that have been damaged by a disease process. This discussion begins with hemostasis and its regulation, to be followed by causes and consequences of thrombosis.

Hemostasis

Hemostasis is a precisely orchestrated process involving platelets, clotting factors, and endothelium that occurs at the site of vascular injury and leads to the formation of a blood clot, which serves to prevent or limit the extent of bleeding. The general sequence of events leading to hemostasis at a site of vascular injury is shown in Fig. 3.5.

- *Arteriolar vasoconstriction* occurs immediately and markedly reduces blood flow to the injured area (see Fig. 3.5A). It is mediated by neurogenic reflexes and augmented by the local secretion of factors such as *endothelin*, a potent endothelium-derived vasoconstrictor. This effect is transient, however, and bleeding resumes without the activation of platelets and coagulation factors.
- *Primary hemostasis: the formation of the platelet plug.* Disruption of the endothelium exposes subendothelial collagen, which binds von Willebrand factor, a molecule that promotes platelet adherence and activation. Activated platelets undergo a dramatic shape change (from small, rounded discs to flat plates with spiky protrusions that markedly increase surface area) and release their secretory granules. Within minutes the secreted products recruit additional platelets, which aggregate to form a *primary hemostatic plug* (see Fig. 3.5B).
- *Secondary hemostasis: deposition of fibrin.* Vascular injury exposes *tissue factor* at the site of injury. Tissue factor is a membrane-bound procoagulant glycoprotein that is normally expressed by subendothelial cells in the vessel wall, such as smooth muscle cells and fibroblasts. Tissue factor binds and activates factor VII (see later), setting in motion a cascade of reactions that lead to *thrombin* generation. Thrombin cleaves circulating fibrinogen into insoluble *fibrin*, creating a fibrin meshwork, and is a potent activator of platelets, leading to additional platelet aggregation at the site of injury.

change and releasing their granule contents. Released adenosine diphosphate (ADP) and thromboxane A₂ (TXA₂) induce additional platelet aggregation through bridging interactions involving fibrinogen and platelet receptor GpIIb-IIIa, leading to formation of the primary hemostatic plug. (C) Activation of the coagulation cascade results in fibrin polymerization, "cementing" the platelets into a secondary hemostatic plug. (D) Platelet contraction and covalent crosslinking of fibrin stabilize the clot.

This sequence, referred to as *secondary hemostasis,* consolidates the platelet plug (see Fig. 3.5C).

- *Clot stabilization.* Polymerized fibrin is crosslinked covalently by factor XIII and platelet aggregates contract, both of which contribute to the formation a solid *permanent plug* that prevents further bleeding (see Fig. 3.5D). The size of the clot is limited by counterregulatory mechanisms (described later) that restrict clotting to the site of injury and eventually lead to clot resorption and tissue repair.

The integrity and function of endothelial cells determine whether clots form, propagate, or dissolve. Healthy endothelial cells express a variety of anticoagulant factors that inhibit platelet aggregation and coagulation and promote fibrinolysis; after endothelial injury or activation, however, this balance shifts to favor clotting (discussed later). Endothelium can be activated by microbial pathogens, hemodynamic forces, and a number of proinflammatory mediators, all of which may increase the risk of thrombosis. We will return to the procoagulant and anticoagulant actions of endothelium after a detailed discussion of the role of platelets and coagulation factors in hemostasis, following the scheme illustrated in Fig. 3.5.

Platelets

Platelets play a critical role in hemostasis by forming the primary plug that initially seals vascular defects and by providing a surface that binds and concentrates activated coagulation factors. Platelets are disc-shaped anucleate cell fragments that are shed from megakaryocytes in the bone marrow into the bloodstream. Their function depends on several glycoprotein receptors, a contractile cytoskeleton, and two types of cytoplasmic granules. *α-Granules* have the adhesion molecule P-selectin on their membranes (Chapter 2) and contain coagulation factors such as fibrinogen, factor V, and vWF as well as protein factors involved in wound healing, such as fibronectin, platelet factor 4 (a heparin-binding chemokine), platelet-derived growth factor (PDGF), and transforming growth factor-β. *Dense* (or δ) *granules* contain adenosine diphosphate (ADP), adenosine triphosphate (ATP), polyphosphate, ionized calcium, serotonin, and epinephrine.

After a traumatic vascular injury, platelets encounter constituents of the subendothelial connective tissue, such as collagen and attached vWF, which is normally present here as well as in the plasma. On contact with these proteins, platelets undergo a sequence of reactions that lead to the formation of a platelet plug (see Fig. 3.5B).

- *Platelet adhesion* is mediated largely by interactions with vWF, which acts as a bridge between the platelet surface receptor glycoprotein Ib (GpIb) and exposed collagen (Fig. 3.6). Notably, genetic deficiencies of vWF (von Willebrand disease, Chapter 10) or GpIb (Bernard-Soulier syndrome) result in bleeding disorders, attesting to the importance of these factors.
- *Platelets rapidly change shape* following adhesion, converting from smooth discs to spiky "sea urchins" with greatly increased surface area. This change is accompanied by alterations in *glycoprotein IIb/IIIa* that increase its affinity for fibrinogen (see later), and by the translocation of *negatively charged phospholipids* (particularly phosphatidylserine) to the platelet surface. These phospholipids bind calcium and serve as nucleation sites for the assembly of coagulation factor complexes.
- *Secretion of granule contents (release reaction)* occurs along with changes in shape; these two events are often referred to together as *platelet activation.* Platelet activation is triggered by a number of factors, including the coagulation factor thrombin and ADP.

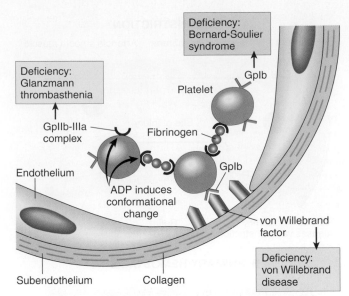

FIG. 3.6 Platelet adhesion and aggregation. Von Willebrand factor (vWF) functions as an adhesion bridge between subendothelial collagen and the glycoprotein Ib (GpIb) platelet receptor. Platelet aggregation is accomplished by fibrinogen binding to platelet GpIIb-IIIa receptors on different platelets. Congenital deficiencies in the various receptors or bridging molecules lead to the diseases indicated in the colored boxes. *ADP,* Adenosine diphosphate.

Thrombin activates platelets by proteolytically cleaving and switching on a special G-protein–coupled receptor referred to as a *protease-activated receptor* (PAR). ADP is a component of dense-body granules; thus, platelet activation and ADP release leads to additional rounds of platelet activation, a phenomenon referred to as *recruitment.* Activated platelets also produce the prostaglandin *thromboxane A2* (TxA2), a potent inducer of platelet aggregation. Aspirin inhibits platelet aggregation and produces a mild bleeding defect by inhibiting cyclooxygenase, a platelet enzyme that is required for TxA2 synthesis. It is thought that growth factors released from platelets such as PDGF contribute to the repair of the vessel wall following injury.

- *Platelet aggregation* follows their activation. The conformational change in glycoprotein IIb/IIIa that occurs with platelet activation allows binding of fibrinogen, a large bivalent plasma protein that forms bridges between activated platelets, leading to their aggregation. Inherited deficiency of GpIIb-IIIa results in a bleeding disorder called *Glanzmann thrombasthenia.* The initial wave of aggregation is reversible, but concurrent activation of thrombin stabilizes the platelet plug by causing further platelet activation and aggregation and by promoting irreversible *platelet contraction.* Platelet contraction is dependent on the cytoskeleton and consolidates the aggregated platelets. In parallel, thrombin converts fibrinogen into insoluble *fibrin* and activates factor XIIIa, which covalently crosslinks fibrin, cementing the platelets in place and creating the definitive *secondary hemostatic plug.* Entrapped red cells and leukocytes are also found in hemostatic plugs, in part due to adherence of leukocytes to P-selectin expressed on activated platelets.

Coagulation Factors

Coagulation factors participate in a series of amplifying enzymatic reactions that lead to the deposition of an insoluble fibrin clot. As discussed later, the dependency of clot formation on various factors differs in the laboratory test tube and in blood vessels in vivo (Fig. 3.7). However, clotting in vitro and in vivo both follow the same general principles, as follows.

The cascade of reactions in the pathway can be likened to a "dance," in which coagulation factors are passed from one partner to the next (Fig. 3.8). Each reaction involves an enzyme (an activated coagulation factor), a substrate (an inactive proenzyme form of a coagulation factor), and a cofactor (a reaction accelerator). These components are assembled on the negatively charged phospholipid surface of activated platelets. Assembly of reaction complexes also depends on calcium, which binds to γ-carboxylated glutamic acid residues that are present in factors II, VII, IX, and X. The enzymatic reactions that produce γ-carboxylated glutamic acid require vitamin K and are antagonized by drugs such as warfarin, which interferes with vitamin K metabolism.

Based on assays performed in clinical laboratories, the coagulation cascade is divided into the *extrinsic* and *intrinsic pathways* (see Fig. 3.7A).

- The *prothrombin time* (PT) assay assesses the function of the proteins in the extrinsic pathway (factors X, VII, V, II [prothrombin], and fibrinogen). In brief, tissue factor, phospholipids, and calcium are added to plasma and the time for a fibrin clot to form is recorded.
- The *partial thromboplastin time* (PTT) assay assesses the function of the proteins in the intrinsic pathway (factors XII, XI, X, IX, VIII, V, II, and fibrinogen). In this assay, clotting of plasma is initiated by the addition of negatively charged particles (e.g., ground glass) that activate factor XII together with phospholipids and calcium, and the time to fibrin clot formation is recorded.

Although the PT and PTT assays are of great utility in evaluating coagulation factor function in patients, they do not recapitulate the events that lead to coagulation in vivo. This point is most clearly made by considering the clinical effects of deficiencies of various coagulation factors. Deficiencies of factors V, VII, VIII, IX, and X are associated with moderate to severe bleeding, and prothrombin deficiency is incompatible with life. By contrast, factor XI deficiency only causes a mild bleeding disorder, and individuals with factor XII deficiency have no bleeding disorder at all. The physiologic role of factor XII is uncertain. Rare individuals with excessive factor XII activity are prone to angioedema, an inflammatory condition that may be triggered by the generation of bradykinin by factor XII through its ability to cleave high-molecular-weight kininogen.

Based on these observations, it is believed that, in vivo, the factor VIIa/tissue factor complex is the most important activator of factor IX and the factor IXa/factor VIIIa complex is the most important activator of factor X (see Fig. 3.7B). The mild bleeding tendency seen in patients with factor XI deficiency is likely explained by the ability of thrombin to activate factor XI, a feedback mechanism that amplifies the coagulation cascade.

Among the coagulation factors, thrombin is the most important because it controls diverse aspects of hemostasis and links clotting to inflammation and repair. Among thrombin's key activities are the following:

- *Conversion of fibrinogen into crosslinked fibrin.* Thrombin converts soluble fibrinogen into fibrin monomers that polymerize into an insoluble fibril and amplifies the generation of fibrin by activating factors V, VIII, and XI. Thrombin also stabilizes fibrin clots by activating factor XIII, which covalently crosslinks fibrin.

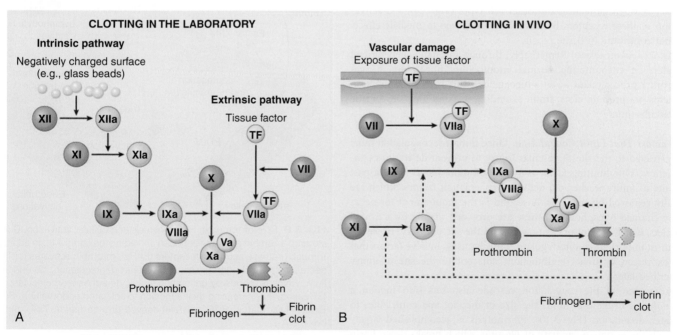

FIG. 3.7 The coagulation cascade in the laboratory and in vivo. (A) Clotting is initiated in the laboratory by adding phospholipids, calcium, and either a negatively charged substance such as glass beads (intrinsic pathway) or a source of tissue factor (extrinsic pathway). (B) In vivo, tissue factor is the major initiator of coagulation, which is amplified by feedback loops involving thrombin *(dotted lines)*. The *red* polypeptides are inactive factors, the *dark green* polypeptides are active factors, and the *light green* polypeptides are cofactors. In addition to exposure through vascular damage, tissue factor may also be expressed on injured or inflamed intact endothelial cells.

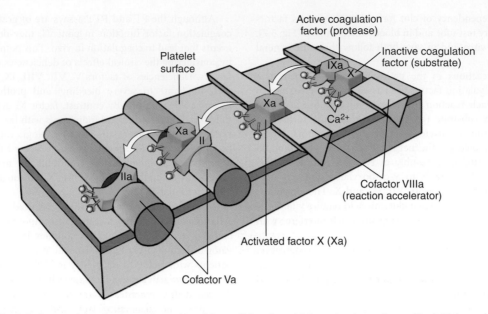

FIG. 3.8 Sequential activation of factor X and factor II (prothrombin) on platelet surfaces. The initial reaction complex consists of a protease (factor IXa), a substrate (factor X), and a reaction accelerator (factor VIIIa) assembled on a negatively charged platelet phospholipid surface. Calcium ions hold the assembled components together and are essential for the reaction. Activated factor Xa then becomes the protease component of the next complex in the cascade, converting prothrombin to thrombin (factor IIa) in the presence of a different cofactor, factor Va.

- *Platelet activation.* Thrombin is a potent inducer of platelet activation, aggregation, and contraction through its ability to activate PARs.
- *Effects on various cell types.* PARs also are expressed on inflammatory cells, endothelium, and other cell types (Fig. 3.9), and activation of these receptors by thrombin is believed to mediate effects that contribute to tissue repair.
- *Anticoagulant effects.* Remarkably, through mechanisms described later, on encountering normal endothelium, thrombin changes from a procoagulant to an anticoagulant; this reversal in function helps to prevent clots from extending beyond the site of the vascular injury.

Factors That Limit Coagulation. Once initiated, coagulation must be restricted to the site of vascular injury to prevent deleterious consequences. One limiting factor is simple dilution: blood flowing past the site of injury washes out activated coagulation factors, which are rapidly removed by the liver. A second is the requirement for negatively charged phospholipids; these are provided mainly by activated platelets, which are not present away from the site of injury. However, the most important counterregulatory mechanisms involve factors that are expressed by intact endothelium adjacent to the site of injury (described later).

Activation of the coagulation cascade also sets into motion a *fibrinolytic cascade* that limits the size of the clot and contributes to its later dissolution (Fig. 3.10). Fibrinolysis is accomplished largely through the enzymatic activity of *plasmin*, which breaks down fibrin and interferes with its polymerization. Elevated levels of breakdown products of fibrinogen (often called fibrin split products), most notably fibrin-derived *D-dimers*, are useful clinical markers of several thrombotic states (described later). Plasmin is generated from *plasminogen*, an inactive circulating precursor, by enzymatic cleavage. The most important plasminogen activator is tissue plasminogen activator

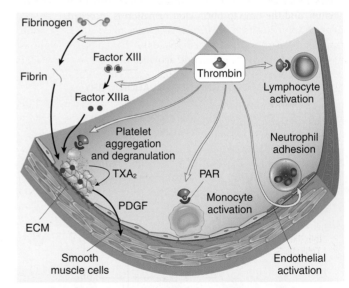

FIG. 3.9 Role of thrombin in hemostasis and cellular activation. During clotting, thrombin cleaves fibrinogen and activates factor XIII. In addition, through protease-activated receptors (PARs), thrombin activates (1) TxA$_2$ secretion, platelet aggregation, and platelet degranulation; (2) endothelium, which responds by generating leukocyte adhesion molecules; and (3) leukocytes, increasing their adhesion to activated endothelium. *ECM,* Extracellular matrix; *PDGF,* platelet-derived growth factor; *TxA$_2$,* thromboxane A$_2$.

(t-PA); it is synthesized principally by endothelium and is most active when bound to fibrin. This characteristic makes t-PA a useful therapeutic agent, since its fibrinolytic activity is largely confined to the site of a clot. Once activated, plasmin is in turn tightly controlled by

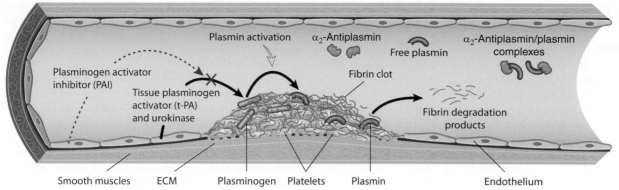

FIG. 3.10 The fibrinolytic system. Circulating plasminogen associates with fibrin clots and undergoes a change in confirmation that makes it susceptible to activation by tissue plasminogen activator and urokinase. Active plasmin degrades fibrin and is in turn subject to inactivation by circulating α_2-antiplasmin. Endothelium is also the source of plasminogen activator inhibitors, negative regulators of plasmin activity.

factors such as α_2-plasmin inhibitor, a plasma protein that binds and rapidly inhibits free plasmin.

Endothelium

The balance between the anticoagulant and procoagulant activities of endothelium often determines whether clot formation, propagation, or dissolution occurs (Fig. 3.11). Normal endothelial cells express a multitude of factors that inhibit the procoagulant activities of platelets and coagulation factors and that augment fibrinolysis. These factors act in concert to prevent thrombosis and to limit clotting to sites of vascular damage. However, if injured or exposed to proinflammatory factors, endothelial cells lose many of their antithrombotic properties. Here, we complete the discussion of hemostasis by focusing on the antithrombotic activities of normal endothelium; we return to the "dark side" of endothelial cells later when discussing thrombosis.

The antithrombotic properties of endothelium can be divided into activities directed at platelets, coagulation factors, and fibrinolysis.

- *Platelet inhibitory effects.* An obvious effect of intact endothelium is to serve as a barrier that shields platelets from subendothelial vWF and collagen. However, normal endothelium also releases a number of factors that inhibit platelet activation and aggregation. Among the most important are *prostacyclin (PGI$_2$), nitric oxide (NO),*

and *adenosine diphosphatase*; the latter degrades ADP, already discussed as a potent activator of platelet aggregation. Prostacyclin and NO are also vasodilators and thus they promote washout of coagulation factors. Finally, endothelial cells bind thrombin and inhibit thrombin's ability to activate platelets.

- *Anticoagulant effects.* Normal endothelium shields coagulation factors from tissue factor in vessel walls and expresses multiple factors that actively oppose coagulation, most notably thrombomodulin, endothelial protein C receptor, heparin-like molecules, and tissue factor pathway inhibitor. *Thrombomodulin* and *endothelial protein C receptor* bind thrombin and protein C, respectively, in complexes on the endothelial cell surface. When bound to thrombomodulin, thrombin loses its ability to activate coagulation factors and platelets and instead cleaves and activates *protein C,* a vitamin K–dependent protease that requires a cofactor, protein S. Activated protein C/protein S complex is a potent inhibitor of coagulation factors Va and VIIIa. *Heparin-like molecules* on the surface of endothelium bind and activate antithrombin III, which then inhibits thrombin and factors IXa, Xa, XIa, and XIIa. The clinical utility of heparin and related drugs is based on their ability to stimulate antithrombin activity. *Tissue factor pathway inhibitor* (TFPI), like protein C, requires protein S as a cofactor and, as the name implies, binds and inhibits tissue factor/factor VIIa complexes.

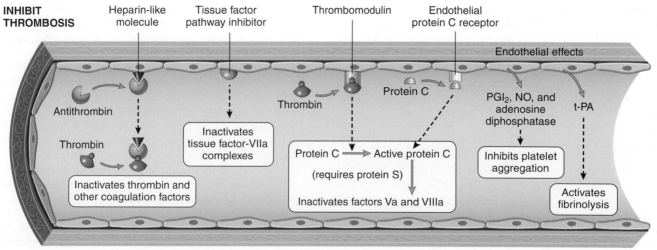

FIG. 3.11 Antithrombotic effects of normal endothelium. See text for details.

- *Fibrinolytic effects.* Normal endothelial cells synthesize t-PA, already discussed as a key component of the fibrinolytic pathway.

Thrombosis

The primary abnormalities that lead to intravascular thrombosis are the so-called "Virchow triad": (1) endothelial injury; (2) stasis or turbulent blood flow; and (3) hypercoagulability of the blood (Fig. 3.12). Thrombosis is one of the scourges of modern man, as it underlies the most serious and common forms of cardiovascular disease. Here, the focus is on its causes and consequences; its role in cardiovascular disorders is discussed in detail in Chapters 8 and 9.

Endothelial Injury

Endothelial injury leading to platelet activation almost inevitably underlies thrombus formation in the heart and the arterial circulation, where the high rates of blood flow otherwise impede clot formation. Notably, cardiac and arterial clots are typically rich in platelets, and it is believed that platelet adherence and activation are necessary prerequisites for thrombus formation under high shear stress, such as exists in arteries. This insight provides part of the reasoning behind the use of aspirin and other platelet inhibitors in coronary artery disease and acute myocardial infarction.

Obviously, severe endothelial injury may trigger thrombosis by exposing vWF and tissue factor. However, inflammation and other noxious stimuli also promote thrombosis by shifting the pattern of gene expression in endothelium to one that is "prothrombotic." This change is sometimes referred to as *endothelial activation* or *dysfunction* and can be produced by diverse exposures, including physical injury, infectious agents, abnormal blood flow, cytokines and other inflammatory mediators, metabolic abnormalities (such as hypercholesterolemia or homocystinemia), and toxins absorbed from cigarette smoke. Endothelial activation is believed to have an important role in triggering arterial thrombotic events.

The role of endothelial activation and dysfunction in arterial thrombosis is further discussed in Chapters 8 and 9. Here it suffices to briefly summarize several of the major prothrombotic alterations:

- *Procoagulant changes.* Activated endothelial cells downregulate the expression of coagulation inhibitors, including thrombomodulin, endothelial protein C receptor, and tissue factor protein inhibitor, and increase expression of tissue factor.

- *Antifibrinolytic effects.* Activated endothelial cells increase their secretion of plasminogen activator inhibitors (PAI), which limit fibrinolysis by antagonizing the activity of t-PA and urokinase.

Abnormal Blood Flow

Turbulence (chaotic blood flow) contributes to arterial and cardiac thrombosis by causing endothelial injury or dysfunction, as well as by forming countercurrents and local pockets of stasis. Stasis is a major factor in the development of venous thrombi. Under conditions of normal laminar blood flow, platelets (and other blood cells) are found mainly in the center of the vessel lumen, separated from the endothelium by a slower-moving layer of plasma. By contrast, stasis and turbulence have the following deleterious effects:

- Both promote endothelial cell activation and enhanced procoagulant activity, in part through flow-induced changes in endothelial gene expression.
- Stasis allows platelets and leukocytes to come into contact with the endothelium.
- Stasis also slows the washout of activated clotting factors and impedes the inflow of clotting factor inhibitors.

Turbulent or static blood flow contributes to thrombosis in a number of clinical settings. Ulcerated atherosclerotic plaques not only expose subendothelial ECM but also cause turbulence. Abnormal aortic and arterial dilations called aneurysms create local stasis and consequently are fertile sites for thrombosis (Chapter 8). Acute myocardial infarction results in focally noncontractile myocardium. Ventricular remodeling after more remote infarction can lead to aneurysm formation. In both cases, cardiac mural thrombi are more easily formed because of the local stasis (Chapter 9). Mitral valve stenosis (e.g., after rheumatic heart disease) results in left atrial dilation. In conjunction with atrial fibrillation (which causes turbulent flow), a dilated atrium also produces stasis and is a prime location for the development of thrombi. Hyperviscosity syndromes (such as polycythemia vera, Chapter 10) predispose to thrombosis in part by increasing resistance to flow and causing small vessel stasis.

Hypercoagulability

Hypercoagulability refers to an abnormally high tendency of the blood to clot and is usually caused by alterations in coagulation factors. It is an important risk factor for venous thrombosis and occasionally contributes to arterial or intracardiac thrombosis. Alterations that lead to hypercoagulability can be divided into primary (genetic) and secondary (acquired) disorders (Table 3.2).

Primary (inherited) hypercoagulability is most often caused by mutations in the factor V and prothrombin genes:

- A factor V mutation, called the Leiden mutation after the Dutch city where it was first described, causes an amino acid substitution in factor V that renders it resistant to proteolysis by protein C. Thus, an important antithrombotic counterregulatory mechanism is lost. Factor V Leiden heterozygotes have a 3- to 4-fold increased risk for venous thrombosis, while homozygotes have a 25- to 50-fold increased risk. Among those with recurrent deep venous thrombosis (DVT), the frequency of *factor V Leiden* approaches 60%. This mutation is seen in approximately 2% to 15% of individuals of European ancestry and is present to varying degrees in other American groups, largely due to population admixture.
- A single-nucleotide substitution in the 3′-untranslated region of the prothrombin gene is found in 1% to 2% of the general population. This variant results in increased prothrombin gene expression and

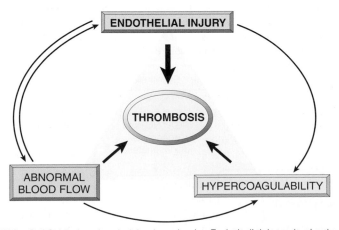

FIG. 3.12 Virchow's triad in thrombosis. Endothelial integrity is the most important factor. Abnormalities of procoagulants or anticoagulants can tip the balance in favor of thrombosis. Abnormal blood flow (stasis or turbulence) can lead to hypercoagulability directly and also indirectly through endothelial dysfunction.

Table 3.2 Hypercoagulable States

Primary (Genetic)
Common (>1% of the Population of the United States)
Factor V mutation (Arg506Glu variant; factor V Leiden)
Prothrombin mutation (G20210A variant)
Increased levels of factor VIII, IX, or XI or fibrinogen
Rare
Antithrombin deficiency
Protein C deficiency
Protein S deficiency
Very Rare
Fibrinolysis defects
Homozygous homocystinuria
Secondary (Acquired)
High Risk for Thrombosis
Prolonged bed rest or immobilization
Myocardial infarction
Atrial fibrillation
Tissue injury (e.g., surgery, fracture, burn)
Cancer
Prosthetic cardiac valves
Disseminated intravascular coagulation
Heparin-induced thrombocytopenia
Antiphospholipid antibody syndrome
Elevated Risk for Thrombosis
Cardiomyopathy
Nephrotic syndrome
Hyperestrogenic states (e.g., pregnancy and postpartum)
Oral contraceptive use
Sickle cell anemia
Smoking

is associated with a nearly 3-fold increased risk for venous thrombosis.

- Less common primary hypercoagulable states include inherited deficiencies of anticoagulants such as antithrombin, protein C, or protein S; affected patients typically present with venous thrombosis and recurrent thromboembolism in adolescence or in early adult life.
- Markedly elevated levels of homocysteine, such as in patients with an inherited deficiency of cystathione β-synthetase, are associated with arterial and venous thrombosis. Studies suggest that more modest elevations of homocysteine, which are seen in 5% to 7% of the population, may also be associated with an increased risk of venous thromboembolism.

Although the risk of thrombosis is only mildly increased in heterozygous carriers of factor V Leiden and the prothrombin gene variant, these aberrations carry added significance for two reasons. First, individuals who are homozygous or compound heterozygous for these variants are not uncommon and are at high risk for thrombosis. Second, the risk in heterozygous individuals is increased significantly when other acquired risk factors, such as pregnancy, prolonged bed rest, and lengthy airplane flights, are also present. Consequently, inherited causes of hypercoagulability should be considered in young patients (<50 years of age), even when acquired risk factors are present. Patients who are heterozygous for factor V Leiden and develop a DVT in the absence of a controllable risk factor are typically anticoagulated for life to prevent recurrent DVT and pulmonary embolism, while

patients who are homozygous and develop a DVT are usually anticoagulated for life even if a controllable risk factor is present.

Although genetic analysis of patients with DVT has proven quite informative, it is worth emphasizing that most patients with DVT lack known genetic risk factors and that most individuals with the most common genetic risk factor (Factor V Leiden) never develop DVT. Thus genetic testing is typically restricted to individuals with a strong family history of DVT or who develop DVT at a young age (<50 years) in the absence of of an acquired risk factor.

Secondary (acquired) hypercoagulability is seen in many settings (see Table 3.2). In some situations (e.g., trauma or cardiac failure), stasis or vascular injury is the most important factor. The hypercoagulability associated with oral contraceptive use and pregnancy may be related to increased hepatic synthesis of coagulation factors and reduced synthesis of antithrombin. In disseminated cancers, release of procoagulant tumor products (e.g., mucin from adenocarcinoma) predisposes to thrombosis. The hypercoagulability seen with advancing age has been attributed to increased platelet aggregation and reduced release of PGI_2 from endothelium. Smoking and obesity promote hypercoagulability by unknown mechanisms.

Among the acquired hypercoagulable states, two are particularly important clinically and deserve special mention:

- *Heparin-induced thrombocytopenia (HIT) syndrome.* This syndrome occurs in up to 5% of patients treated with unfractionated heparin (for therapeutic anticoagulation). It is marked by the development of autoantibodies that bind complexes of heparin and platelet factor-4 (PF4) (Chapter 10). It appears that antibody-PF4-heparin complexes bind to Fc receptors on platelets, leading to their activation, aggregation, and removal from circulation. The net result is a prothrombotic state, even in the face of heparin administration and low platelet counts. Newer low-molecular-weight fractionated heparin preparations induce autoantibodies less frequently but can still cause thrombosis, particularly if antibodies have already formed due to prior exposure to heparin.
- *Antiphospholipid antibody syndrome.* This syndrome (previously called the lupus anticoagulant syndrome) has protean clinical manifestations, including recurrent thromboses, repeated miscarriages, cardiac valve vegetations, and thrombocytopenia. Depending on the vascular bed involved, the clinical presentations can include pulmonary embolism (from deep venous thromboses), pulmonary hypertension (from recurrent pulmonary emboli), stroke, bowel infarction, or renovascular hypertension. Fetal loss does not appear to be explained by thrombosis but rather seems to stem from antibody-mediated interference with the growth and differentiation of trophoblasts, leading to a failure of placentation. Antiphospholipid antibody syndrome is also a cause of renal microangiopathy, resulting in renal failure associated with multiple capillary and arterial thromboses (Chapter 12).

The name antiphospholipid antibody syndrome stems from the presence of antibodies in affected patients that bind phospholipids. This name is misleading, however, as it is believed that the pathologic effects of the antibodies are mediated through binding to epitopes on proteins that are somehow induced or "unveiled" by interaction with phospholipids. Likely antibody targets include β2-glycoprotein I, a plasma protein that associates with the surfaces of endothelial cells and trophoblasts. In vivo, it is suspected that the causative antibodies bind β2-glycoprotein I and perhaps other proteins, thereby inducing a hypercoagulable state through uncertain mechanisms. However, in the clinical laboratory the antibodies neutralize phospholipids and interfere with clotting assays (i.e., they are "anticoagulants"). The antibodies also frequently produce a false-positive serologic test for syphilis because the antigen in the standard assay for syphilis is embedded in the phospholipid cardiolipin.

Antiphospholipid antibody syndrome has primary and secondary forms. Individuals with a well-defined autoimmune disease, such as systemic lupus erythematosus (Chapter 5), are designated as having secondary antiphospholipid syndrome. Historically, because of the association with lupus, these antibodies were referred to as the "lupus anticoagulant." In primary antiphospholipid syndrome, patients exhibit only the manifestations of a hypercoagulable state and lack evidence of other autoimmune disorders. Therapy involves anticoagulation and immunosuppression. Although antiphospholipid antibodies are clearly associated with thrombosis, they have also been identified in 5% to 15% of healthy individuals, implying that they are necessary but not sufficient to cause the full-blown syndrome.

MORPHOLOGY

Thrombi can develop anywhere in the cardiovascular system. Arterial or cardiac thrombi typically arise at sites of endothelial injury or turbulence; venous thrombi characteristically occur at sites of stasis. Thrombi are focally attached to the underlying vascular surface and tend to propagate toward the heart; thus, arterial thrombi grow in a retrograde direction from the point of attachment, whereas venous thrombi extend in the direction of blood flow. The propagating portion of a thrombus tends to be poorly attached and therefore prone to fragmentation and migration through the blood as an **embolus.**

Thrombi can have grossly (and microscopically) apparent laminations called **lines of Zahn**; these represent pale platelet and fibrin layers alternating with darker red cell–rich layers. Such lines are significant in that they are only found in thrombi that form in flowing blood; their presence can therefore distinguish antemortem thrombosis from the bland nonlaminated clots that form in the postmortem state. Although thrombi formed in the "low-flow" venous system superficially resemble postmortem clots, careful evaluation generally shows ill-defined laminations.

Thrombi occurring in heart chambers or in the aortic lumen are called **mural thrombi.** Abnormal myocardial contraction (e.g., arrhythmias, dilated cardiomyopathy, or myocardial infarction) or endomyocardial injury (e.g., myocarditis, catheter trauma) promote cardiac mural thrombi (Fig. 3.13A), whereas ulcerated atherosclerotic plaques and aneurysmal dilation promote aortic thrombosis (Fig. 3.13B).

Arterial thrombi are frequently occlusive. They are typically rich in platelets, as the processes underlying their development (e.g., endothelial injury) lead to platelet activation. They are most commonly found attached to a ruptured atherosclerotic plaque, but other vascular injuries (e.g., vasculitis, trauma) can also trigger thrombosis. **Venous thrombi (phlebothrombosis)** are almost invariably occlusive. They frequently propagate toward the heart, forming a long cast within the vessel lumen that is prone to give rise to emboli. Because these thrombi form in the sluggish venous circulation, they tend to contain more enmeshed red cells, leading to the moniker **red, or stasis, thrombi.** The veins of the lower extremities are most commonly affected (90% of venous thromboses); however, venous thrombi may also occur in the upper extremities, periprostatic plexus, or ovarian and periuterine veins, and under special circumstances, such as in patients with hypercoagulable states, they may be found in the dural sinuses, portal vein, or hepatic vein.

At autopsy, **postmortem clots** can sometimes be mistaken for venous thrombi. However, postmortem clots are gelatinous and because of red cell settling have a dark red dependent portion and a yellow "chicken fat" upper portion. They also are usually not attached to the underlying vessel wall. By contrast, red thrombi typically are firm and focally attached to vessel walls, and they contain gray strands of deposited fibrin.

Thrombi on heart valves are called **vegetations.** Bacterial or fungal bloodborne infections can cause valve damage, leading to the development of large thrombotic masses **(infective endocarditis)** (Chapter 9). Sterile vegetations can also develop on noninfected valves in hypercoagulable states—the lesions of so-called **"nonbacterial thrombotic endocarditis"** (Chapter 9). Less commonly, sterile, **verrucous endocarditis (Libman-Sacks endocarditis)** (eFig. 3.4) can occur in the setting of systemic lupus erythematosus (Chapter 5).

Fates of Thrombi

If a patient survives an initial thrombotic event, during the ensuing days to weeks the thrombus evolves through some combination of the following four processes:

- *Propagation.* The thrombus enlarges through the accretion of additional platelets and fibrin, increasing the odds of vascular occlusion and embolization.
- *Embolization.* Part or all of the thrombus is dislodged and transported elsewhere in the vasculature.
- *Dissolution.* If a thrombus is newly formed, activation of fibrinolytic factors may lead to its rapid shrinkage and complete dissolution. With older thrombi, extensive fibrin polymerization renders the thrombus substantially more resistant to plasmin-induced proteolysis, and lysis is ineffectual. This acquisition of resistance to

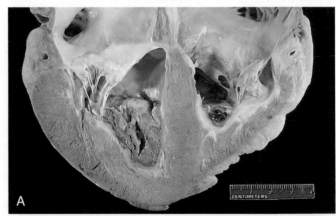
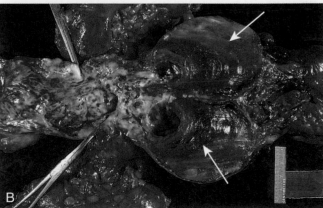

FIG. 3.13 Mural thrombi. (A) Thrombus in the left and right ventricular apices, overlying white fibrous scar. (B) Laminated thrombus *(arrows)* in a dilated abdominal aortic aneurysm. Numerous friable mural thrombi are also superimposed on advanced atherosclerotic lesions of the more proximal aorta *(left side of photograph).*

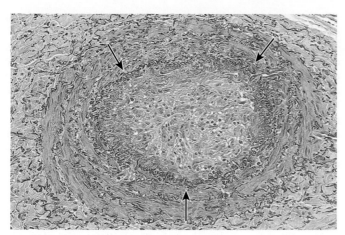

FIG. 3.14 An organized thrombus. Low-power view of a thrombosed artery stained for elastin. The original lumen is delineated by the internal elastic lamina *(arrows)* and is completely filled with organized thrombus.

lysis has clinical significance, as therapeutic administration of fibrinolytic agents (e.g., t-PA in the setting of acute coronary thrombosis) is generally not effective unless given within a few hours of thrombus formation.

- *Organization and recanalization.* Older thrombi become organized by the ingrowth of endothelial cells, smooth muscle cells, and fibroblasts (Fig. 3.14). In time, capillary channels are formed that—to a limited extent—create conduits along the length of the thrombus, thereby reestablishing the patency of the original lumen. Further recanalization can sometimes convert a thrombus into a vascularized mass of connective tissue that is eventually incorporated into the wall of the remodeled vessel. Occasionally, instead of organizing, the center of a thrombus undergoes enzymatic digestion, presumably because of the release of lysosomal enzymes from entrapped leukocytes.

Clinical Features. Thrombi are significant because they cause obstruction of arteries and veins and may give rise to emboli. The site of thrombosis dictates their clinical relevance. Thus, although venous thrombi can cause congestion and edema in vascular beds distal to an obstruction, they are most worrisome because of their potential to embolize to the lungs and cause death. Conversely, while arterial thrombi may also embolize, their tendency to obstruct vessels (e.g., in coronary and cerebral vessels) and cause infarction locally is considerably more important.

Most venous thrombi occur in the superficial or the deep veins of the leg. Superficial venous thrombi usually arise in the saphenous system, particularly in the setting of varicosities; these rarely embolize but they may cause pain, local congestion, and swelling from impaired venous outflow, predisposing the overlying skin to the development of infections and varicose ulcers. Deep venous thromboses (DVTs) in the larger leg veins at or above the knee joint (e.g., popliteal, femoral, and iliac veins) are more serious because they are prone to embolize. Although DVTs may cause local pain and edema, collateral channels often circumvent the venous obstruction. Consequently, DVTs are entirely asymptomatic in approximately 50% of patients and are recognized only after they have embolized to the lungs.

Lower-extremity DVTs are associated with stasis and hypercoagulable states, as described earlier (see Table 3.2). Common predisposing factors include congestive heart failure, bed rest, and immobilization; the latter two factors reduce the milking action of leg muscles and thus slow venous return. Trauma, surgery, and burns not only immobilize a patient but are also associated with vascular injury, procoagulant release, increased hepatic synthesis of coagulation factors, and reduced t-PA production. Many factors contribute to thrombosis during pregnancy; in addition to the potential for amniotic fluid infusion into the circulation at the time of delivery, pressure produced by the enlarging fetus and uterus produce stasis in the veins of the legs, and late pregnancy and the postpartum period are associated with hormone-induced changes in plasma proteins that produce hypercoagulability. Tumor-associated procoagulant release is largely responsible for the increased risk of thromboembolic phenomena in disseminated cancers. These are sometimes referred to as *migratory thrombophlebitis,* because of the tendency to involve several different venous beds transiently, or as *Trousseau syndrome,* named after the physician who both described the disorder and suffered from it. Regardless of the specific clinical setting, the risk of DVT is increased in persons older than 50 years and is greater in males than females.

Atherosclerosis is a major cause of arterial thromboses because it is associated with the loss of endothelial integrity and with abnormal blood flow (see Fig. 3.13B). Myocardial infarction may predispose to mural thrombi by causing dyskinetic myocardial contraction and endocardial injury (see Fig. 3.13A), and rheumatic heart disease may also do so by causing atrial dilation and fibrillation. Both cardiac and aortic mural thrombi are prone to embolization. Although any organ may be affected, the brain, kidneys, and spleen are particularly likely targets because of their rich blood supply.

Disseminated Intravascular Coagulation (DIC)

DIC is widespread thrombosis within the microcirculation that may be of sudden or insidious onset. It may be seen in disorders ranging from obstetric complications to advanced malignancy. To complicate matters, the widespread microvascular thrombosis consumes platelets and coagulation proteins (hence the synonym *consumptive coagulopathy*), and, at the same time, fibrinolytic mechanisms are activated. The net result is that excessive clotting and bleeding may coexist in the same patient. DIC is discussed in greater detail along with other bleeding disorders in Chapter 10.

EMBOLISM

An embolus is a detached intravascular solid, liquid, or gaseous mass that is carried by the blood from its point of origin to a distant site, where it often causes tissue dysfunction or infarction. The vast majority of emboli derive from dislodged thrombi—hence the term thromboembolism. Less commonly, emboli are composed of fat droplets, bubbles of air or nitrogen, atherosclerotic debris (cholesterol emboli), tumor fragments, bits of bone marrow, or amniotic fluid. Inevitably, emboli lodge in vessels too small to permit further passage, resulting in partial or complete vascular occlusion; depending on their origin, emboli may arrest anywhere in the vascular tree. The primary consequence of systemic embolization is ischemic necrosis (infarction) of downstream tissues, whereas embolization in the pulmonary circulation more commonly leads to hypoxia, hypotension, and right-sided heart failure.

Pulmonary Thromboembolism

Pulmonary emboli originate from deep venous thrombi and are responsible for the most common form of thromboembolic disease. Pulmonary embolism (PE) is estimated to cause about 100,000 deaths per year in the United States. The risk factors for PE are the same as those for deep venous thrombosis (see earlier) since more than 95% of cases of venous emboli originate from thrombi within deep leg veins proximal to the popliteal fossa.

Fragmented thrombi from DVTs are carried through progressively larger channels and usually pass through the right side of the heart before arresting in the pulmonary vasculature. Depending on size, a PE can occlude the main pulmonary artery, lodge at the bifurcation of the right and left pulmonary arteries *(saddle embolus)*, or pass into the smaller, branching arterioles (Fig. 3.15). Frequently, multiple emboli occur, either sequentially or as a shower of smaller emboli from a single large thrombus; a patient who has had one PE is at increased risk for having more. Occasionally, a venous embolus passes through an atrial or ventricular defect and enters the systemic circulation *(paradoxical embolism)*. A more complete discussion of PE is found in Chapter 11; the major clinical and pathologic features are the following:

- Most pulmonary emboli (60%–80%) are small and clinically silent. With time, they undergo organization and become incorporated into the vascular wall; in some cases, organization of thromboemboli leaves behind bridging fibrous webs.
- At the other end of the spectrum, a large embolus that blocks a major pulmonary artery can cause sudden death.
- Embolic obstruction of medium-sized arteries does not usually cause pulmonary infarction because the area also receives blood through an intact bronchial arterial circulation (dual circulation). However, a similar embolus in the setting of left-sided cardiac failure (and diminished bronchial artery perfusion) may cause an infarct.
- Embolism to small end-arteriolar pulmonary branches usually causes infarction, which may sometimes be associated with rupture of anoxic capillaries and hemorrhage.
- Multiple recurrent emboli may, over time, cause pulmonary hypertension and right ventricular failure *(cor pulmonale)*.

Systemic Thromboembolism

Most systemic emboli (80%) arise from intracardiac mural thrombi; two-thirds of these are associated with left ventricular infarcts and another 25% with dilated left atria (e.g., secondary to mitral valve disease). The remainder originate from aortic aneurysms, thrombi overlying ulcerated atherosclerotic plaques, fragmented valvular

vegetations, or the venous system (paradoxical emboli); 10% to 15% of systemic emboli are of unknown origin.

In contrast to venous emboli, which lodge primarily in the lung, arterial emboli can travel virtually anywhere; their final resting place depends on their point of origin and the relative flow rates of blood to downstream organs. Common arterial embolization sites include the lower extremities (75%) and central nervous system (10%); the intestines, kidneys, and spleen are less commonly involved. The consequences depend on the caliber of the occluded vessel, the presence or absence of a collateral blood supply, and the affected tissue's vulnerability to anoxia, but infarction is common because arterial emboli often lodge in end arteries.

Fat Embolism

Soft tissue crush injury or rupture of marrow vascular sinusoids (e.g., resulting from a long bone fracture) release microscopic fat globules and associated marrow elements into the circulation. Fat emboli (Fig. 3.16A) are common incidental findings after vigorous cardiopulmonary resuscitation but probably are of little clinical significance. By contrast, a small fraction of individuals with severe

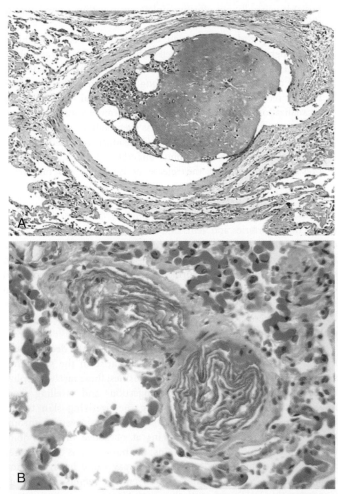

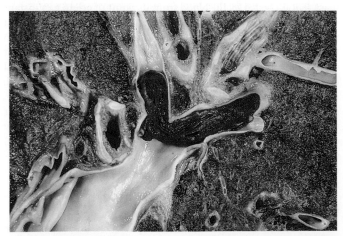

FIG. 3.15 Embolus derived from a lower-extremity deep venous thrombus lodged in a pulmonary artery branch.

FIG. 3.16 Unusual types of emboli. (A) Fat embolus. The embolus is composed of hematopoietic elements and fat cells *(clear spaces)* attached to a thrombus. (B) Amniotic fluid emboli. Two small pulmonary arterioles are packed with laminated swirls of fetal squamous cells. The surrounding lung is edematous and congested. (Courtesy of Dr. Beth Schwartz, Baltimore, MD.)

skeletal injuries develop a fat embolism syndrome characterized by pulmonary insufficiency, neurologic symptoms, anemia, thrombocytopenia, and a diffuse petechial rash. Signs and symptoms appear 1 to 3 days after injury as sudden onset tachypnea, dyspnea, tachycardia, irritability, and restlessness that may progress rapidly to delirium or coma; death occurs in 10% of cases. Thrombocytopenia is attributed to platelet adhesion to fat globules and subsequent aggregation or splenic sequestration; anemia may result from red cell aggregation and/or hemolysis. The petechial rash (seen in 20%—50% of cases) is due to thrombocytopenia and can be a useful diagnostic feature.

The pathogenesis of fat emboli syndrome involves both mechanical obstruction and biochemical alterations. Fat microemboli occlude the pulmonary and cerebral microvasculature, both directly and by triggering platelet aggregation. This deleterious effect is exacerbated by fatty acids release from lipid globules, which causes local endothelial injury. Platelet activation and granulocyte recruitment (with free radical, protease, and eicosanoid release) complete the vascular assault. Because lipids are dissolved by the solvents used during tissue processing, microscopic demonstration of fat microglobules (i.e., in the absence of accompanying marrow elements) requires specialized techniques (e.g., fat stains performed on frozen sections).

Amniotic Fluid Embolism

Amniotic fluid embolism is an uncommon, grave complication of labor and the immediate postpartum period that is caused by the entry of amniotic fluid (and its contents) into the maternal circulation via tears in the placental membranes and/or uterine vein. It occurs in only 1 in 40,000 deliveries but has a mortality rate approaching 80%. It is responsible for 5% to 10% of maternal deaths in the United States; 85% of survivors suffer some form of permanent neurologic deficit. Onset is characterized by sudden severe dyspnea, cyanosis, and shock, followed by seizures and coma. If the patient survives the initial crisis, pulmonary edema usually ensues, and about half of patients develop disseminated intravascular coagulation secondary to release of thrombogenic substances from amniotic fluid.

It is thought that morbidity and mortality result from activation of the coagulation system and the innate immune system by substances in the amniotic fluid rather than mechanical obstruction of pulmonary vessels by the emboli. Histologic examination in fatal cases shows squamous cells shed from fetal skin, lanugo hair, fat from vernix caseosa, and mucin derived from the fetal respiratory or gastrointestinal tracts in the maternal pulmonary microcirculation (Fig. 3.16B). Other findings include marked pulmonary edema, diffuse alveolar damage (Chapter 11), and widespread fibrin thrombi generated by disseminated intravascular coagulation.

Air Embolism

Gas bubbles that enter the circulation can coalesce and obstruct vascular flow and cause distal ischemic injury. Thus, a small volume of air trapped in a coronary artery during bypass surgery or introduced into the cerebral arterial circulation by neurosurgery performed in an upright "sitting position" can occlude flow, with dire consequences. Small venous gas emboli generally have no deleterious effects, but sufficient air can enter the pulmonary circulation inadvertently during obstetric or laparoscopic procedures or as a consequence of a chest wall injury to cause hypoxia, and very large venous gas emboli may arrest in the heart, leading to death.

A particular form of gas embolism called decompression sickness is caused by sudden changes in atmospheric pressure. Scuba divers, underwater construction workers, and persons in unpressurized aircraft who undergo rapid ascent are at risk. When air is breathed at high pressure (e.g., during a deep-sea dive), increased amounts of gas (particularly nitrogen) become dissolved in the blood and tissues. If the individual then moves to a lower pressure environment too rapidly, the nitrogen expands in the tissues and bubbles out of solution in the blood to form gas emboli, which cause tissue ischemia. Rapid formation of gas bubbles within skeletal muscles and supporting tissues in and about joints is responsible for the painful condition called the bends. Gas bubbles in the pulmonary vasculature cause edema, hemorrhages, and focal atelectasis or emphysema, leading to respiratory distress. Bubbles in the central nervous system can cause memory loss, ataxia, visual disturbances, and even the sudden onset of coma. A more chronic form of decompression sickness is called caisson disease (named for pressurized underwater vessels used during bridge construction), in which recurrent or persistent gas emboli in the bones lead to multifocal ischemic necrosis; the heads of the femurs, tibiae, and humeri are most commonly affected.

Placing affected persons in a high-pressure chamber, to force the gas back into solution, treats acute decompression sickness. Subsequent slow decompression permits gradual gas resorption and exhalation so that obstructive bubbles do not re-form.

INFARCTION

An infarct is an area of ischemic necrosis caused by occlusion of the vascular supply of the affected tissue. Infarcts in the heart and the brain are common, important causes of illness. Roughly 40% of deaths in the United States are a consequence of cardiovascular disease, with most stemming from myocardial or cerebral infarction. Pulmonary infarction, bowel infarction, and ischemic necrosis of distal extremities (*gangrene*, mainly seen in patients with diabetes) are also responsible for considerable morbidity and mortality.

Arterial thrombosis or arterial embolism underlies the vast majority of infarctions. Less common causes of arterial obstruction include vasospasm; expansion of an atheroma secondary to intraplaque hemorrhage; and extrinsic compression of a vessel, such as by tumor, a dissecting aortic aneurysm, or edema within a confined space (e.g., in anterior tibial compartment syndrome). Other uncommon causes of tissue infarction include vessel twisting (e.g., in testicular torsion or bowel volvulus), traumatic vascular rupture, and entrapment in a hernia sac. Although venous thrombosis can cause infarction, the more common outcome is simply congestion; typically, bypass channels open and provide sufficient outflow to restore the arterial inflow. Infarcts caused by venous thrombosis thus usually occur only in organs with a single efferent vein (e.g., testis or ovary).

MORPHOLOGY

Infarcts are classified based on their color (reflecting the amount of hemorrhage) and the presence or absence of microbial infection. Thus, infarcts may be either **red (hemorrhagic)** or **white (anemic)** and may be either **septic** or **bland.**

Red infarcts (Fig. 3.17A) occur (1) as a result of venous occlusions (such as in testicular torsion); (2) in tissues with dual circulations such as the lung and small intestine, where partial, albeit inadequate, perfusion by collateral arterial supplies is typical; (3) in previously congested tissues (as a consequence of sluggish venous outflow); and (4) when flow is reestablished after infarction has occurred (e.g., after angioplasty of an arterial obstruction).

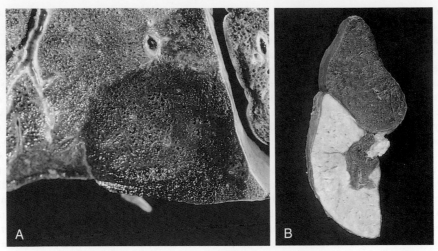

FIG. 3.17 Red and white infarcts. (A) Hemorrhagic, roughly wedge-shaped pulmonary infarct *(red infarct)*. (B) Sharply demarcated pale infarct in the spleen *(white infarct)*.

White infarcts occur with arterial occlusions in solid organs with end-arterial circulations (e.g., heart, spleen, and kidney) (Fig. 3.17B). Infarcts tend to be wedge shaped, with the occluded vessel at the apex and the organ periphery forming the base. When the base is a serosal surface, there is often an overlying fibrinous exudate. Lateral margins may be irregular, reflecting flow from adjacent vessels. The margins of acute infarcts typically are indistinct and slightly hemorrhagic; with time, the edges become better defined by a narrow rim of hyperemia attributable to inflammation.

Infarcts resulting from arterial occlusions in organs without a dual circulation typically become progressively paler and more sharply defined with time (see Fig. 3.17B). By comparison, hemorrhagic infarcts are the rule in the lung and other organs with dual blood supplies (see Fig. 3.17A). Extravasated red cells in hemorrhagic infarcts are phagocytosed by macrophages, and the heme iron is converted to intracellular hemosiderin. Small amounts do not impart any appreciable color to the tissue, but extensive hemorrhages leave a firm, brown residue.

In most tissues, the main histologic finding associated with infarcts is **ischemic coagulative necrosis** (Chapter 1). An inflammatory response begins to develop along the margins of infarcts within a few hours and usually is well defined within 1 to 2 days. Eventually, inflammation is followed by repair (Chapter 2), beginning in the preserved margins. In some tissues, parenchymal regeneration can occur at the periphery of the infarct, where the underlying stromal architecture has been spared. Most infarcts, however, are ultimately replaced by scar (Fig. 3.18). The brain is an exception to these generalizations; ischemic tissue injury in the central nervous system invariably undergoes **liquefactive necrosis** (Chapter 1).

Septic infarcts occur when infected cardiac valve vegetations embolize, or when microbes seed necrotic tissue. In these cases, the infarct is converted into an abscess, with a correspondingly greater inflammatory response and healing by organization and fibrosis (Chapter 2).

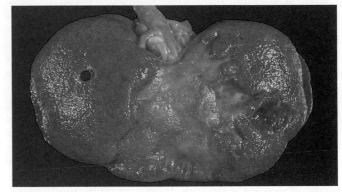

FIG. 3.18 Remote kidney infarct, now replaced by a large fibrotic scar.

Factors That Influence Infarct Development

The effects of vascular occlusion range from inconsequential to tissue necrosis leading to organ dysfunction and sometimes death. The range of outcomes is influenced by the following three variables:

- *Anatomy of the vascular supply.* The presence or absence of an alternative blood supply is the most important factor in determining whether occlusion of an individual vessel causes damage. The dual supply of the lung by the pulmonary and bronchial arteries means that obstruction of the pulmonary arterioles does not cause lung infarction unless the bronchial circulation is also compromised. Similarly, the liver, which receives blood from the hepatic artery and the portal vein, and the hand and forearm, with its parallel radial and ulnar arterial supply, are resistant to infarction. By contrast, the kidney and the spleen both have end-arterial circulations, and arterial obstruction generally leads to infarction in these tissues.

- *Rate of occlusion.* Slowly developing occlusions are less likely to cause infarction because they allow time for the development of collateral blood supplies. For example, small interarteriolar anastomoses, which normally carry minimal blood flow, interconnect the three major coronary arteries. If one coronary artery is slowly occluded (e.g., by an encroaching atherosclerotic plaque), flow in this collateral circulation may increase sufficiently to prevent infarction—even if the original artery becomes completely occluded.

- *Tissue vulnerability to hypoxia.* Different cell types vary in their vulnerability to hypoxic injury mainly because of differences in their basal metabolic needs. Neurons undergo irreversible damage when deprived of their blood supply for only 3 to 4 minutes. Myocardial cells, which are slightly hardier than neurons, die after only 20 to 30 minutes of ischemia. By contrast, fibroblasts remain viable after many hours of ischemia.

SHOCK

Shock is a state in which diminished cardiac output or reduced effective circulating blood volume impairs tissue perfusion and leads to cellular hypoxia. At the outset, the cellular injury is reversible; however, prolonged shock eventually leads to irreversible tissue injury and is often fatal. Shock may complicate severe hemorrhage, extensive trauma or burns, myocardial infarction, pulmonary embolism, and microbial sepsis. Its causes fall into three general categories (Table 3.3):

- *Cardiogenic shock* results from low cardiac output as a result of myocardial pump failure. It may be caused by myocardial damage (infarction), ventricular arrhythmia, extrinsic compression (cardiac tamponade) (Chapter 9), or outflow obstruction (e.g., pulmonary embolism).
- *Hypovolemic shock* results from low cardiac output due to loss of blood or plasma volume (e.g., resulting from hemorrhage or fluid loss from severe burns).
- *Septic shock* is triggered by microbial infections and is associated with severe systemic inflammatory response syndrome (SIRS). In addition to microbes, SIRS may be triggered by burns, trauma, and/or pancreatitis. The common pathogenic mechanism is a massive outpouring of inflammatory mediators from innate and adaptive immune cells that produce arterial vasodilation, vascular leakage, and venous blood pooling. These cardiovascular abnormalities result in tissue hypoperfusion, cellular hypoxia, and metabolic derangements that lead to organ dysfunction and, if severe and persistent, organ failure and death. The pathogenesis of septic shock is discussed in detail below.

Less commonly, shock may result from a loss of vascular tone associated with anesthesia or secondary to a spinal cord injury *(neurogenic shock)*. *Anaphylactic shock* results from systemic vasodilation and increased vascular permeability and is triggered by IgE—mediated hypersensitivity reactions (Chapter 5).

Pathogenesis of Septic Shock

Septic shock is responsible for 2% of all hospital admissions in the United States. Of these, 50% require treatment in intensive care units. The number of cases in the United States exceeds 750,000 per year and the incidence is rising, primarily due to improvements in life support for critically ill patients, as well as the growing ranks of immunocompromised hosts (because of chemotherapy, immunosuppression, advanced age, or human immunodeficiency virus infection) and the increasing prevalence of multidrug-resistant organisms in the hospital setting. Despite improvements in care, the mortality rate remains a staggering 20% to 30%.

Septic shock is most frequently triggered by gram-positive bacterial infections, followed by gram-negative bacteria and fungi. As mentioned in Chapter 2, macrophages, neutrophils, dendritic cells, endothelial cells, and soluble components of the innate immune system (e.g., complement) recognize and are activated by several substances derived from microorganisms. After activation, these cells and factors initiate a number of inflammatory responses that interact in a complex fashion to produce septic shock and multiorgan dysfunction (Fig. 3.19).

Factors believed to play major roles in the pathophysiology of septic shock include the following:

- *Inflammatory and counterinflammatory responses.* In sepsis, various microbial cell wall constituents engage receptors on cells of the innate immune system, triggering proinflammatory responses. These include:
  - Toll-like receptors (TLRs) (Chapter 5), which recognize a host of microbe-derived substances containing so-called "pathogen-associated molecular patterns" (PAMPs)
  - G-protein—coupled receptors, which detect bacterial peptides
  - C-type lectin receptors such as dectins, which recognize fungal cell wall components.

  On activation, innate immune cells produce cytokines such TNF, IL-1, type I interferon, IL-12, and IL-18, as well as other inflammatory mediators, leading to elevated levels of markers of acute inflammation such as C-reactive protein and procalcitonin. Reactive oxygen species and lipid mediators such as prostaglandins are also elaborated. These effector molecules induce endothelial cells (and other cell types) to upregulate adhesion molecule expression and further stimulate cytokine and chemokine production. The complement cascade is also activated by microbial components (Chapter 2), resulting in the production of anaphylatoxins (C3a, C5a), chemotactic fragments (C5a), and opsonins (C3b), all of which contribute to the pro-inflammatory state.

  In addition, microbial components can activate coagulation directly through factor XII and indirectly through altered endothelial function (discussed later). The accompanying widespread activation of thrombin may further augment inflammation by triggering protease-activated receptors on inflammatory cells.

Table 3.3 Major Types of Shock

Type of Shock	Clinical Examples	Principal Pathogenic Mechanisms
Cardiogenic	Myocardial infarction Ventricular rupture Arrhythmia Cardiac tamponade Pulmonary embolism	Failure of myocardial pump resulting from intrinsic myocardial damage, extrinsic pressure, or obstruction to outflow
Hypovolemic	Hemorrhage Water loss (e.g., vomiting, diarrhea, burns)	Inadequate blood or plasma volume

Septic	Overwhelming microbial infections
	    Bacterial sepsis
	    Fungal sepsis
	    Superantigens (e.g., toxic shock syndrome)
		Peripheral vasodilation and pooling of blood; endothelial activation/injury; leukocyte-induced damage; disseminated intravascular coagulation; activation of cytokine cascades

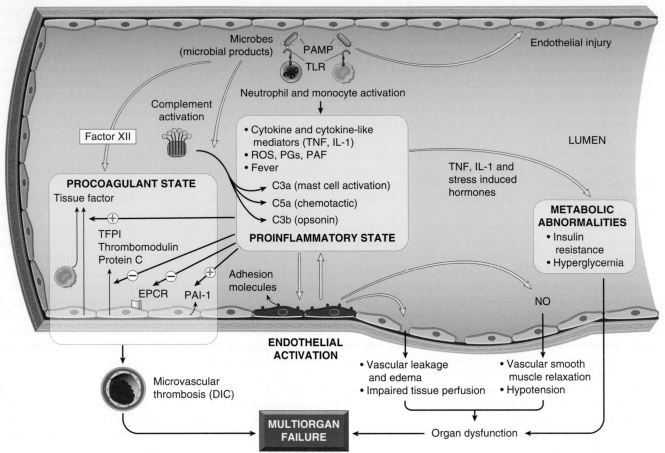

FIG. 3.19 Major pathogenic pathways in septic shock. Microbial products activate endothelial cells and cellular and humoral elements of the innate immune system, initiating a cascade of events that lead to induction of a procoagulant, proinflammatory state accompanied by metabolic changes that if unchecked lead to multiorgan failure. Additional details are provided in the text. *DIC,* Disseminated intravascular coagulation; *EPCR,* endothelial protein C receptor; *IL-1,* interleukin-1; *NO,* nitric oxide; *PAF,* platelet-activating factor; *PAI-1,* plasminogen activator inhibitor-1; *PAMP,* pathogen-associated molecular pattern; *PGs,* prostaglandins; *ROS,* reactive oxygen species; *TFPI,* tissue factor pathway inhibitor; *TLR,* Toll-like receptor; *TNF,* tumor necrosis factor.

With time, the initial hyperinflammatory state initiated by sepsis triggers counterregulatory immunosuppressive mechanisms, which may involve both innate and adaptive immune cells. As a result, septic patients may oscillate between hyperinflammatory and immunosuppressed states during their clinical course. Proposed mechanisms for the immune suppression include a shift from proinflammatory (Th1) to antiinflammatory (Th2) cytokines (Chapter 5), production of antiinflammatory mediators (e.g., soluble TNF receptor, IL-1 receptor antagonist, and IL-10), lymphocyte apoptosis, and the immunosuppressive effects of apoptotic cells.

- *Endothelial activation and injury.* The proinflammatory state and endothelial cell activation associated with sepsis upregulate adhesion molecule expression and lead to widespread vascular leakage and tissue edema, which have deleterious effects on both nutrient delivery and waste removal. One effect of inflammatory cytokines is to loosen endothelial cell tight junctions, making vessels leaky and resulting in the accumulation of protein-rich edema fluid throughout the body. This alteration impedes tissue perfusion and may be exacerbated by attempts to support the patient with intravenous fluids. Activated endothelium also upregulates production of nitric oxide (NO) and other vasoactive inflammatory mediators, which may contribute to vascular smooth muscle relaxation and systemic hypotension.

- *Induction of a procoagulant state.* The derangement in coagulation is sufficient to produce the formidable complication of *disseminated intravascular coagulation* in up to half of septic patients (Chapter 10). Sepsis alters the expression of many factors so as to favor coagulation. Proinflammatory cytokines increase tissue factor production by monocytes and possibly endothelial cells as well, and decrease the production of endothelial anticoagulant factors, such as tissue factor pathway inhibitor, thrombomodulin, and endothelial protein C receptor. They also dampen fibrinolysis by increasing plasminogen activator inhibitor-1 expression (see Fig. 3.10). The vascular leak and tissue edema decrease blood flow at the level of small vessels, producing stasis and diminishing the washout of activated coagulation factors. Acting in concert, these effects lead to systemic activation of thrombin and the deposition of fibrin-rich thrombi in small vessels, often throughout the body, further compromising tissue perfusion. In full-blown disseminated intravascular coagulation, the consumption of coagulation factors and platelets is so great that deficiencies of these factors appear, leading to concomitant bleeding and hemorrhage (Chapter 10).

- *Metabolic abnormalities.* Patients with severe sepsis exhibit insulin resistance and hyperglycemia. Cytokines such as TNF and IL-1, stress-induced hormones (such as glucagon, growth hormone, and glucocorticoids), and catecholamines all drive gluconeogenesis. At the same time, the proinflammatory cytokines suppress insulin release while simultaneously promoting insulin resistance in the liver and other tissues, likely by impairing the surface expression of GLUT-4, a glucose transporter. Although sepsis is initially associated with an acute surge in glucocorticoid production, this phase may be followed by adrenal insufficiency and a functional deficit of glucocorticoids. This may stem from depression of the synthetic capacity of intact adrenal glands or adrenal necrosis *(Waterhouse-Friderichsen syndrome)* resulting from disseminated intravascular dissemination (Chapter 18). Finally, cellular hypoxia and diminished oxidative phosphorylation lead to increased lactate production and lactic acidosis.
- *Organ dysfunction.* Systemic hypotension, interstitial edema, and small vessel thrombosis all decrease the delivery of oxygen and nutrients to the tissues that, because of cellular hypoxia, fail to properly use the nutrients that are delivered. Mitochondrial damage resulting from oxidative stress impairs oxygen use. High levels of cytokines and secondary mediators diminish myocardial contractility and cardiac output. The increased vascular permeability and endothelial injury can also lead to *acute respiratory distress syndrome* (Chapter 11). Ultimately, these factors may conspire to cause the failure of multiple organs, particularly the kidneys, liver, lungs, and heart, culminating in death.

The severity and outcome of septic shock are likely dependent on the extent and virulence of the infection; the immune status of the host; the presence of other comorbid conditions; and the pattern and level of mediator production. The multiplicity of factors and the complexity of the interactions that underlie sepsis explain why attempts to intervene therapeutically with antagonists of specific mediators have not been effective and may even have had deleterious effects in some cases. The standard of care remains antibiotics to treat the underlying infection and intravenous fluids, pressors, and supplemental oxygen to maintain blood pressure and limit tissue hypoxia. Even in the best of clinical centers, septic shock remains an obstinate clinical challenge.

An additional group of secreted bacterial proteins called *superantigens* also cause a syndrome similar to septic shock (e.g., *toxic shock syndrome*). Superantigens are polyclonal T-lymphocyte activators that induce the release of high levels of cytokines, resulting in a variety of clinical manifestations that range from a diffuse rash to vasodilation, hypotension, shock, and death.

Stages of Shock

Shock is a progressive disorder that leads to death if the underlying problems are not corrected. The exact mechanisms of sepsis-related death are still unclear; aside from increased lymphocyte and enterocyte apoptosis, cellular necrosis is minimal. Death typically follows the failure of multiple organs, which usually offer no morphologic clues to explain their dysfunction. For hypovolemic and cardiogenic shock, however, the pathways leading to death are reasonably well understood. Unless the insult is massive and rapidly lethal

(e.g., exsanguination from a ruptured aortic aneurysm), shock tends to evolve through three general (albeit somewhat artificial) stages. These stages have been documented most clearly in hypovolemic shock but are common to other forms as well:

- An initial nonprogressive stage during which reflex compensatory mechanisms are activated and vital organ perfusion is maintained
- A progressive stage characterized by tissue hypoperfusion and onset of worsening circulatory and metabolic derangement, including acidosis
- An irreversible stage in which cellular and tissue injury is so severe that even if the hemodynamic defects are corrected, survival is not possible

In the early nonprogressive phase of shock, various neurohumoral mechanisms maintain cardiac output and blood pressure. These mechanisms include baroreceptor reflexes, release of catecholamines and antidiuretic hormone, activation of the renin-angiotensin-aldosterone axis, and generalized sympathetic stimulation. The net effect is tachycardia, peripheral vasoconstriction, and renal fluid conservation. Cutaneous vasoconstriction causes the characteristic "shocky" skin coolness and pallor (notably, septic shock can initially cause cutaneous vasodilation, so the patient may present with warm, flushed skin). Coronary and cerebral vessels are less sensitive to sympathetic signals and maintain relatively normal caliber, blood flow, and oxygen delivery. Thus, blood is shunted away from the skin to the vital organs such as the heart and the brain.

If the underlying causes are not corrected, next seen is the progressive phase, which is characterized by widespread tissue hypoxia. In the setting of persistent oxygen deficit, intracellular aerobic respiration is replaced by anaerobic glycolysis with excessive production of lactic acid. The resultant lactic acidosis lowers the tissue pH, blunting the vasomotor response of arterioles, which dilate, leading to the pooling of blood in the microcirculation. Peripheral pooling of blood not only lowers cardiac output but also puts endothelial cells at risk for the development of ischemic injury and subsequent DIC. With widespread tissue hypoxia, vital organs begin to fail.

In the absence of intervention, or in severe cases, the process eventually enters an irreversible stage. Widespread cell injury is reflected in lysosomal enzyme leakage, further aggravating cell injury. Myocardial contractile function worsens and the ischemic bowel may allow intestinal flora to enter the circulation; thus, bacteremic shock may be superimposed. Commonly, renal failure occurs as a consequence of ischemic injury of the kidney. Despite therapeutic interventions, this downward spiral often ends in death.

MORPHOLOGY

The pathophysiologic effects of shock are essentially those of hypoxic injury (Chapter 1) and are caused by a combination of **hypoperfusion** and **microvascular thrombosis**. Although any organ may be affected, the brain, heart, kidneys, adrenals, and gastrointestinal tract are most commonly involved. **Fibrin thrombi** may form in any tissue but typically are most readily visualized in kidney glomeruli. **Adrenal cortical cell lipid depletion** is akin to that seen in all forms of stress and reflects increased use of stored lipids for steroid synthesis. Whereas the lungs are resistant to hypoxic injury in hypovolemic shock occurring after hemorrhage, sepsis or trauma can precipitate diffuse alveolar damage (Chapter 11), leading to so-called **"shock lung."** Except for neuronal and cardiomyocyte loss, affected tissues may recover completely if the patient survives.

Clinical Features. The clinical manifestations of shock depend on the precipitating insult. In hypovolemic and cardiogenic shock, patients exhibit hypotension, a weak rapid pulse, tachypnea, and cool, clammy, cyanotic skin. As already noted, in septic shock, the skin may be warm and flushed owing to peripheral vasodilation. The primary threat to life is the underlying initiating event (e.g., myocardial infarction, severe hemorrhage, bacterial infection). However, the cardiac, cerebral, and pulmonary changes rapidly aggravate the situation. If patients survive the initial period, worsening renal function can provoke a phase dominated by progressive oliguria, acidosis, and electrolyte imbalances.

Prognosis varies with the origin of shock and its duration. Thus, more than 90% of young, otherwise healthy patients with hypovolemic shock survive with appropriate management; by comparison, septic or cardiogenic shock is associated with substantially worse outcomes, even with state-of-the-art care.

■ RAPID REVIEW

Edema

- Caused by movement of fluid from the vasculature into the interstitial spaces
- Edema fluid may be protein poor (transudate) or protein rich (exudate).
- Noninflammatory edema may be caused by increased hydrostatic pressure (e.g., heart failure); decreased colloid osmotic pressure resulting from reduced plasma albumin, either due to decreased synthesis (e.g., liver disease, protein malnutrition) or increased loss (e.g., nephrotic syndrome); lymphatic obstruction (e.g., fibrosis or neoplasia); or sodium retention (e.g., renal failure).
- Inflammatory edema is caused by an increase in vascular permeability.

Hemostasis

- Mediated by the adhesion, activation, and aggregation of platelets (primary hemostasis) and coagulation factors (secondary hemostasis)
- Primary hemostasis occurs through the following steps:
  - Vascular injury exposes vWF in the extracellular matrix.
  - Platelets adhere through the binding of platelet GpIb receptors to vWF.
  - Adhesion leads to platelet activation, associated with secretion of platelet granule contents, changes in platelet shape and membrane composition, and conformational changes in GpIIb-IIIa receptors, which bind fibrinogen, leading to platelet aggregation and formation of the primary hemostatic plug.
- Secondary hemostasis occurs through the following steps:
  - Tissue factor exposure at sites of injury initiates the coagulation cascade.
  - In vivo, the most important factors in the coagulation cascade are factors VII, IX, X, II (prothrombin), and fibrinogen, as well as cofactors V and VIII.
  - Thrombin converts fibrinogen into fibrin to form the secondary hemostatic plug and also stabilizes the clot by activating factor XIII, which crosslinks fibrin, and by promoting platelet contraction.
  - Excessive clotting is prevented by several mechanisms, including washout of activated coagulation factors and their removal by the liver; the requirement for phospholipid surfaces provided by activated platelets; the expression of anticoagulant factors on normal endothelium (e.g., thrombomodulin); and the activation of fibrinolytic pathways (e.g., tissue plasminogen activator).

Thrombosis

- Typically caused by one or more components of Virchow triad, consisting of endothelial injury (e.g., by toxins, hypertension, inflammation, or metabolic products); static or turbulent blood flow (e.g., resulting from aneurysms, atherosclerotic plaque); and hypercoagulability, either primary (e.g., factor V Leiden) or secondary (e.g., bed rest)
- Thrombi may propagate, resolve, become organized, or embolize.
- Thrombosis causes tissue injury by local vascular occlusion or by distal embolization.

Embolism

- An embolus is a solid, liquid, or gaseous mass carried by the blood to a distant site from its origin; most are dislodged thrombi.
- Pulmonary emboli (PE) arise primarily from lower-extremity deep vein thrombi.
- The effects of PEs depend on their size, number, and location of arrest.
- The consequences of PE include right-sided heart failure, pulmonary hemorrhage, pulmonary infarction, and sudden death.
- Systemic emboli arise most commonly from cardiac mural or valvular thrombi, aortic aneurysms, and atherosclerotic plaques.
- Whether systemic emboli cause infarction depends on the site of embolization and the presence or absence of an alternative blood supply.
- Fat embolism occurs after crushing injuries to the bones and may cause pulmonary insufficiency and neurologic damage.
- Amniotic fluid embolism is a rare complication of childbirth that is often fatal due to pulmonary and cerebral manifestations.
- Air embolism occurs upon rapid decompression, most commonly in divers, and results from sudden formation of nitrogen gas bubbles.

Infarction

- An infarct is an area of ischemic necrosis that is most commonly caused by arterial occlusion from thrombosis or embolization and rarely by venous occlusion.
- Infarcts are hemorrhagic (red) when caused by venous occlusion or by arterial occlusion in tissues in which the decrease in blood flow is partial or transient.
- White (nonhemorrhagic) infarcts occur in tissues with endarterial blood supplies in which the vascular obstruction is persistent, such that blood cannot seep into the infarcted tissue.
- Whether infarction occurs is influenced by collateral blood supplies, the rate at which an obstruction develops, the intrinsic tissue susceptibility to ischemic injury, and blood oxygenation.

Shock

- Shock is a state of systemic tissue hypoperfusion due to reduced cardiac output and/or reduced circulating blood volume.
- The major types of shock are cardiogenic (e.g., myocardial infarction), hypovolemic (e.g., blood loss), and septic (e.g., infections), all of which may cause hypoxic tissue injury.
- Septic shock is caused by the host response to bacterial or fungal infections.
- Septic shock pathophysiology involves endothelial cell activation and injury, vasodilation, edema in many tissues, disseminated intravascular coagulation, and metabolic derangements.

■ **Laboratory Tests**

Test	Reference Values	Pathophysiology/Clinical Relevance
Activated partial thromboplastin time (aPTT), plasma	25–37 seconds	aPTT assesses the coagulation factors of the intrinsic pathway (factors XII, XI, IX, and VIII) and the common pathway (factors X, V, II, and fibrinogen). Deficiency of any of these factors can cause aPTT elevations. Heparin and antiphospholipid antibodies (lupus anticoagulant) cause isolated aPTT elevation. Since aPTT is a clot-based assay, anticoagulation therapy can result in elevated aPTT.
Activated protein C (aPC) resistance, plasma	Ratio ≥ 2.3	Protein C is a vitamin K–dependent clotting factor synthesized in the liver that is activated by thrombin when thrombin binds thrombomodulin on endothelium. aPC inhibits coagulation by cleaving factor Va and factor VIIIa and by inactivating plasminogen activator inhibitor, leading to fibrinolysis. Resistance to aPC is mainly seen in the context of the factor V Leiden (FVL) mutation, in which an amino acid substitution affecting factor V removes its aPC cleavage site.
Antiphospholipid antibodies (aPL; also known as lupus anticoagulant antibodies), serum	Negative	aPLs are acquired autoantibodies that bind negatively charged phospholipids. They are frequently seen in patients with systemic lupus erythematosus. aPLs prolong the aPTT by binding phospholipids, a necessary cofactor in this test. In vivo, however, aPLs may cause arterial and venous thrombosis and are associated with antiphospholipid syndrome characterized by thrombosis and late-stage spontaneous abortions.
Antithrombin (AT) activity, plasma	Adults: 80%–130%	AT is produced by hepatocytes and binds and inactivates factors IIa, IXa, Xa, XIa, and XIIa. AT deficiency is a risk factor for venous thromboembolism and may be inherited or acquired (e.g., nephrotic syndrome, fulminant hepatic failure, disseminated intravascular coagulation [DIC]). Since heparin acts as an anticoagulant by potentiating the activity of AT, AT deficiency leads to heparin resistance.
D-dimer, plasma	≤500 ng/mL fibrinogen equivalent units (FEU)	D-dimers are a proteolytic byproduct of plasmin-mediated degradation of fibrin and indicate that (1) a fibrin clot was formed and (2) the clot was crosslinked by factor XIIIa then cleaved by plasmin. Elevated D-dimer levels are seen in disorders marked by procoagulant and fibrinolytic activity (e.g., DIC, deep venous thrombosis [DVT], pulmonary embolism [PE], recent surgery, and trauma) and hypercoagulable states (e.g., pregnancy, liver disease, inflammation).
Factor V Leiden (FVL) mutation, blood	Negative	Factor V (FV) is an essential cofactor in the conversion of prothrombin to thrombin by factor Xa. In FVL, a point mutation substitutes arginine for glutamine (R506Q), preventing FVL cleavage by activated protein C (aPC); persistent factor Va produces a hypercoagulable state. This PCR-based test detects the mutation. FVL is the most common cause of inherited venous thromboembolism in individuals of European ancestry but is also seen in other groups due to population admixture. FVL increases the risk of venous thrombosis 25- to 50-fold in homozygotes and 3- to 4-fold in heterozygotes.
Factor VIII (FVIII) activity assay, plasma	55%–200%	FVIII is a coagulation cofactor that is bound to and stabilized by von Willebrand factor (vWF) in the serum. It is an essential cofactor in factor X activation by factor IX. This test measures the activity of FVIII in patient plasma and is reported as a percentage relative to reference normal plasma. Hemophilia A is an X-linked recessive disorder caused by a profound inherited FVIII deficiency; affected patients typically have FVIII activity levels that are less than 5% of normal. It presents with prolonged bleeding following trauma and hemarthoses. Rare patients with homozygous von Willebrand disease may present with low FVIII levels and hemophilia-like bleeding. Autoantibodies to FVIII can inhibit its function, resulting in acquired hemophilia.
Factor IX (FIX) activity assay, plasma	65%–140%	FIX is a protease that is part of the intrinsic coagulation pathway. It is activated by factor XIa or factor VIIa/tissue factor. In the presence of calcium, phospholipids, and factor VIIIa, FIXa activates factor X, which in turn generates thrombin from prothrombin. Inherited FIX deficiency causes hemophilia B, also called Christmas disease, an X-linked recessive disorder that is clinically indistinguishable from hemophilia A.
Fibrinogen, plasma	200–393 mg/dL	Fibrinogen (factor I) is essential for formation of stable clots and thus hemostasis. Fibrinogen links activated platelets via the GpIIb-IIIa receptor and is cleaved by thrombin to form insoluble fibrin polymers. Fibrinogen is an acute phase reactant synthesized by the liver and may be elevated in inflammatory conditions. Decreased levels may be due to underproduction (e.g., intrinsic liver disease, protein malnutrition, rare genetic disorders) or over"consumption" (e.g., DIC).
Heparin-PF4 IgG antibody, serum	Absent	Antibodies to heparin-platelet factor 4 (PF4) complexes form in some patients after heparin therapy, causing heparin-induced thrombocytopenia (HIT), generally beginning 5–10 days after therapy initiation. These patients are at risk for venous and arterial thromboembolism. While the test is sensitive (98%–100%), specificity is limited since not all anti-PF4 antibodies activate or deplete platelets.

| Prothrombin time (PT), plasma | PT: 9.4–12.5 seconds International normalized ratio (INR): 0.9–1.1 | PT assesses the extrinsic pathway of the coagulation cascade and is therefore elevated when there is a quantitative or qualitative abnormality in factors VII, X, II (prothrombin), or I (fibrinogen). PT results may be standardized among laboratories by converting the value into an international normalized ratio (INR), where the normal value is 1. PT/INR is commonly used as a screening test or to monitor patients on warfarin therapy. |
| Von Willebrand factor (vWF) antigen, plasma | 55%–200% | Von Willebrand factor (vWF) is synthesized in endothelial cells and megakaryocytes. In primary hemostasis, vWF binds to platelet receptor GPIb-IX and subendothelial collagen, thereby promoting platelet adhesion to collagen. This test measures vWF quantity and is generally combined with a functional assay of vWF (e.g., vWF:Ristocetin cofactor assay). Decreased levels or decreased function of vWF can be seen in inherited or acquired (autoimmune) forms of von Willebrand disease. |

Adapted from Deyrup AT, D'Ambrosio D, Muir J, et al. Essential Laboratory Tests for Medical Education. *Acad Pathol*. 2022;9. doi: 10.1016/j.acpath.2022.100046.

Genetic and Pediatric Diseases

The contributions of Dr. Anirban Maitra, Department of Translational Molecular Pathology, University of Texas, MD Anderson Cancer Center, Houston, Texas, to this chapter in several previous editions of this book are gratefully acknowledged.

In this chapter we discuss genetic and pediatric diseases together, because many disorders of childhood are of genetic origin. However, it must be borne in mind that not all genetic disorders manifest in infancy and childhood, and, conversely, many pediatric diseases are not of genetic origin. To the latter category belong diseases resulting from immaturity of organ systems.

To facilitate an understanding of the molecular basis of genetic disorders, we begin this chapter with an overview of the architecture of the human genome.

THE GENOME

Remarkable advances have been made in our understanding of the genetic basis of both inherited and acquired human diseases in the past 50 years. This has been brought about by a deeper understanding of the structure of the human genome and the factors that regulate gene expression.

The sequencing of the human genome at the beginning of the 21st century was a landmark achievement of biomedical science. Since then, the rapidly dropping cost of sequencing and the computational capacity to analyze vast amounts of data have revolutionized our understanding of health and disease. At the same time, the emerging information has also revealed a breathtaking level of complexity far beyond the linear sequence of the genome. The potential for these new powerful tools to expand our understanding of pathogenesis and drive therapeutic innovation excites and inspires scientists and the lay public alike. While early studies were focused on discovery of genes that encode proteins, more recent investigations have led to important insights into the role of noncoding DNA in regulating gene expression. We discuss this next.

Protein-Coding and Noncoding DNA

The human genome contains about 3.3 billion DNA base pairs. Yet, within the genome there are only slightly more than 19,000 protein-encoding genes, making up just 1.5% of the genome. The proteins encoded by these genes are the fundamental constituents of cells, functioning as enzymes, structural elements, and signaling molecules. Although 19,000 underestimates the actual number of proteins encoded (many genes produce multiple RNA transcripts that produce distinct protein isoforms), it is nevertheless startling that worms composed of fewer than 1000 cells—and with genomes 30-fold smaller—are also assembled from roughly 20,000 protein-encoding genes. Perhaps even more surprising is that many of these proteins are recognizable homologs of molecules expressed in humans. What then separates humans from worms? The answer is not completely known, but evidence supports the assertion that the difference lies in the 98.5% of the human genome that does not encode proteins. We now know that more than 85% of the human genome is transcribed, with almost 80% being devoted to the regulation of gene expression. It follows that, whereas proteins provide the building blocks and machinery required for assembling cells, tissues, and organisms, it is the noncoding regions of the genome that provide the critical "architectural planning."

The major classes of functional *non—protein-coding DNA sequences* found in the human genome include (Fig. 4.1):

- *Promoter* and *enhancer* regions that bind transcription factors
- Binding sites for proteins that organize and maintain higher-order *chromatin structures*
- *Noncoding regulatory RNAs*. Of the 80% of the genome dedicated to regulatory functions, the vast majority is transcribed into RNAs—micro-RNAs and long noncoding RNAs (described later)—that are never translated into protein but can regulate gene expression
- *Mobile genetic elements* (e.g., *transposons*). Remarkably, more than one-third of the human genome is composed of these "jumping genes," which can move around to various sites in the genome and are implicated in gene regulation and chromatin organization.
- Special structural regions of DNA, including *telomeres* (chromosome ends) and *centromeres* (chromosome "tethers")

Importantly, **many genetic variations (*polymorphisms*) associated with diseases are located in non—protein-coding regions of the genome.** Thus, variation in gene regulation may prove to be more important in disease causation than structural changes in specific proteins. Genome sequencing has shown that any two humans are typically >99.5% DNA identical. Thus, individual variation, including differential susceptibility to diseases and environmental exposures, is encoded in <0.5% of our DNA.

The two most common forms of DNA variation in the human genome are *single-nucleotide polymorphisms (SNPs)* and *copy number variations (CNVs)*.

- SNPs are variants at single nucleotide positions and are almost always *biallelic* (only two choices exist at a given site within the population, such as A or T). More than 6 million human SNPs have been identified, with many showing wide variation in frequency in different populations. The following features are worthy of note:
  - SNPs occur across the genome—within genes and noncoding regions.
  - Roughly 1% of SNPs occur in coding regions, which is about what would be expected by chance, because coding regions constitute about 1.5% of the genome.
  - SNPs located in noncoding regions can occur in regulatory elements in the genome, thereby altering gene expression; in such instances the SNP may have a direct influence on disease susceptibility.
  - SNPs can also be "neutral" variants with no effect on gene function or phenotype.
  - Even "neutral" SNPs may be useful markers if they happen to be coinherited with a disease-associated gene as a result of physical proximity. In other words, the SNP and the causative genetic factor are in *linkage disequilibrium*. Linkage disequilibrium refers to two genetic markers that are found together at frequencies not predicted by their binomial probability. It can result from either positive natural selection favoring one genetic marker, increasing the frequency of all nearby genetic variants, or genetic drift (random association of two alleles due to chance events).
  - The effect of individual SNPs on disease susceptibility is weak, particularly for complex diseases such as diabetes, heart disease, or cancer. This is because many genetic systems are at play and the contributions of individual SNPs are small. It remains to be seen if the identification of such variants, alone or in combination, can be used to better understand pathogenesis or to develop effective strategies for disease prediction or prevention.
- CNVs are a form of genetic variation consisting of different numbers of large contiguous stretches of DNA. These can range from thousands to millions of base pairs. In some instances, these loci are, like SNPs, biallelic and simply duplicated or deleted in a subset of the population. In other instances there are complex rearrangements (inversions) of genomic material, with multiple alleles in the human population. CNVs are responsible for several million base pairs of sequence difference between any two individuals. Approximately 50% of CNVs involve gene-coding sequences; thus, CNVs may underlie a large portion of human phenotypic diversity.

It is important to note that *alterations in DNA sequence cannot by themselves explain the diversity of phenotypes in human populations.* All phenotypes result from a complex interaction between genes, environment, and chance. Moreover, phenotypic variation may be observed even in genetically identical monozygotic twins. In addition,

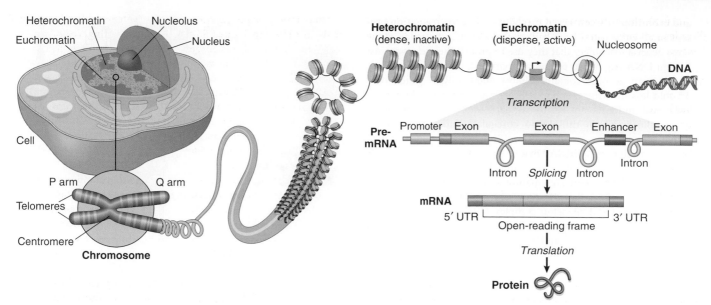

FIG. 4.1 The organization of nuclear DNA. At the light microscopic level, the nuclear genetic material is organized into dispersed, transcriptionally active *euchromatin* or densely packed, transcriptionally inactive *heterochromatin*; some chromatin is bound to the nuclear membrane, and nuclear membrane perturbation can thus influence transcription. Chromosomes (as shown) can only be visualized by light microscopy during cell division. During mitosis, they are organized into paired chromatids connected at *centromeres*; the centromeres act as the locus for the formation of a *kinetochore* protein complex that regulates chromosome segregation at metaphase. The *telomeres* are repetitive nucleotide sequences that cap the termini of chromatids and permit repeated chromosomal replication without loss of DNA at the chromosome ends. The chromatids are organized into short "P" ("petite") and long "Q" ("next letter in the alphabet") arms. The characteristic banding pattern of chromatids has been attributed to relative GC content (less GC content in bands relative to interbands), with genes tending to localize to interband regions. Individual chromatin fibers are composed of a string of *nucleosomes*—DNA wound around octameric histone cores—with the nucleosomes connected via DNA linkers. *Promoters* are noncoding regions of DNA that initiate gene transcription; they are on the same strand and upstream of their associated gene. *Enhancers* are regulatory elements that can modulate gene expression across distances of 100 kB or more by looping back onto promoters and recruiting additional factors that are needed to drive the transcription of pre-messenger RNA (mRNA) species. The intronic sequences are subsequently spliced out of the pre-mRNA to produce mature mRNA, which includes exons that are translated into protein and 5'- and 3'-untranslated regions (UTR) that may have regulatory functions. In addition to the enhancer, promoter, and UTR sequences, noncoding elements are found throughout the genome; these include short repeats, regulatory factor binding regions, noncoding regulatory RNAs, and transposons.

posttranslational modifications such as DNA methylation and histones, have profound impacts on gene expression. We discuss this next.

Epigenetic Changes

Even though virtually all cells in the body have the same genetic composition, differentiated cells have distinct structures and functions arising through lineage-specific programs of gene expression. Such cell type—specific differences in DNA transcription and translation are regulated by *epigenetic* modifications of chromatin that profoundly influence gene expression.

One central mechanism of epigenetic regulation is methylation of cytosine residues in gene promoters—heavily methylated promoters become inaccessible to RNA polymerase, leading to transcriptional silencing. Promoter methylation and silencing of tumor suppressor genes (Chapter 6) are observed in many human cancers, leading to unchecked cell growth. Another major player in epigenetic regulation of transcription involves the family of histone proteins, which are components of structures called nucleosomes, around which DNA is coiled. Histone proteins undergo a variety of reversible modifications such as methylation and acetylation that affect secondary and tertiary DNA structure, and hence gene transcription. As expected, abnormalities in histone modification are observed in many acquired diseases such as cancer, leading to transcriptional dysregulation. Histone deacetylases and inhibitors of DNA methylation are being used in treatment of certain cancers. Physiologic epigenetic silencing during development is called imprinting, and disorders of imprinting are discussed later in this chapter.

Micro-RNA and Long Noncoding RNA

Another mechanism of gene regulation depends on the functions of noncoding RNAs. As the name implies, these are encoded by genes that are transcribed but not translated. Although many distinct families of noncoding RNAs exist, only two examples are discussed here: small RNA molecules called *microRNAs* and *long noncoding RNAs* >200 nucleotides in length.

- *Micro-RNAs (miRNAs)* are relatively short RNAs (22 nucleotides on average) that function primarily to modulate the translation of target mRNAs into their corresponding proteins. **Posttranscriptional silencing of gene expression by miRNA is a fundamental**

and evolutionarily conserved mechanism of gene regulation present in all eukaryotes. Even bacteria have their own version of the same general machinery that they use to protect themselves against foreign DNA (e.g., from phages and viruses).

- The human genome contains almost 6000 miRNA genes, only 3.5-fold less than the number of protein-coding genes. Moreover, individual miRNAs appear to regulate multiple protein-coding genes, allowing each miRNA to coregulate entire programs of gene expression. Transcription of miRNA genes produces a primary transcript (pri-miRNA) that is processed into progressively smaller segments, including trimming by the enzyme *Dicer*, an endonuclease. This generates mature single-stranded miRNAs of 21 to 30 nucleotides that associate with a multiprotein aggregate called RNA-induced silencing complex (RISC) (Fig. 4.2). Subsequent base pairing between the miRNA strand and its target mRNA directs the RISC to either induce mRNA cleavage or repress its translation. In this way, the target mRNA is *posttranscriptionally silenced.*

  Taking advantage of the same pathway, *small interfering RNAs (siRNAs)* are short RNA sequences that can be introduced into cells. These serve as substrates for Dicer and interact with the RISC complex in a manner analogous to endogenous miRNAs. Synthetic siRNAs that can target specific mRNA species are therefore powerful laboratory tools to study gene function (so-called knockdown technology). Several siRNAs are also now in use for treatment of disorders such as macular degeneration.

- *Long noncoding RNA (lncRNA).* lncRNAs modulate gene expression in many ways (Fig. 4.3); for example, they can bind to regions of chromatin, restricting RNA polymerase access to coding genes within the region. The best-known example of a repressive function involves XIST, which is transcribed from the X chromosome and plays an essential role in physiologic X chromosome inactivation. XIST itself escapes X inactivation but forms a repressive "cloak" on the X chromosome from which it is transcribed, resulting in gene silencing. Conversely, it has been appreciated that many enhancers are sites of lncRNA synthesis, with the lncRNAs enhancing transcription from spatially associated gene promoters through a variety of mechanisms (see Fig. 4.3). Ongoing studies are exploring the role of lncRNAs in diseases such as atherosclerosis and cancer.

Gene Editing

Exciting new developments that enable exquisitely specific genome editing are ushering in a biomedical revolution. These advances come from a wholly unexpected source: the discovery of clustered regularly interspaced short palindromic repeats (CRISPRs) and Cas (or CRISPR-associated genes), such as the Cas9 nuclease. These are linked genetic elements that endow prokaryotes with a form of acquired immunity to phages and plasmids. Bacteria use this system to sample the DNA of infecting agents, incorporating it into the host genome as CRISPRs. CRISPRs are transcribed and processed into an RNA sequence that binds and directs the nuclease Cas9 to a sequence (e.g., a phage), leading to its cleavage and the destruction of the phage. Gene editing repurposes this process by using artificial guide RNAs (gRNAs) that bind Cas9 and are complementary to a DNA sequence of interest. Once directed to the target sequence by the gRNA, Cas9 induces double-stranded DNA breaks (Fig. 4.4).

Repair of the resulting highly specific cleavage sites can lead to somewhat random disruptive mutations in the targeted sequences (through nonhomologous end joining [NHEJ]) or the precise introduction of new sequences of interest (by homologous recombination). Both the gRNAs and the Cas9 enzyme can be delivered to cells with a

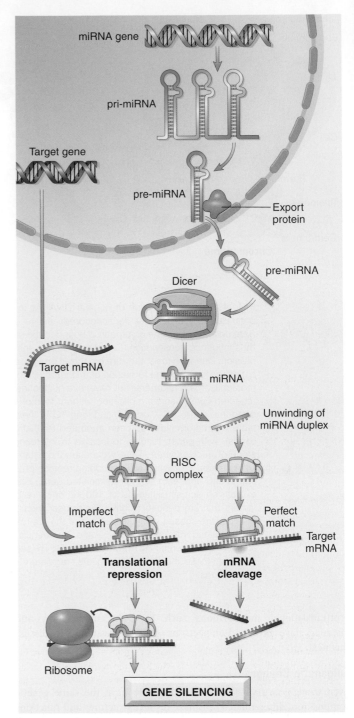

FIG. 4.2 Generation of microRNAs (miRNA) and their mode of action in regulating gene function. miRNA genes are transcribed to produce a primary miRNA (pri-miRNA), which is processed within the nucleus to form precursor miRNA (pre-miRNA) composed of a single RNA strand with secondary hairpin loop structures that form stretches of double-stranded RNA. After this pre-miRNA is exported out of the nucleus via specific transporter proteins, the cytoplasmic enzyme *Dicer* trims the pre-miRNA to generate mature double-stranded miRNAs of 21 to 30 nucleotides. The miRNA subsequently unwinds, and the resulting single strands are incorporated into the multiprotein *RISC*. Base pairing between the single-stranded miRNA and its target mRNA directs RISC to either cleave the mRNA target or to repress its translation. In either case, the target mRNA gene is silenced posttranscriptionally. *RISC*, RNA-induced silencing complex.

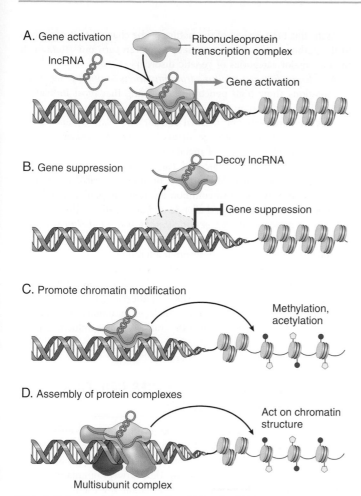

FIG. 4.3 Roles of long noncoding RNAs (lncRNAs). (A) lncRNAs can facilitate transcription factor binding and thus promote gene activation. (B) Conversely, lncRNAs can preemptively bind transcription factors and thus prevent gene transcription. (C) Histone and DNA modification by acetylases or methylases (or deacetylases and demethylases) may be directed by the binding of lncRNAs. (D) In other instances lncRNAs may act as scaffolding to stabilize secondary or tertiary structures and/or multisubunit complexes that influence general chromatin architecture or gene activity. (Adapted from Wang KC, Chang HY: Molecular mechanisms of long noncoding RNAs. *Mol Cell* 43:904, 2011.)

single easy-to-build plasmid. However, the real beauty of the system (and the excitement about its potential for genetic engineering) comes from its impressive flexibility and specificity, which is substantially better than other previous editing systems. Applications include inserting specific mutations into the genomes of cells to model cancers and other diseases and rapidly generating transgenic animals from edited embryonic stem cells. On the flip side, it now is feasible to selectively "correct" mutations that cause hereditable disease, or—perhaps more worrisome—to just eliminate less "desirable" traits. Predictably, the technology has inspired a vigorous debate regarding its application.

GENETIC DISEASES

Before we start a discussion of genetic diseases it is helpful to clarify three commonly used terms: hereditary, familial, and congenital:

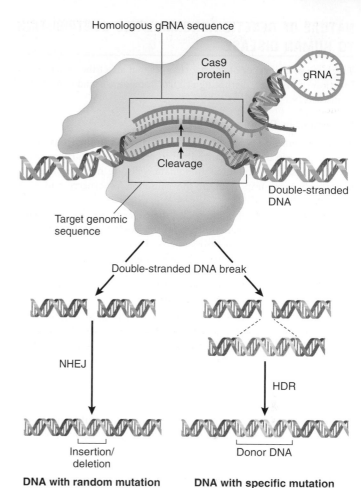

FIG. 4.4 Gene editing with clustered regularly interspersed short palindromic repeats (CRISPRs)/Cas9. In bacteria, DNA sequences consisting of CRISPRs are transcribed into guide RNAs (gRNAs) with a constant region and a variable sequence of about 20 bases. The constant regions of gRNAs bind to Cas9, permitting the variable regions to form heteroduplexes with homologous host cell DNA sequences. The Cas9 nuclease then cleaves the bound DNA, producing a double-stranded DNA break. To perform gene editing, gRNAs are designed with variable regions that are homologous to a target DNA sequence of interest. Coexpression of the gRNA and Cas9 in cells leads to efficient cleavage of the target sequence. In the absence of homologous DNA, the broken DNA is repaired by nonhomologous end joining (NHEJ), an error-prone method that often introduces disruptive insertions or deletions (indels). By contrast, in the presence of a homologous "donor" DNA spanning the region targeted by CRISPR/Cas9, cells instead may use homologous DNA recombination (HDR) to repair the DNA break. HDR is less efficient than NHEJ but has the capacity to introduce precise changes in DNA sequence. *Cas9,* CRISPR-associated protein 9.

- *Hereditary disorders* are transmitted in the parents' gametes and therefore are *familial.*
- *Congenital* simply implies "present at birth." Congenital diseases need not be genetic (e.g., congenital syphilis), and not all genetic diseases are congenital: the symptoms of Huntington disease, for example, begin after the third or fourth decade of life.

NATURE OF GENETIC ABNORMALITIES CONTRIBUTING TO HUMAN DISEASE

There are several types of genetic changes that affect the structure and function of proteins, disrupting cellular homeostasis and contributing to disease.

Mutations in Protein-Coding Genes

The term **mutation** refers to permanent changes in the DNA. Those that affect germ cells are transmitted to progeny and may give rise to inherited diseases. Mutations in somatic cells are not transmitted to progeny but are important in the causation of cancers and some congenital disorders.

Details of specific mutations and their effects are discussed along with the relevant disorders throughout this book. Cited here are some common examples of gene mutations and their effects:

- *Point mutations* result from the substitution of a single nucleotide base by a different base, which may result in the replacement of one amino acid by another in the protein product. For example, a point mutation in the β-globin chain of hemoglobin gives rise to hemoglobin S (HbS), instead of hemoglobin A. The altered properties of HbS produces sickle cell disease. Such mutations are sometimes called *missense* mutations. By contrast, certain point mutations may create a stop codon, resulting in a truncated protein or complete failure of mRNA translation and protein synthesis. Such mutations are referred to as *nonsense* mutations.
- *Frameshift mutations* occur when the insertion or deletion of one or two base pairs alters the reading frame of the DNA strand.
- *Trinucleotide repeat mutations* belong to a special category, because they are characterized by amplification of a sequence of three nucleotides. The specific nucleotide sequence that undergoes amplification varies with different disorders. For example, in fragile X syndrome, prototypical of this category of disorders, there are 200 to 4000 tandem repeats of the sequence CGG within the familial mental retardation-1 gene *(FMR1)*. In unaffected populations, the number of repeats is small, averaging 29. The expansions of the trinucleotide sequences may prevent appropriate expression of the *FMR1* gene, which gives rise to intellectual disability. Another distinguishing feature of trinucleotide repeat mutations is that they are dynamic (i.e., the degree of amplification increases during gametogenesis). These features, discussed in greater detail later in this chapter, influence the pattern of inheritance and the phenotypic manifestations of the diseases caused by this class of mutations.

Alterations in Protein-Coding Genes Other Than Mutations

In addition to alterations in DNA sequence, coding genes also can undergo structural variations, such as copy number changes—*amplifications* or *deletions*—or *translocations* that result in aberrant gain or loss of protein function. As with mutations, structural changes may occur in the germline or be acquired in somatic tissues. In many instances, pathogenic germline alterations involve a contiguous portion of a chromosome rather than a single gene, such as in the 22q microdeletion syndrome, discussed later. With the widespread availability of next-generation sequencing technology for assessing DNA copy number variation at very high resolution genome wide, copy number variants have been linked to a higher risk of developing several disorders, including autism. Cancers often contain somatically acquired structural alterations, including amplifications, deletions, and translocations. The so-called "Philadelphia chromosome"—translocation t(9;22) between the *BCR* and *ABL* genes in chronic myeloid leukemia (Chapter 10)—is a classic example.

With this brief review of the nature of the changes that contribute to the pathogenesis of human diseases, we can turn our attention to the four major categories of genetic disorders:

- *Mendelian disorders resulting from mutations in single genes.* These mutations show high penetrance, meaning that most individuals who inherit the anomaly show phenotypic effects. Mendelian disorders are hereditary and familial and include relatively uncommon conditions, such as storage diseases caused by enzyme defects and other inborn errors of metabolism.
- *Complex disorders involving multiple genes as well as environmental influences.* These are called complex, or multifactorial, diseases. They include some of the most common disorders of mankind, including hypertension, diabetes, and allergic and autoimmune diseases.
- *Diseases arising from changes in chromosomal number or structure.* Several developmental diseases such as Down syndrome are attributable to this type of chromosomal alterations.
- *Other genetic diseases,* which involve single gene mutations but do not follow simple mendelian rules of inheritance. These single-gene disorders with nonclassic inheritance patterns include those resulting from triplet repeat mutations or from mutations in mitochondrial DNA, and those in which the transmission is influenced by an epigenetic phenomenon called genomic imprinting. Each of these four categories is discussed separately.

MENDELIAN DISORDERS: DISEASES CAUSED BY MUTATIONS IN SINGLE GENES

Single-gene mutations follow the well-known mendelian patterns of inheritance (Tables 4.1 and 4.2). Although individually rare, together they are responsible for a significant disease burden. The Online Mendelian Inheritance in Man (OMIM) database (https://www.omim.org/) of the National Center for Biotechnology Information is a useful site for information concerning human genetic diseases. Listed next are a few important tenets and caveats when considering mendelian disorders:

- **Mutations involving single genes follow one of three patterns of inheritance: autosomal dominant, autosomal recessive, or X-linked.**
- A single-gene mutation may have many phenotypic effects *(pleiotropy)* and, conversely, mutations at several genetic loci may produce the same trait *(genetic heterogeneity)*. Marfan syndrome, which results from a structural defect in connective tissue, is associated with widespread effects involving the skeleton, eyes, and cardiovascular system, all of which stem from a mutation in the gene encoding fibrillin, a component of connective tissues. On the other hand, several different types of mutations can cause retinitis pigmentosa, an inherited disorder associated with abnormal retinal pigmentation and consequent visual impairment. Recognition of genetic heterogeneity not only is important in genetic counseling but also feasibility of molecular diagnosis of disorders such as phenylketonuria, discussed later. Although mendelian diseases are rare, elucidation of the genes responsible has been very helpful in understanding normal pathways and the consequences of their disruption in acquired diseases.
- The phenotypic manifestations of mutations affecting a known single gene are influenced by other genetic loci, which are called modifier genes. As discussed later in the section on cystic fibrosis, these modifier loci can affect the severity or extent of disease.
- The use of proactive prenatal genetic screening in high-risk populations (e.g., persons with Ashkenazi Jewish ancestry) has significantly reduced the incidence (see Table 4.1) of certain genetic disorders such as Tay-Sachs disease.

Table 4.1 Estimated Prevalence of Selected Mendelian Disorders Among Live-Born Infants

Disorder	Estimated Prevalence
Autosomal Dominant Inheritance	
Familial hypercholesterolemia	1 in 500
Polycystic kidney disease	1 in 1000
Hereditary spherocytosis	1 in 5000 (U.S. European descent)
Marfan syndrome	1 in 5000
Huntington disease	1 in 10,000
Autosomal Recessive Inheritance	
Sickle cell anemia	1 in 500 (U.S. African descent)[a]
Cystic fibrosis	1 in 3200 (U.S. North European descent)
Tay-Sachs disease	1 in 3500 (U.S. Ashkenazi Jewish ancestry; French Canadians)
Phenylketonuria	1 in 10,000
MPSs—all types	1 in 25,000
Glycogen storage diseases—all types	1 in 50,000
Galactosemia	1 in 60,000
X-Linked Inheritance	
Duchenne muscular dystrophy	1 in 3500 (U.S. males)
Hemophilia	1 in 5000 (U.S. males)

[a]The prevalence of heterozygous sickle cell trait is 1 in 12 for U.S. African descent. Prevalence of sickle cell anemia is increased in areas with evolutionary pressure for malaria including parts of sub-Saharan Africa, southern Europe, the middle East, and India (Chapter 10).

MPS, Mucopolysaccharidosis.

Transmission Patterns of Single-Gene Disorders

Disorders of Autosomal Dominant Inheritance

Disorders of autosomal dominant inheritance are manifested in the heterozygous state, so at least one parent in an index case is usually affected. Both males and females are affected, and both sexes can transmit the condition. When an affected person has a child with an unaffected one, each child has one chance in two of having the disease. The following features also pertain to autosomal dominant diseases:

- *Not all patients have affected parents.* Such patients owe their disorder to new mutations involving either the egg or the sperm from which they were derived. The siblings of these individuals are unaffected.
- *Clinical features can be modified by reduced penetrance and variable expressivity.* Some persons inherit the mutant gene but are phenotypically normal, a phenomenon referred to as *reduced penetrance.* The variables that determine penetrance are not clearly understood. In contrast to penetrance, if a trait is consistently associated with a mutant gene but is expressed differently among persons carrying the gene, the phenomenon is called *variable expressivity.* For example, manifestations of neurofibromatosis 1 range from brownish spots on the skin to multiple tumors and skeletal deformities.
- *In many conditions, the age at onset is delayed, and symptoms and signs do not appear until adulthood.* Examples include Huntington disease and several germline mutations that lead to increased risk of adult-onset cancers.
- *In autosomal dominant disorders, a 50% reduction in the normal gene product is associated with clinical signs and symptoms.* Because a 50% loss of enzyme activity can be compensated for, involved genes in autosomal dominant disorders usually do not encode enzyme proteins but instead fall into several other categories of proteins:
  - Proteins involved in the regulation of complex metabolic pathways, often subject to feedback control (e.g., membrane receptors, transport proteins). An example of this pathogenic

Table 4.2 Biochemical Basis and Inheritance Pattern for Selected Mendelian Disorders

Disease	Abnormal Protein	Protein Type/Function
Autosomal Dominant Inheritance		
Familial hypercholesterolemia	LDL receptor	Receptor transport
Marfan syndrome	Fibrillin	Structural support: extracellular matrix
Ehler-Danlos syndrome[a]	Collagen	Structural support: extracellular matrix
Hereditary spherocytosis	Spectrin, ankyrin, or protein 4.1	Structural support: red cell membrane
Neurofibromatosis, type 1	Neurofibromin-1 (NF-1)	Growth regulation
Adult polycystic kidney disease	Polycystin-1 (PKD-1)	Cell—cell and cell—matrix interactions
Autosomal Recessive Inheritance		
Cystic fibrosis	Cystic fibrosis transmembrane regulator	Ion channel
Phenylketonuria	Phenylalanine hydroxylase	Enzyme
Tay-Sachs disease	Hexosaminidase	Enzyme
Severe combined immunodeficiency[c]	Adenosine deaminase	Enzyme
α- and β-thalassemias[b]	Hemoglobin	Oxygen transport
Sickle cell anemia[b]	Hemoglobin	Oxygen transport
X-Linked Recessive Inheritance		
Hemophilia A	Factor VIII	Coagulation
Duchenne/Becker muscular dystrophy	Dystrophin	Structural support: cell membrane
Fragile X syndrome	FMRP	RNA translation

[a]Some variants of Ehler-Danlos syndrome have an autosomal recessive inheritance pattern.

[b]Although full-blown symptoms require biallelic mutations, heterozygotes for thalassemia and sickle cell anemia may present with mild clinical disease. Thus, these disorders sometimes are categorized as "autosomal codominant."

[c]Some cases of severe combined immunodeficiency are X-linked.

mechanism is found in familial hypercholesterolemia, which results from mutation in the low-density lipoprotein (LDL) receptor gene (discussed later).

- Key structural proteins, such as collagen and components of the red cell membrane skeleton (e.g., spectrin, mutations of which result in hereditary spherocytosis).

The biochemical mechanisms by which a 50% reduction in the levels of structural proteins results in a disease phenotype are not fully understood. In some instances, especially when the gene encodes one subunit of a multimeric protein, the product of the mutant allele is expressed at normal levels but interferes with the assembly of a functionally normal multimer. For example, the collagen molecule is a trimer in which the three collagen chains are arranged in a helical configuration. The presence of mutated collagen chains reduces the assembly of the remaining normal chains, producing a marked deficiency of collagen. In this instance, the mutant allele is called *dominant negative*, because it impairs the function of a wild-type allele. This effect is illustrated in some forms of osteogenesis imperfecta (Chapter 19).

Disorders of Autosomal Recessive Inheritance

Disorders of autosomal recessive inheritance are manifested in the homozygous state. They occur when both alleles at a given gene locus are mutated. Therefore, such disorders are characterized by the following features: (1) the trait does not usually affect the parents, who each carry one mutant allele, but multiple siblings may show the disease; (2) siblings have one chance in four of being affected (i.e., the recurrence risk is 25% for each birth); and (3) if the mutant gene occurs with a low frequency in the population, there is a strong likelihood that the affected patient (the proband) has consanguineous parents. Autosomal recessive disorders make up the largest group of mendelian disorders.

In contrast with the features of autosomal dominant diseases, the following features generally apply to most autosomal recessive disorders:

- *The expression of the defect tends to be more uniform than in autosomal dominant disorders.*
- *Complete penetrance is common.*
- *Onset is frequently early in life.*
- *Although new mutations for recessive disorders do occur, they are rarely detected clinically.* Because an individual carrying the mutation is an asymptomatic heterozygote, several generations may pass before the descendant of such a person mates with another heterozygote and produces affected offspring.
- *In many cases, the affected gene encodes an enzyme.* In heterozygotes, equal amounts of wild-type and affected enzyme are synthesized. Usually the natural "margin of safety" ensures that cells with half of their complement of the enzyme function normally.

X-Linked Disorders

For the most part, sex-linked disorders are X linked. The Y chromosome is home to the testes-determining gene *SRY* as well as several other genes that control spermatogenesis and map to the male specific Y-region (MSY), which directs male sexual differentiation. Males with mutations affecting the Y chromosome are infertile, so no Y chromosome—linked mendelian disorders have been reported. Most X-linked disorders are X-linked recessive and are characterized by the following features:

- *Heterozygous female carriers transmit the trait only to sons, who are hemizygous for the X chromosome.* Sons of heterozygous women have one chance in two of receiving the mutant gene.

- *Heterozygous females rarely express the full phenotypic change, because they have a wild-type allele.* Although one of the X chromosomes in females is inactivated (see further text), this process of inactivation is random, which typically allows sufficient numbers of cells with expression of the wild-type X to emerge.
- *An affected male does not transmit the disorder to sons, but all daughters are carriers.*

Diseases Caused by Mutations in Genes Encoding Structural Proteins

Marfan Syndrome

Marfan syndrome is an autosomal dominant disorder of connective tissues, manifested principally by changes in the skeleton, eyes, and cardiovascular system. It is caused by an inherited defect in an extracellular glycoprotein called *fibrillin*.

Pathogenesis. Fibrillin is secreted by fibroblasts and it is the major component of microfibrils found in the extracellular matrix. Microfibrils serve as scaffolds for the deposition of tropoelastin, an integral component of elastic fibers. Although microfibrils are widely distributed in the body, they are particularly abundant in the aorta, ligaments, and the ciliary zonules that support the ocular lens, precisely the tissues that are affected in Marfan syndrome.

Fibrillin is encoded by the *FBN1* gene, which maps to chromosomal locus 15q21. Mutations in *FBN1* are found in all patients with Marfan syndrome. More than 1000 distinct causative mutations in the very large *FBN1* gene have been found, which complicates diagnosis by DNA sequencing. Therefore the diagnosis is mainly based on clinical findings. Because heterozygotes have clinical symptoms, it is thought that the mutant fibrillin protein acts as a dominant negative, preventing the assembly of normal microfibrils. The prevalence of Marfan syndrome is estimated to be 1 in 5000 worldwide. Approximately 70% to 85% of cases are familial, and the rest are sporadic, arising from de novo *FBN1* mutations in the germ cells of parents.

Although many of the findings in Marfan syndrome can be explained on the basis of the structural defect of connective tissues, some, such as overgrowth of bones, are difficult to relate to simple loss of fibrillin. It is now evident that loss of microfibrils leads to excessive activation of transforming growth factor-β (TGF-β), because normal microfibrils sequester TGF-β, thereby limiting the bioavailability of this cytokine. Excessive TGF-β signaling has deleterious effects on vascular smooth muscle development and the integrity of the extracellular matrix. In support of this hypothesis, mutations in the TGF-β type II receptor give rise to a related syndrome, called Marfan syndrome type 2 (MFS2). Of note, certain angiotensin receptor type II blockers that inhibit the activity of TGF-β are now in clinical use for prevention of cardiovascular disease along with β-adrenergic blocking agents, which lower blood pressure to reduce the risk of cardiovascular catastrophe.

MORPHOLOGY

Skeletal changes are the most evident feature of Marfan syndrome. Patients have a slender, elongated habitus with extremely long legs, arms, and fingers (arachnodactyly); a high-arched palate; and hyperextensibility of joints. A variety of spinal deformities, such as severe kyphoscoliosis, may be present. The chest may exhibit either pectus excavatum (i.e., deeply depressed sternum) or a pigeon-breast deformity. The most characteristic **ocular change** is bilateral dislocation, or subluxation, of the lens secondary to weakness of its suspensory ligaments **(ectopia lentis).** Ectopia lentis, particularly if bilateral, is highly specific for Marfan syndrome and strongly suggests the diagnosis. Most serious, however, is the involvement of the **cardiovascular system.** Fragmentation of the elastic fibers in the tunica media of the aorta predisposes affected patients to aneurysmal dilation and aortic dissection (Chapter 8). These changes, called **cystic medionecrosis,** are not specific for Marfan syndrome; similar lesions occur in hypertension and with aging. Loss of medial support causes dilation of the aortic valve ring, giving rise to aortic incompetence. The cardiac valves, especially the mitral valve, may be excessively distensible and regurgitant **(floppy valve syndrome),** giving rise to mitral valve prolapse and congestive cardiac failure (Chapter 9). Aortic rupture is the most common cause of death and may occur at any age. Less frequently, cardiac failure is the terminal event.

Although the lesions described are typical of Marfan syndrome, they are not seen in all cases. There is much variation in clinical expression, and some patients may exhibit predominantly cardiovascular lesions with minimal skeletal and ocular changes. It is believed that the variable expressivity is related to different mutations in the *FBN1* gene.

Ehlers-Danlos Syndromes

Ehlers-Danlos syndromes (EDSs) are a group of diseases characterized by defects in collagen synthesis or structure. EDSs are caused by mutations in a number of different genes; the most commonly affected genes encode various collagens, and all affected genes, through one mechanism or another, lead to a defect in collagens. All are single-gene disorders, but the mode of inheritance encompasses both autosomal dominant and recessive patterns. There are approximately 30 distinct types of collagen; all have characteristic tissue distributions and are the products of different genes. To some extent, the clinical heterogeneity of EDS can be explained by mutations in different collagen genes.

At least thirteen clinical and genetic variants of EDS are recognized. Although individually rare, the collective frequency of all cases of EDS is 1 in 5000 births worldwide. Since defective collagen is the basis for these disorders, certain clinical features are common to all variants.

- *Tissues rich in collagen, such as skin, ligaments, and joints, are frequently affected in most variants of EDS.* Because the abnormal collagen fibers lack adequate tensile strength, joints are hypermobile. These features permit remarkable hyperflexibility, such as bending the thumb backward to touch the forearm or bending the knee upward to create almost a right angle. Indeed, it is believed that most contortionists have some form of EDS; however, a predisposition to joint dislocation is one of the prices paid for this virtuosity.
- *Skin fragility. The skin is extraordinarily stretchable, extremely fragile, and vulnerable to trauma.* Minor injuries produce gaping defects, and surgical repair or any surgical intervention is accomplished only with great difficulty because of the lack of normal tensile strength.
- *Structural failure of organ or tissues.* The structural defect in connective tissue may lead to *serious internal complications,* including rupture of the colon and large arteries (vascular EDS); ocular fragility, with rupture of the cornea and retinal detachment (kyphoscoliotic EDS); and diaphragmatic hernia (classical EDS), among others.

The molecular bases for three of the more common variants are as follows:

- *Deficient synthesis of type III collagen resulting from mutations affecting the COL3A1 gene.* This variant, vascular EDS, is inherited as an autosomal dominant disorder and is characterized by weakness of tissues rich in type III collagen (e.g., blood vessels, bowel wall), predisposing them to rupture.
- *Deficiency of the enzyme lysyl hydroxylase.* Decreased hydroxylation of lysyl residues in types I and III collagen interferes with the formation of crosslinks among collagen molecules. As might be expected, this variant (kyphoscoliotic EDS), resulting from an enzyme deficiency, is inherited as an autosomal recessive disorder. Patients typically manifest with congenital scoliosis and ocular fragility.
- *Deficient synthesis of type V collagen* resulting from mutations in COL5A1 and COL5A2 is inherited as an autosomal dominant disorder (classical EDS).

Diseases Caused by Mutations in Genes Encoding Receptor Proteins or Channels

Familial Hypercholesterolemia

Familial hypercholesterolemia (FH) is a "receptor disease" caused most commonly (in 80%–85% cases) by loss-of-function mutations in the gene encoding the LDL receptor, which is involved in the transport and metabolism of cholesterol. As a consequence of receptor abnormalities, there is a loss of feedback control that normally holds cholesterol synthesis in check. The resulting elevated levels of cholesterol induce premature atherosclerosis and greatly increase the risk of myocardial infarction. Familial hypercholesterolemia is among the most common of mendelian disorders; the frequency of the heterozygous condition is 1 in 500 in the general population worldwide. The prevalence in those with atherosclerotic cardiovascular disease is 20-fold higher.

Normal Cholesterol Metabolism. Approximately 7% of the body's cholesterol circulates in the plasma, predominantly in the form of LDL. As might be expected, the amount of plasma cholesterol is influenced by its synthesis and catabolism, and the liver plays a crucial role in both these processes, as described later. Cholesterol may be derived from the diet or from endogenous synthesis. Dietary triglycerides and cholesterol are incorporated into chylomicrons in the intestinal mucosa and travel by way of gut lymphatics to the blood. These chylomicrons are hydrolyzed by an endothelial lipoprotein lipase in the capillaries of muscle and fat. The chylomicron remnants, rich in cholesterol, are then delivered to the liver. Some of the cholesterol enters the metabolic pool (to be described), and some is excreted as free cholesterol or as bile acids into the biliary tract.

The endogenous synthesis of cholesterol and LDL begins in the liver (Fig. 4.5). The first step is the secretion of triglyceride-rich very-low-density lipoprotein (VLDL) by the liver into the blood. In the capillary endothelium of adipose tissue and muscle, the VLDL particle undergoes lipolysis and is converted to intermediate-density lipoprotein (IDL). In comparison with VLDL, the content of triglyceride is reduced and that of cholesteryl esters is enriched in IDL, but IDL retains on its surface the VLDL-associated apolipoproteins B-100 and E. Further metabolism of IDL occurs along two pathways: Most of the IDL particles are taken up by the liver through the LDL receptor (described later); others are converted to cholesterol-rich LDL by a further loss of triglycerides and the loss of apolipoprotein E. In the liver cells, IDL is recycled to generate VLDL.

The LDL receptor pathway metabolizes two-thirds of the resultant LDL particles, and the rest is metabolized by a receptor for oxidized LDL (scavenger receptor), to be described later. The LDL receptor binds to apolipoproteins B-100 and E and thus is involved in the transport of both LDL and IDL. Although the LDL receptors are widely distributed, approximately 75% are located on hepatocytes, so

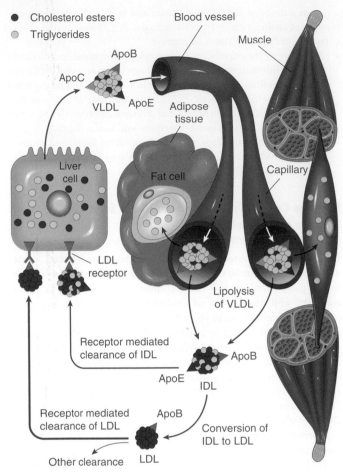

● Cholesterol esters
○ Triglycerides

FIG. 4.5 Low-density lipoprotein (LDL) metabolism and the role of the liver in its synthesis and clearance. Lipolysis of very-low-density lipoprotein (VLDL) by lipoprotein lipase in the capillaries releases triglycerides, which are then stored in fat cells and used as a source of energy in skeletal muscles. IDL (intermediate-density lipoprotein) remains in the blood and is taken up by the liver.

the liver plays an extremely important role in LDL metabolism. The first step in the receptor-mediated transport of LDL involves binding to the cell surface receptor, followed by internalization inside so-called clathrin-coated pits and then into endosomes (Fig. 4.6). Within the cell, the endocytic vesicles fuse with the lysosomes. Here the LDL dissociates from the receptor, which is recycled to the surface. The recycling of LDL receptors is negatively regulated by an enzyme, better known as PCSK9, which degrades the LDL receptor. In the lysosomes LDL molecule is enzymatically degraded, resulting ultimately in the release of free cholesterol into the cytoplasm. The exit of cholesterol from the lysosomes requires the action of two proteins, called NPC1 and NPC2 (described later in the context of Niemann-Pick disease type C). Cholesterol not only is used by the cell for membrane synthesis but also takes part in intracellular cholesterol homeostasis by a sophisticated system of feedback control:

- It suppresses cholesterol synthesis by inhibiting the activity of the enzyme 3-hydroxy-3-methylglutaryl—coenzyme A reductase (HMG-CoA reductase), which is the rate-limiting enzyme in the synthetic pathway.
- It stimulates the formation of cholesterol esters, the storage form of cholesterol.

- It downregulates the synthesis of cell surface LDL receptors, thus preventing excessive accumulation of cholesterol within cells.
- Cholesterol upregulates the expression of the PCSK9, which reduces recycling of LDL receptors by degradation of endocytosed LDL receptors. This provides an additional mechanism of protecting the cells from excessive accumulation of cholesterol.

The transport of LDL by the scavenger receptor, alluded to earlier, seems to occur in cells of the mononuclear phagocyte system and possibly in other cells as well. Monocytes and macrophages have receptors for chemically modified (e.g., acetylated or oxidized) LDLs. The amount catabolized by this scavenger receptor pathway is directly related to the plasma cholesterol level.

Pathogenesis. **In familial hypercholesterolemia, mutations in the LDL receptor protein impair the surface expression and endocytosis of LDL receptors, resulting in the accumulation of LDL cholesterol in the blood.** In addition, the absence of LDL receptors on liver cells impairs the transport of IDL into the liver, so a greater proportion of plasma IDL is converted into LDL. Thus, patients with familial hypercholesterolemia develop excessive levels of blood cholesterol as a result of the combined effects of reduced catabolism and excessive biosynthesis (see Fig. 4.5). This leads to a marked increase of cholesterol uptake by monocytes and macrophages and vascular walls through the scavenger receptor, accounting for the appearance of skin xanthomas and premature atherosclerosis. As mentioned earlier, mutations in the LDL receptor account for 80% to 85% of cases of FH. Less commonly, FH is caused by mutations in two other genes involved in clearance of plasma LDL. Specifically, these mutations consist of (1) loss of function mutations in B-100 (ApoB), the ligand for the LDL receptor on the LDL particle (5% to 10% of cases), and (2) gain of function mutations in the enzyme PCSK9 (1% to 2% of cases), which normally reduces the level of LDL receptor on hepatocytes by dampening their recycling, leading to their degradation in lysosomes. As with mutations in the LDL receptor, these additional types of mutations impair hepatic clearance of LDL and give rise to clinically indistinguishable disease. More than 2000 mutations involving the LDL receptor gene have been identified. One of the most common mutant forms encodes LDL receptor protein that has a folding defect, preventing its expression on the cell surface.

Clinical Features. Familial hypercholesterolemia is an autosomal dominant disease. Heterozygotes have a 2-fold to 3-fold elevation of plasma cholesterol levels, whereas homozygotes may have in excess of a 5-fold elevation. Although their cholesterol levels are elevated from birth, heterozygotes remain asymptomatic until adult life, when they may develop cholesterol deposits (xanthomas) along tendon sheaths and premature atherosclerosis resulting in coronary artery disease. Homozygotes are much more severely affected, developing cutaneous xanthomas in childhood and often dying of myocardial infarction before the age of 20 years.

The discovery of the critical role of LDL receptors in cholesterol homeostasis has led to the rational design of the statin family of drugs that are now widely used to lower plasma cholesterol. They inhibit the activity of HMG-CoA reductase and thus promote greater synthesis of LDL receptors (see Fig. 4.6). However, the upregulation of LDL receptors is accompanied by a compensatory increase in PCSK9 levels, which dampens the effects of statins. Therefore, agents, such as antibodies that antagonize PCSK9 enzymatic function and siRNAs that inhibit transcription of PCSK9, have been developed for treatment of patients with refractory hypercholesterolemia.

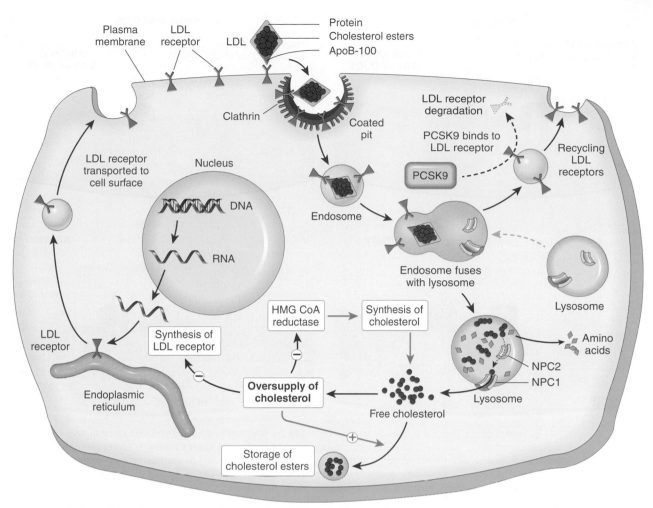

FIG. 4.6 The LDL receptor pathway and regulation of cholesterol metabolism. There are three regulatory functions of free intracellular cholesterol: (1) suppression of cholesterol synthesis by inhibition of HMG-CoA reductase; (2) stimulating the storage of excess cholesterol as esters; and (3) inhibition of synthesis of LDL receptors. PCSK9 causes intracellular degradation of LDL receptors in liver cells, reducing the level of LDL receptors on the cell membrane. NPC1 and NPC2 are required for exit of cholesterol from lysosomes to cytoplasm. *HMG-CoA reductase,* 3-Hydroxy-3-methylglutaryl–coenzyme A reductase; *LDL,* low-density lipoprotein; *NPC1,* Niemann-Pick protein type C1; *NPC2,* Niemann-Pick protein type C2; *PCSK9,* proprotein convertase subtilisin/kexin type 9.

Cystic Fibrosis

Cystic fibrosis (CF) is an inherited disorder of epithelial ion transport affecting fluid secretion in exocrine glands and the epithelial linings of the respiratory, gastrointestinal, and reproductive tracts. The ion transport defects lead to abnormally viscid mucous secretions that block the airways and the pancreatic ducts, which in turn are responsible for the two most important clinical manifestations: (1) recurrent and chronic pulmonary infections and (2) pancreatic insufficiency. In addition, although the exocrine sweat glands are structurally normal (and remain so throughout the course of this disease), *a high level of sodium chloride in the sweat is a consistent, characteristic biochemical finding in CF.* At the same time, it must be remembered that CF can present with a bewilderingly variable set of clinical findings. This variation in phenotype results from diverse mutations in *CFTR,* the gene encoding the CF transmembrane conductance regulator, and the influence of disease modifier genes.

With an incidence of 1 in 2500 live births in the United States, CF is the most common life-limiting genetic disease that affects

individuals of European descent. The carrier frequency in the United States is 1 in 20 among individuals of European descent but significantly lower among individuals of other ancestral origins. CF follows simple autosomal recessive transmission, although even heterozygous carriers have a predisposition toward pulmonary and pancreatic disease at higher rates than the general population.

Pathogenesis. **The primary defect in CF is reduced production or abnormal function of CFTR, an epithelial chloride and bicarbonate channel protein.** Disruptive mutations in *CFTR* render the epithelial membranes relatively impermeable to chloride ions (Fig. 4.7). The impact of this defect on transport function is tissue specific.

- The major function of the CFTR protein in the sweat gland ducts is to reabsorb luminal chloride ions and augment sodium reabsorption through the epithelial sodium channel (ENaC). Therefore, in the sweat ducts, loss of CFTR function leads to decreased

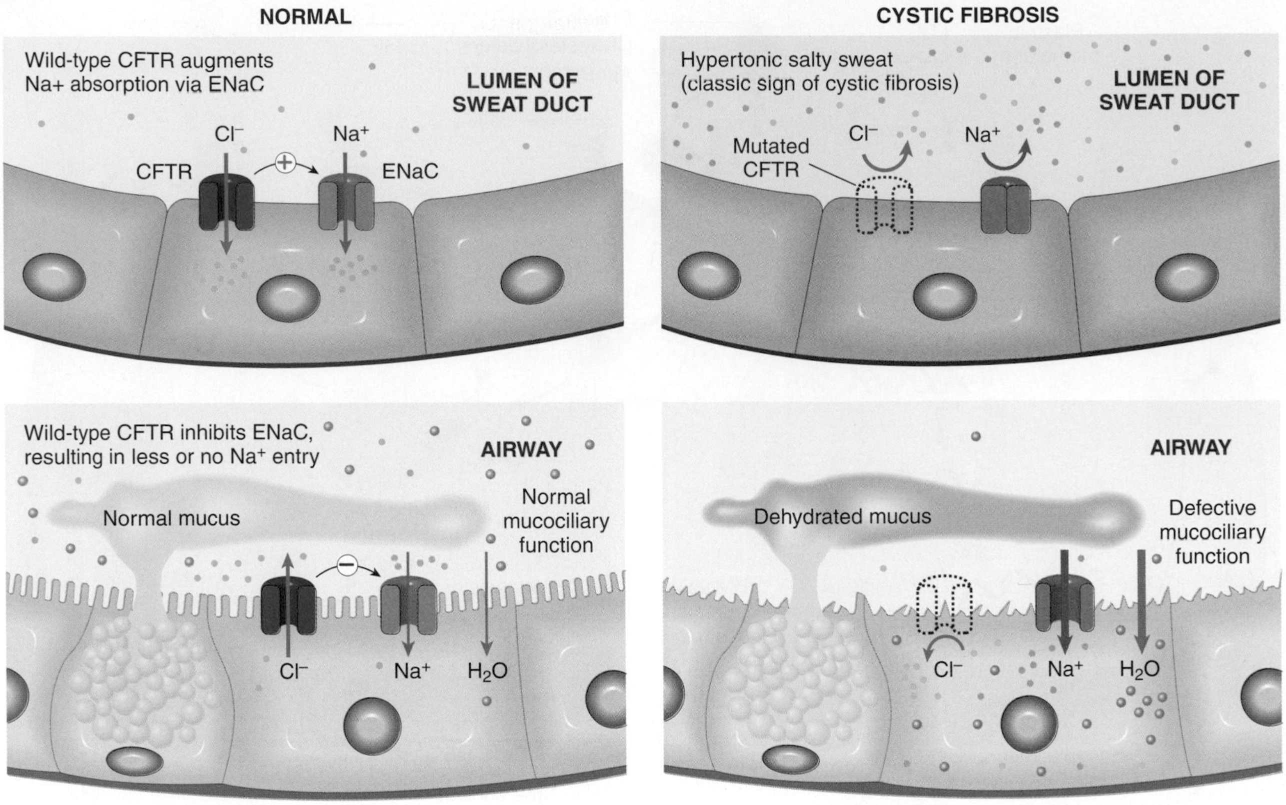

FIG. 4.7 *(Top)* In cystic fibrosis, a chloride channel defect in the sweat duct causes increased chloride and sodium concentration in sweat. *(Bottom)* Patients with cystic fibrosis have decreased chloride secretion and increased sodium and water reabsorption in the airways, leading to dehydration of the mucus layer coating epithelial cells, defective mucociliary action, and mucous plugging. *CFTR,* Cystic fibrosis transmembrane conductance regulator; *ENaC,* epithelial sodium channel.

reabsorption of sodium chloride and production of hypertonic ("salty") sweat (see Fig. 4.7, *top*).

- In contrast to sweat glands, CFTR in the respiratory and intestinal epithelium is one of the most important avenues for active luminal secretion of chloride. At these sites, CFTR mutations result in loss or reduction of chloride secretion into the lumen (see Fig. 4.7, *bottom*). Because of loss of inhibition of the ENaC activity, active luminal sodium absorption through ENaCs is increased, and both of these ion changes increase passive water reabsorption from the lumen, lowering the water content of the surface fluid layer coating mucosal cells. Thus, unlike the sweat ducts, there is no difference in the salt concentration of the surface fluid layer coating the respiratory and intestinal mucosal cells in unaffected individuals and in those with CF. Instead, respiratory and intestinal complications in CF seem to stem from dehydration of the surface fluid layer. In the lungs, this dehydration leads to impaired mucociliary action and the accumulation of concentrated, viscid secretions that obstruct the air passages and predispose to recurrent pulmonary infections. Viscid secretions also may obstruct pancreatic ducts and the vas deferens, leading to pancreatic insufficiency and male infertility, respectively.
- CFTR also regulates the transport of bicarbonate ions in the epithelial cells of the exocrine pancreas, and defective CFTR function therefore leads to reduced bicarbonate secretion and the acidification of pancreatic secretions. This results in precipitation of mucin and diminished activity of digestive enzymes such as trypsin that

function best under alkaline conditions, both of which exacerbate pancreatic insufficiency.

Since *CFTR* was cloned in 1989, more than 2000 disease-causing mutations have been identified. They can be classified on the basis of the clinical features or the nature of the underlying defect. Mechanistically, they may produce disease by reducing the transport of CFTR to the cell surface or by impairing CFTR function. *CFTR* mutations can also be classified as severe or mild, depending on the clinical phenotype. Severe mutations are associated with complete loss of CFTR protein function, whereas mild mutations allow some residual function. The most common *CFTR* mutation is a deletion of three nucleotides coding for phenylalanine at amino acid position 508 (ΔF508) that causes misfolding of CFTR, leading to its degradation within the cell. The small amount of mutated ΔF508 protein that reaches the cell surface is also dysfunctional. Worldwide, the ΔF508 mutation is found in approximately 70% of patients with CF. Although CF remains one of the best-known examples of the "one gene–one disease" axiom, there is increasing evidence that other genes modify the frequency and severity of organ-specific manifestations. Two of these modifier genes encode mannose-binding lectin 2 (MBL2) and transforming growth factor-β1 (TGF-β1). It is postulated that polymorphisms in these genes influence the ability of the lungs to tolerate infections with virulent microbes (see later), thus modifying the natural history of CF.

MORPHOLOGY

Patients with CF can present with a multitude of manifestations (Fig. 4.8). **Pancreatic abnormalities** are present in 85% to 90% of patients. In milder cases, there may be only accumulations of mucus in the small ducts, with some dilation of the exocrine glands. In more advanced cases, usually seen in older children or adolescents, the ducts are totally plugged, causing atrophy of the exocrine glands and progressive fibrosis (Fig. 4.9). The total loss of pancreatic exocrine secretion impairs fat absorption and may lead to vitamin A deficiency. This may contribute to squamous metaplasia of the lining epithelium of the pancreatic ducts, which may exacerbate injury caused by the inspissated mucus secretions. Thick viscid plugs of mucus may also be found in the small intestine of infants. These may cause small bowel obstruction, known as **meconium ileus.**

The **pulmonary changes** are the most serious complications of CF (Fig. 4.10). These changes stem from obstruction of the air passages by viscous mucus secretions of submucosal glands and superimposed infections. The bronchioles are often distended with thick mucus, associated with marked hyperplasia and hypertrophy of the mucus-secreting cells. Superimposed infections give rise to severe chronic bronchitis and bronchiectasis. Development of lung abscesses is common. *Staphylococcus aureus* (including methicillin resistant variants), *Pseudomonas aeruginosa*, and nontuberculous mycobacteria are the three most common organisms responsible for lung infections. Even more sinister is the increasing frequency of infection with another pseudomonad, *Burkholderia cepacia*. *B. cepacia*, originally thought to be a single species, is now known to consist of multiple separate species, collectively known as B. cepacia complex. This opportunistic bacterium is particularly hardy, and infection with this organism has been associated with fulminant illness ("cepacia syndrome"). The **liver involvement** follows the same basic pattern. Bile canaliculi are plugged by mucinous material, accompanied by ductular proliferation and portal inflammation. Hepatic **steatosis** ("fatty liver") is a common finding in liver biopsies. With time, cirrhosis develops, resulting in diffuse hepatic nodularity. Such severe hepatic involvement is encountered in less than 10% of patients. **Azoospermia** and **infertility** are found in 95% of the affected males who survive to adulthood. CF often causes atrophy of the vas deferens during the development of the embryo leading to **bilateral absence of the vas deferens**. In some males, this may be the only feature suggesting an underlying *CFTR* mutation.

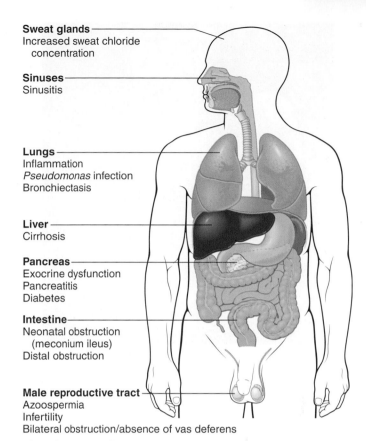

Sweat glands
Increased sweat chloride concentration

Sinuses
Sinusitis

Lungs
Inflammation
Pseudomonas infection
Bronchiectasis

Liver
Cirrhosis

Pancreas
Exocrine dysfunction
Pancreatitis
Diabetes

Intestine
Neonatal obstruction
 (meconium ileus)
Distal obstruction

Male reproductive tract
Azoospermia
Infertility
Bilateral obstruction/absence of vas deferens

FIG. 4.8 Tissues affected in patients with cystic fibrosis. (Adapted from Cutting GR: Cystic fibrosis genetics: from molecular understanding to clinical application. *Nat Rev Genet* 16:45, 2015.)

Clinical Features. Few childhood diseases display clinical manifestations as protean as CF (see Fig. 4.8). Approximately 5% to 10% of the cases come to clinical attention at birth or soon after because of meconium ileus. Exocrine pancreatic insufficiency occurs in 85% to 90% of patients and is associated with "severe" *CFTR* mutations of both alleles (e.g., ΔF508/ΔF508). By contrast, 10% to 15% of patients who have one "severe" and one "mild" *CFTR* mutation or two "mild" *CFTR* mutations have sufficient pancreatic exocrine function to avoid the need for enzyme supplementation (pancreas-sufficient phenotype). Pancreatic insufficiency is associated with malabsorption and increased fecal loss of protein and fat. Manifestations of malabsorption (e.g., large, foul-smelling stools; abdominal distention; poor weight gain) appear during the first year of life. Faulty fat absorption may induce deficiency states of fat-soluble vitamins, resulting in manifestations of vitamin A, D, or K deficiency (Chapter 7). Protein malnutrition may be sufficiently severe to cause hypoproteinemia and generalized edema. Persistent diarrhea may result in rectal prolapse in as many as 10% of children with CF. The pancreas-sufficient phenotype is usually not associated with other gastrointestinal complications, and, in general, these patients

demonstrate excellent growth and development. In contrast to exocrine insufficiency, endocrine insufficiency (i.e., diabetes) is uncommon in CF and occurs late in the course of the disease.

In the United States, in patients who receive follow-up care in CF centers, cardiorespiratory complications, such as chronic cough, persistent lung infections, obstructive pulmonary disease, and cor pulmonale, constitute the most common cause of death (accounting for approximately 80% of fatalities). By 18 years of age, 80% of

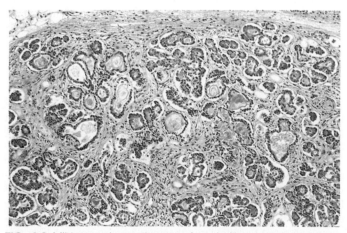

FIG. 4.9 Mild to moderate changes of cystic fibrosis in the pancreas. The ducts are dilated and plugged with eosinophilic mucin, and the parenchymal glands are atrophic and replaced by fibrous tissue.

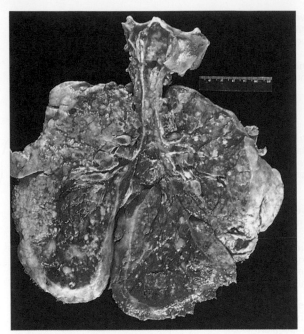

FIG. 4.10 Lungs of a patient who died of cystic fibrosis. Extensive mucous plugging and dilation of the tracheobronchial tree are apparent. The pulmonary parenchyma is consolidated by a combination of both secretions and pneumonia; the greenish discoloration is the product of *Pseudomonas* infections. (Courtesy of Dr. Eduardo Yunis, Children's Hospital of Pittsburgh, Pittsburgh, Pennsylvania.)

patients with severe CF harbor *Pseudomonas aeruginosa*, and a subset also harbor *Burkholderia cepacia*. With the indiscriminate use of antibiotic prophylaxis, there has been an unfortunate resurgence of resistant strains of *Pseudomonas* in many patients. Significant liver disease occurs late in the natural history of CF and is foreshadowed by pulmonary and pancreatic involvement; with increasing life expectancy, liver disease is now the third most common cause of death in patients with CF (after cardiopulmonary and transplant-related complications).

The clinical spectrum of CF is broader than the "classic" multisystem disease described earlier. For example, some patients suffering from recurrent bouts of abdominal pain and pancreatitis since childhood who were previously classified as having "idiopathic" chronic pancreatitis are now known to harbor biallelic *CFTR* variants that are distinct from those seen in "classic" CF. CF carriers were initially thought to be asymptomatic, but studies suggest that they have an increased lifetime risk for chronic lung disease (especially bronchiectasis) and recurrent sinonasal polyps. In most cases, the diagnosis of CF is based on persistently elevated sweat electrolyte concentrations (the mother says her infant "tastes salty"), characteristic clinical findings (sinopulmonary disease and gastrointestinal manifestations), or a family history. Sequencing the *CFTR* gene is the gold standard for diagnosis of CF.

There have been major improvements in the management of acute and chronic complications of CF, including more potent antimicrobial therapies, pancreatic enzyme replacement, and bilateral lung transplantation. These advances have extended the median life expectancy to 40 years, changing a lethal disease of childhood into a chronic disease of adults. Drug therapies are also now available that improve the folding, membrane expression, and function of mutated CFTR molecules. It is too early to determine the impact of these emerging molecular therapies on prognosis and survival.

Diseases Caused by Mutations in Genes Encoding Enzymes

Phenylketonuria (PKU)

PKU results from mutations that cause a severe lack of the enzyme phenylalanine hydroxylase (PAH) leading to hyperphenylalaninemia. It affects 1 in 10,000 live-born infants of European descent, and there are several variants of this disease. The most common form is referred to as classic phenylketonuria; its incidence is higher in European populations and less common in individuals from other geographic regions.

Homozygotes with this autosomal recessive disorder classically have a severe lack of PAH, leading to hyperphenylalaninemia and PKU. They are unaffected at birth but within a few weeks exhibit a rising plasma phenylalanine level, which impairs brain development. Usually, by 6 months of life severe mental disability becomes evident. The vast majority has intelligence quotients (IQs) less than 60. About one-third of these children never walk, and two-thirds cannot talk. Seizures, other neurologic abnormalities, decreased pigmentation of hair and skin, and eczema often accompany the mental disability in untreated children. Hyperphenylalaninemia and the resultant mental disability can be avoided by restricting phenylalanine intake early in life. Hence, several screening procedures are routinely performed to detect PKU in the immediate postnatal period. Dietary treatment is recommended for life.

Female patients with PKU who discontinue dietary treatment in adulthood may appear to be healthy but have marked hyperphenylalaninemia. Between 75% and 90% of children born to such women have severe mental disability and are microcephalic, and 15% have congenital heart disease, even though the infants themselves are heterozygotes. This syndrome, termed maternal PKU, results from the teratogenic effects of phenylalanine or its metabolites that cross the placenta and affect specific fetal organs during development.

Pathogenesis. **The biochemical abnormality in PKU is the inability to convert phenylalanine into tyrosine.** In children with normal PAH activity, less than 50% of the dietary intake of phenylalanine is necessary for protein synthesis. The remainder is converted to tyrosine by the phenylalanine hydroxylase system (Fig. 4.11). When phenylalanine metabolism is blocked because of a lack of PAH enzyme, shunt pathways are activated, yielding several intermediates that are excreted in large amounts in the urine and in the sweat. These impart a strong musty or mousy odor to affected infants. It is believed that excess phenylalanine or its metabolites contribute to the brain damage in PKU. Concomitant lack of tyrosine (see Fig. 4.11), a precursor of melanin, is responsible for the light color of hair and skin.

Approximately 1000 mutant alleles of *PAH* have been identified, only some of which cause a severe deficiency of the enzyme. Infants with mutations resulting in severe PAH deficiency develop classic features of PKU, whereas those with some PAH activity may develop milder disease or may be asymptomatic, a condition referred to as *benign hyperphenylalaninemia*. Because the numerous disease-causing alleles of the *PAH* gene complicate molecular diagnosis, measurement of serum phenylalanine levels is used to differentiate benign hyperphenylalaninemia from PKU; the levels in the latter disorder typically are ≥5 times higher than normal. After a biochemical diagnosis is established, the specific mutation causing PKU can be determined. With this information, carrier testing of at-risk family members can be

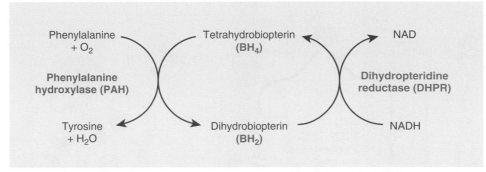

FIG. 4.11 The phenylalanine hydroxylase system. *NADH,* Nicotinamide adenine dinucleotide, reduced form.

performed. Currently, enzyme infusion therapy is being tested in patients with classic PKU. The infused enzyme, known as phenylalanine ammonia lyase (or PAL), converts excess phenylalanine to ammonia and other metabolites, thereby alleviating the toxic effects of phenylalanine.

Galactosemia

Galactosemia is an autosomal recessive disorder of galactose metabolism resulting from a mutation in the gene encoding the enzyme galactose-1-phosphate uridyltransferase (GALT). It affects 1 in 53,000 live-born infants in the United States. Lactase splits lactose, the major carbohydrate of mammalian milk, into glucose and galactose in the intestinal microvilli. Galactose is then converted to glucose in several steps, one of which requires the enzyme GALT. Due to this transferase deficiency, galactose-1-phosphate and other metabolites, including galactitol, accumulate in many tissues, including the liver, spleen, lens of the eye, kidney, cerebral cortex, and red cells.

The liver, eyes, and brain bear the brunt of the damage. The early-onset hepatomegaly results largely from fatty change, but in time widespread scarring that resembles the cirrhosis of excess alcohol use may supervene (Chapter 14). Opacification of the lens (cataract) develops, probably because the lens absorbs water and swells as galactitol (produced by alternative metabolic pathways) accumulates, increasing tonicity. Nonspecific alterations appear in the central nervous system, including loss of nerve cells, gliosis, and edema. There is still no clear understanding of the mechanism of injury to the brain, although elevated galactitol levels in neuronal tissues suggest that this may contribute to the damage.

Almost from birth, affected infants fail to thrive. Vomiting and diarrhea appear within a few days of milk ingestion. Jaundice and hepatomegaly usually become evident during the first week of life. Accumulation of galactose and galactose-1-phosphate in the kidney impairs amino acid transport, resulting in aminoaciduria. Fulminant *Escherichia coli* septicemia occurs with increased frequency. Newborn screening tests are widely utilized in the United States. They depend on fluorometric assay of GALT enzyme activity on a dried blood spot. A positive screening test must be confirmed by quantitative assay of GALT levels in red cells.

Many of the clinical and morphologic changes of galactosemia can be prevented or ameliorated by removal of galactose from the diet for at least the first 2 years of life. If instituted soon after birth, this diet prevents cataracts and liver damage and development is only mildly impaired. Even with dietary restrictions, however, older patients are frequently affected by a speech disorder and gonadal failure (especially premature ovarian failure) and, less commonly, by ataxia.

Lysosomal Storage Diseases

Lysosomes, the digestive system of cells, contain a variety of hydrolytic enzymes that are involved in the breakdown, and subsequent recycling, of complex substrates, such as sphingolipids and mucopolysaccharides, into soluble end products. These substrates may be derived from the turnover of intracellular organelles that enter the lysosomes by *autophagy,* or they may be acquired from outside the cell by endocytosis or phagocytosis. With an inherited lack of a lysosomal enzyme, catabolism of its substrate remains incomplete, leading to accumulation of partially degraded insoluble metabolites within the lysosomes (Fig. 4.12). Stuffed with incompletely digested macromolecules, lysosomes become large and numerous enough to interfere with normal cell functions. Because lysosomal function is also essential for autophagy, impaired autophagy gives rise to *additional storage* of autophagic substrates such as polyubiquitinated proteins and dysfunctional mitochondria. The absence of this quality-control mechanism causes accumulation of defective mitochondria, which can trigger the generation of free radicals and apoptosis.

Approximately 70 lysosomal storage diseases have been identified. These may result from abnormalities of lysosomal enzymes or proteins involved in substrate degradation, endosomal sorting, or lysosomal membrane integrity. Lysosomal storage disorders are divided into categories based on the biochemical nature of the substrates and the accumulated metabolites (Table 4.3). Within each group are several entities, each resulting from the deficiency of a specific enzyme.

Although the combined frequency of lysosomal storage disorders (LSDs) is about 1 in 2500 live births, lysosomal dysfunction may be involved in the etiology of several more-common diseases. For example, an important genetic risk factor for developing Parkinson disease is the carrier state for Gaucher disease, and virtually all Gaucher disease patients develop Parkinson disease. Niemann Pick C is another LSD connected to risk for Alzheimer disease. These associations stem from the multifunctionality of the lysosome. Lysosomes play critical roles in (1) autophagy, resulting from fusion with the autophagosome; (2) immunity, as they fuse with phagosomes; and (3) membrane repair, through fusion with the plasma membrane.

Despite this complexity, certain features are common to most diseases in this group:

- *Autosomal recessive transmission*
- *Patient population consisting of infants and young children*
- *Storage of insoluble intermediates in the mononuclear phagocyte system,* giving rise to hepatosplenomegaly
- *Frequent CNS involvement* with associated neuronal damage
- *Cellular dysfunction caused not only by storage of undigested material but also by a cascade of secondary events,* for example, macrophage activation and release of cytokines

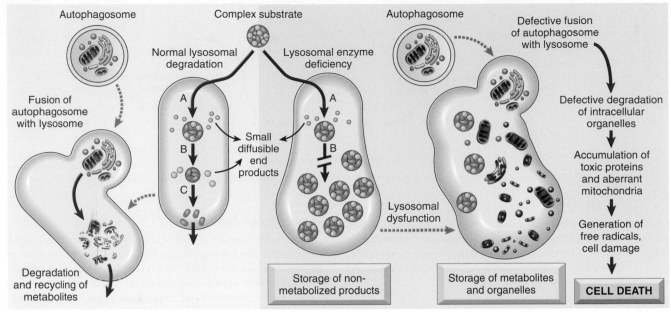

FIG. 4.12 Pathogenesis of lysosomal storage diseases. In this example, a complex substrate is normally degraded by a series of lysosomal enzymes labeled A, B, and C into small soluble end products. If there is a deficiency or malfunction of one of the enzymes (e.g., B), catabolism is incomplete, and insoluble intermediates accumulate in the lysosomes. In addition to this primary storage, secondary storage and toxic effects result from defective autophagy.

Table 4.3 Selected Lysosomal Storage Disorders

Disease	Enzyme Deficiency	Major Accumulating Metabolites
Glycogenosis, type 2-Pompe disease	α-1,4-Glucosidase (lysosomal glucosidase)	Glycogen
Sphingolipidoses		
GM1 gangliosidosis	GM1 ganglioside β-galactosidase	GM1 ganglioside, galactose-containing oligosaccharides
GM2 gangliosidosis		
Tay-Sachs disease	Hexosaminidase A	GM2 ganglioside
Sandhoff disease	Hexosaminidase A and B	GM2 ganglioside, globoside
Sulfatidoses		
Metachromatic leukodystrophy	Arylsulfatase A	Sulfatide
Krabbe disease	Galactosylceramidase	Galactocerebroside
Fabry disease	α-Galactosidase A	Ceramide trihexoside
Gaucher disease	Glucocerebrosidase	Glucocerebroside
Niemann-Pick disease: types A and B	Sphingomyelinase	Sphingomyelin
Mucopolysaccharidoses (MPSs)		
MPS I H (Hurler)	α-L-Iduronidase	Dermatan sulfate, heparan sulfate
MPS II (Hunter)	l-Iduronosulfate sulfatase	
Mucolipidoses (MLs)		
I-cell disease (ML II) and pseudo-Hurler polydystrophy	Deficiency of phosphorylating enzymes essential for the formation of mannose-6-phosphate recognition marker; acid hydrolases lacking the recognition marker cannot be targeted to the lysosomes but are secreted extracellularly	Mucopolysaccharide, glycolipid
Other lysosomal storage diseases		
Wolman disease	Acid lipase	Cholesterol esters, triglycerides
Acid phosphate deficiency	Lysosomal acid phosphatase	Phosphate esters

Most of these conditions are very rare, and their detailed description is better relegated to specialized texts and reviews. Only a few of the more common conditions are considered here.

Tay-Sachs Disease (GM2 Gangliosidosis: Hexosaminidase α-Subunit Deficiency). **Gangliosidoses are characterized by accumulation of gangliosides, principally in the brain, as a result of a deficiency of one of the lysosomal enzymes that catabolize these glycolipids.** Depending on the ganglioside involved, these disorders are subclassified into GM1 and GM2 categories. Tay-Sachs disease, by far the most common of all gangliosidoses, is caused by loss-of-function mutations of the alpha subunit of the enzyme *hexosaminidase A,* which is necessary for the degradation of GM2. More than 100 mutations have been described; most disrupt protein folding or intracellular transport. Due to founder effects, Tay-Sachs disease, similar to other lipid storage disorders, has an increased prevalence among individuals of Ashkenazi Jewish ancestry, among whom the frequency of heterozygous carriers is estimated to be 1 in 30. The Ashkenazim originated in Eastern and Central Europe and constitute more than 90% of the Jewish population in the United States. Heterozygote carriers can be detected by measuring the level of hexosaminidase in serum or by DNA sequencing.

Pathogenesis. In the absence of hexosaminidase A, GM2 ganglioside accumulates in many tissues (e.g., heart, liver, spleen, nervous system), but the **involvement of neurons in the central and autonomic nervous systems and retina dominates the clinical picture.** The accumulation of GM2 occurs within neurons, axon cylinders of nerves, and glial cells throughout the CNS. Affected cells appear swollen and sometimes foamy (Fig. 4.13A). Electron microscopy shows whorled onionskin-like configurations within lysosomes composed of layers of membranes (Fig. 4.13B). These pathologic changes are found throughout the CNS (including the spinal cord), peripheral nerves, and autonomic nervous system. The retina is usually involved as well, where the pallor produced by swollen ganglion cells in the peripheral retina results in a contrasting "cherry red" spot in the relatively unaffected central macula.

The molecular basis for neuronal injury is not fully understood. Because in many cases the mutant protein is misfolded, it induces the so-called "unfolded protein" response (Chapter 1). If such misfolded enzymes are not stabilized by chaperones, they undergo proteasomal degradation, leading to accumulation of toxic substrates and intermediates within neurons. These findings have spurred clinical trials of molecular chaperone therapy for some variants of later-onset Tay-Sachs and other selected lysosomal storage diseases. Such therapy involves the use of synthetic chaperones that can cross the blood—brain barrier, bind to the mutated protein, and enable its proper folding, thereby generating sufficient enzyme activity to restore cellular health.

In the most common acute infantile variant of Tay-Sachs disease, motor weakness begins at 3 to 6 months of age, followed by neurologic impairment, onset of blindness, and progressively more severe neurologic dysfunctions. Death occurs within 2 to 3 years.

Niemann-Pick Disease Types A and B. **Type A and type B Niemann-Pick diseases are related entities characterized by a primary deficiency of *acid sphingomyelinase* and the resultant accumulation of sphingomyelin.** As with Tay-Sachs disease, there is an increased incidence of Niemann-Pick disease types A and B in persons of Ashkenazi Jewish ancestry. The gene for acid sphingomyelinase is one of the imprinted genes that is preferentially expressed from the maternal chromosome as a result of epigenetic silencing of the paternal gene (discussed later).

In type A, characterized by a severe deficiency of sphingomyelinase, the breakdown of sphingomyelin into ceramide and phosphorylcholine is impaired, and excess sphingomyelin accumulates in phagocytic cells and in neurons. Macrophages become stuffed with droplets or particles of the complex lipid, imparting a fine vacuolation or foaminess to the cytoplasm (Fig. 4.14). Electron microscopy shows engorged secondary lysosomes that often contain membranous cytoplasmic bodies resembling concentric lamellated myelin figures, sometimes called "zebra" bodies. Because of their high content of phagocytic cells, the organs most severely affected are the spleen, liver, bone marrow, lymph nodes, and lungs. Splenic enlargement may be striking. In addition, the entire CNS, including the spinal cord and ganglia, is involved in this inexorable process. The affected neurons are enlarged and vacuolated as a result of the accumulation of lipids. This variant manifests in infancy with massive organomegaly and severe neurologic deterioration. Death usually occurs within the first 3 years of life. By comparison, patients with the type B variant, which is associated with mutant sphingomyelinase with some residual activity,

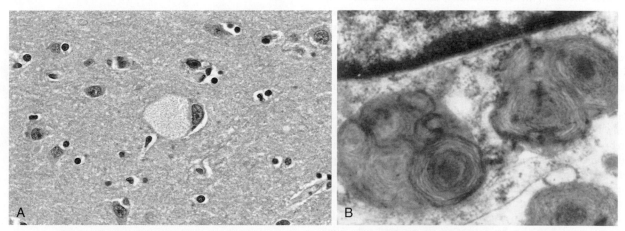

FIG. 4.13 Ganglion cells in Tay-Sachs disease. (A) Under the light microscope, a large neuron has obvious lipid vacuolation. (B) A portion of a neuron under the electron microscope shows prominent lysosomes with whorled configurations just below part of the nucleus. (A, Courtesy of Dr. Arthur Weinberg, Department of Pathology, University of Texas Southwestern Medical Center, Dallas, Texas. B, Courtesy of Dr. Joe Rutledge, Children's Regional Medical Center, Seattle, Washington.)

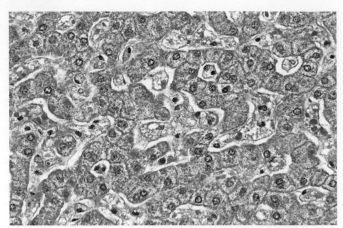

FIG. 4.14 Niemann-Pick type A disease in liver. The hepatocytes and Kupffer cells have a foamy, vacuolated appearance resulting from deposition of lipids. (Courtesy of Dr. Arthur Weinberg, Department of Pathology, University of Texas Southwestern Medical Center, Dallas, Texas.)

have organomegaly but no neurologic manifestations. Estimation of sphingomyelinase activity in the leukocytes can be used for diagnosis of suspected cases, as well as for detection of carriers. Molecular genetic tests are also available for diagnosis at specialized centers.

Niemann-Pick Disease Type C. Although previously considered to be related to type A and type B, Niemann-Pick disease type C (NPC) is molecularly and biochemically distinct and is more common than types A and B combined. Mutations in two related genes, *NPC1* and *NPC2*, give rise to this disorder, with *NPC1* being responsible for a majority of cases. Unlike most other lysosomal storage diseases, NPC results from a primary defect in lipid transport. Both NPC1 and NPC2 are involved in the transport of free cholesterol from the lysosomes to the cytoplasm (see Fig. 4.6). Affected cells accumulate cholesterol as well as gangliosides such as GM1 and GM2. NPC is clinically heterogeneous. The most common form manifests in childhood and is marked by ataxia, vertical supranuclear gaze palsy, dystonia, dysarthria, and psychomotor regression.

Gaucher Disease. **Gaucher disease results from mutations in the gene that encodes *glucocerebrosidase,* and the resultant deficiency of this enzyme leads to an accumulation of glucocerebroside, an intermediate in glycolipid metabolism, in mononuclear phagocytic cells.** There are three autosomal recessive variants of Gaucher disease resulting from distinct allelic mutations. Common to all is deficient activity of glucocerebrosidase, which catalyzes the cleavage of a glucose residue from ceramide. Normally, macrophages, particularly in the liver, spleen, and bone marrow, sequentially degrade glycolipids derived from the breakdown of senescent blood cells. In Gaucher disease, the degradation stops at the level of glucocerebrosides, which accumulate in macrophages. These cells—so-called "Gaucher cells"—become enlarged, with some reaching a diameter as great as 100 μm, because of the presence of distended lysosomes, and they acquire a pathognomonic cytoplasmic appearance resembling "wrinkled tissue paper" (Fig. 4.15). It is now evident that Gaucher disease is caused not just by the burden of storage material but also by activation of macrophages. High levels of macrophage-derived cytokines, such as interleukins (IL-1, IL-6) and tumor necrosis factor (TNF), are found in affected tissues.

One variant, type 1, also called the chronic nonneuronopathic form, accounts for 99% of cases of Gaucher disease. It is characterized by clinical or radiographic bone involvement (osteopenia, focal lytic lesions, and osteonecrosis) in 70% to 100% of cases. Additional features are hepatosplenomegaly and the absence of CNS involvement. The spleen often enlarges to massive proportions, filling the entire abdomen. Gaucher cells are found in the liver, spleen, lymph nodes, and bone marrow. Marrow replacement and cortical erosion may produce radiographically visible skeletal lesions and peripheral blood cytopenias. It is believed that bone changes are caused by the aforementioned macrophage-derived cytokines. Unlike other variants, type 1 is compatible with long life. The carrier frequency of the type 1 in Ashkenazi Jewish population is quite high being close to 1 in 12. By comparison the carrier frequency in non-Jewish population is 1 in 40,000.

Neurologic signs and symptoms characterize types 2 and 3 variants. In type 2, these manifestations appear during infancy (*acute*

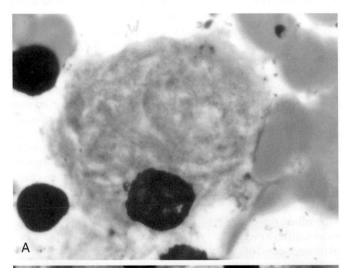

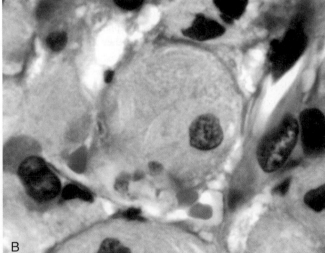

FIG. 4.15 Gaucher disease involving the bone marrow. (A and B) Gaucher cells are plump macrophages that characteristically have the appearance in the cytoplasm of crumpled tissue paper due to accumulation of glucocerebroside. (A) Wright stain; (B) hematoxylin and eosin. (Courtesy of Dr. John Anastasi, Department of Pathology, University of Chicago, Chicago, Illinois.)

infantile neuronopathic form) and are more severe, whereas in type 3, they emerge later and are milder *(chronic neuronopathic form).* Although the liver and spleen also are involved, the clinical features in types 2 and 3 are dominated by neurologic disturbances, including convulsions and progressive mental deterioration.

As mentioned earlier, mutation of the glucocerebroside gene is a strong risk factor for Parkinson disease. Patients with Gaucher disease have a 20-fold higher risk of developing Parkinson disease (compared to controls), and 5% to 10% of patients with Parkinson disease have mutations in the gene encoding glucocerebrosidase. The level of glucocerebrosides in leukocytes or cultured fibroblasts is helpful in diagnosis and in the detection of heterozygote carriers. DNA testing is also available.

Currently, there are two approved therapies for type I Gaucher disease. The first is lifelong *enzyme replacement therapy* via infusion of recombinant glucocerebrosidase. The second, known as *substrate reduction therapy,* involves oral intake of an inhibitor of the enzyme glucosylceramide synthase. This leads to reduced systemic levels of glucocerebroside, the substrate for the defective enzyme in Gaucher disease. Substrate reduction therapy leads to reduced spleen and liver sizes, improved blood counts, and enhanced skeletal function. Other emerging treatments include gene therapy through transplant of hematopoietic stem cells engineered to express normal glucocerebrosidase.

Mucopolysaccharidoses. **Mucopolysaccharidoses (MPSs) are characterized by defective degradation and excessive storage of mucopolysaccharides in various tissues.** Recall that mucopolysaccharides are part of the extracellular matrix and are synthesized by connective tissue fibroblasts. Most mucopolysaccharide is secreted, but a fraction is degraded within lysosomes through a catabolic pathway involving multiple enzymes. Several clinical variants of MPS, classified numerically as MPS I to MPS VII, have been described, each resulting from the deficiency of one specific enzyme in this pathway. The mucopolysaccharides that accumulate within the tissues include dermatan sulfate, heparan sulfate, keratan sulfate, and (in some cases) chondroitin sulfate.

Hepatosplenomegaly; skeletal deformities; lesions of heart valves; subendothelial arterial deposits, particularly in the coronary arteries, and lesions in the brain are features that are seen in all MPSs. Coronary subendothelial lesions lead to myocardial infarction and cardiac decompensation. Most cases are associated with coarse facial features, clouding of the cornea, joint stiffness, and intellectual disability. Urinary excretion of the accumulated mucopolysaccharides is often increased. With all MPSs except one, the mode of inheritance is autosomal recessive; the exception, Hunter syndrome, is an X-linked recessive disease. Of the eleven recognized variants, only two well-characterized syndromes are discussed briefly here.

- *MPS type I, also known as Hurler syndrome, is caused by a deficiency of α-L-iduronidase.* In Hurler syndrome, affected children have a life expectancy of 6 to 10 years, and death is often a result of cardiac complications. Accumulation of mucopolysaccharides is seen in cells of the mononuclear phagocyte system, in fibroblasts, and within endothelium and smooth muscle cells of the vascular wall. The affected cells are swollen and have clear cytoplasm, resulting from the accumulation of stored material within engorged, vacuolated lysosomes. Lysosomal inclusions also are found in neurons, accounting for the intellectual disability.

- *MPS type II, or Hunter syndrome, is caused by a deficiency of L-iduronate sulfatase.* It differs from Hurler syndrome in its mode of inheritance (X-linked), the absence of corneal clouding, and its often milder clinical course. Diagnosis is made by measuring the level of *alpha-L-iduronidase* in leukocytes. DNA diagnosis is not routinely employed because of the large number of distinct causative mutations.

Glycogen Storage Diseases (Glycogenoses)

An inherited deficiency of enzymes involved in glycogen synthesis or degradation can result in excessive accumulation of glycogen or some abnormal form of glycogen in various tissues. The type of glycogen stored, its intracellular location, and the tissue distribution of the affected cells vary depending on the specific enzyme deficiency. Regardless of the tissue or cells affected, the glycogen is most often stored within the cytoplasm. One variant, Pompe disease, is also a form of lysosomal storage disease, because the missing enzyme is localized to lysosomes. Most glycogenoses are autosomal recessive diseases, as is common with "missing enzyme" syndromes.

Approximately a dozen forms of glycogenoses have been described in association with specific enzyme deficiencies. Based on pathophysiologic findings, they can be grouped into three categories (Table 4.4):

- *Hepatic type.* The liver contains several enzymes that synthesize glycogen for storage and break it down into free glucose. Hence, a deficiency of the hepatic enzymes involved in glycogen metabolism is associated with two major clinical effects: enlargement of the liver due to storage of glycogen and hypoglycemia due to a failure of glucose production (Fig. 4.16). *Von Gierke disease* (type I glycogenosis), resulting from a lack of glucose-6-phosphatase, is the most important example of the hepatic form of glycogenosis (see Table 4.4).

- *Myopathic type.* In striated muscle, glycogen is an important source of energy, and most forms of glycogen storage disease affect muscles. When enzymes that are involved in glycolysis are deficient, glycogen storage occurs in muscles and there is an associated muscle weakness due to impaired energy production. Typically, the myopathic forms of glycogen storage diseases are marked by muscle cramps after exercise, myoglobinuria, and failure of exercise to induce an elevation in blood lactate levels because of a block in glycolysis. In this category are included *McArdle disease* (type V glycogenosis), resulting from a deficiency of muscle phosphorylase, and type VII glycogenosis, resulting from a deficiency of muscle phosphofructokinase.

- Type II glycogenosis *(Pompe disease)* is caused by a deficiency of acid alpha glucosidase (lysosomal acid maltase) and is associated with deposition of glycogen in virtually every organ, but cardiomegaly is most prominent (eFig. 4.1). Most affected patients die within 2 years of onset of cardiorespiratory failure. Replacement therapy with glucosidase can reverse cardiac muscle damage and modestly increase longevity.

COMPLEX MULTIGENIC DISORDERS

Complex multigenic disorders—so-called "multifactorial" or "polygenic" disorders—are caused by interactions between genetic variants and environmental factors. A genetic variant that occurs in at least 1% of the population is called a polymorphism. According to

Table 4.4 Principal Subgroups of Glycogenoses

Clinicopathologic Category	Specific Type	Enzyme Deficiency	Morphologic Changes	Clinical Features
Hepatic type	Hepatorenal (von Gierke disease, type I)	Glucose-6-phosphatase	Hepatomegaly: intracytoplasmic accumulations of glycogen and small amounts of lipid; intranuclear glycogen Renomegaly: intracytoplasmic accumulations of glycogen in cortical tubular epithelial cells	In untreated patients, failure to thrive, stunted growth, hepatomegaly, and renomegaly Hypoglycemia resulting from failure of glucose mobilization, often leading to convulsions Hyperlipidemia and hyperuricemia resulting from deranged glucose metabolism; many patients develop gout and skin xanthomas Bleeding tendency caused by platelet dysfunction With treatment (providing continuous source of glucose), most patients survive and develop late complications (e.g., hepatic adenomas)
Myopathic type	McArdle disease (type V)	Muscle phosphorylase	Skeletal muscle only: accumulations of glycogen predominant in subsarcolemmal location	Painful cramps associated with strenuous exercise Myoglobinuria occurs in 50% of cases Onset in adulthood (>20 years) Muscular exercise fails to raise lactate level in venous blood Compatible with normal longevity
Miscellaneous type	Generalized glycogenosis (Pompe disease, type II)	Lysosomal acid alpha glucosidase (acid maltase)	Mild hepatomegaly: ballooning of lysosomes with glycogen creating lacy cytoplasmic pattern Cardiomegaly: glycogen within sarcoplasm as well as membrane bound Skeletal muscle: similar to heart	Massive cardiomegaly, muscle hypotonia, and cardiorespiratory failure before age 2 Milder adult form with only skeletal muscle involvement manifests with chronic myopathy

the common disease—common variant hypothesis, complex multigenic disorders occur when many polymorphisms, each with a modest effect and low penetrance, are coinherited. Three additional important facts have emerged from studies of common complex disorders such as type 1 diabetes:

- Although complex disorders result from the collective inheritance of many polymorphisms, *different polymorphisms vary in significance.* For example, of the 20 to 30 genes implicated in type 1 diabetes, 6 or 7 are most important, and a few HLA alleles contribute more than 50% of the risk (Chapter 18).
- *Some polymorphisms are common to multiple diseases of the same type, whereas others are disease specific.* These associations are well illustrated in immune-mediated inflammatory diseases (Chapter 5).
- *Many of the disease-associated polymorphisms are in noncoding regions,* so they likely affect epigenetic regulation of gene expression.

Several phenotypic characteristics, not associated with disease, are governed by multigenic inheritance, such as hair color, eye color, skin color, height, and intelligence. These characteristics show a continuous variation within, as well as across, all population groups. Environmental influences, however, significantly modify the phenotypic expression of complex traits. For example, type 2 diabetes has many of the features of a complex multigenic disorder. It is well recognized clinically that affected persons often first exhibit

clinical manifestations of this disease after weight gain. Thus, obesity, as well as other environmental influences, unmasks the diabetic genetic trait.

Assigning a disease to this mode of inheritance must be done with caution. Such attribution depends on many factors but first on familial clustering and the exclusion of mendelian and chromosomal modes of transmission. A range of levels of severity of a disease is suggestive of a complex multigenic disorder, but variable expressivity and reduced penetrance of single mutant genes also may account for this phenomenon.

CYTOGENETIC DISORDERS

Chromosomal abnormalities occur much more frequently than is generally appreciated. **It is estimated that approximately 1 in 200 newborn infants has some form of chromosomal abnormality. The figure is much higher in fetuses that do not survive to term; in as many as 50% of first-trimester spontaneous abortions, the fetus may have a chromosomal abnormality.** Cytogenetic disorders result from alterations in the number or structure of chromosomes and may affect autosomes or sex chromosomes.

Before embarking on a discussion of chromosomal aberrations, we review karyotyping as the basic tool of the cytogeneticist. **A karyotype is a digital representation of a stained metaphase spread in which the chromosomes are arranged in order of decreasing length.** A variety of techniques for staining chromosomes have been

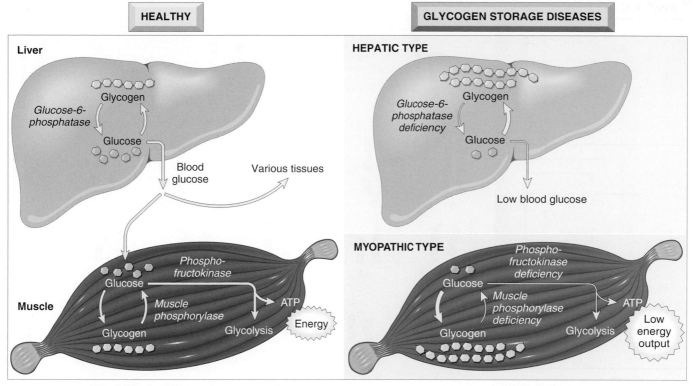

FIG. 4.16 *(Left)* A simplified scheme of normal glycogen metabolism in the liver and skeletal muscles. *(Top right)* The effects of an inherited deficiency of hepatic enzymes involved in glycogen metabolism. *(Bottom right)* The consequences of a genetic deficiency in the enzymes that metabolize glycogen in skeletal muscles.

developed. With the widely used Giemsa stain (G banding) technique, each chromosome displays a distinctive pattern of alternating light and dark bands of variable widths (Fig. 4.17). The use of banding techniques allows identification of each chromosome and can detect and localize structural abnormalities that are large enough to produce changes in banding pattern (described later).

Numeric Abnormalities

In humans, the normal chromosome count in diploid cells is 46 (i.e., 2 each of 22 autosomes and 2 sex chromosomes, sometimes represented as 2n = 46). Any exact multiple of the haploid number (n) is called *euploid*. Chromosome numbers such as 3n and 4n are called *polyploid*. In the fetus, polyploidy generally results in a spontaneous abortion. Any number that is not an exact multiple of n is called *aneuploid*. The chief cause of aneuploidy is nondisjunction of a homologous pair of chromosomes in the zygote at the first meiotic division or a failure of sister chromatids to separate during the second meiotic division. The latter may also occur during mitosis in somatic cells, leading to the production of two aneuploid cells. Failure of pairing of homologous chromosomes followed by random assortment (anaphase lag) also can lead to aneuploidy.

When nondisjunction occurs at the time of meiosis, the gametes formed have either an extra chromosome (n + 1) or one fewer chromosome (n − 1). Fertilization of such gametes by normal gametes would result in two types of zygotes: trisomic, with an extra chromosome (2n + 1), or monosomic (2n − 1). Monosomy involving an autosome is incompatible with life, whereas trisomies of certain autosomes and monosomy involving sex chromosomes are compatible with development through the time of birth and, in the cases of trisomy 21, survival into adulthood.

Mosaicism is a term used to describe the presence of two or more populations of cells with different complements of chromosomes in the same individual. In the context of chromosome numbers, postzygotic mitotic nondisjunction would result in the production of a trisomic and a monosomic daughter cell; the descendants of these cells would then produce a mosaic. As discussed later, mosaicism affecting sex chromosomes is common, whereas autosomal mosaicism is not.

Structural Abnormalities

Structural changes in chromosomes typically result from chromosomal breakage followed by loss or rearrangement of material. Such changes usually are designated using a cytogenetic shorthand in which p (French, petit) denotes the short arm of a chromosome, and q, the long arm. Each arm is then divided into numbered regions (1, 2, 3, and so on) from centromere outward, and within each region the bands are numerically ordered (see Fig. 4.17). Thus, 2q34 indicates chromosome 2, long arm, region 3, band 4. The patterns of chromosomal rearrangement after breakage (Fig. 4.18) are as follows:

- *Translocation* implies transfer of a part of one chromosome to another chromosome. The process is usually reciprocal (i.e., fragments are exchanged between two chromosomes). In genetic shorthand, translocations are indicated by "t" followed by the involved chromosomes in numeric order—for example, 46,XX,t(2;5)(q31;p14). This notation would indicate a reciprocal translocation involving the long arm (q) of chromosome 2 at region 3, band 1, and the short arm of chromosome 5, region 1, band 4. When all the fragments are exchanged, the resulting *balanced reciprocal translocation* (see Fig. 4.18) is not harmful to the carrier, who has the normal number of chromosomes

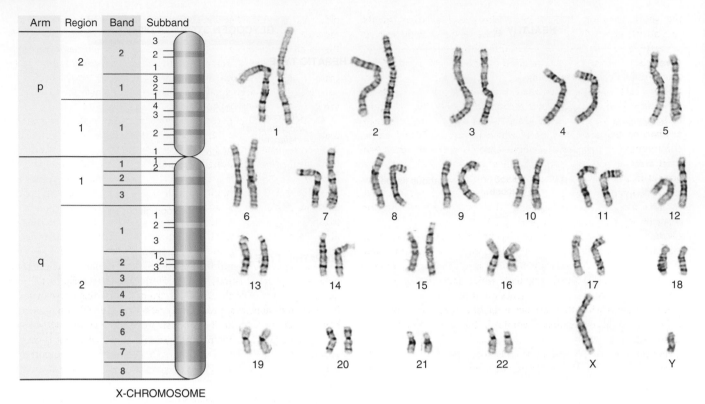

X-CHROMOSOME

FIG. 4.17 G-banded karyotype from a male (46,XY). Also shown is the banding pattern of the X chromosome with nomenclature of arms, regions, bands, and subbands. (Karyotype courtesy of Dr. Stuart Schwartz, Department of Pathology, University of Chicago, Chicago, Illinois.)

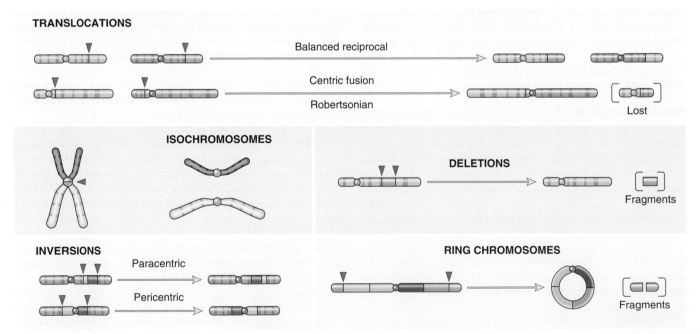

FIG. 4.18 Types of chromosomal rearrangements.

and the full complement of genetic material, unless at least one of the breakpoints involves a critical gene. However, during gametogenesis, abnormal (unbalanced) gametes are formed, resulting in abnormal zygotes. A special pattern of translocation involving two acrocentric chromosomes is called *centric fusion type,* or

Robertsonian, translocation. The breaks typically occur close to the centromere, affecting the short arms of both chromosomes. Transfer of the segments leads to one very large chromosome and one extremely small one (see Fig. 4.18); the latter is subsequently lost, leaving the carrier with 45 chromosomes. Because the short arms of all acrocentric chromosomes carry highly redundant genes (e.g., ribosomal RNA genes), such loss is compatible with survival. However, difficulties arise during gametogenesis, resulting in the formation of unbalanced gametes that could lead to diseased offspring.

- *Isochromosomes* result when there is a homologous exchange of pericentric DNA between sister chromatids, producing two chromosomes composed of two p arms or two q arms, one of which has two centromeres and one of which is acentric. The acentric chromosome is then lost, leaving a chromosome with only two short arms or two long arms. The most common isochromosome present in live births involves the long arm of the X chromosome and is designated i(Xq). When fertilization occurs by a gamete that contains a normal X chromosome, the result is monosomy for genes on Xp and trisomy for genes on Xq.
- *Deletion* involves loss of a portion of a chromosome. A single break may delete a terminal segment. Two interstitial breaks, with union of the proximal and distal segments, may result in loss of an internal segment. The isolated fragment, which lacks a centromere, almost never survives, and thus genes are lost.
- *Inversions* occur when there are two interstitial breaks in a chromosome and the released segment reunites in the opposite orientation of normal.
- A *ring chromosome* is a variant of a deletion. After loss of segments from each end of the chromosome, the arms unite to form a ring.

General Features of Chromosomal Disorders

- Chromosomal disorders may be associated with absence (deletion, monosomy), excess (trisomy), or abnormal rearrangements (translocations) of chromosomes.
- In general, a loss of chromosomal material produces more severe defects than does a gain of chromosomal material.
- Excess chromosomal material may result from a complete chromosome (as in trisomy) or from part of a chromosome (as in Robertsonian translocation).
- Imbalances of sex chromosomes (excess or loss) are tolerated much better than similar imbalances of autosomes.
- Sex chromosomal disorders often produce subtle changes, sometimes not detected at birth. Infertility, a common manifestation, cannot be diagnosed until adolescence.
- In most cases, chromosomal disorders result from de novo changes (i.e., parents are healthy, and risk of recurrence in siblings is low). The translocation form of Down syndrome (described later) exhibits an uncommon but important exception to this principle.

Some specific examples of diseases involving changes in the karyotype are presented next.

Cytogenetic Disorders Involving Autosomes

Three autosomal trisomies (21, 18, and 13) and one deletion syndrome (affecting 22q) occur with sufficient frequency to merit consideration.

Trisomy 21 (Down Syndrome)

Down syndrome, characterized by an extra copy of chromosome 21, is the most common of the chromosomal disorders (Fig. 4.19). About 95% of affected persons have trisomy 21, resulting in a chromosome count of 47. As mentioned earlier, the most common cause of trisomy 21 is meiotic nondisjunction. The parents of such children are unaffected. Maternal age has a strong influence on the incidence of Down syndrome, which occurs in 1 in 1550 live births in women younger than 20 years, in contrast with 1 in 25 live births in women

older than 45 years. The correlation with maternal age suggests that in most cases the meiotic nondisjunction of chromosome 21 occurs in the ovum. Indeed, in 95% of cases the extra chromosome is of maternal origin. The reason for the increased susceptibility of the ovum to nondisjunction with aging is not understood. No effect of paternal age has been found in those cases in which the extra chromosome is derived from the father.

In about 4% of patients with trisomy 21, the extra chromosomal material is present as a translocation of the long arm of chromosome 21 to chromosome 22 or 14. Such cases frequently (but not always) are familial, and the translocated chromosome is inherited from one of the parents, who typically is a carrier of a Robertsonian translocation. Approximately 1% of patients with trisomy 21 are mosaics, usually having a mixture of 46- and 47-chromosome cells. These cases result from mitotic nondisjunction of chromosome 21 during an early stage of embryogenesis. Clinical manifestations in such cases are variable and milder, depending on the proportion of abnormal cells.

The diagnostic clinical features of this condition—flat facial profile, oblique palpebral fissures, and epicanthic folds (see Fig. 4.19)—are usually apparent at birth. Down syndrome is a leading cause of severe intellectual disability; approximately 80% of those with this syndrome have an IQ of 25 to 50. By contrast, some mosaics with Down syndrome have mild phenotypic changes and intelligence that is average or near average. In addition to the phenotypic findings and the intellectual disability already noted, several other clinical features are worthy of mention:

- *Approximately 40% of patients have congenital heart disease,* most commonly defects of the endocardial cushion, including atrial septal defects, atrioventricular valve malformations, and ventricular septal defects (Chapter 9). Cardiac pathology accounts for a majority of the deaths in infancy and early childhood. Several other congenital malformations, including atresias of the esophagus and small bowel, are also common.
- Children with trisomy 21 have a *10- to 20-fold increased risk of developing acute leukemia.* Both acute lymphoblastic leukemias and acute myeloid leukemias occur (Chapter 10).
- Virtually all patients with trisomy 21 older than age 40 develop *neuropathologic changes* characteristic of Alzheimer disease, a degenerative disorder of the brain (Chapter 21).
- Patients with Down syndrome demonstrate *abnormal immune responses* that predispose them to serious infections, particularly of the lungs, and to thyroid autoimmunity (Chapter 18). Although several abnormalities, affecting mainly T cell functions, have been reported, the basis for the immunologic disturbances is not clear.
- In addition, anomalies affecting various other organ systems also occur at a higher frequency than normal. These include gastrointestinal disorders (stenosis of the intestines and Hirschsprung disease); ophthalmologic disorders (cataracts and refractive errors); hearing loss; slow growth rate; and urologic anomalies (cryptorchidism and hypospadias).

Despite these issues, improved medical care has increased the longevity of persons with trisomy 21. Currently the median age at death is 60 years (up from 25 years in 1983). Although the karyotype of Down syndrome has been known for decades, the molecular basis for the disease remains elusive. Extra "doses" of genes located on chromosome 21 have been implicated, such as the gene for amyloid-beta precursor, which is related to Alzheimer disease. In addition, regulation of genes by various micro-RNAs and long noncoding RNAs have been implicated; but causality has not been established for any of these. Several prenatal screening tests are used to diagnose trisomy 21.

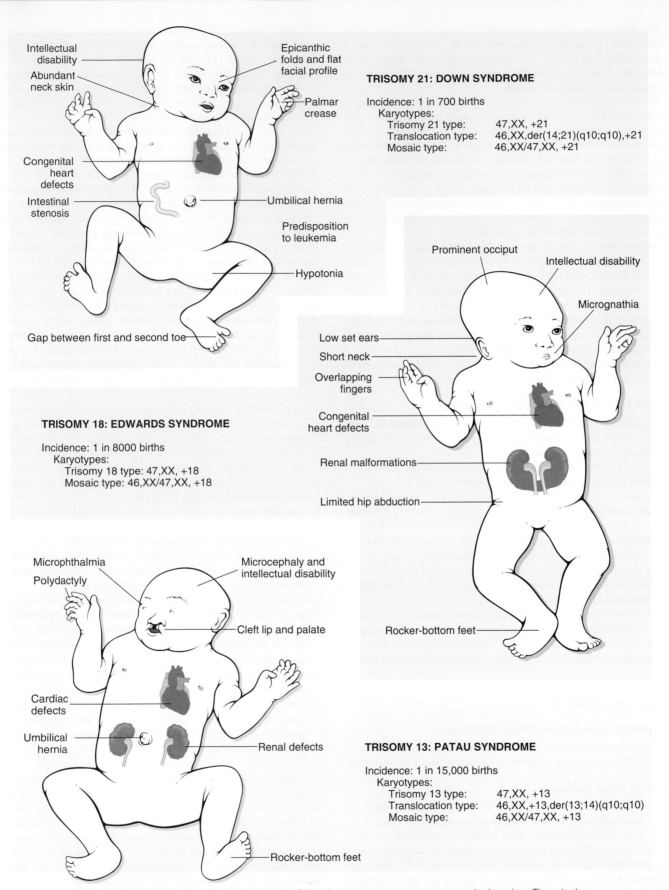

Intellectual disability

Abundant neck skin

Epicanthic folds and flat facial profile

Palmar crease

Congenital heart defects

Intestinal stenosis

Umbilical hernia

Predisposition to leukemia

Hypotonia

Gap between first and second toe

TRISOMY 21: DOWN SYNDROME

Incidence: 1 in 700 births
    Karyotypes:
        Trisomy 21 type: 47,XX, +21
        Translocation type: 46,XX,der(14;21)(q10;q10),+21
        Mosaic type: 46,XX/47,XX, +21

Prominent occiput

Intellectual disability

Micrognathia

Low set ears

Short neck

Overlapping fingers

Congenital heart defects

Renal malformations

Limited hip abduction

Rocker-bottom feet

TRISOMY 18: EDWARDS SYNDROME

Incidence: 1 in 8000 births
    Karyotypes:
        Trisomy 18 type: 47,XX, +18
        Mosaic type: 46,XX/47,XX, +18

Microphthalmia

Polydactyly

Microcephaly and intellectual disability

Cleft lip and palate

Cardiac defects

Umbilical hernia

Renal defects

TRISOMY 13: PATAU SYNDROME

Incidence: 1 in 15,000 births
    Karyotypes:
        Trisomy 13 type: 47,XX, +13
        Translocation type: 46,XX,+13,der(13;14)(q10;q10)
        Mosaic type: 46,XX/47,XX, +13

Rocker-bottom feet

FIG. 4.19 Clinical features and karyotypes of the three most common autosomal trisomies. Though the karyotype is shown with XX chromosomes, individuals may have an XY karyotype.

These include measurement of maternal blood levels of β-HCG (increased) and pregnancy-associated plasma protein A (PAPP) (decreased), and ultrasound assessment of nuchal folds. PAPP is secreted by syncytiotrophoblast, and a low level indicates poor placental function. The basis of high β-HCG levels in Down syndrome is not clear.

Much progress is being made in the molecular diagnosis of Down syndrome prenatally. Approximately 5% to 10% of the total cell-free DNA in maternal blood is derived from the fetus and can be identified by polymorphic genetic markers. By using next-generation sequencing, the gene dosage of chromosome 21-linked genes in fetal DNA can be determined with great precision. This has emerged as a sensitive and specific noninvasive method ("liquid biopsy") for prenatal diagnosis of trisomy 21 as well as other trisomies. Currently, all cases of trisomy 21 identified by the screening tests or by liquid biopsies are confirmed by conventional cytogenetics on fetal cells obtained by amniocentesis.

22q11.2 Deletion Syndrome

The 22q11.2 deletion syndrome encompasses a spectrum of disorders that result from a small interstitial deletion of band 22q11 on the long arm of chromosome 22. The clinical features of this syndrome include congenital heart disease affecting the outflow tracts, abnormalities of the palate, facial dysmorphism, developmental delay, thymic hypoplasia with impaired T-cell immunity (Chapter 5), and parathyroid hypoplasia resulting in hypocalcemia (Chapter 18). Previously, these clinical features were believed to represent two different disorders: DiGeorge syndrome and velocardiofacial syndrome. However, it is now known that both are caused by 22q11.2 deletion. Variations in the size and position of the deletion are thought to be responsible for the differing clinical manifestations. When T-cell immunodeficiency and hypocalcemia are the dominant features, the patients are said to have *DiGeorge syndrome,* whereas patients with the so-called *velocardiofacial syndrome* have mild immunodeficiency and pronounced dysmorphology and cardiac defects. In addition to these malformations, patients with 22q11.2 deletion are at high risk for schizophrenia and bipolar disorder. In fact, it is estimated that schizophrenia develops in approximately 25% of adults with this syndrome. Conversely, deletions of the region are found in 2% to 3% of individuals with childhood-onset schizophrenia. The molecular basis of this syndrome is not fully understood because the affected region of chromosome 11 contains many genes, some encoding proteins and others noncoding (regulatory) RNAs.

The diagnosis may be suspected on clinical grounds but can be established only by detection of the deletion, typically by fluorescence in situ hybridization (FISH) (see later Fig. 4.41B).

Cytogenetic Disorders Involving Sex Chromosomes

A number of abnormal karyotypes involving the sex chromosomes, ranging from 45,X to 49,XXXXY, are compatible with life. Indeed, phenotypically typical males with two and even three Y chromosomes have been identified. Such extreme karyotypic changes are not encountered with the autosomes. In large part, this flexibility relates to two factors: (1) lyonization of X chromosomes and (2) the small amount of genetic information carried by the Y chromosome. Any discussion of lyonization must begin with Mary Lyon, who in 1962 proposed that in females only one X chromosome is genetically active. X inactivation occurs early in fetal life, about 16 days after conception. Either the paternal or the maternal X chromosome is randomly inactivated in each cell of the developing embryo. Once inactivated, the same X chromosome remains inactive in all the progeny of these

cells. Moreover, all but one X chromosome is inactivated, so even a 48,XXXX female has only one active X chromosome. This phenomenon explains why females do not have a double dose (compared with males) of phenotypic attributes encoded on the X chromosome. The Lyon hypothesis also explains why females are mosaics, composed of two cell populations: one with an active maternal X, the other with an active paternal X. The molecular basis of X inactivation involves a long noncoding RNA that is encoded by the *XIST* gene. This noncoding RNA is retained in the nucleus, where it "coats" the X chromosome from which it is transcribed and silences the genes on that chromosome. The other *XIST* allele is switched off in the active X, allowing genes encoded on only one X chromosome to be expressed.

Although essentially accurate, the Lyon hypothesis has been subsequently modified. Most important, the initial presumption that all the genes on the inactive X are "switched off" is incorrect, as roughly 30% of genes on Xp, and a smaller number (3%) on Xq, escape X inactivation. This observation has implications for monosomic X chromosome disorders (Turner syndrome) as discussed later.

Extra Y chromosomes are readily tolerated because the only information known to be carried on the Y chromosome seems to relate to male differentiation. Of note, whatever the number of X chromosomes, the presence of a Y invariably dictates the male phenotype. The gene for male differentiation (*SRY*, sex-determining region of the Y chromosome) is located on the short arm of the Y chromosome.

Described briefly next are two disorders, Klinefelter syndrome and Turner syndrome, which result from aberrations of sex chromosomes.

Klinefelter Syndrome

Klinefelter syndrome is defined by male hypogonadism in an individual with at least two X chromosomes and one or more Y chromosomes. It is one of the most common causes of hypogonadism in males. Most affected patients have a 47,XXY karyotype that results from nondisjunction of sex chromosomes during meiosis. Maternal and paternal nondisjunction contribute equally to the occurrence of Klinefelter syndrome. Approximately 15% of patients show mosaic patterns, including 46,XY/47,XXY, 47,XXY/48,XXXY, and variations on this theme. The presence of a 46,XY line in mosaics is usually associated with a milder clinical condition.

Clinical Features. Klinefelter syndrome is associated with a wide range of clinical manifestations. In some individuals, only hypogonadism is noted, but most patients have a distinctive body habitus with an increase in length between the soles and the pubic bone, which creates the appearance of an elongated body. Reduced facial, body, and pubic hair and gynecomastia are also frequently seen. The testes are markedly reduced in size, sometimes to only 2 cm in greatest dimension. In keeping with the testicular atrophy, the serum testosterone levels are lower than normal, and urinary gonadotropin (FSH) levels are elevated.

Only rarely are patients with the Klinefelter syndrome fertile, and presumably such persons are mosaics with a large proportion of 46,XY cells. Sterility is due to impaired spermatogenesis, sometimes to the extent of total azoospermia. Histologic examination shows hyalinization of tubules, which appear as ghostlike structures in tissue sections. By contrast, Leydig cells are prominent, as a result of either hyperplasia or an apparent increase related to loss of tubules.

Cognitive abilities range from average to below average with modest deficit in verbal skills. Patients with Klinefelter syndrome develop several comorbid conditions. There is an increased incidence of type 2 diabetes and the metabolic syndrome that gives rise to insulin resistance. Patients are also at a higher risk for congenital heart disease, particularly mitral valve prolapse, which is seen in about 50% of adults. They have a 20- to 30-fold higher risk of developing extragonadal germ cell tumors, mostly mediastinal teratomas. In addition, breast cancer and autoimmune diseases such as systemic lupus erythematosus occur more frequently. It should be noted that the physical attributes described here are quite variable; hypogonadism is the only consistent finding.

Turner Syndrome

Turner syndrome, characterized by primary hypogonadism in phenotypic females, results from partial or complete monosomy of the short arm of the X chromosome.

With routine cytogenetic methods, three types of karyotypic abnormalities are seen in individuals with Turner syndrome:

- *Approximately 57% are missing an entire X chromosome, resulting in a 45,X karyotype.* Of the remaining 43%, approximately one-third (14%) have structural abnormalities of the X chromosomes, and two-thirds (29%) are mosaics.
- *The common result of the structural abnormalities is partial monosomy of the X chromosome.* In order of frequency, the structural abnormalities of the X chromosome include (1) an isochromosome of the long arm, 46,X,i(X)(q10), resulting in the loss of the short arm; (2) deletion of portions of both long and short arms, resulting in the formation of a ring chromosome, 46,X,r(X); and (3) deletion of portions of the short or long arm, 46X,del(Xq) or 46X,del(Xp).
- *The patients who are mosaics have a 45,X cell population along with one or more karyotypically normal or abnormal cell types.* Examples of these karyotypes include the following: (1) 45,X/46,XX, (2) 45,X/46,XY, (3) 45,X/47,XXX, or (4) 45,X/46,X,i(X)(q10).
  - 5% to 10% of mosaic patients with Turner syndrome have Y chromosome sequences due to the presence of a complete Y chromosome (e.g., 45,X/46,XY karyotype) or fragments of Y chromosomes translocated on other chromosomes. These patients are at a higher risk for development of a gonadal tumor (gonadoblastoma).

Clinical Features. Typical clinical features associated with 45,X Turner syndrome include growth retardation, leading to abnormally short stature (below the third percentile); swelling of the nape of the neck because of distended lymphatic channels (in infancy) that manifests as webbing of the neck in older children; low posterior hairline; cubitus valgus (an increase in the carrying angle of the arms); shieldlike chest with widely spaced nipples; high-arched palate; lymphedema of the hands and feet; and a variety of congenital malformations such as horseshoe kidney, bicuspid aortic valve, and coarctation of the aorta (Fig. 4.20).

Cardiovascular abnormalities are the most common cause of death in childhood. In adolescence, affected girls fail to develop typical secondary sex characteristics; the genitalia remain infantile, breast development is minimal, and little pubic hair appears. *Most patients have primary amenorrhea, and morphologic examination shows transformation of the ovaries into white streaks of fibrous stroma devoid of follicles.* The intellect of these patients usually is within normal limits, but subtle defects in visual—spatial information processing have been noted. Curiously, hypothyroidism caused by autoantibodies occurs frequently, especially in women with isochromosome Xp. As many as 50% of these patients develop clinical hypothyroidism. In adult patients, a combination of short stature and primary amenorrhea should prompt strong suspicion for Turner syndrome. It is important to appreciate the karyotypic heterogeneity associated with Turner syndrome because it is responsible for

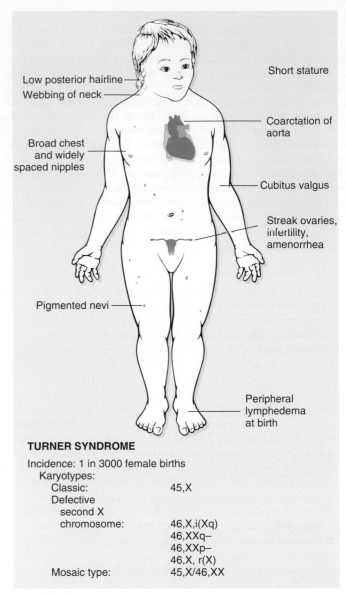

TURNER SYNDROME

Incidence: 1 in 3000 female births

Karyotypes:

Classic:	45,X
Defective second X chromosome:	46,X,i(Xq)
	46,XXq–
	46,XXp–
	46,X, r(X)
Mosaic type:	45,X/46,XX

FIG. 4.20 Clinical features and karyotypes of Turner syndrome.

significant variations in the phenotype. In contrast with the patients with monosomy X, those who are mosaics or have deletion variants may have minimal phenotypic findings and may present only with primary amenorrhea. The diagnosis is established by karyotyping.

Pathogenesis. The pathogenesis of Turner syndrome is not well understood, but studies have begun to shed some light. As mentioned earlier, both X chromosomes are active during oogenesis and are essential for normal development of the ovaries. During normal fetal development, ovaries contain as many as 7 million oocytes. The oocytes gradually disappear so that by menarche their numbers have dwindled to a mere 400,000, and when menopause occurs, fewer than 10,000 remain. In Turner syndrome, fetal ovaries develop normally early in embryogenesis, but the absence of the second X chromosome leads to an accelerated loss of oocytes, which is complete by age 2 years. In a sense, therefore, "menopause occurs before menarche," and the ovaries are reduced to atrophic fibrous strands, devoid of ova and follicles (*streak ovaries*).

Because patients with Turner syndrome also have other (non-gonadal) abnormalities, it follows that genes required for normal growth and development of somatic tissues also must reside on the X chromosome. Among the genes involved in the Turner phenotype is the short stature homeobox *(SHOX)* gene at Xp22.33. This is one of the genes that remains active in both X chromosomes and is unique in having an active homolog on the short arm of the Y chromosome. Thus, both unaffected males and females have two active copies of this gene. Loss of one copy of *SHOX* gives rise to short stature. Indeed, deletions of the *SHOX* gene are noted in 2% to 5% of otherwise un-affected children with short stature. Whereas loss of one copy of *SHOX* can explain the growth deficit in Turner syndrome, it cannot explain other important clinical features such as cardiac malformations and endocrine abnormalities. Clearly, several other genes located on the X chromosome are also involved.

SINGLE-GENE DISORDERS WITH ATYPICAL PATTERNS OF INHERITANCE

Three groups of diseases resulting from mutations affecting single genes do not follow the mendelian rules of inheritance:
- Diseases caused by *triplet repeat mutations*
- Diseases caused by *mutations in mitochondrial genes*
- Diseases associated with *alteration of imprinted regions of the genome*

Triplet Repeat Mutations

Fragile X Syndrome (FXS)

Fragile X syndrome is the prototype of diseases in which the causative mutation occurs in a long repeating sequence of three nucleotides. Other examples of diseases associated with trinucleotide repeat mutations are Huntington disease, myotonic dystrophy, and various forms of spinocerebellar ataxia. This type of mutation is now known to cause about 50 diseases, and all disorders discovered so far are associated with neurodegenerative changes. In each of these conditions, amplification of specific sets of three nucleotides within the gene disrupts its function. Certain unique features of trinucleotide repeat mutations, described later, are responsible for the atypical pattern of inheritance of the associated diseases.

FXS is the most common genetic cause of intellectual disability in males and overall the second most common cause after Down syndrome. It results from a trinucleotide expansion mutation in the *familial mental retardation 1 (FMR1)* **gene.** It has a frequency of 1 in 1550 for males and 1 in 8000 for females. Although discovered initially as the cause of FXS, expansion mutations affecting *FMR1* are now known to be present in two other well-defined disorders—fragile X—associated tremor/ataxia syndrome and fragile X—associated primary ovarian insufficiency.

We begin our discussion of these disorders with consideration of FXS. This syndrome derives its name from the karyotypic appearance of the X chromosome in the original method of diagnosis. Culturing patient cells in a folate-deficient medium typically showed a discontinuity of staining or constriction in the long arm of the X chromosome. This method has now been supplanted by DNA-based analysis of triplet repeat size, as discussed later. Clinically affected males have severe intellectual disability. The typical phenotype includes a long face with a large mandible; large, everted ears; and large testicles *(macroorchidism)*. Hyperextensible joints, a high arched palate, and mitral valve prolapse noted in some patients mimic a connective tissue disorder. Although characteristic of fragile X syndrome, these findings

are not always present or may be quite subtle. The only distinctive physical abnormality that can be detected in at least 90% of post-pubertal males with fragile X syndrome is macroorchidism.

In addition to intellectual disability, several neurologic and neuropsychiatric manifestations have been recognized in patients with FXS. These include epilepsy in 30% of cases, aggressive behavior in 90% of cases, autism spectrum disorder, and anxiety disorder/hyperactivity disorder.

As with all X-linked diseases, fragile X syndrome predominantly affects males. Analysis of several pedigrees, however, shows some patterns of transmission not typically associated with other X-linked recessive disorders (Fig. 4.21). These include the following:
- *Carrier males.* Approximately 20% to 50% of males who, by pedigree analysis and molecular tests, are known to carry a trinucleotide expansion in the *FMR1* gene do not manifest the typical neurologic symptoms. Because carrier males transmit the trait through all their phenotypically normal daughters to affected grandchildren, they are called *normal transmitting males.*
- *Affected females.* Approximately 20% of carrier females are affected (i.e., have intellectual disability as well as other features described below), a number much higher than that in other X-linked recessive disorders.
- *Anticipation.* This term refers to the phenomenon whereby clinical features of fragile X syndrome worsen with each successive generation, as the mutation is transmitted from a man to his grandsons and great-grandsons.
- In addition to these complexities, more recent studies have revealed that a fraction of carrier males and females develop phenotypically and mechanistically distinct disorders—fragile X-associated tremor/ataxia syndrome and fragile X-associated primary ovarian insufficiency. These will be described below.

These unusual features of FXS have been related to the dynamic nature of the mutation. In unaffected individuals, the number of repeats of the sequence CGG in the *FMR1* gene is small, averaging around 29, whereas affected persons have 200 to 4000 repeats. These so-called "full mutations" are believed to arise through an intermediate stage of premutations characterized by 52 to 200 CGG repeats. Carrier males and females have premutations. During oogenesis (but not spermatogenesis), premutations can be converted to full mutations by further amplification of the CGG repeats, which can then be transmitted to both the sons and the daughters of the carrier female. These observations provide an explanation for why some carrier males are unaffected (they have premutations), and certain carrier females are affected (they inherit full mutations).

Pathogenesis. The molecular basis for fragile X syndrome is related to the silencing of the product of the *FMR1* gene, familial mental retardation protein (FMRP). The normal *FMR1* gene contains CGG repeats in its 5′ untranslated region. When the number of trinucleotide repeats exceeds approximately 230, the DNA of the 5′ region of the gene becomes hypermethylated, including the promoter region, resulting in transcriptional suppression of *FMR1*. FMRP is widely expressed in normal tissues, but higher levels are found in the brain and the testis. It is an RNA-binding protein that is transported from the cytoplasm to the nucleus, where it binds specific mRNAs and transports them to the axons and dendrites (Fig. 4.22). It is in the synapses that FMRP—mRNA complexes perform critical roles in regulating the translation of specific mRNAs involved in control of synaptic functions. A reduction in FMRP results in increased translation of the bound mRNAs at synapses. This leads to an

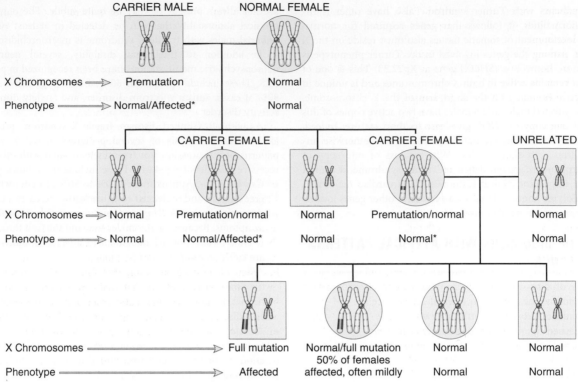

FIG. 4.21 Fragile X pedigree. X and Y chromosomes are shown. Note that in the first generation, all sons are healthy and all females are carriers (harbor a premutation). During oogenesis in the carrier female, premutation expands to full mutation; hence, in the next generation, all males who inherit the X with full mutation are affected. However, only 50% of females who inherit the full mutation are affected, and often only mildly. *As mentioned in the text 50% of carrier males develop a tremor/ataxia syndrome and 20% of carrier females develop premature ovarian failure. (Based on an original sketch courtesy of Dr. Nancy Schneider, Department of Pathology, University of Texas Southwestern Medical School, Dallas, Texas.)

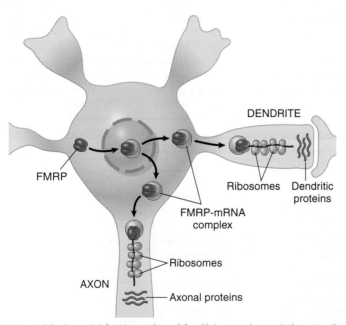

FIG. 4.22 A model for the action of familial mental retardation protein (FMRP) in neurons. FMRP plays a critical role in regulating the translation of proteins from bound RNAs at synaptic junctions. These locally produced proteins, in turn, regulate synaptic plasticity which is important for learning and memory. (Adapted from Hin P, Warren ST: New insights into fragile X syndrome: from molecules to neurobehavior. *Trends Biochem Sci* 28:152, 2003.)

imbalance in the production of proteins at the synapses and results in loss of synaptic plasticity—the ability of synapses to change and adapt in response to specific signals, which is essential for learning and memory.

Fragile X—Associated Tremor/Ataxia Syndrome and Fragile X—Associated Primary Ovarian Failure

CGG premutations in the *FMR1* gene can also cause two disorders that are phenotypically different from FXS and occur through a distinct mechanism involving a toxic gain of function. These entities were discovered when it was noted that approximately 20% of females carrying the premutation (carrier females) have premature ovarian failure (before the age of 40 years). This condition is called *fragile X—associated primary ovarian failure.* Affected women have menstrual irregularities and decreased fertility. Approximately 50% of premutation-carrying males (transmitting males) exhibit a progressive neurodegenerative syndrome starting in their sixth decade. This syndrome, referred to as *fragile X—associated tremor/ataxia*, is characterized by intention tremors and cerebellar ataxia and may progress to parkinsonism.

Pathogenesis. How do premutations cause disease? In a subset of carrier females and transmitting male patients, the *FMR1* gene instead of being methylated and silenced continues to be transcribed. CGG-containing *FMR1* mRNAs so formed are "toxic." They recruit RNA-binding proteins and impair their function by sequestration from their normal locales. In affected males, the expanded *FMR1* mRNA and the sequestered RNA-binding proteins aggregate in the nucleus and form intranuclear inclusions in both the central and the peripheral nervous systems. The pathogenesis of fragile X—associated primary ovarian insufficiency is less well understood. Aggregates containing *FMR1* mRNA have been detected in granulosa cells and ovarian stromal cells. Perhaps these aggregates cause premature death of ovarian follicles.

As noted earlier, many other neurodegenerative diseases related to trinucleotide repeat expansions are recognized. Some general principles follow:

- In all cases, gene functions are altered by an expansion of the repeats, but the precise threshold at which premutations are converted to full mutations differs with each disorder.
- Whereas the expansion of premutation to full mutation in fragile X syndrome occurs during oogenesis, in other disorders such as Huntington disease, premutations are converted to full mutations during spermatogenesis.
- The expansion may involve any part of the gene, and the range of possibilities can be divided into two broad categories: those that affect untranslated regions (as in fragile X syndrome) and those that affect coding regions (as in Huntington disease) (Fig. 4.23). Typically, when mutations affect noncoding regions, there is "loss of function," because protein synthesis is suppressed (e.g., FMRP). By contrast, mutations involving translated parts of the gene give rise to misfolded proteins (e.g., Huntington disease). Many of these so-called "toxic gain-of-function" mutations involve CAG repeats that encode polyglutamine tracts, and the resultant diseases, which primarily affect the nervous system, are sometimes referred to as polyglutamine diseases. Accumulation of misfolded proteins in aggregates within the cytoplasm is a common feature of such diseases.

Diseases Caused by Mutations in Mitochondrial Genes

The mitochondrial genome contains several genes that encode enzymes involved in oxidative phosphorylation. Inheritance of mitochondrial DNA differs from that of nuclear DNA in that the former is associated with maternal inheritance since ova contain the normal complement of mitochondria within their abundant cytoplasm, whereas spermatozoa contain few, if any, mitochondria. The mitochondrial DNA of the zygote is therefore derived entirely from the ovum. Thus, only mothers transmit mitochondrial genes to their offspring, both male and female.

Diseases caused by mutations in mitochondrial genes are rare. Because mitochondrial DNA encodes enzymes involved in oxidative phosphorylation, diseases caused by mutations in such genes preferentially affect the tissues that are most dependent on oxidative phosphorylation (e.g., CNS, skeletal muscle, cardiac muscle, liver, and kidney). *Leber hereditary optic neuropathy* is the prototypical disorder in this group. This neurodegenerative disease manifests as progressive bilateral loss of central vision that leads in due course to blindness.

Diseases Caused by Alterations of Imprinted Regions: Prader-Willi and Angelman Syndromes

All humans inherit two copies of each autosome, carried on homologous maternal and paternal chromosomes. It was long assumed that there was no difference between normal homologous genes derived from the mother and the father. Indeed, this is true for most genes. It has been established, however, that functional differences exist between the paternal and the maternal copies of some genes. **The differences arise from an epigenetic process called *genomic imprinting*, whereby certain homologous genes are differentially "inactivated" during paternal and maternal gametogenesis.** Maternal imprinting refers to transcriptional silencing of the maternal allele, whereas paternal imprinting indicates that the paternal allele is inactivated. At the molecular level, imprinting is associated with methylation of the gene promoter and modification of DNA-binding histone proteins, which act together to silence the gene. Imprinting occurs in ova or sperm and is then stably transmitted to all somatic cells derived from the zygote.

Genomic imprinting is best illustrated by considering two uncommon genetic disorders, Prader-Willi syndrome and Angelman syndrome.

Intellectual disability, short stature, hypotonia, obesity, small hands and feet, and hypogonadism characterize Prader-Willi syndrome. In 60% to 75% of cases, an interstitial deletion of band q12 in the long arm of chromosome 15—del(15)(q11;q13)—is detected. In such cases, the deletion affects the paternally derived chromosome 15. In contrast to Prader-Willi syndrome, patients with the phenotypically distinct Angelman syndrome are born with a deletion of the same

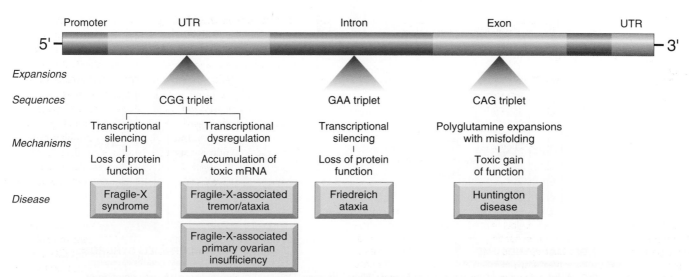

FIG. 4.23 Sites of expansion and the affected sequence in selected diseases caused by nucleotide repeat mutations. *UTR,* Untranslated region.

chromosomal region derived from their mothers. **Patients with Angelman syndrome also have intellectual disability, but in addition they present with ataxic gait, seizures, and inappropriate laughter.** A comparison of these two syndromes clearly demonstrates the "parent-of-origin" effects on gene function. If all the paternal and maternal genes contained within chromosome 15 were expressed in an identical fashion, clinical features resulting from these deletions would be expected to be identical regardless of the parental origin of chromosome 15.

Pathogenesis. The molecular basis of these two syndromes can be understood in the context of imprinting (Fig. 4.24). A set of genes on the maternal chromosome at 15q12 is imprinted (and hence silenced), so the paternal chromosome provides the only functional alleles. When these are lost as a result of a deletion in the paternal chromosome, the patient develops Prader-Willi syndrome. Among the set of genes that are deleted in Prader-Willi syndrome, the most likely culprit is believed to be a gene cluster encoding multiple distinct small nucleolar RNAs (snoRNAs), which are involved in messenger RNA processing. Conversely, a distinct gene, *UBE3A*, that also maps to the same region of chromosome 15 is imprinted on the paternal chromosome. *UBE3A* encodes for a ubiquitin ligase, a family of enzymes that targets other cellular proteins for proteasomal degradation through the addition of ubiquitin moieties. Only the maternally derived allele of the gene normally is active. Deletion of this maternal gene on chromosome 15 gives rise to Angelman syndrome. The neurologic manifestations of Angelman are principally due to a lack of *UBE3A* expression in specific regions of the brain.

Molecular studies of patients with Prader-Willi syndrome who have no cytogenetic abnormalities have shown that in some cases both of the structurally normal copies of chromosome 15 are derived from the mother. Inheritance of both chromosomes of a pair from one parent is called *uniparental disomy.* The net effect is the same as in patients with chromosome 15 deletions; functional copies of the implicated snoRNA genes are absent. Angelman syndrome, as might be expected, sometimes results from uniparental disomy of paternal chromosome 15.

PEDIATRIC DISEASES

As mentioned earlier and as illustrated by several examples, many diseases of infancy and childhood are of genetic origin. Others, although not genetic, either are unique to children or take distinctive forms in this patient population and thus merit the designation pediatric diseases.

Each stage of development of the infant and child is susceptible to a somewhat different group of disorders: (1) the neonatal period (the first 4 weeks of life); (2) infancy (the first year of life); (3) 1 to 4 years of age; and (4) 5 to 14 years of age. Congenital anomalies, prematurity and low birth weight, sudden infant death syndrome, and maternal complications and injuries are the leading causes of death in the first 12 months of life. Once the infant survives the first year of life, the outlook brightens measurably. In the next two age groups—1 to 4 years and 5 to 9 years—unintentional injuries resulting from accidents are the leading cause of death. Among the natural diseases, in order of importance, congenital anomalies and malignant neoplasms assume major significance. In the 10- to 14-year age group, firearm related injuries, accidents, malignancies, suicide, homicide, and congenital malformations are the leading causes of death. The following

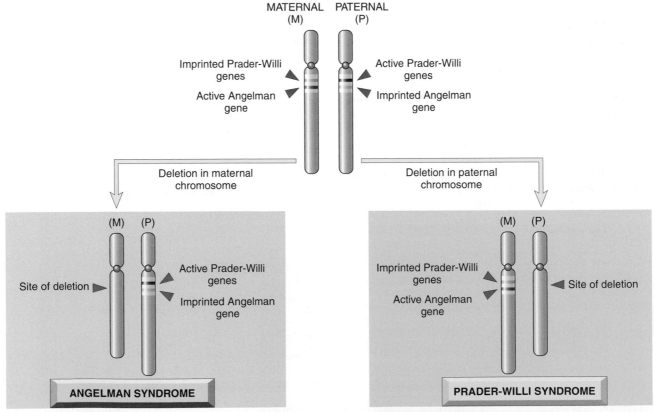

FIG. 4.24 Genetics of Angelman and Prader-Willi syndromes. Depicted is chromosome 15 with deletion of 15q.12.

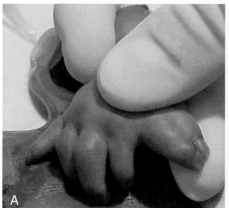 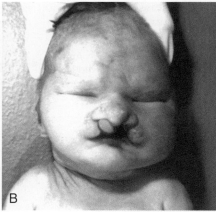 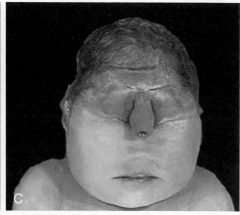

FIG. 4.25 Examples of malformations. Malformations range in severity from the incidental to the lethal. (A) Polydactyly (one or more extra digits) and syndactyly (fusion of digits) have little functional consequence when they occur in isolation. (B) Similarly, cleft lip, with or without associated cleft palate, is compatible with life when it occurs as an isolated anomaly; in this case, however, the child had an underlying malformation syndrome (trisomy 13) and expired because of severe cardiac defects. (C) Stillbirth associated with a lethal malformation, in which the midface structures are fused or ill formed; in almost all cases, this degree of external dysmorphogenesis is associated with severe internal anomalies, such as maldevelopment of the brain and cardiac defects. (A and C, Courtesy of Dr. Reade Quinton, Department of Pathology, University of Texas Southwestern Medical Center, Dallas, Texas. B, Courtesy of Dr. Beverly Rogers, Department of Pathology, University of Texas Southwestern Medical Center, Dallas, Texas.)

discussion looks at specific conditions encountered during the various stages of infant and child development.

CONGENITAL ANOMALIES

Congenital anomalies are structural defects that are present at birth, although some, such as cardiac defects and renal anomalies, may not become clinically apparent until years later. As will be evident from the ensuing discussion, the term congenital does not imply or exclude a genetic basis. It is estimated that about 120,000 babies are born with a birth defect each year in the United States, an incidence of 1 in 33. Congenital anomalies are an important cause of infant mortality. Moreover, they continue to be a significant source of illness, disability, and death throughout the early years of life.

Before considering the etiology and pathogenesis of congenital anomalies, we must define some of the terms used to describe errors in morphogenesis.

- *Malformations are primary errors of morphogenesis.* There is an intrinsically abnormal developmental process. Malformations are usually multifactorial, rather than the result of a single gene or chromosomal defect. They may manifest in any of several patterns. In some presentations, such as congenital heart diseases, single body systems may be involved, whereas in others, multiple malformations involving many organs and tissues may coexist (Fig. 4.25).
- *Disruptions result from secondary destruction of an organ or body region that was previously normal in development*; thus, in contrast with malformations, disruptions arise from an extrinsic disturbance in morphogenesis. Amniotic bands, stemming from rupture of amnion with resultant formation of "bands" that encircle, compress, or attach to parts of the developing fetus, constitute the classic example of a disruption (Fig. 4.26). A variety of environmental agents may cause disruptions (see later). Disruptions are not heritable, of course, and thus are not associated with risk of recurrence in subsequent pregnancies.

- *Deformations, like disruptions, also represent an extrinsic disturbance of development rather than an intrinsic error of morphogenesis.* Deformations are common, affecting approximately 2% of newborn infants to various degrees. They are caused by localized or generalized compression of the growing fetus by abnormal biomechanical forces, leading eventually to a variety of structural abnormalities. The most common cause of deformations is uterine constraint. Between weeks 35 and 38 of gestation, rapid increase in the size of the fetus outpaces the growth of the uterus, and the relative amount of amniotic fluid (which normally acts as a cushion) also decreases. Thus, even the healthy fetus is subjected to some

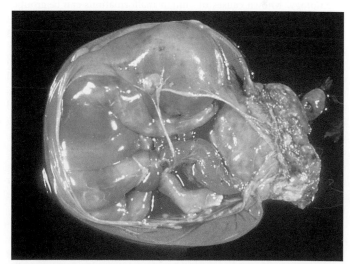

FIG. 4.26 Disruption due to amniotic bands. In the specimen shown, the placenta is at the right, and the band of amnion extends from the top portion of the amniotic sac to encircle the leg of the fetus. (Courtesy of Dr. Theonia Boyd, Children's Hospital of Boston, Boston, Massachusetts.)

degree of uterine constraint. However, several variables increase the likelihood of excessive compression of the fetus, including maternal conditions such as first pregnancy, small uterus, malformed (bicornuate) uterus, and leiomyomas. Causes relating to the fetus, such as presence of multiple fetuses, oligohydramnios, and abnormal fetal presentation, also may be involved.

- *Sequence refers to multiple congenital anomalies that result from secondary effects of a single localized aberration in organogenesis.* The initiating event may be a malformation, deformation, or disruption. An excellent example is the oligohydramnios (or Potter) sequence (Fig. 4.27A). Oligohydramnios (decreased amniotic fluid) may be caused by a variety of maternal, placental, or fetal abnormalities, including chronic leakage of amniotic fluid because of rupture of the amnion; uteroplacental insufficiency resulting from maternal hypertension or severe toxemia; and renal agenesis in the fetus (because fetal urine is a major constituent of amniotic fluid). The fetal compression associated with oligohydramnios results in a classic phenotype in the newborn infant consisting of flattened face and positional abnormalities of the hands and feet (Fig. 4.27B). The hips may be dislocated. Growth of the chest wall and the lungs is also compromised, sometimes to the extent that survival is not possible. If the embryologic connection between these defects and the initiating event is not recognized, a sequence may be mistaken for a malformation syndrome.

- *Malformation syndrome refers to the presence of several defects that cannot be explained on the basis of a single localizing initiating error in morphogenesis.* Syndromes most often arise from a single causative condition (e.g., viral infection or a specific chromosomal abnormality) that simultaneously affects several tissues.

- *In addition to these global definitions, some general terms are applied to organ-specific malformations.* Agenesis refers to the complete absence of an organ or its anlage, whereas aplasia and hypoplasia indicate incomplete development and underdevelopment, respectively. *Atresia* describes the absence of an opening, usually of a hollow visceral organ or duct such as the intestine or bile duct.

Etiology. Known causes of human malformations can be grouped into three major categories: genetic, environmental, and multifactorial (Table 4.5). The cause is not identified in nearly half of the reported cases.

Genetic causes of malformations include all the previously discussed mechanisms of genetic disease. Virtually all chromosomal syndromes are associated with congenital malformations. Examples are Down syndrome and other trisomies, Turner syndrome, and Klinefelter syndrome. Most chromosomal disorders arise during gametogenesis and hence are not familial. Single-gene mutations, characterized by mendelian inheritance, may underlie major malformations. For example, holoprosencephaly, the most common developmental defect of the forebrain and midface in humans (see Chapter 21), is associated with loss-of-function mutations that affect the Hedgehog signaling pathway in familial cases.

Environmental influences, such as viral infections, drugs, and radiation to which the mother was exposed during pregnancy, may cause fetal malformations (the appellation of "malformation" is used loosely in this context because, technically, these anomalies represent disruptions). Among the viral infections listed in Table 4.5, rubella was a major scourge of the 19th and early 20th centuries; however, maternal rubella and the resultant embryopathy have been virtually eliminated in higher-income countries due to vaccination. Maternal infection

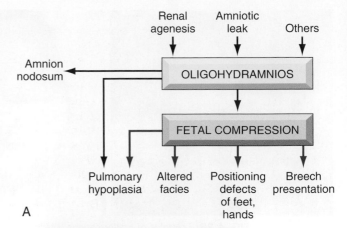

A

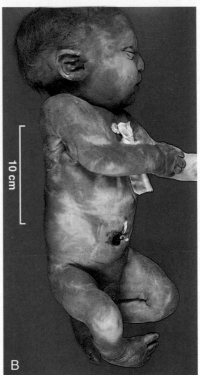

B

FIG. 4.27 (A) Pathogenesis of the oligohydramnios (Potter) sequence. (B) Amnion nodosum is a nodule found on the amnion. It composed of squamous cell aggregates derived from the vernix caseosa on the fetal skin. It occurs due to abrasion of amnion with fetal skin that occurs in oligohydramnios. Infant with oligohydramnios (Potter) sequence. Note flattened facial features and deformed foot (talipes equinovarus).

with Zika virus can give rise to severe malformations of the central nervous system (see later). A variety of drugs and chemicals are teratogenic, but perhaps less than 1% of congenital malformations are caused by these agents. The list includes thalidomide, alcohol, anticonvulsants, warfarin (oral anticoagulant), and 13-cis-retinoic acid, which is used in the treatment of severe acne. Thalidomide, formerly used as a tranquilizer in Europe and currently used for treatment of certain cancers, causes an extremely high incidence (50% to 80%) of limb malformations. Alcohol is an important environmental teratogen: infants born to mothers who consume alcohol excessively while pregnant can show prenatal and postnatal growth retardation, facial anomalies (microcephaly, short palpebral fissures, maxillary

Table 4.5 Causes of Congenital Malformations in Humans

Cause	Frequency of Malformations[a] (%)
Genetic	
Chromosomal aberrations	10–15
Mendelian inheritance	2–10
Environmental	
Maternal/placental infections	2–3
Rubella	
Toxoplasmosis	
Syphilis	
Cytomegalovirus infection	
Human immunodeficiency virus infection	
Zika virus infection	
Maternal disease states	6–8
Diabetes	
Phenylketonuria	
Endocrinopathies	
Drugs and chemicals	~1
Alcohol	
Folic acid antagonists	
Androgens	
Phenytoin	
Thalidomide	
Warfarin	
13-Cis-retinoic acid	
Others	
Irradiation	~1
Multifactorial	**20–25**
Unknown	**40–60**

[a]Live births.

Data from Stevenson RE, Hall JG, Goodman RM, editors: *Human Malformations and Related Anomalies,* New York, 1993, Oxford University Press, p 115.

hypoplasia), and psychomotor disturbances (fetal alcohol syndrome), depending on the amount of alcohol consumed and the gestational age at the time of consumption. Although nicotine from tobacco smoking has not been convincingly demonstrated to be a teratogen, there is a high incidence of spontaneous abortions, premature labor, and placental abnormalities among pregnant smokers, and babies born to mothers who smoke often have a low birth weight and may be prone to sudden infant death syndrome (SIDS). In light of these findings, it is best to avoid tobacco smoke exposure during pregnancy. Among maternal conditions listed in Table 4.5, diabetes is a common entity, and despite advances in antenatal obstetric monitoring and glucose control, the incidence of major malformations in infants of mothers with diabetes remains between 6% and 10% in most reported series. Maternal hyperglycemia–induced fetal hyperinsulinemia results in fetal macrosomia (organomegaly and increased body fat and muscle mass); cardiac anomalies, neural tube defects, and other CNS malformations are some of the major anomalies seen in diabetic embryopathy.

Multifactorial inheritance, which implies the interaction of environmental influences with two or more genes of small effect, is the most common genetic cause of congenital malformations. Included in this category are some relatively common malformations such as cleft lip and palate and neural tube defects. The importance of environmental contributions to multifactorial inheritance is underscored by the dramatic reduction in the incidence of neural tube defects by periconceptional intake of folic acid. The recurrence risks and mode of transmission of multifactorial disorders were described earlier in this chapter.

Pathogenesis. The pathogenesis of congenital anomalies is complex and still poorly understood, but two general principles are relevant regardless of the etiologic agent:

1. *The timing of the prenatal teratogenic insult has an important impact on the occurrence and the type of anomaly produced.* The intrauterine development of humans can be divided into two phases: (1) the embryonic period, occupying the first 9 weeks of pregnancy, and (2) the fetal period, terminating at birth.
    - In the *early embryonic period* (first 3 weeks after fertilization), an injurious agent may damage only a few cells, allowing the embryo to recover without deficits, or sufficient cells to cause death and abortion. *Between the third and the ninth weeks, the embryo is extremely susceptible to teratogenesis,* with the peak sensitivity occurring between the fourth and the fifth weeks. During this period organs are being crafted out of the germ-cell layers.
    - The *fetal period* that follows organogenesis is marked chiefly by further organ growth and maturation, with greatly reduced susceptibility to teratogenic agents. However, the fetus is susceptible to growth retardation or injury to already formed organs. Therefore, a given agent may produce different anomalies depending on the time of exposure.
2. The complex interplay between environmental teratogens and intrinsic genetic defects is exemplified by the fact that features of dysmorphogenesis caused by environmental insults can often be recapitulated by genetic defects in the pathways targeted by these teratogens. Some representative examples follow:
    - *Valproic acid* is an antiepileptic and a recognized teratogen. It disrupts expression of a family of highly conserved developmentally critical transcription factors known as *homeobox (HOX)* proteins. In vertebrates, HOX proteins have been implicated in the patterning of limbs, vertebrae, and craniofacial structures. Not surprisingly, mutations in the *HOX* gene family are responsible for congenital anomalies that mimic features observed in *valproic acid embryopathy*.
    - The vitamin A (retinol) derivative *all-trans-retinoic acid* is essential for normal development and differentiation, and its absence during embryogenesis results in a constellation of malformations affecting multiple organ systems, including the eyes, genitourinary system, cardiovascular system, diaphragm, and lungs (see Chapter 7 for vitamin A deficiency in the postnatal period). Conversely, in utero exposure to excessive retinoic acid (a treatment for acne) is also teratogenic. Retinoic acid embryopathy is characterized by CNS, cardiac, and craniofacial defects (e.g., cleft lip and cleft palate). The last entity may stem from retinoic acid–mediated deregulation of components of the transforming growth factor-β (TGF-β) signaling pathway, which is involved in palatogenesis.

PERINATAL INFECTIONS

Infections of the fetus and neonate may be acquired transcervically or transplacentally.
- *Transcervical (ascending) infections* are caused by microbial spread from the cervicovaginal canal and may be acquired in utero or

during birth. Most bacterial infections (e.g., α-hemolytic strepto-coccal infection) and a few viral infections (e.g., herpes simplex) are acquired in this manner. The organism is passed to the fetus by "inhaling" infected amniotic fluid into the lungs or by passing through an infected birth canal during delivery. This mode of spread is typical for pneumonia and, in severe cases, sepsis and meningitis. *In utero* fetal infection is a common cause of preterm birth.

- *Transplacental (hematogenous) infections* gain access to the fetal bloodstream by crossing the placenta via the chorionic villi and may occur at any time during gestation or occasionally at the time of delivery via maternal-to-fetal transfusion (e.g., hepati-tis B, human immunodeficiency virus). Most parasitic (e.g., toxoplasma, malaria) and viral infections and a few bacterial infections (e.g., *Listeria, Treponema*) follow this mode of hema-togenous transmission. The clinical manifestations of these infec-tions are highly variable, depending largely on the gestational timing and the microorganism involved. The most important transplacental infections can be remembered by the acronym *TORCH*. The elements of the TORCH complex are *Toxoplasma* (T), rubella virus (R), cytomegalovirus (C), herpesvirus (H), and any of a number of other (O) microbes, such as *Treponema pal-lidum*. These agents are grouped together because they may evoke similar clinical and pathologic manifestations. TORCH infections occurring early in gestation may cause chronic sequelae in the child, including growth restriction, intellectual disability, cata-racts, and congenital cardiac anomalies, whereas infections later in pregnancy result primarily in tissue injury accompanied by inflammation (e.g., encephalitis, chorioretinitis, hepatosplenome-galy, pneumonia, and myocarditis). Zika virus has emerged as another agent that can be transmitted by pregnant females to their offspring with devastating consequences, including microcephaly and brain damage.

PREMATURITY AND FETAL GROWTH RESTRICTION

Prematurity

Prematurity is defined by a gestational age less than 37 weeks. It is the second most common cause of neonatal mortality (second only to congenital anomalies). Infants born before completion of gestation weigh less than normal (<2500 gm). The major risk factors for pre-maturity include the following:

- *Preterm premature rupture of membranes* (PPROM) and *premature rupture of membranes* (PROM): PPROM complicates about 3% of all pregnancies and is responsible for as many as one-third of all preterm deliveries. Rupture of membranes (ROM) before the onset of labor can be spontaneous or induced. PPROM refers to sponta-neous ROM occurring *before* 37 weeks of gestation (hence the annotation "preterm"). By contrast, PROM refers to spontaneous ROM occurring *after* 37 weeks of gestation. This distinction is important because after 37 weeks the associated risk to the fetus is considerably decreased.
- *Intrauterine infection:* This is a major cause of preterm labor (approximately 25% of cases) and is usually associated with inflam-mation of the placental membranes (chorioamnionitis) and inflam-mation of the umbilical cord (funisitis). Microorganisms implicated in intrauterine infections leading to preterm labor are *Ureaplasma urealyticum, Mycoplasma hominis, Gardnerella vaginalis, Tricho-monas, Neisseria gonorrhea,* and *Chlamydia.*
- *Uterine, cervical, and placental structural abnormalities:* Uterine distortion (e.g., uterine fibroids), compromised structural support

of the cervix, placenta previa, and abruptio placentae (Chapter 17) are associated with an increased risk of prematurity. The imma-turity of organ systems in preterm infants makes them especially vulnerable to several important complications: *neonatal respiratory distress syndrome* (also called hyaline membrane disease), *necro-tizing enterocolitis, sepsis, and intraventricular and germinal matrix hemorrhage* (Chapter 21).

Fetal Growth Restriction

Although birth weight is low in preterm infants, it is usually appro-priate after adjustment for gestational age. By contrast, as many as one-third of infants who weigh less than 2500 gm are born at term and are therefore undergrown (small-for-gestational age, SGA) due to *fetal growth restriction.* Fetal growth restriction may result from fetal, maternal, or placental abnormalities, although in many cases the specific cause is unknown.

- *Maternal factors:* This category comprises by far the most common causes of the growth deficit in SGA infants. Important examples are vascular diseases such as *preeclampsia* (Chapter 17) and *chronic hy-pertension.* Hypercoagulability, either acquired or inherited, is increasingly being recognized as a factor in fetal growth restriction (Chapter 3). Some of the avoidable causes are maternal narcotic use, alcohol intake, and heavy cigarette smoking. They contribute to growth restriction, as well as to the pathogenesis of congenital anomalies. Both teratogenic (e.g., phenytoin) and nonteratogenic drugs have been implicated in fetal growth restriction. Maternal malnutrition (in particular, prolonged hypoglycemia) also may affect fetal growth.
- *Fetal abnormalities:* This category consists of conditions that reduce fetal growth potential despite an adequate supply of nutri-ents from the mother. These include chromosomal disorders, congenital anomalies, and congenital infections. Fetal infection should be considered in all growth-restricted neonates, with the TORCH group of infections (see earlier) being a common cause. When the causation is intrinsic to the fetus, fetal growth restriction is symmetric (i.e., all organs are equally affected).
- *Placental abnormalities:* Placental causes include any factor that compromises the uteroplacental blood supply, such as placenta pre-via (low implantation of the placenta), placental abruption (separa-tion of the placenta from the decidua by a retroplacental clot), or placental infarction. With placental (and maternal) abnormalities, the fetal growth restriction is asymmetric (i.e., the brain is spared relative to visceral organs such as the liver).

Not only is the growth-restricted infant challenged in the perinatal period, but the deficits persist into childhood and adult life. Affected persons are thus more likely to have cerebral dysfunction, learning disabilities, and sensory (i.e., visual and hearing) impairment.

NEONATAL RESPIRATORY DISTRESS SYNDROME

The most common cause of respiratory insufficiency in the newborn is *respiratory distress syndrome (RDS),* also known as *hyaline membrane disease* because of the formation of "mem-branes" in the peripheral air spaces observed in infants who suc-cumb to this condition. RDS is primarily a disorder of premature infants: it occurs in about 60% of infants born at less than 28 weeks' gestation, 30% of those born between 28 to 34 weeks' gestation, and less than 5% of those born after 34 weeks' gestation. Additional as-sociations include male gender, maternal diabetes, and delivery by cesarean section. Less common causes of neonatal respiratory distress include excessive sedation of the mother, fetal head injury during delivery, aspiration of blood or amniotic fluid, and intrauterine hypoxia secondary to cord compression due to coiling of the umbilical cord about the neck.

Pathogenesis. **The fundamental defect in RDS is the inability of the immature lung to synthesize sufficient surfactant.** Surfactant is a complex of surface-active phospholipids, principally dipalmitoyl-phosphatidylcholine (lecithin) and at least two groups of surfactant-associated proteins. The importance of surfactant-associated proteins in normal lung function can be gauged by the occurrence of severe respiratory failure in neonates with a congenital deficiency of surfactant caused by loss of function mutations in the corresponding genes. Surfactant is synthesized by type II pneumocytes and, with the healthy newborn's first breath, rapidly coats the surface of alveoli, reducing surface tension and thus decreasing the pressure required to keep the alveoli open. Without surfactant, alveoli tend to collapse, and a greater inspiratory effort is required with each breath to open the alveoli. The infant rapidly tires from breathing and generalized atelectasis sets in. The resulting hypoxia sets into motion a sequence of events that leads to epithelial and endothelial damage and eventually to the formation of hyaline membranes (Fig. 4.28). This sequence is greatly modified by surfactant treatment.

Hormones regulate surfactant synthesis. Corticosteroids stimulate the formation of surfactant lipids and associated proteins. Therefore, conditions associated with intrauterine stress and fetal growth restriction, which increase corticosteroid release, lower the risk of developing RDS. Conversely, the compensatory high blood levels of insulin in infants of mothers with diabetes can suppress surfactant synthesis; infants of mothers with diabetes are at increased risk for developing RDS. Labor stimulates surfactant synthesis; thus, cesarean section performed before the onset of labor may also increase risk.

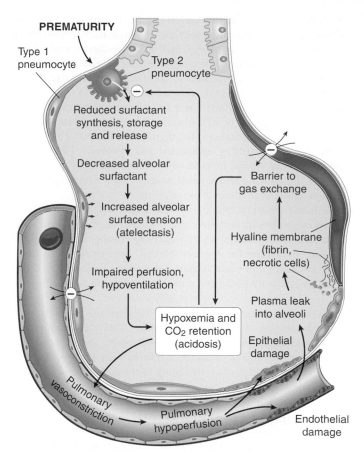

FIG. 4.28 Pathophysiology of respiratory distress syndrome (see text).

MORPHOLOGY

The lungs in infants with RDS are of normal size but are heavy and relatively airless. They have a mottled purple color; on microscopic examination the tissue appears solid, with poorly developed, generally collapsed (atelectatic) alveoli. If the infant dies within the first several hours of life, only necrotic cellular debris is present in the terminal bronchioles and alveolar ducts. Later in the course, characteristic **eosinophilic hyaline membranes** line the respiratory bronchioles, alveolar ducts, and alveoli (Fig. 4.29). These "membranes" contain necrotic type II pneumocytes admixed with extravasated plasma proteins, mainly fibrinogen which gives rise to fibrin. There is a paucity of neutrophilic inflammatory reaction associated with these membranes. The lesions of hyaline membrane disease are not seen in stillborn infants or in live-born infants who die within a few hours of birth. If an infant with RDS dies after several days, evidence of reparative changes, including proliferation of type II pneumocytes and interstitial fibrosis, is present.

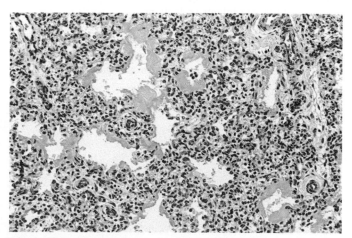

FIG. 4.29 Hyaline membrane disease (hematoxylin-eosin stain). Alternating atelectasis and dilation of the alveoli can be seen. Note the eosinophilic thick hyaline membranes lining the dilated alveoli.

Clinical Features. The classic clinical presentation before the era of treatment with exogenous surfactant was described earlier. Currently, the clinical course and prognosis for neonatal RDS vary, depending on the maturity and birth weight of the infant and the promptness of therapy. Control of RDS focuses on prevention, either by delaying labor until the fetal lung reaches maturity or by inducing maturation of the lung in the at-risk fetus by antenatal steroids. Critical to these objectives is the ability to assess fetal lung maturity accurately. Because

pulmonary secretions are discharged into the amniotic fluid, analysis of amniotic fluid phospholipids provides a good estimate of the level of surfactant in the alveolar lining. Prophylactic administration at birth of exogenous surfactant to extremely premature infants (born before 28 weeks' gestational age) is very beneficial, and it is now uncommon for infants to die of acute RDS.

In uncomplicated cases, recovery begins within 3 or 4 days. Ventilator-administered oxygen is part of treatment, though its use at high concentrations for prolonged periods is associated with two well-known complications: retinopathy of prematurity (also called retrolental fibroplasia) of the eyes and bronchopulmonary dysplasia. Both complications are now less common due to gentler ventilation techniques, antenatal glucocorticoid therapy, and prophylactic surfactant treatments. They are described briefly:

- *Retinopathy of prematurity* has a two-phase pathogenesis. During the hyperoxic phase of RDS therapy (phase I), expression of the proangiogenic vascular endothelial growth factor (VEGF) is markedly decreased, causing endothelial cell apoptosis. VEGF levels rebound after return to relatively hypoxic room air ventilation (phase II), inducing retinal vessel proliferation (*neovascularization*) characteristic of the lesions in the retina.
- The major abnormality in *bronchopulmonary dysplasia* is a striking decrease in alveolar septation (manifested as large, simplified alveolar structures) and a dysmorphic capillary configuration. Multiple factors—hyperoxemia, hyperventilation, prematurity, inflammatory cytokines, and vascular maldevelopment—contribute to bronchopulmonary dysplasia and probably synergize to promote injury.

Infants who recover from RDS are at increased risk for a variety of other complications associated with preterm birth, including *patent ductus arteriosus, intraventricular hemorrhage, and necrotizing enterocolitis.* Although technologic advances help save the lives of many infants with RDS, they also bring to the surface the fragility of the immature neonate.

NECROTIZING ENTEROCOLITIS

Necrotizing enterocolitis (NEC) most commonly occurs in premature infants, with the incidence of the disease being inversely proportional to the gestational age. It occurs in approximately 1 of 10 very-low-birth-weight infants (<1500 gm).

Pathogenesis. The pathogenesis of NEC is multifactorial, and implicated factors include (1) immaturity of the intestinal mucosal barrier and immune system; (2) alterations in the gut microbiome and resultant increased growth of potentially pathogenic bacteria; and (3) an exaggerated inflammatory host response with release of cytokines and chemokines. Many inflammatory mediators have been associated with the pathogenesis of NEC. In particular, platelet-activating factor may increase mucosal permeability by promoting enterocyte apoptosis and compromising intercellular tight junctions, thereby "adding fuel to the fire." In addition to prematurity, most cases are associated with milk feeding, suggesting that some postnatal insult (such as the introduction of bacteria) sets in motion the cascade, culminating in tissue destruction.

MORPHOLOGY

NEC typically involves the terminal ileum, cecum, and right colon, although any part of the small or large intestine may be involved. The involved segment typically is distended, friable, and congested (Fig. 4.30), or it may be gangrenous; intestinal perforation with accompanying peritonitis may be seen. On microscopic examination, mucosal or transmural coagulative necrosis, ulceration, bacterial colonization, and submucosal gas bubbles are all features associated with NEC. Evidence of reparative changes, such as granulation tissue and fibrosis, may be seen shortly after resolution of the acute episode.

Clinical Features. The clinical course is fairly typical, with the onset of bloody stools, abdominal distention, and circulatory instability. Abdominal radiographs often demonstrate gas within the intestinal wall (*pneumatosis intestinalis*). When detected early, NEC can often be managed conservatively, but many cases (20% to 60%) require operative intervention including resection of the necrotic segments of the bowel. NEC is associated with high perinatal mortality; infants who survive often develop post-NEC strictures from fibrosis caused by the healing process.

SUDDEN INFANT DEATH SYNDROME (SIDS)

According to the National Institute of Child Health and Human Development, *SIDS is defined as* "**the sudden death of an infant**

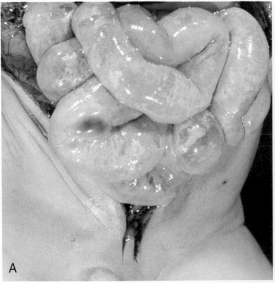
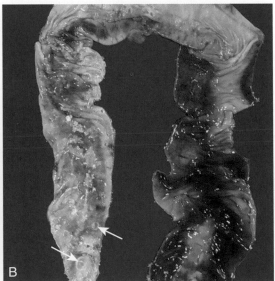

FIG. 4.30 Necrotizing enterocolitis. (A) At postmortem examination in a severe case, the entire small bowel was markedly distended and perilously thin (usually this appearance implies impending perforation). (B) The congested portion of the ileum corresponds to areas of hemorrhagic infarction and transmural necrosis. Submucosal gas bubbles (pneumatosis intestinalis) can be seen in several areas *(arrows)*.

under 1 year of age which remains unexplained after a thorough case investigation, including performance of a complete autopsy, examination of the death scene, and review of the clinical history." Many cases of sudden death in infancy are found to have an anatomic or biochemical basis at autopsy (Table 4.6). These cases should not be labeled as SIDS, but rather as sudden unexpected infant death (SUID). The Centers for Disease Control and Prevention estimates that SIDS accounts for approximately half of the cases of SUID in the United States. An aspect of SIDS that is not stressed in the definition is that the infant usually dies while asleep—hence the lay terms crib death and cot death.

SIDS is the leading cause of death between the ages of 1 month and 1 year in U.S. infants, and the third leading cause of death overall in this age group, after congenital anomalies and diseases of prematurity and low birth weight. In 90% of cases, the infant is younger than 6 months; most are between the ages of 2 and 4 months. SIDS in an earlier sibling is associated with a 5-fold relative risk of recurrence; traumatic child abuse must be carefully excluded in all cases.

Table 4.6 Factors Associated With Sudden Infant Death Syndrome (SIDS)

Parental
Young maternal age (age younger than 20 years)
Maternal smoking during pregnancy
Drug use in *either* parent, specifically paternal marijuana and maternal opiate, cocaine use
Short intergestational intervals
Late or no prenatal care
Low socioeconomic group

Infant
Brain stem abnormalities, associated with delayed development of arousal and cardiorespiratory control
Prematurity and/or low birth weight
Male sex
Product of a multiple birth
SIDS in a previous sibling

Environment
Prone or side sleep position
Sleeping on a soft surface
Hyperthermia

Postmortem Abnormalities Detected in Cases of Sudden Unexpected Infant Death (SUID)[a]
Infections
Viral myocarditis
Bronchopneumonia
Unsuspected congenital anomaly
Congenital aortic stenosis
Anomalous origin of the left coronary artery from the pulmonary artery
Traumatic child abuse
Intentional suffocation (filicide)
Genetic and metabolic defects
Long QT syndrome e.g., *SCN5A* and *KCNQ1* mutations
Fatty acid oxidation disorders e.g., *MCAD* mutations

[a]SIDS is not the only cause of SUIDs, but rather is a *diagnosis of exclusion*. Therefore, performance of an autopsy may often show findings that would explain the cause of an SUID. These cases should *not*, strictly speaking, be labeled as "SIDS."
KCNQ1, Potassium voltage-gated channel, KQT-like subfamily, member 1; *MCAD*, medium-chain acyl coenzyme A dehydrogenase; *SCN5A*, sodium channel, voltage-gated, type V, alpha polypeptide.

Pathogenesis. SIDS is a multifactorial condition, with a mixture of contributing causes in any given case. Three interacting variables have been proposed: (1) a vulnerable infant; (2) delayed development of cardiorespiratory control; and (3) one or more exogenous stressors. According to this model, several factors increase vulnerability during the critical developmental period (i.e., 1 month to 1 year). These factors may be specific to the parents or the infant, whereas the exogenous stressor or stressors are attributable to the environment (Table 4.6). Although numerous factors have been proposed to account for a vulnerable infant, the most compelling hypothesis is that SIDS is associated with a delayed development of arousal and cardiorespiratory control. The brain stem and, in particular, the medulla oblongata play a critical role in the body's "arousal" response to noxious stimuli such as episodic hypercarbia, hypoxia, and thermal stress encountered during sleep. The serotonergic (5-HT) system of the medulla is implicated in these "arousal" responses as well as regulation of other critical homeostatic functions such as respiratory drive, blood pressure, and upper airway reflexes. Abnormalities in serotonin-dependent signaling in the brain stem may be the underlying basis for SIDS in some infants.

Among the potential environmental causes, prone sleeping position, sleeping on soft surfaces, and thermal stress are the most important modifiable risk factors for SIDS. Many studies have clearly shown increased risk for SIDS in infants who sleep in a prone position, prompting the **American Academy of Pediatrics to recommend placing healthy infants on their backs when laying them down to sleep. This "Back to Sleep" campaign has resulted in substantial decreases in SIDS-related deaths since its inception in 1994.** The prone position increases the infant's vulnerability to one or more recognized noxious stimuli (i.e., hypoxia, hypercarbia, and thermal stress) during sleep and is associated with decreased arousal responsiveness compared with the supine position.

SIDS is a diagnosis of exclusion, requiring careful examination of the death scene and a complete postmortem examination. The latter can show an unsuspected cause of sudden death in as many as 20% or more of babies presumed to have died of SIDS (see Table 4.6). Infections (e.g., viral myocarditis or bronchopneumonia) are the most common causes of SUID, followed by a congenital anomaly. Several genetic causes of SUID have emerged. Fatty acid oxidation disorders, characterized by defects in mitochondrial fatty acid oxidative enzymes, may be responsible for as many as 5% of sudden deaths in infancy; of these, a deficiency in medium-chain acyl-coenzyme A dehydrogenase is the most common. Retrospective analyses in cases of sudden infant death originally designated SIDS have also revealed mutations of cardiac sodium and potassium channels, which result in a form of cardiac arrhythmia characterized by prolonged QT intervals; these cases account for fewer than 1% of SUIDs.

MORPHOLOGY

Anatomic studies of victims have yielded inconsistent histologic findings. **Multiple petechiae,** usually of the thymus, visceral and parietal pleura, and epicardium, are the most common autopsy finding (approximately 80% of cases). The lungs are typically congested, and vascular engorgement with or without **pulmonary edema** is present in a majority of cases. Quantitative brain stem abnormalities such as **hypoplasia of the arcuate nucleus** or a subtle decrease in brain stem neuronal populations have been noted, but these observations are not uniform and the use of such studies is not feasible in most "routine" autopsy procedures.

Table 4.7 Major Causes of Fetal Hydrops

Cardiovascular
Malformations
Tachyarrhythmia
High-output failure
Chromosomal
Turner syndrome
Trisomy 21, trisomy 18
Thoracic Causes
Diaphragmatic hernia
Fetal Anemia
Homozygous α-thalassemia
Parvovirus B19
Immune hydrops (Rh and ABO)
Twin Gestation
Twin-to-twin transfusion
Infection (excluding parvovirus)
Cytomegalovirus
Syphilis
Toxoplasmosis

ªThe cause of fetal hydrops may be undetermined ("idiopathic") in up to 20% of cases.

Data from Machin GA: Hydrops, cystic hygroma, hydrothorax, pericardial effusions, and fetal ascites. In Gilbert-Barness E, et al, editors: *Potter's Pathology of the Fetus, Infant, and Child,* St. Louis, 2007, Mosby, pp 33.

FETAL HYDROPS

Fetal hydrops **refers to the accumulation of edema fluid in at least two serous cavities combined with subcutaneous edema during intrauterine growth.** The causes of fetal hydrops are manifold; the most important are listed in Table 4.7. In the past, hemolytic anemia caused by Rh blood group incompatibility between mother and fetus (immune hydrops) was the most common cause, but with successful prophylaxis of this disorder (see later), causes of nonimmune hydrops have emerged as the principal culprits. The fluid accumulation can be quite variable, ranging in degree from progressive, generalized edema of the fetus *(hydrops fetalis),* a usually lethal condition, to more localized and less marked edematous processes, such as pleural and peritoneal effusions or postnuchal fluid collections *(cystic hygroma),* that often are compatible with life (Fig. 4.31). The mechanism of immune hydrops is discussed first, followed by other important causes of fetal hydrops.

Immune Hydrops

Immune hydrops results from an antibody-induced hemolytic anemia in the newborn that is caused by blood group incompatibility between mother and fetus. Such an incompatibility occurs when the fetus inherits red cell antigenic determinants from the father that are foreign to the mother. The most common clinically relevant antigens are the Rh and ABO blood group antigens. Of the numerous Rh antigens, only the D antigen is a major cause of Rh incompatibility. Fetal red cells may reach the maternal circulation

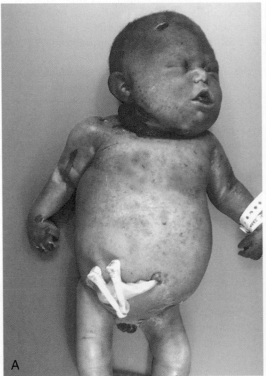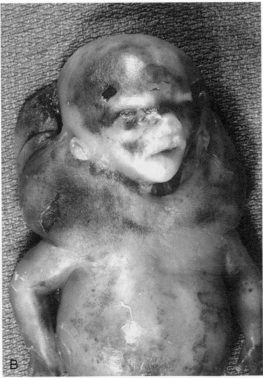

FIG. 4.31 Hydrops fetalis. (A) Generalized accumulation of fluid in the fetus. (B) Fluid accumulation particularly prominent in the soft tissues of the neck. This condition has been termed *cystic hygroma.* Cystic hygromas are characteristically seen with, but not limited to, constitutional chromosomal anomalies such as 45,X karyotypes. (Courtesy of Dr. Beverly Rogers, Department of Pathology, University of Texas Southwestern Medical Center, Dallas, Texas.)

during the last trimester of pregnancy, when the cytotrophoblast is no longer present as a barrier, or during childbirth itself (fetomaternal bleed). The mother becomes sensitized to the foreign antigen and produces anti-Rh IgG antibodies that, in future pregnancies, can freely traverse the placenta to the fetus and cause red cell destruction. With initiation of immune hemolysis, progressive anemia in the fetus leads to tissue ischemia, intrauterine cardiac failure, and peripheral pooling of fluid (edema). As discussed later, cardiac failure may be the final pathway by which edema occurs in many cases of nonimmune hydrops as well.

Several factors influence the immune response to Rh-positive fetal red cells that reach the maternal circulation:

- Concurrent *ABO incompatibility* protects the mother against Rh immunization, because the fetal red cells are promptly coated by isohemagglutinins (preformed anti-A or anti-B IgM antibodies) and removed from the maternal circulation.
- The antibody response depends on the *dose of immunizing antigen*: hemolytic disease develops only with a significant transplacental bleed (more than 1 mL of Rh-positive red cells).
- The *antibody isotype* is important: IgG, but not IgM, antibodies are able to cross the placenta. At initial exposure to Rh antigen, IgM antibodies are formed, so Rh disease is very uncommon with the first pregnancy. Exposure in subsequent pregnancies generally leads to a brisk IgG antibody response.

Therapeutic control is attained by giving Rh immune globulin (RhIg) to Rh-negative mothers at 28 weeks of pregnancy and within 72 hours after delivery of an Rh-positive baby. The RhIg masks the antigenic sites on the fetal red cells that may have leaked into the maternal circulation during childbirth, thus preventing long-lasting sensitization to Rh antigens.

Because of the success of this intervention, fetomaternal ABO incompatibility is now the most common cause of immune hemolytic disease of the newborn. Although ABO incompatibility occurs in approximately 20% to 25% of pregnancies, hemolysis develops in only a small fraction of infants born subsequently. The disease is usually much milder than Rh incompatibility, in part because the expression of A and B antigens on many cells other than red cells that act like a sponge for the transferred antibody. **ABO hemolytic disease occurs almost exclusively in infants of blood group A or B who are born to mothers of blood group O.** The normal anti-A and anti-B isohemagglutinins in group O mothers usually are of the IgM type and therefore do not cross the placenta. However, for reasons not well understood, some group O women possess IgG antibodies directed against group A or B antigens (or both) even without previous sensitization. Therefore, the firstborn may be affected. There is no effective method of preventing hemolytic disease resulting from ABO incompatibility.

Nonimmune Hydrops

The major causes of nonimmune hydrops include disorders associated with cardiovascular defects, chromosomal anomalies, and fetal anemia.

- *Structural cardiovascular defects and functional abnormalities* (e.g., arrhythmias) may result in intrauterine cardiac failure and hydrops. Among the chromosomal anomalies, 45,X karyotype (Turner syndrome) and trisomies 21 and 18 are associated with fetal hydrops; the basis for this disorder usually is the presence of underlying structural cardiac anomalies, although in Turner syndrome there may be an abnormality of lymphatic drainage from the neck leading to postnuchal fluid accumulation (resulting in *cystic hygromas*).

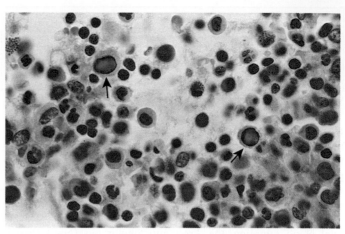

FIG. 4.32 Bone marrow from an infant infected with parvovirus B19. The *arrows* point to two erythroid precursors with large homogeneous intranuclear inclusions and a surrounding peripheral rim of residual chromatin.

- *Fetal anemias* resulting from causes other than Rh or ABO incompatibility also may result in hydrops. In fact, in some parts of the world (e.g., Southeast Asia), severe fetal anemia caused by homozygous α-thalassemia is probably the most common cause of fetal hydrops.
- *Transplacental infection* by parvovirus B19 is increasingly recognized as an important cause of fetal hydrops. The virus infects erythroid precursors (normoblasts), where it replicates. The ensuing apoptosis of the normoblasts causes red cell aplasia. Parvoviral intranuclear inclusions can be seen within erythroid precursors (Fig. 4.32).

The basis for hydrops in fetal anemia of immune and nonimmune causes is tissue ischemia with secondary myocardial dysfunction and circulatory failure. Secondary liver failure may also occur, with loss of synthetic function contributing to hypoalbuminemia, reduced plasma osmotic pressure, and edema.

MORPHOLOGY

The anatomic findings in fetuses with intrauterine fluid accumulation vary according to the severity of the disease and the underlying etiology. **Hydrops fetalis** is the most severe and generalized manifestation (see Fig. 4.31), and lesser degrees of edema such as isolated pleural, peritoneal, or postnuchal fluid collections can occur. Infants may be stillborn, die within the first few days, or recover completely. The presence of dysmorphic features suggests underlying constitutional chromosomal abnormalities; postmortem examination may show a cardiac anomaly. In hydrops associated with fetal anemia, both fetus and placenta are pale, and in most cases, the liver and spleen are enlarged as a consequence of **cardiac failure** and congestion. Additionally, the bone marrow shows compensatory hyperplasia of erythroid precursors (parvovirus-associated red cell aplasia being a notable exception), and **extramedullary hematopoiesis** is present in the liver, the spleen, and possibly other tissues such as the kidneys, lungs, lymph nodes, and even the heart (Fig. 4.33). The increased erythropoietic activity accounts for the presence in the peripheral circulation of large numbers of erythroid progenitors, including normoblasts and even more immature erythroblasts **(erythroblastosis fetalis)**.

Hemolysis due to Rh or ABO incompatibility is associated with the added complication of increased circulating bilirubin from red cell breakdown. The CNS may be damaged when hyperbilirubinemia is marked (usually greater than 20 mg/dL in full-term infants, but often less in premature infants). Circulating unconjugated bilirubin is taken up in the brain, where it exerts a toxic effect. The basal ganglia and brain stem are particularly prone to deposition of bilirubin pigment, which imparts a characteristic yellow hue to the parenchyma **(kernicterus)** (Fig. 4.34).

Clinical Features. Early recognition of fetal hydrops is imperative, because even severe cases can sometimes be salvaged with timely therapy. Immune hydrops that results from Rh incompatibility can be predicted with reasonable certainty, since its severity correlates well with rapidly rising Rh antibody titers in the mother during pregnancy. Antenatal identification and management of the at-risk fetus have been facilitated by amniocentesis and chorionic villus and fetal blood sampling: the direct antiglobulin test (direct Coombs test) (Chapter 10) using fetal cord blood is positive if the red cells have been coated by maternal antibody. Fetal Rh status can be determined by sequencing fetal DNA in maternal blood or amniotic fluid. Cases of severe intrauterine hemolysis may be treated by fetal intravascular transfusions via the umbilical cord and early delivery. Postnatally, phototherapy is helpful, because visible light converts bilirubin to readily excreted dipyrroles. As already discussed, in an overwhelming majority of cases, administration of RhIg to the mother prevents the occurrence of immune hydrops in subsequent pregnancies. Group ABO hemolytic disease is more difficult to predict but is readily anticipated by awareness of the blood incompatibility between mother and father and by hemoglobin and bilirubin determinations in the vulnerable newborn. In fatal cases of fetal hydrops, a thorough postmortem examination is imperative to determine the cause and to exclude a potentially recurring cause such as a chromosomal abnormality.

TUMORS AND TUMORLIKE LESIONS OF INFANCY AND CHILDHOOD

Malignant neoplasms constitute the second most common cause of death in children between the ages of 4 and 14 years; only accidents exact a higher toll. Benign tumors are even more common than malignancies.

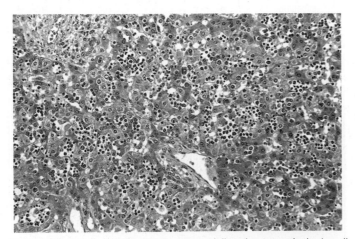

FIG. 4.33 Numerous islands of extramedullary hematopoiesis *(small blue cells)* are scattered among mature hepatocytes in this histologic preparation from an infant with nonimmune hydrops fetalis.

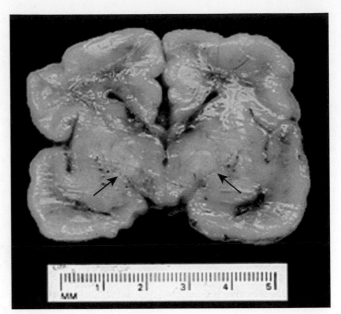

FIG. 4.34 Kernicterus. Severe hyperbilirubinemia in the neonatal period—for example, secondary to immune hydrolysis—results in deposition of bilirubin pigment *(arrows)* in the brain parenchyma. This occurs because the blood–brain barrier is less developed in the neonatal period than it is in adulthood. Infants who survive develop long-term neurologic sequelae.

It can be difficult to segregate, on morphologic grounds, true neoplasms from tumorlike lesions in the infant and child. In this context, two special categories of tumorlike lesions should be recognized:

- *Heterotopia* or *choristoma* refers to microscopically normal cells or tissues that are present in abnormal locations. Examples are an ectopic pancreatic tissue nodule found in the wall of the stomach or small intestine and a small mass of adrenal cells found in the kidney, lungs, ovaries, or elsewhere. Heterotopic rests usually are of little clinical significance, but they can be confused with neoplasms.
- *Hamartoma* refers to an excessive but focal overgrowth of cells and tissues native to the organ in which it occurs. Although these mature cellular elements are identical to those found in the remainder of the organ, they do not demonstrate normal architectural features. The line of demarcation between a hamartoma and a benign neoplasm is often unclear because both lesions can be clonal. Hemangiomas, lymphangiomas, rhabdomyomas of the heart, and adenomas of the liver are examples of lesions that blur the distinction between hamartomas and neoplasms. Though histologically benign, they can cause serious complications because of their size or location.

Benign Neoplasms

Virtually any neoplasm may be encountered in the pediatric age group, but three—hemangiomas, lymphangiomas, and teratomas—deserve special mention here.

Hemangioma **is the most common neoplasm of infancy.** Both cavernous and capillary hemangiomas may be encountered (Chapter 8); the latter are often more cellular than those seen in adults and thus may appear deceptively worrisome. In children, most hemangiomas are located in the skin, particularly on the face and scalp, where they are irregular, erythematous to violaceous lesions that range from flat to plaque to nodular forms (Fig. 4.35). Hemangiomas may enlarge as

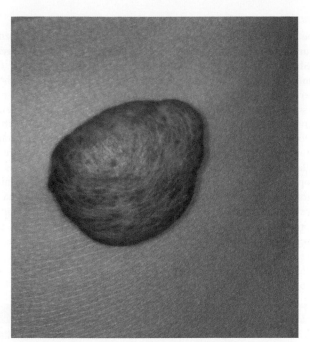

FIG. 4.35 Nodular capillary hemangioma from the back of an 18-month-old girl. (Courtesy of Dr. Jane Bellet, Duke University School of Medicine, Durham, North Carolina.)

Malignant Neoplasms

The organ systems involved most commonly by malignant neoplasms in infancy and childhood are the hematopoietic system, nervous system, and soft tissues (Table 4.8). This distribution is in sharp contrast with cancer in adults, in whom epithelial tumors of the lung, breast, prostate, and colon are most common. Malignant neoplasms of infancy and childhood also differ biologically and histologically from those in adults. The main differences are as follows:

- *Relatively frequent demonstration of a close relationship between abnormal development (teratogenesis) and tumor induction (oncogenesis)*, suggesting a common stem cell defect
- *Prevalence of germline mutations that predispose to cancer*, whereas somatic mutations are more common in cancers in adults
- *Tendency of fetal and neonatal malignancies to regress spontaneously or to undergo "differentiation" into mature elements*
- *Improved survival or cure of many childhood tumors*, such that much attention is now paid to minimizing the adverse delayed effects of chemotherapy and radiotherapy in survivors, including the development of second malignancies

Many malignant pediatric neoplasms are histologically unique. In general, they tend to exhibit a primitive *(embryonal)* rather than pleomorphic-anaplastic microscopic appearance (Chapter 6) and frequently exhibit features of organogenesis specific to the site of

the child ages, but in many instances they spontaneously regress (Fig. 4.36). The vast majority of superficial hemangiomas have no more than a cosmetic significance; rarely, they may be a manifestation of a hereditary disorder associated with disease within internal organs, such as von Hippel-Lindau syndrome resulting from homozygous loss of the *VHL* tumor suppressor gene (Chapter 8). A subset of CNS cavernous hemangiomas are familial; affected families harbor mutations in one of three *cerebral cavernous malformation* (CCM) genes.

Lymphangiomas **represent the lymphatic counterpart of hemangiomas.** Microscopic examination shows cystic and cavernous spaces lined by endothelial cells and surrounded by lymphoid aggregates; the spaces usually contain pale fluid. They may occur on the skin but, more importantly, they are also encountered in the deeper regions of the neck, axilla, mediastinum, and retroperitoneum. Although histologically benign, they tend to enlarge after birth and may encroach on mediastinal structures or nerve trunks in the axilla.

Teratomas **are neoplasms that include tissues derived from all three germ cell layers: ectoderm, endoderm, and mesoderm. They include benign, well-differentiated cystic lesions (mature teratomas), lesions of indeterminate potential (immature teratomas), and unequivocally malignant tumors** (Chapter 17). Sacrococcygeal teratomas are the most common teratomas of childhood, accounting for 40% or more of cases (Fig. 4.37). In view of the overlap in the mechanisms underlying congenital malformations and oncogenesis, it is interesting that approximately 10% of sacrococcygeal teratomas are associated with congenital anomalies, primarily defects of the hindgut and cloacal region and other midline defects (e.g., meningocele, spina bifida) that cannot be attributed to local effects of the tumor. Approximately 75% of these tumors are mature teratomas with a benign course, and about 12% are unmistakably malignant. The remainder are designated immature teratomas, and their malignant potential correlates with the amount of immature tissue elements present. In younger infants (4 months of age or younger), most teratomas are benign, whereas children with malignant lesions tend to be somewhat older.

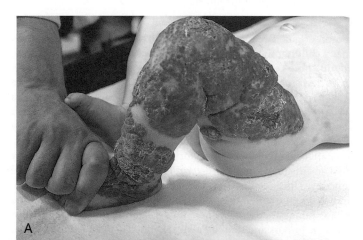

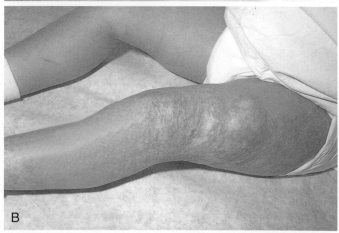

FIG. 4.36 Congenital capillary hemangioma (A) at birth and (B) at 2 years of age after the lesion had undergone spontaneous regression. (Courtesy of Dr. Eduardo Yunis, Children's Hospital of Pittsburgh, Pittsburgh, Pennsylvania.)

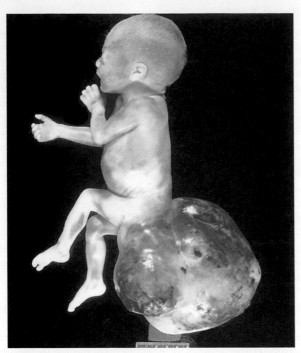

FIG. 4.37 Sacrococcygeal teratoma. Note the size of the lesion compared with that of the infant.

tumor origin. **Because of their primitive histologic appearance, many childhood tumors have been collectively referred to as small, round, blue-cell tumors.** Sheets of cells with small, round nuclei characterize these tumors, which include neuroblastoma, lymphoma (Chapter 10), rhabdomyosarcoma (Chapter 19), Ewing sarcoma (Chapter 19), medulloblastoma (Chapter 21), retinoblastoma, and some cases of Wilms tumor. Sufficient distinctive features are usually present to permit definitive diagnosis on the basis of histologic examination alone, but confirmatory molecular studies are routinely used for diagnosis and for determining the prognosis of childhood cancers. Three common tumors—neuroblastoma, retinoblastoma, and Wilms tumor—are worthy of discussion. Neuroblastoma and Wilms tumor are described here to highlight the differences between pediatric tumors and those in adults. Retinoblastoma is considered in Chapter 21.

Table 4.8 Common Malignant Neoplasms of Infancy and Childhood

0–4 Years of Age	5–9 Years of Age	10–14 Years of Age
Leukemia	Leukemia	Leukemia
Retinoblastoma	Retinoblastoma	Hepatocellular
Neuroblastoma	Neuroblastoma	carcinoma
Wilms tumor	Hepatocellular	Soft tissue
Hepatoblastoma	carcinoma	sarcoma
Soft tissue sarcoma	Soft tissue	Osteosarcoma
(especially	sarcoma	Thyroid carcinoma
rhabdomyosarcoma)	Ewing sarcoma	Hodgkin lymphoma
Teratomas	CNS tumors	
CNS tumors	Lymphoma	

CNS, Central nervous system.

Neuroblastoma

The term neuroblastic includes tumors derived from primordial neural crest cells that populate sympathetic ganglia and adrenal medulla; neuroblastoma is the most important member of this family. It is the second most common solid malignancy of childhood after brain tumors, accounting for 7% to 10% of all pediatric neoplasms, and as many as 50% of malignancies diagnosed in infancy. Neuroblastomas demonstrate several unique features in their natural history, including spontaneous regression and spontaneous or therapy-induced maturation. Most occur sporadically, but 1% to 2% are familial, with autosomal dominant transmission, and in such cases the neoplasms may involve both adrenal glands or multiple primary autonomic sites. Germline mutations in the anaplastic lymphoma kinase *(ALK)* gene have been linked to the familial predisposition to neuroblastoma. Somatic gain-of-function *ALK* mutations are also observed in 8% to 10% of sporadic neuroblastomas and are markers of adverse prognosis. Clinical trials using inhibitors that target the mutated ALK tyrosine kinase are underway. Some lung cancers also harbor *ALK* mutations and respond to ALK inhibitors (Chapter 11).

MORPHOLOGY

In childhood, about 40% of neuroblastomas arise in the **adrenal medulla.** The remainder occur anywhere along the sympathetic chain, with the most common locations being the paravertebral region of the abdomen (25%) and posterior mediastinum (15%). Macroscopically, neuroblastomas range from clinically silent minute nodules (in situ lesions) to large masses weighing more than 1 kg. The great majority of the silent lesions spontaneously regress, possibly because they have not accumulated enough mutations to become fully transformed. Some neuroblastomas are sharply demarcated, but others are infiltrative and invade surrounding structures, including the kidneys, renal vein, and vena cava, sometimes enveloping the aorta. On transection, they are composed of soft, gray-tan tissue. Larger tumors have areas of necrosis, softening, and hemorrhage.

Histologically, neuroblastomas are composed of sheets of small, primitive-appearing cells with dark nuclei, scant cytoplasm, and poorly defined cell borders (Fig. 4.38A). Mitotic activity, nuclear breakdown (karyorrhexis), and pleomorphism may be prominent. The background often demonstrates faintly eosinophilic fibrillary material (neuropil) that corresponds to neuritic processes of the primitive neuroblasts. Typically, so-called **Homer-Wright pseudorosettes** can be found in which the tumor cells are concentrically arranged about a central space filled with neuropil (the absence of an actual central lumen garners the designation *pseudo*). Other helpful features include immunochemical detection of neural markers, such as **neuron-specific enolase,** and demonstration of small, membrane-bound, cytoplasmic catecholamine-containing secretory granules by electron microscopy.

Some neoplasms show signs of **maturation,** either spontaneous or therapy induced. Larger cells having more abundant cytoplasm with large vesicular nuclei and a prominent nucleolus, representing **ganglion cells** in various stages of maturation, may be found in tumors admixed with primitive neuroblasts **(ganglioneuroblastoma).** Lesions that are even better differentiated contain many more large cells resembling mature ganglion cells in the absence of residual neuroblasts; such neoplasms merit the designation **ganglioneuroma** (Fig. 4.38B). Maturation of neuroblasts into ganglion cells is usually accompanied by the appearance of Schwann cells and predicts a better prognosis.

Clinical Features. Many factors influence prognosis, but the most important are the stage of the tumor and the age of the patient.

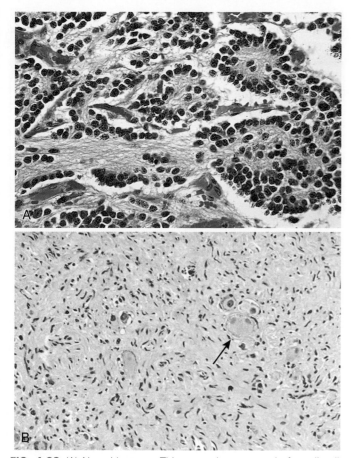

FIG. 4.38 (A) Neuroblastoma. This tumor is composed of small cells embedded in a finely fibrillar matrix (neuropil). A Homer-Wright pseudorosette (tumor cells arranged concentrically around a central core of neuropil) is seen in the upper right corner. (B) Ganglioneuroma, arising from spontaneous or therapy-induced maturation of neuroblastoma, is characterized by clusters of large ganglion cells with vesicular nuclei and abundant eosinophilic cytoplasm *(arrow)*. Spindle-shaped Schwann cells are present in the background stroma.

- *Staging.* The international neuroblastoma staging system is of great importance in establishing a prognosis. Four stages (1–4) are defined on the basis of local, regional, and distant spread. Particular note should be taken of stage 4S (S means *special*), because the outlook for these patients is excellent, despite wide spread of disease. Typically, such tumors are localized but with metastatic spread limited to liver, skin, and bone marrow, without bone involvement. The biologic basis for this welcome behavior is not clear.
- *Age.* The outlook for children younger than 18 months is much more favorable than for older children. Most neoplasms diagnosed in children during the first 18 months of life are stage 1 or 2, or stage 4S ("low" risk category), whereas neoplasms in older children fall into the "intermediate" or "high" category of risk based on other prognostic markers discussed below.
- *Histology* is an independent prognostic variable in neuroblastic tumors: evidence of Schwannian stroma and gangliocytic differentiation is indicative of a favorable prognosis.
- *Amplification of the MYCN* oncogene has a profound impact on prognosis. *MYCN* amplification is present in about 25% to 30% of primary tumors. The greater the number of copies, the worse

the prognosis. Amplification of *MYCN* is not seen as chromosomal gain at the site of the gene (2p23-24), but rather as extrachromosomal double minute chromosomes or homogeneously staining regions on other chromosomes (Fig. 4.39). **MYCN amplification is currently the most important genetic abnormality used in risk stratification of neuroblastic tumors and automatically renders a tumor as "high" risk, regardless of stage or age.** In one large study children with *MYCN*-amplified tumors had event-free survival of 50% versus 90%, compared with those without *MYCN* amplification.

- *DNA ploidy* is another prognostic factor: tumors that are hyperdiploid (with whole chromosome gains) have more favorable prognosis than tumors that are diploid.

Children younger than 2 years with neuroblastomas generally present with a protuberant abdomen resulting from an abdominal mass, fever, and weight loss. In older children the tumor may remain unnoticed until metastases cause hepatomegaly, ascites, and bone pain. Neuroblastomas may metastasize widely through the hematogenous and lymphatic systems, particularly to liver, lungs, bones, and the bone marrow. In neonates, disseminated neuroblastomas may manifest with multiple cutaneous metastases associated with deep blue discoloration of the skin. About 90% of neuroblastomas, regardless of location, produce catecholamines (similar to the catecholamines associated with pheochromocytomas), which constitutes an important diagnostic feature (i.e., elevated blood levels of catecholamines and elevated urine levels of catecholamine metabolites such as vanillylmandelic acid [VMA] and homovanillic acid [HVA]). Despite the elaboration of catecholamines, hypertension is much less frequent with these neoplasms than with pheochromocytomas (Chapter 18).

Retinoblastoma

Retinoblastoma is the most common primary intraocular malignancy of children. The molecular genetics of retinoblastoma is discussed in Chapter 6. Approximately 40% of the tumors are associated with a germline mutation in the *RB* gene and are therefore heritable.

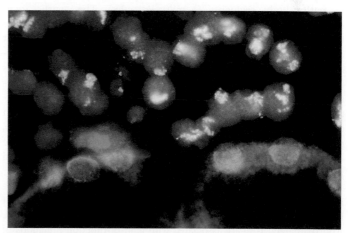

FIG. 4.39 FISH using a fluorescein-labeled probe for *MYCN* on a tissue section containing kidney with neuroblastoma. Note the neuroblastoma cells in the upper half of the field with large areas of staining *(yellow-green)*; this corresponds to amplified *MYCN* in the form of homogeneously staining regions. Renal tubular epithelial cells in the lower half of the field show no nuclear staining and background *(green)* cytoplasmic staining. (Courtesy Dr. Timothy Triche, Children's Hospital, Los Angeles, California.)

The remaining tumors develop sporadically, and these have somatic *RB* gene mutations. Familial cases are typically associated with development of multiple bilateral tumors, although they may be unifocal and unilateral. Sporadic tumors are unilateral and unifocal. Patients with familial retinoblastoma are also at increased risk for the development of osteosarcoma and other soft tissue tumors. The morphology and clinical features of retinoblastoma are discussed in Chapter 21.

Wilms Tumor

Wilms tumor, or nephroblastoma, is the most common primary tumor of the kidney in children, with most cases occurring in children between 2 and 5 years of age. This tumor illustrates several important concepts of childhood tumors: the relationship between congenital malformation and increased risk of tumors; the histologic similarity between the tumor and developing organ; and, finally, the remarkable success in the treatment of childhood tumors. Each of these concepts is presented in the following discussion.

Three groups of congenital malformations are associated with an increased risk for Wilms tumor. These are *WAGR syndrome* (Wilms tumor, aniridia, genital abnormalities, and mental retardation), *Denys-Drash syndrome (DDS)*, and *Beckwith-Wiedemann syndrome (BWS)*. Approximately one in three patients with WAGR syndrome will develop this tumor. Those with DDS have an even higher risk of developing Wilms tumor (approximately 90%). DDS is characterized by gonadal dysgenesis and early onset nephropathy. Both of these conditions are associated with abnormalities of the Wilms tumor 1 *(WT1)* gene, located on chromosome 11p13. The nature of the genetic aberration differs, however: patients with WAGR syndrome demonstrate loss of genetic material (i.e., deletions) of *WT1,* while individuals with DDS harbor a dominant negative inactivating mutation in *WT1* that interferes with the function of normal WT1 protein encoded by the other *WT1* allele. *WT1* is critical for normal renal and gonadal development and constitutional inactivation of one copy of this gene results in genitourinary abnormalities in humans.

A third group of patients, those with BWS, are also at increased risk for the development of Wilms tumor. These patients exhibit enlargement of individual body organs (e.g., tongue, kidneys, or liver) or entire body segments (hemihypertrophy). The genetic locus implicated in BWS maps to subband p15.5 of chromosome 11 distal to the *WT1* locus. This region contains several genes, including one that encodes insulin-like growth factor-2 (IGF2). The *IGF2* gene is normally expressed from the paternal allele, whereas the maternal allele is imprinted. In some Wilms tumors, loss of imprinting (i.e., reexpression of *IGF2* by the maternal allele) occurs, leading to overexpression of the IGF-2 protein, which is postulated to result in both organ enlargement and tumorigenesis. In addition to Wilms tumors, patients with BWS are also at increased risk for the development of hepatoblastoma, adrenocortical tumors, rhabdomyosarcoma, and pancreatic tumors.

In contrast to syndromic Wilms tumors, the molecular abnormalities underlying sporadic (i.e., nonsyndromic) tumors, which account for 90% of cases overall in children, are only recently being elucidated. Approximately, 10% are associated with gain-of-function mutations of the gene encoding β-catenin (Chapter 6). In 15% to 20% of cases recurrent mutations occur in genes encoding proteins involved in microRNA processing; these lead to reduced levels of many mature microRNAs, in particular those involved in "mesenchymal to epithelial transformation" during renal morphogenesis. The lack of mesenchymal to epithelial transformation likely leads to persistent blastemal "rests" in the kidney (see the following), which can evolve into Wilms tumors.

Finally, tumors with *TP53* mutations are associated with an especially poor prognosis and often have a distinctive anaplastic histologic appearance, described later.

MORPHOLOGY

Wilms tumor typically is a large, solitary, well-circumscribed mass, although 10% are either bilateral or multicentric at the time of diagnosis. On cut section, the tumor is soft, homogeneous, and tan to gray, with occasional foci of hemorrhage, cystic degeneration, and necrosis (Fig. 4.40).

On microscopic examination, Wilms tumors are characterized by recognizable attempts to recapitulate different stages of nephrogenesis. The classic **triphasic combination** of blastemal, stromal, and epithelial cell types is observed in most lesions, although the percentage of each component varies (Fig. 4.41A). Sheets of small blue cells, with few distinctive features, characterize the **blastemal component.** Epithelial "differentiation" usually takes the form of **abortive tubules or glomeruli.** Stromal cells are usually fibroblastic or myxoid in nature, although skeletal muscle "differentiation" is not uncommon. Approximately 5% of tumors contain foci of **anaplasia** (cells with large, hyperchromatic, pleomorphic nuclei and abnormal mitoses) (Fig. 4.41B). The presence of anaplasia correlates with the presence of acquired *TP53* mutations and the emergence of resistance to chemotherapy.

Nephrogenic rests are putative precursor lesions of Wilms tumors and are sometimes present in the renal parenchyma adjacent to the tumor. Nephrogenic rests contain a mixture of cells resembling those seen in Wilms tumor with occasional admixed immature tubules or glomeruli. It is important to document the presence of nephrogenic rests in the resected specimen, because these patients are at an increased risk for the development of Wilms tumor in the contralateral kidney.

Clinical Features. Patients typically present with a palpable abdominal mass, which may extend across the midline and down into the pelvis. Less often, the presenting features are fever and abdominal pain,

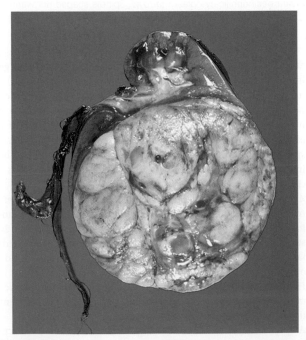

FIG. 4.40 Wilms tumor in the lower pole of the kidney with the characteristic tan to gray color and well-circumscribed margins.

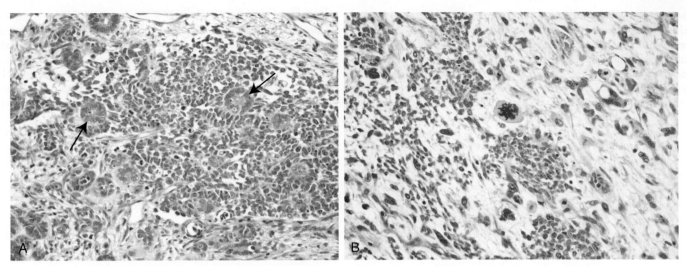

FIG. 4.41 (A) Wilms tumor with tightly packed blue cells consistent with the blastemal component and interspersed primitive tubules *(arrows)*, representing the epithelial component. (B) Focal anaplasia was present in other areas within this Wilms tumor, characterized by cells with hyperchromatic, pleomorphic nuclei, and an abnormal mitosis (center of field). Predominance of blastemal morphology and diffuse anaplasia are associated with specific molecular lesions (see text).

hematuria or, occasionally, intestinal obstruction as a result of pressure from the tumor. The prognosis for Wilms tumor is generally very good, and excellent results are obtained with a combination of nephrectomy and chemotherapy. Diffuse anaplasia is an indicator of adverse prognosis.

MOLECULAR DIAGNOSIS OF GENETIC DISORDERS

Several factors have enabled the rapid expansion of molecular diagnostics from the realm of research to clinical pathology laboratories. These include (1) the sequencing of the human genome and availability of these data in publicly available databases; (2) the availability of numerous "off-the-shelf" polymerase chain reaction (PCR) kits tailor-made for the identification of specific genetic disorders; (3) the availability of high-resolution microarrays ("gene chips") that can interrogate both DNA and RNA on a genomewide scale using a single platform; and, finally, (4) the emergence of automated, high-throughput, next-generation ("NextGen") sequencing (NGS) technologies. The last two advances have been especially useful in the context of new research to elucidate the genetic basis for both mendelian and complex disorders. Although a detailed discussion of molecular diagnostics is beyond the scope of this book, some of the better-known approaches are highlighted in the ensuing paragraphs. Regardless of the technique used, the genetic aberration being queried can be either in the germline (i.e., present in each and every cell of the affected person, as with a *CFTR* mutation in a patient with CF) or somatic (i.e., restricted to specific tissue types or lesions, as with *MYCN* amplification in neuroblastoma cells). This consideration determines the nature of the sample (e.g., peripheral blood lymphocytes, saliva, tumor tissue) used for the assay.

Indications for Genetic Analysis

In general, indications for genetic analysis can be divided into inherited conditions and acquired conditions. Within inherited conditions, genetic testing can be offered at either the prenatal or postnatal stages. It may involve conventional cytogenetics, FISH, molecular diagnostics, or a combination of these techniques.

Prenatal genetic analysis should be offered to all patients who are at risk of having children with cytogenetic abnormalities. It can be performed on cells obtained by amniocentesis, on chorionic villus biopsy material, or cell-free fetal DNA from maternal blood. Some important indications are the following:

- *Advanced maternal age* (beyond 34 years), which is associated with greater risk of trisomies
- *Confirmed carrier status* for a balanced reciprocal translocation, Robertsonian translocation, or inversion (in such cases, the gametes may be unbalanced, so the progeny would be at risk for chromosomal disorders)
- *Fetal abnormalities* observed on ultrasound, or an abnormal result on routine maternal blood screening
- *A chromosomal abnormality or mendelian disorder affecting a previous child*
- *Determination of fetal sex* when the patient or partner is a confirmed carrier of an X-linked genetic disorder

Postnatal genetic analysis is usually performed on peripheral blood lymphocytes. Indications are as follows:

- *Multiple congenital anomalies*
- *Suspicion of a metabolic syndrome*
- *Unexplained intellectual disability* and/or developmental delay
- *Suspected aneuploidy* (e.g., features of Down syndrome) or other syndromic chromosomal abnormality (e.g., deletions, inversions)
- *Suspected sex chromosomal abnormality* (e.g., Turner syndrome)
- *Suspected fragile X syndrome*
- *Infertility* to rule out sex chromosomal abnormality
- *Multiple spontaneous abortions* to rule out balanced translocation in a parent

Acquired genetic alterations, such as somatic mutations in cancer, are increasingly becoming a focus area in molecular diagnostics laboratories, especially with the advent of targeted therapies. Although single gene tests (mutations of *EGFR* or *BRAF*, amplification of *HER2*) have been used for years to inform treatment decisions, the advent of cost-effective next-generation sequencing approaches now allows interrogation of large numbers of coding genes (often in the 100s), as well as cancer-relevant translocations, in a single assay. The clinical team typically receives a "genomic report" on the patient's cancer, including potential molecularly targeted treatment recommendations. Another major focus of molecular diagnostics has been the rapid identification of infectious diseases, such as suspected tuberculosis or virulent pathogens such as SARS-CoV-2, using DNA-based approaches. In general, these approaches have reduced the time required for diagnosis from weeks to a matter of days. Besides de novo identification of pathogens, molecular diagnostics laboratories can also contribute to the identification of treatment resistance (e.g., acquired mutations in influenza viruses that render them resistant to antiviral medications), and to the monitoring of treatment efficacy using assays for "viral load" in the blood. Similar parameters (measuring efficacy of therapy and emergence of resistance) are also widely used in patients with cancer.

Because of the rapid advances in molecular diagnostics, terms such as "personalized therapy" and "precision medicine" are being increasingly used to indicate therapy tailored to the needs of the individual patient.

Molecular Tests and Their Application

The field of testing for genetic disorders is rapidly evolving. A brief review of current testing modalities and their use for the diagnosis of genetic disorders is offered below and is summarized in Table 4.9. Tests that are used to confirm the diagnosis of various genetic disorders are designed to identify the causative genetic abnormality or, in some instances, the effect of the abnormality on proteins encoded by mutated genes. These tests can be broadly divided into several categories:

Tests That Detect Structural Abnormalities of Chromosomes

Historically, these were identified by *karyotype analysis*, which is only capable of identifying microscopically evident structural abnormalities. Increasingly, karyotyping has been replaced by array-based *comparative genomic hybridization* (CGH), in which DNA from a patient and a control specimen are labeled with two different fluorescent dyes. The DNAs are mixed and hybridized to an array of probes displayed as distinct spots on a slide that span the genome. Over- or underrepresentation of patient DNA corresponding to a particular genomic region is scored as a change in the ratio of fluorescent tag 1 to fluorescent tag 2. Array CGH has several advantages over karyotyping: It does not require cell culture, is easy to interpret, and also has much greater resolution, which is limited only by the number of discrete probes that are present in the array.

Fluorescence In Situ Hybridization. Fluorescence in situ hybridization (FISH) uses DNA probes that recognize sequences specific to chromosomal regions of tens to hundreds of kilobases, which defines the limit of resolution with this technique for identifying chromosomal changes. Such probes are labeled with fluorescent dyes and are applied to metaphase spreads or interphase nuclei. The probe hybridizes to its complementary sequence on the chromosome and thus labels the specific chromosomal region, which is then visualized under a fluorescence microscope. The ability of FISH to circumvent the need for dividing cells is invaluable when a rapid diagnosis is needed (e.g., in a critically ill infant suspected of having an underlying genetic disorder). Such analyses can be performed on prenatal samples (e.g., cells obtained by amniocentesis, chorionic villus biopsy, or umbilical cord blood), peripheral blood lymphocytes, and even archival tissue sections. FISH is used for the detection of numeric abnormalities

Table 4.9 Testing Modalities for Genetic Disorders

Test Type	Applications and Examples
Biochemical Assays	
Quantitative assays for metabolites or electrolytes	Detection of abnormal metabolite levels in metabolic disorders (e.g., phenylketonuria); detection of high chloride levels in sweat (cystic fibrosis)
Assay of enzyme activity	Detection of enzyme deficiencies (e.g., acid maltase in Pompe disease; G6PD deficiency)
Hemoglobin electrophoresis	Detection of abnormal hemoglobins (e.g., sickle hemoglobin)
Cytogenetic Assays	
Karyotyping	Grossly evident structural changes in chromosomes (e.g., trisomy 21 in Down syndrome)
Fluorescence in situ hybridization (FISH)	Subtle/submicroscopic structural changes in chromosomes (e.g., 22.q11.2 del syndrome)
"Molecular" Cytogenetic Assays	
Multiplex ligation-dependent probe amplification	Small deletions and insertions (e.g., partial deletion of *BRCA1* in familial breast cancer)
Array-based genomic hybridization	Copy number changes (e.g., trisomy 21 in Down syndrome)
Next-generation sequencing (NGS)	Copy number changes, translocations (mainly used clinically to identify somatic copy number changes and translocations in cancer cells)
Genetic Assays	
Allele-specific PCR and related techniques	Specific base pair changes (single, e.g., sickle hemoglobin mutation, or multiple, e.g., *CFTR* mutations in cystic fibrosis)
Sanger DNA sequencing	Mutations in individual genes (e.g., glucose-6-phosphatase mutations in von Gierke disease)
Next-generation sequencing (NGS)	Mutations in many genes and/or in noncoding regions (used clinically to identify somatic mutations in cancer cells and in research to discover mutations responsible for unusual phenotypes)

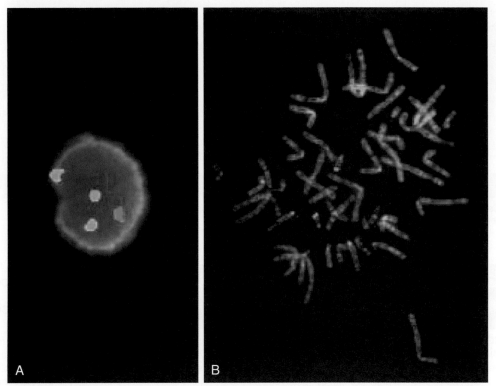

FIG. 4.42 FISH. (A) Interphase nucleus from a male patient with suspected trisomy 18. Three different fluorescent probes have been used in a "FISH cocktail"; the green probe hybridizes to the X chromosome centromere *(one copy),* the red probe to the Y chromosome centromere *(one copy),* and the aqua probe to the chromosome 18 centromere *(three copies).* (B) A metaphase spread in which two fluorescent probes have been used, one hybridizing to chromosome region 22q13 *(green)* and the other hybridizing to chromosome region 22q11.2 *(red).* There are two 22q13 signals. One of the two chromosomes does not stain with the probe for 22q11.2, indicating a microdeletion in this region. This abnormality gives rise to the 22q11.2 deletion syndrome (DiGeorge syndrome). (Courtesy of Dr. Nancy R. Schneider and Jeff Doolittle, Cytogenetics Laboratory, University of Texas Southwestern Medical Center, Dallas, Texas.)

of chromosomes (aneuploidy) (Fig. 4.42A), subtle microdeletions (Fig. 4.42B) and complex translocations not indentifiable by routine karyotyping, and gene amplification (e.g., *MYCN* amplification in neuroblastomas).

Liquid Biopsy

Molecular tests also have been developed that use cell-free fetal DNA found in maternal blood *(liquid biopsy)* to assess whole-chromosome numbers in the developing fetus. Current applications include identification of fetal sex and the detection of copy number changes in sex chromosomes and autosomes, including trisomies 13, 18, and 21. Liquid biopsy is also being used for diagnosis and management of certain cancers since cell-free tumor DNA can be found in the circulation of patients with cancer.

Tests That Detect Mutations in Single Genes

If a mutation in a particular gene is suspected, that region can be amplified by *polymerase chain reaction* (PCR), sequenced, and compared with a normal reference sequence. PCR analysis, which involves exponential amplification of DNA, is now widely used in molecular diagnosis. If RNA is used as the substrate, it is first reverse-transcribed to obtain cDNA and then amplified by PCR. This method involving *reverse transcription* (RT) often is abbreviated RT-PCR. To amplify a DNA segment of interest, two primers that bind to the 3′ and 5′ ends of the normal sequence are designed. By using appropriate DNA polymerases and thermal cycling, the target DNA is greatly amplified, producing millions of copies of the DNA sequence between the two primer sites. The DNA sequence of the PCR product can then be analyzed in several ways.

It is becoming easier to sequence many genes, even the entire genome, by capturing genomic DNA through hybridization to a set of known nucleotide oligomers (baits) and sequencing the subsequently immobilized DNA template. This method, called *next-generation sequencing* (NGS), is becoming increasingly affordable and is used widely, but interpretation of the results is complex and requires specially trained individuals. The principle of NGS is illustrated in Fig 4.43.

Even in this era of molecular testing, in many single-gene disorders, it is easier, cheaper, or faster to test for alterations in mutated proteins or their functions than to identify the underlying DNA mutation directly. Examples include sweat chloride testing in cystic fibrosis; serum phenylalanine levels in phenylketonuria; electrophoresis of hemoglobin in sickle cell disease; and identification of enzyme deficiencies in a wide variety of disorders.

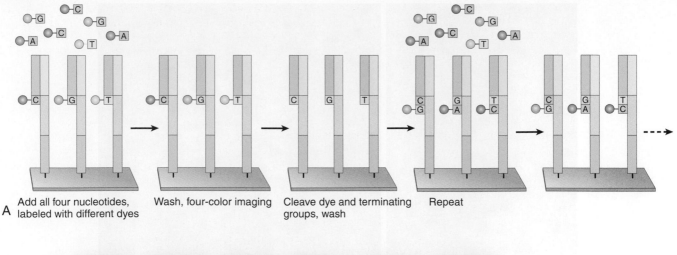

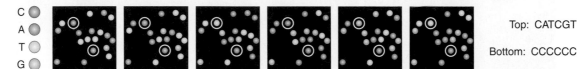

Top: CATCGT

Bottom: CCCCCC

FIG. 4.43 Principle of next-generation sequencing. Several alternative approaches are currently available for "Next generation" sequencing, and one of the more commonly used platforms is illustrated. (A) Short fragments of genomic DNA ("template") between 100 and 500 base pairs in length are immobilized on a solid phase platform such as a glass slide, using universal capture primers that are complementary to adapters that have previously been added to ends of the template fragments. The addition of fluorescently labeled complementary nucleotides, one per template DNA per cycle, occurs in a "massively parallel" fashion, at millions of templates immobilized on the solid phase at the same time. A four-color imaging camera captures the fluorescence emanating from each template location (corresponding to the specific incorporated nucleotide), following which the fluorescent dye is cleaved and washed away, and the entire cycle is repeated. (B) Powerful computational programs can decipher the images to generate sequences complementary to the template DNA at the end of one "run," and these sequences are then mapped back to the reference genomic sequence, to identify alterations. (Reproduced with permission from Metzker M: Sequencing technologies—the next generation. *Nat Rev Genet* 11:31–46, 2010, © Nature Publishing Group.)

■ RAPID REVIEW

Transmission Patterns of Single-Gene Disorders

- Autosomal dominant disorders are characterized by phenotypic expression in the heterozygous state; they affect both sexes equally, and both sexes can transmit the disorder.
- Autosomal dominant disorders often involve dysfunctional receptors, structural proteins, and tumor suppressor genes.
- Autosomal recessive diseases occur when both copies of a gene are mutated and frequently involve enzymes. Both sexes are affected equally.
- X-linked disorders are transmitted by heterozygous females to their sons, who manifest the disease. Female carriers are usually unaffected because of random inactivation of one X chromosome.

Marfan Syndrome

- Marfan syndrome is caused by a mutation in the *FBN1* gene encoding fibrillin, which is required for structural integrity of connective tissues and activation of TGF-β.
- The major tissues affected are the skeleton, eyes, and cardiovascular system.

- Clinical features may include tall stature, long fingers, bilateral subluxation of the lens, mitral valve prolapse, aortic aneurysm, and aortic dissection.
- Prevention of cardiovascular disease involves the use of drugs that lower blood pressure and inhibit TGF-β signaling.

Ehlers-Danlos Syndromes

- There are thirteen variants of EDS, all characterized by defects in collagen synthesis or assembly. Each of the variants is caused by a distinct mutation.
- Clinical features may include fragile, hyperextensible skin that is vulnerable to trauma, hypermobile joints, and ruptures involving the colon, cornea, or large arteries. Wound healing is poor.

Familial Hypercholesterolemia

- Familial hypercholesterolemia is an autosomal dominant disorder caused most often by mutations in the gene encoding the LDL receptor. Less commonly mutations affecting ApoB-100 (ligand for LDL receptor) and activating mutations of PCSK9, which degrades LDL receptors, also cause a similar phenotype.
- Patients develop hypercholesterolemia as a consequence of impaired transport of LDL into the cells.

- In heterozygotes, elevated serum cholesterol greatly increases the risk of atherosclerosis and resultant coronary artery disease; homozygotes have an even greater increase in serum cholesterol and a higher frequency of ischemic heart disease. Cholesterol also deposits along tendon sheaths to produce xanthomas.

Cystic Fibrosis (CF)

- Cystic fibrosis is an autosomal recessive disease caused by mutations in the *CFTR* gene encoding a transmembrane regulator (CFTR).
- CFTR is an ion channel that regulates the transport of chloride, sodium, and bicarbonate ions. The defect in chloride ion transport results in high salt concentrations in sweat and in viscous luminal secretions in respiratory and gastrointestinal tracts. Defective bicarbonate transport in pancreatic ducts contributes to obstruction due to precipitation of mucin.
- *CFTR* mutations can be severe (e.g., ΔF508), resulting in multisystem disease, or mild, with limited disease extent and severity.
- Cardiopulmonary complications constitute the most common cause of death; pulmonary infections, especially with resistant *Pseudomonas* or *Burkholderia* species, are frequent. Bronchiectasis and right-sided heart failure are long-term sequelae.
- Pancreatic insufficiency is extremely common; infertility caused by congenital bilateral absence of vas deferens is a characteristic finding in adult males with CF.
- Liver disease, including cirrhosis, is increasing in frequency as life expectancy increases.
- Molecular therapies that enhance the transport or stability of mutant CFTR protein are useful in patients who harbor certain CFTR alleles.

Phenylketonuria

- PKU is an autosomal recessive disorder caused by a lack of the enzyme phenylalanine hydroxylase and a consequent inability to metabolize phenylalanine.
- Clinical features of untreated PKU may include severe mental disability, seizures, and decreased pigmentation of skin, all of which can be avoided by restricting the intake of phenylalanine in the diet.
- Females with PKU who discontinue dietary treatment have high phenylalanine levels and can give birth to children with neurologic deficits resulting from transplacental passage of phenylalanine metabolites.

Galactosemia

- Galactosemia is an autosomal recessive disorder caused by lack of the galactose-1-phosphate uriydyltransferase, an enzyme required for conversion of galactose to glucose. Its absence leads to the accumulation of galactose-1-phosphate and its metabolites in tissues.
- Clinical features may include jaundice, liver damage, cataracts, neural damage, vomiting and diarrhea, and *E. coli* sepsis. Dietary restriction of galactose can prevent at least some of the more severe complications.

Lysosomal Storage Diseases

- Inherited mutations leading to defective lysosomal enzyme functions give rise to accumulations and storage of complex substrates in the lysosomes and defective autophagy resulting in cellular injury.
- Tay-Sachs disease is caused by an inability to metabolize GM2 gangliosides because of a lack of lysosomal hexosaminidase A. GM2 gangliosides accumulate in the CNS and cause severe intellectual disability, blindness, motor weakness, and death by 2 to 3 years of age.
- Niemann-Pick disease types A and B are caused by a deficiency of sphingomyelinase. In the more severe, type A variant, accumulation of sphingomyelin in the nervous system results in neuronal damage. Sphingomyelin is also stored in phagocytes within the liver, spleen, bone marrow, and lymph nodes, causing their enlargement. In type B, neuronal damage is not present.
- Niemann-Pick disease type C is caused by a defect in cholesterol transport and resultant accumulation of cholesterol and gangliosides in the nervous system. Affected children exhibit ataxia, dysarthria, and psychomotor regression.
- Gaucher disease results from lack of the lysosomal enzyme glucocerebrosidase and accumulation of glucocerebroside in mononuclear phagocytic cells. In the most common, type 1 variant, affected phagocytes become enlarged (Gaucher cells) and accumulate in liver, spleen, and bone marrow, causing hepatosplenomegaly and bone erosion. Types 2 and 3 are characterized by variable neuronal involvement. Gaucher disease is a risk factor for Parkinson disease.
- Mucopolysaccharidoses result from accumulation of mucopolysaccharides in many tissues including liver, spleen, heart, blood vessels, brain, cornea, and joints. Affected patients in all forms have coarse facial features. Manifestations of Hurler syndrome include corneal clouding, coronary arterial and valvular deposits, and death in childhood. All MPSs are autosomal recessive disorders except Hunter syndrome, which is X-linked and associated with a milder clinical course.

Glycogen Storage Diseases

- Inherited deficiency of enzymes involved in glycogen metabolism can result in storage of normal or abnormal forms of glycogen.
- In the hepatic form (von Gierke disease), liver cells store glycogen because of a lack of hepatic glucose-6-phosphatase.
- There are several myopathic forms, including McArdle disease, in which lack of muscle phosphorylase gives rise to storage in skeletal muscles and cramps after exercise.
- In Pompe disease there is lack of lysosomal acid maltase, and all organs are affected, but heart involvement is predominant.

Cytogenetic Disorders Involving Autosomes

- Down syndrome is associated with an extra copy of genes on chromosome 21, most commonly due to trisomy 21 and less frequently from translocation of extra chromosomal material from chromosome 21 to other chromosomes or from mosaicism.
- Patients with Down syndrome have severe intellectual disability, flat facial profile, epicanthic folds, cardiac malformations, higher risk of leukemia and infections, and premature development of Alzheimer disease.
- Deletion of genes at chromosomal locus 22q11.2 gives rise to malformations affecting the face, heart, thymus, and parathyroids. The resulting disorders are recognized as (1) DiGeorge syndrome (thymic hypoplasia with diminished T-cell immunity and parathyroid hypoplasia with hypocalcemia) and (2) velocardiofacial syndrome (congenital heart disease involving outflow tracts, facial dysmorphism, and developmental delay).

Cytogenetic Disorders Involving Sex Chromosomes

- In females, one X chromosome, maternal or paternal, is randomly inactivated during development (lyonization).
- In Klinefelter syndrome, there are two or more X chromosomes with one Y chromosome as a result of nondisjunction of sex chromosomes. Patients have testicular atrophy, sterility, reduced body hair, and gynecomastia. It is the most common cause of male sterility.
- In Turner syndrome, there is partial or complete monosomy of genes on the short arm of the X chromosome, most commonly caused by the absence of one X chromosome (45,X) and less commonly by mosaicism, or by deletions involving the short arm of the X chromosome. Short stature, webbing of the neck, cubitus valgus, cardiovascular malformations, amenorrhea, lack of secondary sex characteristics, and fibrotic ovaries are typical clinical features.

Fragile X Syndrome, Fragile X—Associated Tremor/Ataxia Syndrome, and Fragile X—Associated Primary Ovarian Failure

- Pathologic amplification of trinucleotide repeats causes loss of function (fragile X syndrome [FXS]) or toxic gain-of-function (Huntington disease) mutations. Most such mutations produce neurodegenerative disorders.
- FXS results from loss of *FMR1* gene function and is characterized by severe intellectual disability and a variety of neuropsychiatric conditions such as autism spectrum disorders.
- In the healthy population, there are about 29 to 55 CGG repeats in the *FMR1* gene. The genomes of carrier males and females contain premutations with 55 to 200 CGG repeats that can expand up to 4000 repeats (full mutations) during oogenesis. When full mutations are transmitted to progeny, FXS occurs.
- Carriers of premutations develop fragile X—associated tremor/ataxia (males) and fragile X—associated primary ovarian failure (females) due to toxic gain of function by the abnormal *FMR1* mRNA.

Genomic Imprinting

- Imprinting involves transcriptional silencing of the paternal or maternal copies of certain genes during gametogenesis. For such genes only one functional copy exists in the individual. Loss of the functional allele (not imprinted) by deletions or uniparental disomy gives rise to diseases.
- Prader-Willi syndrome results from loss of paternal chromosomal region 15q12 and is characterized by intellectual disability, short stature, hypotonia, obesity, and hypogonadism.
- Angelman syndrome results from loss of maternal chromosomal region 15q12 and is characterized by intellectual disability, ataxia, seizures, and inappropriate laughter.

Congenital Anomalies

- Congenital anomalies result from intrinsic abnormalities (malformations) as well as extrinsic disturbances (deformations, disruptions).
- Congenital anomalies can result from genetic (chromosomal abnormalities, gene mutations), environmental (infections, drugs, alcohol), and multifactorial causes.
- The timing of the in utero insult has profound influence on the extent of congenital anomalies, with earlier events usually having greater impact.

- The interplay between genetic and environmental causes of anomalies is emphasized by the fact that teratogens often target signaling pathways in which mutations have been reported as a cause for the same anomalies.

Neonatal Respiratory Distress Syndrome

- Neonatal RDS (hyaline membrane disease) is a disease of prematurity; most cases occur in neonates born before 28 weeks' gestational age.
- The fundamental abnormality in RDS is insufficient pulmonary surfactant, which results in failure of lungs to inflate after birth.
- The characteristic morphologic pattern in RDS is the presence of hyaline membranes (consisting of necrotic epithelial cells and plasma proteins) lining the airways.
- RDS can be ameliorated by prophylactic administration of steroids, surfactant therapy, and improved ventilation techniques.
- Long-term sequelae associated with RDS therapy include retinopathy of prematurity and bronchopulmonary dysplasia; the incidence of both complications has decreased with improvements in management of RDS.

Sudden Infant Death Syndrome

- SIDS is a disorder of unknown cause, defined as the sudden death of an infant younger than 1 year of age that remains unexplained after a thorough case investigation including performance of an autopsy. Most SIDS deaths occur between the ages of 2 and 4 months.
- The most likely basis for SIDS is a delayed development of arousal reflexes and cardiorespiratory control.
- Numerous environmental risk factors have been proposed, of which the prone sleeping position is best recognized—hence the success of the "Back to Sleep" program in reducing the incidence of SIDS.

Fetal Hydrops

- Fetal hydrops refers to the accumulation of edema fluid in the fetus during intrauterine growth.
- The degree of fluid accumulation is variable, from generalized hydrops fetalis to localized cystic hygromas.
- The most common causes of fetal hydrops are nonimmune (chromosomal abnormalities, cardiovascular defects, and fetal anemia), since immune hydrops has become less frequent as a result of Rh antibody prophylaxis.
- Erythroblastosis fetalis (circulating immature erythroid precursors) is a characteristic finding of fetal anemia-associated hydrops.
- Hemolysis-induced hyperbilirubinemia can result in bilirubin toxicity (kernicterus) in the basal ganglia and brain stem, particularly in premature infants.

Neuroblastoma

- Neuroblastomas and related tumors arise from neural crest—derived cells in the sympathetic ganglia and adrenal medulla.
- Neuroblastomas are undifferentiated, whereas ganglioneuroblastomas and ganglioneuromas demonstrate evidence of differentiation (Schwannian stroma and ganglion cells). Homer-Wright pseudorosettes are characteristic of neuroblastomas.

- Age, stage, and *MYCN* amplification and ploidy are the most important prognostic features; children younger than 18 months usually have a better prognosis than older children, whereas children with higher-stage tumors or *MYCN* amplification fare worse.
- Neuroblastomas secrete catecholamines, whose metabolites (VMA/HVA) can be used for screening patients.

Wilms Tumor

- Wilms tumor is the most common renal neoplasm of childhood.
- Patients with three syndromes are at increased risk for Wilms tumors: Denys-Drash syndrome, Beckwith-Wiedemann syndrome, and WAGR syndrome (Wilms tumor, aniridia, genital abnormalities, and mental retardation).
- WAGR syndrome and DDS are associated with *WT1* gene inactivation, whereas Beckwith-Wiedemann arises through imprinting abnormalities principally involving the *IGF2* gene.
- The morphologic components of Wilms tumor include blastemal (small, round, blue cells) and epithelial and stromal elements.
- Nephrogenic rests are precursor lesions of Wilms tumors.

■ Laboratory Tests

Test	Normal Value	Pathophysiology/Clinical Relevance
CFTR (cystic fibrosis transmembrane conductance regulator) gene mutation	Negative	More than 2000 disease-causing mutations have been identified in the *CFTR* gene that encodes an anion channel which regulates transport of multiple ions, primarily chloride and bicarbonate. Cystic fibrosis is an autosomal recessive disease in which defective chloride, sodium, and bicarbonate transport gives rise to increased NaCl in sweat and dehydrated mucus in the airspaces and pancreatic acini. The most common *CFTR* mutation is ΔF508 (about 67% worldwide, higher in patients of Northern European descent). Diagnosis is based on persistently elevated sweat electrolyte concentrations and molecular testing for *CFTR* mutations.
Hexosaminidase A activity, serum	≤15 years old: 20%–90% of total hexosaminidase activity	Hexosaminidase A levels are decreased in the lysosomal storage disorder, Tay-Sachs disease, a GM2 gangliosidosis caused by deficiency of the α subunit of hexosaminidase A. Hexosaminidase A and hexosaminidase B are isoenzymes. This test measures activity of total hexosaminidase (A and B) using an artificial substrate. This test can also be used to detect carrier status.
TORCH IgG, serum	*Toxoplasma* antibody, negative Rubella antibody: vaccinated, positive unvaccinated, negative CMV antibody, negative HSV1 and HSV2 antibodies, negative	TORCH infections occurring early in gestation may cause chronic sequelae in the child, including growth restriction, intellectual disability, cataracts, and congenital cardiac anomalies, whereas infections later in pregnancy result primarily in tissue injury accompanied by inflammation (e.g., encephalitis, chorioretinitis, hepatosplenomegaly, pneumonia, and myocarditis)

References values from https://www.mayocliniclabs.com/ by permission of Mayo Foundation for Medical Education and Research. All rights reserved.

Adapted from Deyrup AT, D'Ambrosio D, Muir J, et al. Essential Laboratory Tests for Medical Education. *Acad Pathol.* 2022;9. doi: 10.1016/j.acpath.2022.100046.

5

Diseases of the Immune System

Immunity refers to protection against infections. The immune system is the collection of cells and molecules that are responsible for defending the body against the countless pathogens that individuals encounter. Defects in the immune system are the cause of *immunodeficiency diseases,* which render individuals easy prey to infections. But the immune system is itself capable of causing tissue injury and disease, called *hypersensitivity disorders.*

This chapter is devoted to diseases caused by too little immunity or too much immunologic reactivity. We also consider amyloidosis, a disease in which an abnormal protein, usually derived from fragments of antibodies or produced during chronic inflammatory disorders, is deposited in tissues. First, we review some important features of normal immune responses that are relevant to our understanding of immunologic diseases.

THE NORMAL IMMUNE RESPONSE

Defense against pathogens consists of two types of reactions (Fig. 5.1). **Innate immunity** (also called *natural,* or *native,* immunity) **is mediated by cells and proteins that are always present** (hence the term *innate*), **poised to react against infectious pathogens.** These mechanisms are called into action immediately in response to infection and thus provide the first line of defense. Some of these mechanisms are also involved in clearing damaged cells and tissues.

Many pathogens have evolved to resist innate immunity, and protection against these infections requires the more specialized and powerful mechanisms of **adaptive immunity** (also called *acquired,* or *specific,* immunity). **Adaptive immunity is normally quiescent and responds** (or *adapts*) **to the presence of infectious agents by generating potent mechanisms for neutralizing and eliminating the pathogens.** By convention, the terms *immune system* and *immune response* usually refer to adaptive immunity. The adaptive immune response typically takes 3 to 7 days to become fully active; innate immune mechanisms provide host defense during this critical early window after an infection.

Innate Immunity

The major components of innate immunity are epithelial barriers that block the entry of microbes, phagocytic cells (mainly neutrophils and macrophages), dendritic cells (DCs), natural killer (NK) cells and other innate lymphoid cells, and several plasma proteins, including the proteins of the complement system (Chapter 2).

Tissue-resident phagocytes, dendritic cells, and many other cells, such as epithelial cells, express receptors that detect the presence of infectious agents and substances released from dead cells. The microbial structures recognized by these receptors are called *pathogen-associated molecular patterns (PAMPs)*; they are shared among microbes of the same type, and they are essential for the survival and

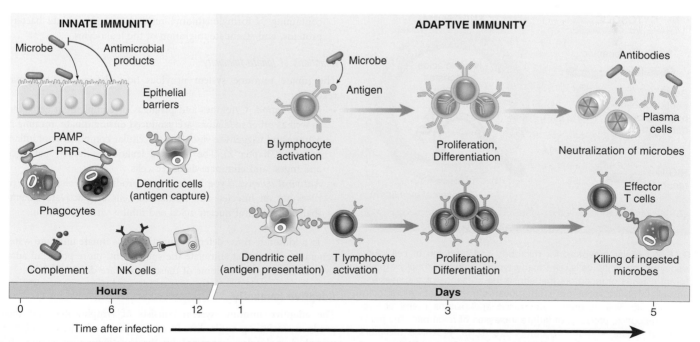

FIG. 5.1 The principal components and kinetics of innate and adaptive immune responses. *NK cells,* Natural killer cells. *PAMP,* Pathogen-associated molecular pattern; *PRR,* pattern recognition receptor.

infectivity of the microbes (so the microbes cannot evade innate immune recognition by mutating these molecules). The substances released from injured and necrotic cells are called *damage-associated molecular patterns (DAMPs)*. The cellular receptors that recognize these molecules are called *pattern recognition receptors*. It is estimated that innate immunity uses about 100 different receptors to recognize a few thousand molecular patterns.

Receptors of Innate Immunity

Pattern recognition receptors are located in all the cellular compartments where pathogens may be present: plasma membrane receptors detect extracellular pathogens, endosomal receptors detect ingested microbes, and cytosolic receptors detect microbes in the cytoplasm (Fig. 5.2). Several classes of these receptors have been identified.

Toll-Like Receptors. The best known of the pattern recognition receptors are the Toll-like receptors (TLRs). The plasma membrane TLRs recognize bacterial products such as lipopolysaccharide (LPS), and endosomal TLRs recognize RNA and DNA from viruses and bacteria that are phagocytosed into endosomes. Recognition of microbes by TLRs activates transcription factors that stimulate the production of mediators of inflammation (e.g., cytokines), antiviral cytokines called interferons (IFNs), and proteins such as costimulators (discussed later) that promote lymphocyte activation and the more potent adaptive immune responses.

NOD-Like Receptors and the Inflammasome. NOD-like receptors (NLRs) are cytosolic receptors named after the founding members of this group, NOD-1 and NOD-2. They recognize a wide variety of substances, including products of necrotic cells (e.g., uric acid and released ATP); ion disturbances (e.g., loss of K$^+$), which indicate cell damage; and some microbial products. Several of the NLRs signal via a cytosolic multiprotein complex called the *inflammasome*, which activates an enzyme (caspase-1) that cleaves a precursor form of the cytokine interleukin-1 (IL-1) to generate the biologically active form. As discussed in Chapter 2, IL-1 is a mediator of inflammation that recruits leukocytes and induces fever. Gain-of-function mutations in the NLRs result in systemic inflammatory disorders called autoinflammatory syndromes, which, as expected, respond well to treatment with IL-1 antagonists. The NLR-inflammasome pathway may also play a role in a number of chronic disorders marked by inflammation. For example, recognition of urate crystals by a class of NLRs underlies the inflammation associated with gout.

Other Receptors for Microbial Products. Other receptor families that play a role in innate immunity include the following.

- C-type lectin receptors expressed on the plasma membrane of macrophages and DCs detect microbial (bacterial and fungal) polysaccharides and stimulate phagocytosis and inflammatory reactions.
- Several types of receptors detect the nucleic acids of viruses that replicate in the cytoplasm of infected cells and stimulate the production of type I IFNs. Some of these receptors also recognize host DNA if it accumulates in the cytosol, which is often an indication of nuclear damage, leading to an inflammatory response that clears the injured cell. Excessive activation of these receptors may occur because of genetic defects in their regulation or defects in endonucleases that allow self DNA to accumulate. The resulting unregulated production of interferon causes systemic inflammatory diseases that are called interferonopathies.
- G protein–coupled receptors on neutrophils, macrophages, and most other types of leukocytes recognize short bacterial peptides containing N-formylmethionyl residues, which initiate bacterial proteins, and stimulate migration of the leukocytes.

Reactions of Innate Immunity

The innate immune system provides host defense by two main reactions:

- *Inflammation.* Cytokines and products of complement activation, as well as other mediators, are produced during innate immune reactions and trigger the vascular and cellular components of inflammation (Chapter 2). The recruited leukocytes destroy pathogens and ingest and eliminate damaged cells.
- *Antiviral defense.* Type I interferons produced in response to viruses act on infected and uninfected cells and activate enzymes that degrade viral nucleic acids and inhibit viral replication.

In addition to these defensive functions, the innate immune system generates signals that stimulate the subsequent, more powerful adaptive immune response. Some of these signals are described later.

Adaptive Immunity

The adaptive immune system consists of lymphocytes and their products, including antibodies. In contrast to the limited number of microbial molecules recognized by the innate immune system, the adaptive immune system can recognize a vast array of foreign substances.

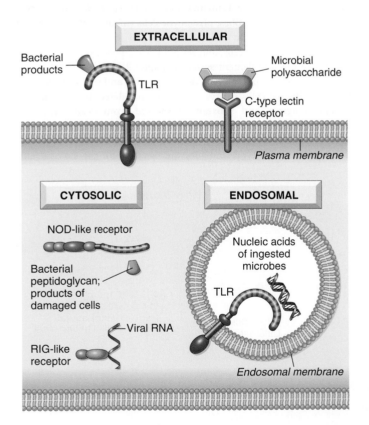

FIG. 5.2 Cellular receptors for microbes and products of cell injury. Phagocytes, dendritic cells, and many types of epithelial cells express different classes of receptors that sense the presence of microbes and dead cells. Toll-like receptors (TLRs) located in different cellular compartments, as well as other cytoplasmic and plasma membrane receptors, recognize products of different classes of microbes. The major classes of innate immune receptors are TLRs, NOD-like receptors (NLRs), C-type lectin receptors, RIG-like receptors for viral RNA, named after the founding member RIG-I, and cytosolic DNA sensors.

There are two types of adaptive immunity: **humoral immunity,** mediated by soluble proteins called **antibodies** that are produced by **B lymphocytes** (also called **B cells**), and **cell-mediated (or cellular) immunity,** mediated by **T lymphocytes** (also called **T cells**). Antibodies provide protection against extracellular pathogens in the blood, mucosal organs, and tissues. T lymphocytes are important in defense against microbes that have adapted to survive and replicate inside cells. They work by either directly killing infected cells (the function of cytotoxic T lymphocytes) or by activating phagocytes to kill ingested microbes, through the production of *cytokines* such as IFN-γ (made by helper T cells).

CELLS OF THE IMMUNE SYSTEM

The cells of the immune system consist of lymphocytes, most of which have specific receptors for antigens and mount adaptive immune responses; specialized antigen-presenting cells (APCs), which capture and display microbial and other antigens to lymphocytes; and various other cells such as phagocytes and eosinophils. We next discuss the major cell types involved in adaptive immune responses (Fig. 5.3).

T Lymphocytes

T lymphocytes, so called because they mature in the thymus, develop into the effector cells of cellular immunity following their activation and also stimulate B cells to produce antibodies against protein antigens. T cells constitute 60% to 70% of the lymphocytes in peripheral blood and are the major lymphocyte population in splenic periarteriolar sheaths and lymph node interfollicular zones. T cells cannot recognize free or circulating antigens; instead, the vast majority (>95%) of T cells see only peptide fragments of intracellular proteins displayed by molecules of the major histocompatibility complex (MHC), discussed in more detail later.

There are two major classes of T cells that are distinguished by the expression of CD4 or CD8 on their surfaces. CD4+ T cells are called *helper T cells* because they secrete soluble molecules (cytokines) that stimulate (help) B cells to produce antibodies and help macrophages to destroy phagocytosed microbes. The central role of CD4+ helper cells in immunity is highlighted by the severe immune defects that result from destruction of these cells by human immunodeficiency virus (HIV) infection (described later). The most important function of CD8+ T cells is to directly kill virus-infected cells and tumor cells; hence, they are called *cytotoxic T lymphocytes (CTLs).*

Peptide antigens presented by MHC molecules are recognized by the *T-cell receptor (TCR),* a heterodimer that in most T cells is composed of disulfide-linked α and β protein chains (Fig. 5.4A). Each chain has a variable region that participates in binding a particular peptide antigen and a constant region that interacts with associated signaling molecules. The sequence diversity of the antigen-binding portions is a consequence of the rearrangement and assembly of a multitude of TCR gene segments into functional TCR genes. T cells also express a number of other molecules that serve important

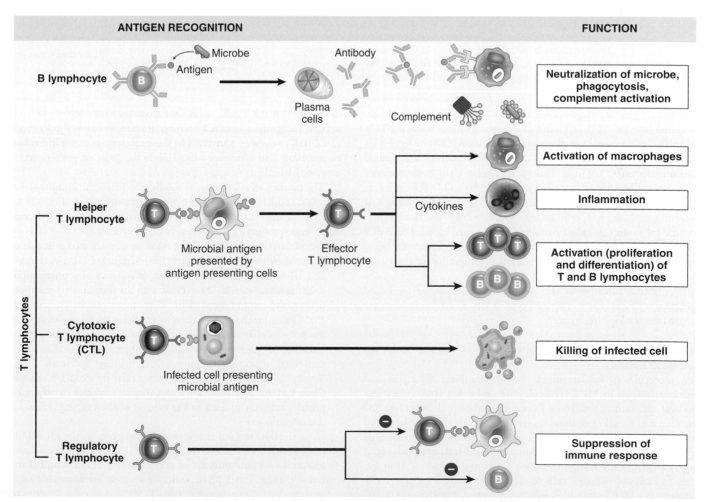

FIG. 5.3 The principal classes of lymphocytes and their functions in adaptive immunity.

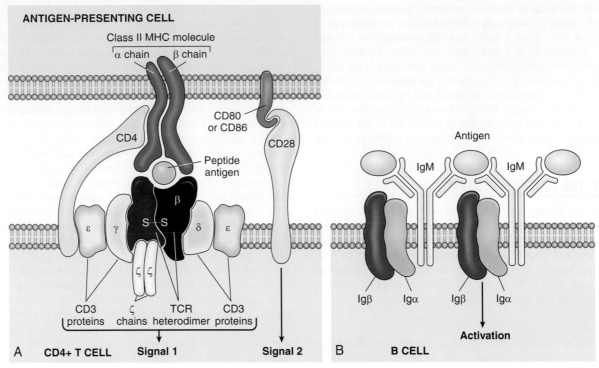

FIG. 5.4 Antigen receptors of T and B lymphocytes. (A) The T-cell receptor (TCR) complex and other molecules involved in T-cell activation. The TCR heterodimer, consisting of an α chain and a β chain, recognizes antigen (in the form of peptide-MHC complexes expressed on antigen-presenting cells), and the linked CD3 complex and ζ chains initiate activating signals. CD4 and CD28 are also involved in T-cell activation; CD28 recognizes the costimulators CD80 and CD86 (also called B7 molecules). (Note that some T cells express CD8 and not CD4; these molecules serve analogous roles.) The sizes of the molecules are not drawn to scale. (B) The B-cell antigen receptor complex is composed of membrane immunoglobulin M (IgM; or IgD, *not shown*), which recognizes antigens, and the associated signaling proteins Igα and Igβ. *MHC,* Major histocompatibility complex.

functions in immune responses. The CD3 complex is noncovalently associated with the TCR and initiates activating signals following TCR recognition of antigen. During antigen recognition, CD4 molecules on T cells bind to invariant portions of class II MHC molecules (described later) on selected APCs; in an analogous fashion, CD8 binds to class I MHC molecules. CD4 is expressed on 60% to 70% of T cells, whereas CD8 is expressed on about 30% to 40% of T cells. Other important invariant proteins on T cells include CD28, which functions as the receptor for molecules called *costimulators* that are induced on APCs by microbes, and various adhesion molecules that strengthen the bond between the T cells and APCs and control the migration of the T cells to different tissues.

T cells that function to suppress immune responses are called *regulatory T lymphocytes*. This cell type is described later, when we discuss immunologic tolerance.

Major Histocompatibility Complex Molecules: The Peptide Display System of Adaptive Immunity

MHC molecules are fundamental to T-cell recognition of antigens, and genetic variations in MHC molecules are associated with graft rejection and autoimmune diseases; hence, it is important to review the structure and function of these molecules. The MHC was discovered on the basis of studies of graft rejection and acceptance (tissue, or *"histo,"* compatibility). **The normal function of MHC molecules is to display peptides for recognition by CD4+ and CD8+ T lymphocytes.** In each individual, T cells recognize only peptides displayed by that person's MHC molecules, which, of course, are the only MHC

molecules that the T cells normally encounter. This property of T-cell antigen recognition is called *MHC restriction*. Because T cells recognize MHC molecules, variations in these molecules among individuals elicit strong immune responses. This is the basis of graft rejection, described later.

The human MHC, known as the human leukocyte antigen (HLA) complex, consists of a cluster of genes on chromosome 6 (Fig. 5.5). On the basis of their chemical structure, tissue distribution, and function, MHC gene products fall into two main categories:

- *Class I MHC* molecules are expressed on all nucleated cells and are encoded by three closely linked loci, designated HLA-A, HLA-B, and HLA-C. Each of these molecules consists of a polymorphic α chain noncovalently associated with an invariant β_2-microglobulin polypeptide (encoded by a separate gene on chromosome 15). The extracellular portion of the α chain contains a cleft where the polymorphic residues are located and where foreign peptides bind to MHC molecules for presentation to T cells, and a conserved region that binds CD8, ensuring that only CD8+ T cells can respond to peptides displayed by class I molecules. Class I MHC molecules bind and display peptides derived from protein antigens present in the cytosol of the cell (e.g., viral and tumor antigens).

- *Class II MHC* molecules are encoded by genes in the HLA-D region, which contains three subregions: DP, DQ, and DR. Class II molecules are heterodimers of noncovalently linked α and β subunits. Unlike class I MHC molecules, which are expressed on all nucleated cells, expression of class II MHC molecules is restricted

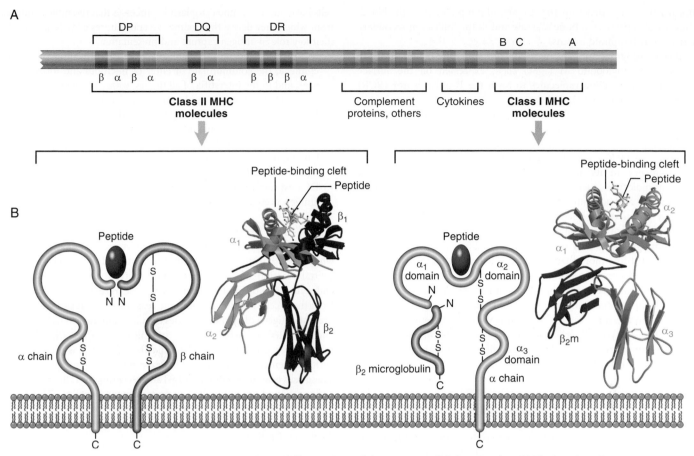

FIG. 5.5 The human leukocyte antigen (HLA) complex and the structure of HLA molecules. (A) The location of genes in the HLA complex. The relative locations, sizes, and distances between genes are not to scale. Genes that encode several proteins involved in antigen processing (the TAP transporter, components of the proteasome, and HLA-DM) are located in the class II region *(not shown)*. (B) Schematic diagrams and crystal structures of class I and class II HLA molecules. N and C refer to amino and carboxy termini, respectively, and S-S to disulfide bonds. *MHC,* Major histocompatibility complex. (Crystal structures are courtesy of Dr. P. Bjorkman, California Institute of Technology, Pasadena, California.)

to a few cell types, mainly APCs (notably, dendritic cells), macrophages, and B cells. The extracellular portion of class II MHC molecules contains a cleft for the binding of antigenic peptides and a region that binds CD4. In general, class II MHC molecules bind peptides derived from extracellular proteins, for example, from microbes that are ingested and then broken down inside the cell. This property allows CD4+ T cells to recognize the presence of extracellular pathogens.

HLA genes are highly polymorphic; that is, there are alternative forms (alleles) of each gene at each locus (estimated to number over 10,000 for all HLA genes and over 3500 for HLA-B alleles alone). Each individual expresses only one set of HLA genes, and each MHC molecule can display only one peptide at a time. The many MHC variants in the population evolved to display the multitude of microbial peptides that could be encountered in the environment. As a result of this polymorphism, a vast number of combinations of HLA molecules exist in the population. HLA genes are closely linked, so they are passed from parent to offspring *en bloc* and behave like a single locus with respect to their inheritance patterns. Each set of maternal and paternal HLA genes is referred to as an *HLA haplotype.* Because of this mode of inheritance, the probability that siblings will

inherit the same HLA alleles is 25%. By contrast, the probability that an unrelated donor will share the same HLA genes is very low. The implications of HLA polymorphism for transplantation are obvious; because each person has HLA alleles that differ to some extent from those of every other unrelated individual, grafts from unrelated donors will elicit immune responses in the recipient and be rejected unless the T cell response is suppressed (see discussion later). Only identical twins can accept grafts from one another without fear of rejection.

The inheritance of particular MHC alleles influences both protective and harmful immune responses. The ability of any given MHC allele to bind the peptide antigens generated from a particular pathogen will determine whether a specific individual's T cells can recognize and mount a protective response to that pathogen. Conversely, if the antigen is an allergen and the response is an allergic reaction, inheritance of some HLA alleles may make individuals susceptible to the allergic reaction. Many autoimmune diseases are associated with particular HLA alleles. We return to a discussion of these associations when we consider autoimmunity.

B Lymphocytes

B lymphocytes, so-called because they mature in the bone marrow, are the cells that produce antibodies, the mediators of humoral

immunity. B cells make up 10% to 20% of lymphocytes in the blood. They are also present in bone marrow and in the follicles of secondary (peripheral) lymphoid organs.

B cells recognize antigens by means of membrane-bound antibody of the immunoglobulin M (IgM) class, expressed on the surface together with signaling molecules to form the B-cell receptor (BCR) complex (see Fig. 5.4B). Whereas T cells recognize only MHC-associated peptides, B cells recognize and respond to many more chemical structures, including soluble or cell-associated proteins, lipids, polysaccharides, nucleic acids, and small chemicals, without requiring the MHC. As with TCRs, each antibody has a unique amino acid sequence in its antigen-binding site. B cells express several invariant molecules, such as Igα and Igβ, that are responsible for signal transduction and activation following antigen recognition by the BCR.

After stimulation, B cells differentiate into *plasma cells,* which secrete large amounts of antibodies. There are five classes, or isotypes, of immunoglobulins that differ in their constant regions: IgG, IgM, and IgA constitute more than 95% of circulating antibodies (IgG being at the highest concentration); IgA is the major isotype in mucosal secretions; IgE is present in the circulation at very low concentrations and is found attached to the surfaces of tissue mast cells; and IgD is expressed on the surfaces of B cells but is virtually undetectable in the blood. These isotypes differ in their ability to activate complement and recruit inflammatory cells and thus have different roles in host defense and disease states.

Natural Killer Cells

Natural killer (NK) cells are lymphocytes that arise from the same common lymphoid progenitor that gives rise to T lymphocytes and B lymphocytes. **NK cells are innate immune cells, as they are functional without prior activation and do not express highly variable receptors for antigens.** The activation of NK cells is regulated by signals from two types of receptors. *Inhibitory receptors* recognize self class I MHC molecules, which are expressed on all healthy cells, whereas *activating receptors* recognize molecules that are expressed at high levels on stressed or infected cells. Normally, signals from inhibitory receptors dominate over those of activating receptors, preventing spontaneous activation of the NK cells and killing of normal host cells. Infections (especially viral infections) and stress are associated with reduced expression of class I MHC molecules and increased expression of proteins that engage activating receptors, resulting in activation of NK cells and elimination of the infected or stressed cells. NK cells also secrete cytokines such as interferon-γ (IFN-γ), thus providing early defense against intracellular microbial infections.

Innate lymphoid cells (ILCs) are lymphocytes related to NK cells that are not cytotoxic but produce many of the same cytokines that helper T cells do. ILCs do not express antigen receptors but respond to cytokines produced as a result of cell injury and stress. Because ILCs are always present in tissues, they may be early responders to microbes that damage tissues. However, their role in host defense in humans is not established.

Antigen-Presenting Cells

Numerous cell types are specialized to capture antigens and display them to lymphocytes. Of these, dendritic cells play a major role in displaying protein antigens to naïve T cells. Several other cell types present antigens to lymphocytes at various stages of immune responses.

Dendritic Cells

Dendritic cells (DCs) are the most important antigen-presenting cells (APCs) for initiating T-cell responses against protein antigens. These cells have numerous fine cytoplasmic processes that resemble dendrites, from which they derive their name. Several features of DCs account for their key role in antigen capture and presentation.

- DCs are located at the right place to capture antigens—under epithelia, the common site of entry of microbes and foreign antigens, and in the interstitia of all tissues, where antigens may be produced. DCs within the epidermis are called *Langerhans cells.*
- DCs express receptors for capturing and responding to microbes (and other antigens), including TLRs and C-type lectin receptors.
- In response to microbes, DCs migrate to the T-cell zones of lymphoid organs, where they are ideally positioned to present antigens to T cells.
- DCs express high levels of MHC and other molecules needed for antigen presentation and activation of T cells.

Other Antigen-Presenting Cells

Macrophages present antigens of phagocytosed microbes to T cells, which then activate the phagocytes to destroy the microbes. This is a central reaction of cell-mediated immunity. B lymphocytes present endocytosed antigens to helper T cells and receive activating signals from the T cells in humoral immune responses. All nucleated cells can present antigens of cytosolic viruses or tumor antigens to CD8+ T cells and are killed by these T cells. A specialized fibroblast with dendritic morphology, called the *follicular dendritic cell (FDC),* is present in the germinal centers of lymphoid follicles in the spleen and lymph nodes. These cells bear Fc receptors for IgG and receptors for C3b and can trap antigen bound to antibodies or complement proteins. These cells display antigens to B lymphocytes in lymphoid follicles and promote antibody responses but are not involved in capturing antigens for display to T cells.

Lymphoid Tissues

The tissues of the immune system consist of the *generative* (also called *primary,* or *central*) *lymphoid organs,* in which T lymphocytes and B lymphocytes mature and become competent to respond to antigens, and the *secondary* (or *peripheral*) *lymphoid organs,* in which adaptive immune responses to microbes are initiated. The principal generative lymphoid organs are the thymus, where T cells develop, and the bone marrow, the site of production of all blood cells and where B lymphocytes mature (described in Chapter 10). The major peripheral organs are briefly described next.

Secondary Lymphoid Organs

The secondary lymphoid organs are organized to concentrate antigens, APCs, and lymphocytes in a way that optimizes interactions among these cells and the development of adaptive immune responses. Most of the body's lymphocytes are located in these organs (Table 5.1).

Table 5.1 Distribution of Lymphocytes in Tissues[a]

Tissue	Number of Lymphocytes $\times 10^9$
Lymph nodes	190
Spleen	70
Bone marrow	50
Blood	10
Skin	20
Intestines	50
Liver	10
Lungs	30

[a]Approximate numbers of lymphocytes in different tissues in a healthy adult.

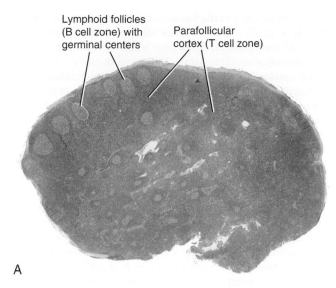

Lymphoid follicles (B cell zone) with germinal centers

Parafollicular cortex (T cell zone)

A

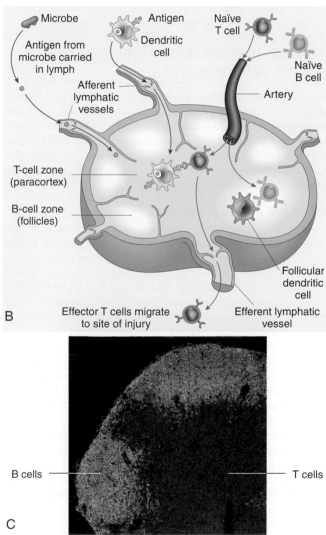

Microbe

Antigen from microbe carried in lymph

Antigen

Dendritic cell

Naïve T cell

Naïve B cell

Afferent lymphatic vessels

Artery

T-cell zone (paracortex)

B-cell zone (follicles)

Follicular dendritic cell

B

Effector T cells migrate to site of injury

Efferent lymphatic vessel

C

B cells

T cells

FIG. 5.6 Morphology of a lymph node. (A) Light micrograph shows a cross section of a lymph node illustrating the T cell and B cell zones. The B cell zones contain numerous follicles in the cortex, some of which contain lightly stained central areas (germinal centers). (B) The segregation of B cells and T cells in different regions of the lymph node, illustrated schematically. (C) The location of B cells (*stained green,* using the immunofluorescence technique) and T cells (*stained red*) in a lymph node. (A, Courtesy of Robert Ohgami, MD, PhD, and Kaushik Sridhar, MS Department of Pathology, University of California San Francisco; C, Courtesy of Drs. Kathryn Pape and Jennifer Walter, University of Minnesota School of Medicine, Minneapolis, Minnesota.)

- *Lymph nodes* are encapsulated, organized collections of lymphocytes, dendritic cells, and macrophages that are located along lymphatic channels throughout the body (Fig. 5.6A). As lymph passes through lymph nodes, resident APCs are able to sample antigens that are carried to the node in lymph from the interstitial fluids of tissues. In addition, DCs transport antigens from nearby epithelial surfaces and tissues by migrating through lymphatic vessels to the lymph nodes. Thus, antigens (e.g., of microbes that enter through epithelia or colonize tissues) become concentrated in draining lymph nodes.
- The *spleen* is organized into white pulp, which is where lymphocytes reside, and red pulp, which contains a network of sinusoids (through which blood flows). It plays an important role in immune responses to bloodborne antigens. Blood entering the spleen flows through the sinusoids where bloodborne antigens are trapped by resident DCs and macrophages.
- The *cutaneous and mucosal lymphoid systems* are located under the epithelia of the skin and the gastrointestinal and respiratory tracts, respectively. They respond to antigens that enter through breaches in the epithelium. Pharyngeal tonsils and Peyer's patches of the intestine are two anatomically defined mucosal lymphoid tissues. The large number of lymphocytes in mucosal organs (second only to lymph nodes) reflects the huge surface area of these organs.

In the secondary lymphoid organs, T lymphocytes and B lymphocytes are segregated into different regions (Fig. 5.6B, C). In lymph nodes, the B cells are concentrated in discrete structures, called *follicles,* located at the periphery, or cortex, of each node. If the B cells in a follicle have recently responded to an antigen, the follicle develops a central pale-staining region called a *germinal center.* T lymphocytes are concentrated in the parafollicular cortex. The follicles contain the FDCs that are involved in the activation of B cells, and the paracortex contains the DCs that present antigens to T lymphocytes. In the spleen, T lymphocytes are concentrated in periarteriolar lymphoid sheaths surrounding small arterioles, and B cells reside in the follicles.

Cytokines: Messenger Molecules of the Immune System

Cytokines are secreted proteins that mediate immune and inflammatory reactions. Molecularly defined cytokines are called *interleukins,* a name implying a role in communication between leukocytes. Most cytokines have a wide spectrum of actions, and some are produced by several different cell types. The majority of cytokines act on the cells that produce them or on neighboring cells, but some (like IL-1) also have systemic effects.

Different cytokines contribute to specific types of immune responses.

- In innate immune responses, cytokines are produced rapidly after microbes and other stimuli are encountered, and function to induce inflammation and inhibit virus replication. These cytokines include TNF, IL-1, IL-12, type I IFNs, IFN-γ, and chemokines (Chapter 2). They are produced primarily by macrophages, DCs, ILCs, and NK cells but can also be secreted by endothelial and epithelial cells.
- In adaptive immune responses, cytokines are produced principally by CD4+ T lymphocytes activated by antigen and other signals. They function to promote lymphocyte proliferation and differentiation

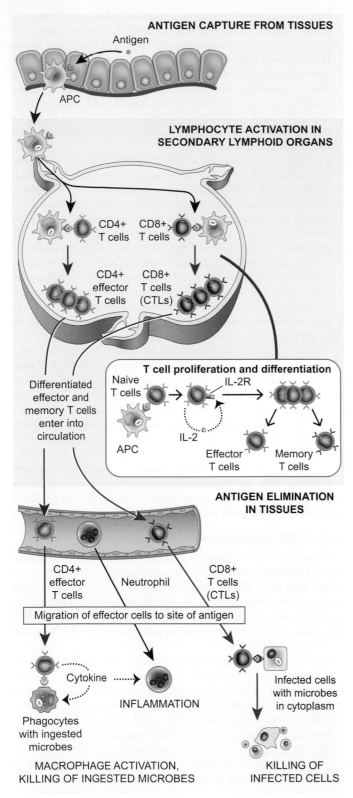

ANTIGEN CAPTURE FROM TISSUES

Antigen

APC

LYMPHOCYTE ACTIVATION IN SECONDARY LYMPHOID ORGANS

CD4+ T cells   CD8+ T cells

CD4+ effector T cells   CD8+ T cells (CTLs)

Differentiated effector and memory T cells enter into circulation

T cell proliferation and differentiation

Naïve T cells   IL-2R

APC   IL-2   Effector T cells   Memory T cells

ANTIGEN ELIMINATION IN TISSUES

CD4+ effector T cells   Neutrophil   CD8+ T cells (CTLs)

Migration of effector cells to site of antigen

Cytokine

INFLAMMATION

Phagocytes with ingested microbes

Infected cells with microbes in cytoplasm

MACROPHAGE ACTIVATION, KILLING OF INGESTED MICROBES

KILLING OF INFECTED CELLS

FIG. 5.7 Cell-mediated immunity. Dendritic cells (DCs) capture microbial antigens from epithelia and tissues and transport the antigens to lymph nodes. During this process, the DCs mature and express high levels of MHC molecules and costimulators. Naïve T cells recognize MHC-associated peptide antigens displayed on DCs. The T cells are activated to proliferate and to differentiate into effector and memory cells, which migrate to sites of infection and serve various functions in cell-mediated immunity. CD4+ effector T cells of the Th1 subset recognize the antigens of microbes ingested by phagocytes and activate

and to activate effector cells. The main cytokines in this group are IL-2, IL-4, IL-5, IL-17, and IFN-γ; their roles in immune responses are described later. Some cytokines serve mainly to limit and terminate immune responses; these include TGF-β and IL-10.

- Other cytokines stimulate hematopoiesis and are called *colony-stimulating factors* because they stimulate formation of blood cell colonies from bone marrow progenitors (Chapter 10), which increases leukocyte numbers during immune and inflammatory responses and replaces leukocytes that are consumed during such responses. They are produced by marrow stromal cells, T lymphocytes, macrophages, and other cells. Examples include IL-3, IL-7, and granulocyte-colony-stimulating factor.

The knowledge gained about cytokines has numerous practical therapeutic applications. Inhibiting cytokine production or actions can control the harmful effects of inflammation. For example, patients with rheumatoid arthritis often show dramatic responses to TNF antagonists. Other cytokine antagonists are now used to treat various inflammatory disorders. Conversely, administration of cytokines is used to boost reactions that are normally dependent on these proteins, such as hematopoiesis (e.g., following stem cell transplantation).

OVERVIEW OF LYMPHOCYTE ACTIVATION AND ADAPTIVE IMMUNE RESPONSES

Adaptive immune responses proceed in steps, consisting of antigen recognition; activation, proliferation and differentiation of specific lymphocytes into effector and memory cells; elimination of the antigen; and decline of the response, with memory cells being the long-lived survivors. The major events in each step are summarized next; these general principles apply to protective responses against microbes as well as pathologic responses that injure the host.

Capture and Display of Antigens

Microbes and other foreign antigens can enter the body virtually anywhere, and it is obviously impossible for lymphocytes of every specificity to patrol every possible portal of antigen entry. To overcome this problem, microbes and their protein antigens in epithelia and other tissues are captured by dendritic cells, which then carry their antigenic cargo to draining lymph nodes through which T cells constantly recirculate (Fig. 5.7). Here, the antigens are processed and complexed with MHC molecules for display on the cell surface, where the antigens are recognized by T cells. Similarly, soluble antigens are captured and concentrated in follicles in lymph nodes and the spleen, where they may be recognized by B cells via their antigen receptors.

Even before microbial antigens are recognized by T lymphocytes and B lymphocytes, the microbe activates innate immune cells expressing pattern recognition receptors. In the case of immunization with a protein antigen, as in a vaccine, a microbial mimic called an *adjuvant* that stimulates innate immune responses is given with the antigen. As part of the innate response, the microbe or adjuvant activates APCs to express molecules called *costimulators* and to secrete cytokines that stimulate the proliferation and differentiation of T

the phagocytes to kill the microbes; other subsets of effector cells enhance leukocyte recruitment and stimulate different types of immune responses. CD8+ cytotoxic T lymphocytes (CTLs) kill infected cells harboring microbes in the cytoplasm. Some activated T cells remain in the lymphoid organs and help B cells to produce antibodies, and some T cells differentiate into long-lived memory cells *(not shown)*. *APC,* Antigen-presenting cell.

lymphocytes. The principal costimulators for T cells are the B7 proteins (CD80 and CD86), which are expressed on APCs and are recognized by the CD28 receptor on naïve T cells.

The reactions and functions of T lymphocytes and B lymphocytes differ in important ways and are best considered separately.

Cell-Mediated Immunity: Activation of T Lymphocytes and Elimination of Intracellular Microbes

Naïve T lymphocytes are activated by antigen and costimulators in secondary lymphoid organs and proliferate and differentiate into effector cells that migrate to the site where the antigen (microbe) is present (see Fig. 5.7). One of the earliest responses of CD4+ helper T cells is secretion of the cytokine IL-2 and expression of high-affinity receptors for IL-2. IL-2 is a growth factor that acts on these T lymphocytes and stimulates their proliferation, leading to an increase in the number of antigen-specific lymphocytes. **The functions of helper T cells are mediated by the combined actions of CD40-ligand (CD40L) and cytokines.** CD40 is a member of the TNF-receptor family, and CD40L is a membrane protein homologous to TNF. When CD4+ helper T cells recognize antigens being displayed by macrophages or B lymphocytes, the T cells express CD40L, which engages CD40 on the macrophages or B cells and activates these cells. Mutations in the *CD40L* gene are the cause of *X-linked hyper-IgM syndrome,* in which both humoral and cell-mediated immunity are compromised (discussed later).

Some of the activated CD4+ T cells differentiate into effector cells that secrete different sets of cytokines and perform different functions (Fig. 5.8). The three best-defined subsets are the following:

- *Th1 cells* secrete the cytokine IFN-γ, which is a potent macrophage activator. The combination of CD40- and IFN-γ—mediated activation results in "classical" macrophage activation (Chapter 2), leading to the induction of microbicidal substances in macrophages and the destruction of ingested microbes.
- *Th2 cells* produce IL-4, which stimulates B cells to differentiate into IgE-secreting plasma cells; IL-5, which activates eosinophils; and IL-13, which activates mucosal epithelial cells to secrete mucus, and induces the "alternative" pathway of macrophage activation,

which is associated with tissue repair and fibrosis (Chapter 2). Eosinophils destroy pathogens such as helminthic parasites.
- *Th17 cells,* so called because the signature cytokine of these cells is IL-17, recruit neutrophils and monocytes, which destroy some extracellular bacteria and fungi and are involved in certain inflammatory diseases.

Activated CD8+ T lymphocytes differentiate into CTLs that kill cells harboring cytoplasmic microbes, thereby eliminating otherwise hidden reservoirs of infection. The principal mechanism of killing by CTLs depends on the perforin—granzyme system. Perforin and granzymes are stored in the granules of CTLs and are rapidly released when CTLs engage their targets (cells bearing the appropriate class I MHC—bound peptides). Perforin binds to the plasma membrane of the target cells and promotes the entry of granzymes, proteases that specifically cleave and thereby activate cellular caspases (Chapter 1), which induce the apoptosis of target cells.

T-cell responses are regulated by a balance between costimulatory and inhibitory receptors. The major costimulatory receptor is CD28, mentioned earlier. Other proteins of the CD28 family include two "coinhibitory" receptors, CTLA-4, which blocks and removes B7 molecules and thus reduces CD28 engagement, and PD-1, which inhibits signals from the TCR and from CD28 and thus terminates T-cell responses. Blocking these coinhibitors has proved to be a powerful approach for enhancing antitumor immune responses (Chapter 6).

Humoral Immunity: Activation of B Lymphocytes and Elimination of Extracellular Microbes

Upon activation, B lymphocytes proliferate and then differentiate into plasma cells that secrete different classes of antibodies with distinct functions. There are two major pathways of B-cell activation.
- *T cell—dependent.* The response of B cells to protein antigens requires help from CD4+ T cells. B cells also act as APCs—they ingest protein antigens, degrade them, and display peptides bound to class II MHC molecules for recognition by helper T cells (Fig. 5.9). The helper T cells express CD40L, which engages CD40 expressed on B cells, and secrete cytokines, which work together to activate the B cells.

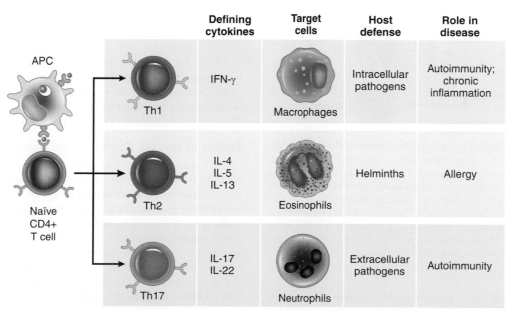

	Defining cytokines	Target cells	Host defense	Role in disease
Th1	IFN-γ	Macrophages	Intracellular pathogens	Autoimmunity; chronic inflammation
Th2	IL-4 IL-5 IL-13	Eosinophils	Helminths	Allergy
Th17	IL-17 IL-22	Neutrophils	Extracellular pathogens	Autoimmunity

FIG. 5.8 Subsets of helper T (Th) cells. In response to stimuli (mainly cytokines) present at the time of antigen recognition, naïve CD4+ T cells may differentiate into populations of effector cells that produce distinct sets of cytokines that act on different cells (indicated as target cells) and mediate different functions. The roles of these subsets in host defense and immunologic diseases are summarized. Some activated T cells produce multiple cytokines and do not fall into a distinct subset. *APC,* Antigen-presenting cell; *IFN-γ,* interferon-gamma; *IL,* interleukin.

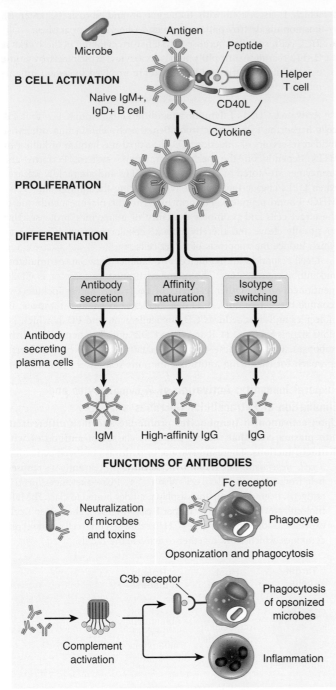

FIG. 5.9 Humoral immunity. Naïve B lymphocytes recognize antigens, and under the influence of Th cells and other stimuli *(not shown)*, the B cells are activated to proliferate and to differentiate into antibody-secreting plasma cells. Some of the activated B cells undergo heavy-chain class switching and affinity maturation, and some become long-lived memory cells. Antibodies of different heavy-chain classes (isotypes) perform different effector functions. Note that the antibodies shown are IgG; these and IgM activate complement; and the specialized functions of IgA (mucosal immunity) and IgE (mast cell and eosinophil activation) are *not shown*.

- *T cell–independent.* Many polysaccharide and lipid antigens have multiple identical antigenic determinants (epitopes) that can cross-link several antibody molecules on each B cell and initiate the process of B-cell activation without a requirement for T-cell help.

Some of the progeny of the expanded B-cell clones differentiate into antibody-secreting plasma cells. Each plasma cell secretes antibodies with the same specificity as the cell surface antibodies (B-cell antigen receptors) that first recognized the antigen. Polysaccharides and lipids stimulate secretion mainly of IgM antibody. Protein antigens, by virtue of CD40L- and cytokine-mediated helper T-cell actions, induce the production of antibodies of different classes (IgG, IgA, IgE). Production of functionally different antibodies relies on *heavy-chain class (isotype) switching*, which results from DNA breaks adjacent to constant region genes followed by joining to downstream constant regions. This process changes the Fc regions of antibodies, thus increasing the range of functions that antibodies serve. The isotype-specific functions of antibodies are described later. Helper T cells also stimulate the production of antibodies with higher affinity for the antigen. This process, called *affinity maturation*, results from somatic mutations in the antigen-binding regions of Ig molecules followed by selection of cells that express high-affinity receptors; thus, the process improves the quality of the humoral immune response. Some activated B cells migrate into follicles and form germinal centers, which are the sites of isotype switching and affinity maturation. The helper T cells that stimulate these processes in B lymphocytes also migrate to and reside in the germinal centers and are called *T follicular helper (Tfh) cells*.

The humoral immune response combats microbes in numerous ways (see Fig. 5.9).
- High-affinity antibodies of all classes bind to microbes and prevent them from infecting cells, thereby neutralizing the microbes.
- IgG antibodies coat (opsonize) microbes and target them for phagocytosis by neutrophils and macrophages, which express receptors for the Fc tails of IgG molecules.
- IgG and IgM activate the complement system by the classical pathway, and complement products promote phagocytosis and destruction of microbes.
- IgA is secreted in mucosal tissues and neutralizes microbes in the lumens of the respiratory and gastrointestinal tracts (and other mucosal tissues).
- IgG is actively transported across the placenta and protects the newborn until the immune system becomes mature. This is a form of *passive immunity*.
- IgE activates mast cells and is involved in defense against helminths.

Circulating IgG antibodies have half-lives of about 3 weeks, which is much longer than the half-lives of most blood proteins, as a consequence of special mechanisms for recycling IgG and reducing its catabolism. Some antibody-secreting plasma cells migrate to the bone marrow and live for years, continuing to produce low levels of antibodies.

Decline of Immune Responses and Immunologic Memory

The majority of effector lymphocytes induced by an infectious pathogen die by apoptosis after the microbe is eliminated, thus returning the immune system to its basal resting state. The initial activation of lymphocytes generates long-lived *memory cells*, which may survive for years after the infection. Memory cells are an expanded pool of antigen-specific lymphocytes (more numerous than the naïve cells specific for any antigen that are present before encounter with that antigen) that respond faster and more effectively when reexposed to the antigen than do naïve cells. Generation of memory cells is therefore an important goal of vaccination.

This brief introduction to normal immune responses provides a background for our discussion of disorders of the immune system.

HYPERSENSITIVITY: IMMUNOLOGICALLY MEDIATED TISSUE INJURY

Immune responses that normally are protective are also capable of causing tissue injury. Injurious immune reactions are grouped under *hypersensitivity,* and the resulting diseases are called *hypersensitivity diseases.* This term originated from the idea that persons who mount immune responses against an antigen are sensitized to that antigen, so pathologic or excessive reactions are manifestations of a hypersensitive state. A system of checks and balances has evolved to optimize the eradication of infecting organisms without serious injury to host tissues. However, immune responses may be inadequately controlled or directed against normally harmless antigens or inappropriately targeted to host tissues, and in such situations, the normally beneficial response is the cause of disease. In this section, we describe the causes and general mechanisms of hypersensitivity diseases and then discuss specific situations in which the immune response is responsible for the disease.

Causes of Hypersensitivity Reactions

Pathologic immune responses may be directed against different types of antigens.

- *Autoimmunity: reactions against self antigens.* Normally, the immune system does not react against one's own antigens. This phenomenon is called *self-tolerance,* implying that the body "tolerates" its own antigens. On occasion, self-tolerance fails, resulting in reactions against one's own cells and tissues called *autoimmunity*; diseases caused by autoimmunity are referred to as *autoimmune diseases.* We will return to the mechanisms of self-tolerance and autoimmunity later in this chapter.
- *Reactions against microbes.* There are many types of reactions against microbial antigens that may cause disease. In some cases, the reaction is excessive or the microbial antigen is unusually persistent. T-cell responses against persistent microbes, such as *Mycobacterium tuberculosis,* may give rise to severe inflammation, sometimes with the formation of granulomas (Chapter 2); this is the cause of tissue injury in tuberculosis and some other infections. If antibodies are produced against microbial antigens, the antibodies may bind to the antigens to produce immune complexes, which deposit in tissues and trigger inflammation; this is the underlying mechanism of postinfectious glomerulonephritis (Chapter 12). Rarely, antibodies or T cells reactive with a microbe cross-react with a host tissue; such cross-reactivity is believed to be the basis for rheumatic heart disease (Chapter 9). The SARS-CoV-2 coronavirus can induce a systemic inflammatory reaction that is an important cause of morbidity in COVID-19.
- *Reactions against environmental antigens.* In higher-income countries, 20% or more of the population is allergic to common environmental substances (e.g., pollens, animal dander, and dust mites), as well as some metal ions and therapeutic drugs. Such individuals are predisposed to make unusual immune responses to noninfectious, typically harmless, antigens to which all persons are exposed but against which only some react.

In all these conditions, tissue injury is caused by the same mechanisms that normally function to eliminate infectious pathogens—namely, antibodies, effector T lymphocytes, and various other cells such as macrophages and eosinophils. The fundamental problem in these diseases is that the immune response is triggered and maintained inappropriately. Because the stimuli for these abnormal immune responses are difficult or impossible to eliminate (e.g., self antigens, persistent microbes, or environmental antigens), and the immune system has many intrinsic positive feedback loops (which normally promote protective immunity), once a hypersensitivity reaction starts, it is difficult to control or terminate it. Therefore, these diseases tend to be chronic and debilitating and are therapeutic challenges.

Classification of Hypersensitivity Reactions

Hypersensitivity reactions can be subdivided into four types based on the principal immune mechanism responsible for injury; three are variations on antibody-mediated injury, and the fourth is T cell mediated (Table 5.2). The rationale for this classification is that the mechanism of immune injury is often a good predictor of the clinical manifestations and may help to guide therapy.

The main types of hypersensitivity reactions are as follows:

- In *immediate (type I) hypersensitivity,* also called *allergy,* the injury is caused by Th2 cells, IgE antibodies, and mast cells and other leukocytes. Mast cells release mediators that act on blood vessels and smooth muscle as well as cytokines that recruit and activate inflammatory cells.
- *Antibody-mediated disorders (type II hypersensitivity)* are caused by secreted IgG and IgM antibodies that bind to antigens in tissue or on a cell surface. Antibodies injure cells by promoting their phagocytosis or lysis and injure tissues by inducing inflammation. Antibodies may also interfere with cellular functions and cause disease without cell or tissue injury.
- In *immune complex—mediated disorders (type III hypersensitivity),* IgG and IgM antibodies bind antigens, usually in the circulation, and form antigen-antibody complexes that deposit in vascular beds and induce inflammation. The leukocytes that are recruited (neutrophils and monocytes) damage tissues by releasing lysosomal enzymes and generating toxic free radicals.
- *T cell—mediated (type IV) hypersensitivity disorders* are caused mainly by immune responses in which T lymphocytes of the Th1 and Th17 subsets produce cytokines that induce inflammation and activate neutrophils and macrophages, which are responsible for tissue injury. CD8+ CTLs may also contribute to injury by directly killing host cells.

Immediate (Type I) Hypersensitivity

Immediate hypersensitivity is a tissue reaction that occurs rapidly (typically within minutes) after the interaction of antigen with IgE antibody bound to the surface of mast cells. The reaction is initiated by entry of an antigen, which is called an *allergen* because it triggers allergy. Many allergens are environmental substances against which some individuals are predisposed to mounting Th2 and IgE responses, which are responsible for the clinical and pathologic manifestations of the reaction. Immediate hypersensitivity may occur as a mild reaction (e.g., seasonal rhinitis, hay fever), or it can be severely debilitating (e.g., asthma) or even fatal (e.g., anaphylaxis).

Sequence of Events in Immediate Hypersensitivity Reactions

Most immediate hypersensitivity reactions follow a stereotypic sequence of cellular responses (Fig. 5.10):

- *Activation of Th2 cells and production of IgE antibody.* Only a subset of individuals exposed to common environmental antigens make strong Th2 and IgE responses. The factors that contribute to this propensity are discussed later. Th2 cells secrete several cytokines, including IL-4, IL-5, and IL-13, which are responsible for the reactions of immediate hypersensitivity. IL-4 and IL-13 stimulate allergen-specific B cells to undergo heavy-chain class switching to IgE. IL-5 activates eosinophils that are recruited to the reaction,

Table 5.2 Mechanisms of Hypersensitivity Reactions

Type	Immune Mechanisms	Histopathologic Lesions	Prototypical Disorders
Immediate (type I) hypersensitivity	Production of IgE antibody → immediate release of vasoactive amines and other mediators from mast cells; later recruitment of inflammatory cells	Vascular dilation, edema, smooth muscle contraction, mucus production, tissue injury, inflammation	Anaphylaxis; allergies; bronchial asthma (atopic forms)
Antibody-mediated (type II) hypersensitivity	Production of IgG, IgM → binds to antigen on target cell or tissue → phagocytosis or lysis of target cell by activated complement or Fc receptors; recruitment of leukocytes	Phagocytosis and lysis of cells; inflammation; in some diseases, functional derangements without cell or tissue injury	Autoimmune hemolytic anemia; Goodpasture syndrome
Immune complex—mediated (type III) hypersensitivity	Deposition of antigen-antibody complexes → complement activation → recruitment of leukocytes by complement products and Fc receptors → release of enzymes and other toxic molecules	Inflammation, necrotizing vasculitis (fibrinoid necrosis)	Systemic lupus erythematosus; some forms of glomerulonephritis; serum sickness; Arthus reaction
Cell-mediated (type IV) hypersensitivity	Activated T lymphocytes → (1) release of cytokines, inflammation and macrophage activation; (2) T cell—mediated cytotoxicity	Perivascular cellular infiltrates; edema; granuloma formation; cell destruction	Contact dermatitis; multiple sclerosis; type 1 diabetes; tuberculosis

Ig, Immunoglobulin.

and IL-13 stimulates mucus secretion from epithelial cells. Th2 cells are often recruited to the site of allergic reactions in response to locally produced chemokines; one of these chemokines, eotaxin, also recruits eosinophils to the same site.

- *Sensitization of mast cells by IgE antibody.* Mast cells are derived from precursors in the bone marrow and widely distributed in tissues, often residing near blood vessels and nerves and in subepithelial locations. Mast cells express a high-affinity receptor for the Fc portion of the ε heavy chain of IgE, called *FcεRI.* Although the serum concentration of IgE is very low (in the range of 0.1 to 10 μg/mL), the affinity of the mast cell FcεRI receptor is so high that the receptors are always occupied by IgE. These antibody-bearing mast cells are sensitized to react if the specific antigen (the allergen) binds to the antibody molecules. Basophils, circulating cells that resemble mast cells, also express FcεRI, may be recruited into tissues, and may contribute to immediate hypersensitivity reactions.
- *Activation of mast cells and release of mediators.* When a person who has been sensitized by exposure to an allergen is reexposed to that allergen, the allergen binds to antigen-specific IgE molecules on mast cells, usually at or near the site of allergen entry. Cross-linking of these IgE molecules triggers a series of biochemical signals from the associated FcεRI receptor that culminate in the secretion of various mediators from the mast cells.

Three groups of mediators are important in different immediate hypersensitivity reactions:

- *Vasoactive amines* released from granule stores. The granules of mast cells contain *histamine,* which is released within seconds or minutes of activation. Histamine causes vasodilation, increased vascular permeability, smooth muscle contraction, and increased mucus secretion. Other rapidly released mediators include neutral proteases (e.g., tryptase), which may damage tissues and also

generate kinins and cleave complement components to produce additional chemotactic and inflammatory factors (e.g., C5a) (Chapter 2). The granules also contain acidic proteoglycans (e.g., heparin, chondroitin sulfate), which seem to serve as a storage matrix for the amines.
- Newly synthesized *lipid mediators.* Mast cells synthesize and secrete prostaglandins and leukotrienes by the same pathways as do other leukocytes (Chapter 2). These lipid mediators have several actions that are important in immediate hypersensitivity reactions. Prostaglandin D2 (PGD$_2$) is the most abundant mediator generated by the cyclooxygenase pathway in mast cells. It causes intense bronchospasm as well as increased mucus secretion. The leukotrienes LTC$_4$ and LTD$_4$ are the most potent vasoactive and spasmogenic agents known; on a molar basis, they are several thousand times more active than histamine in increasing vascular permeability and in causing bronchial smooth muscle contraction. LTB$_4$ is highly chemotactic for neutrophils, eosinophils, and monocytes.
- *Cytokines.* Activated mast cells secrete several cytokines that are important for the late-phase reaction. These include TNF and chemokines, which recruit and activate leukocytes (Chapter 2).

The reactions of immediate hypersensitivity did not evolve to cause human discomfort and disease. The Th2 response plays an important protective role in combating parasitic infections, mainly by destruction of helminths by eosinophil granule proteins. Mast cells are also involved in defense against bacterial infections and animal venoms.

Development of Allergies

Susceptibility to immediate hypersensitivity reactions is genetically determined. An increased propensity to develop immediate hypersensitivity reactions is called *atopy.* Atopic individuals tend to have higher serum IgE levels and more IL-4—producing Th2 cells than does the general population. A positive family history of allergy is found in

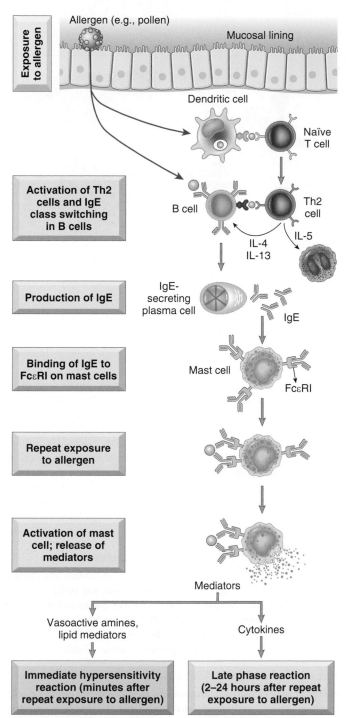

FIG. 5.10 Sequence of events in immediate (type I) hypersensitivity. Immediate hypersensitivity reactions are initiated by the introduction of an allergen, which stimulates Th2 responses and IgE production in genetically susceptible individuals. IgE binds to Fc receptors (FcεRI) on mast cells, and subsequent exposure to the allergen activates the mast cells to secrete the mediators that are responsible for the pathologic manifestations of immediate hypersensitivity.

50% of atopic individuals. Genes that are implicated in susceptibility to asthma and other atopic disorders include those encoding HLA molecules (which may confer immune responsiveness to particular allergens), cytokines (which may control Th2 responses), a component

of the FcεRI receptor, and ADAM33, a metalloproteinase that may be involved in tissue remodeling in the airways.

Environmental factors are also important in the development of allergic diseases. Exposure to environmental pollutants, all too common in industrialized societies, is an important predisposing factor for allergy. Dogs and cats living in the same environment as humans can develop allergies, whereas chimps living in the wild do not despite their much closer genetic similarity to humans. This simple observation suggests that environmental factors may be more important in the development of allergic disease than genetics. Viral infections of the airways are important triggers for bronchial asthma, an allergic disease affecting the lungs (Chapter 11). Bacterial skin infections are strongly associated with atopic dermatitis.

It is estimated that 20% to 30% of immediate hypersensitivity reactions are triggered by nonantigenic stimuli such as temperature extremes and exercise and do not involve Th2 cells or IgE. It is believed that in these cases of nonatopic allergy, mast cells are abnormally sensitive to activation by various nonimmune stimuli.

The incidence of many allergic diseases is increasing in higher-income countries, perhaps related to a decrease in infections during early life. This observation has led to an idea, called the *hygiene hypothesis,* that early childhood and even prenatal exposure to microbial antigens educates the immune system such that subsequent pathologic responses against common environmental allergens are prevented. Thus, too little exposure to potential allergens and, perhaps, microbes in childhood may predispose individuals to allergies later in life. This idea has received support from clinical studies demonstrating that exposing infants to peanuts reduces the incidence of peanut allergy later in life.

Clinical and Pathologic Manifestations of Allergic Diseases

Often, the IgE-triggered reaction has two well-defined phases (Fig. 5.11).

- The *immediate response,* usually evident within 5 to 30 minutes after exposure to an allergen and subsiding by 60 minutes, is stimulated by mast cell granule contents and lipid mediators. It is characterized by vasodilation, vascular leakage, and smooth muscle spasm.
- A second, *late-phase reaction* usually begins 2 to 8 hours later and may last for several days. It is stimulated mainly by cytokines and is characterized by inflammation as well as tissue injury, such as mucosal epithelial cell damage. The dominant inflammatory cells in the late-phase reaction are neutrophils, eosinophils, and lymphocytes, especially Th2 cells. Neutrophils are recruited by various chemokines; their roles in inflammation were described in Chapter 2. Eosinophils, which are recruited by eotaxin and other chemokines released from epithelium, produce granule proteins that are toxic to epithelial cells as well as leukotrienes and other factors that promote inflammation. Th2 cells produce cytokines that have multiple actions, as described earlier. These recruited leukocytes can amplify and sustain the injurious inflammatory response, even in the absence of continuous allergen exposure. Because inflammation is a major component of many allergic diseases, notably asthma and atopic dermatitis, therapy includes antiinflammatory drugs such as corticosteroids.

Immediate hypersensitivity reactions may occur as systemic disorders or as local reactions (Table 5.3). The route of antigen exposure often determines the nature of the reaction. Exposure to protein antigens (e.g., in bee venom) or drugs (e.g., penicillin) that enter the circulation may result in systemic *anaphylaxis.* Within

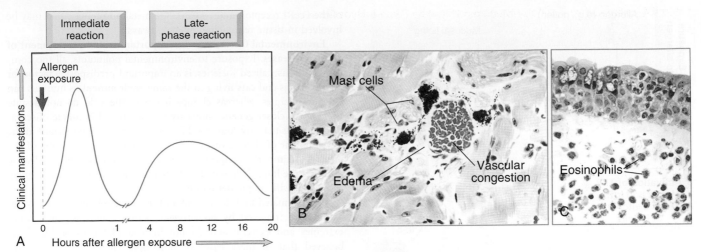

FIG. 5.11 Phases of immediate hypersensitivity reactions. (A) Kinetics of the immediate and late-phase reactions. The immediate vascular and smooth muscle reaction to allergen develops within minutes after challenge (allergen exposure in a previously sensitized individual), and the late-phase reaction develops 2 to 24 hours later. The immediate reaction (B) is characterized by vasodilation, congestion, and edema, and the late-phase reaction (C) is characterized by an inflammatory infiltrate rich in eosinophils, neutrophils, and T cells. (Courtesy of Dr. Daniel Friend, Department of Pathology, Brigham and Women's Hospital, Boston, Massachusetts.)

minutes of the exposure in a sensitized host, itching, urticaria (hives), and skin erythema appear, followed rapidly by profound respiratory difficulty caused by pulmonary bronchoconstriction and hypersecretion of mucus. Laryngeal edema may exacerbate matters by causing upper airway obstruction. In addition, the musculature of the entire gastrointestinal tract may be affected, with resultant vomiting, abdominal cramps, and diarrhea. Without immediate intervention, there may be systemic vasodilation with a fall in blood pressure (anaphylactic shock), and the patient may progress to circulatory collapse and death within minutes.

Local reactions generally occur when the antigen is confined to a particular site, such as the skin (following contact), the gastrointestinal tract (following ingestion), or the lung (following inhalation). *Atopic dermatitis (eczema), food allergies, allergic rhinitis (hay fever),* and certain forms of *asthma* are examples of localized allergic reactions. However, ingestion or inhalation of allergens also can trigger systemic reactions if the allergen is absorbed into the circulation, as happens in

cases of peanut allergy. Sometimes, infants develop atopic dermatitis, followed, later in life, by allergic rhinitis and asthma. These three disorders are grouped under the *atopic triad*, and their sequential development has been called the *atopic march*.

Therapy for allergies relies on corticosteroids (to reduce inflammation) and agents to counteract the effects of mediators (such as antihistamines, leukotriene antagonists, bronchodilators for asthma, and epinephrine to correct the drop in blood pressure in anaphylaxis). Antibodies that block Th2 cytokines or their receptors or neutralize IgE are now used for the treatment of asthma, atopic dermatitis, and peanut allergy.

Antibody-Mediated Diseases (Type II Hypersensitivity)

Antibody-mediated (type II) hypersensitivity disorders are caused by antibodies directed against target antigens on the surface of cells or other tissue components. The antigens may be normal molecules intrinsic to cell membranes or in the extracellular matrix, or they may be adsorbed exogenous antigens (e.g., a drug metabolite). These reactions are the cause of several important diseases (Table 5.4).

Mechanisms of Antibody-Mediated Diseases

In type II hypersensitivity, antibodies cause disease by targeting cells for phagocytosis, activating the complement system, or interfering with normal cellular functions (Fig. 5.12). The antibodies that are responsible are typically high-affinity IgG and IgM antibodies capable of activating complement and, for IgG, binding to phagocyte Fc receptors.

- *Opsonization and phagocytosis.* When circulating cells, such as red cells or platelets, are coated (opsonized) with autoantibodies, with or without complement proteins, the cells become targets for phagocytosis by neutrophils and macrophages (see Fig. 5.12A). These phagocytes express receptors for the Fc tails of IgG antibodies and for breakdown products of the C3 complement protein and use these receptors to bind and ingest opsonized particles. Opsonized blood cells are usually eliminated by macrophages in the spleen, which is why splenectomy is of clinical benefit in some antibody-mediated diseases.

Table 5.3 Examples of Disorders Caused by Immediate Hypersensitivity

Clinical Syndrome	Clinical and Pathologic Manifestations
Anaphylaxis (may be caused by drugs, bee sting, food)	Fall in blood pressure (shock) caused by vascular dilation; airway obstruction due to laryngeal edema
Bronchial asthma	Airway obstruction caused by bronchial smooth muscle hyperactivity; inflammation and tissue injury caused by late-phase reaction
Allergic rhinitis, sinusitis (hay fever)	Increased mucus secretion; inflammation of upper airways and sinuses
Food allergies	Increased peristalsis due to contraction of intestinal muscles, resulting in vomiting and diarrhea

Table 5.4 Examples of Antibody-Mediated Diseases (Type II Hypersensitivity)

Disease	Target Antigen	Mechanisms of Disease	Clinicopathologic Manifestations
Autoimmune hemolytic anemia	Red cell membrane proteins	Opsonization and phagocytosis of red cells	Hemolysis, anemia
Autoimmune thrombocytopenic purpura	Platelet membrane proteins (Gpllb:Illa integrin)	Opsonization and phagocytosis of platelets	Bleeding
Pemphigus vulgaris	Proteins in intercellular junctions of epidermal cells (desmogleins)	Antibody-mediated activation of proteases, disruption of intercellular adhesions	Skin vesicles (bullae)
Vasculitis caused by ANCA	Neutrophil granule proteins, presumably released from activated neutrophils	Neutrophil degranulation and inflammation	Vasculitis
Goodpasture syndrome	Protein in basement membranes of kidney glomeruli and lung alveoli	Complement- and Fc receptor–mediated inflammation	Nephritis, lung hemorrhage
Acute rheumatic fever	Streptococcal cell wall antigen; antibody cross-reacts with myocardial antigen	Inflammation, macrophage activation	Myocarditis, arthritis
Myasthenia gravis	Acetylcholine receptor	Antibody inhibits acetylcholine binding; complement-mediated injury	Muscle weakness, paralysis
Graves disease (hyperthyroidism)	TSH receptor	Antibody-mediated stimulation of TSH receptors	Hyperthyroidism
Pernicious anemia	Intrinsic factor of gastric parietal cells	Neutralization of intrinsic factor, decreased absorption of vitamin B_{12}	Abnormal erythropoiesis, anemia

ANCA, Antineutrophil cytoplasmic antibodies; *TSH,* thyroid-stimulating hormone.

Antibody-mediated cell destruction occurs in the following clinical situations: (1) transfusion reactions, in which cells from an incompatible donor react with preformed antibody in the host (Chapter 10); (2) hemolytic anemia of the fetus and newborn (erythroblastosis fetalis), in which IgG anti–red cell antibodies from the mother cross the placenta and cause destruction of fetal red cells (Chapter 4); (3) autoimmune hemolytic anemia, neutropenia, and thrombocytopenia, in which individuals produce antibodies to their own blood cells (Chapter 10); and (4) certain drug reactions, in which a drug attaches to plasma membrane proteins of red cells and antibodies are produced against the drug-protein complex.

- *Inflammation.* Antibodies bound to tissue antigens activate the complement system by the classical pathway (see Fig. 5.12B). Products of complement activation serve several functions (Chapter 2), one of which is to recruit neutrophils and monocytes, triggering inflammation in tissues. Leukocytes may also be activated by engagement of Fc receptors, which recognize the bound antibodies. Antibody-mediated inflammation is responsible for tissue injury in some forms of glomerulonephritis, vascular rejection in organ grafts, and other disorders.

- *Antibody-mediated cellular dysfunction.* In some cases, antibodies directed against an essential protein impair or dysregulate important functions without directly causing cell injury or inflammation. In pernicious anemia, antibodies against intrinsic factor, which is required for absorption of vitamin B_{12} in the stomach, lead to a deficiency of this vitamin and abnormal hematopoiesis; antibody-mediated damage to gastric epithelial cells may also contribute. Previously, it was thought that in myasthenia gravis, antibodies specific for the acetylcholine receptor in neuromuscular junctions of motor end plates of skeletal muscles inhibited neuromuscular transmission, resulting in muscle weakness, but without injury. However, recent clinical studies have shown benefit with complement inhibition therapies, suggesting that antibody- and complement-mediated damage

to motor end plates may be involved in disease pathogenesis. Antibodies can also stimulate excessive cellular responses; e.g., in Graves disease, antibodies against the thyroid-stimulating hormone receptor stimulate thyroid epithelial cells to secrete thyroid hormones, resulting in hyperthyroidism (see Fig. 5.12C).

Immune Complex–Mediated Diseases (Type III Hypersensitivity)

Antigen–antibody (immune) complexes that are formed in the circulation may deposit in blood vessels, leading to complement activation and acute inflammation. In some cases, the complexes may be formed at sites where antigen has been "planted" previously *(in situ immune complexes).* The antigens that form immune complexes may be exogenous, such as a foreign protein that is injected or produced by an infectious microbe, or endogenous, if the individual produces antibody against self antigens (autoimmunity) (Table 5.5). Immune complex–mediated diseases tend be systemic because the complexes can deposit in blood vessels anywhere in the body, but often preferentially involve the kidney (glomerulonephritis), joints (arthritis), and small blood vessels (vasculitis), all of which are common sites of immune complex deposition.

Pathogenesis. The pathogenesis of immune complex diseases can be divided into three phases (Fig. 5.13).

Formation of Immune Complexes. Protein antigens trigger immune responses that result in the formation of antibodies, typically about 1 week after the introduction of the antigen. These antibodies are secreted into the blood, where they react with the antigen still present in the circulation and form immune complexes.

Deposition of Immune Complexes. In the next phase, the circulating antigen-antibody complexes are deposited in various tissues. The factors that determine whether immune complex formation will lead to tissue deposition and disease are not fully understood, but

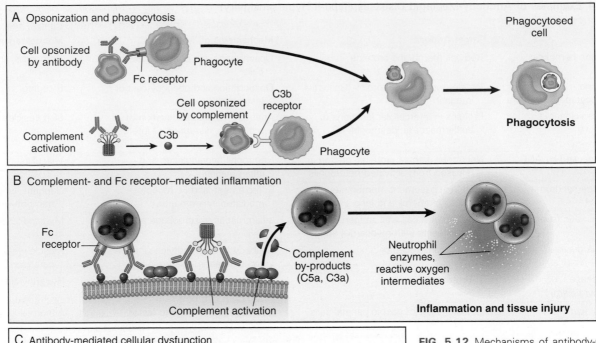

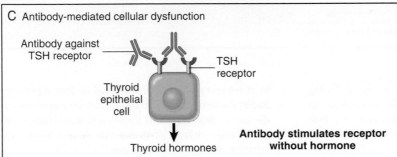

FIG. 5.12 Mechanisms of antibody-mediated injury. (A) Opsonization of cells by antibodies and complement components and ingestion by phagocytes. (B) Inflammation induced by antibody binding to Fc receptors of leukocytes and by complement breakdown products. (C) Antireceptor antibodies disturb the normal function of receptors. In the example shown, antibodies against the thyroid-stimulating hormone (TSH) receptor activate thyroid cells in Graves disease.

the major influences seem to be the characteristics of the complexes and the features of the vasculature. In general, the most pathogenic immune complexes are those that are produced in amounts and size that are not efficiently cleared by phagocytes in the spleen and liver. Organs where blood is filtered at high pressure to form other fluids, like urine and synovial fluid, are sites where immune complexes become concentrated and deposit; hence, immune complex disease often affects glomeruli and joints. The endothelium in these tissues is also often fenestrated, promoting passage of immune complexes between endothelial cells.

Inflammation and Tissue Injury. Once deposited in tissues, immune complexes initiate an acute inflammatory reaction via complement activation and engagement of leukocyte Fc receptors. Typically, the antibodies are IgG or IgM, both of which activate complement by the classical pathway. Deposition of complement proteins can be detected at the site of injury. Consumption of

Table 5.5 Examples of Immune Complex–Mediated Diseases (Type III Hypersensitivity)

Disease	Antigen Involved	Clinicopathologic Manifestations
Systemic lupus erythematosus	Nuclear antigens (circulating or "planted" in kidney)	Nephritis, skin lesions, arthritis, others
Poststreptococcal glomerulonephritis	Streptococcal cell wall antigen(s); may be "planted" in glomerular basement membrane	Nephritis
Polyarteritis nodosa	Hepatitis B virus antigens in some cases	Systemic vasculitis
Reactive arthritis	Bacterial antigens (e.g., *Yersinia*)	Acute arthritis
Serum sickness	Various proteins (e.g., foreign serum protein such as horse antithymocyte globulin)	Arthritis, vasculitis, nephritis
Arthus reaction (experimental)	Various foreign proteins	Cutaneous vasculitis

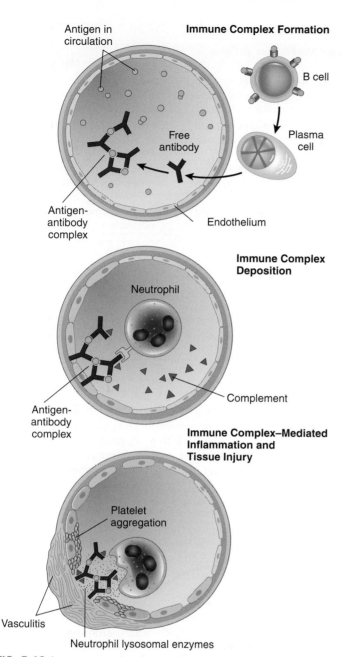

Immune Complex Formation

Antigen in circulation

Free antibody

B cell

Plasma cell

Antigen-antibody complex

Endothelium

Immune Complex Deposition

Neutrophil

Antigen-antibody complex

Complement

Immune Complex–Mediated Inflammation and Tissue Injury

Platelet aggregation

Vasculitis

Neutrophil lysosomal enzymes

FIG. 5.13 Immune complex disease. The sequential phases in the induction of systemic immune complex–mediated diseases (type III hypersensitivity).

vessel wall and variable neutrophilic infiltration (Chapter 2). When deposited in kidney glomeruli, the complexes cause **glomerulonephritis** and can be seen on immunofluorescence microscopy as granular deposits of immunoglobulin and complement and on electron microscopy as electron-dense deposits along the glomerular basement membrane (Chapter 12).

Systemic Immune Complex Disease

Much of what we know about systemic immune complex disease is derived from studies of *acute serum sickness,* which was once a complication of the administration of large amounts of foreign protein (e.g., in serum from immunized horses used for protection against diphtheria). In modern times, the disease is infrequent and is usually seen in individuals who receive antibodies from other individuals or species, e.g., horse or rabbit antithymocyte globulin administered to deplete T cells in recipients of organ grafts.

Acute serum sickness induced by administration of a single large dose of antigen is characterized by fever, rash, and arthritis; the lesions tend to resolve as the complexes are cleared by phagocytes. A form of *chronic serum sickness* results from repeated or prolonged exposure to an antigen. This occurs in several diseases, such as systemic lupus erythematosus (SLE), which is associated with persistent antibody responses to autoantigens. In many diseases, the morphologic changes and other findings suggest immune complex deposition, but the inciting antigens are unknown. Included in this category are several vasculitides, such as polyarteritis nodosa.

Local Immune Complex Disease (Arthus Reaction)

A model of local immune complex diseases is the *Arthus reaction,* in which an area of tissue necrosis appears as a result of acute immune complex vasculitis. The reaction is produced experimentally by injecting an antigen into the skin of a previously immunized animal. Immune complexes form as the antigen diffuses into the vascular wall at the site of injection and binds to preformed antibody, triggering the same inflammatory reaction and histologic appearance as in systemic immune complex disease. Within a few hours, the injection site develops edema and hemorrhage, occasionally followed by ulceration.

T Cell–Mediated Diseases (Type IV Hypersensitivity)

Several autoimmune disorders, as well as pathologic reactions to environmental chemicals and persistent microbes, are known to be caused by T cells (Table 5.6). Two types of T-cell reactions are capable of causing tissue injury and disease (Fig. 5.14). The most frequent is cytokine-mediated inflammation, in which the cytokines are produced mainly by CD4+ T cells. Direct cell cytotoxicity mediated by CD8+ T cells may also contribute to tissue injury. This group of diseases is of great clinical interest because T-cell reactions are increasingly recognized as the basis of chronic inflammatory diseases, and many of the new rationally designed therapies for these diseases have been developed to target T cells.

CD4+ T Cell–Mediated Inflammation

In CD4+ T cell–mediated hypersensitivity reactions, cytokines produced by the T cells induce inflammation that may be chronic and destructive. The prototype of T cell–mediated inflammation is *delayed-type hypersensitivity (DTH),* a tissue reaction to antigens given to individuals who are already sensitized. In this setting, an antigen administered into the skin results in a detectable cutaneous reaction within 24 to 48 hours (hence the term *delayed,* in contrast to *immediate* hypersensitivity).

complement during the active phase of the disease decreases serum levels of C3, which can be used as a marker for disease activity, e.g., in systemic lupus erythematosus (SLE). During this phase (approximately 10 days after antigen administration), clinical manifestations such as fever, urticaria, joint pain (arthralgia), lymph node enlargement, and proteinuria appear. Wherever complexes deposit, the tissue damage is similar. The resultant inflammatory lesion is termed *vasculitis* if it occurs in blood vessels, *glomerulonephritis* if it occurs in renal glomeruli, *arthritis* if it occurs in the joints, and so on.

MORPHOLOGY

The principal morphologic manifestation of immune complex deposition in blood vessels is **acute vasculitis,** associated with fibrinoid necrosis of the

Table 5.6 Examples of T Cell–Mediated Diseases (Type IV Hypersensitivity)

Disease	Specificity of Pathogenic T Cells	Principal Mechanisms of Tissue Injury	Clinicopathologic Manifestations
Rheumatoid arthritis	Collagen? Citrullinated self proteins?	Inflammation mediated by Th17 (and Th1?) cytokines; role of antibodies and immune complexes?	Chronic arthritis with inflammation, destruction of articular cartilage
Multiple sclerosis	Protein antigens in myelin (e.g., myelin basic protein)	Inflammation mediated by Th1 and Th17 cytokines; myelin destruction by activated macrophages	Demyelination in CNS with perivascular inflammation; paralysis
Type 1 diabetes	Antigens of pancreatic islet β cells (insulin, glutamic acid decarboxylase, others)	T cell–mediated inflammation, destruction of islet cells by CTLs	Insulitis (chronic inflammation in islets), destruction of β cells; diabetes
Inflammatory bowel disease	Enteric bacteria; self antigens?	Inflammation mediated by Th1 and Th17 cytokines	Chronic intestinal inflammation, obstruction
Psoriasis	Unknown	Inflammation mediated mainly by Th17 cytokines	Plaques in the skin
Contact sensitivity	Various environmental chemicals (e.g., urushiol from poison ivy or poison oak, therapeutic drugs)	Inflammation mediated by Th1 (and Th17?) cytokines	Epidermal necrosis, dermal inflammation, causing skin rash and blisters

Examples of human T cell–mediated diseases are listed. In many cases, the specificity of the T cells and the mechanisms of tissue injury are inferred based on the similarity with experimental animal models of the diseases.

CTLs, Cytotoxic T lymphocytes.

As described earlier, naïve T cells are activated in secondary lymphoid organs by recognition of peptide antigens displayed by dendritic cells and the T cells differentiate into effector cells. Classical T cell–mediated hypersensitivity is a reaction of Th1 effector cells, but Th17 cells also may contribute, especially when neutrophils are prominent in the inflammatory infiltrate. Th1 cells secrete cytokines, mainly IFN-γ, which are responsible for many of the manifestations of delayed-type hypersensitivity. IFN-γ–activated (so-called classically activated, or M1) macrophages produce substances that destroy microbes and damage tissues and mediators that promote inflammation

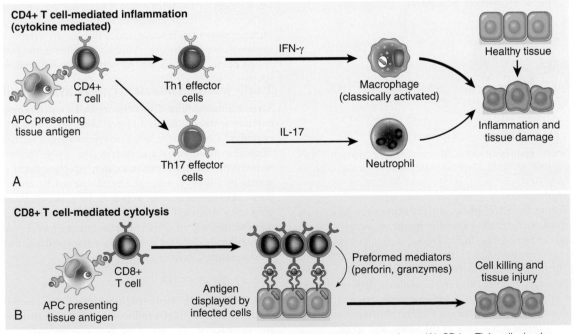

FIG. 5.14 Mechanisms of T cell–mediated (type IV) hypersensitivity reactions. (A) CD4+ Th1 cells (and sometimes CD8+ T cells, *not shown*) respond to tissue antigens by secreting cytokines that stimulate inflammation and activate phagocytes, leading to tissue injury. CD4+ Th17 cells contribute to inflammation by recruiting neutrophils (and, to a lesser extent, monocytes). (B) In some diseases, CD8+ cytotoxic T lymphocytes (CTLs) directly kill tissue cells expressing intracellular antigens (shown as *orange bars* inside cells). *APC,* Antigen-presenting cell.

(Chapter 2). Activated Th17 cells secrete cytokines that recruit neutrophils and monocytes.

Clinical Examples of CD4+ T Cell—Mediated Inflammatory Reactions

The classic example of DTH is the *tuberculin reaction* (known in clinical medicine as the *PPD skin test*), which is produced by the intracutaneous injection of purified protein derivative (PPD, also called *tuberculin*), containing protein antigens of the *Mycobacterium tuberculosis* bacillus. In a previously exposed individual, reddening and induration of the site appear in 8 to 12 hours, reach a peak in 24 to 72 hours, and then slowly subside. Morphologically, delayed-type hypersensitivity is characterized by the accumulation of mononuclear cells, mainly CD4+ T cells and macrophages, around venules, producing perivascular "cuffing" (Fig. 5.15). Prolonged DTH reactions against persistent microbes or other stimuli may result in a special pattern of reaction called *granulomatous inflammation* (eFig. 5.1), described in Chapter 2. The release of IFN-γ from blood cells stimulated with mycobacterial antigens in vitro is another widely used test for tuberculosis.

Contact dermatitis is a common example of tissue injury resulting from DTH reactions. It may be evoked by contact with urushiol, the antigenic component of poison ivy and poison oak, and presents as a vesicular dermatitis. It is thought that in these reactions, the environmental chemical binds to and structurally modifies self proteins, and peptides derived from these modified proteins are recognized by T cells that elicit the reaction. The same mechanism is responsible for many *drug reactions,* among the most common hypersensitivity reactions of humans. The responsible drug (often a reactive chemical) alters self proteins, including MHC molecules, and these neoantigens are recognized as foreign by T cells, leading to cytokine production and inflammation. Drug reactions often manifest as skin rashes.

CD4+ T cell—mediated inflammation is the basis of tissue injury in many organ-specific and systemic autoimmune diseases, such as rheumatoid arthritis and multiple sclerosis, as well as diseases probably caused by uncontrolled reactions to bacterial commensals, such as inflammatory bowel disease (see Table 5.6).

CD8+ T Cell—Mediated Cytotoxicity

In this type of T cell—mediated reaction, CD8+ CTLs kill antigen-expressing target cells. Tissue destruction by CTLs may be a component of some T cell—mediated diseases, such as type 1 diabetes. CTLs directed against cell surface histocompatibility antigens play an important role in organ transplant rejection, which is discussed later. They also play a role in reactions against viruses. In a virus-infected cell, viral peptides are displayed by class I MHC molecules and the complex is recognized by the TCR of CD8+ T lymphocytes. The killing of infected cells leads to elimination of the infection but, in some cases, causes cell damage (e.g., in viral hepatitis). CD8+ T cells also produce cytokines, notably IFN-γ, and are involved in inflammatory reactions resembling DTH, especially following virus infections and exposure to some contact sensitizing agents.

Now that we have described how the immune system can cause tissue damage, we turn to autoimmune disorders, which are the result of failure of tolerance to self antigens and in which disease is caused by hypersensitivity reactions.

AUTOIMMUNE DISEASES

Autoimmunity refers to immune reactions against self ("auto") antigens. Autoimmune diseases are fairly common, estimated to affect 5% to 8% of the U.S. population. Autoimmune diseases may be *organ-specific,* in which the immune responses are directed against one particular organ or cell type and result in localized tissue damage, or *systemic,* characterized by lesions in many organs (Table 5.7). In systemic diseases that are caused by immune complexes and autoantibodies, the lesions principally affect the connective tissues and blood vessels of involved organs. Therefore, these diseases are often referred to as *collagen vascular diseases* or *connective tissue diseases,* even though the immunologic reactions are not specifically directed against constituents of connective tissue or blood vessels.

Normally, individuals are unresponsive (tolerant) to their own (self) antigens, and autoimmunity results from a failure of self-tolerance. Therefore, understanding the pathogenesis of autoimmunity requires familiarity with the mechanisms of normal immunologic tolerance.

Immunologic Tolerance

During the generation of a highly diverse repertoire of lymphocytes, it is inevitable that some of the antigen receptors that are expressed are specific for self antigens, yet healthy individuals do not react against their own antigens. This feature of the immune system is known as *tolerance.* Although many mechanisms of self-tolerance have been described, mostly based on experimental models, the following are the ones known to be most important in humans (Fig. 5.16).

- *Elimination of self-reactive lymphocytes during their development in the thymus and bone marrow.* The generation of mature lymphocytes from their precursors occurs in the thymus for T cells and the bone marrow for B cells. When cells that have not completed their maturation encounter self antigens, the immature cells die, a process called *deletion* or *negative selection.* The expression of many self antigens in the thymus is controlled by a protein called AIRE (autoimmune regulator). Mutations in the *AIRE* gene cause an autoimmune disease called *autoimmune polyglandular syndrome* that affects endocrine and other tissues, because in the absence of AIRE, many self antigens are not expressed in the thymus and

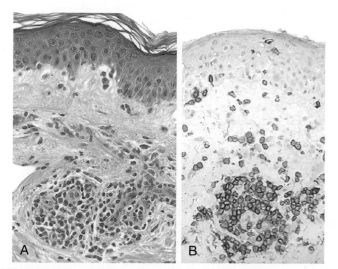

FIG. 5.15 Delayed hypersensitivity reaction in the skin. (A) Perivascular accumulation ("cuffing") of mononuclear inflammatory cells (lymphocytes and macrophages), with associated dermal edema and fibrin deposition. (B) Immunoperoxidase staining reveals that the perivascular infiltrate consists mainly of CD4+ T cells. (Courtesy of Dr. Louis Picker, Department of Pathology, Oregon Health Sciences University, Portland, Oregon.)

Table 5.7 Autoimmune Diseases

Organ-Specific	Systemic
Diseases Mediated by Antibodies	
Autoimmune hemolytic anemia	Systemic lupus
Autoimmune thrombocytopenia	erythematosus
Autoimmune atrophic gastritis of	ANCA-associated
pernicious anemia	vasculitis
Myasthenia gravis	
Graves disease	
Goodpasture syndrome	
Diseases Mediated by T Cells[a]	
Type 1 diabetes mellitus	Rheumatoid arthritis
Multiple sclerosis	Systemic sclerosis
	(scleroderma)[b]
	Sjögren syndrome[b]
Diseases Postulated to Be Autoimmune	
Inflammatory bowel diseases	Polyarteritis nodosa[b]
(Crohn disease, ulcerative colitis)[c]	
Primary biliary cholangitis[b]	
Autoimmune (chronic active) hepatitis	

ANCA, Antineutrophil cytoplasmic antibody.

[a]A role for T cells has been demonstrated in these disorders, but antibodies may also be involved in tissue injury.

[b]An autoimmune basis of these disorders is suspected, but not proven.

[c]These disorders may result from excessive immune responses to commensal enteric microbes, autoimmunity, or a combination of the two.

self-reactive immature T cells cannot be deleted. In the B lymphocyte lineage, immature cells that recognize self antigens in the bone marrow can produce a new antigen receptor, a process called receptor editing. If editing fails, the self-reactive B cells are deleted. Because of negative selection, the mature repertoire of T and B lymphocytes is purged of many self-reactive cells. The process, however, is imperfect, in part because not all self antigens may be expressed in the thymus and bone marrow. Other "fail safe" mechanisms, described below, prevent the activation of self-reactive lymphocytes that mature and populate peripheral tissues.

- *Suppression by regulatory T cells (Treg).* Treg are a population of CD4+ T cells that are generated by recognition of self or foreign antigens and function to block lymphocyte activation. The development and function of Treg require the transcription factor FoxP3; mutations in the *FOXP3* gene are the cause of a severe systemic autoimmune disease called *IPEX* (for immune dysregulation, polyendocrinopathy, enteropathy, X-linked). Treg express CTLA-4, which blocks and removes B7 costimulators from APCs, preventing T-cell activation. Treg express high levels of the receptor for IL-2, an essential growth-inducing cytokine for T cells, and outcompete responding T cells for this growth factor. Some Treg secrete immunosuppressive cytokines such as IL-10 and TGF-β. Mutations in the genes encoding CTLA4, the IL-2 receptor α chain, IL-10, or the IL-10 receptor impair Treg function and cause autoimmunity.
- *Inhibition of lymphocyte activation by inhibitory receptors.* Activated T cells express the coinhibitors CTLA-4 and PD-1, both of which suppress continuing T-cell activation and thus impose

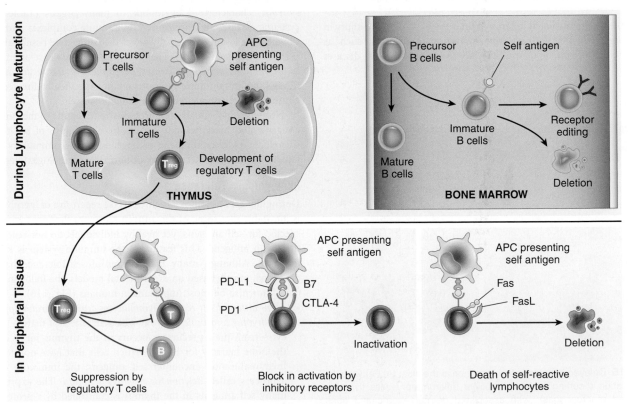

FIG. 5.16 Mechanisms of immunologic tolerance to self antigens. Self-tolerance in T cells and B cells may be induced in the generative lymphoid organs (thymus and bone marrow) and in peripheral tissues. *APC,* Antigen-presenting cell; *CTLA-4,* Cytotoxic T-lymphocyte-associated antigen 4; *PD1,* programmed cell death protein 1; *PD-L1,* programmed cell death–ligand 1.

checkpoints in immune responses. Many cancer patients treated with antibodies that block these receptors, in order to stimulate antitumor immunity, develop autoimmune diseases. B cells express inhibitory receptors called FcγRII and CD22, which also block the activation of these cells. The role of these receptors in self-tolerance has been demonstrated in experimental models and, in some cases, in humans as well.

- *Death of self-reactive lymphocytes.* Activation of lymphocytes results in the coexpression of the death receptor Fas and its ligand; engagement of Fas induces apoptotic death of the cells. Mutations in *FAS* are the cause of an autoimmune disease called *autoimmune lymphoproliferative syndrome (ALPS),* characterized by lymphoproliferation and the production of multiple autoantibodies.

The importance of these mechanisms of self-tolerance has been established by studying rare autoimmune diseases caused by mutations affecting these pathways and, in some cases, by identifying autoimmune diseases that develop as an adverse effect of therapeutic blockade of these pathways. However, it still is not known which of these mechanisms fail in common autoimmune diseases.

Mechanisms of Autoimmunity: General Principles

Now that we have summarized the principal mechanisms of self-tolerance, we can ask how these mechanisms might break down to give rise to pathologic autoimmunity. Unfortunately, the underlying causes of most human autoimmune diseases remain to be determined. The best hypothesis is that **breakdown of self-tolerance and development of autoimmunity result from the combined effects of** **susceptibility genes, which influence lymphocyte tolerance, and environmental factors, such as infections or tissue injury, that alter the display of and responses to self antigens** (Fig. 5.17).

Genetic Factors in Autoimmunity

Most autoimmune diseases are complex multigenic disorders. There is abundant evidence that inherited genes play a role in the development of autoimmune diseases.

- Autoimmune diseases tend to cluster in families, and there is a greater incidence of the same disease in monozygotic than in dizygotic twins.
- Several autoimmune diseases are linked to the HLA locus, especially alleles of HLA-DR and HLA-DQ. The frequency of a disease in individuals with a particular trait compared with those who do not have that trait is called the *odds ratio* or *relative risk.* The relative risk for individuals with particular HLA alleles developing autoimmunity ranges from 3 or 4 for rheumatoid arthritis (RA) in HLA-DR4-positive individuals to 100 or more for ankylosing spondylitis and HLA-B27. The association of most autoimmune diseases, such as SLE, type 1 diabetes, and multiple sclerosis, with different HLA alleles is weak (low odds ratios). Most individuals with a susceptibility-related MHC allele never develop disease, and, conversely, individuals without the relevant MHC gene may be affected. Thus, the disease-associated MHC alleles may increase susceptibility to disease development but are not causal by themselves.
- Genome-wide association studies (GWAS) have revealed many other genetic polymorphisms that are associated with different

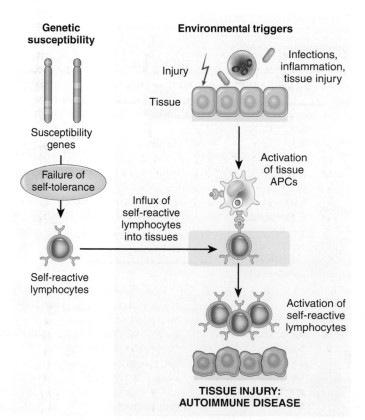

FIG. 5.17 Pathogenesis of autoimmunity. Autoimmunity results from multiple factors, including susceptibility genes that may interfere with self-tolerance and environmental triggers (such as infections, tissue injury, and inflammation) that promote lymphocyte entry into tissues, activation of self-reactive lymphocytes, and tissue damage.

autoimmune diseases. Some of these genetic variants are disease specific, but many of the associations are with genes involved in immune activation and regulation and are seen in multiple disorders, suggesting that they affect general mechanisms of self-tolerance. Interestingly, many of these variants are located in noncoding regions of genes, suggesting that they influence gene expression. However, these associations are generally weak, and the mechanisms by which most of these genetic variants contribute to particular autoimmune diseases are not established.

Role of Infections, Tissue Injury, and Other Environmental Factors

A variety of microbes, including bacteria, mycoplasmas, and viruses, have been implicated as triggers for autoimmunity. Microbes may induce autoimmune reactions by several mechanisms (Fig. 5.18):

- Microbial infections and associated tissue necrosis and inflammation can stimulate expression of costimulatory molecules on APCs and the production of cytokines that activate T cells, thus favoring a breakdown of T-cell tolerance and subsequent T cell–mediated tissue injury.
- Viruses and other microbes may share cross-reacting epitopes with self antigens, and, as a result, responses induced by the microbes may extend to self tissues, a phenomenon called *molecular mimicry*. The best example of a pathogenic immunologic cross-reaction is rheumatic heart disease, in which an antibody produced against streptococci reacts with cardiac antigens. It is not known if mimicry has a role in most common autoimmune diseases.

There is great interest in the idea that the development of autoimmunity is influenced by the normal gut and skin *microbiome* (the diverse collection of commensal microbes that live with us in a symbiotic relationship). It is possible that different commensal microbes affect the relative proportions of effector and regulatory T cells and shape the host response toward or away from aberrant activation. However, it is still not clear which commensal microbes contribute to specific diseases in humans or if the microbiome can be manipulated to prevent or treat these disorders.

Adding to the complexity of the link between microbes and autoimmunity are recent observations suggesting that infections paradoxically protect individuals from some autoimmune diseases, notably type 1 diabetes, multiple sclerosis, and Crohn disease. The possible mechanisms underlying this effect are not understood.

In addition to infections, the display of tissue antigens may be altered by a variety of environmental factors. As discussed later, *ultraviolet (UV) radiation* causes cell death and may lead to the exposure of nuclear antigens, which elicit pathologic immune responses in lupus; this mechanism is the proposed explanation for the association of SLE flares with exposure to sunlight. *Smoking* is a risk factor for rheumatoid arthritis, perhaps because it leads to chemical modification of self antigens. Local tissue injury for any reason may lead to the release of normally sequestered self antigens (such as antigens in the eye and testis) and autoimmune responses.

Finally, there is a strong *gender bias* of autoimmunity, with many of these diseases being more common in women than in men (Fig. 5.19). The underlying mechanisms are not well understood but may involve the effects of hormones on immune cells and other factors.

An autoimmune response may itself promote further autoimmune attack. Tissue injury caused by an autoimmune response or any other cause may lead to exposure of previously concealed self antigen

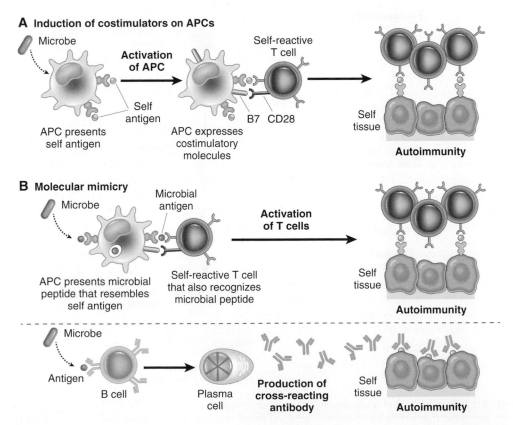

A **Induction of costimulators on APCs**

Microbe

Activation of APC

Self-reactive T cell

Self antigen

APC presents self antigen

APC expresses costimulatory molecules

B7   CD28

Self tissue

Autoimmunity

B **Molecular mimicry**

Microbe

Microbial antigen

Activation of T cells

APC presents microbial peptide that resembles self antigen

Self-reactive T cell that also recognizes microbial peptide

Self tissue

Autoimmunity

Microbe

Antigen

B cell

Plasma cell

Production of cross-reacting antibody

Self tissue

Autoimmunity

FIG. 5.18 Postulated role of infections in autoimmunity. Infections may promote activation of self-reactive lymphocytes by inducing the expression of costimulators (A), or microbial antigens may mimic self antigens and activate self-reactive lymphocytes as a cross-reaction (B).

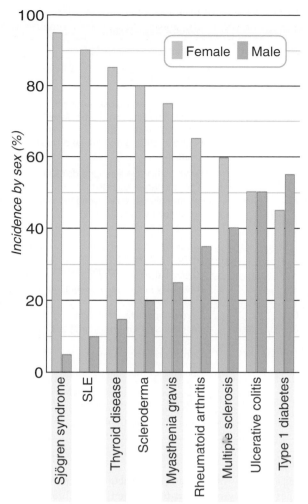

FIG. 5.19 Gender distribution of major autoimmune diseases. The percentages are approximations based on incidence data until the year 2000. *SLE,* Systemic lupus erythematosus. (From Whitacre CC. Sex differences in autoimmune diseases. *Nat Immunol* 2001;2:777. With permission of the publishers.)

epitopes that are presented to T cells in an immunogenic form. The activation of such autoreactive T cells is called *epitope spreading,* because the immune response spreads to epitopes that were not recognized initially. This is one of the mechanisms that may contribute to the chronicity of autoimmune diseases.

Having discussed the general principles of tolerance and autoimmunity, we proceed to a discussion of some of the most common autoimmune diseases. Although each disease is discussed separately, there is considerable overlap in their clinical and morphologic features and underlying pathogenesis. Here we cover the systemic autoimmune diseases; autoimmune diseases that affect single organ systems are discussed in chapters that deal with the relevant organs.

Systemic Lupus Erythematosus

Systemic lupus erythematosus (SLE) is an autoimmune disease involving multiple organs, characterized by the production of autoantibodies, particularly antinuclear antibodies (ANAs). In SLE, injury is caused mainly by deposition of immune complexes and binding of antibodies to various cells and tissues. Injury to the skin,

joints, kidneys, and serosal membranes is prominent, but virtually every organ in the body may be affected. The clinical presentation of the disease is extremely variable and heterogeneous. SLE is a fairly common disease, with a prevalence that may be as high as 400 per 100,000 in certain populations. Although it often presents when a person is in their twenties or thirties, it may manifest at any age, even in early childhood. Similar to many autoimmune diseases, SLE predominantly affects women, with a female-to-male ratio of 9 : 1 for the reproductive age group of 17 to 55 years. By comparison, the female-to-male ratio is only 2 : 1 for disease developing during childhood or after 65 years of age. The prevalence and severity of the disease are higher in African-Americans and Latin-Americans than in European-Americans in the United States.

Spectrum of Autoantibodies in SLE

The hallmark of SLE is the production of autoantibodies. Some antibodies recognize nuclear and cytoplasmic components, while others are directed against cell surface antigens of blood cells. Apart from their value in the diagnosis and management of patients with SLE, these autoantibodies are of major pathogenic significance, as, for example, in the immune complex—mediated glomerulonephritis typical of this disease. Autoantibodies are also found in other autoimmune diseases, many of which tend to be associated with specific types of autoantibodies (Table 5.8).

Antinuclear Antibodies (ANAs). ANAs can be grouped into four categories: (1) antibodies to DNA; (2) antibodies to histones; (3) antibodies to nonhistone proteins bound to RNA; and (4) antibodies to nucleolar antigens. A widely used method for detecting ANAs is immunofluorescent staining of a cell line with antibodies from patient serum. This method identifies the presence of antibodies that react with the nuclear antigens cited above (collectively called generic ANAs). The pattern of nuclear staining suggests the specificity of the antibody present in the patient's serum (eFig. 5.2). However, the staining patterns are often not easy to interpret because many autoantibodies may be present, and combinations of patterns are frequent. Attempts are ongoing to replace microscopic assays with quantitative assays for antibodies against specific nuclear and other antigens. Indeed, antibodies to double-stranded DNA and the so-called "Smith (Sm) antigen," a nonhistone nuclear protein, can be detected by more quantitative assays and are virtually diagnostic of SLE.

Other Autoantibodies. In addition to ANAs, patients with SLE have a host of other autoantibodies. Some are directed against blood cells, such as red cells, platelets, and lymphocytes. Antiphospholipid antibodies are present in 30% to 40% of patients with SLE. They are actually specific for epitopes of various plasma proteins that are revealed when the proteins are in complex with phospholipids. Antibodies against the phospholipid—β_2-glycoprotein complex also bind to cardiolipin antigen, which is used in serologic tests for syphilis; as a result patients with SLE may have a false-positive test result for syphilis. Because these antibodies bind to phospholipids, they prolong the partial thromboplastin time, an in vitro clotting test that requires phospholipids. For this reason, these antibodies were previously called lupus anticoagulant. Despite the observed clotting delay in vitro, patients with antiphospholipid antibodies have complications related to excessive clotting (a hypercoagulable state), such as thrombosis (Chapter 3).

Pathogenesis. **The fundamental defect in SLE is a failure of the mechanisms that maintain self-tolerance.** Although what causes this failure of self-tolerance remains unknown, as is true of most autoimmune diseases, both genetic and environmental factors play a role.

Table 5.8 Autoantibodies in Systemic Autoimmune Diseases

Disease	Specificity of Autoantibody	% Positive	Disease Associations
Systemic lupus erythematosus (SLE)	Double-stranded DNA	40–60	Nephritis; specific for SLE
	U1-RNP	30–40	
	Smith (Sm) antigen (core protein of small RNP particles)	20–30	Specific for SLE
	Ro (SS-A) nucleoprotein	30–50	Congenital heart block; neonatal lupus
	Phospholipid-protein complexes (anti-PL)	30–40	Antiphospholipid syndrome (in ~10% of patients with SLE)
	Multiple nuclear antigens ("generic ANAs")	95–100	Found in other autoimmune diseases, not specific
Systemic sclerosis	DNA topoisomerase 1	30–70	Diffuse skin disease, lung disease; specific for systemic sclerosis
	Centromeric proteins (CENPs) A, B, C	20–40	Limited skin disease, ischemic digital loss, pulmonary hypertension
	RNA polymerase III	15–20	Acute onset, scleroderma renal crisis, cancer
Sjögren syndrome	Ro/SS-A	75	More sensitive for Sjogren syndrome
	La/SS-B	50	More specific for Sjogren syndrome
Autoimmune myositis	Histidyl aminoacyl-tRNA synthetase, Jo1	25	Interstitial lung disease, Raynaud phenomenon
	Mi-2 nuclear antigen	5–10	Dermatomyositis, skin rash
	MDA5 (cytoplasmic receptor for viral RNA)	20–35 (Japanese)	Vascular skin lesions, interstitial lung disease
	TIF1γ nuclear protein	15–20	Dermatomyositis, cancer
Rheumatoid arthritis	Peptides from various citrullinated proteins	60–80	Specific for rheumatoid arthritis
	Rheumatoid factor	60–70	Not specific

"Generic" antinuclear antibodies (ANAs), which may react against many nuclear antigens, are positive in a large fraction of patients with SLE but are also positive in other autoimmune diseases. *% positive* refers to the approximate % of patients who test positive for each antibody.
Table compiled with the assistance of Dr. Antony Rosen, Johns Hopkins University, and Dr. Andrew Gross, University of California San Francisco.

Genetic Factors. Many lines of evidence support a genetic predisposition to SLE.

- *Familial association.* Family members have an increased risk for the development of SLE, and up to 20% of unaffected first-degree relatives have autoantibodies. There is a higher rate of concordance in monozygotic twins (25%) than in dizygotic twins (1%–3%).
- *HLA association.* The odds ratio (relative risk) for persons with HLA-DR2 or HLA-DR3 is 2 to 3, and if both haplotypes are present, the relative risk is about 5.
- *Other genes.* Genetic deficiencies of classical pathway complement proteins, especially C1q, C2, or C4, are seen in about 10% of patients with SLE. The complement deficiencies may result in defective clearance of immune complexes and apoptotic cells, and failure of B-cell tolerance. A polymorphism in the inhibitory Fc receptor, FcγRIIb, has been described in some patients; this may contribute to inadequate control of B-cell activation. Additional genes have been implicated by genome-wide association studies, but their contribution to the development of the disease remains unclear.

Environmental Factors. There are many indications that environmental factors are also involved in the pathogenesis of SLE.

- Exposure to UV light exacerbates the disease in many individuals. UV irradiation may induce apoptosis and may alter DNA, rendering it immunogenic, perhaps by enhancing its recognition by TLRs. In addition, UV light may modulate the immune response, for example, by stimulating keratinocytes to produce IL-1, a cytokine that promotes inflammation.

- The gender bias of SLE has been attributed to actions of sex hormones and may be related to genes on the X chromosome, but the underlying mechanisms remain unclear.
- Drugs such as hydralazine, procainamide, and D-penicillamine can induce an SLE-like disorder.

Immunologic Factors. Recent studies in animal models and patients have revealed several immunologic aberrations that collectively may result in the persistent and uncontrolled activation of self-reactive lymphocytes.

- Failure of self-tolerance in B cells results from defective receptor editing or elimination of self-reactive B cells in the bone marrow or defects in peripheral tolerance mechanisms.
- CD4+ helper T cells specific for nucleosomal antigens also escape tolerance and contribute to the production of high-affinity pathogenic autoantibodies. The autoantibodies in SLE show characteristics of T cell–dependent antibodies produced in germinal centers, and increased numbers of follicular helper T cells have been detected in the blood of patients with SLE.
- Type I interferons. Blood cells show a molecular signature that indicates exposure to interferon-α (IFN-α), a type I interferon that is produced mainly by a subset of DCs called plasmacytoid DCs. Some studies have shown that such cells from SLE patients produce abnormally large amounts of IFN-α.
- TLR signals. Studies in animal models have shown that TLRs that recognize DNA and RNA, notably the DNA-recognizing TLR9 and the RNA-recognizing TLR7, produce signals that regulate responses of B cells specific for self nuclear antigens.

- Other cytokines that may play a role in unregulated B-cell activation include the TNF family member BAFF, which promotes survival of B cells. In some patients and animal models, increased production of BAFF has been reported, and this has led to modest success of an antibody that blocks BAFF as a therapy for SLE.

A Model for the Pathogenesis of SLE. Although we still don't know why SLE develops, we can attempt to synthesize results from human studies and animal models into a hypothetical model of its pathogenesis (Fig. 5.20). Abnormalities in B lymphocytes and T lymphocytes are responsible for defective tolerance, because of which self-reactive lymphocytes survive and remain functional. UV irradiation and other environmental factors lead to the apoptosis of cells. Inadequate clearance of the nuclei of these cells results in a large burden of nuclear antigens. Self-reactive lymphocytes are stimulated by nuclear self antigens, and antibodies are produced against the

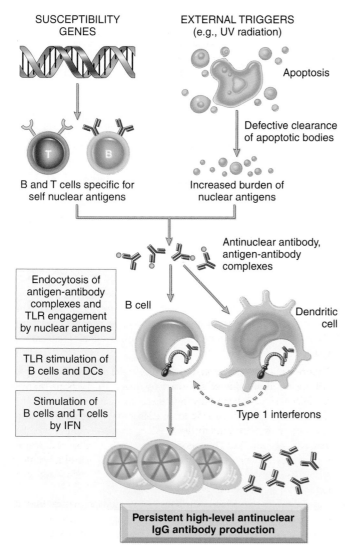

FIG. 5.20 Pathogenesis of systemic lupus erythematosus. In this hypothetical model, susceptibility genes interfere with the maintenance of self-tolerance, and external triggers lead to persistence of nuclear antigens. The result is an antibody response against self nuclear antigens, which is amplified by the action of nucleic acids on dendritic cells (DCs) and B cells, and the production of type I interferons. *TLRs,* Toll-like receptors.

antigens. Complexes of the antigens and antibodies bind to Fc receptors on B cells and dendritic cells and may be internalized. The nucleic acid components engage TLRs and stimulate B cells to produce more autoantibodies. TLR stimuli also activate dendritic cells to produce interferons and other cytokines, which further enhance the immune response and cause apoptosis. The net result is a cycle of antigen release and immune activation resulting in the production of high-affinity autoantibodies.

Mechanisms of Tissue Injury. A variety of autoantibodies cause most of the lesions of SLE.

- **Most of the systemic lesions are caused by immune complexes (type III hypersensitivity).** DNA-anti-DNA complexes can be detected in the glomeruli and small blood vessels. Low levels of serum complement (secondary to consumption of complement proteins) and granular deposits of complement and immunoglobulins in the glomeruli further support the immune complex nature of the disease. T-cell infiltrates are also frequently seen in the kidneys, but the role of these cells in tissue damage is not established.
- **Autoantibodies of different specificities contribute to the pathology and clinical manifestations of SLE (type II hypersensitivity).** For example, autoantibodies specific for red cells, leukocytes, and platelets opsonize these cells and promote their phagocytosis, resulting in cytopenias.
- *Antiphospholipid antibody syndrome.* Patients with antiphospholipid antibodies may develop venous and arterial thromboses, which may cause recurrent spontaneous miscarriages and focal cerebral or ocular ischemia. This constellation of clinical features, in association with lupus, is referred to as the *secondary antiphospholipid antibody syndrome.* The mechanisms of thrombosis are not defined, and antibodies against clotting factors, platelets, and endothelial cells have all been proposed as being responsible for thrombosis (Chapter 3). Some patients develop these autoantibodies and the clinical syndrome without associated SLE. They are said to have the *primary antiphospholipid antibody syndrome* (Chapter 3).
- The *neuropsychiatric manifestations* of SLE have been attributed to antibodies that cross the blood–brain barrier and react with neurons or receptors for various neurotransmitters. However, this is not established in all cases, and mechanisms involving other immune factors, such as cytokines, may underlie the cognitive dysfunction and other CNS abnormalities that are associated with SLE.

MORPHOLOGY

The morphologic changes in SLE are extremely variable. The frequency of individual organ involvement is shown in Table 5.9. The most characteristic lesions result from immune complex deposition in blood vessels, kidneys, connective tissue, and skin.

Blood Vessels. An acute necrotizing vasculitis involving capillaries, small arteries, and arterioles may be present in any tissue. The arteritis leads to fibrinoid necrosis of the vessel walls. In chronic stages, vessels undergo fibrous thickening with luminal narrowing.

Kidney. Up to 50% of patients with SLE have clinically significant renal involvement, and the kidney virtually always shows evidence of abnormality if examined by electron microscopy and immunofluorescence. Renal involvement takes a number of forms, all of which are associated with the deposition of immune complexes within the glomeruli. Lupus nephritis is described in Chapter 12, where we discuss diseases of the kidney.

Skin. Characteristic erythema affects the face along the bridge of the nose and cheeks (the **butterfly rash**) in approximately 50% of patients, but a similar rash may also be seen on the extremities and trunk. Urticaria, bullae, maculopapular lesions, and ulcerations also occur. Exposure to sunlight incites or accentuates the erythema. Histologically the involved areas show vacuolar degeneration of the basal layer of the epidermis (Fig. 5.21A). In the dermis, there is variable edema and perivascular inflammation. Vasculitis with fibrinoid necrosis may be prominent. Immunofluorescence microscopy shows deposits of immunoglobulin and complement along the dermoepidermal junction (Fig. 5.21B); these may also be present in uninvolved skin. This finding is not diagnostic of SLE and is sometimes seen in scleroderma and dermatomyositis.

Joints. Joint involvement is typically a nonerosive synovitis with little deformity, which contrasts with rheumatoid arthritis.

Central Nervous System. Significant vasculitis is rarely present. Instead, noninflammatory occlusion of small vessels by intimal proliferation is sometimes noted, which may be due to endothelial damage caused by autoantibodies or immune complexes.

Pericarditis and Other Serosal Cavity Involvement. Inflammation of the serosal lining membranes may be acute, subacute, or chronic. During the acute phase, the mesothelial surfaces are sometimes covered with fibrinous exudate. Later they become thickened, opaque, and coated with shaggy fibrous tissue that may lead to partial or total obliteration of the serosal cavity. Pleural and pericardial effusions may be present.

Cardiovascular system involvement may manifest as damage to any layer of the heart. Histologically, pericardial involvement is present in up to 50% of patients. Myocarditis is less common and may cause resting tachycardia and electrocardiographic abnormalities. **Valvular** (so-called Libman-Sacks) **endocarditis** was more common prior to the widespread use of steroids. This sterile endocarditis appears as single or multiple 1- to 3-mm verrucous deposits, which may form on either surface of the leaflets, a distinctive feature (eFig. 5.3). By comparison, the vegetations in infective endocarditis are larger, while those in rheumatic heart disease (Chapter 9) are smaller and confined to the lines of closure of the valve leaflets. Ischemic heart disease is an increasingly frequent cause of death.

Spleen. Splenomegaly, capsular thickening, and follicular hyperplasia are common features. Central penicilliary arteries may show concentric intimal and smooth muscle cell hyperplasia, producing so-called **onion-skin lesions.**

Lungs. In addition to pleuritis and accompanying pleural effusions, some cases are complicated by chronic interstitial fibrosis and secondary pulmonary hypertension.

Other Organs and Tissues. Lymph nodes may be enlarged due to hyperplasia of B cell follicles or even demonstrate necrotizing lymphadenitis due to vasculitis.

Table 5.9 Clinical and Pathologic Manifestations of Systemic Lupus Erythematosus

Clinical Manifestation	Prevalence in Patients (%)[a]
Hematologic	100
Arthritis, arthralgia, or myalgia	80–90
Skin	85
Fever	55–85
Fatigue	80–100
Weight loss	60
Renal	50–70
Neuropsychiatric	25–35
Pleuritis	45
Pericarditis	25
Gastrointestinal	20
Raynaud phenomenon	15–40
Ocular	5–15
Peripheral neuropathy	15

[a]Percentages are approximate and may vary with age, ethnicity, and other factors. Table compiled with the assistance of Dr. Meenakshi Jolly, Rush Medical Center, Chicago, IL.

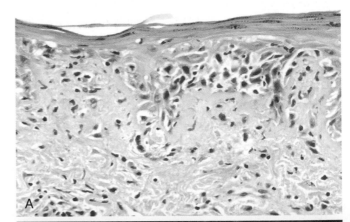
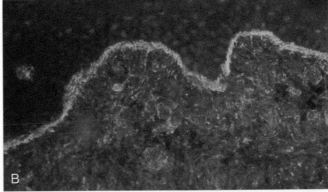

FIG. 5.21 Systemic lupus erythematosus involving the skin. (A) An H&E-stained section shows liquefactive degeneration of the basal layer of the epidermis and edema at the dermoepidermal junction. (B) An immunofluorescence micrograph stained for IgG reveals deposits of Ig along the dermoepidermal junction. (A, Courtesy of Dr. Jag Bhawan, Boston University School of Medicine, Boston, Massachusetts. B, Courtesy of Dr. Richard Sontheimer, Department of Dermatology, University of Texas Southwestern Medical School, Dallas, Texas.)

Clinical Features. SLE is a highly variable multisystem disease, and its diagnosis relies on a constellation of clinical, serologic, and morphologic findings. It may be acute or insidious in its onset. Often, the patient is a young woman with some or all of the following features: a butterfly rash on the face; fever; pain without deformity in one or more joints; pleuritic chest pain; and photosensitivity. In many patients, however, the presentation is subtle and puzzling, taking forms such as fever of unknown origin, abnormal urinary findings, or joint disease masquerading as rheumatoid arthritis or rheumatic fever. Generic ANAs, detected by immunofluorescence assays, are found in virtually 100% of patients but are not specific, whereas antibodies to double-stranded DNA are specific for SLE. Renal involvement may produce a variety of findings, including hematuria, red cell casts, proteinuria, and nephrotic syndrome (Chapter 12). Anemia or thrombocytopenia are presenting manifestations in some patients and may be the dominant clinical problems. In others, neuropsychiatric manifestations, including psychosis or convulsions, or coronary artery disease may be prominent. Infections are also common, presumably due to immune dysfunction and treatment with immunosuppressive drugs.

The course of SLE is unpredictable. Rare acute cases result in death within weeks to months. More often, with appropriate therapy, SLE follows a relapsing and remitting course over a period of years or decades. During acute flares, increased formation of immune complexes results in complement activation, often leading to hypocomplementemia. Disease flares are usually treated with corticosteroids or other immunosuppressive drugs. Even without therapy, in some patients the disease runs an indolent course for years with relatively mild manifestations, such as skin changes and mild hematuria. The overall 5-year and 10-year survivals are approximately 90% and 80%, respectively. The most common causes of death are renal failure and intercurrent infections. An increasing number of patients are affected by coronary artery disease manifesting as angina or myocardial infarction. This complication may be seen in young patients with long-standing disease and is especially prevalent in those who have been treated with corticosteroids. The pathogenesis of accelerated coronary atherosclerosis is unclear but is probably multifactorial. Risk factors for atherosclerosis, including hypertension, obesity, and hyperlipidemia, are more commonly present in patients with SLE than in the population at large. In addition, immune complexes and antiphospholipid antibodies may cause endothelial damage and promote atherosclerosis.

As mentioned earlier, involvement of skin along with multisystem disease is fairly common in SLE. The following section describes two syndromes in which cutaneous involvement is the exclusive or most prominent feature.

Chronic Discoid Lupus Erythematosus and Subacute Cutaneous Lupus Erythematosus

Chronic discoid lupus erythematosus is a disease in which the skin manifestations may mimic SLE, but systemic manifestations are rare. It is characterized by the presence of skin plaques with elevated erythematous borders, most often on the face and scalp, showing varying degrees of edema, erythema or hyperpigmentation, scaliness, follicular plugging, and skin atrophy. It progresses to SLE in 5% to 10% of patients, usually after many years. Conversely, some patients with SLE may have prominent discoid lesions in the skin. Approximately 35% of patients have a positive test for generic ANAs, but antibodies to double-stranded DNA are rarely present. Immunofluorescence studies of skin biopsy specimens show deposition of immunoglobulin and C3 at the dermoepidermal junction similar to that in SLE.

Subacute cutaneous lupus erythematosus refers to a group intermediate between SLE and lupus erythematosus localized to skin. The skin rash in this entity tends to be widespread and superficial. Most patients have mild systemic symptoms similar to those in SLE.

Drug-Induced Lupus Erythematosus

An SLE-like syndrome may develop in patients receiving a variety of drugs, including hydralazine, procainamide, isoniazid, and D-penicillamine. Anti-TNF therapy, which is effective in rheumatoid arthritis and other autoimmune diseases, can also cause drug-induced lupus. Many of these drugs are associated with the development of ANAs, especially antibodies specific for histones. The disease remits after withdrawal of the offending drug.

Rheumatoid Arthritis and Related Disorders

Rheumatoid arthritis is an autoimmune disease that primarily affects the joints but may also involve extraarticular tissues such as the skin, blood vessels, lungs, and heart. Because the principal manifestations of the disease are in the joints, it is discussed in Chapter 19.

Arthritis is also seen in association with other immunologic diseases, including psoriasis (Chapter 19). *Spondyloarthritis* mainly affects cervical vertebral joints and is usually seronegative. *Reactive arthritis* is a variant of spondyloarthritis that develops after infections, e.g., of the urinary tract.

Sjögren Syndrome

Sjögren syndrome is a chronic disease characterized by dry eyes (keratoconjunctivitis sicca) and dry mouth (xerostomia) resulting from immunologically mediated destruction of the lacrimal and salivary glands. It occurs as an isolated disorder (primary form), also known as the *sicca syndrome,* but in about 60% of patients, it is present in association with another autoimmune disease (secondary form). Rheumatoid arthritis is the most commonly associated disorder, but other associations include SLE, polymyositis, systemic sclerosis, vasculitis, mixed connective tissue disease, or autoimmune thyroid disease.

The lacrimal and salivary glands characteristically show dense lymphocytic infiltration consisting mainly of activated CD4+ helper T cells and some B cells, including plasma cells. Serologic studies frequently reveal autoantibodies. Antibodies against two ribonucleoprotein antigens, SS-A (Ro) and SS-B (La) (see Table 5.8), can be detected in as many as 90% of patients by sensitive techniques. High titers of antibodies to SS-A are associated with early disease onset, longer disease duration, and extraglandular manifestations, such as cutaneous vasculitis, nephritis, and pulmonary fibrosis. These autoantibodies are also present in a smaller percentage of patients with SLE and hence are not diagnostic of Sjögren syndrome. In addition, about 75% of patients have rheumatoid factor (an antibody reactive with self IgG), and 50% to 80% of patients have ANAs.

Pathogenesis. The pathogenesis of Sjögren syndrome remains obscure, but the pathology and serology, as well as an association, albeit weak, with certain HLA alleles, all point to activation of autoreactive T cells and B cells. The initiating trigger may be a viral infection of the salivary glands, which causes local cell death and release of tissue self antigens. In genetically susceptible individuals, CD4+ T cells and B cells specific for these self antigens may escape tolerance and participate in immune reactions that lead to tissue damage and, eventually, fibrosis. However, the role of particular cytokines or T-cell subsets, and the nature of the autoantigens recognized by these lymphocytes, remain unknown.

MORPHOLOGY

Lacrimal and salivary glands are the major targets of the disease, but other exocrine glands, including those lining the respiratory and gastrointestinal tracts and the vagina, also may be involved. The earliest histologic finding in the major and minor salivary glands is periductal and perivascular lymphocytic infiltration. With time, the lymphocytic infiltrate becomes extensive (Fig. 5.22), and in the larger salivary glands, lymphoid follicles with germinal centers may be seen. The epithelial cells lining the ducts may become hyperplastic and obstruct the ducts. Later there is atrophy of the acini, fibrosis, and hyalinization; still later in the course, the atrophic parenchyma may be replaced with

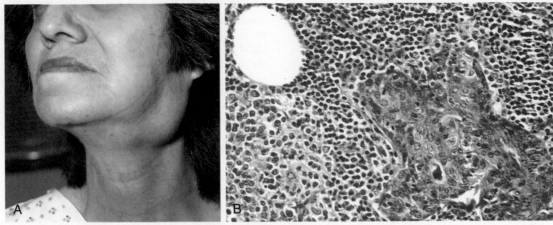

FIG. 5.22 Sjögren syndrome. (A) Enlargement of the salivary gland. (B) Intense lymphocytic and plasma cell infiltration with ductal epithelial hyperplasia in a salivary gland. (A, Courtesy of Dr. Richard Sontheimer, Department of Dermatology, University of Texas Southwestern Medical School, Dallas, Texas. B, Courtesy of Dr. Dennis Burns, Department of Pathology, University of Texas Southwestern Medical School, Dallas, Texas.)

fat. In some cases, the lymphoid infiltrate may be so intense as to give the appearance of a lymphoma. Indeed, these patients are at high risk for development of B-cell lymphomas of the salivary gland and other extranodal sites (Chapter 10). The histologic findings are not specific or diagnostic and may be mimicked by chronic sialadenitis caused by ductal obstruction due to calculi.

Lack of tears leads to drying of the corneal epithelium, which becomes inflamed, eroded, and ulcerated; the oral mucosa may atrophy, with inflammatory fissuring and ulceration; and dryness and crusting of the nose may lead to ulcerations and even perforation of the nasal septum.

Clinical Features. Sjögren syndrome occurs most commonly in women between 50 and 60 years of age. Symptoms relate mainly to inflammatory destruction of the exocrine glands. Keratoconjunctivitis results in blurred vision, burning and itching of the eyes, and the accumulation of thick secretions in the conjunctival sac. Xerostomia causes difficulty in swallowing solid foods, decreased taste sensation, cracks and fissures in the mouth, and dryness of the buccal mucosa. Parotid gland enlargement is present in half the patients; dryness of the nasal mucosa, epistaxis, recurrent bronchitis, and pneumonitis are other symptoms. Manifestations of extraglandular disease are seen in one-third of patients and include synovitis, pulmonary fibrosis, and peripheral neuropathy. In contrast to SLE, glomerular lesions are rare in Sjögren syndrome. Defects of tubular function, however, including renal tubular acidosis, uricosuria, and phosphaturia, are often seen and may be associated with tubulointerstitial nephritis (Chapter 12).

Systemic Sclerosis (Scleroderma)

Systemic sclerosis is an immunologic disorder characterized by excessive fibrosis in multiple tissues, obliterative vascular disease, and evidence of autoimmunity, mainly the production of multiple autoantibodies. Although the term *scleroderma* is ingrained in clinical medicine, the name *systemic sclerosis* is preferred because excessive fibrosis is seen in multiple organs. Cutaneous involvement is the usual presenting manifestation and eventually appears in approximately 95% of cases, but it is the visceral involvement—of the gastrointestinal tract, lungs, kidneys, heart, and skeletal muscles—that is responsible for most of the morbidity and mortality. Disease limited to the skin is also called *localized scleroderma.*

Systemic sclerosis is classified into two groups on the basis of its course:

- *Diffuse systemic sclerosis,* characterized by initial widespread skin involvement, with rapid progression and early visceral involvement
- *Limited systemic sclerosis,* with relatively mild skin involvement, often confined to the fingers and face, and late involvement of viscera. This presentation is also called *CREST syndrome* because of its frequent features of calcinosis, Raynaud phenomenon, esophageal dysmotility, sclerodactyly, and telangiectasia.

Pathogenesis. The cause of systemic sclerosis is not known, but **the disease likely results from three interrelated processes—autoimmune responses, vascular damage, and collagen deposition.**

- *Autoimmunity.* It is proposed that CD4+ T cells responding to an as yet unidentified antigen accumulate in the skin and release cytokines that activate inflammatory cells and fibroblasts. Several cytokines, including IL-13 produced by Th2 cells and TGF-β produced by alternatively activated macrophages and other cell types, are known to stimulate synthesis of collagen and extracellular matrix proteins in fibroblasts. The presence of various autoantibodies, notably ANAs, provides diagnostic and prognostic information. There is no evidence that these antibodies stimulate fibrosis.
- *Vascular damage.* Microvascular disease is consistently present early in the course of systemic sclerosis. However, the cause of the vascular injury is unknown; it could be the initiating event or the result of chronic inflammation, with the production of mediators from inflammatory cells that damage the microvascular endothelium. Repeated cycles of endothelial injury followed by platelet aggregation lead to release of platelet and endothelial factors (e.g., PDGF, TGF-β) that trigger endothelial proliferation and intimal and perivascular fibrosis. Eventually, widespread narrowing of the microvasculature leads to ischemic injury and scarring. The pulmonary vasculature is frequently involved, and the resulting pulmonary hypertension is a serious complication of the disease.
- *Fibrosis.* The progressive fibrosis characteristic of the disease may be the culmination of multiple abnormalities, including the

accumulation of alternatively activated macrophages, actions of fibrogenic cytokines produced by infiltrating leukocytes, hyperresponsiveness of fibroblasts to these cytokines, and scarring following ischemic damage caused by the vascular lesions.

MORPHOLOGY

In systemic sclerosis, the most prominent changes occur in the skin, gastrointestinal tract, musculoskeletal system, and kidney, but lesions also are often present in the blood vessels, heart, lungs, and peripheral nerves.

Skin. Most patients have diffuse fibrosis of the skin and associated atrophy, which usually begins in the fingers and distal regions of the upper extremities and extends proximally to involve the upper arms, shoulders, neck, and face. Edema and perivascular infiltrates containing CD4+ T cells are seen, together with swelling and degeneration of collagen fibers, which become eosinophilic. Capillaries and small arteries (150–500 μm in diameter) may show thickening of the basal lamina, endothelial damage, and partial occlusion. With disease progression, there is increasing fibrosis of the dermis, which becomes tightly bound to subcutaneous structures. Fibrosis is often accompanied by thinning of the epidermis, loss of rete pegs, atrophy of the dermal appendages, and hyaline thickening of the walls of dermal arterioles and capillaries (Fig. 5.23B). Subcutaneous calcifications may develop, especially in patients with CREST syndrome. In advanced stages the fingers take on a tapered, clawlike appearance and have limited joint mobility, and the face becomes taut and masklike. Loss of blood supply may lead to cutaneous ulcerations and atrophic changes (Fig. 5.23C) or even autoamputation of the terminal phalanges.

Gastrointestinal (GI) Tract. The GI tract is affected in approximately 90% of patients. Progressive atrophy and fibrous replacement of the muscularis may develop at any level of the gut but are most severe in the esophagus. The lower two-thirds of the esophagus often develops a rubber-hose—like inflexibility. The associated dysfunction of the lower esophageal sphincter gives rise to gastroesophageal reflux and its complications, including Barrett metaplasia (Chapter 13) and strictures. The mucosa is thinned and may ulcerate, and there is excessive collagenization of the lamina propria and submucosa. Loss of villi and microvilli in the small bowel may cause a malabsorption syndrome.

Musculoskeletal System. Inflammation of the synovium, associated with synoviocyte hypertrophy, is common in the early stages; fibrosis later ensues. These changes are reminiscent of rheumatoid arthritis, but joint destruction is not common in systemic sclerosis. A small subset of patients (approximately 10%) develop an inflammatory myositis.

Kidneys. Renal abnormalities occur in two-thirds of patients; vascular lesions are the most prominent feature. Interlobular arteries show intimal thickening due to deposition of mucinous material containing glycoproteins and acid mucopolysaccharides and concentric proliferation of intimal cells. These changes resemble those seen in severe hypertension, but in systemic sclerosis the alterations are restricted to vessels 150 to 500 μm in diameter and are not always associated with hypertension. Hypertension, however, does occur in 30% of patients, in whom vascular alterations are more pronounced and often associated with fibrinoid necrosis of arterioles that can lead to thrombosis and infarction. Such patients often die of renal failure, which accounts for about 50% of deaths. There are no specific glomerular changes.

Lungs. The lungs are affected in more than 50% of cases. This involvement may manifest as pulmonary hypertension and interstitial fibrosis. Pulmonary vasospasm secondary to endothelial dysfunction is considered a factor in the pathogenesis of pulmonary hypertension. Pulmonary fibrosis, when present, is indistinguishable from that seen in idiopathic pulmonary fibrosis (Chapter 11).

Heart. Pericarditis with effusion, myocardial fibrosis, and thickening of intramyocardial arterioles occur in one-third of patients. Right ventricular hypertrophy and failure (cor pulmonale) secondary to pulmonary changes are frequent.

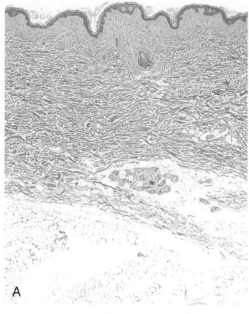

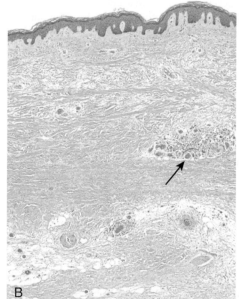

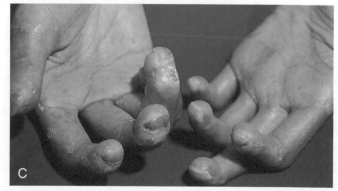

FIG. 5.23 Systemic sclerosis. (A) Normal skin. (B) Skin biopsy from a patient with systemic sclerosis. Note the extensive deposition of dense collagen in the dermis, the virtual absence of appendages (e.g., hair follicles), and foci of inflammation *(arrow)*. (C) The extensive subcutaneous fibrosis has virtually immobilized the fingers, creating a clawlike flexion deformity. Loss of blood supply has led to cutaneous ulcerations. (C, Courtesy of Dr. Richard Sontheimer, Department of Dermatology, University of Texas Southwestern Medical School, Dallas, Texas.)

Clinical Features. Systemic sclerosis has a female-to-male ratio of 3 : 1 and a peak incidence in the 50- to 60-year age group. Although systemic sclerosis shares features with SLE, rheumatoid arthritis (Chapter 19), and polymyositis (Chapter 20), it is distinguished by the striking cutaneous changes, notably skin thickening. Raynaud phenomenon, caused by episodic vasoconstriction of the arteries and arterioles of the extremities, is seen in virtually all patients and precedes other symptoms in 70% of cases. Progressive collagen deposition in the skin leads to increasing stiffness, especially of the hands, with eventually complete immobilization of the joints. Nailfold capillary loops are distorted early in the disease and later disappear. Dysphagia attributable to esophageal fibrosis and its resultant hypomotility are present in more than 50% of patients. Eventually, fibrosis of the esophageal wall leads to atony and dilation, especially distally. Abdominal pain, intestinal obstruction, or malabsorption syndrome reflects involvement of the small intestine. Respiratory difficulties caused by the pulmonary fibrosis may result in right-sided cardiac dysfunction, and myocardial fibrosis may cause either arrhythmias or cardiac failure. Proteinuria occurs in as many as 30% of patients but is rarely severe enough to cause nephrotic syndrome. The most ominous manifestation is severe hypertension, with the subsequent development of renal failure (Chapter 12), but in its absence progression of the disease may be slow. In most patients the disease steadily worsens over many years, although life span is improving with better treatment of the complications. As therapy for the renal complications has improved, pulmonary and cardiac involvement has become the major cause of death.

Virtually all patients have ANAs that react with a variety of nuclear antigens (see Table 5.8). Two ANAs are strongly associated with systemic sclerosis. One directed against DNA topoisomerase I (anti-Scl 70) is highly specific and is associated with a greater likelihood of pulmonary fibrosis and peripheral vascular disease. The other, an anticentromere antibody, is associated with a higher likelihood of CREST syndrome. Patients with this syndrome have relatively limited skin disease, often confined to fingers, forearms, and face, and subcutaneous calcifications. Involvement of the viscera, including esophageal lesions and pulmonary hypertension, may not occur at all or occur late. In general, these patients live longer than those with systemic sclerosis with diffuse visceral involvement from the outset.

Inflammatory Myopathies

Inflammatory myopathies comprise an uncommon, heterogeneous group of disorders characterized by injury and inflammation of mainly the skeletal muscles that are probably immunologically mediated. Based on clinical, morphologic, and immunologic features, several disorders—polymyositis, immune-mediated necrotizing myopathy, dermatomyositis, and inclusion body myositis—have been described. Each may occur alone or with other immune-mediated diseases, particularly systemic sclerosis. These diseases are described in Chapter 20, along with other disorders affecting muscles.

Mixed Connective Tissue Disease

Mixed connective tissue disease is a disorder with clinical features that overlap those of SLE, systemic sclerosis, and polymyositis. The disease is characterized serologically by high titers of antibodies to U1 ribonucleoprotein. It typically presents with synovitis of the fingers, Raynaud phenomenon, and mild myositis. Renal involvement is modest, and there is a favorable response to corticosteroids, at least in the short term. Because these clinical features are shared with other diseases, mixed connective tissue disease may not be a distinct entity, and in fact it may evolve over time into classic SLE or systemic sclerosis. However, progression to other autoimmune disorders is not universal, and there may be a form of mixed connective tissue disease that is distinct from other autoimmune diseases. Serious complications of mixed connective tissue disease include pulmonary hypertension, interstitial lung disease, and renal disease.

Polyarteritis Nodosa and Other Vasculitides

Polyarteritis nodosa belongs to a group of disorders characterized by necrotizing inflammation of the walls of blood vessels that show strong evidence of an immunologic basis. Any type of vessel may be involved—arteries, arterioles, veins, or capillaries. These vasculitides are discussed in Chapter 8.

IgG4-Related Disease

IgG4-related disease (IgG4-RD) is characterized by tissue infiltrates rich in IgG4 antibody–producing plasma cells and lymphocytes, particularly T cells, associated with fibrosis and obliterative phlebitis (Fig. 5.24). Increased numbers of IgG4-producing plasma cells in tissue are a sine qua non of this disorder, and serum IgG4 is often, but not always, elevated. IgG4-related disease has now been described in virtually every organ system. Many conditions long viewed as disorders of single organs are now part of the IgG4-RD spectrum. These include *Mikulicz syndrome* (enlargement and fibrosis of salivary and lacrimal glands), *Riedel thyroiditis, idiopathic retroperitoneal fibrosis, autoimmune pancreatitis,* and *inflammatory pseudotumors* of the orbit, lungs, and kidneys, to name a few. The disease most often affects middle-aged and older men.

The pathogenesis of this condition is not understood, and although IgG4 production in lesions is a hallmark of the disease, it is not known if this antibody type contributes to the pathology. The key role of B cells is supported by clinical trials in which depletion of B cells by anti–B-cell agents such as rituximab provided clinical benefit.

IMMUNOLOGY OF TRANSPLANTATION

A major barrier to transplantation is the process of *rejection,* in which the recipient's immune system recognizes the graft as foreign and attacks it. The key to successful transplantation has been the development of therapies that prevent or minimize rejection. Transplant rejection is discussed here because it involves several of the immunologic reactions that underlie hypersensitivity disorders.

Recognition and Rejection of Allografts

Rejection is a process in which T lymphocytes and antibodies produced against graft antigens react with and destroy the grafts. Like other immune responses, this process proceeds in steps, which include recognition of the graft as foreign to the host, activation of T and B lymphocytes by the foreign antigens of the graft, and destruction of the graft by the immune response.

Recognition of Graft Alloantigens

The major graft antigens that are recognized by the recipient as foreign are HLA molecules. Grafts exchanged between individuals of the same species are called *allografts.* Because HLA genes are highly polymorphic, there are differences between the HLA

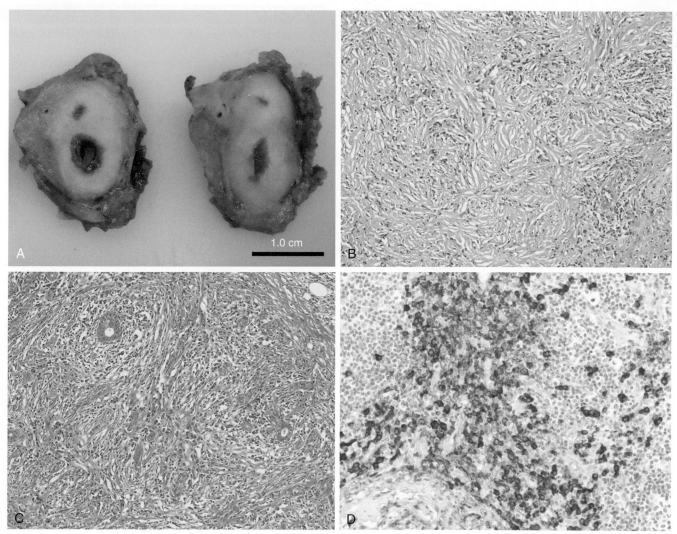

FIG. 5.24 IgG4-related disease: representative lesions. (A) Bile duct showing sclerosing cholangitis. (B) Sclerotic area of the bile duct with storiform fibrosis. (C) Submandibular gland with infiltrates of lymphocytes and plasma cells and whorls of fibrosis. (D) Section of an involved lacrimal gland stained with an antibody against IgG4, showing large numbers of IgG4-producing plasma cells. (From Kamisawa T, Zen Y, Pillai S, et al: IgG4-related disease. *Lancet* 385:1460, 2015.)

molecules of individuals (except, of course, identical twins; 25% of siblings may also inherit the same HLA alleles). Following transplantation, the recipient's T cells recognize donor HLA antigens from the graft (the allogeneic antigens, or alloantigens) by two pathways. The graft antigens are either presented directly to recipient T cells by graft APCs, or the graft antigens are picked up by host APCs, processed (like any other foreign antigen), and presented to host T cells. These are called the direct and indirect pathways of recognition of alloantigens, respectively. Both lead to the activation of CD8+ T cells, which develop into CTLs, and CD4+ T cells, which become cytokine-producing effector cells, mainly Th1 cells. The direct pathway may be most important for CTL-mediated acute rejection, while the indirect pathway may play a greater role in chronic rejection, described later. The production of anti-HLA antibodies is an example of indirect recognition because donor HLA antigens are picked up by host B cells and presented to helper T cells, resulting in production of alloantibodies specific for donor HLA.

The frequency of T cells that can recognize the foreign HLA antigens in a graft is much higher than the frequency of T cells specific for any microbe. For this reason, immune responses to allografts are stronger than responses to pathogens. Predictably, these strong reactions can destroy grafts rapidly, and their control requires powerful immunosuppressive agents.

Mechanisms of Graft Rejection

Graft rejection is classified into hyperacute, acute, or chronic on the basis of clinical and pathologic features. This classification was devised by nephrologists and pathologists based on rejection of kidney allografts and has stood the test of time remarkably well. Each type of rejection is mediated by a particular kind of immune response. In the following discussion, the description of the morphology of rejection is limited to kidney allografts, but similar changes are seen in other solid organ transplants.

- **Hyperacute rejection is mediated by preformed antibodies specific for antigens on graft endothelial cells.** The preformed antibodies may be natural IgM antibodies specific for blood group antigens or may be antibodies specific for allogeneic HLA molecules that were induced by prior exposure through blood transfusions, pregnancy, or organ transplantation. Immediately after the graft is implanted and blood flow is restored, the antibodies bind to antigens on the graft endothelium and activate the complement and clotting systems, leading to endothelial injury, thrombus formation, and ischemic necrosis of the graft (Fig. 5.25A). Hyperacute rejection is now uncommon because all donors and recipients are matched for blood type, and potential recipients are tested for antibodies against the cells of the prospective donor, a test called a *cross-match.*

MORPHOLOGY

In hyperacute rejection, the affected kidney rapidly becomes cyanotic, mottled, and anuric. Virtually all arterioles and arteries exhibit acute fibrinoid necrosis of their walls and narrowing or complete occlusion of their lumens by thrombi (Fig. 5.25B). Neutrophils rapidly accumulate within arterioles, glomeruli, and peritubular capillaries. As these changes intensify and become diffuse, the glomerular capillaries also undergo thrombotic occlusion, and eventually the kidney cortex undergoes necrosis because of infarction. Affected kidneys are nonfunctional and must be removed.

- **Acute rejection is mediated by T cells and antibodies that are activated by alloantigens in the graft.** It occurs within days or weeks after transplantation and is the principal cause of early graft failure. It also may appear suddenly months or even years later, after immunosuppression is tapered or terminated. Based on the role of T cells or antibodies, acute rejection is divided into two types, although in most rejecting grafts, both patterns are present.

  In *acute cellular rejection,* CD8+ CTLs directly destroy graft cells, or CD4+ cells secrete cytokines and induce inflammation, which damages the graft (Fig. 5.26A). T cells may also react against graft vessels, leading to vascular damage. Current immunosuppressive therapy is designed mainly to prevent and reduce acute rejection by blocking the activation of alloreactive T cells.

MORPHOLOGY

Acute cellular (T cell—mediated) rejection may produce two different patterns of injury.

- In the *tubulointerstitial pattern,* there is extensive interstitial inflammation and tubular inflammation (tubulitis) associated with focal tubular injury (Fig. 5.26B). As might be expected, the inflammatory infiltrates contain activated CD4+ and CD8+ T lymphocytes.
- The *vascular pattern* shows inflammation of vessels (Fig. 5.26C) and sometimes necrosis of vessel walls. The affected vessels have swollen endothelial cells, and at places lymphocytes are seen between the endothelium and the vessel wall, a finding termed *endotheliitis* or *intimal arteritis.* The recognition of cellular rejection is important because, in the absence of accompanying humoral rejection, most patients respond well to immunosuppressive therapy.

In acute *antibody-mediated (vascular* or *humoral) rejection,* antibodies bind to vascular endothelium and activate complement via the classical pathway (Fig. 5.27A). The resultant inflammation and endothelial damage cause graft failure.

MORPHOLOGY

Acute antibody-mediated rejection is manifested mainly by damage to glomeruli and small blood vessels. Typically, there is inflammation of glomeruli and peritubular capillaries (Fig. 5.27B) associated with deposition of complement products, which is due to activation of the complement system by the antibody-dependent classical pathway (Fig. 5.27C). Small vessels may also show focal thrombosis.

- **Chronic rejection is an indolent form of graft damage that occurs over months or years, leading to progressive loss of graft function.** Chronic rejection manifests as interstitial *fibrosis* and gradual narrowing of graft blood vessels *(graft arteriosclerosis).* In both lesions, the culprits are believed to be T cells that react against graft alloantigens and secrete cytokines, which stimulate the proliferation and activities of fibroblasts and vascular smooth muscle

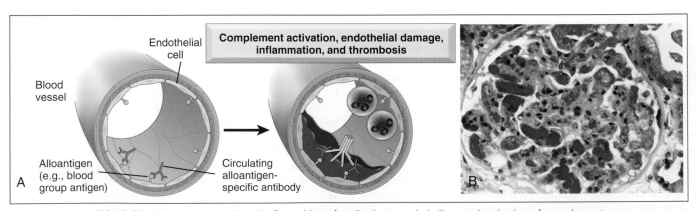

FIG. 5.25 Hyperacute rejection. (A) Deposition of antibody on endothelium and activation of complement causes thrombosis. (B) Hyperacute rejection of a kidney allograft showing platelet fibrin thrombi and ischemic injury in a glomerulus. (Courtesy of Dr. David Howell, Department of Pathology, Duke University School of Medicine, Durham, NC.)

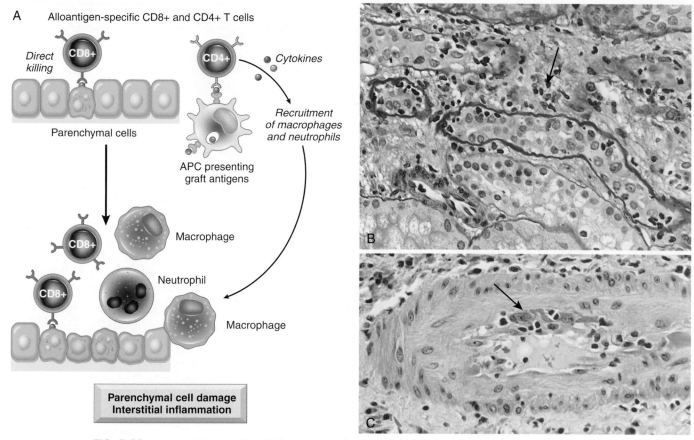

FIG. 5.26 Acute cellular rejection. (A) Destruction of graft cells by T cells. Acute T cell—mediated rejection involves direct killing of graft cells by CD8+ CTLs and inflammation caused by cytokines produced by CD4 T cells. (B) Acute cellular rejection of a kidney graft, manifested by inflammatory cells in the interstitium *(arrow)* and between epithelial cells of the tubules (tubulitis). Collapsed tubules are outlined by wavy basement membranes. (C) Acute vascular rejection in a kidney graft. An arteriole is shown with inflammatory cells attacking and undermining the endothelium (endotheliitis) *(arrow)*. (B, C, Courtesy of Drs. Zoltan Laszik and Kuang-Yu Jen, Department of Pathology, University of California, San Francisco, California.)

cells in the graft (Fig. 5.28A). Alloantibodies also contribute to chronic rejection. Although treatments to prevent or curtail acute rejection have steadily improved, chronic rejection is refractory to most therapies and is becoming the principal cause of graft failure.

MORPHOLOGY

Chronic rejection is dominated by vascular changes, often with intimal thickening and vascular occlusion (Fig. 5.28B). Chronically rejecting kidney grafts show glomerulopathy, with duplication of the basement membrane, likely secondary to chronic endothelial injury (Fig. 5.28C), and peritubular capillaritis with multilayering of peritubular capillary basement membranes. Interstitial fibrosis and tubular atrophy with loss of renal parenchyma may occur secondary to the vascular lesions (Fig. 5.28D). Interstitial mononuclear cell infiltrates are typically sparse.

Methods of Increasing Graft Survival

Because HLA molecules are the major antigens targeted in transplant rejection, HLA matching of the donor and the recipient improves graft survival. HLA matching is more beneficial for living related kidney transplants than for other types of organ transplants, and survival improves with increasing number of loci matched. However, due to improvements in immunosuppressive drugs, HLA matching is no longer done for heart, lung, liver, and islet transplantation; in such instances, the recipient often needs a transplant urgently and other considerations, such as anatomic compatibility (i.e., size), are of greater importance.

Immunosuppression of the recipient is a necessity in all organ transplantation, except in the case of identical twins. At present, combinations of several drugs are used. Cyclosporine and tacrolimus suppress T cell—mediated immunity by inhibiting transcription of cytokine genes, in particular the gene for IL-2, and rapamycin inhibits T-cell proliferative responses to IL-2. Although immunosuppression has made transplantation of many organs feasible, it creates its own problems. Suppression of the immune system results in increased susceptibility to opportunistic fungal, viral, and other infections. Reactivation of latent viruses, such as cytomegalovirus (CMV) and polyomavirus, are frequent complications. Immunosuppressed patients are also at increased risk for developing virus-induced tumors, such as Epstein-Barr virus (EBV)—associated lymphomas and human papillomavirus (HPV)—induced squamous cell carcinomas. Attempts

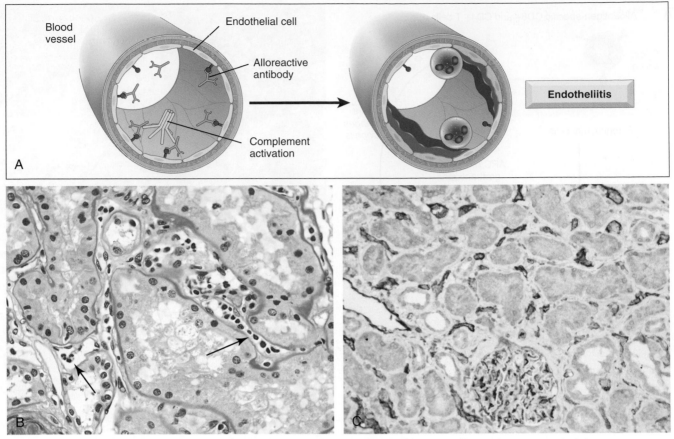

FIG. 5.27 Acute antibody-mediated (humoral) rejection. (A) Graft damage caused by antibody deposition in vessels. (B) Light micrograph showing inflammation (capillaritis) in peritubular capillaries *(arrows)* in a kidney graft. (C) Immunoperoxidase stain shows complement deposition in peritubular capillaries and a glomerulus. (Courtesy of Dr. Zoltan Laszik, Department of Pathology, University of California, San Francisco, California.)

to induce donor-specific tolerance in host T cells, which would reduce reactions to graft antigens but leave intact other immune responses, have not yet succeeded.

Transplantation of Hematopoietic Stem Cells

Use of hematopoietic stem cell (HSC) transplants to treat hematologic malignancies, bone marrow failure syndromes (such as aplastic anemia), and disorders caused by inherited HSC defects (such as sickle cell anemia, thalassemia, and primary immunodeficiencies) is increasing in number each year. Transplantation of hematopoietic stem cells obtained from affected patients and "engineered" to replace defective genes may be useful in treating inherited forms of immunodeficiency. Historically, HSCs were obtained from the bone marrow, but now they are usually harvested from peripheral blood after they are mobilized from the bone marrow by administration of hematopoietic growth factors, or from the umbilical cord blood of newborn infants, a rich source of HSCs. In most of the conditions in which HSC transplantation is indicated, the recipient is irradiated or treated with chemotherapy to destroy the immune system (and, sometimes, cancer cells) and to "open up" niches in the microenvironment of the marrow that nurture HSCs, thus allowing the transplanted HSCs to engraft. These treatments often lead to a period of immune deficiency before the transplanted HSCs can generate a functional immune system. *Graft-versus-host disease* is a major complication of this form of transplantation that distinguishes it from organ transplants.

Graft-Versus-Host Disease

Graft-versus-host disease (GVHD) occurs when immunologically competent cells or their precursors are transplanted into immunologically depleted recipients, and the transferred cells recognize alloantigens in the host and attack host tissues. It is seen most commonly in the setting of HSC transplantation but, rarely, may occur following transplantation of organs rich in lymphoid cells (e.g., the liver or intestine). T cells present in the donor graft perceive the host's tissue as foreign and react against it. This results in the activation of donor CD4+ and CD8+ T cells, ultimately causing inflammation and killing recipient cells. To minimize GVHD, the donor and recipient of HSC transplants are carefully HLA-matched using DNA sequencing.

There are two forms of GVHD:

- *Acute GVHD* (occurring days to weeks after transplantation) is characterized by epithelial cell necrosis in three principal organs: liver, skin, and GI tract. Destruction of small bile ducts gives rise to jaundice, and mucosal ulceration of the gut results in bloody diarrhea. Cutaneous involvement is characterized by lymphocyte infiltration (Fig. 5.29A) and apoptosis of epidermal cells (Fig. 5.29B). It manifests clinically as a rash, usually appearing first on the neck, ears, and palms of the hands and soles of the feet and then becoming generalized.
- *Chronic GVHD* may follow the acute syndrome or may occur insidiously. Patients develop skin lesions with dermal fibrosis (Fig. 5.29C)

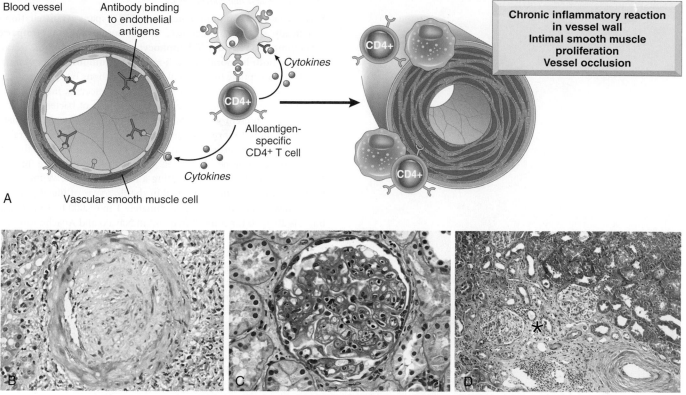

FIG. 5.28 Chronic rejection. (A) Graft arteriosclerosis caused by T-cell cytokines and antibody deposition. (B) Graft arteriosclerosis in a cardiac transplant. (C) Transplant glomerulopathy, the characteristic manifestation of chronic antibody-mediated rejection in the kidney. The glomerulus shows inflammatory cells within the capillary loops (glomerulitis), accumulation of mesangial matrix, and duplication of the capillary basement membrane. (D) Interstitial fibrosis and tubular atrophy, resulting from arteriosclerosis of arteries and arterioles in a chronically rejecting kidney allograft. In this trichrome stain, the blue area *(asterisk)* shows fibrosis, contrasted with the healthy kidney *(top right)*. An artery showing prominent arteriosclerosis is shown *(bottom right)*. (B, Courtesy of Dr. Richard Mitchell, Department of Pathology, Brigham and Women's Hospital, Boston, Massachusetts. C and D, Courtesy of Dr. Zoltan Laszik, Department of Pathology, University of California, San Francisco, California.)

resembling those of systemic sclerosis (discussed earlier) and manifestations mimicking other autoimmune disorders.

Because GVHD is mediated by T lymphocytes in the transplanted donor cells, depletion of donor T cells before transplantation virtually eliminates the disease. This approach, however, is a mixed blessing: GVHD is reduced, but the recurrence of tumor in patients with leukemia, as well as the incidence of graft failures and EBV-related B-cell lymphoma, increase.

IMMUNODEFICIENCY SYNDROMES

Immune deficiencies can be divided into *primary* (or *congenital*) *immunodeficiencies*, which are caused by genetic defects (usually mutations), and *secondary* (or *acquired*) *immunodeficiencies*, which may arise as complications of cancers, infections, or malnutrition, or side effects of immunosuppression, irradiation, or chemotherapy for cancer and other diseases. **Immunodeficiencies are manifested clinically by increased infections, which may be newly acquired or reactivation of latent infections.** The primary immunodeficiency syndromes are accidents of nature that provide valuable insights into some of the

molecules required for the development and function of the immune system. Paradoxically, several immunodeficiencies are also associated with autoimmune disorders, which are the consequences of excessive and aberrant immune responses, perhaps because the deficiency results in loss of regulatory mechanisms or persistence of infections that promote autoimmunity. Here we briefly discuss the more important and best-defined primary immunodeficiencies, to be followed by a more detailed description of acquired immunodeficiency syndrome (AIDS), a devastating example of secondary immunodeficiency.

Primary (Congenital) Immunodeficiencies

Primary immunodeficiency diseases are inherited genetic disorders that impair mechanisms of innate immunity (phagocytes, NK cells, or complement) or the humoral and/or cellular arms of adaptive immunity (mediated by B lymphocytes and T lymphocytes, respectively). These immunodeficiencies are usually detected in infancy, between 6 months and 2 years of age, due to recurrent infections. With advances in genetic analyses, the mutations responsible for many of these diseases are now known (Fig. 5.30). We first discuss the more common defects in the maturation and activation of B lymphocytes and T lymphocytes, followed by disorders of innate immunity.

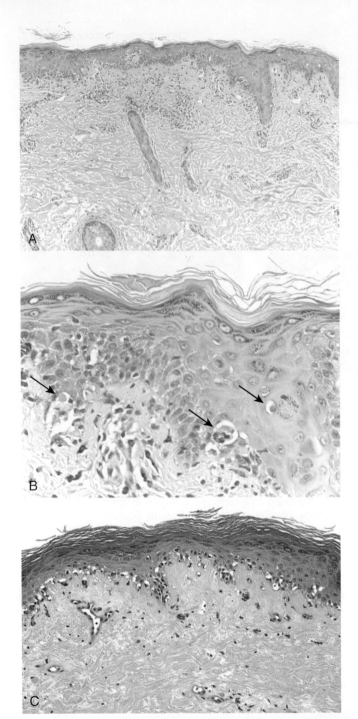

FIG. 5.29 Graft-versus-host disease (GVHD) involving the skin. *Acute GVHD.* Low-power (A) and high-power (B) photomicrographs are shown of a skin biopsy from a patient with acute GVHD. A sparse lymphocytic infiltrate can be seen at the dermoepidermal junction, and damage to the epithelial layer is manifested by spaces at the dermoepidermal junction (vacuolization), cells with abnormal keratin staining (dyskeratosis), apoptotic keratinocytes *(arrows)*, and disorganization of maturation of keratinocytes from the basal layer to the surface. *Chronic GVHD.* (C) Chronic GVHD showing a sparse lymphocytic infiltrate at the dermoepidermal junction, which has resulted in occasional damaged keratinocytes. The epidermis is thinned due to atrophy. The underlying dermis shows thick collagen bundles, indicative of sclerosis. (A and B, Courtesy Dr. Scott Grantor, Department of Pathology, Brigham and Women's Hospital and Harvard Medical School, Boston, Massachusetts. C, Courtesy Dr. Jarish Cohen, Department of Pathology, University of California San Francisco.)

Severe Combined Immunodeficiency

Severe combined immunodeficiency (SCID) spans a constellation of genetically distinct syndromes, all having in common impaired development of mature T lymphocytes and/or B lymphocytes and defects in both humoral and cell-mediated immunity. Children with SCID are susceptible to recurrent, severe infections by a wide range of pathogens, including *Candida albicans, Pneumocystis jirovecii, Pseudomonas,* cytomegalovirus, varicella, and a host of bacteria. Affected infants often present with thrush (oral candidiasis), persistent diaper rash, and failure to thrive. Some affected infants develop a generalized rash shortly after birth because maternal T cells that enter the fetal circulation cannot be eliminated by the baby's defective immune system and attack the fetus, causing a form of GVHD. Without HSC transplantation, death occurs within the first year of life. The overall prevalence of the disease is approximately 1 in 65,000 to 1 in 100,000, but it is 20 to 30 times more frequent in Navajo and Apache American Indian populations.

Despite the common clinical manifestations of different forms of SCID, the underlying genetic defects are quite varied. Often, the defect affects the T-cell compartment; the impairment of humoral immunity in the setting of normal B cells is due to lack of T-cell help. There are two major forms of SCID.

- *X-linked SCID.* **Approximately half of the cases of SCID are X-linked; these are caused by mutations in the gene encoding the common γ (γc) chain shared by the receptors for the cytokines IL-2, IL-4, IL-7, IL-9, and IL-15.** Defective IL-7 signaling is the underlying basis of this disease because this cytokine is responsible for stimulating the survival and expansion of immature T-cell precursors in the thymus.
- *Autosomal recessive SCID.* **Another 40% to 50% of SCID cases follow an autosomal recessive pattern of inheritance, with approximately half of these caused by mutations in adenosine deaminase (ADA), an enzyme involved in purine metabolism.** ADA deficiency results in accumulation of adenosine and deoxyadenosine triphosphate metabolites, which inhibit DNA synthesis and are especially toxic to proliferating lymphocyte progenitors. Other autosomal recessive forms of SCID result from defects in genes encoding the recombinase responsible for the rearrangement of lymphocyte antigen-receptor genes and various other rare mutations affecting lymphocyte maturation.

MORPHOLOGY

The thymus is small and devoid of lymphoid cells. In X-linked SCID, the thymus contains lobules of undifferentiated epithelial cells resembling fetal thymus, whereas in SCID caused by ADA deficiency, remnants of Hassall corpuscles can be found. In both diseases, secondary lymphoid tissues are hypoplastic as well, with marked depletion of T-cell areas and in some cases both T-cell and B-cell zones.

Currently, HSC transplantation is the mainstay of treatment. X-linked SCID is the first disease in which gene therapy has been successful. For gene therapy, a normal γc gene is expressed using a viral vector in HSCs taken from patients, and the cells are then transplanted back into the patients. The clinical experience remains small, but some patients have shown beneficial levels of reconstitution of their immune systems for more than a decade after therapy. However, about 20% of patients who received a first-generation viral vector developed T-cell acute lymphoblastic leukemia (T-ALL) (Chapter 10), highlighting the dangers of this particular approach to

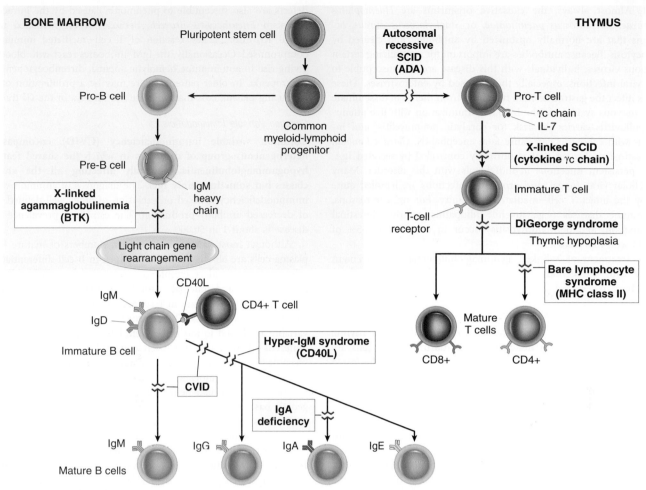

FIG. 5.30 Primary immunodeficiencies. Shown are the principal pathways of lymphocyte development and the blocks in these pathways in selected primary immune deficiency diseases. The affected genes are indicated in parentheses for some of the disorders. *ADA,* Adenosine deaminase; *BTK,* Bruton tyrosine kinase; *CD40L,* CD40 ligand (also known as *CD154*); *CVID,* common variable immunodeficiency; *SCID,* severe combined immunodeficiency.

gene therapy. The neoplastic proliferation in this instance is the result of the virus integrating into the genome close to an oncogene, leading to oncogene activation. Current protocols use new vectors with safety features built in. Patients with ADA deficiency have also been treated with HSC transplantation, and with administration of the enzyme or gene therapy involving the introduction of a normal ADA gene into T-cell precursors.

X-Linked Agammaglobulinemia

X-linked agammaglobulinemia (XLA), or Bruton disease, is characterized by the failure of pre-B cells to differentiate into mature B cells and a resultant absence of antibodies (gamma globulin) in the blood. It is one of the more common forms of primary immunodeficiency, occurring at a frequency of about 1 in 100,000 male infants. During normal B-cell maturation, immunoglobulin (Ig) heavy chain genes are rearranged first in developing B cells called pre-B cells, followed by light chain genes. At each stage, signals are received from the expressed components of the antigen receptor that drive maturation to the next stage; these signals act as quality controls to ensure that the correct receptor proteins are being produced. In XLA, B-cell maturation stops after the initial heavy chain gene rearrangement

because of mutations in a gene encoding a tyrosine kinase called *Bruton tyrosine kinase (BTK)*. BTK is associated with the receptor of pre-B cells, and is involved in signal transduction. When BTK is nonfunctional, the pre-B cell receptor cannot signal the cells to proceed along the maturation pathway. As a result, Ig light chains are not produced, and the complete Ig molecule containing heavy and light chains cannot be assembled and transported to the cell membrane, although free heavy chains can be found in the cytoplasm. Because the *BTK* gene is on the X chromosome, the disorder is only seen in males. Rare cases with similar features have been described in females, possibly due to mutations in other genes that function in the same pathway.

Classically, the disease is characterized by a profound reduction in the number of B cells in the blood and secondary lymphoid organs and an absence of germinal centers and plasma cells in these organs. T-cell numbers and responses may be normal. The disease does not usually become apparent until about 6 months of age, as transplacental transfer of maternal antibodies provides adequate protection for a time. In most cases, recurrent bacterial infections of the respiratory tract, such as acute and chronic pharyngitis, sinusitis, otitis media, bronchitis, and pneumonia, call attention to the underlying immune defect. Almost always, the causative organisms are *Haemophilus influenzae, Streptococcus pneumoniae,* or *Staphylococcus aureus,* organisms that are normally opsonized by antibodies and cleared by phagocytosis. Because antibodies are important for neutralizing certain infectious viruses, individuals with this disease are also susceptible to some viral infections, especially those caused by enteroviruses. These viruses infect the gastrointestinal tract, and from there can disseminate to the nervous system via the blood. Immunization with live attenuated poliovirus carries the risk for paralytic poliomyelitis, and infections with echovirus can cause fatal encephalitis. *Giardia lamblia,* an intestinal protozoan that is normally controlled by secreted IgA, causes persistent infections in individuals with this disorder. Many intracellular viral, fungal, and protozoal infections are handled quite well by the intact T cell–mediated immunity. For unclear reasons, autoimmune diseases (e.g., juvenile idiopathic arthritis, intestinal inflammation, and dermatomyositis) occur in as many as 35% of patients with this disease.

The treatment of X-linked agammaglobulinemia is replacement therapy with intravenous immunoglobulin (IVIG) produced from pooled human serum.

DiGeorge Syndrome (Thymic Hypoplasia)

DiGeorge syndrome is caused by a congenital defect in thymic development resulting in deficient T-cell maturation. T cells are absent in the lymph nodes, spleen, and peripheral blood, and affected infants are extremely vulnerable to viral, fungal, and protozoal infections. Patients are also susceptible to infection with intracellular bacteria due to defective T cell–mediated immunity. B cells and serum immunoglobulins are generally unaffected.

The disorder is a consequence of a malformation affecting the third and fourth pharyngeal pouches, structures that give rise to the thymus, parathyroid glands, and portions of the face and aortic arch. Thus, in addition to the thymic and T-cell defects, there may be parathyroid gland hypoplasia, resulting in hypocalcemic tetany, as well as additional midline developmental abnormalities (velocardiofacial syndrome). In 90% of cases of DiGeorge syndrome, there is a deletion affecting chromosomal region 22q11 (22q11.2 deletion syndrome; Chapter 4). Transplantation of thymic tissue has successfully treated some infants with complete DiGeorge syndrome, but in the majority of patients, immunity tends to improve spontaneously with age and such therapy is not necessary.

Hyper-IgM Syndrome

This disease is characterized by the production of normal (or even supranormal) levels of IgM antibodies and decreased levels of IgG, IgA, and IgE isotypes; the underlying defect is an inability of T cells to activate B cells and macrophages. Many of the functions of CD4+ helper T cells require the engagement of CD40 on B cells, macrophages, and dendritic cells by CD40L (also called CD154) expressed on antigen-activated T cells. This interaction triggers Ig class switching and affinity maturation in B cells and stimulates the microbicidal functions of macrophages. Approximately 70% of individuals with hyper-IgM syndrome have the X-linked form of the disease caused by mutations in the gene encoding CD40L. In the remaining patients, the disease is inherited in an autosomal recessive pattern and is caused by loss-of-function mutations involving genes encoding either CD40 or the enzyme called *activation-induced deaminase (AID),* a DNA-editing enzyme that is required for Ig class switching and affinity maturation.

Patients present with recurrent pyogenic infections due to low levels of opsonizing IgG antibodies. Those with CD40L or CD40

defects are also susceptible to pneumonia caused by the intracellular organism *Pneumocystis jirovecii,* because CD40L-mediated macrophage activation, a key reaction of T cell–mediated immunity, is compromised. Occasionally, the IgM antibodies react with blood cells, giving rise to autoimmune hemolytic anemia, thrombocytopenia, and neutropenia. In older patients, there may be a proliferation of IgM-producing plasma cells that infiltrate the mucosa of the GI tract.

Common Variable Immunodeficiency

Common variable immunodeficiency (CVID) encompasses a heterogeneous group of disorders in which the shared feature is hypogammaglobulinemia, generally affecting all the antibody classes but sometimes only IgG. The diagnosis of common variable immunodeficiency is based on exclusion of other well-defined causes of decreased antibody production. The estimated prevalence of the disease is about 1 in 50,000.

Although most patients have normal numbers of mature B cells, plasma cells are absent, suggesting a block in B-cell differentiation. B cell areas of secondary lymphoid organs (i.e., lymphoid follicles in nodes, spleen, and mucosal tissues) are often hyperplastic, perhaps because B cells proliferate in response to antigens but do not differentiate into plasma cells. The defective antibody production has been variably attributed to intrinsic B-cell defects or deficient T-cell help. Different genetic causes have been identified, including mutations in a receptor for B cell–activating cytokines and in a molecule called ICOS (inducible costimulator), a homolog of CD28 that contributes to the function of T follicular helper cells. However, in >90% of cases, the genetic basis is unknown.

Patients typically present with recurrent sinopulmonary bacterial infections. About 20% have recurrent herpesvirus infections, and serious enterovirus infections causing meningoencephalitis may occur. Individuals with this disorder are also prone to the development of persistent diarrhea caused by *G. lamblia.* In contrast to X-linked agammaglobulinemia, common variable immunodeficiency affects both sexes equally, and the onset of symptoms is later, in childhood or adolescence. As in X-linked agammaglobulinemia, these patients have a high frequency of autoimmune diseases (approximately 20%), including rheumatoid arthritis. The risk for lymphoid malignancy is also increased, and an increase in gastric cancer has been reported.

Isolated IgA Deficiency

This is the most common primary immune deficiency disease; it affects about 1 in 700 individuals of European descent and occurs worldwide. As noted previously, IgA is the major immunoglobulin in mucosal secretions and is thus involved in defending the airways and the gastrointestinal tract. Weakened mucosal defenses due to IgA deficiency predispose patients to recurrent sinopulmonary and intestinal infections, although the majority of patients are asymptomatic. About 2% of patients have celiac disease. The pathogenesis of IgA deficiency seems to involve a block in the terminal differentiation of IgA-secreting B cells to plasma cells; IgM and IgG subclasses of antibodies are present in normal or even supranormal levels. When transfused with blood containing normal IgA, some patients develop an anaphylactic reaction since the host immune system views the transfused IgA as a foreign protein. The molecular basis for this defect is not defined.

Other Defects in Lymphocyte Activation

Many rare cases of lymphocyte activation defects have been described that affect antigen receptor signaling and various biochemical pathways. Defects in Th1 responses are associated with atypical mycobacterial infections, and defective Th17 responses are the cause of chronic mucocutaneous candidiasis as well as bacterial infections of the skin (a disorder called *Job syndrome*).

Immunodeficiencies Associated With Systemic Diseases

In some inherited systemic disorders, immune deficiency is a prominent clinical problem. Two representative examples of such diseases are described next.

- *Wiskott-Aldrich syndrome* is an X-linked disease characterized by thrombocytopenia, eczema, and a marked vulnerability to recurrent infection that results in early death. The thymus is normal early in the disease course, but there is progressive loss of T lymphocytes from the blood and the T-cell zones (paracortical areas) of lymph nodes, with variable defects in cellular immunity. Patients do not make antibodies to polysaccharide antigens, and the response to protein antigens is poor. IgM levels in the serum are low, but levels of IgG are usually normal and, paradoxically, IgA and IgE are often elevated. The syndrome is caused by mutations in an X-linked gene encoding Wiskott-Aldrich syndrome protein (WASP). WASP belongs to a family of signaling proteins that link membrane receptors, such as antigen receptors, to cytoskeletal elements. The WASP protein is involved in cytoskeleton-dependent responses, including cell migration and signal transduction, but how this contributes to the functions of lymphocytes and platelets is unclear. The only treatment is HSC transplantation.

- *Ataxia telangiectasia* is an autosomal recessive disorder characterized by abnormal gait (ataxia), vascular malformations (telangiectasias), neurologic deficits, increased incidence of tumors, and immunodeficiency. The immunologic defects are of variable severity and may affect both B cells and T cells. The most prominent humoral immune abnormalities are defective production of isotype-switched antibodies, mainly IgA and IgG2. The T-cell defects are usually less pronounced and may be associated with thymic hypoplasia. Patients experience upper and lower respiratory tract bacterial infections, multiple autoimmune phenomena, and increasingly frequent cancers, particularly lymphoid tumors, with advancing age. The gene responsible for this disorder encodes a protein called ATM (ataxia telangiectasia mutated), a sensor of DNA damage that activates cell cycle checkpoints and apoptosis in cells with damaged DNA. Lack of ATM also leads to abnormalities in Ig and TCR gene recombination (and therefore defects in the generation of antigen receptors) and abnormal immunoglobulin class switching, processes that require regulated breakage and rejoining of antigen receptor genes.

Defects in Innate Immunity

Inherited defects in the early innate immune response typically affect leukocyte functions or the complement system and lead to increased vulnerability to infections (Table 5.10).

Defects in Leukocyte Function

- *Leukocyte adhesion deficiencies (LADs)* stem from inherited defects in adhesion molecules that impair leukocyte recruitment to sites of infection, resulting in recurrent bacterial infections. LAD1 is caused by defects in the β_2 chain that is shared by the integrins LFA-1 and Mac-1, while LAD2 is caused by a defect in a fucosyl transferase that is required to synthesize functional sialyl-Lewis X, the ligand for E- and P-selectins (Chapter 2).

Table 5.10 Inherited Immune Deficiencies of Phagocytic Leukocytes and the Complement System

Disease	Defect
Defects in Leukocyte Function	
Leukocyte adhesion deficiency 1	Defective leukocyte adhesion because of mutations in the β chain of CD11/CD18 integrins
Leukocyte adhesion deficiency 2	Defective leukocyte adhesion because of mutations in fucosyl transferase required for synthesis of sialylated oligosaccharide (receptor for selectins)
Chédiak-Higashi syndrome	Decreased leukocyte functions because of mutations affecting protein involved in lysosomal membrane traffic
Chronic granulomatous disease	Decreased oxidative burst
X-linked	Phagocyte oxidase (membrane component)
Autosomal recessive	Phagocyte oxidase (cytoplasmic components)
Myeloperoxidase deficiency	Decreased microbial killing because of defective MPO-H_2O_2 system
Defects in the Complement System	
C2, C4 deficiency	Defective classical pathway activation; results in reduced resistance to infection and reduced clearance of immune complexes
C3 deficiency	Defects in all complement functions
Deficiency of complement regulatory proteins	Excessive complement activation; clinical syndromes include angioedema, paroxysmal hemoglobinuria, and others

Modified in part from Gallin JI: Disorders of phagocytic cells. In Gallin JI, et al, editors: *Inflammation: Basic Principles and Clinical Correlates*, ed 2, New York, 1992, Raven Press, pp 860—861.

- *Chronic granulomatous disease* results from inherited defects in the genes encoding components of phagocyte oxidase, the phagolysosomal enzyme that generates ROS such as superoxide, resulting in defective bacterial killing and susceptibility to recurrent bacterial infection. The name of this disease comes from the macrophage-rich chronic inflammatory reaction that appears at sites of infection when the initial neutrophil response is inadequate. These collections of activated macrophages form granulomas in an effort to wall off the microbes. There are two variants, X-linked and autosomal recessive, in which distinct proteins are affected (see Table 5.10).

- *Chédiak-Higashi syndrome* is characterized by defective fusion of lysosomes, resulting in poor phagocyte clearance of microbes and increased susceptibility to infections. The main leukocyte abnormalities are neutropenia, impaired degranulation, and delayed microbial killing. The affected leukocytes contain giant granules, which are readily seen in peripheral blood smears and are thought to result from aberrant phagolysosome fusion. In addition, there are abnormalities in melanocytes (leading to albinism), cells of the nervous system (associated with nerve defects), and platelets (causing bleeding disorders). They have a high risk of developing hemophagocytic lymphohistiocytosis (Chapter 10). The gene associated with this disorder encodes a large cytosolic protein called LYST, which is believed to regulate lysosomal trafficking.

- *TLR defects* are rare but informative. Defects in TLR3, a receptor for viral RNA, result in recurrent herpes simplex encephalitis, and defects in MyD88, an adaptor protein needed for signaling downstream of multiple TLRs, are associated with destructive bacterial pneumonias.
- *Cytokine defects* may be caused by mutations in genes encoding cytokines or by autoantibodies produced against cytokines. Defects affecting the antiviral cytokines type I interferons are associated with viral infections, including severe forms of COVID-19. Mutations affecting the receptor for IL-12, a Th1-inducing cytokine, or for IFN-γ, the effector cytokine of Th1 cells, result in increased susceptibility to infections with intracellular bacteria such as environmental mycobacteria, which are of low virulence and do not cause disease in healthy individuals. The disorder is called *Mendelian susceptibility to mycobacterial disease.*

Deficiencies Affecting the Complement System

Inherited deficiencies of several complement proteins give rise to immune deficiencies or other diseases.

- Deficiency of several *complement components* have been described, with C2 deficiency being the most common. Deficiencies of C2 or C4, early components of the classical pathway, are associated with increased bacterial or viral infections; however, many patients are asymptomatic, presumably because the alternative complement pathway is able to control most infections. Surprisingly, in some patients with C2, C4, or C1q deficiency, the dominant manifestation is an SLE-like autoimmune disease, possibly because these classical complement pathway proteins are involved in clearance of immune complexes. C3 deficiency is rare. It is associated with severe pyogenic infections as well as immune complex—mediated glomerulonephritis (presumably the result of antibodies eliciting inflammation by engaging Fc receptors since complement activation is defective). *Neisseria* bacteria (gonococci and meningococci) are typically cleared by the membrane attack complex (C5 to C9) since their thin cell walls are especially susceptible to the lytic actions of complement; when there is a deficiency of these late components, patients have an increased susceptibility to recurrent infections by these organisms.
- Defects in *complement regulatory proteins* result in excessive inflammation or cell injury. A deficiency of C1 inhibitor (C1 INH) gives rise to an autosomal dominant disorder called *hereditary angioedema*. C1 INH is an inhibitor of many proteases, including kallikrein and coagulation factor XII, which are involved in the production of vasoactive peptides such as bradykinin. Therefore, defective C1 INH activity leads to overproduction of bradykinin, which is a potent vasodilator. Affected patients have episodes of edema affecting skin and mucosal surfaces such as the larynx and the gastrointestinal tract. Deficiencies of other complement regulatory proteins are the cause of *paroxysmal nocturnal hemoglobinuria* (Chapter 10) and some cases of *hemolytic uremic syndrome* (Chapter 12).

Secondary (Acquired) Immunodeficiencies

Secondary (acquired) immune deficiencies may be encountered in individuals with cancer, particularly those that replace normal bone marrow (e.g., leukemia), diabetes and other metabolic diseases, or malnutrition, and in patients receiving chemotherapy or radiation therapy for cancer or immunosuppressive drugs to prevent graft rejection or to treat autoimmune diseases (Table 5.11). As a group, the secondary immune deficiencies are more common than the primary disorders of genetic origin. Discussed next is perhaps the most important secondary immune deficiency disease, AIDS, which remains one of the great scourges of humankind.

ACQUIRED IMMUNODEFICIENCY SYNDROME

Acquired immunodeficiency syndrome (AIDS) is caused by the retrovirus human immunodeficiency virus (HIV) and is characterized by profound immunosuppression that leads to opportunistic infections, secondary neoplasms, and neurologic manifestations. Although AIDS was first recognized as a distinct entity only in the 1980s, more than 34 million deaths are attributable to it, with almost 1 million deaths annually. Of the estimated 38 million HIV-infected individuals worldwide, about 70% are in Africa and 20% in Asia. Effective antiretroviral drugs and preexposure prophylaxis have been developed, but the infection continues to spread in parts of the world where these therapies are not widely available. As the population of people living with HIV increases, care must be taken to prevent the spread of infection. Neither a cure nor a vaccine has been developed to date.

The enormous medical and social burden of AIDS has led to an explosion of research aimed at understanding this modern plague and its ability to disable host defenses. The literature on HIV and AIDS is vast. Here we summarize the currently available data on the epidemiology, pathogenesis, and clinical features of HIV infection.

Epidemiology

Transmission of HIV occurs under conditions that facilitate exchange of blood or body fluids containing the virus or virus-infected cells. It is acquired by introduction into mucosal tissues or by injection. HIV does not have animal reservoirs and cannot persist in aerosols, so infection does not occur by inhalation, ingestion, or contact with the skin. The main routes of transmission are the following.

- *Sexual transmission* is the most common route of infection. In the United States, this is seen mostly in men who have sex with men (about 70% of new infections), but also among heterosexuals (about 20%). In Africa and Asia, heterosexual transmission is

Table 5.11 Causes of Secondary (Acquired) Immunodeficiencies

Cause	Mechanism
Human immunodeficiency virus infection	Depletion of CD4+ helper T cells
Involvement of bone marrow by cancers (e.g., leukemias)	Reduced leukocyte development due to loss of normal leukocyte progenitors
Immunosuppression for graft rejection, autoimmune diseases	Impaired responses of mature lymphocytes and other immune cells
Irradiation and chemotherapy treatments for cancer	Decreased bone marrow precursors for all leukocytes
Severe acute malnutrition	Metabolic derangements inhibit lymphocyte maturation and function
Removal of spleen	Decreased phagocytosis of microbes

dominant, and because of the high rates of infection in these areas, it accounts for >80% of new infections worldwide. High viral load in the source, the type of sexual activity, and other concurrent sexually transmitted infections are risk factors for this form of transmission.

- *Parenteral transmission* in the United States occurs primarily in *intravenous substance users* due to sharing of contaminated needles and syringes. This is responsible for 6% of new cases in the United States. Transmission by transfusion of blood and blood products has largely been eliminated by current screening protocols.
- *Mother-to-infant transmission* is the major cause of pediatric AIDS, accounting for 2% of all cases. This occurs most often during delivery through the birth canal but can also occur from infected milk. Antiviral therapy given to pregnant women who are infected has greatly reduced this mode of transmission. Delivery via cesarean section, prior to onset of labor and rupture of placental membranes, also reduces the risk of transmission.
- In approximately 5% of cases, risk factors cannot be determined.

Properties of HIV

HIV is a nontransforming human retrovirus belonging to the lentivirus family. There are two related but genetically different forms of HIV, HIV-1 and HIV-2. HIV-1 is the type most commonly associated with AIDS in the United States, Europe, and Central Africa, whereas HIV-2 causes a similar disease principally in West Africa and India. The ensuing discussion relates primarily to HIV-1 but is generally applicable to HIV-2 as well.

Structure of HIV

Similar to most retroviruses, the HIV-1 virion is spherical and contains an electron-dense, cone-shaped core surrounded by a lipid envelope derived from the host cell membrane (Fig. 5.31). The virus core contains (1) the major capsid protein p24; (2) nucleocapsid protein p7/p9; (3) two copies of viral RNA; and (4) three viral enzymes (protease, reverse transcriptase, and integrase). p24 is the most abundant viral antigen and is detected by the assay widely used to diagnose HIV infection. The viral core is surrounded by a matrix protein called p17, which lies underneath the virion envelope. Studding the viral envelope are two viral glycoproteins, gp120 and gp41, which are critical for HIV infection of cells.

The HIV-1 RNA genome contains the *gag, pol,* and *env* genes, which are typical of retroviruses. The *gag* gene encodes nucleocapsid proteins; the *pol* gene encodes reverse transcriptase, integrase, and protease, enzymes that are essential for the viral life cycle; and the *env* gene encodes p160, which is cleaved to produce gp120 and gp41. HIV contains several other genes, including *tat, rev, vif, nef, vpr,* and *vpu,* which regulate the synthesis and assembly of infectious viral particles and the pathogenicity of the virus. The envelope proteins, especially gp120, show great variability among viral isolates due to a high frequency of *env* gene mutation, making it difficult to produce gp120 vaccines.

Pathogenesis of HIV Infection and AIDS

Profound immune deficiency, primarily affecting cell-mediated immunity, is the hallmark of AIDS. This results chiefly from infection and subsequent loss of CD4+ T cells. We first describe the mechanisms involved in viral entry into T cells and macrophages and the replicative cycle of the virus within cells.

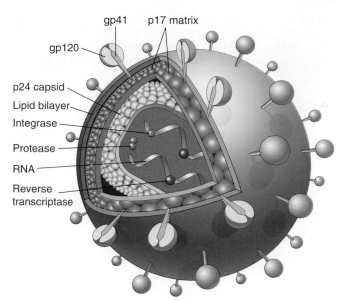

FIG. 5.31 The structure of the human immunodeficiency virus-1 virion. The viral particle is covered by a lipid bilayer derived from the host cell and studded with viral glycoproteins gp41 and gp120.

Life Cycle of HIV

The life cycle of HIV consists of infection of cells, integration of the provirus into the host cell genome, viral replication, and production and release of infectious virus (Fig. 5.32).

Infection of Cells by HIV. **HIV infects cells by using the CD4 molecule as a receptor and various chemokine receptors as coreceptors.** Binding of HIV gp120 to CD4 is essential for infection and accounts for the tropism of the virus for CD4+ T cells. However, binding to CD4 is not sufficient for infection, as HIV gp120 must also bind to other cell surface molecules (coreceptors) for entry into the cell. Chemokine receptors, particularly CCR5 and CXCR4, serve this role. HIV isolates can be distinguished by their use of these coreceptors: R5 strains use CCR5, X4 strains use CXCR4, and some strains (R5X4) can use either. R5 strains preferentially infect cells of the monocyte/macrophage lineage and are thus referred to as *M-tropic,* whereas X4 strains are *T-tropic,* preferentially infecting T cells, but these distinctions are not absolute. The infection is spread mainly by T-tropic strains. Polymorphisms in the gene encoding CCR5 are associated with altered susceptibility to HIV infection. About 1% of Americans of European descent inherit two mutated copies of the *CCR5* gene and are resistant to R5 HIV isolates. About 20% of individuals are heterozygous for this protective *CCR5* allele; these individuals are not protected from AIDS, but the onset of their disease after infection is delayed. Only rare homozygotes for the mutation have been found in African and East Asian populations.

Molecular details of the interaction between HIV glycoproteins and their cell surface receptors have been elucidated. The initial step in infection is the binding of the gp120 envelope glycoprotein to CD4 molecules, which leads to a conformational change that creates a new recognition site on gp120 for the coreceptors CCR5 or CXCR4. Binding to the coreceptors induces conformational changes in gp41 that exposes a hydrophobic region at the tip of gp41 called the fusion peptide. This peptide inserts into the cell membrane of the target cells,

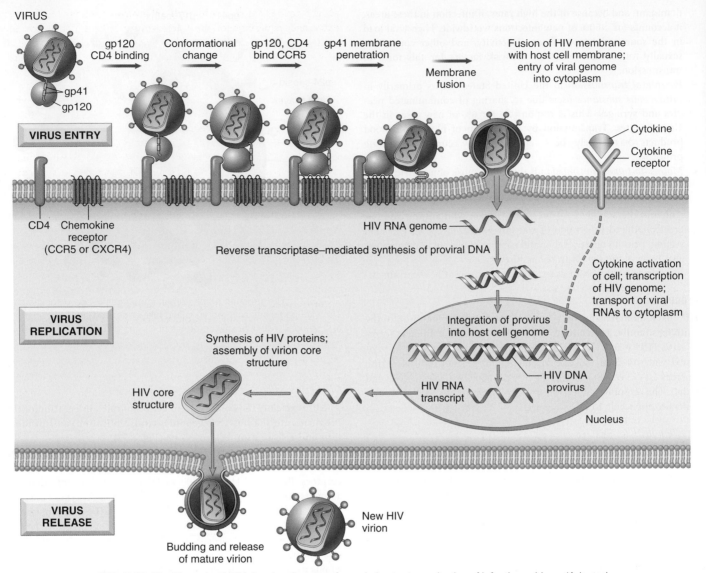

FIG. 5.32 The life cycle of HIV showing the steps from viral entry to production of infectious virions. (Adapted from Wain-Hobson S: HIV. One on one meets two. *Nature* 384:117, 1996.)

leading to fusion of the virus with the host cell. After fusion, the virus core containing the HIV genome enters the cytoplasm of the cell.

Viral Replication. Once internalized, the RNA genome of the virus undergoes reverse transcription, leading to the synthesis of double-stranded DNA, called proviral DNA. In quiescent (unactivated, nondividing) T cells, the proviral DNA may remain in the cytoplasm in a linear episomal form. In activated, proliferating T cells, the DNA circularizes, enters the nucleus, and is then integrated into the host genome. After integration, the provirus may be silent for months or years, a form of *latent infection.* Alternatively, proviral DNA may be transcribed, leading to the expression of viral proteins that are required for the formation of complete viral particles. HIV infects memory cells and activated T cells but is inefficient at productively infecting naïve (resting) T cells.

Completion of the viral life cycle in latently infected cells occurs only after cell activation, and in the case of most CD4+ T cells, virus activation results in death of the infected cells. Activation of T cells by antigens or cytokines upregulates several transcription factors, including NF-κB, which moves from the cytosol into the nucleus. In the nucleus, NF-κB binds to regulatory sequences within several genes, including genes for cytokines and other immune mediators, promoting their transcription. The long-terminal-repeat sequences that flank the HIV genome also contain NF-κB–binding sites, so binding of the transcription factor activates viral gene expression. When a latently infected CD4+ cell encounters an environmental antigen, induction of the transcription factor NF-κB in such a cell (a physiologic response) activates the transcription of HIV proviral DNA (a pathologic outcome) and leads ultimately to the production of virions and to cell death. Furthermore, TNF and other cytokines produced by activated macrophages also stimulate NF-κB activity and thus lead to production of HIV RNA. Thus, it seems that HIV thrives when the host T cells and macrophages are physiologically activated, a situation that can be described as "subversion from within." Such activation in vivo may result from antigenic stimulation by HIV itself or by other infecting microorganisms. Individuals who are HIV positive are at increased risk for recurrent infections, which leads to increased lymphocyte activation and production of proinflammatory cytokines. These, in turn, stimulate more HIV production, loss of additional CD4+ T cells, and more infections. Thus, HIV infection sets up a vicious cycle that culminates in inexorable destruction of the immune system.

Mechanism of T-Cell Depletion in HIV Infection

Loss of CD4+ T cells is mainly caused by the direct cytopathic effects of the replicating virus. In individuals who are infected, approximately 100 billion new viral particles are produced and 1 to 2 billion CD4+ T cells die each day. Death of these cells is a major cause of the relentless, and eventually profound, T cell immunodeficiency. Up to a point, the immune system can replace the dying T cells, but as the disease progresses, renewal of CD4+ T cells cannot keep up with their loss. Possible mechanisms by which the virus directly kills infected cells include increased plasma membrane permeability associated with budding of virus particles and defects in protein synthesis stemming from interference by viral proteins involved in viral replication.

In addition to direct killing of cells by the virus, other mechanisms may contribute to the loss or functional impairment of T cells. These include:

- Chronic activation of uninfected cells responding to HIV itself or to infections that are common in individuals with AIDS, leading to apoptosis of these cells
- HIV infection of cells in lymphoid organs (i.e., spleen, lymph nodes, and tonsils), altering the architecture and cellular composition of lymphoid tissues
- Fusion of infected and uninfected cells, leading to formation of syncytia (giant cells). In tissue culture the gp120 expressed on productively infected cells binds to CD4 molecules on uninfected T cells, followed by cell fusion. Fused cells usually die within a few hours.
- Qualitative defects in T-cell function. Even in asymptomatic individuals with HIV, defects have been reported, including a reduction in antigen-induced T-cell proliferation, a decrease in Th1-type responses relative to the Th2 type, defects in intracellular signaling, and many more. The loss of Th1 responses results in deficient cell-mediated immunity. Because HIV infection often starts in mucosal tissues (the site of viral entry) and these tissues contain a large number of memory lymphocytes, there is also a selective loss of the memory subset of CD4+ helper T cells early in the course of the disease, which explains poor recall responses to previously encountered antigens.

Low-level chronic or latent infection of T cells is an important feature of HIV infection. Integrated provirus, without viral gene expression (latent infection), can persist in cells for months or years. Even with potent antiviral therapy, latent virus lurks within CD4+ T cells and macrophages in lymph nodes. According to some estimates, 0.05% of CD4+ T cells in the lymph nodes are latently infected. Because most of these infected T cells are memory cells, they are long lived, with a life span of months to years, and thus provide a persistent reservoir of virus.

HIV Infection of Non—T Immune Cells

In addition to infection and loss of CD4+ T cells, infection of macrophages and DCs is also important in the pathogenesis of HIV infection.

Macrophages. In certain tissues, such as the lungs and brain, as many as 10% to 50% of macrophages are infected, mainly by phagocytosis of the virus. Although cell division is required for nuclear entry and replication of most retroviruses, HIV-1 can infect and multiply in terminally differentiated nondividing macrophages, which may contain large numbers of virus particles. Even though macrophages allow viral replication, they are more resistant to the cytopathic effects of HIV than are CD4+ T cells. Thus, macrophages may be reservoirs of infection, and in late stages of HIV infection, when CD4+ T-cell numbers decline greatly, macrophages may be an important site of continued viral replication.

Dendritic Cells. Mucosal DCs may internalize the virus and transport it to regional lymph nodes, where the virus is transmitted to CD4+ T cells. Follicular dendritic cells (FDCs) in the germinal centers of lymph nodes bind antibody-coated virus particles and are also potential reservoirs of HIV. Although some FDCs may be susceptible to HIV infection, most of the virus is found on the surface of their dendritic processes.

B Cell Function in HIV Infection. Although B cells cannot be infected by HIV, they may show profound abnormalities. Paradoxically, there is spontaneous B-cell activation and hypergammaglobulinemia in association with an inability to mount antibody responses to newly encountered antigens. The defective antibody responses may be due to lack of T-cell help as well as acquired defects in B cells.

Pathogenesis of Central Nervous System Involvement

The central nervous system is a target of HIV infection. It is believed that HIV is carried into the brain by infected monocytes. In keeping with this, HIV isolates from the brain are almost exclusively M-tropic. Because neurons are not infected and the neuropathologic changes are often less than might be expected from the severity of neurologic symptoms, most experts believe that the neurologic deficit is caused indirectly by viral products and by soluble factors produced by infected macrophages, such as cytokines.

Natural History and Course of HIV Infection

HIV disease begins with acute infection, which is only partly controlled by the host immune response, and advances to chronic progressive infection of peripheral lymphoid tissues (Figs. 5.33 and 5.34).

- *Acute phase.* **HIV typically enters through mucosal surfaces, and acute (early) infection is characterized by infection of memory CD4+ T cells (which express CCR5) in mucosal lymphoid tissues, followed by the death of many of these infected cells.** At this stage, few infected cells are detectable in the blood and other tissues.

  Mucosal infection is followed by dissemination of the virus and the development of host immune responses. DCs in epithelia at sites of virus entry capture the virus and then migrate into the lymph nodes. Once in lymphoid tissues, DCs pass HIV on to CD4+ T cells through direct cell—cell contact. Within days after the first exposure to HIV, viral replication can be detected in lymph nodes. This replication leads to viremia, during which high numbers of HIV particles are present in the patient's blood. The virus disseminates throughout the body and infects helper T cells, macrophages, and DCs in peripheral lymphoid tissues.

  Within 3 to 6 weeks of initial infection, 40% to 90% of individuals develop an *acute HIV syndrome,* which is triggered by the initial spread of the virus and the host response. This phase is associated with a self-limited acute illness with nonspecific symptoms, including sore throat, myalgias, fever, weight loss, and

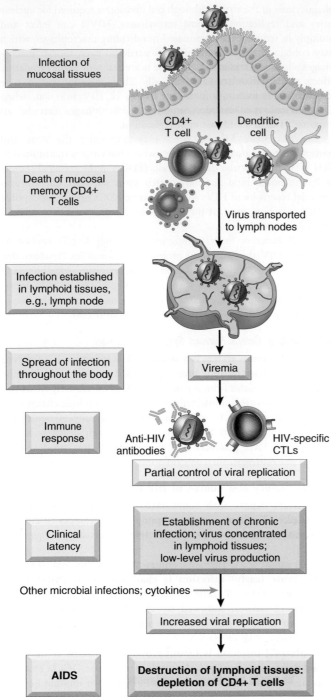

FIG. 5.33 Pathogenesis of HIV-1 infection. The initial infection starts in mucosal tissues, involving mainly memory CD4+ T cells and dendritic cells, and spreads to lymph nodes. Viral replication leads to viremia and widespread seeding of lymphoid tissue. The viremia is controlled by the host immune response, and the patient then enters a phase of clinical latency. During this phase, viral replication in both T cells and macrophages continues unabated, but there is some immune containment of virus (not shown). A gradual erosion of CD4+ cells continues, and, ultimately, CD4+ T-cell numbers decline and the patient develops clinical symptoms of full-blown AIDS. *CTL*, Cytotoxic T lymphocyte.

As the infection spreads, the individual mounts antiviral humoral and cell-mediated immune responses. These responses are evidenced by seroconversion (usually within 3 to 7 weeks of presumed exposure) and by the appearance of virus-specific CD8+ cytotoxic T cells. HIV-specific CD8+ T cells are detected in the blood at about the time viral titers begin to fall and are most likely responsible for the initial containment of HIV infection. These immune responses partially control the infection and viral production, resulting in a drop in viremia to low but detectable levels by about 12 weeks after the initial exposure.

- *Chronic phase.* **In the next, chronic phase of the disease, lymph nodes and the spleen are sites of continuous HIV replication and cell destruction.** During this period of the disease, few or no clinical manifestations of the HIV infection are present; therefore, this phase of disease is called the *clinical latency period.* Although few peripheral blood T cells harbor the virus, destruction of CD4+ T cells within lymphoid tissues continues during this phase, and the number of circulating blood CD4+ T cells steadily declines.

- *AIDS.* **The final phase is progression to AIDS, characterized by a breakdown of host defense, a dramatic increase in viremia, and severe, life-threatening clinical disease.** Typically, the patient presents with long-lasting fever (>1 month), fatigue, weight loss, and diarrhea. After a variable period, opportunistic infections, secondary neoplasms, or neurologic disease (grouped under the rubric *AIDS indicator diseases* or *AIDS-defining illnesses,* discussed later) emerge, and the patient is said to have developed AIDS.

The extent of viremia, measured as HIV-1 RNA levels in the blood, is a useful marker of HIV disease progression and is of value in the management of patients with HIV. The viral load at the end of the acute phase reflects the equilibrium reached between the virus and the host response, and in a given patient it may remain fairly stable for several years. This level of steady-state viremia, called the *viral set point,* is a predictor of the rate of decline of CD4+ T cells and, therefore, progression of HIV disease. Because the loss of immune containment is associated with declining CD4+ T-cell counts, the Centers for Disease Control and Prevention (CDC) classification of HIV infection stratifies patients into three groups based on CD4+ cell counts: 500 cells/μL or greater, 200 to 499 cells/μL, and fewer than 200 cells/μL.

In the absence of treatment, most patients with HIV infection progress to AIDS after a chronic phase lasting from 7 to 10 years, but there are exceptions. In *rapid progressors,* the middle, chronic phase is telescoped to 2 to 3 years after primary infection. About 5% to 15% of infected individuals are *long-term nonprogressors,* defined as untreated individuals with HIV who remain asymptomatic for 10 years or more, with stable CD4+ T-cell counts and low levels of viremia (usually <500 viral RNA copies/mL). Remarkably, about 1% of infected individuals have undetectable plasma virus (<50 to 75 RNA copies/mL); these have been called *elite controllers.* Individuals with such an uncommon clinical course have attracted great attention in the hope that studying them may shed light on host and viral factors that influence disease progression. Studies thus far indicate that this group is heterogeneous with respect to the variables that influence the course of the disease. In most cases, the viral isolates do not show qualitative abnormalities, suggesting that the uneventful course cannot be attributed to a "weak" virus. In all cases, there is evidence of a vigorous anti-HIV immune response, but the immune correlates of protection are still unknown. Some of these individuals have high levels of HIV-specific CD4+ and CD8+ T-cell responses, and these

fatigue, resembling a flulike syndrome. Rash, lymphadenopathy, diarrhea, and vomiting may also occur. This syndrome typically resolves spontaneously in 2 to 4 weeks.

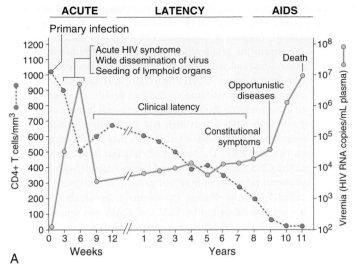

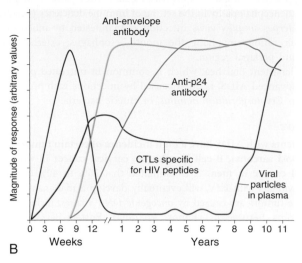

FIG. 5.34 Clinical course of HIV infection. (A) During the early period after primary infection, there is dissemination of virus, development of an immune response to HIV, and often an acute viral syndrome. During the period of clinical latency, viral replication continues and the CD4+ T-cell count gradually decreases, until it reaches a critical level below which there is a substantial risk for AIDS-associated diseases. (B) Immune response to HIV infection. A cytotoxic T-lymphocyte (CTL) response to HIV is detectable by 2 to 3 weeks after the initial infection, and it peaks by 9 to 12 weeks. Marked expansion of virus-specific CD8+ T-cell clones occurs during this time, and up to 10% of a patient's CTLs may be HIV specific at 12 weeks. The humoral immune response to HIV peaks at about 12 weeks. (A, Redrawn from Fauci AS, Lane HC: Human immunodeficiency virus disease: AIDS and related conditions. In Fauci AS, et al, editors: *Harrison's Principles of Internal Medicine*, ed 14, New York, 1997, McGraw-Hill, p 1791.)

levels are maintained over the course of infection. The inheritance of particular *HLA* alleles seems to correlate with resistance to disease progression, perhaps reflecting the ability to mount antiviral T-cell responses.

Clinical Features of AIDS

In the United States, the typical untreated adult patient with AIDS presents with fever, weight loss, diarrhea, generalized lymphadenopathy, multiple opportunistic infections, neurologic disease, and, in many cases, secondary neoplasms. Patients frequently develop anemia, neutropenia, and thrombocytopenia, perhaps because HIV infects hematopoietic progenitor cells. As we will discuss later, the morbidity and mortality associated with the infection have been markedly reduced by the use of highly active antiretroviral therapy (HAART), which relies on a combination of three or four drugs that block different steps of the HIV life cycle.

Opportunistic Infections

Opportunistic infections account for the majority of deaths in untreated patients with AIDS. Many of these infections represent reactivation of latent infections, which are normally kept in check by a robust immune system but are not completely eradicated because the infectious agents have evolved to coexist with their hosts.

- Approximately 15% to 30% of individuals with untreated HIV develop *pneumonia* caused by the fungus *Pneumocystis jirovecii* at some time during the course of the disease. Before the advent of HAART, this infection was the presenting feature in about 20% of cases, but the incidence is much less in patients who respond to HAART.
- *Candidiasis* is the most common fungal infection in patients with AIDS, and infection of the oral cavity, vagina, and esophagus are

its most frequent clinical manifestations. In individuals who are infected with HIV, oral candidiasis is a sign of immunologic decompensation and often heralds the transition to AIDS. Invasive candidiasis is infrequent in patients with AIDS; it usually occurs when there is drug-induced neutropenia or use of indwelling catheters.

- *Cytomegalovirus* (CMV) may cause disseminated disease but more commonly affects the eye and gastrointestinal tract. Chorioretinitis used to be common but has decreased dramatically after the initiation of HAART. CMV retinitis occurs almost exclusively in patients with CD4+ T-cell counts less than 50 per microliter. Gastrointestinal CMV infection, seen in 5% to 10% of cases, manifests as esophagitis and colitis, the latter associated with multiple mucosal ulcerations.
- Disseminated infection with *Mycobacterium tuberculosis* and *nontuberculous,* or *atypical, mycobacteria* (mainly *Mycobacterium avium complex*) also occur late, in the setting of severe immunosuppression. Coincident with the AIDS epidemic, the incidence of tuberculosis has risen dramatically. Worldwide, almost one-third of all deaths in patients with AIDS are attributable to tuberculosis, but this complication remains uncommon in the United States. Both reactivation of latent pulmonary disease and new primary infection contribute to this toll. As with tuberculosis in other settings, the infection may be confined to the lungs or may involve multiple organs. Most worrisome are reports indicating that a growing number of isolates are resistant to multiple antimycobacterial drugs.
- *Cryptococcosis* occurs in about 10% of patients with AIDS, its major clinical manifestation being meningitis.
- *Toxoplasma gondii,* another frequent invader of the CNS in AIDS, causes encephalitis.

- *JC virus,* a human papovavirus, causes progressive multifocal leukoencephalopathy in the setting of immune deficiency (Chapter 21).
- *Herpes simplex virus* infection is manifested by mucocutaneous ulcerations involving the mouth, esophagus, external genitalia, and perianal region.
- Persistent diarrhea, which is common in untreated patients with advanced AIDS, is often caused by infections with protozoa, such as *Cryptosporidium hominis,* or enteric bacteria.

Tumors

Patients with AIDS have a high incidence of certain tumors, notably Kaposi sarcoma, B-cell lymphoma, cervical cancer in women, and anal cancer in men. It is estimated that 25% to 40% of untreated individuals with HIV will eventually develop a malignancy. Many of these tumors are caused by *oncogenic DNA viruses,* including Kaposi sarcoma herpesvirus (Kaposi sarcoma), Epstein-Barr virus (B-cell lymphoma), and human papillomavirus (cervical and anal carcinoma). These viruses establish latent infections that are kept in check in healthy individuals by a competent immune system. The increased risk for malignancy in patients with AIDS exists mainly because of failure to contain the infection following reactivation of the viruses and decreased cellular immunity against virally infected cells undergoing malignant transformation. Individuals infected with HIV are also more susceptible to tumors that occur in the general population, such as lung and skin cancers and certain forms of lymphoma. The incidence of many of these tumors, especially Kaposi sarcoma, has decreased as treatment has improved and patients have less immune compromise.

Kaposi Sarcoma. Kaposi sarcoma (KS), a vascular tumor that is otherwise rare in the United States, is considered an AIDS-defining malignancy. The pathogenesis and morphology of KS and its occurrence in patients not infected with HIV are discussed in Chapter 8. At the onset of the AIDS epidemic, up to 30% of infected men who had sex with men had KS, but with use of antiviral therapy there has been a dramatic decline in its incidence. In contrast, in areas of sub-Saharan Africa where HIV infection is both frequent and often untreated, Kaposi sarcoma is one of the most common tumors.

The lesions of KS are characterized by a proliferation of spindle-shaped cells that express endothelial cell markers. KS is caused by the *KS herpesvirus (KSHV),* also called *human herpesvirus 8 (HHV8).* However, KSHV infection, while necessary for KS development, is not sufficient, and additional cofactors are needed. In the AIDS-related form, that cofactor is clearly HIV. HIV-mediated immune suppression may aid in dissemination of KSHV in the host. Clinically, AIDS-associated KS is quite different from the sporadic form. In individuals with HIV, the tumor is usually widespread, affecting the skin, mucous membranes, gastrointestinal tract, lymph nodes, and lungs. These tumors also tend to be more locally aggressive than sporadic KS.

Lymphomas. Lymphoma occurs at a markedly increased rate in individuals with AIDS, making it another AIDS-defining tumor. Roughly 5% of untreated patients with AIDS present with lymphoma, and approximately another 5% develop lymphoma during their subsequent course. Even in the era of HAART, lymphoma continues to occur in individuals infected with HIV at an incidence that is at least 10-fold greater than the population average. Based on molecular characterization of HIV-associated lymphomas and the epidemiologic considerations above, at least two mechanisms appear to underlie the increased risk for B-cell tumors in individuals infected with HIV: (1) oncogenic viruses and (2) germinal center B-cell reactions.

- *Tumors Induced by Oncogenic Viruses.* T-cell immunity is required to restrain the proliferation of B cells latently infected with oncogenic viruses such as EBV and KSHV. With the severe T-cell depletion in the course of HIV infection, this control is lost, and the infected B cells undergo unchecked proliferation that predispose to mutations and the development of B-cell tumors. As a result, patients with AIDS are at high risk for developing aggressive B-cell lymphomas composed of tumor cells infected by oncogenic viruses, particularly EBV. The tumors often occur in extranodal sites, such as the CNS, GI tract, orbit, and lungs. Patients with AIDS are also prone to rare lymphomas that present as malignant effusions (so-called "primary effusion lymphoma"), in which the tumor cells are usually coinfected by EBV and KSHV, an unusual example of cooperativity between two oncogenic viruses.
- *Germinal Center B-Cell Reactions.* The majority of the lymphomas that arise in patients with preserved CD4 T-cell counts are not associated with EBV or KSHV. The increased risk for lymphoma in these patients may be related to the germinal center B-cell hyperplasia that occurs in HIV infection. The high level of proliferation and somatic mutations that occur in germinal center B cells set the stage for chromosomal translocations and mutations involving tumor-causing genes. In fact, the aggressive B-cell tumors that arise outside the setting of severe T-cell depletion in HIV-infected individuals, such as Burkitt lymphoma and diffuse large B-cell lymphoma, are often associated with translocations involving immunoglobulin genes and oncogenes such as *MYC* and *BCL6,* which likely occur during the attempted rearrangement of immunoglobulin genes in germinal center B cells (Chapter 10).

Several other EBV-related proliferations also merit mention. *Hodgkin lymphoma,* an unusual B-cell tumor (Chapter 10), occurs at increased frequency in individuals infected with HIV. In virtually all instances of HIV-associated Hodgkin lymphoma, the characteristic tumor cells (Reed-Sternberg cells) are infected with EBV. EBV infection is also responsible for oral hairy leukoplakia (white plaques on the tongue), which results from EBV-driven squamous cell proliferation of the oral mucosa (Chapter 13).

Other Tumors. In addition to KS and lymphomas, patients with AIDS also have an increased occurrence of *carcinoma of the uterine cervix* and *anal cancer.* Both of these tumors are strongly associated with *human papillomavirus* infection, which is poorly controlled in the setting of immunodeficiency.

Central Nervous System Disease

Involvement of the CNS is a common and important manifestation of AIDS. Ninety percent of patients demonstrate some form of neurologic involvement at autopsy, and 40% to 60% have clinically apparent neurologic dysfunction. Importantly, in some patients, neurologic manifestations may be the sole or earliest presenting feature of HIV infection. Lesions include a self-limited presumed viral meningoencephalitis or aseptic meningitis, vacuolar myelopathy, peripheral neuropathies, and, most commonly, a progressive encephalopathy called *HIV-associated neurocognitive disorder* (Chapter 21).

Effect of Antiretroviral Drug Therapy on the Course of HIV Infection

The advent of new drugs that target the viral reverse transcriptase, protease, and integrase enzymes and other proteins has changed the clinical course of AIDS. When a combination of at least three effective drugs is used appropriately, HIV replication is reduced to below the threshold of detection (<50 RNA copies/mL) and remains there while the patient adheres to therapy. Once the virus is suppressed, the progressive loss of CD4+ T cells is halted, and the peripheral CD4+ T-cell count slowly increases, often returning to a normal level. With the use of these drugs, the annual death rate from AIDS in the United States has decreased from a peak of 16 to 18 per 100,000 individuals in 1995–1996 to less than 4 per 100,000 currently. Many AIDS-associated disorders, such as opportunistic infections with *P. jirovecii* and Kaposi sarcoma, now are uncommon. Antiretroviral therapy has also reduced the transmission of the virus, especially from infected mothers to newborns.

Despite these dramatic improvements, several new complications associated with HIV infection and its treatment have emerged. Some patients with advanced disease who are given antiretroviral therapy develop a paradoxical clinical deterioration during the period of recovery of the immune system despite increasing CD4+ T-cell counts and decreasing viral load. This disorder, called *immune reconstitution inflammatory syndrome,* is not understood but is postulated to be a poorly regulated host response to the antigenic burden of persistent microbes. In addition, significant adverse side effects are associated with long-term antiretroviral therapy. These include lipoatrophy (loss of facial fat), lipoaccumulation (excess fat deposition centrally), lipodystrophy (changes in fat distribution, often accompanied by metabolic abnormalities), elevated lipids, insulin resistance, peripheral neuropathy, and premature cardiovascular, kidney, and liver disease. Finally, major causes of morbidity are cancer and accelerated cardiovascular disease. The mechanism for these complications is not known, but persistent inflammation and T-cell dysfunction may have a role.

MORPHOLOGY

Tissue changes are neither specific nor diagnostic. Common pathologic features of AIDS include opportunistic infections, Kaposi sarcoma, and B-cell lymphomas. Most of these lesions are discussed elsewhere, because they also occur in individuals who do not have HIV infection. Lesions in the central nervous system are described in Chapter 21.

Biopsy specimens from enlarged lymph nodes in the early stages of HIV infection reveal a marked **hyperplasia of B-cell follicles,** which often take on unusual, serpiginous shapes. The mantle zones that surround the follicles are attenuated, and the germinal centers impinge on interfollicular T-cell areas. This hyperplasia of B cells is the morphologic reflection of the polyclonal B-cell activation and hypergammaglobulinemia seen in individuals infected with HIV.

With disease progression B-cell proliferation subsides and **lymphoid involution** begins. The lymph nodes are depleted of lymphocytes, and the organized network of follicular dendritic cells is disrupted. The germinal centers disappear or sometimes become hyalinized. During this advanced stage, viral burden in the nodes is reduced, in part because of loss of cells that carry the virus. These "burnt-out" lymph nodes are atrophic and small and may harbor numerous opportunistic pathogens, often within macrophages. Because of profound immunosuppression, the inflammatory response to infections in the lymph nodes and at extranodal sites may be sparse or atypical. For example, mycobacteria often fail to evoke granuloma formation because CD4+ cells are deficient, and the presence of these and other infectious agents may not be apparent without special stains. As might be expected, lymphoid involution is not confined to the nodes; in later stages of AIDS, the spleen and thymus are virtually devoid of lymphocytes.

Although with effective drug therapy the mortality rate has declined in the United States, treated patients still carry viral DNA in their lymphoid tissues. Truly curative therapy remains elusive. Similarly, although considerable effort has been mounted to develop a protective vaccine, this has yet to become a reality. Recent attempts have focused on producing broadly neutralizing antibodies against relatively invariant portions of HIV proteins. At present, therefore, prevention, public health measures and antiretroviral drugs remain the mainstays in the fight against AIDS.

AMYLOIDOSIS

Amyloidosis is a condition associated with a number of disorders in which extracellular deposits of fibrillar proteins are responsible for tissue damage and dysfunction. These abnormal fibrils are produced by the aggregation of improperly folded proteins (which are soluble in their normal folded configuration). The fibrillar deposits bind a wide variety of proteoglycans and glycosaminoglycans, which contain charged sugar groups that give the deposits staining characteristics thought to resemble those of starch (amylose). Therefore, the deposits were called *amyloid,* a name that is firmly entrenched, although the deposits are unrelated to starch.

Pathogenesis of Amyloid Deposition

Amyloid deposits can occur in a variety of conditions. Although the morphologic appearance is the same regardless of the underlying disorder, the protein composition varies. In fact, at least 30 different proteins can aggregate to form fibrils with the appearance of amyloid. About 95% of amyloid deposits are composed of nonbranching fibrils, each formed of intertwined polypeptides in a β-pleated sheet conformation (Fig. 5.35). The remaining 5% of the deposits are various glycoproteins, such as the serum amyloid P (SAP) component.

The three most common forms of amyloid are the following:
- *AL (amyloid light chain) amyloid* is made up of complete immunoglobulin light chains, the amino-terminal fragments of light chains, or both.
- *AA (amyloid-associated) amyloid* is composed of an 8500-dalton protein derived by proteolysis of serum amyloid-associated (SAA) protein, which is synthesized in the liver (Chapter 2).
- *β-amyloid protein (Aβ)* is a 4000-dalton peptide that is derived from the transmembrane glycoprotein called *amyloid precursor protein.*

Many other proteins can also deposit as amyloid in a variety of clinical settings. Some of the most clinically important examples are mentioned in the following section.

Classification of Amyloidosis and Mechanisms of Amyloid Formation

Amyloidosis results from abnormal folding of proteins, which assume a β-pleated sheet conformation, aggregate, and deposit as fibrils in extracellular tissues. Normally, intracellular misfolded proteins are degraded in proteasomes and extracellular protein aggregates are taken up and degraded by macrophages. In amyloidosis, these quality control mechanisms fail and fibrillar proteins accumulate outside of cells. The proteins that form amyloid fall into two general categories (Fig. 5.36): (1) normal proteins that have an inherent tendency to self-associate and form fibrils, particularly when produced in increased amounts, and (2) mutant

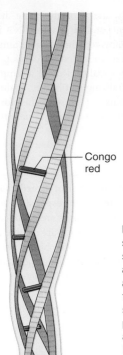

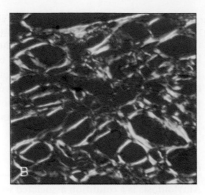

FIG. 5.35 Structure of amyloid. (A) A schematic diagram of an amyloid fiber showing four fibrils (there can be as many as six in each fiber) wound around one another with regularly spaced binding of the Congo red dye. (B) Congo red staining shows apple-green birefringence under polarized light, a diagnostic feature of amyloid. (From Merlini G, Bellotti V: Molecular mechanisms of amyloidosis. *N Engl J Med* 349:583–596, 2003.)

proteins that are prone to misfolding and aggregation. The mechanisms of deposition of different types of amyloid are discussed next along with classification.

Because a given form of amyloid (e.g., AA) may be associated with diverse clinical settings, we will follow a classification that takes into account clinical and biochemical features (Table 5.12). Amyloid may be systemic (generalized), involving several organ systems, or it may be localized to a single organ, such as the heart. The systemic pattern is subclassified into primary amyloidosis when it is associated with a clonal plasma cell proliferation, or secondary amyloidosis when it occurs as a complication of an underlying chronic inflammatory process. Hereditary or familial amyloidosis constitutes a separate, heterogeneous group with several distinctive patterns of organ involvement.

Primary Amyloidosis: Plasma Cell Proliferations Associated With Amyloidosis. Amyloid in this category is of the *AL type* and is usually systemic in distribution. This is the most common form of amyloidosis, with approximately 2000 to 3000 new cases each year in the United States. It is caused by a *clonal proliferation of plasma cells* that synthesize abnormal Ig molecules. The AL type of systemic amyloidosis occurs in 5% to 15% of individuals with multiple myeloma, a plasma-cell tumor characterized by excessive production of free immunoglobulin light chains (Chapter 10). The free, unpaired κ or λ light chains (referred to as *Bence Jones protein*) tend to aggregate and deposit in tissues as amyloid. However, not all free light chains are equally prone to producing amyloid; probably due to structural differences, λ light chains are approximately six times more likely to deposit as amyloid than κ light chains.

Most persons with AL amyloid do not have multiple myeloma or any other overt B-cell neoplasm; such cases have been traditionally classified as primary amyloidosis, because their clinical features derive

solely from the effects of amyloid deposition rather than formation of tumor masses. In virtually all such cases, however, monoclonal immunoglobulins or free light chains, or both, can be found in the blood or urine. Most of these patients also have a modest increase in the number of plasma cells in the bone marrow, which presumably secrete the precursors of AL protein.

Reactive Systemic Amyloidosis. The amyloid deposits in this pattern are systemic in distribution and composed of *AA protein*. This category was previously referred to as secondary amyloidosis because it is *secondary to an associated inflammatory condition*. At one time, tuberculosis, bronchiectasis, and chronic osteomyelitis were the most frequent underlying conditions, but these infections usually now resolve with antibiotic treatment and less often lead to amyloidosis. Currently, reactive systemic amyloidosis more commonly complicates rheumatoid arthritis, other connective tissue disorders such as ankylosing spondylitis, and inflammatory bowel disease, particularly Crohn disease and ulcerative colitis. Among these, the most frequently associated condition is rheumatoid arthritis. Amyloidosis is reported to occur in approximately 3% of patients with rheumatoid arthritis and is clinically significant in one-half of those affected. Long-term subcutaneous heroin injection can also lead to generalized AA amyloidosis, thought to be secondary to chronic skin infections. Reactive systemic amyloidosis may also occur in association with certain cancers, the most common being renal cell carcinoma and Hodgkin lymphoma.

In AA amyloidosis, SAA synthesis by liver cells is stimulated by cytokines such as IL-6 and IL-1 that are produced during inflammation; thus, long-standing inflammation leads to a sustained elevation of SAA levels. While SAA levels are increased in all cases of inflammation, only a small subset develop amyloidosis. It seems that in some patients SAA breakdown produces intermediates that are prone to forming fibrils.

Heredofamilial Amyloidosis. A variety of familial forms of amyloidosis have been described. Most are rare and occur in limited geographic areas. The most common and best studied is an autosomal recessive condition called *familial Mediterranean fever* (FMF), which is encountered largely in individuals of Armenian, Sephardic Jewish, and Arabic origins. However, due to population admixture and migration, FMF is not restricted to these populations; it is also found with a lower prevalence in parts of Asia and Southern Europe. FMF is an "autoinflammatory" syndrome associated with excessive production of the cytokine IL-1. It is characterized by intermittent fevers accompanied by inflammation of serosal surfaces that manifests as peritonitis, pleuritis, and synovitis. The gene for FMF encodes a protein called pyrin that is involved in the activation of inflammasomes and production of proinflammatory cytokines, mainly IL-1. The amyloid seen in this disorder is of the AA type, suggesting that it is related to the recurrent bouts of inflammation.

In contrast to FMF, a group of autosomal dominant familial disorders is characterized by deposition of amyloid made up of fibrils derived from mutant *transthyretin* (TTR), a transporter of the hormone thyroxine. Remarkably, specific TTR mutant polypeptides tend to form amyloid in different organs; thus, in some families, deposits are seen mainly in peripheral nerves (familial amyloidotic polyneuropathies), whereas in others cardiac deposits predominate. A variant of the *TTR* gene that leads to cardiac amyloidosis is carried by approximately 4% of the African-American population in the United States; restrictive cardiomyopathy has been identified in both homozygous and heterozygous patients. The origin of the allele in this population appears to be in West African regions where much of the

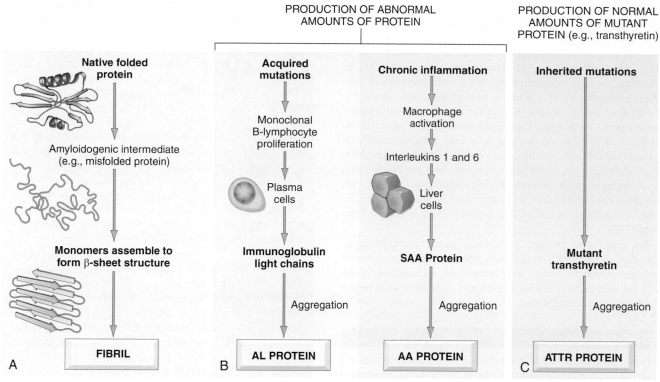

PRODUCTION OF ABNORMAL AMOUNTS OF PROTEIN

PRODUCTION OF NORMAL AMOUNTS OF MUTANT PROTEIN (e.g., transthyretin)

FIG. 5.36 Pathogenesis of amyloidosis. (A) General mechanism of formation of amyloid fibrils. (B) Formation of amyloid from excessive production of proteins prone to misfolding. (C) Formation of amyloid from mutant protein. *AA*, Amyloid A; *AL*, amyloid light chain; *ATTR*, amyloid transthyretin; *SAA*, serum amyloid A.

African-American population of the United States originated. Penetrance of this variant differs substantially among individuals, leading to severe disease in some and no disease in others.

Localized Amyloidosis. Amyloid deposits may be limited to a single organ or tissue. The deposits may produce grossly detectable nodular masses or be evident only on microscopic examination.

Nodular deposits of amyloid are most often encountered in the lung, larynx, skin, urinary bladder, tongue, and the region about the eye. Frequently, there are infiltrates of lymphocytes and plasma cells associated with these amyloid masses. At least in some cases, the amyloid consists of AL protein and may therefore represent a localized form of plasma cell–derived amyloid.

Table 5.12 Classification of Amyloidosis

Clinicopathologic Category	Associated Diseases	Major Fibril Protein	Chemically Related Precursor Protein
Systemic (Generalized) Amyloidosis			
Plasma cell proliferations with amyloidosis (primary amyloidosis)	Multiple myeloma and other monoclonal plasma cell proliferations	AL	Immunoglobulin light chains, chiefly λ type
Reactive systemic amyloidosis (secondary amyloidosis)	Chronic inflammatory conditions (e.g., rheumatoid arthritis, Crohn disease)	AA	SAA
Hemodialysis-associated amyloidosis[a]	Chronic renal failure	Aβ₂m	β₂-microglobulin
Hereditary Amyloidosis			
Familial Mediterranean fever		AA	SAA
Familial amyloidotic neuropathies (several types); cardiac amyloidosis		ATTR	Transthyretin (mutated)
Systemic senile amyloidosis		ATTR	Transthyretin (wild-type)
Localized Amyloidosis			
Senile cerebral	Alzheimer disease	Aβ	APP
Endocrine	Type 2 diabetes		
	Medullary carcinoma of thyroid	A Cal	Calcitonin
	Islets of Langerhans	AIAPP	Islet amyloid peptide
Isolated atrial amyloidosis		AANF	Atrial natriuretic factor

[a]Now rarely seen because of improved dialysis membranes.

Endocrine Amyloid. Microscopic deposits of localized amyloid may be found in certain endocrine tumors, such as medullary carcinoma of the thyroid gland, islet tumors of the pancreas, pheochromocytomas, and undifferentiated carcinomas of the stomach, and in the islets of Langerhans in individuals with type 2 diabetes mellitus. In these settings, the amyloidogenic proteins are sometimes derived from polypeptide hormones (e.g., calcitonin in medullary carcinoma).

Amyloid of Aging. Several well-documented forms of amyloid deposition occur with aging. Senile systemic amyloidosis refers to the systemic deposition of amyloid in elderly patients (usually in their seventies and eighties). Because of the dominant involvement and related dysfunction of the heart, this form was previously called *senile cardiac amyloidosis.* Those who are symptomatic present with a restrictive cardiomyopathy and arrhythmias (Chapter 9). The amyloid in this form, in contrast to familial forms, is derived from wild-type TTR.

In the past, some patients on chronic hemodialysis developed amyloid deposits derived from β_2-microglobulin, because this protein did not pass through dialysis membranes and accumulated in the blood. This complication has been essentially eliminated with the use of improved dialysis membranes.

MORPHOLOGY

There are no consistent or distinctive patterns of organ or tissue distribution of amyloid deposits in any of the categories cited, but a few generalizations can be made. In AA amyloidosis secondary to chronic inflammatory disorders, kidneys, liver, spleen, lymph nodes, adrenal glands, thyroid glands, and many other tissues are typically affected. Although AL amyloidosis associated with plasma cell proliferations cannot reliably be distinguished from the AA form by its organ distribution, it more often involves the heart, gastrointestinal tract, respiratory tract, peripheral nerves, skin, and tongue. The localization of amyloid deposits in the hereditary syndromes is varied. In familial Mediterranean fever, the amyloidosis is of the AA type and accordingly may be widespread, involving the kidneys, blood vessels, spleen, respiratory tract, and (rarely) liver.

Amyloid may be appreciated macroscopically when it accumulates in large amounts. The organ is frequently enlarged, and the tissue appears gray and has a waxy, firm consistency. Histologically, the amyloid deposition is always extracellular and begins between cells, often closely adjacent to basement membranes (Fig. 5.37). As the amyloid accumulates, it encroaches on the cells, in time surrounding and destroying them. In the form associated with plasma cell proliferation, perivascular and vascular deposits are common.

The diagnosis of amyloidosis is based on histopathology. With the light microscope and hematoxylin and eosin stains, amyloid appears as an amorphous, eosinophilic, hyaline, extracellular substance. To differentiate amyloid from other hyaline materials (e.g., collagen, fibrin), a variety of histochemical stains is used. The most widely used is the **Congo red stain,** which under ordinary light gives a pink or red color to tissue deposits, but far more striking and specific is the green birefringence of the stained amyloid when observed by polarizing microscopy (see Fig. 5.37B). This staining reaction is shared by all forms of amyloid and is imparted by the crossed β-pleated sheet configuration of amyloid fibrils. The specific type of amyloid can be defined by immunohistochemistry in some cases (best for AA and TTR-associated amyloid), but definitive identification, especially of AL amyloid, requires mass spectroscopy or protein sequencing.

The pattern of organ involvement in different forms of amyloidosis is variable.

Kidney. Amyloidosis of the kidney is the most common and potentially the most serious form of organ involvement. Grossly, the kidneys may be of normal size and color, or in advanced cases they may be shrunken because of ischemia due to vascular narrowing induced by the deposition of amyloid within arterial

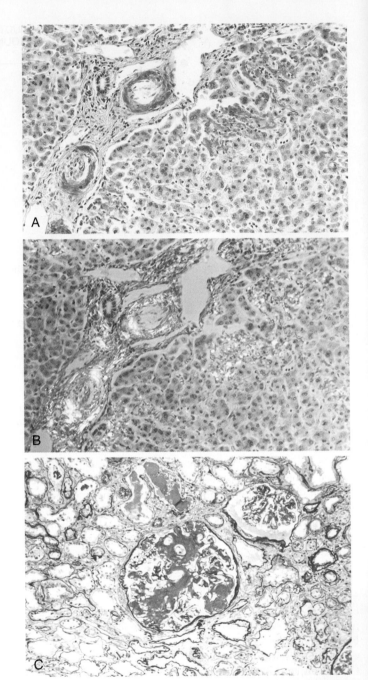

FIG. 5.37 Amyloidosis. (A) A section of the liver stained with Congo red reveals pink-red deposits of amyloid in the walls of blood vessels and along sinusoids. (B) Note the yellow-green birefringence of the deposits when observed by polarizing microscope. (C) Amyloidosis of the kidney. The glomerular architecture is almost totally obliterated by the massive accumulation of amyloid. (A, B, Courtesy of Dr. Trace Worrell and Sandy Hinton, Department of Pathology, University of Texas Southwestern Medical School, Dallas, Texas.)

and arteriolar walls. Histologically, the amyloid is deposited primarily in the glomeruli, but the interstitial peritubular tissue, arteries, and arterioles are also affected (see Fig. 5.37C). The glomerular deposits occur in the mesangium and along the basement membranes and cause capillary narrowing and distortion of the glomerular vascular tuft. With progression of glomerular amyloidosis, the capillary lumens are obliterated and the obsolescent glomerulus is replaced by confluent masses or interlacing broad ribbons of amyloid.

Spleen. Amyloidosis of the spleen may be inapparent grossly or may cause moderate to marked splenomegaly. For unknown reasons, two distinct patterns of deposition are seen. In one, the deposits are largely limited to the splenic follicles. In the other pattern, the amyloid involves the walls of the splenic sinuses and connective tissue framework in the red pulp.

Liver. The deposits may be inapparent grossly or may cause moderate to marked hepatomegaly. Amyloid appears first in the space of Disse and then progressively encroaches on adjacent hepatic parenchymal cells and sinusoids (see Fig. 5.37A). In time, deformity, pressure atrophy, and disappearance of hepatocytes occur, causing total replacement of large areas of liver parenchyma. Vascular involvement and deposits in Kupffer cells are frequent. Liver function is usually preserved despite sometimes quite extensive involvement.

Heart. Amyloidosis of the heart (Chapter 9) may occur in any form of systemic amyloidosis. It is also the major organ involved in senile systemic amyloidosis. The heart may be enlarged and firm, but more often it shows no appreciable change on gross inspection. Histologically, the deposits begin as focal subendocardial accumulations between the muscle fibers of the myocardium. Expansion of these myocardial deposits eventually causes pressure atrophy of myocardial fibers. Subendocardial deposits may impinge on the conduction system and give rise to arrhythmias.

Other Organs. Nodular depositions in the **tongue** may cause macroglossia, giving rise to the designation tumor-forming amyloid of the tongue. The **respiratory tract** may be involved focally or diffusely from the larynx down to the smallest bronchioles. A distinct form of amyloid is found in the **brains** of patients with Alzheimer disease. It is present in plaques as well as blood vessels (Chapter 21). Amyloidosis of peripheral and autonomic **nerves** is a feature of several familial amyloidotic neuropathies.

Clinical Features. Amyloidosis may be found as an unsuspected anatomic change, having produced no clinical manifestations, or it may cause serious clinical problems and even death. The symptoms depend on the abundance of the deposits and on the sites or organs affected. At first, clinical manifestations are often entirely nonspecific, such as weakness, weight loss, lightheadedness, or syncope. More specific findings appear later and most often relate to renal, cardiac, and gastrointestinal involvement.

Renal involvement gives rise to proteinuria that may be severe enough to cause the nephrotic syndrome (Chapter 12). Progressive obliteration of glomeruli in advanced cases ultimately leads to renal failure. Cardiac amyloidosis may present insidiously as congestive heart failure. The most serious aspects of cardiac amyloidosis are conduction disturbances and arrhythmias, which may prove fatal. Occasionally, cardiac amyloidosis produces a restrictive pattern of cardiomyopathy and masquerades as hypertensive cardiomyopathy (but without hypertension) or chronic constrictive pericarditis (Chapter 9). Gastrointestinal amyloidosis may be asymptomatic, or it may present in a variety of ways. Amyloidosis of the tongue may cause sufficient enlargement and inelasticity to hamper speech and swallowing. Depositions in the stomach and intestine may lead to malabsorption, diarrhea, and disturbances in digestion. Vascular amyloidosis causes vascular fragility that may lead to bleeding, sometimes massive, that can occur spontaneously or following seemingly trivial trauma. In some cases AL amyloid binds and inactivates factor X, a critical coagulation factor, leading to a life-threatening bleeding disorder.

The diagnosis of amyloidosis often relies on the histologic demonstration of Congo red—positive deposits in tissues. The most commonly biopsied sites are the kidney, when renal manifestations are present, or rectal or gingival tissues in patients suspected of having systemic amyloidosis. Examination of abdominal fat aspirates stained with Congo red can also be used for the diagnosis of systemic amyloidosis. The test is quite specific, but its sensitivity is low. In suspected cases of AL amyloidosis, serum and urine protein electrophoresis and immunoelectrophoresis are performed. Bone marrow examination in such cases often shows a monoclonal population of plasma cells, even in the absence of overt multiple myeloma. Scintigraphy with radiolabeled SAP component is a rapid and specific test, since SAP binds to amyloid deposits and reveals their presence. It also gives a measure of the extent of amyloidosis and can be used to follow patients undergoing treatment, but it is available only in some centers. Mass spectroscopy is a useful tool for identification of the protein component of amyloid. It can be performed on paraffin-embedded tissues.

The prognosis for individuals with generalized amyloidosis is poor. Those with AL amyloidosis without multiple myeloma have a median survival of 2 years after diagnosis. Individuals with myeloma-associated amyloidosis have an even poorer prognosis. The outlook for individuals with reactive systemic amyloidosis is somewhat better and depends to some extent on the control of the underlying condition. Resorption of amyloid after treatment of the associated condition has been reported, but this is a rare occurrence. New drugs that reduce TTR synthesis and stabilize TTR tetramers have been developed that slow the progression of this type of amyloidosis.

■ RAPID REVIEW

The Normal Immune Response

- Innate immunity provides early rapid defense against microbes and clears damaged and dead cells; adaptive immunity provides the later and more effective defense.
- Components of the innate immune system include epithelial barriers, phagocytes, NK cells, and plasma proteins (e.g., complement). Innate immune reactions are often manifested as inflammation.
- The innate immune system uses several families of receptors, such as Toll-like receptors, to recognize molecules present in various types of microbes and produced by damaged cells.
- Lymphocytes are the mediators of adaptive immunity and the only cells that produce specific and diverse receptors for antigens.
- The antigen receptors of T (thymus-derived) lymphocytes, called T-cell receptors (TCRs), recognize peptide fragments of protein antigens displayed by MHC molecules on the surface of antigen-presenting cells.
- B (bone marrow—derived) lymphocytes express membrane-bound antibodies that recognize a wide variety of antigens. B cells are activated to become plasma cells, which secrete antibodies.
- Natural killer (NK) cells kill cells that are infected by some microbes or are stressed and damaged beyond repair. NK cells express inhibitory receptors that recognize MHC molecules that are normally expressed on healthy cells and are thus prevented from killing normal cells.
- The cells of the immune system are organized in tissues, some of which are the sites of production of mature lymphocytes (the generative lymphoid organs, namely the bone marrow and thymus), and others are the sites of immune responses (the secondary lymphoid organs, including lymph nodes, spleen, and mucosal lymphoid tissues).
- Microbes and other foreign antigens are captured by dendritic cells (DCs) and transported to lymph nodes, where the antigens are recognized by naïve lymphocytes. The lymphocytes are activated to proliferate and differentiate into effector and memory cells.

- Cell-mediated immunity is the reaction of T lymphocytes, designed to combat cell-associated microbes (e.g., phagocytosed microbes and microbes in the cytoplasm of infected cells). Humoral immunity is mediated by antibodies and is effective against extracellular microbes (in the circulation and mucosal lumens).
- CD4+ helper T cells help B cells to make antibodies, activate macrophages to destroy ingested microbes, stimulate recruitment of leukocytes, and regulate all immune responses to protein antigens. The functions of CD4+ T cells are mediated by secreted proteins called *cytokines*.
- CD8+ cytotoxic T lymphocytes kill cells that express antigens in the cytoplasm that are seen as foreign (e.g., virus-infected and tumor cells) and can also produce cytokines.
- Antibodies secreted by plasma cells neutralize microbes and block their infectivity and promote the phagocytosis and destruction of pathogens. Antibodies also confer passive immunity to neonates.

Immediate (Type I) Hypersensitivity (Allergy)

- Induced by environmental antigens (allergens) that stimulate strong Th2 responses and IgE production in genetically susceptible individuals.
- IgE coats mast cells by binding to the FcεRI receptor; reexposure to the allergen leads to cross-linking of the IgE and FcεRI, activation of mast cells, and release of mediators.
- Principal mediators: histamine, proteases, and other granule contents; prostaglandins and leukotrienes; and cytokines.
- Mediators are responsible for the immediate vascular and smooth muscle reactions and the late-phase reaction (inflammation).
- The clinical manifestations may be local or systemic and range from mild rhinitis to fatal anaphylaxis.

Diseases Caused by Antibodies and Immune Complexes (Types II and III Hypersensitivity)

- Antibodies can coat (opsonize) cells, with or without complement proteins, and target these cells for phagocytosis by phagocytes (macrophages), which express receptors for the Fc tails of IgG and for complement proteins. The result is depletion of the opsonized cells.
- Antibodies and immune complexes may deposit in tissues or blood vessels, and elicit an acute inflammatory reaction by activating complement or by engaging Fc receptors of leukocytes. The inflammatory reaction causes tissue injury.
- Antibodies can bind to cell surface receptors or other essential molecules and cause functional derangements (either inhibition or unregulated activation) without cell injury.

T Cell—Mediated Hypersensitivity Reactions (Type IV Hypersensitivity)

- *Cytokine-mediated inflammation:* CD4+ T cells are activated by exposure to a protein antigen and differentiate into Th1 and Th17 effector cells. Subsequent exposure to the antigen results in the secretion of cytokines. IFN-γ activates macrophages to produce substances that cause tissue damage, and IL-17 and other cytokines recruit leukocytes, thus promoting inflammation.
- The classical T cell—mediated inflammatory reaction is *delayed-type hypersensitivity*. Chronic Th1 reactions associated with macrophage activation often lead to granuloma formation.

- *T cell—mediated cytotoxicity:* CD8+ cytotoxic T lymphocytes (CTLs) specific for an antigen recognize cells expressing the target antigen and kill these cells. CD8+ T cells also secrete IFN-γ.

Autoimmunity

- Autoimmunity is the result of failure of tolerance to self antigens.
- Self-tolerance is maintained by numerous mechanisms:
  - Death of immature T and B lymphocytes that recognize self antigens in the generative lymphoid organs (thymus and bone marrow); in the B-cell lineage, some of the self-reactive lymphocytes switch to new antigen receptors that are not self-reactive.
  - Mature lymphocytes that recognize self antigens in peripheral tissues are suppressed by regulatory T lymphocytes, engage inhibitory receptors (such as CTLA-4 and PD-1) that block activation, or die by apoptosis.
- The factors that lead to a failure of self-tolerance and the development of autoimmunity include (1) inheritance of susceptibility genes that disrupt different tolerance pathways, and (2) infections and tissue injury that expose self antigens and activate APCs and lymphocytes in the tissues.

Systemic Lupus Erythematosus

- SLE is a systemic autoimmune disease caused by autoantibodies produced against numerous self antigens and the formation of immune complexes.
- The major autoantibodies, and the ones responsible for the formation of circulating immune complexes, are directed against nuclear antigens. Other autoantibodies react with red cells, platelets, and various phospholipid-protein complexes.
- Disease manifestations include nephritis, skin lesions and arthritis (caused by the deposition of immune complexes), hematologic abnormalities (caused by antibodies against red cells, white cells, and platelets), and neurologic abnormalities (caused by obscure mechanisms).
- The underlying cause of the breakdown in self-tolerance in SLE is unknown. Possibilities include excessive generation or persistence of nuclear antigens (e.g., secondary to cell death caused by UV irradiation), abnormal signaling by nucleic acid-recognizing TLRs, and excessive production of type I interferons.

Sjögren Syndrome

- Sjögren syndrome is an inflammatory disease that primarily affects the salivary and lacrimal glands, causing dryness of the mouth and eyes.
- The disease is believed to be caused by an autoimmune T-cell reaction against an unknown self antigen expressed in these glands, or immune reactions against the antigens of a virus that infects the tissues.

Systemic Sclerosis

- Systemic sclerosis (commonly called *scleroderma*) is characterized by progressive fibrosis involving the skin, gastrointestinal tract, and other tissues.
- Fibrosis may be the result of activation of fibroblasts by cytokines produced by T cells and macrophages, but what triggers T-cell responses is unknown.
- Endothelial injury and microvascular disease are commonly present in the lesions of systemic sclerosis, perhaps causing chronic ischemia, but the pathogenesis of vascular injury is not known.

Immunology of Transplantation

- Rejection of solid organ transplants is initiated mainly by host T cells that recognize the foreign HLA antigens of the graft, either directly (on APCs in the graft) or indirectly (after uptake and presentation by host APCs).
- Types and mechanisms of rejection of solid organ grafts are as follows:
  - *Hyperacute rejection:* Preformed antidonor antibodies bind to graft endothelium immediately after transplantation, leading to thrombosis, ischemic damage, and rapid graft failure.
  - *Acute cellular rejection:* T cells destroy graft parenchyma (and vessels) by cytotoxicity and inflammatory reactions.
  - *Acute antibody-mediated (humoral) rejection:* Antibodies damage graft vasculature.
  - *Chronic rejection:* Dominated by arteriosclerosis and ischemic injury, caused by activated T cells and antibodies. The T cells may secrete cytokines that induce proliferation of vascular smooth muscle cells, and the antibodies cause endothelial injury. The ischemic damage and T-cell reactions cause parenchymal fibrosis.
- Treatment of graft rejection relies on immunosuppressive drugs, which inhibit immune responses against the graft but make patients susceptible to infections and cancers.
- Transplantation of hematopoietic stem cells (HSCs) requires careful matching of donor and recipient and may be complicated by graft-versus-host disease (GVHD).

Primary (Inherited) Immune Deficiency Diseases

- These diseases are caused by inherited mutations in genes involved in lymphocyte maturation or function, or in innate immunity.
- Some of the more common disorders affecting lymphocytes and the adaptive immune response are:
  - *X-SCID:* Failure of T-cell and B-cell maturation; mutation in the common γ chain of a cytokine receptor, leading to failure of IL-7 signaling and defective lymphopoiesis; inheritance is X-linked.
  - *Autosomal recessive SCID:* Failure of T-cell development; secondary defect in antibody responses; approximately 50% of cases caused by mutation in the gene encoding adenosine deaminase (ADA), leading to accumulation of toxic metabolites during lymphocyte maturation and proliferation
  - *X-linked agammaglobulinemia (XLA):* Failure of B-cell maturation, absence of antibodies; caused by mutations in the *BTK* gene, which encodes B-cell tyrosine kinase, required for maturation signals from the pre—B-cell and B-cell receptors
  - *DiGeorge syndrome:* Failure of development of thymus, with T-cell deficiency
  - *X-linked hyper-IgM syndrome:* Failure to produce isotype-switched high-affinity antibodies (IgG, IgA, IgE); mutations in genes encoding CD40L or activation-induced cytosine deaminase
  - *Common variable immunodeficiency:* Defects in antibody production; cause unknown in most cases
  - *Selective IgA deficiency:* Failure of IgA production; cause unknown
- Deficiencies in innate immunity include defects of leukocyte function, complement, and innate immune receptors.
- These diseases present clinically with increased susceptibility to infections in early life.

Human Immunodeficiency Virus Life Cycle and the Pathogenesis of AIDS

- *Virus entry into cells:* Requires CD4 and coreceptors, which are receptors for chemokines; involves binding of viral gp120 and fusion with the cell mediated by viral gp41 protein; main cellular targets: CD4+ helper T cells; macrophages and DCs may also be infected
- *Viral replication:* Integration of provirus genome into host cell DNA; triggering of viral gene expression by stimuli that activate infected cells (e.g., infectious microbes, cytokines produced during normal immune responses)
- *Progression of infection:* Acute infection of mucosal T cells and DCs; viremia with dissemination of virus; latent infection of cells in lymphoid tissue; continuing viral replication and progressive loss of CD4+ T cells
- *Mechanisms of immune deficiency:*
  - Loss of CD4+ T cells: T-cell death during viral replication and budding (similar to other cytopathic infections); apoptosis occurring as a result of chronic stimulation; decreased thymic output; functional defects
  - Defective macrophage and DC functions
  - Destruction of architecture of lymphoid tissues (late)

Clinical Course and Complications of HIV Infection

- *Progression of disease.* HIV infection progresses through phases.
  - *Acute HIV infection.* Manifestations of acute viral illness
  - *Chronic (latent) phase.* Dissemination of virus, host immune response, progressive destruction of immune cells
  - *AIDS.* Severe immune deficiency
- *Clinical features.* Full-blown AIDS manifests with several complications, mostly resulting from immune deficiency.
  - Opportunistic infections
  - Tumors, especially tumors caused by oncogenic viruses
  - Neurologic complications of unknown pathogenesis
- Antiretroviral therapy has greatly decreased the incidence of opportunistic infections and tumors but also has numerous complications.

Amyloidosis

- Amyloidosis is a disorder characterized by the extracellular deposits of proteins that are prone to aggregate and form insoluble fibrils.
- The deposition of these proteins may result from excessive production of proteins that are prone to aggregation; mutations that produce proteins that cannot fold properly and tend to aggregate; defective or incomplete proteolytic degradation of extracellular proteins.
- Amyloidosis may be localized or systemic. It is seen in association with a variety of primary disorders, including monoclonal B-cell proliferations (in which the amyloid deposits consist of immunoglobulin light chains); chronic inflammatory diseases such as rheumatoid arthritis (deposits of amyloid A protein, derived from an acute-phase protein produced in inflammation); familial conditions in which the amyloid deposits consist of mutated proteins (e.g., transthyretin in familial amyloid polyneuropathies); and Alzheimer disease (amyloid β protein).
- Amyloid deposits cause tissue injury and impair normal function by causing pressure on cells and tissues. They do not evoke an inflammatory response.

■ **Laboratory Tests**[c]

Test	Reference Values	Pathophysiology/Clinical Relevance
Anticentromere antibody[a], serum	<1.0 U	Anticentromere antibodies are present in approximately 80% of cases of limited cutaneous scleroderma/CREST syndrome (calcinosis, Reynaud phenomenon, esophageal dysmotility, sclerodactyly, and telangiectasia). These antibodies are not specific and can also be present in systemic sclerosis and systemic lupus erythematosus (SLE).
Anticitrullinated peptide Ab, serum	<20 U/mL	Citrullinated proteins represent posttranslational modifications that can be associated with inflammation, particularly in synovial tissues. In rheumatoid arthritis (RA), autoantibodies are induced against a number of citrullinated antigens. These anticitrullinated peptide antibodies (ACPA) have been identified in the synovial fluid of some patients with RA and may play a pathogenic role by triggering proinflammatory cytokines and bone destruction via osteclastogenesis. ACPA can be found in 60%–80% of patients with RA, and ELISA-based serum tests show specificity ranging from 85%–99%. There is also evidence that ACPA may precede the development of RA several years prior to disease presentation. Some groups have suggested that levels of ACPA may be associated with disease progression and response to anti–tumor necrosis factor (TNF) antibody treatment.
Anti-DNA topoisomerase I (Scl-70)[a], serum	<1.0 U	DNA topoisomerase I is present in the nucleolus and nucleoplasm and its function is to cleave and relax supercoiled DNA. Anti-DNA topoisomerase antibodies produce a speckled nuclear or nucleolar ANA pattern. Anti-DNA topoisomerase antibodies are found in 20%–60% of patients with systemic sclerosis/scleroderma. They are associated with the diffuse variant of the disease, pulmonary fibrosis, and poor prognosis.
Antidouble-stranded (ds) DNA[a], serum	<30 IU/mL	Anti-dsDNA antibodies produce a peripheral or diffuse staining pattern. Anti-dsDNA antibodies form immune complexes that deposit in glomeruli, fix complement, and cause renal damage. Anti-dsDNA antibodies are seen in 40%–60% cases of SLE and are quite specific. Anti-dsDNA IgG levels appear to correlate with disease activity and severity of renal involvement in SLE. Anti-dsDNA antibodies are rare in other rheumatologic diseases.
Antihistone[a], serum	<100 AU/mL[b]	Antihistone antibodies produce a diffuse staining pattern and are positive in both drug-induced lupus (DIL) and SLE. Patients with low levels of the acetyltransferase that acetylates and detoxifies some drugs (e.g., hydralazine, procainamide) are at increased risk for DIL following exposure.
Anti-Jo antibody, serum	<1.0 U	Anti-Jo1 antibody recognizes the transfer RNA synthetase that catalyzes the binding of the amino acid histidine to its cognate tRNA. It is identified in up to 20% of adult patients with idiopathic inflammatory myopathies.
Antinuclear antibodies (ANAs)[a], serum	≤1.0 U	Different autoantibodies produce different ANA patterns by indirect immuno-fluorescence assays (e.g., homogeneous, speckled, centromere, nucleolar). ELISA is more specific but is less sensitive. ANAs are present in many autoimmune diseases but are not specific; they can be seen in other conditions (e.g., infection, malignancy) or in otherwise healthy individuals. The American College of Rheumatology generally recommends against testing for antibodies against specific nuclear antigens (including anti-dsDNA, anti-Smith, anti-RNP, anti-SSA, anti-SSB, anti-Scl-70, anticentromere) if ANA is negative.
Antinucleosome antibody (antichromatin)[a], serum	<1.0 Negative AI	Nucleosomes are subunits of the histone-DNA complex. Antinucleosome antibodies are positive in up to 75% of patients with systemic lupus erythematosus (SLE) and up to 100% of drug-induced lupus patients; in the former, they are associated with renal disease. Antibody titer correlates with disease severity.
Anti-Ro/anti-SSA antibody, serum	<1.0 U	These antibodies are a type of antinuclear autoantibodies. Depending on the technique used for detection, these antibodies are present in 40%–80% of patients with primary Sjögren syndrome and are seen in 50% of patients with SLE.
Anti-Smith antigen[a], serum	<1.0 U	Smith antigen is part of a group of nuclear proteins that include SSA, SSB, and ribonuclear protein. Anti-Smith antibodies are associated with a speckled ANA pattern and are fairly specific for SLE; they are positive in 20%–30% of patients with SLE.
C3 complement, serum	75–175 mg/dL	Complement proteins are plasma proteins that are activated directly by microbes or by antibodies bound to antigens, and mediate important functions (opsonization, inflammation, lysis of some cells). Complement activation pathways converge on cleavage of the C3 protein, the central component of the complement system. Widespread complement activation leads to consumption of these proteins and decreased plasma levels. C3 is measured by immunoassay and is evaluated in the workup of autoimmune diseases (e.g., SLE, membranoproliferative glomerulonephritis); levels often correlate with disease activity (e.g., levels decrease in active immune complex disease). Low levels of both C3 and C4 indicate classical pathway activation. Low serum level of C3 with normal C4 level indicates alternative pathway activation.

Test	Reference	Description
C4 complement, serum	14–40 mg/dL	C4 is part of the classical complement pathway, which is activated by antibodies bound to antigens; levels are low when this pathway is activated. C4 complement is measured by immunoassay and is evaluated in the workup of autoimmune diseases (e.g., SLE). Levels may help determine disease activity.
CD4 count, blood	Adults: 400–1400 CD4+ cells/μL[b]; Pediatric ranges vary by age	CD4 counts may be directly measured by flow cytometry or the absolute count may be calculated by measuring percentage of CD4+ T cells by flow cytometry (CD4+ T cell % × WBC count). CD4+ T-cell counts correlate with current immune competence in patients with HIV and are used for disease staging, to assess risk for certain complications and the need for prophylaxis, and to evaluate response to antiretroviral therapy. Key clinical indicators include CD4 counts <200 cells/μL (*P. jirovecii* prophylaxis indicated) and <50/μL (*M. avium* complex prophylaxis indicated).
HIV antibody/antigen, plasma	Negative	Third-generation IgM and IgG tests can detect the presence of antibodies 20 to 30 days after HIV exposure and are often the initial screening test used for HIV infection. Combination HIV antigen/antibody tests detect IgG and IgM antibodies as well as the HIV p24 antigen and can become positive 15 to 20 days after exposure. By comparison, HIV RNA tests can be positive 10 to 15 days after exposure. First-time positive tests should be confirmed by another method (e.g., HIV RNA, HIV-1/HIV-2 differentiation assay). Combination tests can detect p24 antigen before seroconversion (the "window period"). Rapid antibody tests have >99% specificity and sensitivity in chronic infection but are less sensitive in acute infection.
HIV DNA, plasma	Undetected	Diagnosis of HIV infection is primarily serologic (i.e., detection of HIV-specific antibodies). However, in neonates (who have immature immune systems and who may have maternal anti-HIV antibodies), in early HIV infection (<30 days from exposure) or in individuals with equivocal serologic results, assays for HIV proviral DNA and HIV RNA are useful adjuncts. These tests are typically informative 10 to 14 days after infection.
HIV NAT (nucleic acid test), plasma	Undetected	NAT is used to detect a particular nucleic acid sequence to identify a specific organism (e.g., HIV, *Neisseria gonorrhoeae*). Quantitative assays can be used to guide antiretroviral therapy, while qualitative assays are used for HIV diagnosis. NAT can detect infection 10 to 33 days after exposure, compared to antigen/antibody tests (18 to 45 days after exposure) and antibody tests (23 to 90 days). The NAT qualitative test is mainly used at donor centers to confirm safety of blood products and for early diagnosis in infants born to mothers who are HIV positive.
HIV RNA (HIV viral load)	Undetected	More than 99% of HIV cases worldwide are due to HIV-1. Therefore, this is the viral type most commonly assessed. HIV viral load (number of HIV-1 RNA copies/mL of plasma) correlates with disease stage and, combined with CD4+ T-cell numbers, is useful in monitoring response to treatment. This test determines how actively virus is replicating in a person with HIV infection. US Health and Human Services defines <200 copies/mL as virologic failure. When 2 tests performed at least 2 to 4 weeks apart show virologic failure, drug-drug interactions and patient adherence to the regimen should be evaluated. At determined levels (e.g., 500 copies/mL), testing for drug resistance genotypes may be warranted.
Rheumatoid factor, serum	<15 IU/mL	Rheumatoid factors are antibodies that react with the Fc portion of other immunoglobulin G antibodies. Despite its name, RF lacks specificity for RA and can be seen in other autoimmune diseases, particularly Sjögren syndrome. High titers are associated with increased disease severity and worse prognosis. RF has a sensitivity and specificity of about 70% and 85% for RA, respectively. Combination of RF and anticitrullinated peptide antibodies is more informative diagnostically.

[a]Autoantibodies against nuclear antigens are found in many systemic autoimmune diseases. These antibodies arise because of a failure of immune tolerance combined with ineffective clearance of nuclear fragments, typically from apoptotic cells. Antinuclear antibodies are measured by an indirect immunofluorescence assay (IFA) in which binding of serial dilutions of serum antibodies to nuclei of a cultured hepatocyte cell line is defined. Different binding patterns indicate the specificity of the antibodies for different nuclear components. Attempts are being made to replace some of these assays with more specific and quantitative ELISA.

[b]Duke University Health Systems Clinical Laboratories reference values: https://testcatalog.duke.edu/.

[c]Assistance of Dr. Pankti D. Reid and Dr. Bauer Ventura, Department of Medicine, University of Chicago, is gratefully acknowledged for their help in reviewing this table.

Reference values from https://www.mayocliniclabs.com/ by permission of Mayo Foundation for Medical Education and Research. All rights reserved.

Adapted from Deyrup AT, D'Ambrosio D, Muir J, et al. Essential Laboratory Tests for Medical Education. *Acad Pathol.* 2022;9. doi: 10.1016/j.acpath.2022.100046.

6

Neoplasia

Cancer is the second leading cause of death in the United States; only cardiovascular diseases exact a higher toll. Cancer is not one disease but many, all sharing a profound dysregulation of growth. Some types of cancer are curable, while others are virtually always fatal. Advances in diagnosis, treatment, and prognosis will depend on a deeper understanding of the molecular and cellular basis of each type of cancer.

This chapter deals with the basic biology of neoplasia—the nature of benign and malignant neoplasms and the molecular basis of neoplastic transformation. The host response to tumors and the clinical features of neoplasia are also discussed. Before turning to the defining characteristics of cancer cells and the mechanisms of carcinogenesis, we first summarize the fundamental and shared features of all cancers:

- **Cancer is a genetic disorder caused by DNA mutations.** Pathogenic mutations may occur due to exposure to mutagens, may occur spontaneously due to error-prone processes in cells, or may be inherited. In addition, cancers frequently show epigenetic alterations (e.g., altered DNA methylation and histone modification). In concert, these genetic and epigenetic abnormalities alter the expression or function of key genes that regulate fundamental cellular processes, such as growth, survival, and senescence.
- **Genetic alterations in cancer cells are heritable, being passed to daughter cells upon cell division; as a result, cells harboring these mutations are subject to Darwinian selection (survival of the fittest).** Cells bearing mutations that provide a growth or survival advantage outcompete their neighbors and thus come to dominate the population. At the time of tumor initiation, these selective advantages are conferred on a single cell and, as a result, individual tumors are *clonal* (i.e., the progeny of one cell). However, beyond the point of initiation Darwinian selection continues to shape the clonal evolution of cancers by favoring the proliferation of genetically distinct subclones with more aggressive characteristics, a concept referred to as *tumor progression.*
- **Mutations and epigenetic alterations impart to cancer cells a set of properties that are referred to collectively as *cancer hallmarks*.** These properties produce the cellular phenotypes that dictate the natural history of cancers as well as their response to various therapies. The molecular underpinnings of each hallmark of cancer are discussed later.

Basic research has elucidated many of the cellular and molecular abnormalities that give rise to cancer and govern its behavior. These insights are in turn leading to a revolution in the diagnosis and treatment of cancer, an evolving triumph of biomedical science.

NOMENCLATURE

Neoplasia means "new growth," and neoplastic cells are said to be "transformed" because they replicate incessantly as a result of resistance to the regulatory influences that control normal cells. Neoplasms therefore enjoy a degree of autonomy, but some important dependencies remain. All neoplasms, for example, depend on the host for their nutrition and blood supply, and neoplasms derived from hormone responsive tissues often require endocrine support. As we will discuss, such dependencies can sometimes be exploited therapeutically.

In common medical usage, a neoplasm is often referred to as a *tumor,* and the study of tumors is called *oncology* (from *oncos,* "tumor," and *logos,* "study of"). Tumors are generally categorized as benign or malignant, an assessment that is central to the accurate prediction of a tumor's behavior and prognosis.

- *A tumor is said to be* benign *when its microscopic and gross characteristics indicate that it will remain localized and is amenable to local surgical removal.* Patients with benign tumors can generally be cured of their disease. However, not all benign tumors are easily excised, and some produce significant morbidity or are even lethal, particularly if they are located near a vital structure or organ.
- *Malignant, as applied to a neoplasm, implies that the lesion may be locally invasive and has the capacity to spread to distant sites (metastasize).* Malignant tumors are collectively referred to as *cancers,* derived from the Latin word for "crab," as they infiltrate and seize upon normal tissues in an obstinate manner, similar to a crab's behavior. Not all cancers pursue an aggressive course, and, paradoxically, some of the most aggressive are also highly curable, but the designation *malignant* constitutes a red flag.

All tumors, benign and malignant, have two basic components: (1) *parenchyma,* made up of transformed or neoplastic cells and (2) *stroma,* the supporting host-derived, nonneoplastic connective tissue, inflammatory cells, and blood vessels. Even leukemias, neoplasms in which the malignant cells circulate in the blood (Chapter 10), depend on stromal interactions to support the growth of the tumor cells. The parenchyma of the neoplasm largely determines its biologic behavior, and it is this component from which the tumor derives its name. However, the stroma is crucial to the growth of the neoplasm, since it provides the blood supply. Moreover, stromal cells and tumor cells carry on a two-way conversation that influences the behavior and growth pattern of tumor cells.

Benign Tumors

In general, benign tumors are designated by attaching the suffix -*oma* to the cell type from which the tumor arises. For example, a benign tumor of fibroblasts is a *fibroma*; a benign cartilaginous tumor is a *chondroma*. More complex nomenclature is used for benign epithelial tumors.

- *Adenoma* is applied to most benign epithelial neoplasms, including those that produce glandlike structures and those that do not.
- *Papilloma* refers to a benign epithelial neoplasm that produces microscopic or macroscopic fingerlike fronds (eFig. 6.1).
- *Polyp* refers to a mass that projects above a mucosal surface to form a macroscopically visible structure (Fig. 6.1). Although this term is commonly used for benign tumors, some malignant tumors may grow as polyps, and other polyps (such as nasal polyps) are not neoplastic but inflammatory in origin.
- *Cystadenoma* refers to hollow cystic mass; these are most common in the ovary (Chapter 17).

Malignant Tumors

The nomenclature of malignant tumors essentially follows that of benign tumors, with certain additions and exceptions. Although the nomenclature of neoplasms is complex (and sometimes inconsistent), students must be familiar with it because it is the means by which a tumor's nature and significance are conveyed by physicians.

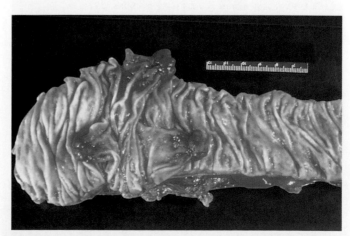

FIG. 6.1 Colonic polyps. Several pedunculated "velvety" polyps are seen in this segment of colon.

- Malignant neoplasms arising in "solid" mesenchymal tissue or its derivatives are named *sarcomas,* whereas those arising from the cells of the blood are called *leukemias* or *lymphomas.* Sarcomas are designated based on their principal cell type. Thus, a malignant neoplasm comprising fatlike cells is a *lipo*sarcoma, and a malignant neoplasm composed of chondrocyte-like cells is a *chondro*sarcoma.

- Although epithelia may be derived from all three germ cell layers, malignant neoplasms of epithelial cells are called *carcinomas* regardless of the tissue of origin. Thus, malignant neoplasms arising in the renal tubular epithelium (mesoderm), the skin (ectoderm), or lining epithelium of the gut (endoderm) are all considered carcinomas.

- Carcinomas are subdivided further. Carcinomas that grow in a glandular pattern are called *adenocarcinomas,* and those that produce squamous cells are called *squamous cell carcinomas.* Sometimes the tissue or organ of origin is specified, as in the designation of renal cell carcinoma. Tumors may show little or no differentiation; these are referred to as *poorly differentiated* or *undifferentiated carcinoma.*

The neoplastic cells in a tumor, whether benign or malignant, usually resemble each other, consistent with their origin from a single transformed progenitor cell. In some unusual instances, however, the tumor cells undergo divergent differentiation, creating so-called "mixed tumors." Mixed tumors are clonal, but the progenitor cell in such tumors has the capacity to differentiate along more than one lineage. One example is mixed tumor of the salivary gland, commonly referred to as *pleomorphic adenoma.* This benign tumor has epithelial components dispersed throughout a fibromyxoid stroma, sometimes harboring islands of cartilage or bone (Fig. 6.2). *Teratoma* is a special type of mixed tumor that contains recognizable mature or immature cells or tissues derived from more than one germ cell layer, and sometimes all three. Teratomas originate from totipotent germ cells, which normally reside in the ovary and testis and may be present in midline embryonic rests. Germ cells have the capacity to differentiate

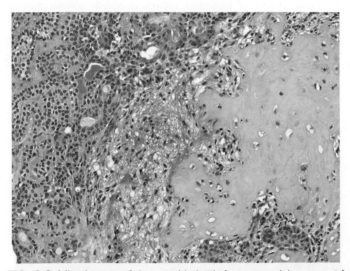

FIG. 6.2 Mixed tumor of the parotid gland. Areas containing nests of epithelial cells (on the left) and myxoid stroma forming cartilage and bone (an unusual feature, on the right) are present in this field. (From Fletcher CD: *Diagnostic Histopathology of Tumors,* ed 5, Philadelphia, 2021, Elsevier, Fig. 7.11.)

into any of the cell types found in the adult body; therefore, they may give rise to neoplasms that contain elements resembling bone, epithelium, muscle, fat, nerve, and other tissues, mixed together in a helter-skelter fashion (eFig. 6.2).

The specific names of the more common neoplasms are presented in Table 6.1. Some glaring inconsistencies may be noted. For example, the terms *lymphoma, mesothelioma, melanoma,* and *seminoma* are used for malignant neoplasms. Unfortunately for students, these exceptions are firmly entrenched in medical terminology. There are also other instances of confusing terminology:

- *Hamartoma* is a mass of disorganized tissue resembling the involved site, such as the lung or the liver. Although historically thought of as developmental malformations, hamartomas have clonal chromosomal aberrations that are acquired through somatic mutations and are best considered unusual benign neoplasms.

- *Choristoma* is a congenital anomaly consisting of a heterotopic nest of cells. For example, a small nodule of pancreatic tissue may be found in the submucosa of the stomach, duodenum, or small intestine. The designation *-oma,* connoting a neoplasm, gives these lesions an undeserved gravity, as they are usually trivial.

CHARACTERISTICS OF BENIGN AND MALIGNANT NEOPLASMS

Three features can be used to distinguish between most benign and malignant tumors: differentiation and anaplasia; local invasion; and metastasis. In general, rapid growth also signifies malignancy, but some malignant tumors grow slowly and as a result growth rate is not a reliable discriminator. Although some neoplasms defy easy characterization, in most instances the determination of benign versus malignant is made with remarkable accuracy using long-established criteria.

Differentiation and Anaplasia

Differentiation refers to the extent to which neoplasms resemble their cells of origin; lack of differentiation is called *anaplasia.* In general, benign neoplasms are composed of well-differentiated cells that closely resemble their normal counterparts. A lipoma is made up of mature fat cells laden with cytoplasmic lipid vacuoles, and a chondroma is made up of mature cartilage cells that synthesize cartilaginous matrix—evidence of morphologic and functional differentiation (eFig. 6.3). In well-differentiated benign tumors, mitoses are usually rare and are of normal configuration.

By contrast, most malignant neoplasms exhibit morphologic alterations that demonstrate their malignant nature. In well-differentiated cancers (Fig. 6.3), these features may be quite subtle. For example, well-differentiated adenocarcinoma of the thyroid gland may contain normal-appearing follicles, its malignant potential being revealed only by invasion into adjacent tissues or metastasis. In addition, cancers may induce stromal responses that are not seen in benign tumors. For example, certain cancers induce a dense, abundant fibrous stroma *(desmoplasia),* making them hard, "scirrhous" tumors.

Tumors composed of undifferentiated cells are said to be *anaplastic,* a feature that is a reliable indicator of malignancy. The term *anaplasia* literally means "backward formation"—implying dedifferentiation, or loss of the structural and functional differentiation of normal cells. In some instances, dedifferentiation of apparently mature cells occurs during carcinogenesis. However, other cancers arise from stem cells in tissues; in these tumors, failure of

Table 6.1 Nomenclature of Selected Tumors

Tissue of Origin	Benign	Malignant
Tumors Composed Predominantly of a Single Cell Type		
Connective tissue and derivatives	Fibroma	Fibrosarcoma
	Lipoma	Liposarcoma
	Chondroma	Chondrosarcoma
	Osteoma	Osteosarcoma
Endothelium and related cell types		
Blood vessels	Hemangioma	Angiosarcoma
Lymph vessels	Lymphangioma	Lymphangiosarcoma
Mesothelium		Mesothelioma
Brain coverings	Meningioma	Invasive meningioma
Blood cells and related cell types		
Hematopoietic cells		Leukemias
Lymphoid tissue		Lymphomas
Muscle		
Smooth	Leiomyoma	Leiomyosarcoma
Striated	Rhabdomyoma	Rhabdomyosarcoma
Skin		
Stratified squamous	Squamous cell papilloma	Squamous cell or epidermoid carcinoma
Basal cells of skin or adnexa		Basal cell carcinoma
Tumors of melanocytes	Nevus	Melanoma
Epithelial lining of glands or ducts	Adenoma	Adenocarcinoma
	Papilloma	Papillary carcinomas
	Cystadenoma	Cystadenocarcinoma
Lung	Bronchial adenoma	Bronchogenic carcinoma
Kidney	Renal tubular adenoma	Renal cell carcinoma
Liver	Hepatic adenoma	Hepatocellular carcinoma
Bladder	Urothelial papilloma	Urothelial carcinoma
Placenta	Hydatidiform mole	Choriocarcinoma
Testicle		Seminoma Embryonal carcinoma
Ovary	Serous cystadenoma, mucinous cystadenoma	Serous cystadenocarcinoma, mucinous cystadenocarcinoma
Tumors Composed of Multiple Cell Types Normally Derived From the Same Germ Cell Layer		
Salivary glands	Pleomorphic adenoma (mixed tumor of salivary gland)	Malignant mixed tumor of salivary gland
Renal anlage		Wilms tumor
Tumors Composed of Multiple Cell Types Normally Derived From More Than One Germ Cell Layer		
Totipotential cells in gonads or in embryonic rests	Mature teratoma, dermoid cyst	Immature teratoma, teratocarcinoma

differentiation of transformed stem cells, rather than dedifferentiation of specialized cells, accounts for their anaplastic appearance. Anaplastic cells often display the following features:

- *Cellular and nuclear pleomorphism.* Tumor cells and their nuclei show great variation in shape and size (Fig. 6.4). In addition nuclei show hyperchromasia (dark staining), or unusually prominent single or multiple nucleoli. Enlargement of nuclei may result in an increased nuclear-to-cytoplasmic ratio that approaches 1 : 1 instead of the normal 1 : 4 or 1 : 6. Nucleoli may attain astounding sizes, sometimes approaching the diameter of normal lymphocytes.

- *Tumor giant cells* may be formed. These are considerably larger than neighboring cells and may possess either one enormous nucleus or several nuclei (see Fig. 6.4).
- *Atypical mitoses,* which may be numerous. Multiple spindles may produce tripolar or quadripolar mitotic figures (Fig. 6.5).
- *Loss of polarity,* such that cells grow in sheets, with loss of normal orientation and absence of identifiable growth patterns, such as glands or stratified squamous architecture

Well-differentiated tumor cells are likely to retain the functional capabilities of their normal counterparts, whereas anaplastic tumor

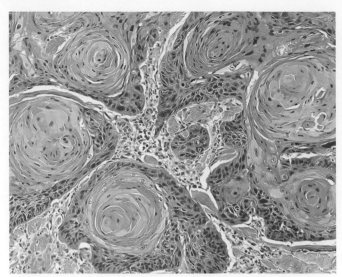

FIG. 6.3 Well-differentiated squamous cell carcinoma of the skin. Note the terminal differentiation of the tumor cells, which are forming keratin pearls. (From Fletcher CD: *Diagnostic Histopathology of Tumors,* ed 5, Philadelphia, 2021, Elsevier, Fig. 23.42.)

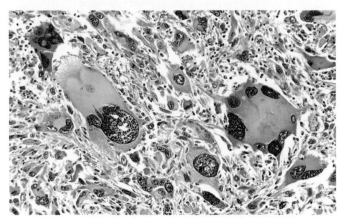

FIG. 6.4 Pleomorphic malignant tumor (rhabdomyosarcoma). Note the marked variation in cell and nuclear sizes, the hyperchromatic nuclei, and the presence of tumor giant cells. (Courtesy of Dr. Trace Worrell, Department of Pathology, University of Texas Southwestern Medical School, Dallas, Texas.)

cells are much less likely to have specialized functional activities. For example, benign neoplasms and even well-differentiated cancers of endocrine glands frequently elaborate the hormones characteristic of their cell of origin. Similarly, well-differentiated squamous cell carcinomas produce keratin (see Fig. 6.3), just as well-differentiated hepatocellular carcinomas secrete bile. In other instances, unanticipated functions emerge. Some cancers express fetal proteins not produced by comparable cells in the adult. Cancers of nonendocrine origin may also produce so-called "ectopic hormones." For example, certain lung carcinomas secrete adrenocorticotropic hormone (ACTH), parathyroid hormone—like hormone, insulin, glucagon, and others. More is said about these so-called "paraneoplastic" phenomena later.

Also relevant in the discussion of differentiation and anaplasia is *dysplasia,* referring to disorderly proliferation. **Dysplastic epithelium is recognized by loss of uniformity of individual cells and disturbed architectural orientation.** Dysplastic cells exhibit pleomorphism and

often possess abnormally large, hyperchromatic nuclei. Mitotic figures are more abundant than usual and frequently appear in the superficial epithelium, an abnormal location. In addition, there is architectural disarray. For example, the usual progressive maturation of tall cells in the basal layer to flattened squames on the surface of squamous epithelium may be lost, such that the epithelium consists of a disordered mixture of dark basal-appearing cells. When dysplastic changes are severe and involve the entire thickness of the epithelium, the lesion is referred to as *carcinoma in situ,* a preinvasive stage of cancer (Fig. 6.6).

It is important to appreciate that dysplasia is not synonymous with cancer. Mild to moderate dysplasia sometimes regresses completely, particularly if inciting causes are removed. However, dysplasia is often present adjacent to frankly malignant neoplasms (e.g., in lung carcinomas arising in the context of cigarette smoking) and as a general rule marks a tissue as being at increased risk for cancer development.

Local Invasion

The growth of cancers is accompanied by progressive infiltration, invasion, and destruction of surrounding tissues, whereas most benign tumors grow as cohesive expansile masses that remain localized. Because benign tumors grow and expand slowly, they usually develop a rim of compressed fibrous tissue, often called the capsule (Fig. 6.7). The capsule consists of extracellular matrix that is deposited by stromal cells such as fibroblasts, which may be activated by the mechanical stress created by compression of normal tissue by the expanding tumor. Encapsulation creates a tissue plane that makes the tumor discrete, moveable (nonfixed), and readily excisable by surgical enucleation. However, not all benign neoplasms are encapsulated. For example, uterine leiomyoma is discretely demarcated from the surrounding smooth muscle by a zone of compressed and attenuated normal myometrium but lacks a capsule. A few benign tumors are neither encapsulated nor discretely defined; lack of demarcation is particularly likely in benign vascular neoplasms such as hemangiomas, which may be difficult to excise. These exceptions are pointed out only to emphasize that, although encapsulation is the rule in benign tumors, the lack of a capsule does not mean a tumor is malignant.

Next to the development of metastases, invasiveness is the feature that most reliably distinguishes cancers from benign tumors (Fig. 6.8). Cancers lack well-defined capsules. There are instances in which a slowly growing malignant tumor, such as follicular carcinoma

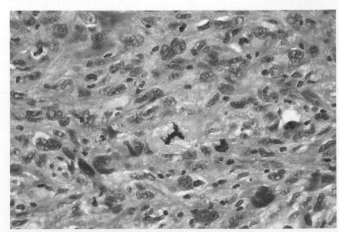

FIG. 6.5 High-power detailed view of anaplastic tumor cells shows cellular and nuclear variation in size and shape. The prominent cell in the center field has an abnormal tripolar spindle.

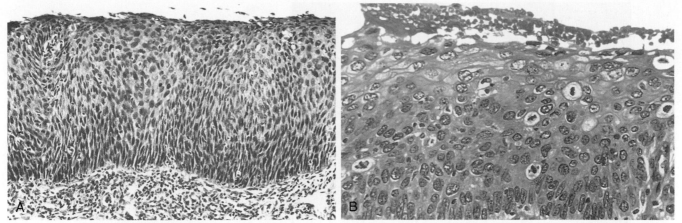

FIG. 6.6 Carcinoma in situ. (A) Low-power view shows that the entire thickness of the epithelium is replaced by atypical dysplastic cells. There is no orderly differentiation of squamous cells. The basement membrane is intact, and there is no tumor in the subepithelial stroma. (B) High-power view of another region shows failure of normal differentiation, marked nuclear and cellular pleomorphism, and numerous mitotic figures extending toward the surface. The intact basement membrane *(below)* is not seen in this section.

of thyroid, appears to be encased by a capsule, but careful microscopic examination reveals tiny tongues of tumor penetrating the margin and infiltrating adjacent structures. This infiltrative mode of growth makes it necessary to remove a wide margin of surrounding normal tissue when complete excision of a malignant tumor is attempted. Pathologists carefully examine the margins of resected tumors to ensure they are devoid of cancer cells *(clean surgical margins)*.

Metastasis

Metastasis is defined by the spread of a tumor to sites that are physically discontinuous with the primary tumor and is one of the hallmarks of malignant tumors. The invasiveness of cancers permits them to penetrate blood vessels, lymphatics, and body cavities, providing opportunities for spread (Fig. 6.9). Overall, approximately 30% of patients with newly diagnosed solid tumors (excluding skin cancers other than melanomas) present with clinically evident metastases, and an additional 20% have occult metastases at the time of diagnosis.

In general, large anaplastic neoplasms are more likely to have metastasized at diagnosis, but there are exceptions. Extremely small cancers may metastasize; conversely, some large and ominous-looking lesions may not. While all malignant tumors can metastasize, some do so very infrequently. For example, basal cell carcinomas of the skin and most primary tumors of the central nervous system are locally invasive but rarely metastasize. It is evident then that the properties of local invasion and metastasis are separable.

A special circumstance involves so-called "blood cancers," the leukemias and lymphomas. These tumors are derived from blood-forming cells that normally have the capacity to enter the bloodstream and travel to distant sites; as a result, with only rare exceptions, leukemias and lymphomas are assumed to be disseminated at diagnosis and are always considered to be malignant.

Malignant neoplasms disseminate by one of three pathways: (1) seeding within body cavities; (2) lymphatic spread; or (3) hematogenous spread. *Spread by seeding* occurs when neoplasms invade a body cavity. This mode of dissemination is particularly

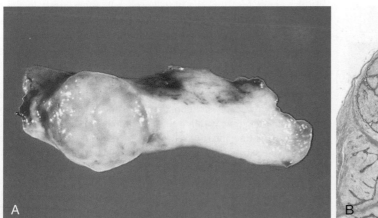

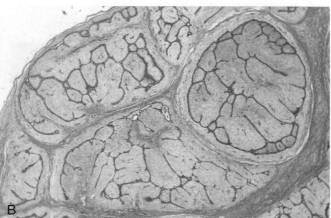

FIG. 6.7 Fibroadenoma of the breast. (A) The tan, encapsulated tumor is sharply demarcated from surrounding white breast tissue. (B) A microscopic view shows cords of entrapped dark staining epithelium compressed by a loose fibrous stroma surrounded by bands of collagen. (B, From Fletcher CD: *Diagnostic Histopathology of Tumors,* ed 5, Philadelphia, 2021, Elsevier, Fig. 16.15A.)

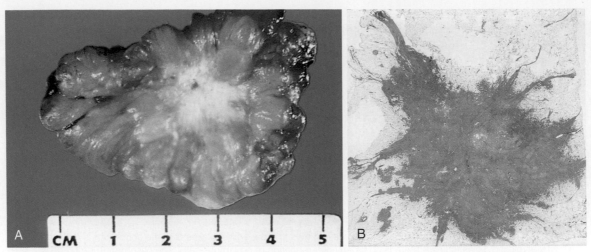

FIG. 6.8 Invasive ductal carcinoma of the breast. (A) Cut section shows that the stony-hard lesion is retracted and infiltrates the surrounding breast substance. (B) A microscopic view shows invasion of breast stroma and fat by nests and cords of tumor cells. Note the absence of a well-defined capsule. (Courtesy of Dr. Susan Lester, Brigham and Women's Hospital, Boston, Massachusetts.)

characteristic of cancers of the ovary, which often cover the peritoneal surfaces widely yet may not invade the underlying tissues. In this instance, the ability to implant and grow at distant sites seems to be separable from the capacity to invade. Neoplasms of the central nervous system, such as a medulloblastoma or ependymoma, may penetrate the cerebral ventricles and be carried by the cerebrospinal fluid until they implant on the meningeal surfaces surrounding the brain or spinal cord.

Lymphatic spread is more typical of carcinomas, whereas hematogenous spread is favored by sarcomas. There are numerous interconnections, however, between the lymphatic and vascular systems, so all forms of cancer may disseminate through either or both systems. The pattern of lymph node involvement depends on the site of the primary neoplasm and the pathways of local lymphatic drainage. Lung carcinomas arising in the respiratory passages metastasize first to the regional bronchial lymph nodes and then to the tracheobronchial and hilar nodes. Carcinoma of the breast usually arises in the upper outer quadrant and spreads first to the axillary nodes; however, medial breast lesions may drain to the nodes along the internal mammary artery. Thereafter, in both instances, the supraclavicular and infraclavicular nodes may be seeded. In some cases, cancer cells travel in lymphatic channels through the immediately proximal nodes only to be trapped in subsequent lymph nodes, producing so-called "skip metastases." The cells may also traverse all the lymph nodes and reach the vascular compartment by way of the thoracic duct.

A **"sentinel lymph node" is the first regional lymph node that receives lymph flow from a primary tumor.** It can be identified by injection of dyes or radiolabeled tracers near the primary tumor. Biopsy of sentinel lymph nodes allows determination of the extent of tumor spread and can be used to plan treatment. Of note, although enlargement of nodes near a primary neoplasm should raise concern of metastatic spread, it does not always indicate cancerous involvement. The necrotic cells of the neoplasm and tumor antigens often evoke immunologic responses in draining nodes that lead to reactive hyperplasia *(lymphadenitis)*. Thus, biopsy is necessary to determine if an enlarged lymph node is involved by tumor.

Hematogenous spread of cancers is most likely to occur through the penetration of thin-walled veins instead of thick-walled arteries. With venous invasion, the bloodborne cells often arrest in the first capillary bed they encounter. Since the portal system flows to the liver and caval blood flows to the lungs, the liver and lungs are the most frequent sites of hematogenous dissemination. Cancers arising in organs near the vertebral column such as the thyroid and prostate often embolize through the paravertebral plexus, possibly explaining the proclivity of these cancers to spread to the spine. Other carcinomas, particularly renal cell carcinoma and hepatocellular carcinoma, have a propensity to grow within veins in a snakelike fashion, sometimes extending up the inferior vena cava to the right side of the heart. Remarkably, such intravenous growth may not be accompanied by widespread dissemination.

In addition to the stepwise spread of cancers to the next draining lymph node or capillary bed, other cancers frequently spread to noncontiguous organs. For example, prostatic carcinoma preferentially spreads to bone, bronchogenic carcinoma tends to involve the adrenal glands and the brain, neuroblastoma spreads to the liver and bones, and uveal melanoma spreads to the liver. Conversely, other tissues such as skeletal muscle, although rich in capillaries, are rarely sites of

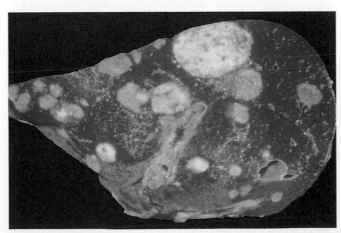

FIG. 6.9 A liver studded with metastatic cancer.

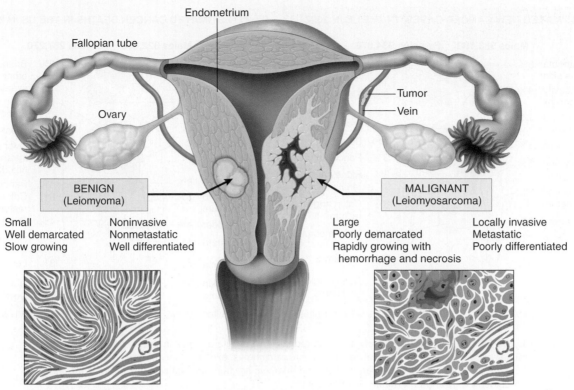

FIG. 6.10 Comparison between a benign tumor of the myometrium (leiomyoma) and a malignant tumor of similar origin (leiomyosarcoma).

tumor metastases. The molecular basis of such tissue-specific homing of tumor cells is discussed later.

Thus, numerous features of tumors (summarized in Fig. 6.10) usually permit the differentiation of benign and malignant neoplasms.

EPIDEMIOLOGY

Major insights into the causes of cancer have been obtained by identifying associations between particular environmental, hereditary, or cultural influences and specific neoplasms. The well-established causal association of cigarette smoking with lung cancer arose primarily from epidemiologic studies. A comparison of the incidence rates for colon cancer and dietary patterns in the Western world and in Africa led to the recognition that dietary fat and fiber content may contribute significantly to the causation of this cancer. Certain diseases associated with an increased risk for cancer also provide clues to cancer pathogenesis. Next, we first summarize the overall magnitude of cancer incidence and then review factors relating to the patient and the environment that influence the predisposition to cancer.

Cancer Incidence

For the year 2018, it is estimated that there were over 17 million cases of cancer and 9.6 million deaths due to cancer worldwide (approximately 26,300 deaths per day). Moreover, due to increasing population size, it is projected that the numbers of cancer cases and deaths worldwide will increase to 24 million and 14.6 million, respectively, by the year 2035. Additional perspective on the prevalence of specific cancers can be gained from national incidence and mortality data. In the United States, it is estimated that the year 2022 will be marked by 1.9 million new cases of cancer and 609,000 cancer deaths. Recent incidence data for the most common forms of cancers in the United States, with the major killers identified, are presented in Fig. 6.11.

The death rates for certain cancers in the United States have changed over several decades. Since 1995, the cancer death rate has decreased by roughly 20% in men and 10% in women. Among men, 80% of the decrease is attributed to lower death rates for cancers of the lung, prostate, and colon; among women, nearly 60% of the decrease is due to reductions in death rates from breast and colorectal cancers. Decreased use of tobacco products is responsible for the reduction in lung cancer deaths, while improved detection and treatment are responsible for the decrease in death rates for colorectal, female breast, and prostate cancers.

The last half-century has also seen a sharp decline in death rates from cervical cancer and gastric cancer in the United States. The decrease in cervical cancer is directly attributable to widespread use of the Papanicolaou (Pap) test for early detection of this tumor and its precursor lesions. The widespread deployment of the human papillomavirus (HPV) vaccine may nearly eliminate this cancer in coming years. The cause of the decline in death rates for cancer of the stomach is obscure; it may be related to decreasing exposure to unknown dietary carcinogens.

Environmental Factors

Environmental exposures are dominant risk factors for many common cancers, suggesting that many cancers are preventable. This notion is supported by the geographic variation in death rates from specific cancers, which is thought to stem mainly from differences in environmental exposures. For instance, death rates from breast cancer are about four to five times higher in the United States and Europe than in Japan. Conversely, the death rate for gastric carcinoma in men and women is about seven times higher in Japan than

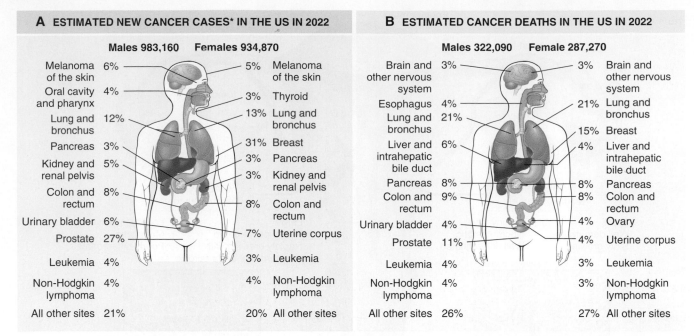

FIG. 6.11 Estimated cancer incidence (A) and mortality (B) by site and sex in the United States. Excludes basal cell and squamous cell skin cancers and in situ carcinomas, except urinary bladder. The most common tumors are denoted by red text. (Data and derived numbers are from the National Cancer Institute - Surveillance Epidemiology and End Result [SEER] program.)

in the United States. Hepatocellular carcinoma is the most lethal cancer in many parts of Africa. Most evidence suggests that these geographic differences have environmental origins. For example, Nisei (second-generation Japanese living in the United States) have mortality rates for certain forms of cancer that are intermediate between those in natives of Japan and in Americans who have lived in the United States for many generations. The two rates come closer with each passing generation.

There is no paucity of environmental factors that contribute to cancer. They are present in the ambient environment, in the workplace, in food, and in personal practices. Some are universal (e.g., sunlight) whereas others are largely restricted to urban settings (e.g., asbestos) or particular occupations (Table 6.2). The most important environmental exposures linked to cancer include the following:

- *Diet.* Certain features of diet have been implicated as predisposing influences. More broadly, obesity, currently epidemic in the United States and other parts of the world, is associated with a modestly increased risk for developing many cancers.
- *Smoking,* particularly of cigarettes, is linked to cancer of the mouth, pharynx, larynx, esophagus, pancreas, bladder, and, most significantly, the lung, as 90% of lung cancer deaths are related to smoking.
- *Alcohol consumption.* Excess alcohol intake is an independent risk factor for cancers of the oropharynx, larynx, esophagus, breast, and (due to alcoholic cirrhosis) liver. Moreover, alcohol and tobacco smoking act synergistically to increase the risk for developing cancers of the upper airways and upper digestive tract.
- *Reproductive history.* There is strong evidence that lifelong cumulative exposure to estrogen stimulation, particularly if unopposed by progesterone, increases the risk for developing cancers of the endometrium and breast, both of which are estrogen-responsive tissues.
- *Infectious agents* are estimated to cause approximately 15% of cancers worldwide (discussed later).

Age and Cancer

In general, the frequency of cancer increases with age. Most cancer deaths occur between 55 and 75 years of age; the rate declines, along with the population base, after 75 years of age. The rising incidence with age is explained by the accumulation of somatic mutations in cells that drive the emergence of malignant neoplasms (discussed later), and by the decline in immune surveillance that accompanies aging.

Although cancer preferentially affects older adults, it is also responsible for slightly more than 10% of all deaths among children younger than 15 years of age (Chapter 5). The major lethal cancers in children are tumors of the central nervous system, leukemias, lymphomas, and soft tissue and bone sarcomas. As discussed later, study of childhood tumors such as retinoblastoma has provided fundamental insights into the pathogenesis of malignant transformation.

Acquired Predisposing Conditions

Acquired conditions that predispose to cancer include chronic inflammatory disorders, immunodeficiency states, and precursor lesions. Many chronic inflammatory conditions create a fertile "soil" for the development of malignant tumors (Table 6.3). Tumors arising in the context of chronic inflammation are mostly carcinomas but also include mesothelioma and several kinds of lymphoma. By contrast, immunodeficiency states mainly predispose to virus-induced cancers, including specific types of lymphoma and carcinoma and some sarcoma-like proliferations.

Precursor lesions are characterized by disturbances of epithelial differentiation that are associated with an elevated risk of carcinoma. They may arise secondary to chronic inflammation or hormonal imbalances (in endocrine-sensitive tissues) or occur spontaneously. Molecular analyses have shown that precursor lesions often possess some of the same genetic lesions that are found in their associated cancers (discussed later). However, progression to cancer is not

Table 6.2 Occupational Cancers

Agents or Groups of Agents	Human Cancers for Which Reasonable Evidence Is Available	Typical Use or Occurrence
Arsenic and arsenic compounds	Lung carcinoma, skin carcinoma	By-product of metal smelting; component of alloys, electrical and semiconductor devices, medications and herbicides, fungicides, and animal dips
Asbestos	Lung carcinoma, mesothelioma	Formerly used for many applications because of fire, heat, and friction resistance; still found in existing construction as well as fire-resistant textiles, friction materials (i.e., brake linings), underlayment and roofing papers, and floor tiles
Benzene	Acute myeloid leukemia	Principal component of light oil; despite known risk, many applications exist in printing and lithography, paint, rubber, dry cleaning, adhesives and coatings, and detergents; formerly widely used as solvent and fumigant
Cadmium and cadmium compounds	Prostate carcinoma	Uses include yellow pigments and phosphors; found in solders; used in batteries and as alloy and in metal platings and coatings
Chromium compounds	Lung carcinoma	Component of metal alloys, paints, pigments, and preservatives
Nickel compounds	Lung and oropharyngeal carcinoma	Nickel plating; component of ferrous alloys, ceramics, and batteries; by-product of stainless-steel arc welding
Radon and its decay products	Lung carcinoma	From decay of minerals containing uranium; potentially serious hazard in quarries and underground mines
Vinyl chloride	Hepatic angiosarcoma	Refrigerant; monomer for vinyl polymers; adhesive for plastics; formerly inert aerosol propellant in pressurized containers

Modified from Stellman JM, Stellman SD: Cancer and the workplace, *CA Cancer J Clin* 46:70–92, 1996, with permission from Lippincott Williams & Wilkins.

inevitable, and it is important to recognize precursor lesions because their removal or reversal lowers cancer risk.

Many different precursor lesions have been described; among the most common are the following:
- *Squamous metaplasia and dysplasia of bronchial mucosa,* seen in habitual smokers—a risk factor for lung carcinoma (Chapter 11)
- *Endometrial hyperplasia and dysplasia,* seen in women with unopposed estrogenic stimulation, is a risk factor for endometrial carcinoma (Chapter 17)
- *Leukoplakia of the oral cavity, vulva, and penis,* which may progress to squamous cell carcinoma (Chapters 13, 16, and 17)

- *Villous adenoma of the colon* is associated with a high risk for progression to colorectal carcinoma (Chapter 13)

In this context it also may be asked, "What is the risk for malignant change in a benign neoplasm?"—or, stated differently, "Are benign tumors precancers?" In general, the answer is no but, inevitably, there are exceptions; it may be better to say that each type of benign tumor is associated with a particular level of risk, ranging from high to virtually nonexistent. For example, adenomas of the colon undergo malignant transformation in up to 50% of cases, whereas malignant change is extremely rare in uterine leiomyomas.

Table 6.3 Chronic Inflammatory States and Cancer

Pathologic Condition	Associated Neoplasm(s)	Etiologic Agent
Asbestosis, silicosis	Mesothelioma, lung carcinoma	Asbestos fibers, silica particles
Inflammatory bowel disease	Colorectal carcinoma	
Lichen sclerosis	Vulvar squamous cell carcinoma	
Pancreatitis	Pancreatic carcinoma	Chronic alcohol use, germline mutations (e.g., in the trypsinogen gene)
Chronic cholecystitis	Gallbladder cancer	Bile acids, bacteria, gallbladder stones
Reflux esophagitis, Barrett esophagus	Esophageal adenocarcinoma	Gastric acid
Sjögren syndrome, Hashimoto thyroiditis	Extranodal marginal zone lymphoma	
Opisthorchis, cholangitis	Cholangiocarcinoma, colon carcinoma	Liver flukes (*Opisthorchis viverrini*)
Gastritis/ulcers	Gastric adenocarcinoma, extranodal marginal zone lymphoma	*Helicobacter pylori*
Hepatitis	Hepatocellular carcinoma	Hepatitis B and/or C virus
Osteomyelitis	Carcinoma in draining sinuses	Bacterial infection
Chronic cystitis	Bladder carcinoma	Schistosomiasis

Adapted from Tlsty TD, Coussens LM: Tumor stroma and regulation of cancer development, *Ann Rev Pathol Mech Dis* 1:119, 2006.

Interactions Between Environmental and Genetic Factors

Certain cancers are hereditary, usually due to germline mutations that affect the function of a gene that suppresses cancer (a so-called "tumor suppressor gene," discussed later). What then can be said about the influence of heredity on "sporadic" malignant neoplasms, which constitute roughly 95% of the cancers in the United States? While the evidence suggests that sporadic cancers are largely attributable to environmental factors or acquired predisposing conditions, it may be difficult to tease out hereditary and genetic contributions because environmental and genetic factors often interact. Such interactions may be particularly complex when tumor development is affected by small contributions from multiple genes. Furthermore, genetic factors may alter the risk for developing environmentally induced cancers. Instances where this holds true often involve inherited variation in enzymes such as components of the cytochrome P-450 system that metabolize procarcinogens to active carcinogens. Conversely, environmental factors can influence the risk for developing cancer, even in individuals who inherit well-defined "cancer genes."

CANCER GENES

Cancer is a disease caused by mutations that alter the function of a finite subset of the 20,000 or so human genes. For simplicity, we will refer to these genes as cancer genes. **Cancer genes can be defined as genes that are recurrently affected by genetic aberrations in cancers, presumably because they contribute directly to the malignant behavior of cancer cells.** Causative mutations that give rise to cancer genes may be acquired by the action of environmental agents (such as chemicals, radiation, or viruses), may occur spontaneously, or may be inherited in the germline. If such mutations drive carcinogenesis, a key prediction is that each cell in an individual tumor should share mutations that were present in the founding cell at the time of transformation. This expectation has been realized in all tumors that have been systematically analyzed by genomic sequencing, providing strong support for the hypothesis that cancer is at its root a genetic disease.

Cancer genes number in the hundreds and new ones are still being discovered. They fall into one of four major functional classes:

- *Oncogenes* induce a transformed phenotype when expressed in cells by promoting increased cell growth. Oncogenes are mutated or overexpressed versions of normal cellular genes, which are called *proto-oncogenes*. Most oncogenes encode transcription factors, factors that trigger progrowth signaling pathways, or factors that enhance cell survival. They are considered dominant genes because a mutation involving a single allele is sufficient to produce an oncogenic effect.
- *Tumor suppressor genes* normally prevent uncontrolled growth and, when mutated or lost from a cell, allow the transformed phenotype to develop. In most instances, both normal alleles of tumor suppressor genes must be damaged or silenced for transformation to occur. Tumor suppressor genes can be placed into two general groups: those that act as important brakes on cellular proliferation and those that are responsible for sensing genomic damage. The latter genes may initiate and choreograph a complex "damage control response" that leads to the cessation of proliferation or, if the damage is too great to be repaired, induce apoptosis.
- *Genes that regulate apoptosis* primarily influence cell survival, rather than stimulating proliferation. Understandably, genes of this class that protect against apoptosis are often overexpressed in cancer cells, whereas those that promote apoptosis tend to be underexpressed or functionally inactivated by mutations.
- To this list may now be added *genes that regulate interactions between tumor cells and host cells,* as these genes are also recurrently mutated or functionally altered in certain cancers. Particularly important are genes that enhance or inhibit recognition of tumor cells by the host immune system.

In most instances, the specific mutations that give rise to cancer genes are acquired during life and are confined to the cancer cells. However, specific causative mutations are sometimes inherited in the germline and are therefore present in every cell in the body, placing the affected individual at high risk for particular cancers (Table 6.4). We will touch on important familial cancer syndromes and associated genes and cancers later in this chapter.

Presented next is a discussion of the varied genetic lesions that underlie altered cancer gene expression and function.

GENETIC LESIONS IN CANCER

The genetic changes found in cancers vary from point mutations involving single nucleotides to abnormalities large enough to produce gross changes in chromosome structure. In certain neoplasms, genetic abnormalities are nonrandom and highly characteristic. Specific chromosomal abnormalities have been identified in many leukemias and lymphomas and in an increasing number of nonhematopoietic tumors, while other tumors are characterized by particular point mutations. These recurrent genetic changes alter the activity of one or more cancer genes in a fashion that gives the affected cells a selective advantage, presumably by contributing to one or more of the hallmarks of cancer.

Table 6.4 Inherited Predisposition to Cancer

Inherited Predisposition	Gene(s)
Autosomal Dominant Cancer Syndromes	
Retinoblastoma	*RB*
Li-Fraumeni syndrome (various tumors)	*TP53*
Melanoma	*CDKN2A*
Familial adenomatous polyposis/ colon cancer	*APC*
Neurofibromatosis 1 and 2	*NF1, NF2*
Breast and ovarian tumors	*BRCA1, BRCA2*
Multiple endocrine neoplasia 1 and 2	*MEN1, RET*
Hereditary nonpolyposis colon cancer	*MSH2, MLH1, MSH6*
Nevoid basal cell carcinoma syndrome	*PTCH1*
Autosomal Recessive Syndromes of Defective DNA Repair	
Xeroderma pigmentosum	Diverse genes involved in nucleotide excision repair
Ataxia-telangiectasia	*ATM*
Bloom syndrome	*BLM*
Fanconi anemia	Diverse genes involved in repair of DNA cross-links

Driver and Passenger Mutations

Driver mutations are mutations that alter the function of cancer genes and thereby directly contribute to the development or progression of cancer. They are usually acquired, but as mentioned earlier, occasionally inherited. By contrast, *passenger mutations* are acquired mutations that are neutral in terms of fitness and do not affect cellular behavior. Because they occur at random, passenger mutations are sprinkled throughout the genome, whereas driver mutations tend to be tightly clustered within cancer genes. It is now appreciated that passenger mutations may greatly outnumber driver mutations, particularly in cancers caused by carcinogen exposure, such as melanoma and smoking-related lung cancer.

Although apparently innocuous in nature, passenger mutations are important in several ways:

- In carcinogen-associated cancers, analysis of passenger mutations has provided definitive evidence that most genomic damage is directly caused by the carcinogen in question. For example, before sequencing of melanoma genomes, the causative role of sun exposure in this cancer was debated. This is no longer so, as most melanomas have thousands of passenger mutations of a type that is specifically linked to damage caused by ultraviolet light.
- One effect of passenger mutations is that they create genetic variants that, while initially neutral, may provide tumor cells with a selective advantage in the setting of therapy. The evidence for this comes from DNA sequence analyses of tumors at the time of recurrence after drug therapy. In many instances, mutations that lead directly to drug resistance are found in most tumor cells, generally in the target of the drug (e.g., a tyrosine kinase like BCR-ABL, described later). Generally, the same resistance mutations can also be found before therapy, but only in a very small fraction of cells. In such instances, it appears that the selective pressure of therapy "converts" a neutral passenger mutation into a driver mutation, contributing to tumor progression.
- Passenger mutations produce altered proteins that elicit host immune responses. The significance of this will become apparent when we discuss cancer immunity and immunotherapy.

Point Mutations

Point mutations can either activate or inactivate the protein products of the affected genes depending on their precise position and consequence. Point mutations that convert proto-oncogenes into oncogenes generally produce a gain of function by altering amino acid residues in a domain that normally holds the protein's activity in check. A cardinal example is point mutations that convert the proto-oncogene *RAS* into a cancer gene, one of the most common events in human cancers. By contrast, point mutations in tumor suppressor genes reduce or disable the function of the encoded protein. The tumor suppressor gene that is most commonly affected by point mutations in cancer is *TP53*, a prototypical tumor suppressor gene (discussed later).

Gene Rearrangements

Gene rearrangements may be produced by chromosomal translocations, inversions, deletions, or other more complex genetic events. Specific gene rearrangements are highly associated with certain malignancies, particularly neoplasms derived from hematopoietic cells and other kinds of mesenchymal cells. These rearrangements can activate proto-oncogenes in two ways:

- **Some gene rearrangements result in overexpression of proto-oncogenes by removing them from their normal regulatory elements and placing them under control of a highly active**

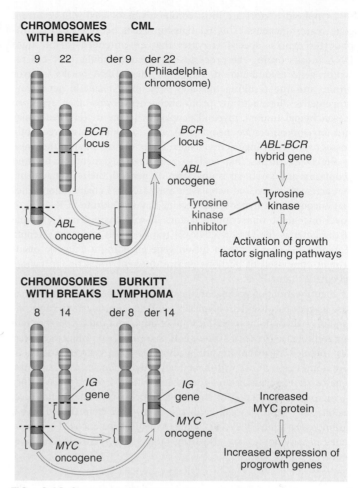

FIG. 6.12 Chromosomal translocations, involved oncogenes, and downstream oncogenic activities in chronic myeloid leukemia (CML) and Burkitt lymphoma. *der*, Derivative.

promoter or enhancer. Two different types of B-cell lymphoma provide illustrative examples of this mechanism. In more than 90% of cases of *Burkitt lymphoma,* the cells have a balanced reciprocal translocation, usually between chromosomes 8 and 14, that leads to overexpression of the *MYC* gene on chromosome 8 by juxtaposition of *MYC* with immunoglobulin heavy chain gene regulatory elements on chromosome 14 (Fig. 6.12). In *follicular lymphoma,* a balanced reciprocal translocation between chromosomes 14 and 18 leads to overexpression of the antiapoptotic gene *BCL2* on chromosome 18, also driven by immunoglobulin gene regulatory elements.

- **Other oncogenic gene rearrangements create fusion genes encoding novel chimeric proteins.** Most notable is the Philadelphia (Ph) chromosome in chronic myeloid leukemia (Chapter 10), which is usually created by a balanced reciprocal translocation between chromosomes 9 and 22 (see Fig. 6.12). This cytogenetic change is seen in more than 90% of cases of chronic myeloid leukemia and results in the fusion of portions of the *BCR* gene on chromosome 22 and the *ABL* gene on chromosome 9. The few Philadelphia chromosome–negative cases harbor cryptic (karyotypically invisible) *BCR-ABL* fusion genes, the presence of which is the *sine qua non* of chronic myeloid leukemia. As discussed later, the *BCR-ABL* fusion gene encodes a novel tyrosine kinase with potent transforming activity.

Lymphoid tumors are most commonly associated with recurrent gene rearrangements. This relationship exists because normal lymphocytes express special enzymes that are intended to introduce DNA breaks during the processes of immunoglobulin or T-cell receptor gene recombination. Repair of these DNA breaks is error prone, and the resulting mistakes sometimes result in gene rearrangements that activate proto-oncogenes. Two other types of mesenchymal tumors, myeloid neoplasms (acute myeloid leukemias and myeloproliferative neoplasms) and sarcomas, also frequently possess gene rearrangements. Unlike lymphoid neoplasms, the cause of the DNA breaks that lead to gene rearrangements in myeloid neoplasms and sarcomas is unknown. In general, the rearrangements that are seen in myeloid neoplasms and sarcomas create fusion genes that encode either hyperactive tyrosine kinases (akin to BCR-ABL) or novel oncogenic transcription factors. A well-characterized example of the latter is the (11;22)(q24;q12) translocation in Ewing sarcoma (Chapter 19) that creates a fusion gene encoding a chimeric oncoprotein composed of portions of two different transcription factors called EWS and FLI1.

Identification of pathogenic gene rearrangements in carcinomas has lagged because karyotypically evident translocations and inversions (which point to the location of important oncogenes) are rare in carcinomas. However, widespread sequencing of cancer genomes has revealed recurrent cryptic pathogenic gene rearrangements in carcinomas as well. As with hematologic malignancies and sarcomas, gene rearrangements in carcinoma contribute to carcinogenesis either by increasing expression of an oncogene or by generation of a novel fusion gene. Examples will be discussed in other chapters. As with a fusion gene such as BCR-ABL, some of the proteins encoded by fusion genes in carcinomas are also drug targets (e.g., EML-ALK in lung cancer; Chapter 11).

Deletions

Recurrent deletion of specific regions of chromosomes in cancer cells usually results in the loss of particular tumor suppressor genes. Tumor suppressive functions generally require inactivation of both alleles before antioncogenic activities are lost. A common mechanism is for an inactivating point mutation to occur in one allele and a deletion to occur in the other. As discussed later, deletions involving chromosome 13q14, the site of the RB gene, are associated with retinoblastoma, and deletion of chromosome 17p is associated with loss of TP53, perhaps the most important tumor suppressor gene.

Gene Amplifications

Proto-oncogenes may be converted to oncogenes by gene amplification, with consequent overexpression and hyperactivity of otherwise normal proteins. Such amplification may produce up to several hundred copies of a gene, a change in copy number that is readily detected by molecular hybridization with appropriate DNA probes. In some cases, the amplified genes produce chromosomal changes that can be identified microscopically. Two patterns are seen: (1) multiple small, extrachromosomal structures called *double minutes* and (2) *homogeneously staining regions*. The latter derive from the insertion of the amplified genes into new chromosomal locations, which may be distant from the normal location of the involved genes. Because regions containing amplified genes lack normal banding, they have a homogeneous staining pattern in a G-banded karyotype. Two clinically important examples of amplification involve the MYCN gene in neuroblastoma and the HER2 gene in breast cancers. In 25% to 30% of neuroblastomas, MYCN is amplified, a feature that is associated

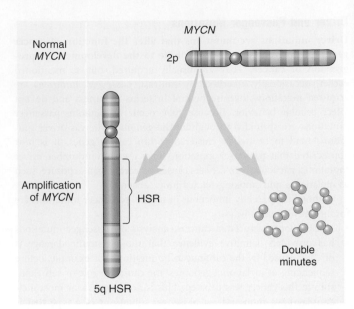

FIG. 6.13 Amplification of the *MYCN* gene in human neuroblastoma. The *MYCN* gene, present normally on chromosome 2p, becomes amplified and is seen either as extrachromosomal double minutes or as a chromosomally integrated homogeneous-staining region (HSR). (Modified from Brodeur GM, Seeger RC, Sather H, et al: Clinical implications of oncogene activation in human neuroblastomas. *Cancer* 58:541, 1986. Reprinted by permission of Wiley-Liss, Inc, a subsidiary of John Wiley & Sons, Inc.)

with poor prognosis (Fig. 6.13). HER2 (also known as *ERBB2*) amplification occurs in about 20% of breast cancers, and therapy directed against the receptor encoded by the HER2 gene is highly effective in this subset of tumors.

Aneuploidy

***Aneuploidy* is defined as a number of chromosomes that is not a multiple of the haploid state; for humans, that is any chromosome number that is not a multiple of 23.** Aneuploidy is remarkably common in cancers and was proposed as a cause of carcinogenesis over 100 years ago. It frequently results from errors of the mitotic checkpoint, a major cell cycle control mechanism that prevents mistakes in chromosome segregation by inhibiting the transition to anaphase until all of the replicated chromosomes have attached to spindle microtubules.

Mechanistic data establishing aneuploidy as a cause of carcinogenesis, rather than a consequence, have been difficult to generate. However, detailed analysis of cancer cells suggests that aneuploidy increases the copy number of key oncogenes and decreases the copy number of potent tumor suppressors. For example, chromosome 8, which is almost never lost and is often present in increased copies in tumor cells, is where the MYC oncogene is located. By contrast, portions of chromosome 17, where the TP53 gene is located, are often lost and infrequently gained. Thus, tumor development and progression may be molded by changes in chromosome numbers that enhance the dosage of oncogenes or decrease the dosage of tumor suppressor genes.

MicroRNAs and Cancer

As discussed in Chapter 4, microRNAs (miRNAs) are short, noncoding, single-stranded RNAs that function as negative regulators of genes. They inhibit gene expression posttranscriptionally by repressing translation or, in some cases, by promoting the cleavage of messenger RNA (mRNA). In view of their important functions in control of cell growth, differentiation, and survival, it is not surprising that miRNAs can also contribute to carcinogenesis. Specifically, if the target of a miRNA is a tumor suppressor gene, then overactivity of the miRNA can reduce the activity of the encoded tumor suppressor protein. Such miRNAs are sometimes referred to as *oncomirs*. Conversely, if a miRNA normally inhibits the translation of an oncogene, a reduction in the quantity or function of that miRNA will lead to overproduction of the oncogene product. Such relationships have been established by miRNA profiling of several human tumors. For example, down-regulation or deletion of certain miRNAs in some leukemias and lymphomas results in increased expression of *BCL2*, an antiapoptotic gene. Dysregulation of other miRNAs that control the expression of the *RAS* and *MYC* oncogenes has also been detected in lung tumors and in certain B-cell leukemias, respectively.

Epigenetic Modifications and Cancer

You will recall from Chapter 4 that epigenetics refers to reversible, heritable changes in gene expression that occur without mutation. Such changes involve posttranslational modifications of histones and DNA methylation, both of which affect gene expression. In normal, differentiated cells, a large portion of the genome is not expressed. These regions of the genome are silenced by DNA methylation and histone modifications. On the other hand, cancer cells are characterized by global DNA hypomethylation and selective promoter-localized hypermethylation. Indeed, it has become evident that tumor suppressor genes are sometimes silenced by hypermethylation of promoter sequences, rather than by mutation. In addition, genome-wide hypomethylation has been shown to cause chromosomal instability and to induce tumors in mice. Thus, epigenetic changes may influence carcinogenesis in many ways. As an added wrinkle, deep sequencing of cancer genomes has identified mutations in genes that regulate epigenetic modifications in many cancers. Thus, certain genetic changes in cancers may be selected because they lead to epigenetic alterations (e.g., DNA methylation and histone modifications) that favor cancer growth and survival.

CARCINOGENESIS: A MULTISTEP PROCESS

Carcinogenesis is a multistep process resulting from the accumulation of multiple genetic alterations that collectively give rise to the transformed phenotype and all of its associated hallmarks, discussed later. As mentioned earlier, the presence of driver mutations in some nonneoplastic precursor lesions suggests the need for additional mutations for transition to a full-blown cancer and thus supports this model.

Beyond tumor initiation from a single founding cell, it is important to recognize that cancers continue to undergo Darwinian selection and therefore continue to evolve (Fig. 6.14). It is well established that during their course cancers generally become more aggressive and acquire greater malignant potential, a phenomenon referred to as *tumor progression*. At the molecular level, tumor progression most likely results from mutations that accumulate independently in different cells. Some of these mutations may be lethal, but others may affect the function of cancer genes, thereby making the affected cells more adept at growth, survival, invasion, metastasis, or immune evasion. Due to this selective advantage, subclones that acquire these mutations may come to dominate one area of a tumor, either at the primary site or at sites of metastasis. **As a result of continuing mutation and Darwinian selection, even though malignant tumors are monoclonal in origin they are typically genetically heterogeneous by the time of their clinical presentation.** In advanced tumors exhibiting genetic instability, the extent of genetic heterogeneity may be enormous.

Genetic evolution shaped by Darwinian selection can explain the two most pernicious properties of cancers: the tendency over time for cancers to become both more aggressive and less responsive to therapy. Thus, genetic heterogeneity has implications not only for cancer progression but also for response to therapy. Experience has shown that when tumors recur after chemotherapy, the recurrent tumor is almost always resistant to the original drug regimen if it is given again. Experimental data suggest that this acquired resistance stems from the outgrowth of subclones that have, by chance, mutations (or epigenetic alterations) that confer drug resistance.

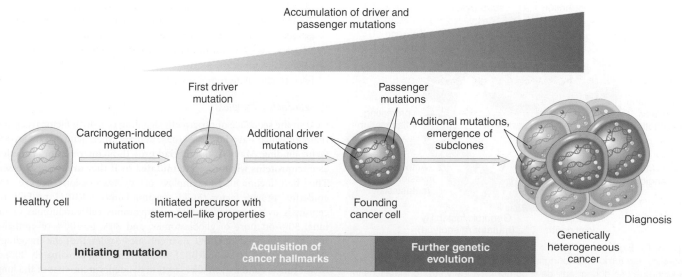

FIG. 6.14 Development of cancer through stepwise accumulation of complementary driver mutations. The order in which various driver mutations occur is usually unknown and may vary from tumor to tumor.

HALLMARKS OF CANCER

As mentioned earlier, bona fide cancer genes number in the hundreds, at a minimum. While it is traditional to describe the function of cancer genes one gene at a time, the blizzard of mutated genes emerging from the sequencing of cancer genomes has blanketed the landscape and revealed the limitations of trying to grasp the fundamental properties of cancer gene by gene. A more tractable and conceptually satisfying way to think about the biology of cancer is to consider the common phenotypic and biologic properties of cancer cells. It appears that **all cancers display several fundamental changes in cell physiology, which are considered the hallmarks of cancer.** These changes, illustrated in Fig. 6.15, consist of the following:

- *Self-sufficiency in growth signals*
- *Insensitivity to growth-inhibitory signals*
- *Altered cellular metabolism*
- *Evasion of apoptosis*
- *Limitless replicative potential (immortality)*
- *Sustained angiogenesis*
- *Invasion and metastasis*
- *Evasion of immune surveillance*

The acquisition of the genetic and epigenetic alterations that confer these hallmarks may be accelerated by *cancer-promoting inflammation* and by *genomic instability*. These are considered enabling characteristics because they aid and abet cellular transformation and subsequent tumor progression.

Mutations in genes that regulate some or all these cellular traits are seen in every cancer; accordingly, these traits form the basis of the following discussion of the molecular origins of cancer. Of note, by convention, gene symbols are italicized but their protein products are not (e.g., *RB* gene and RB protein, *TP53* and p53, *MYC* and MYC).

Self-Sufficiency in Growth Signals

The self-sufficiency in growth that characterizes cancer cells generally stems from gain-of-function mutations that convert proto-oncogenes to oncogenes. Oncogenes encode proteins called oncoproteins that promote cell growth even in the absence of normal growth-promoting signals. To appreciate how oncogenes drive inappropriate cell growth, it is helpful to review the sequence of events that characterize normal cell proliferation. Under physiologic conditions, signals that drive cell proliferation can be resolved into the following steps:

1. Binding of a growth factor to its specific receptor on the cell membrane
2. Transient and limited activation of the growth factor receptor, which in turn activates several signal-transducing proteins on the inner leaflet of the plasma membrane
3. Transmission of the transduced signal across the cytosol to the nucleus by second messengers or a cascade of signal transduction molecules
4. Induction and activation of nuclear regulatory factors that initiate and regulate DNA transcription and thus the biosynthesis of other cellular components that are needed for cell division, such as organelles, membrane components, and ribosomes
5. Entry and progression of the cell into the cell cycle, resulting ultimately in cell division

The mechanisms that endow cancer cells with the ability to proliferate can be grouped according to their role in the growth factor–induced signal transduction cascade and cell cycle regulation. Indeed, each one of the steps listed above is susceptible to perturbation in cancer cells.

Growth Factors

Cancers may secrete their own growth factors or induce stromal cells in the tumor microenvironment to produce growth factors. Most growth factors are made by one cell type and act on a neighboring cell of a different type to stimulate proliferation (paracrine action). Normally, cells that produce the growth factor do not express that factor's receptor, preventing the formation of positive feedback loops within the same cell. This "rule" is broken by certain cancers in several ways.

- Some cancer cells acquire the ability to synthesize the same growth factors to which they are responsive. For example, many glioblastomas secrete platelet-derived growth factor (PDGF) and have amplifications of the PDGF receptor gene, and many sarcomas secrete transforming growth factor-α (TGF-α) and express its receptor. Similar autocrine loops are fairly common in other types of cancer as well.
- In other cancers, the tumor cells send signals that induce normal cells in the supporting stroma to produce growth factors that feedback to stimulate tumor growth.

Growth Factor Receptors

Next in the sequence of progrowth signaling is growth factor receptors, many of which have intrinsic kinase activity when activated by growth factor binding. **Many of the myriad growth factor receptors function as oncoproteins when they are mutated or if they are overexpressed.** The best-documented examples of overexpression involve the epidermal growth factor (EGF) receptor family. ERBB1, the EGF receptor, is overexpressed in 80% of squamous cell carcinomas of the lung, 50% or more of glioblastomas, and 80% to 100% of epithelial tumors of the head and neck. As mentioned earlier, the gene encoding a related receptor, HER2 (ERBB2), is amplified in approximately 20% of breast cancers and in a smaller fraction of adenocarcinomas of the lung, ovary, stomach, and salivary glands. The significance of HER2 in the pathogenesis of breast cancers is illustrated dramatically by the clinical

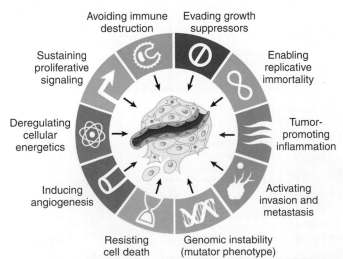

FIG. 6.15 Eight cancer hallmarks and two enabling factors (genomic instability and tumor-promoting inflammation). Most cancer cells acquire these properties during their development, typically due to mutations in critical genes. (From Hanahan D, Weinberg RA: Hallmarks of cancer: the next generation. *Cell* 144:646, 2011.)

benefit derived from blocking the extracellular domain of this receptor with anti-HER2 antibodies, an elegant example of "bench to bedside" medicine. In other instances, the tyrosine kinase activity of the receptors is stimulated by point mutations or small insertions or deletions that lead to subtle but functionally important changes in protein structure, or by gene rearrangements that create fusion genes encoding chimeric receptors. In each of these cases, the mutated receptors are either constitutively active, delivering mitogenic signals to cells even in the absence of growth factors, or are hyperresponsive to growth factors.

Downstream Signal-Transducing Proteins

Cancer cells often acquire growth autonomy as a result of mutations in genes that encode components of signaling pathways downstream of growth factor receptors. The signaling proteins that couple growth factor receptors to their nuclear targets are activated by ligand binding to growth factor receptors. Two particularly important oncogenic signaling molecules are RAS and ABL, which are discussed next.

RAS. RAS is the most commonly mutated oncogene in human tumors. Approximately 20% of all human tumors contain mutated *RAS* genes, and the frequency is even higher in specific cancers (e.g., pancreatic adenocarcinoma). RAS is a member of a family of small G proteins that bind guanosine nucleotides (guanosine triphosphate

[GTP] and guanosine diphosphate [GDP]). The activity of RAS is regulated by the relative binding of GDP and GTP.

- *Normally, RAS flips back and forth between an excited signal-transmitting state and a quiescent state.* RAS is inactive when bound to GDP; stimulation of cells by growth factors such as EGF and PDGF leads to exchange of GDP for GTP and subsequent conformational changes that activate RAS (Fig. 6.16). This excited signal-emitting state is short lived, however, because an intrinsic guanosine triphosphatase (GTPase) activity of activated RAS hydrolyzes GTP to GDP, releasing a phosphate group and returning the protein to its quiescent GDP-bound state. The GTPase activity of activated RAS is magnified dramatically by a family of GTPase-activating proteins (GAPs) that act as molecular brakes that prevent uncontrolled RAS activation by favoring hydrolysis of GTP to GDP.
- *Activated RAS stimulates downstream regulators of proliferation by several interconnected pathways that converge on the nucleus and alter the expression of genes that regulate growth, such as* MYC. While details of the signaling cascades (some illustrated in Fig. 6.16) downstream of RAS are not discussed here, an important point is that mutational activation of these signaling intermediates mimics the growth-promoting effects of activated RAS. For

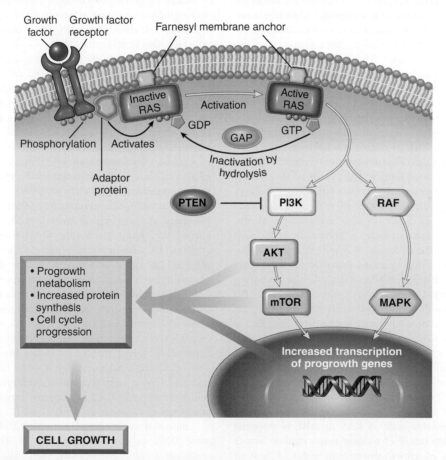

FIG. 6.16 Model for action of RAS. When a normal cell is stimulated through a growth factor receptor, inactive (GDP-bound) RAS is activated to a GTP-bound state. This activation is normally transient, due to an intrinsic GTPase activity in RAS and GTPase activating proteins (GAPs), which accelerate the breakdown of GTP. Activated RAS transduces proliferative, progrowth signals to the cell along two pathways: the so-called "RAF/MAP kinase pathway" and the "PI3K/AKT kinase" pathway. There are several closely related members of each component of the PI3K/AKT and RAF/MAP kinase pathways; one that is frequently mutated in cancer (BRAF) is discussed in the text. GAPs and a protein called PTEN, an inhibitor of PI3 kinase, act as important brakes on signaling downstream of activated RAS. *GDP,* Guanosine diphosphate; *GTP,* guanosine triphosphate; *MAPK,* mitogen-activated protein kinase; *mTOR,* mammalian target of rapamycin; *PI3K,* phosphatidylinositol 3-kinase.

example, BRAF, which is part of the so-called "RAF/ERK/MAP kinase pathway," is mutated in more than 60% of melanomas and is associated with unregulated cell proliferation. Mutations of phosphatidylinositol-3 kinase (PI3 kinase) in the PI3K/AKT pathway also occur with high frequency in some tumor types, with similar consequences.

RAS most commonly becomes constitutively activated as a result of point mutations in amino acid residues that are either within the GTP-binding pocket or in the enzymatic region that carries out GTP hydrolysis. Both types of mutations interfere with the breakdown of GTP so RAS stays in the GTP-bound active form and the cell receives continuous progrowth signals. It follows logically that the consequences of activating mutations in RAS should be mimicked by loss-of-function mutations in GAPs, which would also lead to decreased GTP hydrolysis. Indeed, the GAP neurofibromin-1 (NF1) is mutated in the cancer-prone familial disorder neurofibromatosis type 1 (Chapter 20) and is a bona fide tumor suppressor.

ABL. Several non–receptor tyrosine kinases function as signal transducing molecules. In this group, ABL is the best defined with respect to carcinogenesis.

The ABL proto-oncoprotein has tyrosine kinase activity that is dampened by internal negative regulatory domains. As discussed earlier (see Fig. 6.12), in chronic myeloid leukemia and certain acute leukemias, part of the *ABL* gene is translocated from its normal site on chromosome 9 to chromosome 22, where it fuses with part of the breakpoint cluster region (*BCR*) gene. This fusion gene encodes a BCR-ABL hybrid protein that contains the ABL tyrosine kinase domain and a BCR domain that self-associates, an event that mimics the effect of ligand binding and results in constitutive tyrosine kinase activity. Of interest, the BCR-ABL protein activates all the signals that are downstream of RAS, making it a potent stimulator of cell growth.

The crucial role of BCR-ABL in cancer has been confirmed by the dramatic clinical response of patients with chronic myeloid leukemia to BCR-ABL kinase inhibitors. The prototype of this kind of drug, imatinib mesylate, galvanized interest in the design of drugs that target specific molecular lesions found in various cancers (so-called "targeted therapy"). BCR-ABL is also an example of the concept of *oncogene addiction*, wherein a tumor is profoundly dependent on a single signaling molecule. *BCR-ABL* fusion gene formation is an early, perhaps initiating, event that drives leukemogenesis. Development of leukemia probably requires other collaborating mutations, but the transformed cell continues to depend on BCR-ABL for signals that mediate growth and survival. BCR-ABL signaling can be likened to a central pillar around which the transformed state is "built." If the pillar is removed by inhibition of the BCR-ABL kinase, the structure collapses. In view of this level of dependency, it is not surprising that acquired resistance of tumors to BCR-ABL inhibitors is often due to the outgrowth of a subclone with a mutation that prevents binding of the drug to the BCR-ABL protein.

Nuclear Transcription Factors. **The ultimate consequence of signaling through oncoproteins such as RAS or ABL is inappropriate and continuous stimulation of nuclear transcription factors that drive the expression of growth-promoting genes.** A host of oncoproteins, including products of the *MYC, MYB, JUN, FOS,* and *REL* oncogenes, function as transcription factors that regulate the expression of growth-promoting genes. Of these, MYC is involved most commonly in human tumors.

MYC. **Dysregulation of MYC promotes tumorigenesis by simultaneously promoting the progression of cells through the cell cycle and enhancing alterations in metabolism that support cell growth.** MYC primarily functions by activating the transcription of other genes, including several growth-promoting genes, such as cyclin-dependent kinases (CDKs), whose products drive cells into the cell cycle (discussed next), and genes that control metabolic pathways that produce the building blocks (e.g., amino acids, lipids, nucleotides) that are needed for cell growth and division. As mentioned earlier (see Fig. 6.12), in Burkitt lymphoma dysregulation of *MYC* results from a (8;14) translocation. In breast, colon, lung, and many other cancers *MYC* is amplified, while in neuroblastomas and small cell cancers of the lung, the related *MYCN* and *MYCL* genes are amplified, respectively.

Control of the Cell Cycle

The ultimate outcome of growth-promoting stimuli is the entry of quiescent cells into the cell cycle, a complex process that regulates cellular proliferation. In addition to mutations in growth factor signaling pathways (discussed earlier), cancer cells are often freed of the normal requirements for growth factors by mutations or other alterations in genes that encode components of the cell cycle machinery. To understand how these alterations contribute to carcinogenesis, we must first briefly review the cell cycle and its key regulators.

Following entry into the cell cycle, normal cells undergo a tightly choreographed sequence of events that lead to DNA replication and ultimately cell division. These events occur in four distinct phases called G_1 (Gap1), S (synthesis), G_2 (Gap2), and M (mitosis); quiescent cells that are not actively proliferating are in the G_0 state. Cells can enter G_1 either from the G_0 quiescent cell pool or after completing a round of mitosis. Each stage requires completion of the previous step as well as the activation of stage-specific factors (described next); the failure to complete DNA replication or a deficiency of essential cofactors results in the arrest of cells at the various transition points between cell cycle phases.

Cyclins, Cyclin-Dependent Kinases, and Cyclin-Dependent Kinase Inhibitors. **The cell cycle is regulated by numerous activators and inhibitors.** Cell-cycle progression is driven by proteins called *cyclins*—named for the cyclical rise and fall in their levels—and cyclin-associated enzymes called *cyclin-dependent kinases* (CDKs). CDKs acquire the ability to phosphorylate protein substrates (i.e., kinase activity) by forming complexes with specific cyclin partners (Fig. 6.17), an event that activates the CDK. Active CDKs phosphorylate multiple substrate proteins, altering their activity in a way that promotes cell cycle progression. Importantly, other factors are also activated that lead to cyclin degradation, albeit with a time delay, leading to the transient accumulation of cyclins in cells. More than 15 cyclins have been identified; cyclins D, E, A, and B appear sequentially during the cell cycle and bind to one or more CDKs. The cell cycle thus resembles a relay race in which each leg is regulated by a distinct set of cyclin/CDK complexes: as one collection of cyclin/CDK complexes leaves the track, the next set takes over.

Embedded in the cell cycle are surveillance mechanisms primed to sense DNA or chromosomal damage. These sensing mechanisms constitute quality-control *checkpoints,* which act to ensure that cells with genetic imperfections do not go forward in the cell cycle. Thus, the G_1-S checkpoint monitors the health of the cell and the integrity of its DNA before committing cellular resources to DNA replication and cell division. Later in the cell cycle, the G_2-M checkpoint ensures that the DNA has been accurately replicated before the cell actually divides. When cells do detect DNA irregularities, checkpoint activation delays cell-cycle progression and triggers DNA repair mechanisms. If the

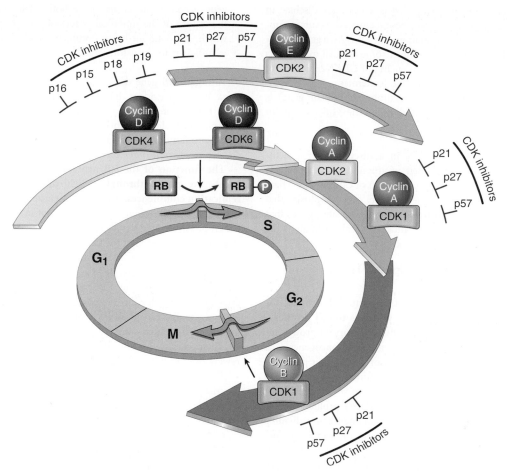

FIG. 6.17 Role of cyclins, CDKs, and CDK inhibitors in regulating the cell cycle. *Shaded arrows* represent the phases of the cell cycle during which specific cyclin-CDK complexes are active. Cyclin D-CDK4, cyclin D-CDK6, and cyclin E-CDK2 promote passage through the G_1-S checkpoint by phosphorylating the RB protein (RB-P). Cyclin A-CDK2 and cyclin A-CDK1 are active in S phase. Cyclin B-CDK1 is essential for the transition from G_2 to M phase. Two families of CDK inhibitors can block the activity of CDKs and progression through the cell cycle. The inhibitors, p15, p16, p18, and p19, act on cyclin D-CDK4 and cyclin D-CDK6. Inhibitors belonging to the other family, p21, p27, and p57, can inhibit all CDKs. *CDK,* Cyclin dependent kinase.

genetic derangement is too severe to be repaired, the cells either undergo apoptosis or enter a nonreplicative state called *senescence*—primarily through p53-dependent mechanisms (see later).

Enforcing the cell-cycle checkpoints is the job of *CDK inhibitors (CDKIs)*; they accomplish this by modulating CDK-cyclin complex activity. Defective CDKI checkpoint proteins allow cells with damaged DNA to divide, resulting in mutated daughter cells at risk for malignant transformation. There are several different CDKIs:

- One family of CDKIs—composed of three proteins called p21, p27, and p57—broadly inhibits multiple CDKs
- Another family of CDKIs has selective effects on cyclin CDK4 and cyclin CDK6; these proteins are called p15, p16, p18, and p19

An equally important aspect of cell growth and division is the biosynthesis of other cellular components needed to make two daughter cells, such as membranes and organelles. Thus, when growth factor receptor signaling stimulates cell-cycle progression, it also activates events that promote changes in cellular metabolism that support growth. Chief among these is the Warburg effect (discussed later), which is marked by increased cellular uptake of glucose and glutamine,

increased glycolysis, and (counterintuitively) decreased oxidative phosphorylation.

Dysregulation of the Cell Cycle in Cancer Cells. **Of the two main cell cycle checkpoints, the G1-S checkpoint is particularly likely to be lost in cancer cells.** Once cells pass through the G_1/S checkpoint, they are generally committed to undergo cell division, and thus cells with defects in this checkpoint proliferate excessively. Indeed, virtually all cancers appear to harbor genetic lesions that disable the G_1/S checkpoint, causing cells to continually reenter the S phase. For unclear reasons, particular lesions vary widely in frequency across tumor types, but they fall into two major categories.

- *Gain-of-function mutations involving CDK4 or D cyclins.* Changes increasing the expression of cyclin D or CDK4 are common events in neoplastic transformation. The cyclin D genes are overexpressed in many cancers, including those affecting the breast, esophagus, and liver, as well as a subset of lymphomas and plasma cell tumors. Amplification of the *CDK4* gene occurs in melanomas, sarcomas, and glioblastomas. Mutations affecting the genes encoding cyclins B and E and other CDKs also occur, but they are much less frequent than those affecting the genes encoding D cyclins and CDK4.

- *Loss-of-function mutations involving CDKIs.* CDKIs are disabled in many human malignancies, in which these factors act as tumor suppressors. For example, germline mutations of *CDKN2A*, a gene encoding the CDK inhibitor p16, are present in some familial melanomas and acquired deletion or epigenetic silencing of *CDKN2A* is seen in many gliomas, carcinomas, sarcomas, and leukemias.
- Loss of function mutations in *RB* (a tumor suppressor gene) is another oncogenic mechanism that disables the G$_1$S checkpoint (discussed below).

A final consideration of importance in a discussion of growth-promoting signals is that the increased production of oncoproteins does not, by itself, lead to sustained proliferation of cancer cells. There are two built-in mechanisms, cell senescence and apoptosis, that oppose oncogene-mediated cell growth. As discussed later, genes that regulate these two braking mechanisms must be disabled to allow the action of oncogenes to proceed unopposed.

Insensitivity to Growth Inhibitory Signals: Tumor Suppressor Genes

Whereas oncogenes encode proteins that promote cell growth, the products of tumor suppressor genes apply brakes to cell proliferation. Disruption of such genes renders cells refractory to growth inhibition and mimics the growth-promoting effects of oncogenes. The following discussion describes tumor suppressor genes, their products, and possible mechanisms by which loss of their function contributes to unregulated cell growth.

In principle, antigrowth signals can prevent cell proliferation by several complementary mechanisms. The signal may cause dividing cells to enter G$_0$ (quiescence), where they remain until external cues prod their reentry into the proliferative pool. Alternatively, the cells may enter a postmitotic, differentiated pool and lose replicative potential. Nonreplicative senescence, alluded to earlier, is another mechanism of escape from sustained cell growth. Finally, the cells may be programmed to die by apoptosis.

RB: Governor of the Cell Cycle

RB, a key negative regulator of the cell cycle, is directly or indirectly inactivated in most human cancers. The retinoblastoma gene *(RB)* was the first tumor suppressor gene to be discovered and is now considered the prototype of this family of cancer genes. As with many advances in medicine, the discovery of tumor suppressor genes was accomplished by the study of a rare disease—in this case, retinoblastoma, an uncommon childhood tumor. Approximately 60% of retinoblastomas are sporadic, while the remainder are familial, in which the hereditary predisposition to develop the tumor is transmitted as an autosomal dominant trait. To account for the sporadic and familial occurrence of an identical tumor, Knudson, in 1974, proposed his two-hit hypothesis, which in molecular terms can be stated as follows:

- *Both normal alleles of the RB locus must be inactivated* (hence the two hits) for the development of retinoblastoma (Fig. 6.18).
- *In familial cases, children inherit one defective copy of the RB gene in the germline;* the other copy is wild-type. Retinoblastoma develops when the wild-type *RB* gene is rendered dysfunctional in retinoblasts by a somatic mutation. Because a single germline mutation is sufficient to transmit disease risk in familial retinoblastoma, the trait has an autosomal dominant inheritance pattern.
- *In sporadic cases, both wild-type RB alleles are functionally inactivated by somatic mutation* in a retinoblast. The end result is the same: a retinal cell that has lost both wild-type copies of the *RB*

gene becomes cancerous. Since both alleles must be inactivated, the nature of the mutation is recessive (as opposed to oncogenes which, as mentioned, are dominant since a single mutated allele is sufficient for transformation).

Although *RB* gene defects were initially discovered in retinoblastoma, it is now evident that biallelic loss of this gene is a fairly common feature of several sporadic tumors, including osteosarcoma, breast cancer, bladder cancer, and small cell cancer of the lung. Patients with familial retinoblastoma are also at greatly increased risk for developing certain other cancers, particularly osteosarcoma.

The function of the RB protein is to regulate the G$_1$/S checkpoint, the portal through which cells must pass before DNA replication commences. As already mentioned, the transition from G$_1$ to S is a particularly important checkpoint in the cell cycle "clock." In the G$_1$ phase, diverse signals are integrated to determine whether a cell should progress through the cell cycle and divide or exit the cell cycle and differentiate. RB is a DNA-binding protein that serves as a point of integration for these diverse signals, which act by altering the phosphorylation state of RB. Specifically, signals that promote cell cycle progression lead to the phosphorylation and inactivation of RB, while those that block cell cycle progression maintain RB in an active hypophosphorylated state.

To appreciate this crucial role of RB in the cell cycle, it is helpful to review the mechanisms that enforce the G$_1$/S transition.

- *The initiation of DNA replication (S phase) requires the activity of cyclin E/CDK2 complexes,* and expression of cyclin E is dependent on the E2F family of transcription factors. Early in G$_1$, the hypophosphorylated, active form of RB binds and inhibits the function of E2F factors in at least two ways (Fig. 6.19). First, it sequesters E2F factors, preventing them from interacting with transcriptional activators. Second, RB recruits enzymes such as histone deacetylases and histone methyltransferases that modify the chromatin of genes such as cyclin E, rendering them less sensitive to E2F factors.
- *The inhibitory effect of RB is overcome by mitogenic signals that hyperphosphorylate RB.* Growth factor signaling leads to cyclin D expression and formation of cyclin D–CDK4/6 complexes. The effects of mitogens may be opposed by inhibitory inputs from factors such as TGF-α and p53 (described later), which upregulate CDKIs such as p16. If the balance of progrowth stimuli is stronger, cyclin D-CDK4/6 complexes phosphorylate and inactivate RB, releasing E2F to induce the transcription of genes such as cyclin E. Cyclin E/CDK complexes then stimulate DNA replication and progression through the cell cycle. Once cells enter S phase, they are committed to divide without additional growth factor stimulation. During the ensuing M phase, the phosphate groups are removed from RB by cellular phosphatases, regenerating the active, hypophosphorylated form of RB.

In view of the centrality of RB to the control of the cell cycle, one might expect that *RB* would be mutated in every cancer. In fact, mutations in other genes that control RB phosphorylation can mimic the effect of RB loss and are commonly found in many cancers that have wild-type *RB* genes. For example, mutational activation of CDK4 and overexpression of cyclin D favor cell proliferation by facilitating RB phosphorylation and inactivation. Cyclin D is overexpressed in many tumors because of amplification or translocation of D cyclin genes. Mutational inactivation of genes encoding CDKIs may also drive proliferation by removing important brakes on cyclin/CDK activity. As mentioned earlier, the *CDKN2A* gene, which encodes the

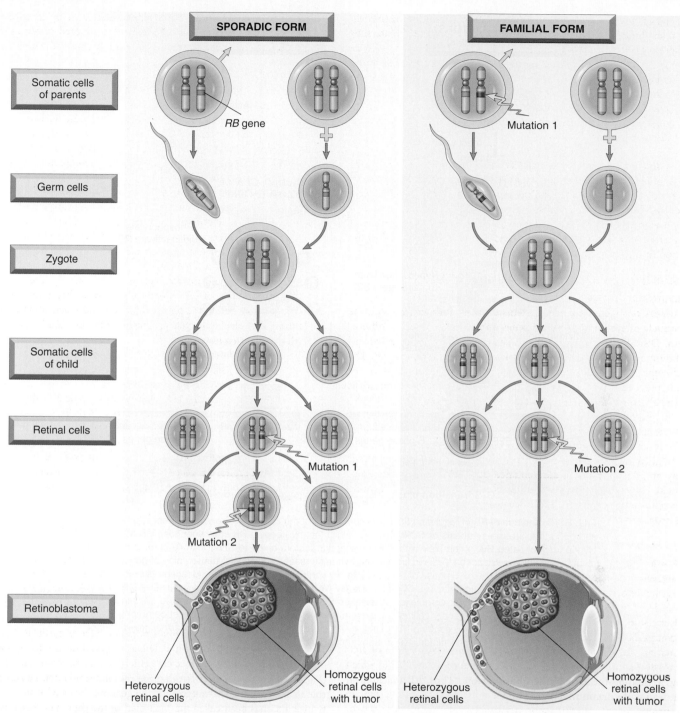

FIG. 6.18 Pathogenesis of retinoblastoma. Loss of function of both alleles of the *RB* locus, on chromosome 13q14, leads to neoplastic proliferation of the retinal cells. In the sporadic form, both *RB* mutations in the tumor-founding retinal cell are acquired. In the familial form, all somatic cells inherit one mutant *RB* gene from a carrier parent, and as a result only one additional *RB* mutation in a retinal cell is required for complete loss of *RB* function. Hence in the sporadic form all the somatic cells, including retinal cells, initially have two functional copies of *RB* (green cells), and in the familial form all somatic cells including nontransformed retinal cells have only one functional copy of *RB* (red-green cells).

CDK inhibitor p16, is an extremely common target of deletion or mutational inactivation in human tumors. It should be evident that *CDKN2A* acts as a tumor suppressor gene.

It is now accepted that loss of normal cell cycle control is central to malignant transformation and that at least one of the four key **regulators of the cell cycle (p16, cyclin D, CDK4, RB) is mutated in most human cancers.** Notably, in cancers caused by certain oncogenic viruses (discussed later), this is achieved through direct targeting of RB by viral proteins. For example, the human papillomavirus (HPV) E7 protein binds to the hypophosphorylated form of RB, preventing it

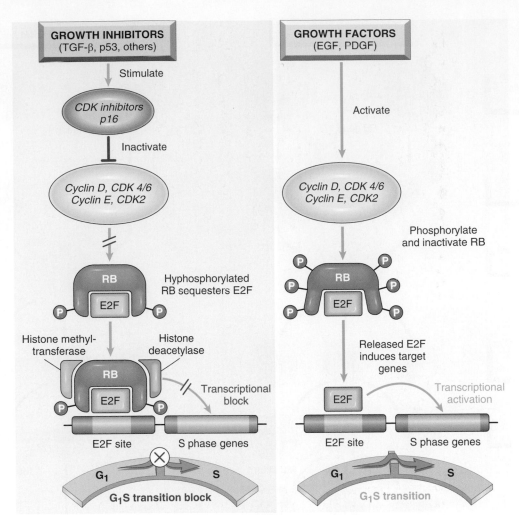

FIG. 6.19 The role of RB in regulating the G_1–S checkpoint of the cell cycle. Growth inhibitors such as TGF-β and p53 stimulate the synthesis of CDK inhibitors, which act by keeping RB in a hypophosphorylated state. Hypophosphorylated RB in complex with E2F transcription factors binds to DNA, recruits chromatin remodeling factors (histone deacetylases and histone methyltransferases), and inhibits transcription of genes whose products are required for the S phase of the cell cycle. By contrast, growth factors bind receptors that transmit signals that lead to activation of cyclin-CDK complexes. When RB is phosphorylated by cyclin D–CDK4, cyclin D–CDK6, and cyclin E–CDK2 complexes, it releases E2F factors, which then activate the transcription of S-phase genes. Virtually all cancer cells show dysregulation of the G_1–S checkpoint, most commonly as the result of mutations in genes encoding RB, CDK4, cyclin D, or CDKN2A [p16]. *EGF*, Epidermal growth factor; *PDGF*, platelet-derived growth factor; *TGF-β*, transforming growth factor-β.

from inhibiting the E2F transcription factors. Thus, RB function is lost, leading to uncontrolled growth.

TP53: Guardian of the Genome

The p53-encoding tumor suppressor gene *TP53* is the most commonly mutated gene in human cancer. The p53 protein is a transcription factor that thwarts neoplastic transformation by three complementary mechanisms: activation of temporary cell cycle arrest (*quiescence*); induction of permanent cell cycle arrest (*senescence*); and triggering of programmed cell death (*apoptosis*). If RB is a "sensor" of external signals, p53 can be viewed as a monitor of internal stress, directing stressed cells toward one of these pathways.

p53 is activated by stresses such as DNA damage and promotes DNA repair by causing G_1 arrest and inducing the expression of DNA repair genes. A cell with damaged DNA that cannot be repaired is directed by p53 to either enter senescence or undergo apoptosis

(Fig. 6.20). By managing DNA damage responses, p53 plays a central role in maintaining the integrity of the genome. In view of these activities, p53 has been called the "guardian of the genome." Responses dependent on p53 are triggered by a variety of stresses in addition to DNA damage, including anoxia and inappropriate progrowth stimuli (e.g., unbridled MYC or RAS activity).

In nonstressed, healthy cells, p53 has a short half-life (20 minutes) because of its association with MDM2, a protein that targets p53 for destruction. When the cell is stressed (for example, by DNA damage), "sensors" that include protein kinases such as ATM (ataxia telangiectasia mutated) are activated. These activated sensors catalyze posttranslational modifications in p53 that release it from MDM2, increasing its half-life and enhancing its ability to drive the transcription of target genes. The transcription of hundreds of genes is stimulated by p53. These genes suppress neoplastic transformation by three mechanisms:

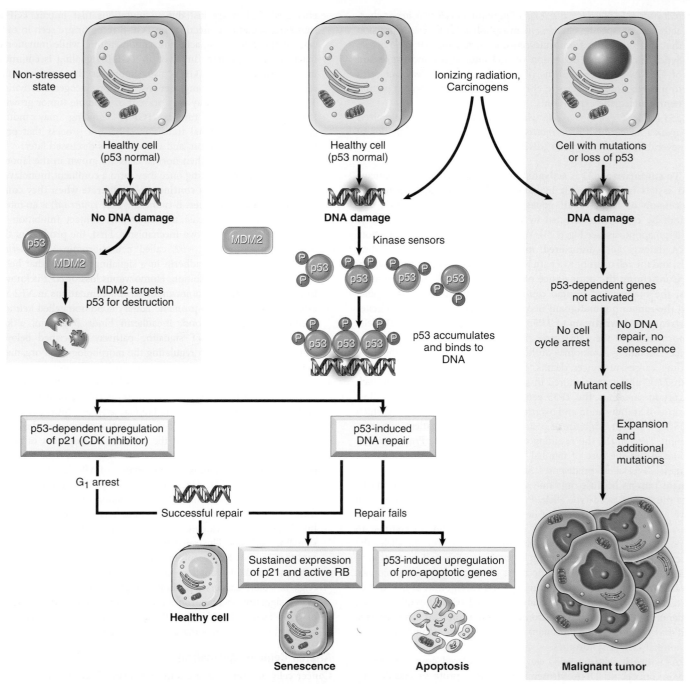

FIG. 6.20 The role of p53 in maintaining the integrity of the genome. Levels of p53 protein are low in nonstressed healthy cells due to the action of factors such as MDM2, which forms a complex that degrades p53 *(left panel)*. When healthy cells suffer DNA damage *(middle panel),* kinases that participate in pathways that sense DNA damage phosphorylate p53, protecting it from degradation and allowing p53 to accumulate. This leads to cell cycle arrest in G$_1$ and induction of DNA repair. Successful repair of DNA allows cells to proceed with the cell cycle; if DNA repair fails, p53 triggers either apoptosis or senescence. In cells with loss of p53 function *(right panel),* DNA damage does not induce cell cycle arrest or DNA repair, and genetically damaged cells proliferate, eventually giving rise to malignant neoplasms.

- *p53-mediated cell cycle arrest in response to DNA damage* (see Fig. 6.20). This occurs late in the G$_1$ phase and is caused mainly by p53-dependent transcription of *CDKN1A*, a gene that encodes the CDKI p21. p21 inhibits cyclin–CDK complexes and prevents phosphorylation of RB, thereby arresting cells in the G$_1$ phase. Such a pause gives the cells "breathing time" to repair DNA damage. The p53 protein also induces expression of DNA damage repair genes. If DNA damage is repaired successfully, p53 upregulates transcription of MDM2, leading to its own destruction and release of the cell cycle block. If the damage cannot be repaired, the cell may enter p53-induced senescence or undergo p53-directed apoptosis.

- *p53-induced senescence is a form of permanent cell cycle arrest* characterized by specific changes in morphology and gene expression that differentiate it from quiescence or reversible cell cycle arrest. Senescence requires activation of p53 and/or RB and expression of CDKIs. The mechanisms of senescence are unclear but seem to involve global changes in chromatin that drastically and permanently alter gene expression.
- *p53-induced apoptosis of cells with irreversible DNA damage protects against neoplastic transformation.* It is mediated by upregulation of several proapoptotic genes (discussed later).

To summarize, p53 is activated by stresses such as DNA damage and assists in DNA repair by causing G₁ arrest and inducing the expression of DNA repair genes. A cell with damaged DNA that cannot be repaired is directed by p53 to either enter senescence or undergo apoptosis (see Fig. 6.20). With loss of p53 "guardian" function, DNA damage goes unrepaired, mutations become fixed in dividing cells, and the cell turns onto a path leading to malignant transformation.

Confirming the importance of *TP53* in controlling carcinogenesis, the majority of human cancers have mutations in this gene, and the remaining malignant neoplasms often have defects in genes upstream or downstream of *TP53* that impair p53 function. Biallelic abnormalities of the *TP53* gene are found in virtually every type of cancer, including carcinomas of the lung, colon, and breast—the three leading causes of cancer deaths. In most cases, mutations affecting both *TP53* alleles are acquired in somatic cells. In other tumors, such as certain sarcomas, the *TP53* gene is intact but p53 function is lost because of amplification and overexpression of the *MDM2* gene, which encodes a potent inhibitor of p53. Less commonly, patients inherit a mutant *TP53* allele; the resulting disorder is called *Li-Fraumeni syndrome*. As in the case of familial retinoblastoma, inheritance of one mutant *TP53* allele predisposes affected individuals to develop malignant tumors because only one additional "hit" is needed to inactivate the second, wild-type allele. Patients with Li-Fraumeni syndrome have a much greater chance of developing a malignant tumor by 50 years of age compared with the general population. In contrast to tumors developing in patients who inherit a mutant *RB* allele, the spectrum of tumors that develop in patients with Li-Fraumeni syndrome is much more varied; the most common types are sarcomas, breast cancer, leukemias, brain tumors, and carcinomas of the adrenal cortex. Compared with individuals diagnosed with sporadic tumors, patients with Li-Fraumeni syndrome develop tumors at a younger age and may develop multiple primary tumors, which is a common feature of familial cancer syndromes.

As with RB, wild-type p53 can also be rendered nonfunctional by certain oncogenic DNA viruses. Specifically, proteins encoded by oncogenic HPVs and certain polyoma viruses bind to p53 and nullify its protective function. Thus, transforming DNA viruses subvert two of the best-understood tumor suppressors, RB and p53.

Other Growth Inhibitors

Several components of signaling pathways act to inhibit cell growth, and unsurprisingly some of these factors function as tumor suppressors. Among the most important are the following:

- *Transforming growth factor-β signaling.* Although TGF-β was discovered as a growth factor for tumor cells in vitro, in most normal epithelial, endothelial, and hematopoietic cells, it is a potent inhibitor of proliferation. Binding of TGF-β to its receptor enhances the transcription of growth-suppressive CDKIs and represses the transcription of growth-promoting genes such as *MYC* and *CDK4*. In many forms of cancer, the growth-inhibiting

effects of TGF-β are lost due to mutations that impair TGF-β signaling. Mutations affecting the TGF-β receptor are seen in cancers of the colon, stomach, and endometrium, while mutational inactivation of proteins involved in TGF-β signaling is common in pancreatic cancer. TGF-β also suppresses the host immune response and promotes angiogenesis, both prooncogenic activities. Thus, the TGF-β pathway may prevent or promote tumor growth. Indeed, in late-stage tumors TGF-β signaling may induce epithelial-to-mesenchymal transition (EMT), a process that promotes migration, invasion, and metastasis, as discussed later.

- *E-cadherin and NF2.* When normal cells are grown in the laboratory, they stop proliferating once they form a confluent monolayer. By contrast, **cancer cells continue to proliferate when they come in contact with each other.** E-cadherin (E for *epithelial*) is an intercellular adhesion molecule that maintains contact inhibition in normal cells by at least two mechanisms. First, the product of the tumor suppressor gene *NF2*, called neurofibromin-2 or *merlin*, acts downstream of E-cadherin in a signaling pathway that helps to maintain contact inhibition. Homozygous loss of *NF2* is known to cause certain neural tumors, and germline mutations in *NF2* are associated with a tumor-prone hereditary condition called *neurofibromatosis type 2*. Second, E-cadherin binds β-catenin, a key component of the WNT signaling pathway (described below), which has broad roles in regulating the morphology and organization of epithelial cells lining structures such as the gut.
- *APC, a negative regulator of WNT signaling.* Loss-of-function mutations in the *APC* (adenomatous polyposis coli) gene is the cause of the rare hereditary disease familial adenomatous polyposis, which is characterized by the development of numerous adenomatous polyps in the colon and the eventual development of carcinoma. *APC* mutations are also seen in 70% to 80% of sporadic colon cancers, highlighting the importance of APC loss in this cancer type (Chapter 13). *APC* encodes a cytoplasmic protein whose dominant role is to promote the degradation of the transcription factor β-catenin, which has several functions. In addition to binding E-cadherin, β-catenin is a key component of the WNT signaling pathway (illustrated in Fig. 6.21). WNTs are soluble factors that bind WNT receptors and create signals that prevent the APC-mediated degradation of β-catenin. With loss of APC (e.g., in colon cancers), β-catenin degradation is prevented and WNT signaling is inappropriately activated even in the absence of WNT factors. In colonic epithelium this leads to increased transcription of genes encoding growth-promoting factors.

Altered Cellular Metabolism

Cancer cells demonstrate a distinctive form of cellular metabolism characterized by high levels of glucose and glutamine uptake and increased conversion of glucose to lactate (fermentation) via the glycolytic pathway, even in the presence of ample oxygen. This pathway of aerobic glycolysis, also called the *Warburg effect*, has been recognized for many years (indeed, Otto Warburg received the Nobel Prize in 1931 for its discovery). Clinically, this "glucose-hunger" is visualized via positron emission tomography (PET) scanning, in which patients are injected with ^{18}F-fluorodeoxyglucose, a glucose derivative that is preferentially taken up into tumor cells (as well as normal, actively dividing tissues such as the bone marrow). Most tumors are PET-positive, and rapidly growing ones are markedly so.

Metabolic pathways (like signaling pathways) in normal and cancer cells are still being elucidated and the details are complex, but at the heart of the Warburg effect lies a simple question: why is it advantageous for a cancer cell to rely on seemingly inefficient glycolysis

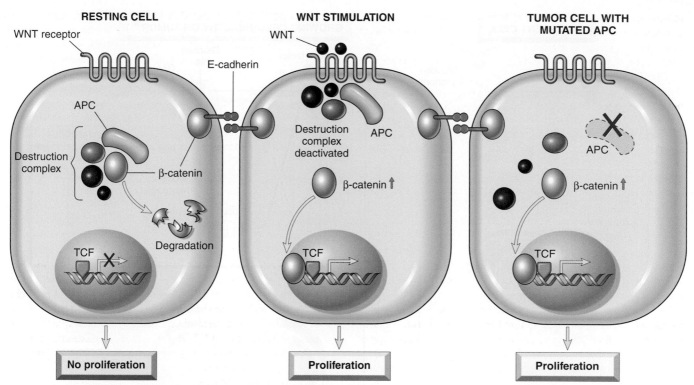

FIG. 6.21 The role of APC in regulating the stability and function of β-catenin. APC and β-catenin are components of the WNT signaling pathway. In resting cells (not exposed to WNT), β-catenin binds a macromolecular complex containing the APC protein that destroys β-catenin, keeping intracellular levels of β-catenin low. When cells are stimulated by secreted WNT molecules, the destruction complex is deactivated, β-catenin degradation does not occur, and cytoplasmic levels of β-catenin rise. β-catenin then translocates to the nucleus, where it binds to TCF, a transcription factor that activates several genes involved in cell proliferation. When APC is mutated or absent, the destruction of β-catenin cannot occur, and cells behave as if they are under constant stimulation by the WNT pathway, leading to abnormal growth and proliferation. *APC,* Adenomatous polyposis coli; *TCF,* T-cell factor (a misnomer, since this factor is expressed in many cell types).

(which generates two molecules of ATP per molecule of glucose) instead of oxidative phosphorylation (which generates up to 36 molecules of ATP per molecule of glucose)?

The answer is simple: **aerobic glycolysis provides rapidly dividing tumor cells with metabolic intermediates that are needed for the synthesis of cellular components, whereas mitochondrial oxidative phosphorylation does not.** Notably, rapidly proliferating healthy cells also rely on aerobic glycolysis; thus, "Warburg metabolism" is not cancer specific but instead is a general property of growing cells that is utilized by cancer cells. A growing cell has a strict biosynthetic requirement; it must duplicate all its cellular components—DNA, RNA, proteins, lipids, and organelles—before it can divide and produce two daughter cells. While "pure" oxidative phosphorylation yields abundant ATP, it fails to produce any carbon moieties that can be used to build the cellular components needed for growth (e.g., proteins, lipids, and nucleic acids). Even cells that are not actively growing must shunt some metabolic intermediates away from oxidative phosphorylation in order to synthesize macromolecules that are needed for cellular maintenance.

By contrast, in actively growing cells only a fraction of the cellular glucose is shunted through the oxidative phosphorylation pathway, such that on average each molecule of glucose metabolized produces approximately four molecules of ATP. Presumably, this balance (biased toward aerobic fermentation, with a bit of oxidative phosphorylation) is optimal for growth. It follows that growing cells do rely on mitochondrial metabolism. However, in addition to generating ATP, a major function of mitochondria in growing cells is the synthesis of metabolic intermediates that serve as precursors in the synthesis of cellular building blocks. Most of the carbon moieties found in these building blocks are derived from glucose and glutamine, both of which are taken up avidly by rapidly growing cells.

So how is this reprogramming of metabolism, the Warburg effect, triggered in proliferating normal and malignant cells, and how does it get hard-wired in cancer cells? **Metabolic reprogramming is produced by signaling cascades downstream of growth factor receptors, the very same pathways that are deregulated by mutations in oncogenes and tumor suppressor genes in cancers.** Thus, whereas aerobic glycolysis ceases in normal cells when they are no longer growing, in cancer cells this reprogramming persists due to the action of oncogenes and the loss of tumor suppressor gene function. Some of the important points of crosstalk between progrowth signaling factors and cellular metabolism are shown in Fig. 6.22 and include the following:

- *Growth factor receptor signaling.* In addition to transmitting growth signals to the nucleus, signals from growth factor receptors also influence metabolism by upregulating glucose uptake and inhibiting the activity of pyruvate kinase (PK, in Fig. 6.22), which catalyzes the last step in the glycolytic pathway, the conversion of phosphoenolpyruvate to pyruvate. This leads to the buildup of upstream glycolytic intermediates such as glucose-6-phosphate, which are used to synthesize DNA, RNA, and protein.

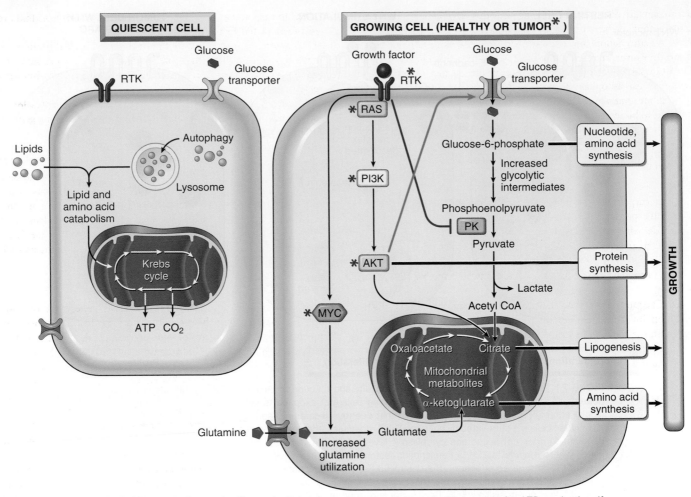

FIG. 6.22 Metabolism and cell growth. Quiescent cells rely mainly on the Krebs cycle for ATP production; if starved, autophagy (self-eating) is induced to provide a source of fuel. When stimulated by growth factors, healthy cells markedly upregulate glucose and glutamine uptake, which provide carbon sources for synthesis of nucleotides, proteins, and lipids. This diagram shows a subset of the key molecules and connections that underlies progrowth metabolism. In cancers, oncogenic gain-of-function mutations involving proteins in progrowth signaling pathways deregulate these metabolic pathways, leading to increased, unregulated cell growth. Examples of gene products that are frequently mutated are identified with an asterisk. *ATP,* Adenosine triphosphate; *PK,* pyruvate kinase; *RTK,* receptor tyrosine kinase.

- *RAS signaling.* Signals downstream of RAS along the PI3K/AKT pathway upregulate the expression and activity of glucose transporters and glycolytic enzymes, thus increasing glycolysis; they promote shunting of mitochondrial intermediates to pathways leading to lipid biosynthesis; and they activate factors that stimulate protein synthesis.
- *MYC.* As mentioned earlier, progrowth pathways upregulate expression of the transcription factor MYC, which drives changes in gene expression that support anabolic metabolism and cell growth. Among the MYC-regulated genes are those for several glycolytic enzymes and glutaminase, which is required for mitochondrial utilization of glutamine, a key source of carbon moieties needed for biosynthesis of cellular building blocks.

By contrast, many tumor suppressors can inhibit metabolic pathways that support growth. We have already discussed the "braking" effect of the tumor suppressors NF1 and PTEN on signals downstream of growth factor receptors and RAS, allowing them to oppose the

Warburg effect. Moreover, p53, arguably the most important tumor suppressor, inhibits the expression of many genes that are involved in the synthesis of cellular building blocks. Thus, the functions of many oncoproteins and tumor suppressors are inextricably intertwined with cellular metabolism.

Beyond the Warburg effect, there are two other links between metabolism and cancer that are of sufficient importance to merit brief mention, autophagy and an unusual set of oncogenic mutations that lead to the creation of *oncometabolites,* small molecules that appear to directly contribute to the transformed state.

Autophagy

Autophagy is a state of severe nutrient deficiency in which cells not only arrest their growth but also consume their own organelles, proteins, and membranes as carbon sources for energy production (Chapter 1). If this adaptation fails, the cells die. Tumor cells often seem to be able to grow under marginal environmental conditions without triggering autophagy, suggesting that the pathways that induce autophagy are disrupted. In keeping with this, several genes that promote autophagy have been observed to have tumor suppressive activities. Whether autophagy is always bad from the vantage point of the tumor, however, remains a matter of active investigation and debate. For example, under conditions of severe nutrient deprivation, tumor cells may use autophagy to become "dormant," a state of metabolic hibernation that allows cells to survive for long periods. Such cells are believed to be resistant to therapies that kill actively dividing cells and could therefore be responsible for therapeutic failures. Thus, autophagy may impart either an advantage or a disadvantage to tumor cells depending on their environmental circumstances.

Oncometabolism

Another surprising group of genetic alterations are mutations in enzymes that participate in the Krebs cycle. Of these, mutations in isocitrate dehydrogenase (IDH) are of particular interest, as they have revealed a new mechanism of oncogenesis termed *oncometabolism* (Fig. 6.23).

The proposed steps in the oncogenic pathway involving IDH are as follows:

- *IDH* acquires a mutation that leads to a specific amino acid substitution involving residues in the active site of the enzyme. As a result, the mutated protein loses its ability to function as an isocitrate dehydrogenase and acquires a new enzymatic activity that catalyzes the production of 2-hydroxyglutarate (2-HG).

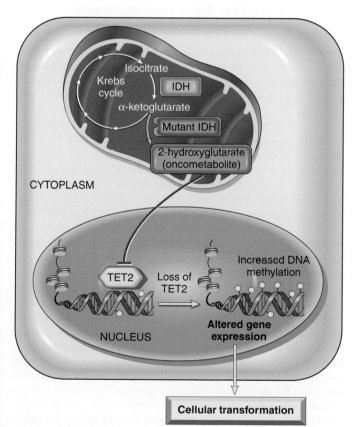

FIG. 6.23 Proposed action of the oncometabolite 2-hydroxyglutarate (2-HG) in cancer cells with mutated isocitrate dehydrogenase (mIDH). One key effect of 2-HG is inhibition of the enzyme TET2, which leads to altered DNA methylation and changes in gene expression that can promote the transformation of certain types of cells. *TET2*, Tet methylcytosine dioxygenase 2.

- 2-HG in turn acts as an inhibitor of several other enzymes that are members of the TET family, including TET2.
- TET2 is one of several factors that regulate DNA methylation, an epigenetic modification that controls normal gene expression and often goes awry in cancer. Loss of TET2 activity leads to abnormal patterns of DNA methylation.
- Abnormal DNA methylation in turn leads to aberrant expression of cancer genes, which drive cellular transformation and oncogenesis.

According to this scenario, mutated IDH acts as an oncoprotein by producing 2-HG, a prototypical *oncometabolite*. Oncogenic *IDH* mutations have now been described in a diverse collection of cancers, including a sizable fraction of cholangiocarcinomas, gliomas, acute myeloid leukemias, and sarcomas. Since the mutated IDH proteins have an altered structure, it has been possible to develop drugs that inhibit mutated IDH and not the normal IDH enzyme. These drugs are now approved for treatment of certain *IDH*-mutated cancers such as acute myeloid leukemia.

Evasion of Cell Death

Tumor cells frequently contain mutations in genes that regulate apoptosis, making the cells resistant to cell death. As discussed in Chapter 1, apoptosis is a form of regulated cell death characterized by orderly dismantling of cells into component pieces, which are then efficiently consumed by phagocytes without stimulating inflammation. There are two pathways that lead to apoptosis: the extrinsic pathway, triggered by the death receptor FAS and FAS-ligand, and the intrinsic pathway (also known as the *mitochondrial pathway*), initiated by perturbations such as loss of growth factors and DNA damage. Cancer cells are subject to a number of intrinsic stresses that can initiate apoptosis, particularly DNA damage, metabolic disturbances stemming from dysregulated growth, and hypoxia caused by insufficient blood supply. These stresses are enhanced manyfold when tumors are treated with chemotherapy or radiation therapy, which mainly kill tumor cells by activating the intrinsic pathway of apoptosis. Thus, there is strong selective pressure, both before and during therapy, for cancer cells to develop resistance to intrinsic stresses that induce apoptosis. Accordingly, **evasion of apoptosis by cancer cells occurs mainly by way of acquired mutations and changes in gene expression that disable key components of the intrinsic pathway, or that reset the balance of regulatory factors so as to favor cell survival in the face of intrinsic stresses (Fig. 6.24).**

Before delving into modes of resistance to apoptosis, we briefly review the intrinsic pathway. Activation of this pathway leads to permeabilization of the mitochondrial outer membrane and release of molecules, such as cytochrome c, that initiate apoptosis. The integrity of the mitochondrial outer membrane is determined by a delicate balancing act between proapoptotic and antiapoptotic members of the BCL2 protein family. The proapoptotic proteins BAX and BAK are required for apoptosis and directly promote mitochondrial permeabilization. Their action is inhibited by the antiapoptotic members of this family, which are exemplified by BCL2 and BCL-X_L. A third set of factors that belong to the "BH3 domain only" members of the BCL2 family, which include BAD, BID, and PUMA, shift the balance between the proapoptotic and antiapoptotic family members so that the activity of the proapoptotic factors BAX and BAK is enhanced. When the activities of BAX and BAK predominate they form pores in the mitochondrial membrane that allow mitochondrial cytochrome c to leak into the cytosol, where it associates with a cofactor called APAF-1 and triggers a series of reactions that activate caspase-9 and executioner caspases such as caspase-3. Another group of factors that

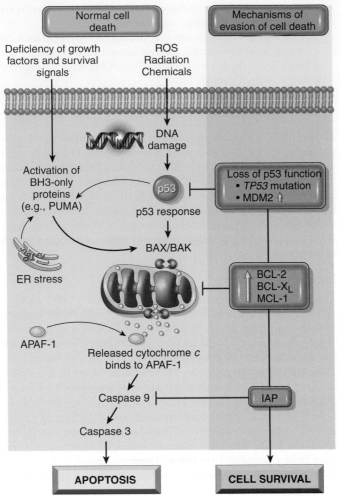

FIG. 6.24 Intrinsic pathway of apoptotic cell death and mechanisms used by tumor cells to evade apoptotic cell death. The most important evasion mechanisms are loss of p53 function, either through mutation of the *TP53* gene or overexpression of MDM2, which leads to the destruction of p53; or upregulation of antiapoptotic proteins of the BCL-2 family. Less commonly, increased expression of members of the inhibitor of apoptosis (IAP) family protects cancer cells from apoptosis. *APAF-1,* Apoptotic protease activating factor-1.

function as negative regulators of the intrinsic pathway are known as *inhibitor of apoptosis proteins (IAPs),* which bind caspase-9 and prevent apoptosis.

Within this framework, it is possible to illustrate the major mechanisms by which apoptosis is evaded by cancer cells (see Fig. 6.24). These mainly involve loss of p53, a key component of early steps in the intrinsic pathway, and increased expression of antiapoptotic members of the BCL2 family.

- *Loss of p53 function.* As already discussed, *TP53* is commonly mutated in cancers at diagnosis. Moreover, the frequency of *TP53* mutations is even higher in tumors that relapse after cytotoxic therapy. Loss of p53 function prevents the upregulation of PUMA, a proapoptotic member of the BCL2 family that is a direct target of p53. As a result, cells survive levels of DNA damage and cell stress that would otherwise result in their death.
- *Overexpression of antiapoptotic members of the BCL2 family.* Overexpression of BCL2 is a common event that protects tumor cells from apoptosis and occurs through several mechanisms. One of the best-understood examples is follicular lymphoma (Chapter 10), a B-cell

tumor carrying a characteristic (14;18)(q32;q21) translocation that fuses the *BCL2* gene (located at 18q21) to the transcriptionally active immunoglobulin heavy chain gene (located at 14q32). The resulting overabundance of BCL2 protects lymphocytes from apoptosis and increases their survival. Because BCL2-overexpressing follicular lymphomas arise in large part through reduced cell death rather than explosive cell proliferation, they tend to be indolent (slow-growing). In other tumors such as chronic lymphocytic leukemia (Chapter 10), it appears that BCL2 is upregulated through loss of expression of specific micro-RNAs that normally dampen *BCL2* expression. Many other mechanisms leading to overexpression of antiapoptotic members of the BCL2 family have been described, particularly in the setting of chemotherapy resistance.

Recognition of the mechanisms by which cancers evade cell death has stimulated several lines of targeted drug development. Restoration of p53 function in *TP53*-mutated tumors is a daunting problem (because of the inherent difficulty of "fixing" defective genes) but is possible in tumors in which p53 is inactive because of overexpression of its inhibitor, MDM2. Indeed, inhibitors of MDM2 that reactivate p53 and induce apoptosis in tumors with *MDM2* gene amplification, such as certain types of sarcoma, are being tested in clinical trials. More impressive are results that have been achieved with drugs that inhibit the function of antiapoptotic members of the BCL2 family, particularly BCL2 itself. These drugs have potent activity against tumors characterized by BCL2 overexpression (such as chronic lymphocytic leukemia) and are now used routinely to treat a number of cancers.

Limitless Replicative Potential (Immortality)

Tumor cells, unlike normal cells, are capable of limitless replication. As discussed previously in the context of cellular aging (Chapter 1), most normal human cells are capable of at most 70 doublings. Thereafter, the cells lose the ability to divide and enter replicative senescence. This phenomenon has been ascribed to progressive shortening of telomeres at the ends of chromosomes. Markedly eroded telomeres are recognized by the DNA repair machinery as double-stranded DNA breaks, leading to cell cycle arrest and senescence, mediated by p53 and RB. In cells in which p53 or RB are disabled by mutations, the nonhomologous end-joining pathway is activated in a final effort to save the cell, joining the shortened ends of two chromosomes. This inappropriately activated repair system results in dicentric chromosomes that are pulled apart at anaphase, resulting in new double-stranded DNA breaks. The resulting genomic instability from the repeated bridge—fusion—breakage cycles eventually produces mitotic catastrophe and death by apoptosis.

It follows that for tumors to acquire the ability to grow indefinitely, loss of growth restraints is not enough; cellular senescence and mitotic catastrophe must also be avoided (Fig. 6.25). If a cell manages to reactivate telomerase, the bridge—fusion—breakage cycles cease, and the cell is able to avoid death. However, during the period of genomic instability that precedes telomerase activation, numerous mutations may accumulate, increasing the progression toward malignancy. Telomerase, active in normal stem cells, is present at very low levels or absent in most somatic cells. By contrast, telomere maintenance is seen in virtually all types of cancers. In 85% to 95% of cancers, this is due to upregulation of the enzyme telomerase. How telomerase expression is regained is incompletely understood, but many tumors have mutations in the promoter of the gene *TERT*, which encodes a subunit of telomerase; these mutations lead to high levels of *TERT* expression. The remaining 5% to 15% of tumors lacking telomerase maintain

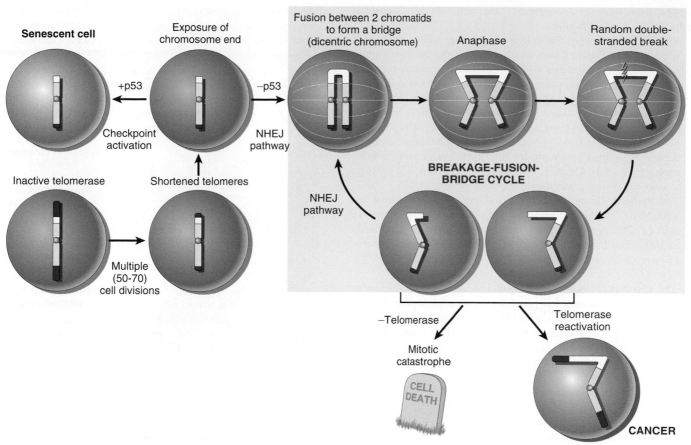

FIG. 6.25 Escape of cells from replicative senescence and mitotic catastrophe caused by telomere shortening. Erosion of telomeres over the course of many cell divisions eventually leaves a "naked" chromosome end that is sensed as a double-stranded DNA break. In cells with functional p53, this leads to upregulation of genes that drive cells into a nonreplicative senescent state. In the absence of p53, cell division occurs unabated and the ends of chromosomes without telomeres may be joined through an error-prone repair process called nonhomologous end joining (NHEJ). The resulting dicentric chromosome is prone to random breakage followed by additional rounds of chromosome fusion, a process referred to as the breakage-fusion-bridge cycle. Eventually, due to extensive chromosome damage, multiple rounds of breakage-fusion-bridge cycle leads to mitotic catastrophe and cell death. However, such cells can be rescued if telomerase is reactivated, and the altered expression of cancer genes in these damaged cells may lead to the development of cancer.

their telomeres through a different mechanism termed *alternative lengthening of telomeres,* an incompletely understood process that depends on DNA recombination.

Sustained Angiogenesis

Even if a solid tumor possesses all of the genetic aberrations that are required for malignant transformation, it cannot enlarge beyond 1 to 2 mm in diameter unless it has a blood supply. Thus the capacity to induce angiogenesis is an important hallmark of all cancers. Presumably the 1- to 2-mm zone represents the maximal distance across which oxygen, nutrients, and waste can diffuse to and from blood vessels. Growing cancers stimulate neoangiogenesis, during which new vessels sprout from previously existing capillaries. Neovascularization has a dual effect on tumor growth: perfusion supplies needed nutrients and oxygen, and newly formed endothelial cells stimulate the growth of adjacent tumor cells by secreting growth factors, such as insulin-like growth factors (IGFs) and PDGF. While the resulting tumor vasculature is effective at delivering nutrients and removing wastes, it is not normal; intratumoral vessels are leaky and dilated and have a haphazard pattern of connection, features that can

be appreciated on angiograms. These abnormal vessels further contribute to metastatic potential.

How do growing tumors develop a blood supply? The current paradigm is that **angiogenesis is controlled by a balance between angiogenesis promoters and inhibitors; in angiogenic tumors this balance is skewed in favor of promoters.** Early in their development, most tumors do not induce angiogenesis. Starved of nutrients, these tumors remain small or in situ, possibly for years, until an *angiogenic switch* terminates this stage of vascular quiescence. The molecular basis of the angiogenic switch involves increased production of angiogenic factors and/or loss of angiogenic inhibitors. These factors may be produced by the tumor cells themselves or by inflammatory cells (e.g., macrophages) or resident stromal cells (e.g., tumor-associated fibroblasts). Proteases, either elaborated by the tumor cells or by stromal cells in response to the tumor, are also involved in regulating the balance between angiogenic and antiangiogenic factors. Many proteases can release proangiogenic basic fibroblast growth factor that is stored in the ECM; conversely, the angiogenesis inhibitors angiostatin and endostatin are produced by proteolytic cleavage of plasminogen and collagen, respectively.

The local balance of angiogenic and antiangiogenic factors is influenced by several factors:

- Relative lack of oxygen due to hypoxia stabilizes HIF1α, an oxygen-sensitive transcription factor, which then activates the transcription of proangiogenic cytokines such as VEGF. These factors create an angiogenic gradient that stimulates the proliferation of endothelial cells and guides the growth of new vessels toward the tumor.
- Mutations involving tumor suppressors and oncogenes in cancers also tilt the balance in favor of angiogenesis. For example, p53 stimulates the expression of antiangiogenic molecules such as thrombospondin-1 and represses the expression of proangiogenic molecules such as VEGF. Thus, loss of p53 in tumor cells provides a more permissive environment for angiogenesis.
- The transcription of VEGF is also influenced by signals from the RAS-MAP kinase pathway, and gain-of-function mutations in *RAS* or *MYC* upregulate the production of VEGF. Elevated levels of VEGF can be detected in the serum and urine of a significant fraction of cancer patients.

The idea that angiogenesis is essential for solid tumors to grow to clinically significant sizes has provided a powerful impetus for the development of therapeutic agents that block angiogenesis. These agents are now a part of the armamentarium that oncologists use against cancers; a cardinal example is bevacizumab, a monoclonal antibody that neutralizes VEGF activity and is approved for use in the treatment of multiple cancers. However, angiogenesis inhibitors have not been nearly as effective as was originally hoped; they can prolong life but usually for only a few months and at high financial cost. The mechanisms that underlie the persistence and ultimate progression of cancers in the face of therapy with angiogenesis inhibitors are complex and may involve a switch to angiogenic factors other than VEGF that are not inhibited by the anti-VEGF therapy or changes in tumor behavior, such as adoption of a more locally invasive phenotype. The modest benefit of antiangiogenic therapy highlights the ability of advanced cancers to circumvent therapies directed at genetically stable stromal support cells, such as endothelium.

Invasion and Metastasis

Invasion and metastasis, the major causes of cancer-related morbidity and mortality, are due to complex interactions involving cancer cells, stromal cells, and the extracellular matrix (ECM). These interactions can be broken down into a series of steps consisting of local invasion, penetration of blood and lymph vessels, transit through the vasculature, extravasation from the vessels, formation of micrometastases, and growth of micrometastases into macroscopic tumors (Fig. 6.26). This sequence of steps may be interrupted at any stage by either host-related or tumor-related factors. For the purpose of discussion, the metastatic cascade can be subdivided into two phases: (1) invasion of ECM and (2) vascular dissemination and homing of tumor cells.

Invasion of Extracellular Matrix

Human tissues are organized into a series of compartments separated from each other by two types of ECM: basement membranes and interstitial connective tissue. Although organized differently, both types of ECM are composed of collagens, glycoproteins, and proteoglycans. Tumor cells must interact with the ECM at several stages in the metastatic cascade (see Fig. 6.26). A carcinoma cell must first breach the underlying basement membrane, then traverse the interstitial connective tissue, and ultimately gain access to the circulation

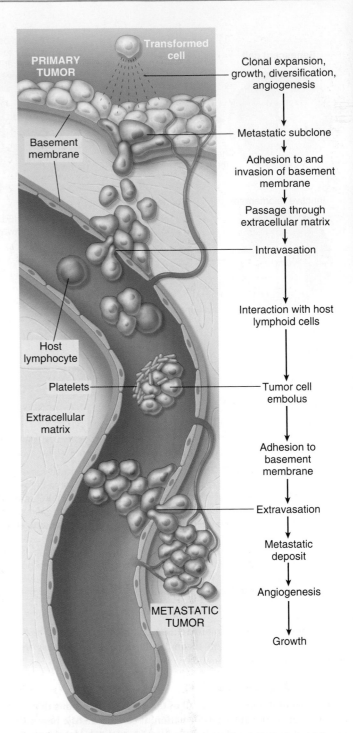

FIG. 6.26 The metastatic cascade: the sequential steps involved in the hematogenous spread of a tumor.

by penetrating the vascular basement membrane. This process is repeated in reverse when tumor cell emboli extravasate at a distant site. Invasion of the ECM initiates the metastatic cascade and is an active process that can be resolved into several sequential steps (Fig. 6.27):

- *Loosening of intercellular connections between tumor cells.* As mentioned earlier, E-cadherins act as intercellular glues, and their cytoplasmic portions bind to β-catenin (see Fig. 6.21). Adjacent E-cadherin molecules keep the cells together; in addition, as

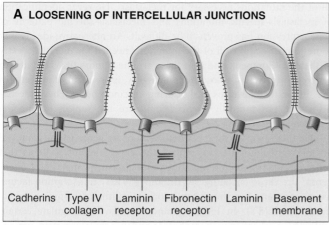

A LOOSENING OF INTERCELLULAR JUNCTIONS

Cadherins | Type IV collagen | Laminin receptor | Fibronectin receptor | Laminin | Basement membrane

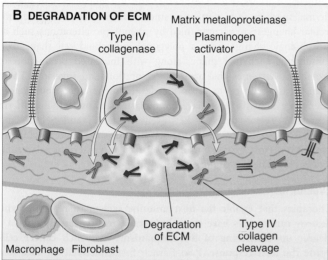

B DEGRADATION OF ECM

Type IV collagenase | Matrix metalloproteinase | Plasminogen activator

Macrophage Fibroblast | Degradation of ECM | Type IV collagen cleavage

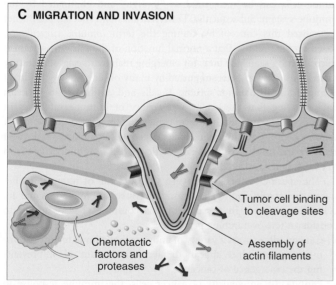

C MIGRATION AND INVASION

Tumor cell binding to cleavage sites

Chemotactic factors and proteases | Assembly of actin filaments

FIG. 6.27 Sequence of events in the invasion of epithelial basement membranes by tumor cells. (A) Tumor cells detach from each other because of reduced expression of adhesion molecules such as cadherins and (B) produce a number of proteases that digest the basement membrane extracellular matrix (ECM). Under the influence of chemotactic factors produced by inflammatory cells and stromal cells (C), which also produce additional proteases, tumor cells adopt an invasive phenotype, tracking along binding sites that are created in part by cleavage of the ECM.

discussed earlier, E-cadherin can transmit antigrowth signals by sequestering β-catenin. E-cadherin function is decreased in many epithelial cancers by mutational inactivation of E-cadherin genes, activation of β-catenin genes, or inappropriate expression of the SNAIL and TWIST transcription factors, which suppress E-cadherin expression.

- *Local degradation of the basement membrane and interstitial connective tissue.* Tumor cells may secrete proteolytic enzymes themselves or induce stromal cells (e.g., fibroblasts and inflammatory cells) to elaborate proteases. Multiple different proteases such as matrix metalloproteinases (MMPs), cathepsin D, and urokinase plasminogen activator have been implicated in tumor cell invasion. MMPs regulate tumor invasion not only by remodeling insoluble components of the basement membrane and interstitial matrix but also by releasing ECM-sequestered growth factors, which have chemotactic, angiogenic, and growth-promoting effects. For example, MMP-9 is a gelatinase that cleaves type IV collagen in the epithelial and vascular basement membranes and stimulates release of VEGF from ECM-sequestered pools. Benign tumors of the breast, colon, and stomach show little type IV collagenase activity, whereas their malignant counterparts overexpress this enzyme. Concurrently, the levels of metalloproteinase inhibitors are reduced so that the balance is tilted toward tissue degradation. Overexpression of MMPs and other proteases has been reported for many malignant tumors.

- *Changes in attachment of tumor cells to ECM proteins.* Normal epithelial cells have receptors such as integrins for basement membrane laminin and collagens that are localized to their basal surfaces; these receptors help to maintain the cells in a polarized, resting, differentiated state. Loss of adhesion in normal cells leads to induction of apoptosis, but tumor cells are resistant to this form of cell death. Additionally, the matrix in cancers itself is modified in ways that promote invasion and metastasis. For example, cleavage of the basement membrane proteins collagen IV and laminin by MMP-2 and MMP-9 generates novel sites that bind to receptors on tumor cells and stimulate migration.

- *Locomotion* is the final step of invasion, propelling tumor cells through the degraded basement membranes and proteolyzed ECM. Migration is a complex, multistep process that involves many families of receptors and signaling proteins that eventually impinge on the actin cytoskeleton. Such movement seems to be potentiated and directed by stromal cell–derived cytokines; the latter includes hepatocyte growth factor/scatter factor (HGF/SCF), which binds to receptors on tumor cells. HGF/SCF levels are elevated at the advancing edges of highly invasive cancers such as the brain tumor glioblastoma, supporting their role in motility. Certain cleavage products of matrix components (e.g., collagen, laminin), and some growth factors (e.g., insulin-like growth factors 1 and 2) also have chemotactic activity for tumor cells.

It has also become clear that the stromal cells surrounding tumor cells participate in reciprocal signaling events that enable multiple cancer hallmarks (discussed later). For example, a variety of studies have demonstrated that tumor-associated fibroblasts exhibit altered expression of genes that encode ECM molecules, proteases, protease inhibitors, and various growth factors and chemokines/cytokines, all of which can influence tumor invasion and extravasation as well as the host immune response. Infiltrating immune cells have similarly complex roles. The most successful tumors may be those that can co-opt the activities of stromal cells.

Vascular Dissemination and Homing of Tumor Cells

Because of their invasive properties, tumor cells frequently escape their sites of origin and enter the circulation. It is now recognized from studies of "liquid biopsies" (blood samples taken from patients with solid tumors) that millions of tumor cells are shed daily from even small cancers; hence, both tumor cells and tumor-derived DNA can be detected in circulation. Most of these tumor cells circulate as single cells, while others form emboli by aggregating and adhering to circulating blood elements, particularly platelets.

Given the ease with which tumor cells access the circulation, it is apparent that the ability of cancer cells to leave the circulation, invade, and grow to clinically significant tumor sizes at other sites in the body is highly inefficient. Several factors seem to limit the metastatic potential of circulating tumor cells. While in the circulation, tumor cells are vulnerable to destruction by host immune cells (discussed later), and the process of adhesion to normal vascular beds and invasion of normal distant tissues may be much more difficult than the escape of tumor cells from the cancer. Even following extravasation, tumor cells may find it difficult to grow in a site different from their origin due to lack of critical stromal support or due to recognition and suppression by resident immune cells. Indeed, the concept of tumor dormancy, referring to the prolonged survival of micrometastases without progression, is well described in melanoma and in breast and prostate carcinoma. Dormancy of tumor cells at distant sites may be the last defense against clinically significant metastatic disease.

espite these limiting factors, if neglected, virtually all malignant tumors will eventually produce macroscopic metastases. **The site at which metastases appear is related to two factors: the anatomic location and vascular drainage of the primary tumor and the tropism of particular tumors for specific tissues.** As mentioned earlier, most metastases occur in the first capillary bed available to the tumor, hence the frequency of metastases to liver and lung. However, natural pathways of drainage do not wholly explain the distribution of metastases, particularly in the case of specific tumors that tend to metastasize to particular tissues. Although the molecular mechanisms of colonization of distant sites by tumor cells are still being unraveled, a consistent theme seems to be that tumor cells secrete cytokines, growth factors, and proteases that act on the resident stromal cells, which in turn make the metastatic site habitable for the cancer cell.

Metastasis

Of central importance in oncology is the question, why do some tumors only invade locally whereas others metastasize? Even in tumors that metastasize, there are differences in the frequency and extent of metastases. Satisfying answers are still lacking. Some variation in metastasis clearly relates to inherent differences in the behavior of particular tumors; for example, small cell carcinoma of the lung virtually always metastasizes to distant sites, whereas some tumors, such as basal cell carcinoma, rarely do so. In general, large tumors are more likely to metastasize than small tumors, presumably because (all other things being equal) large tumors will have been present in the patient for longer periods of time, providing additional chances for metastasis to occur. However, tumor size and type cannot adequately explain the behavior of individual cancers, and it is still open to question whether metastasis is merely probabilistic (a matter of chance multiplied by tumor cell number and time) or reflects inherent differences in metastatic potential from tumor to tumor (a deterministic model).

The deterministic model proposes that metastasis is inevitable with certain tumors because as tumor cells grow, they randomly accumulate all of the mutations necessary for metastasis. However, identification of metastasis-specific mutations and metastasis-specific patterns of gene expression has proven to be difficult. An alternative idea is that some tumors acquire all of the mutations needed for metastasis early in their development, and that these are the tumors that are fated to progress. Metastasis, according to this view, is an intrinsic property of the tumor that develops early during carcinogenesis. These mechanisms are not mutually exclusive and are the subject of ongoing research.

Another open question is whether there are genes whose principal or sole contribution is to control the expression of proteins that promote metastasis. Among candidates for such "metastasis oncogenes" are those encoding SNAIL and TWIST, transcription factors whose primary function is to promote epithelial-to-mesenchymal transition (EMT). In EMT, carcinoma cells downregulate certain epithelial markers (e.g., E-cadherin) and upregulate certain mesenchymal markers (e.g., vimentin, smooth muscle actin). These molecular changes are accompanied by phenotypic alterations such as morphologic change from a polygonal epithelioid cell shape to a spindly mesenchymal shape, along with increased production of proteolytic enzymes that promote migration and invasion. These changes are believed to favor the development of a promigratory phenotype that is essential for metastasis. Loss of E-cadherin expression seems to be a key event in EMT, and SNAIL and TWIST are transcriptional repressors that downregulate E-cadherin expression. How expression of these master transcriptional regulators is stimulated in tumors is not clear.

Evasion of Immune Surveillance

Therapies that enable the host immune system to recognize and destroy cancer cells have recently become reality, largely due to a clearer understanding of the mechanisms by which cancer cells evade the host response. Paul Ehrlich first conceived the idea that tumor cells can be recognized as "foreign" and eliminated by the immune system. Subsequently, Lewis Thomas and Macfarlane Burnet formalized this concept by coining the term *immune surveillance,* based on the premise that a normal function of the immune system is to constantly "scan" the body for emerging malignant cells and destroy them. This idea has been supported by many observations—the direct demonstration of tumor-specific T cells and antibodies in patients; data showing that the extent and quality of immune infiltrates in cancers often correlate with outcome; the increased incidence of certain cancers in immunodeficient people and mice; and most recently and most directly, the dramatic success of immunotherapy in the treatment of several cancers.

The specific factors that govern the outcome of interactions between tumor cells and the host immune system are numerous and are still being defined. In the face of this complexity, it is helpful to consider a few overarching principles:

- Cancer cells express a variety of antigens that stimulate the host immune system, which appears to have an important role in preventing the emergence of cancers.
- Despite the antigenicity of cancer cells, the immune response to established tumors is ineffective, and in some instances may actually promote cancer growth, due to acquired changes that allow cancer cells to evade antitumor immune responses and foster protumor immune responses.
- Defining mechanisms of immune evasion and "immuno-manipulation" by cancer cells has led to effective new immunotherapies that work by reactivating latent host immune responses.

Tumor Antigens

Cancers express various types of antigens that may be recognized by the immune system as foreign. Several sources of these tumor antigens are recognized.

- *Neoantigens* generated by the varied mutations found in cancers are protein sequences that the immune system has not seen and therefore is not tolerant of and can react to. Mutations that may give rise to neoantigens include not only driver mutations but also passenger mutations, which are particularly abundant in cancers that are caused by mutagenic exposures (e.g., sunlight, smoking). Of the many new protein sequences that are produced by mutated genes, the only ones that function as antigens are those that bind to that particular patient's HLA molecules and thus can be displayed to that patient's T cells.
- *Unmutated proteins* expressed by tumor cells can also stimulate the host immune response. One such antigen is *tyrosinase*, an enzyme involved in melanin biosynthesis that is expressed only in normal melanocytes and melanomas. It may be surprising that the immune system is able to respond to this normal self antigen. The probable explanation is that tyrosinase is normally produced in such small amounts and in so few normal cells that it is not recognized by the immune system and fails to induce tolerance. Another group of tumor antigens, the *cancer-testis antigens,* are encoded by genes that are silent in all adult tissues except germ cells in the testis—hence their name. Although the protein is present in the testis it is not expressed on the cell surface in a form that can be recognized by CD8+ T cells, because sperm do not express MHC class I molecules. Thus, for all practical purposes these antigens are tumor specific and are therefore capable of stimulating antitumor immune responses.
- *Viral proteins* that are expressed in cancer cells transformed by oncogenic viruses are another important class of tumor antigens. The most potent of these antigens are proteins produced by cells that are latently infected with DNA viruses, the most important of which are human papillomavirus (HPV) and Epstein-Barr virus (EBV). There is abundant evidence that cytotoxic T lymphocytes (CTLs) recognize viral antigens and play important roles in surveillance against virus-induced tumors through their ability to recognize and kill virus-infected cells. Most notably, multiple cancers associated with oncogenic viruses, including HPV-associated cervical carcinoma and EBV-related B-cell lymphomas, occur at significantly higher rates in individuals with defective T-cell immunity, such as patients infected with HIV.

Effective Immune Responses to Tumor Antigens

The principal immune mechanism of tumor eradication is killing of tumor cells by cytotoxic T lymphocytes specific for tumor antigens. It appears likely that immune reactions to cancers are initiated by the death of individual cancer cells, which occurs at some frequency in all cancers due to dysregulated growth, metabolic stresses, and hypoxia due to insufficient blood supply. When tumor cells die, they release "danger signals" (damage associated molecular patterns, see Chapter 5) that stimulate innate immune cells, including resident phagocytes and antigen-presenting cells. It is believed that some of the dead cells are phagocytosed by dendritic cells, which migrate to draining lymph nodes and present tumor neoantigens in the context of MHC class I molecules. The displayed tumor antigens are recognized by antigen-specific cytotoxic T lymphocytes (CTLs), which become activated, proliferate, and travel to the site of the tumor, where they recognize and kill tumor cells presenting tumor antigens in the context of their own MHC class I molecules (Fig. 6.28).

IFN-γ-producing T helper cells of the Th1 subset, which may also be induced by recognition of tumor antigens, can activate macrophages and thus contribute to the destruction of tumors.

As will be discussed shortly, some of the strongest evidence for the importance of CTL responses in immunosurveillance stems from the characterization of established human cancers, which often feature acquired mutations that prevent CTLs from recognizing tumor cells as "foreign." It has also been noted in large studies of a wide variety of human tumors that high levels of infiltrating CTLs and Th1 cells correlate with better clinical outcomes. While other cell types such as natural killer cells have been implicated in antitumor responses, the quality and strength of CTL responses are believed to be of preeminent importance.

Immune Evasion by Cancers

Immune responses often fail to check tumor growth because cancers evade immune recognition or resist immune effector mechanisms. Since the immune system is capable of recognizing and eliminating nascent cancers, it follows that tumors that reach clinically

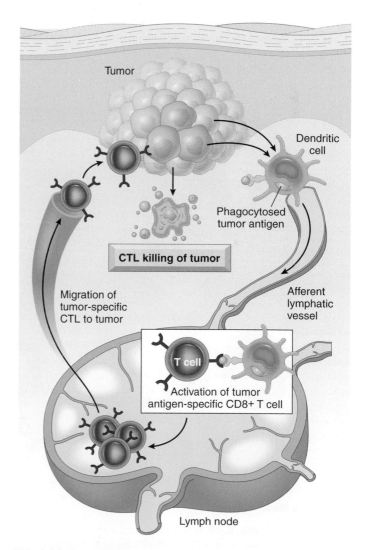

FIG. 6.28 Recognition of tumor antigens and induction of CD8+ cytotoxic T-cell antitumor response. *CTL,* Cytotoxic T-lymphocyte. (Modified from Abbas AK, Lichtman AH, Pillai S: *Cellular and Molecular Immunology,* ed 9, Philadelphia, 2018, Elsevier.)

significant sizes must be composed of cells that are either invisible to the host immune system or that express factors that actively suppress host immunity. The term *cancer immunoediting* has been used to describe the ability of the immune system to promote the Darwinian selection of tumor subclones that are most able to avoid host immunity or even manipulate the immune system. Since CTL responses appear to be the most important defense that the host has against tumors, it should come as no surprise that tumor cells show a variety of alterations that abrogate CTL responses. These include acquired mutations in β_2-microglobulin that prevent the assembly of functional MHC class I molecules, and increased expression of a variety of proteins that inhibit CTL activation or function. These proteins work by triggering what is referred to as *immune checkpoints*, inhibitory pathways that normally are crucial for maintaining self-tolerance and controlling the size and duration of immune responses so as to minimize collateral tissue damage.

One of the best-characterized immune checkpoints involves a protein called PD-L1 (programmed cell death ligand 1), which is often expressed on the surface of tumor cells and on myeloid cells such as macrophages in the tumor infiltrate (Fig. 6.29). When PD-L1 engages its receptor, PD-1, on CTLs, the CTLs become unresponsive and lose their ability to kill tumor cells. Experimental studies have identified several other immune checkpoint pathways involving different ligands

and receptors that also have been implicated in immunoevasion by tumors. One is CTLA-4, a receptor expressed on T cells that inhibits T-cell activation. T-cells responding to tumor antigens increase their expression of PD-1 and CTLA-4, both normal regulatory events that serve to dampen immune responses.

The discovery of checkpoints that shut off antitumor immunity has led to the development of antibodies that block these checkpoints and release the brakes on the immune response. Current checkpoint blockade therapies against targets such as CTLA-4, PD-1, and PD-L1 have resulted in response rates of 10% to 30% in a variety of solid tumors (e.g., melanoma, lung cancer, bladder cancer), and even higher rates in some hematologic malignancies such as Hodgkin lymphoma (Chapter 10). Because these checkpoints evolved to prevent responses to self antigens (Chapter 5), patients treated with checkpoint inhibitors develop various autoimmune manifestations, such as colitis and other types of systemic inflammation. Most of these reactions can be controlled with antiinflammatory agents, but sometimes they are sufficiently severe that the treatment must be discontinued. Checkpoint blockade therapy has the potential to induce long-lived remissions and even cures because when the immune response is unleashed, it leads to the development of memory lymphocytes that continue to provide protection for long periods. One of the challenges with checkpoint blockade therapy is that despite its enormous

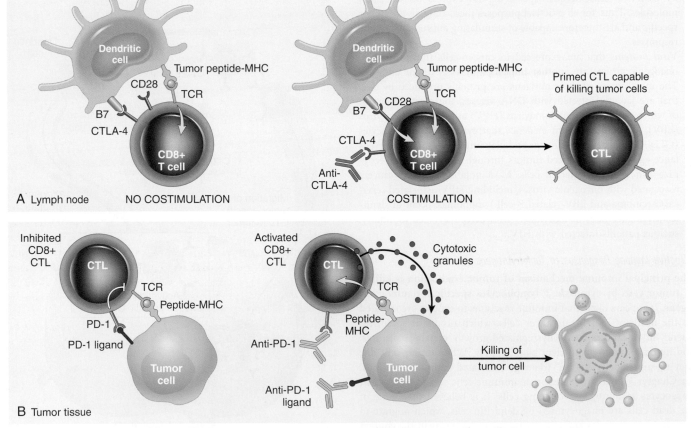

FIG. 6.29 Activation of host antitumor immunity by checkpoint inhibitors. (A) Blockade of the CTLA4 surface molecule with an inhibitor antibody allows cytotoxic CD8+ T cells (CTLs) to engage B7 family coreceptors, leading to T-cell activation. (B) Blockade of PD-1 receptor or PD-1 ligand by inhibitory antibodies abrogates inhibitory signals transmitted by PD-1, again leading to activation of CTLs. *CTLA-4*, Cytotoxic T-lymphocyte-associated protein-4; *MHC*, major histocompatibility complex; *PD-1*, programmed cell death-1; *PD-L1*, programmed cell death ligand 1; *TCR*, T-cell receptor. (Reprinted from Abbas AK, Lichtman AH, Pillai S: *Cellular and Molecular Immunology*, ed 9, Philadelphia, 2018, Elsevier.)

promise, only a minority of tumors respond. Much effort is being devoted to understand why this is so and how the frequency of responding tumors can be increased. Predictably, tumors with high mutation rates (often secondary to mismatch repair and DNA polymerase defects, discussed later) produce abundant neoantigens and are more responsive, on average, to checkpoint blockade. In fact, this therapy is approved for all recurrent or metastatic cancers with mismatch repair defects regardless of the histologic features or cell of origin—the first example of a cancer therapy based solely on the mutational signature of the tumor.

The remarkable response of advanced cancers to immune checkpoint inhibitors has energized other work focused on harnessing the immune system to combat cancer. These include efforts to develop personalized tumor vaccines using neoantigens identified in the tumors of individual patients as well as new kinds of adoptive immunotherapy. The most advanced of the latter are patient-derived CTLs engineered to express chimeric antigen receptors (CARs). CARs have extracellular domains consisting of antibodies that bind tumor antigens and intracellular domains that deliver signals that activate CTLs following their engagement with antigen on the surface of tumor cells. CAR-T cells are potent killers of tumor cells and have produced long-term remissions in patients with certain hematologic malignancies, such as B-cell acute lymphoblastic leukemia (Chapter 10). However, CAR-T cells are also associated with serious complications related to cytokines released from the activated CTLs and for now remain second-line therapies for patients when conventional treatments fail. Also, though successful against hematologic malignancies, CAR-T-cell therapy that is effective against solid tumors has yet to be developed.

Beyond complications of immunotherapy, it should also be recognized that the host immune response to tumors is a double-edged sword. For example, tumors release factors that alter the function of certain immune cells such as macrophages and Th2 lymphocytes in a fashion that is suspected of promoting angiogenesis, tissue fibrosis, and the accumulation of alternatively activated (M2) macrophages, which you will recall from Chapter 2 are associated with suppression of the inflammatory response during wound healing. These types of responses are suspected of promoting tumor growth.

To summarize, while the future is bright for cancer immunotherapy, important hurdles remain to be cleared. At present, response and resistance to immune checkpoint inhibitors are unpredictable. Why do only a subset of tumors such as melanoma and lung cancer respond to checkpoint blockade? New biomarkers are needed to better tailor therapies for individual patients.

Genomic Instability as an Enabler of Malignancy

Aberrations that increase mutation rates are common in cancers and facilitate the acquisition of driver mutations that lead to transformation and tumor progression. The preceding section identified the eight defining features of malignancy, all of which appear to be produced by genetic alterations involving cancer genes. How do these mutations arise? Although environmental agents that are mutagenic (e.g., chemicals, radiation, sunlight) are common, cancers are relatively rare outcomes of these encounters. This state of affairs results from the ability of normal cells to sense and repair DNA damage.

The importance of DNA repair in maintaining the integrity of the genome is highlighted by inherited disorders in which DNA repair is defective, placing affected individuals at greatly increased risk of cancer. Defects in several DNA repair systems—mismatch repair, nucleotide excision repair, homologous recombination, and DNA polymerase proofreading—underlie these inherited disorders,

which we discuss later. In addition, we will briefly mention several situations in which other special types of acquired genomic instability contribute to cancer development.

Hereditary Nonpolyposis Colorectal Cancer Syndrome. Hereditary nonpolyposis colorectal syndrome (HNPCC, also known as Lynch syndrome) dramatically illustrates the role of DNA repair genes in predisposition to cancer. This disorder, characterized by familial carcinomas of the colon affecting predominantly the cecum and proximal colon (Chapter 13), results from defects in genes involved in DNA mismatch repair. When a strand of DNA is being replicated, the products of mismatch repair genes act as "spell checkers." For example, if there is an erroneous pairing of G with T, rather than the normal A with T, the mismatch repair genes correct the defect. Without these "proofreaders," errors accumulate at an increased rate.

Mutations in at least four mismatch repair genes have been found to underlie HNPCC (Chapter 13). Each affected individual inherits one defective copy of one of these DNA mismatch repair genes and acquires the second "hit" in colonic epithelial cells. Thus, altered DNA repair genes affect cell growth only indirectly—by allowing mutations in other genes during the process of normal cell division. A characteristic finding in the genome of tumors with mismatch repair defects is *microsatellite instability* (MSI). Microsatellites are tandem repeats of one to six nucleotides found throughout the genome. In wild-type tumors, the length of these microsatellites remains constant. By contrast, in tumors with HNPCC, these satellites are unstable and increase or decrease in length. While HNPCC accounts for only 2% to 4% of all colonic cancers, MSI is also detected in about 15% of sporadic cancers that typically have acquired mutations in mismatch repair genes.

Xeroderma Pigmentosum. Xeroderma pigmentosum is an autosomal recessive disorder caused by a defect in DNA repair that is associated with a greatly increased risk for cancers of sun-exposed skin. Ultraviolet (UV) rays in sunlight cause cross-linking of pyrimidine residues, preventing normal DNA replication. Such DNA damage is repaired by the nucleotide excision repair system. Several proteins are involved in nucleotide excision repair, and the inherited loss of any one of these can give rise to xeroderma pigmentosum.

Diseases Caused by Defects in Repair of DNA by Homologous Recombination. The autosomal recessive disorders *Bloom syndrome, ataxia-telangiectasia,* and *Fanconi anemia* are characterized by hypersensitivity to DNA-damaging agents such as ionizing radiation (in Bloom syndrome and ataxia-telangiectasia) or to DNA cross-linking agents such as certain chemotherapy drugs (in Fanconi anemia). Their phenotype is complex and includes, in addition to predisposition to cancer, features such as neurological symptoms (in ataxia-telangiectasia), anemia (in Fanconi anemia), and developmental defects (in Bloom syndrome). The gene mutated in ataxia-telangiectasia is *ATM*, which encodes a protein kinase that is important in "sensing" DNA damage caused by ionizing radiation and in activating p53 to initiate the DNA damage response, as described earlier.

Evidence for the role of DNA repair genes in the origin of cancer also comes from the study of hereditary breast cancer. **Germline mutations in two genes involved in repair of DNA by homologous recombination, *BRCA1* and *BRCA2*, account for 50% of cases of familial breast cancer.** In addition to breast cancer, women with *BRCA1* mutations have a substantially higher risk of epithelial ovarian cancers, and men have a slightly higher risk of prostate cancer. Likewise, germline mutations in the *BRCA2* gene increase the risk of breast cancer in both men and women, as well as cancers originating from the ovary, prostate, pancreas, bile ducts, stomach, melanocytes, and B lymphocytes. Cells lacking normal BRCA1 or BRCA2 proteins are prone to develop chromosomal rearrangements and severe aneuploidy due to defects in homologous recombination, which is required to repair certain types of DNA damage. Both copies of *BRCA1* and *BRCA2* must be inactivated for cancer to develop.

Genomic Instability Caused by DNA Polymerase Mutations. Under normal circumstances, cellular DNA polymerases involved in DNA replication have a very low rate of error, defined as addition of a nucleotide that does not match its partner on the template strand of DNA. This fidelity stems from an inherent exonuclease activity that allows DNA polymerase to pause, excise mismatched bases, and insert the proper nucleotide before proceeding down the template strand. Subsets of certain cancers, most often endometrial carcinomas and colon cancers, harbor mutations in DNA polymerase that result in loss of this "proofreading" function and the accumulation of numerous point substitutions. Cancers with DNA polymerase mutations (mainly endometrial and colorectal cancers) are among the most heavily mutated of all human cancers and, presumably because of a high burden of neoantigens, have excellent responses to immune checkpoint inhibitors.

Regulated Genomic Instability in Lymphoid Cells. Adaptive immunity relies on the ability of B cells and T cells to diversify their antigen receptor genes (Chapter 5). Immature B cell and T cell progenitors express a pair of gene products, RAG1 and RAG2, that carry out antigen receptor gene recombination, permitting the assembly of functional immunoglobulin and T-cell receptor genes. In addition, after encountering antigen, mature B cells express a specialized enzyme called *activation-induced cytosine deaminase (AID)*, which catalyzes both immunoglobulin gene class switch recombination and immunoglobulin diversification through somatic hypermutation. Both antigen receptor gene assembly and immunoglobulin gene class switching and diversification involve DNA breaks and ligation, and errors in these processes are responsible for many of the mutations that cause lymphoid neoplasms, discussed in detail in Chapter 10.

Tumor-Promoting Inflammation as an Enabler of Malignancy

Infiltrating cancers provoke a chronic inflammatory reaction. In patients with advanced cancers, this inflammatory reaction can be so extensive as to cause systemic signs and symptoms, such as anemia (the so-called "anemia of chronic inflammation"), fatigue, and cachexia. However, studies carried out on cancers in animal models suggest that inflammatory cells also modify the tumor microenvironment to enable many of the hallmarks of cancer. These effects may stem from direct interactions between inflammatory cells and tumor cells, or through indirect effects of inflammatory cells on other resident stromal cells, particularly fibroblasts and endothelial cells. Proposed cancer-enabling effects of inflammatory cells and resident stromal cells include the following:

- *Release of factors that promote proliferation.* Infiltrating leukocytes and activated stromal cells have been shown to secrete a wide variety of growth factors, such as EGF, and proteases that can liberate growth factors from the extracellular matrix (ECM).
- *Removal of growth suppressors.* As mentioned earlier, the growth of epithelial cells is suppressed by cell—cell and cell—ECM interactions. Proteases released by inflammatory cells can degrade the adhesion molecules that mediate these interactions, removing a barrier to growth.
- *Enhanced resistance to cell death.* Detachment of epithelial cells from basement membranes and from cell—cell interactions can

lead to a particular form of programmed cell death. Tumor-associated macrophages may prevent this type of cell death by expressing adhesion molecules such as integrins that promote direct physical interactions with tumor cells.

- *Angiogenesis.* Inflammatory cells release numerous factors, including VEGF, that stimulate angiogenesis.
- *Invasion and metastasis.* Proteases released from macrophages foster tissue invasion by remodeling the ECM, while factors such as TNF and EGF may directly stimulate tumor cell motility. As mentioned earlier, other factors released from stromal cells such as TGF-β may promote epithelial-mesenchymal transition (EMT), which may be a key event in the process of invasion and metastasis.
- *Evasion of immune destruction.* A variety of soluble factors released by macrophages and other stromal cells are believed to contribute to an immunosuppressive tumor microenvironment. The leading candidates for mediating such effects include TGF-β and other factors that either favor the recruitment and development of immunosuppressive T regulatory cells and so-called myeloid-derived suppressor cells (MDSCs) or suppress the function of CTLs. Furthermore, there is abundant evidence in cancer models and emerging evidence in human disease that advanced cancers contain mainly alternatively activated (M2) macrophages (Chapter 2). M2 macrophages produce cytokines that promote angiogenesis, fibroblast proliferation, and collagen deposition, all of which are commonly observed in invasive cancers as well as in healing wounds.

Important clinical considerations emerge from the principles presented in the foregoing discussion of the hallmarks of cancer: These hallmarks provide a road map for the development of new therapeutic agents for the treatment of cancer (Fig. 6.30).

ETIOLOGY OF CANCER: CARCINOGENIC AGENTS

Carcinogenic agents inflict genetic damage, which lies at the heart of carcinogenesis. Three classes of carcinogenic agents have been identified: (1) chemicals, (2) radiant energy, and (3) microbes. Chemicals and radiant energy are documented causes of cancer in humans, and oncogenic viruses are involved in the pathogenesis of tumors in several animal models and some human tumors. In the following discussion, each class of agents is considered separately; of note, however, several may act in concert or sequentially to produce the multiple genetic abnormalities characteristic of neoplastic cells.

Chemical Carcinogens

More than 200 years ago, the London surgeon Sir Percival Pott attributed scrotal skin cancer in chimney sweeps to chronic exposure to soot. On the basis of this observation, the Danish Chimney Sweeps Guild ruled that its members must bathe daily. This simple public health measure resulted in the disappearance of scrotal cancer, proving Sir Percival correct. Subsequently, hundreds of chemicals have been shown to be carcinogenic in animals. A few comments on several of these are offered next.

Direct-Acting Agents

Direct-acting agents require no metabolic conversion to be carcinogenic. They are typically weak carcinogens; however, some of them are cancer chemotherapy drugs (e.g., alkylating agents) used in regimens that may treat certain types of cancer (e.g., Hodgkin lymphoma) only to evoke a subsequent, second form of cancer, usually leukemia. This situation also applies to the use of such agents for nonneoplastic

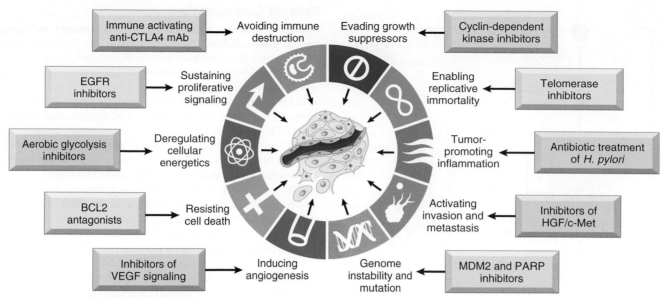

FIG. 6.30 Therapeutic targeting of the hallmarks of cancer. Selected examples of drugs targeting each hallmark that are approved or under development are shown. *CTLA-4,* Cytotoxic T-lymphocyte-associated protein-4; *EGFR,* epidermal growth factor receptor; *HGF,* hepatocyte growth factor; *MDM2,* mouse double minute 2 homolog; *PARP,* poly (ADP-ribose) polymerase; *VEGF,* vascular endothelial growth factor. (From Hanahan D, Weiberg RA: The hallmarks of cancer: the next generation. *Cell* 144:646, 2011.)

disorders, such as rheumatoid arthritis or granulomatosis with poly-angiitis. The associated risk for induced cancer is low, but its existence dictates judicious use of such agents.

Indirect-Acting Agents

The designation *indirect acting* refers to chemicals that require metabolic conversion to produce the ultimate carcinogen. Some of the most potent indirect chemical carcinogens are polycyclic hydro-carbons that are created by burning fossil fuels, plants, and animal materials. For example, benzo[a]pyrene and other carcinogens formed during the combustion of tobacco are implicated in the causation of lung cancer. Polycyclic hydrocarbons may also be pro-duced from animal fats during broiling of meats and are present in smoked meats and fish. In the body, benzo[a]pyrene is metabolized to epoxides, which form covalent adducts (addition products) with DNA, RNA, and proteins.

The aromatic amines and azo dyes constitute another class of indirect-acting carcinogens. Before its carcinogenicity was recognized, β-naphthylamine exposure caused a 50-fold increased incidence of bladder cancers in workers in the aniline dye and rubber industries. Because indirect-acting carcinogens require metabolic activation for their conversion to DNA-damaging agents, much interest is focused on the enzymatic pathways that are involved, particularly the cyto-chrome P-450—dependent monooxygenases. The genes that encode these enzymes are polymorphic, and enzyme activity varies among individuals, a factor that may lead to different levels of risk. For example, various P-450 isoforms that differ in their ability to convert benzo[a]pyrene into carcinogenic metabolites are associated with different levels of lung cancer risk in smokers.

A few other agents merit brief mention. Aflatoxin B_1 is of interest because it is a naturally occurring agent produced by some strains of *Aspergillus,* a mold that grows on improperly stored grains and nuts. A strong correlation has been found between the dietary level of this food contaminant and the incidence of hepatocellular carcinoma in parts of

Africa and Southeast Asia. Additionally, vinyl chloride, arsenic, nickel, chromium, insecticides, fungicides, and polychlorinated biphenyls are potential carcinogens in the workplace and in the home. Finally, nitrites used as food preservatives cause nitrosylation of amines contained in food; the nitrosamines thus formed are carcinogenic.

Mechanisms of Action of Chemical Carcinogens

Malignant transformation results from mutations, and it should therefore not be surprising that most chemical carcinogens are mutagenic. All direct and ultimate carcinogens contain highly reactive electrophile groups that form chemical adducts with DNA. Any gene may be the target of chemical carcinogens, but it is the mutation of important cancer genes, such as *RAS* and *TP53,* that is responsible for carcinogenesis. Of interest, one specific chemical carcinogen, aflatoxin B_1, produces a characteristic mutation in *TP53,* such that detection of this mutation points toward aflatoxin as the causative agent. Specific "mutational signatures" also exist for cancers caused by UV light, tobacco smoke, and certain other envi-ronmental carcinogens and are proving to be useful tools in epidemiologic studies of carcinogenesis.

Carcinogenicity of some chemicals is augmented by subsequent administration of *promoters* (e.g., phorbol esters, hormones, phenols, certain drugs), which are by themselves nontumorigenic. To be effec-tive, repeated or sustained exposure to the promoter must follow the application of the mutagenic chemical, or *initiator* (Fig. 6.31). The initiation-promotion sequence of chemical carcinogenesis raises an important question: Since promoters are not mutagenic, how do they contribute to tumorigenesis? Although the effects of tumor promoters are pleiotropic, **induction of cell proliferation is a *sine qua non* of tumor promotion.** It seems most likely that while the application of an initiator may cause the mutational activation of an oncogene such as *RAS,* subsequent application of promoters leads to clonal expansion of initiated (mutated) cells. Stimulated to proliferate, the initiated clone of cells accumulates additional mutations, eventually developing into a

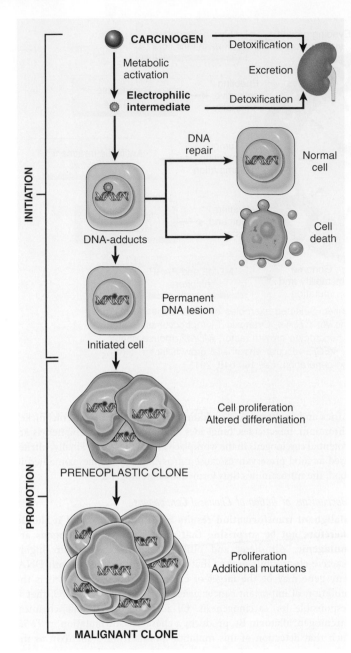

FIG. 6.31 Initiation and promotion of cancer by chemical carcinogens. Note that carcinogens that act as promoters cause clonal expansion of the initiated cell, thus producing a preneoplastic clone. Further proliferation induced by promoters or other factors causes accumulation of additional mutations and emergence of a malignant tumor.

malignant tumor. Indeed, the concept that sustained cell proliferation increases the risk for mutagenesis, and hence promotes neoplastic transformation is also applicable to human carcinogenesis. For example, endometrial hyperplasia (Chapter 17) and increased regenerative activity that accompanies chronic liver cell injury are associated with the development of cancer in these organs. Were it not for the DNA repair mechanisms discussed earlier, the incidence of chemically induced cancers would in all likelihood be much higher. As mentioned previously, the rare hereditary disorders of DNA repair, including xeroderma pigmentosum, are associated with greatly increased risk for developing cancers induced by UV light and certain chemicals.

Radiation Carcinogenesis

Radiation, whatever its source (UV rays of sunlight, radiographs, nuclear fission, radionuclides), is carcinogenic. Unprotected miners of radioactive elements have a 10-fold increased incidence of lung cancers. A follow-up study of survivors of the atomic bombs dropped on Hiroshima and Nagasaki disclosed a markedly increased incidence of leukemia after an average latent period of about 7 years, as well as increased mortality rates for thyroid, breast, colon, and lung carcinomas. The nuclear power accident at Chernobyl in the former Soviet Union continues to exact its toll in the form of high cancer incidence in the surrounding areas. Therapeutic irradiation of the head and neck can also give rise to papillary thyroid cancers years later.

The oncogenic properties of ionizing radiation are related to its mutagenic effects; it causes chromosome breakage, chromosomal rearrangements such as translocations and inversions, and, less frequently, point mutations. Double-stranded DNA breaks seem to be the most mutagenic form of DNA damage caused by ionizing radiation.

The oncogenic effect of UV rays merits special mention because it highlights the importance of DNA repair in carcinogenesis. Natural UV radiation derived from the sun can cause skin cancers (e.g., melanomas, squamous cell carcinomas, and basal cell carcinomas). At greatest risk are fair-skinned people who live in locales that receive a great deal of sunlight (e.g., Australia). Nonmelanoma skin cancers are associated with total cumulative exposure to UV radiation, whereas melanomas are associated with intense intermittent exposure—as occurs with sunbathing or tanning beds. UV light has several biologic effects on cells. Of particular relevance to carcinogenesis is DNA damage resulting in the formation of pyrimidine dimers, which is typically repaired by the nucleotide excision repair pathway. With extensive exposure to UV light, the repair systems may be overwhelmed, resulting in skin cancer. As mentioned earlier, patients with the inherited disease *xeroderma pigmentosum* have a defect in the nucleotide excision repair pathway and have a greatly increased predisposition to skin cancers.

Viral and Microbial Oncogenesis

Many DNA and RNA viruses have proved to be oncogenic in animals as disparate as frogs and primates. Despite intense scrutiny, only a few viruses have been causally linked with human cancer. Conversely, however, some of these viruses, particularly human papillomavirus, Epstein-Barr virus, and hepatitis viruses B and C, are collectively associated with up to 15% to 20% of cancers worldwide. The following discussion focuses on human oncogenic viruses. Also discussed is the role of the bacterium *Helicobacter pylori* in gastric cancer.

Oncogenic RNA Viruses

Although the study of animal retroviruses has provided spectacular insights into the molecular basis of cancer, including the discovery of oncogenes, only one human retrovirus, human T-cell leukemia virus type 1 (HTLV-1), is firmly implicated in the pathogenesis of cancer in humans.

HTLV-1 causes *adult T-cell leukemia/lymphoma* (ATLL), a tumor that is endemic in certain parts of Japan, the Caribbean basin, South America, and Africa, and found sporadically elsewhere, including the United States. Worldwide, it is estimated that 15 to 20 million people are infected with HTLV-1. Similar to the human immunodeficiency virus (HIV), which causes AIDS, HTLV-1 has tropism for CD4+ T cells, and hence this subset of T cells is the major target for neoplastic transformation. Human infection requires transmission of infected T cells via sexual intercourse, blood products, or breastfeeding. Leukemia develops in only 3% to 5% of the infected individuals, typically after a long latent period of 40 to 60 years.

There is little doubt that HTLV-1 infection of T lymphocytes is necessary for leukemogenesis, but the molecular mechanisms of transformation are not certain. In contrast to several murine retroviruses, HTLV-1 does not contain an oncogene, and no consistent pattern of proviral integration next to a proto-oncogene has been discovered. In leukemic cells, however, viral integration shows a clonal pattern: although the site of viral integration in host chromosomes is random (the viral DNA is found at different locations in different cancers), the site of integration is identical within all cells of a given cancer. This would not occur if HTLV-1 were merely a passenger that infects cells after transformation; rather, it means that HTLV-1 must have been present at the moment of transformation.

The HTLV-1 genome contains the *gag, pol, env,* and long-terminal-repeat regions typical of all retroviruses but, in contrast to other leukemia viruses, it contains another gene referred to as *tax*. Tax protein is essential for viral replication, because it stimulates transcription of viral RNA from the 5′ long-terminal repeat. However, Tax also alters the transcription of several host cell genes and interacts with certain host cell signaling proteins, including the progrowth PI3-kinase pathway and the transcription factor NF-κB, which promotes the growth and survival of lymphocytes.

The precise steps that lead to the development of adult T-cell leukemia/lymphoma are not known, but a plausible scenario is as follows. Infection by HTLV-1 causes the expansion of a nonmalignant polyclonal cell population through stimulatory effects of Tax on cell proliferation. The proliferating T cells are at increased risk for mutations and genomic instability due to the effects of Tax and possibly other viral factors as well. This instability allows the accumulation of oncogenic mutations and eventually a monoclonal neoplastic T-cell population emerges.

Oncogenic DNA Viruses

Five DNA viruses—HPV, Epstein-Barr virus (EBV), Kaposi sarcoma herpesvirus (KSHV, also called human herpesvirus-8 [HHV-8]), a polyoma virus called Merkel cell virus, and hepatitis B virus (HBV)—are strongly associated with human cancer. KSHV and Kaposi sarcoma are discussed in Chapter 8. Merkel cell virus is associated with a particular cancer, Merkel cell carcinoma, that is too rare to merit further discussion. The others are presented here. We also briefly touch on the oncogenic effects of hepatitis C virus, an RNA virus, during our discussion of HBV, since both viruses share an association with chronic liver injury and liver cancer.

Human Papillomavirus. Scores of genetically distinct types of HPV have been identified. Some types (e.g., 1, 2, 4, and 7) cause benign squamous papillomas (warts) in humans (Chapter 22). Genital warts are associated with low-risk HPVs, predominantly HPV-6 and HPV-11, which have minimal malignant potential. By contrast, high-risk HPVs (e.g., types 16 and 18) cause several cancers, particularly squamous cell carcinoma of the cervix, anogenital region, and oropharynx.

The oncogenic potential of HPV can be related to the products of two viral genes, E6 and E7 (Fig. 6.32), each of which has several activities that are prooncogenic.

- *Oncogenic activities of E6.* The E6 protein binds to and mediates the degradation of p53 and stimulates the expression of TERT, the catalytic subunit of telomerase, which contributes to the immortalization of cells. E6 from high-risk HPV types has a higher affinity for p53 than E6 from low-risk HPV types, a property that likely contributes to oncogenesis.
- *Oncogenic activities of E7.* The E7 protein has effects that complement those of E6, all of which are centered on speeding cells through the G_1-S cell cycle checkpoint. It binds to the RB protein, releasing the E2F transcription factors that are normally sequestered by RB, promoting progression through the cell cycle. As with E6 proteins and p53, E7 proteins from high-risk HPV types have a higher affinity for RB than do E7 proteins from low-risk HPV types. E7 also inactivates the CDK inhibitor p21, another activity that promotes cell cycle progression.

An additional factor that contributes to the oncogenic potential of HPVs is viral integration into the host genome. In precursor cervical lesions, the HPV genome is maintained in a nonintegrated episomal form, while in cancers, the HPV genome is randomly integrated into the host genome. Integration interrupts a negative regulatory region in the viral DNA, resulting in overexpression of the E6 and E7 oncoproteins. Furthermore, cells in which the viral genome has integrated show significantly more genomic instability, which may contribute to acquisition of prooncogenic mutations in host cancer genes.

To summarize, **high-risk HPVs encode oncogenic proteins that inactivate RB, p53, and the cyclin-dependent kinase inhibitor p21 and upregulate telomerase, thereby promoting immortalization, cellular proliferation, and resistance to cell death.** Thus, it is evident that HPV proteins promote many of the hallmarks of cancer. The

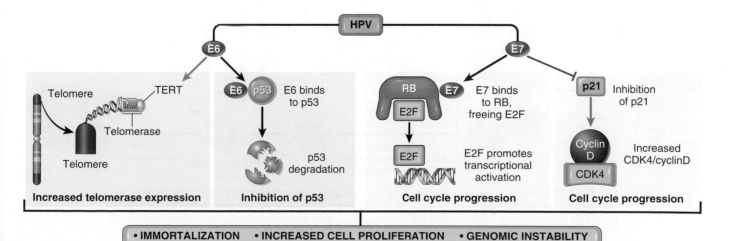

FIG. 6.32 Transforming effects of HPV E6 and E7 proteins. The net effect of HPV E6 and E7 proteins is to immortalize cells, protect cells from cell death, and remove the restraints on cell proliferation. *CDK,* Cyclin dependent kinase; *HPV,* human papillomavirus; *RB,* retinoblastoma; *TERT,* telomerase reverse transcriptase.

primacy of HPV infection in the causation of cervical cancer is confirmed by HPV vaccines, which are highly effective in preventing cervical cancer. However, infection with HPV itself is not sufficient for carcinogenesis, as the acquisition of mutations in host cancer genes (e.g., *RAS*) is required for full transformation. A significant proportion of women infected with HPV clear the infection by immunologic mechanisms, but others do not, some because of acquired immune abnormalities, such as those that result from HIV infection. Women who are coinfected with high-risk HPV types and HIV are at particularly high risk for developing cervical cancer.

Epstein-Barr Virus. **EBV, a member of the herpesvirus family, was the first virus linked to a human tumor, Burkitt lymphoma.** Burkitt lymphoma is an aggressive tumor that is endemic in certain parts of Africa and occurs sporadically elsewhere. In endemic areas, the tumor cells in virtually all affected patients carry the EBV genome. Since its discovery in Burkitt lymphoma, more than 50 years ago, EBV has been detected within the cells of a surprisingly diverse list of other tumors, including most nasopharyngeal carcinomas and a subset of T-cell lymphomas, NK cell lymphomas, Hodgkin lymphoma, gastric carcinomas, and, in rare instances, smooth muscle tumors, mainly in patients who are immunosuppressed.

The manner in which EBV causes B-cell tumors such as Burkitt lymphoma is complex and incompletely understood but best appreciated by considering its effects on normal B cells. EBV uses the complement receptor CD21 to attach to and infect B cells. In vitro, such infection leads to polyclonal B-cell proliferation and generation of immortal B lymphoblastoid cell lines. One EBV-encoded gene, *LMP1* (latent membrane protein 1), acts as an oncogene, as proven by its ability to induce B-cell lymphomas in transgenic mice. LMP1 promotes B-cell proliferation, mimicking the effects of a key surface receptor known as CD40. CD40 is normally activated by interaction with CD40 ligand expressed on helper T cells. By contrast, LMP1 is constitutively active and stimulates signaling through the NF-κB and

JAK/STAT pathways, both of which promote B-cell proliferation and survival. Thus, the virus "borrows" a normal B-cell activation pathway to promote its own replication by expanding the pool of infected cells. Another EBV-encoded protein, EBNA2, activates the expression of other genes that promote the growth of the infected B cells, including cyclin D and proto-oncogenes of the *SRC* family. In immunologically healthy persons, the EBV-driven polyclonal B-cell proliferation is readily controlled by CTLs, and the affected patient either remains asymptomatic or experiences a self-limited episode of infectious mononucleosis. However, a small number of EBV-infected B cells downregulate expression of immunogenic viral proteins such as LMP-1 and EBNA2 and remain in a long-lived pool of memory B cells that persist throughout life.

Given these observations, how then does EBV contribute to the genesis of endemic Burkitt lymphoma? One possibility is shown in Fig. 6.33. In regions of the world where Burkitt lymphoma is endemic, concomitant infections such as malaria impair immune competence, allowing sustained B-cell proliferation. Eventually, CTLs eliminate most of the EBV-infected B cells, but a small number survive. It appears that lymphoma cells emerge from this residual population following the acquisition of specific mutations, most notably translocations involving the *MYC* oncogene. In nonendemic areas, 80% of Burkitt lymphomas are unrelated to EBV, but virtually all endemic and sporadic tumors possess the (8;14) translocation or other translocations that dysregulate *MYC*. Thus, although sporadic Burkitt lymphomas are triggered by mechanisms other than EBV infection, they appear to develop through similar oncogenic pathways.

The oncogenic role played by EBV is more direct in EBV-positive B-cell lymphomas in immunosuppressed patients. Some individuals with AIDS or who receive immunosuppressive therapy to prevent allograft rejection develop EBV-positive B-cell tumors, often at multiple sites. These proliferations are polyclonal at the outset but can evolve into monoclonal neoplasms. In contrast to Burkitt lymphoma,

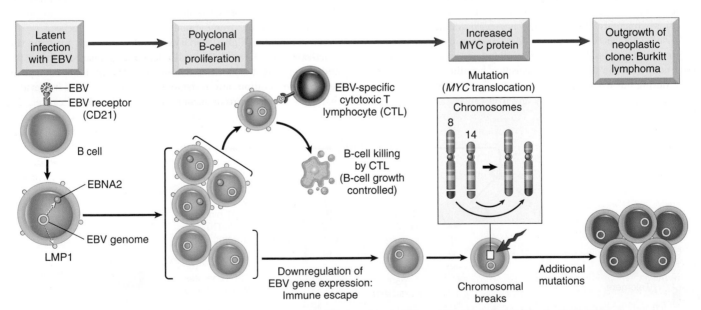

FIG. 6.33 Possible evolution of EBV-induced Burkitt lymphoma. After establishing a latent infection in B cells, EBV initially expresses gene products such as EBNA2 and LMP1 that drive the proliferation of the infected cells. This proliferation is usually controlled by cytotoxic T cells, an immune response that sometimes produces systemic symptoms (infectious mononucleosis). A small number of infected B cells escape from the host immune response by downregulating the expression of immunogenic viral proteins, and if these cells acquire a chromosomal translocation involving the *MYC* gene on chromosome 8, an aggressive B-cell tumor (Burkitt lymphoma) may emerge. *EBNA2,* Epstein-Barr virus nuclear antigen 2; *EBV,* Epstein-Barr virus; *LMP1,* latent membrane protein 1.

the tumors in immunosuppressed patients usually lack *MYC* translocations and uniformly express LMP-1 and EBNA2, which, as discussed, are antigenic and can be recognized by cytotoxic T cells. These potentially lethal proliferations can be subdued if T-cell function is restored, as may be achieved through withdrawal of immunosuppressive drugs in transplant recipients.

Nasopharyngeal carcinoma is also associated with EBV infection. This tumor is endemic in southern China, parts of Africa, and the Inuit population of the Arctic. In contrast to Burkitt lymphoma, nasopharyngeal carcinomas in all parts of the world are EBV associated. The integration site of the viral genome is identical (clonal) in the tumor cells within individual tumors, excluding the possibility that EBV infection occurred after tumor development. The uniform association of EBV with nasopharyngeal carcinoma suggests that EBV has a central role in the genesis of the tumor, but (as with Burkitt lymphoma) the restricted geographic distribution indicates that genetic or environmental cofactors (or both) also contribute to tumor development. Unlike Burkitt lymphoma, LMP-1 is expressed in nasopharyngeal carcinoma cells and, as in B cells, activates the NF-κB pathway. NF-κB, in turn, upregulates the expression of factors such as VEGF and matrix metalloproteases that may contribute to oncogenesis.

The relationship of EBV to the pathogenesis of Hodgkin lymphoma, yet another EBV-associated tumor, is discussed in Chapter 10.

Hepatitis B and Hepatitis C Viruses. **It is estimated that 70% to 85% of hepatocellular carcinomas worldwide are caused by HBV or HCV.** The epidemiologic evidence linking chronic HBV and hepatitis C virus (HCV) infection with hepatocellular carcinoma is strong (Chapter 16). However, the mode of action of these viruses in tumorigenesis is not fully elucidated. The oncogenic effects of HBV and HCV are likely multifactorial, but the dominant effect seems to be immunologically mediated chronic inflammation associated with hepatocyte death, leading to regeneration and (with time) genomic damage. Although the immune system is generally thought to be protective against cancer, recent work has demonstrated that in the setting of unresolved chronic inflammation, as occurs in viral hepatitis or chronic gastritis caused by *H. pylori* (see later), the immune response may become maladaptive, promoting tumorigenesis.

As with any cause of hepatocellular injury, chronic viral infection leads to the compensatory proliferation of hepatocytes. This regenerative process is aided and abetted by a plethora of growth factors, cytokines, chemokines, and other bioactive substances produced by activated immune cells that promote cell survival, tissue remodeling, and angiogenesis. A key molecular step seems to be activation of the nuclear factor-κB (NF-κB) pathway in hepatocytes caused by mediators derived from the activated immune cells. Activation of NF-κB blocks apoptosis, allowing the dividing hepatocytes to incur genotoxic stress and to accumulate mutations.

HCV, an RNA virus, is also strongly linked to the pathogenesis of liver cancer. The molecular mechanisms used by HCV are even less well defined than those for HBV, but chronic inflammation and reparative proliferation of hepatocytes again are felt to have central roles.

Helicobacter pylori. ***H. pylori*** **infection is implicated in the genesis of both gastric adenocarcinomas and gastric lymphomas.** First identified as a cause of peptic ulcers, *H. pylori* now has acquired the distinction of being the first bacterium classified as a carcinogen.

The scenario for the development of gastric adenocarcinoma is similar to that for HBV- and HCV-induced liver cancer. It involves increased epithelial cell proliferation on a background of chronic inflammation. As in viral hepatitis, the inflammatory milieu is a witches brew containing numerous genotoxic agents, such as reactive oxygen species. The sequence of histopathologic changes consists of initial development of chronic inflammation/gastritis, followed by gastric atrophy, intestinal metaplasia of the lining cells, dysplasia, and cancer. This sequence takes decades to complete and occurs in only 3% of infected patients.

As mentioned earlier, *H. pylori* is associated with an increased risk for the development of a gastric lymphoma referred to as extranodal marginal zone lymphoma. These lymphomas are of B-cell origin, and because the transformed B cells grow in a pattern resembling that of normal mucosa-associated lymphoid tissue (MALT), they have also been referred to as *MALT lymphomas* (Chapter 10). Their molecular pathogenesis seems to involve strain-specific *H. pylori* factors, as well as host genetic factors such as polymorphisms in the promoters of inflammatory cytokines such as IL-1β and tumor necrosis factor (TNF). It is thought that *H. pylori* infection leads to the activation of *H. pylori*–reactive T cells, which in turn stimulate a polyclonal B-cell proliferation. In time, a monoclonal B-cell tumor emerges from the proliferating B cells, perhaps as a result of accumulation of mutations in growth regulatory genes. Consistent with this model, early in the course of disease, eradication of *H. pylori* with antibiotics causes regression of the lymphoma by removing the antigenic stimulus for T cells. These lymphomas are thus a remarkable example of a tumor that depends on signals elicited by interactions with host immune cells for its continued growth and survival.

CLINICAL ASPECTS OF NEOPLASIA

Although malignant tumors have a greater potential for harm than benign tumors, morbidity and mortality may be associated with any tumor, even one that is benign. The following discussion considers the effects of a tumor on the patient, the grading and clinical staging of cancer, and the laboratory diagnosis of neoplasms.

Effects of Tumor on the Host

Malignant and benign tumors may cause injury through (1) damage of healthy tissues due to compression, invasion, and replacement by tumor; (2) ulceration of surfaces, leading to bleeding and infection; (3) release of substances such as hormones and procoagulants with systemic effects; (4) alteration of immune function, leading to infection and certain paraneoplastic syndromes; and (5) cachexia or wasting. Less commonly, benign or malignant neoplasms that protrude into the gut lumen may become caught in the peristaltic pull of the gut, causing intussusception (Chapter 13) and intestinal obstruction or infarction.

Location is crucial in both benign and malignant tumors. For example, a small (1-cm) pituitary adenoma can compress and destroy the surrounding normal gland, giving rise to hypopituitarism. A 0.5-cm leiomyoma in the wall of the renal artery may encroach on the blood supply, leading to renal ischemia and hypertension. A comparably small carcinoma within the common bile duct may induce fatal biliary tract obstruction.

Signs and symptoms related to hormone production are often seen in patients with benign and malignant neoplasms arising in endocrine glands. Adenomas and carcinomas arising in the beta cells of the pancreatic islets of Langerhans can produce hyperinsulinism, which may be fatal. Similarly, adenomas and carcinomas of the adrenal cortex may disrupt homeostatic mechanisms by elaborating steroid hormones (e.g., aldosterone, which induces sodium retention, hypertension, and hypokalemia). Such hormonal activity is more likely with a well-differentiated benign tumor than with a corresponding carcinoma.

Cancer Cachexia

Many patients with cancer experience progressive loss of body fat and lean body mass, accompanied by profound weakness, anorexia, and anemia—a condition referred to as *cachexia*. There is some correlation between the size and extent of spread of the cancer and the severity of the cachexia. However, cachexia is not caused by the nutritional demands of the tumor. Although patients with cancer are often anorexic, cachexia results from the action of soluble factors such as cytokines produced by the tumor and the host, not simply reduced food intake. In patients with cancer, calorie expenditure remains high and basal metabolic rate is increased, despite reduced food intake. This is in contrast with the lower metabolic rate that occurs as an adaptive response in starvation. The basis of these metabolic abnormalities is not fully understood. It is suspected that TNF and other cytokines produced by macrophages in response to tumor cells or by the tumor cells themselves mediate cachexia. TNF suppresses appetite and inhibits the action of lipoprotein lipase, preventing the release of free fatty acids from lipoproteins. There is no effective treatment for cancer cachexia other than removal of the underlying cause, the tumor.

Paraneoplastic Syndromes

Symptom complexes that occur in patients with cancer that cannot be explained by local or distant spread of the tumor or by the elaboration of hormones typical to the tissue of tumor origin are referred to as *paraneoplastic syndromes*. They appear in 10% to 15% of patients with cancer, and their clinical recognition is important for several reasons:

- Such syndromes may represent the earliest manifestation of an occult neoplasm.
- In affected patients, they may produce significant clinical illness or even be lethal.
- The symptom complex may mimic metastatic disease, thereby confounding treatment.

Paraneoplastic syndromes are diverse and are associated with many different tumors (Table 6.5). **The most common paraneoplastic syndromes are hypercalcemia, Cushing syndrome, and nonbacterial thrombotic endocarditis,** and the neoplasms most often associated with these and other syndromes are lung and breast cancers and

Table 6.5 Paraneoplastic Syndromes

Clinical Syndrome	Major Forms of Neoplasia	Causal Mechanism(s)/Agent(s)
Endocrinopathies		
Cushing syndrome	Small cell carcinoma of lung Pancreatic carcinoma Neural tumors	ACTH or ACTH-like substance
Syndrome of inappropriate antidiuretic hormone secretion	Small cell carcinoma of lung Intracranial neoplasms	Antidiuretic hormone
Hypercalcemia	Squamous cell carcinoma of lung Breast carcinoma Renal cell carcinoma Adult T-cell leukemia/lymphoma	Parathyroid hormone–related protein, TGF-α
Hypoglycemia	Fibrosarcoma Other sarcomas Ovarian carcinoma	Insulin or insulin-like substance
Polycythemia	Renal cell carcinoma Cerebellar hemangioma Hepatocellular carcinoma	Erythropoietin
Nerve and Muscle Syndrome		
Myasthenia	Bronchogenic carcinoma, thymoma	Immunologic
Disorders of the central and peripheral nervous systems	Breast carcinoma, teratoma	Immunologic
Dermatologic Disorders		
Acanthosis nigricans	Gastric carcinoma Lung carcinoma Uterine carcinoma	Secretion of epidermal growth factor or other growth factors
Dermatomyositis	Bronchogenic and breast carcinoma	Immunologic
Osseous, Articular, and Soft-Tissue Changes		
Hypertrophic osteoarthropathy and clubbing of the fingers	Bronchogenic carcinoma	Unknown
Vascular and Hematologic Changes		
Venous thrombosis (Trousseau phenomenon)	Pancreatic carcinoma Lung carcinoma Other cancers	Tumor products (mucins that activate clotting)
Nonbacterial thrombotic endocarditis	Advanced cancers	Hypercoagulability
Red cell aplasia	Thymoma	Immunologic
Others		
Nephrotic syndrome	Various cancers	Tumor antigens, immune complexes

ACTH, Adrenocorticotropic hormone; *IL-1,* interleukin-1; *TGF-α,* transforming growth factor-α; *TNF,* tumor necrosis factor.

hematologic malignancies. Hypercalcemia in cancer patients is multifactorial, but the most important paraneoplastic mechanism is the secretion of a parathyroid hormone—related protein (PTHrP) by tumor cells. Also implicated are other tumor-derived factors, such as TGF-α and the active form of vitamin D. Cushing syndrome arising as a paraneoplastic phenomenon is usually related to ectopic production of ACTH or ACTH-like polypeptides by cancer cells, as occurs in small cell carcinoma of the lung.

Paraneoplastic syndromes may also manifest as hypercoagulability, leading to venous thrombosis and nonbacterial thrombotic endocarditis (Chapter 9). Other manifestations are clubbing of the fingers and hypertrophic osteoarthropathy in patients with lung carcinomas (Chapter 11). Still others are discussed when we consider cancers of the various organs of the body.

Grading and Staging of Cancer

Methods to quantify the probable clinical aggressiveness of a given neoplasm and its extent and spread are necessary to predict prognosis accurately and to compare the results of various treatment protocols. For instance, the treatment plan and prognosis differ substantially between well-differentiated thyroid adenocarcinomas localized to the thyroid gland and anaplastic thyroid cancers that have invaded the neck organs. Systems have been developed to express the level of differentiation, or *grade,* and extent of spread of a cancer within the patient, or *stage,* as measures of the clinical gravity of the disease. Notably, **staging has proved to be of greater clinical value than tumor grading.**

- *Grading.* Grading of a cancer is based on the degree of differentiation of the tumor cells and, in some cancers, the number of mitoses, extent of tumor necrosis, and the presence of certain architectural features (e.g., loss of gland formation and replacement by solid sheets of cells). Increased mitotic activity and the extent of necrosis (which relates to a tumor outgrowing its blood supply) correlate with the pace of tumor growth, while loss of the normal architecture is a reflection of increasingly dysregulated gene expression. Grading schemes have evolved for each type of malignancy and generally range from two categories (low grade and high grade) to five categories. Criteria for the individual grades vary according to tumor type and so are not detailed here. All attempt, in essence, to judge the extent to which the tumor cells resemble or fail to resemble their normal counterparts and their tendency toward rapid growth.

- *Staging.* The staging of solid cancers is based on the size of the primary lesion, the extent of its spread to regional lymph nodes, and the presence or absence of metastases. The major staging system currently in use is the American Joint Committee on Cancer Staging. This system uses a classification called the *TNM system—T* for primary tumor, *N* for lymph node involvement, and *M* for metastases. TNM staging varies for specific forms of cancer but follows certain general principles. The primary lesion is characterized as T1 to T4 based on increasing size and invasion of adjacent structures. T0 is used to indicate an in situ lesion which is still bounded by the basement membrane. N0 signifies no nodal involvement, whereas N1 to N3 denotes involvement of an increasing number and range of nodes. M0 signifies no distant metastases, whereas M1 or sometimes M2 reflects the presence and estimated number of metastases.

In modern practice, grading and staging of tumors are being augmented by molecular characterization, described later.

Laboratory Diagnosis of Cancer

Every year the approach to laboratory diagnosis of cancer becomes more complex, more sophisticated, and more specialized. For virtually every neoplasm mentioned in this text, experts have characterized several diagnostic subcategories. Each of the following sections attempts to present the state of the art, avoiding details of technologies.

Morphologic Methods

In most instances, the laboratory diagnosis of cancer is not difficult. The two ends of the benign—malignant spectrum pose no problems; between these two extremes, however, accurate diagnosis may be challenging. Clinical and radiologic data are invaluable for optimal pathologic diagnosis. Radiation-induced changes in the skin or mucosa may resemble those of cancer. Sections taken from a healing fracture can mimic an osteosarcoma. The laboratory evaluation of a lesion is only as good as the submitted specimen, which must be adequate in size, representative, and properly preserved.

Several means to sample tumors are used clinically, including excision or biopsy, fine-needle aspiration, and cytologic smears. When excision is not possible, biopsy of the mass is required. A rapid *frozen section* diagnosis performed on freshly removed tissue is sometimes used to direct immediate surgical decisions, as, for example, in determining the nature of a mass or in evaluating regional lymph nodes in a patient with cancer for possible metastases. This method, in which a sample is quick-frozen and sectioned, permits histologic evaluation within minutes. In experienced, competent hands, frozen section diagnosis is accurate, but there are instances in which the superior histologic detail provided by more time-consuming routine methods is needed. In such instances, it is better to wait a few days, despite the drawbacks, than to perform incorrect, inadequate, or unnecessary surgery.

Fine-needle aspiration of tumors is a minimally invasive approach that can be performed in the clinic setting. It involves aspiration of cells from a mass, followed by cytologic examination of the cells (described below) after they have been spread out on a slide. This procedure is used most commonly with readily palpable lesions affecting the breast, thyroid gland, lymph nodes, and salivary glands. Current imaging techniques permit extension of the method to deeper structures, such as the liver, pancreas, and pelvic lymph nodes. Use of this diagnostic modality obviates surgery and its attendant risks. Although it entails some difficulties such as small sample size and sampling errors, in experienced hands it can be rapid, reliable, and useful.

Cytologic (Papanicolaou) tests provide another method for the detection of cancer. Historically, this approach has been used most widely to detect neoplasia of the uterine cervix, but it is now used in many other settings, including the evaluation of suspected endometrial, bronchogenic, bladder, prostate, and gastric carcinomas and the identification of tumor cells in abdominal, pleural, joint, and cerebrospinal fluids. Neoplastic cells are less cohesive than normal and are readily shed into fluids or secretions (Fig. 6.34). The shed cells are evaluated for features of anaplasia indicative of their origin from a tumor. The control of cervical cancer is the best testament to the value of the cytologic method.

Immunohistochemistry offers a powerful adjunct to routine histologic examination by enabling accurate identification of tissue types. Detection of cytokeratin by stains performed with specific monoclonal antibodies points to a diagnosis of undifferentiated carcinoma rather than lymphoma. Similarly, detection of prostate-specific antigen (PSA) in metastatic deposits allows definitive diagnosis of a primary tumor in the prostate gland, while immunohistochemical detection of estrogen receptor allows prognostication and directs therapeutic intervention in breast cancers.

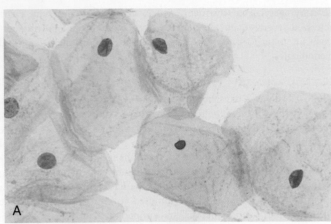

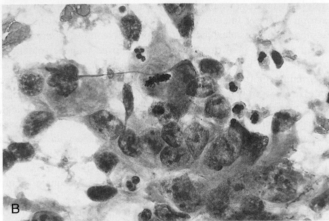

FIG. 6.34 (A) Normal Papanicolaou smear from the uterine cervix. Large, flat cells with small nuclei are typical. (B) Abnormal smear containing a sheet of malignant cells with large hyperchromatic nuclei. Nuclear pleomorphism is evident, and one cell is in mitosis. A few interspersed neutrophils, much smaller in size and with compact, lobate nuclei, are seen. (Courtesy of Dr. Richard M. DeMay, Department of Pathology, University of Chicago, Chicago, Illinois.)

Flow cytometry is used routinely in the classification of leukemias and lymphomas. In this method, fluorescently labeled antibodies against cell surface molecules and differentiation antigens are used to obtain the phenotype of the malignant cells (Chapter 10).

Tumor Markers

Biochemical assays for tumor-associated enzymes, hormones, and other tumor markers in the blood cannot be utilized for definitive diagnosis of cancer; however, they are used with varying success as screening tests and have utility in monitoring the response to therapy or detecting disease recurrence. The application of these assays is discussed in other chapters, so only a few examples suffice here. Prostate specific antigen (PSA) is one of the most frequently used tumor markers in clinical practice. Prostatic carcinoma can be suspected when elevated levels of PSA are found in the blood. However, PSA screening also highlights problems encountered with use of virtually every tumor marker. Although PSA levels are often elevated in cancer, PSA levels also may be elevated in benign prostatic hyperplasia (Chapter 16). Furthermore, prostate cancer may be present even when PSA levels are within the normal range. Thus, the PSA test suffers from both low sensitivity and low specificity, and its use as a screening tool has become controversial. The PSA assay is extremely valuable, however, for detecting residual disease or recurrence following treatment for prostate cancer. Other tumor markers used in clinical practice include carcinoembryonic antigen (CEA), which is elaborated by carcinomas of the colon, pancreas, stomach, and breast; alpha fetoprotein (AFP), which is produced by hepatocellular carcinomas, yolk sac tumors, and occasionally embryonal carcinomas; cancer antigen 125 (CA-125), which is produced by cancers of the fallopian tube, ovary, and colon; and cancer antigen 19-9 (CA-19-9), which is produced by cancers of the pancreas, gastrointestinal and hepatobiliary tracts, and ovary. Like PSA, CEA, AFP, CA19-9, and CA-125 can be elevated in a variety of non-neoplastic conditions and thus also lack the specificity and sensitivity required for early detection of cancers but are similarly useful in monitoring disease once the diagnosis is established. With successful resection of the tumor, these markers disappear from the serum; their reappearance almost always signifies recurrence. CEA is further discussed in Chapter 13 and alpha fetoprotein in Chapter 14.

Molecular Diagnosis

An increasing number of molecular techniques are being used for the diagnosis of tumors and for predicting their behavior.

- *Diagnosis of malignancy.* Because each T cell and B cell has unique antigen receptor gene rearrangements, polymerase chain reaction (PCR)—based detection of rearranged T-cell receptor or immunoglobulin genes allows monoclonal (neoplastic) and polyclonal (reactive) lymphocytic proliferations to be distinguished. Many hematopoietic neoplasms as well as a few solid tumors are defined by particular translocations, so detection of such translocations are required for diagnosis. For example, fluorescence in situ hybridization (FISH) or PCR analysis (Chapter 4) can be used to detect translocations characteristic of Ewing sarcoma and several leukemias and lymphomas. PCR-based detection of *BCR-ABL* transcripts can confirm the diagnosis of chronic myeloid leukemia (Chapter 10). Finally, certain hematologic malignancies are now defined by the presence of point mutations in particular oncogenes. For example, the diagnosis of *polycythemia vera*, another myeloid neoplasm, requires the identification of specific mutations in *JAK2*, a gene that encodes a nonreceptor tyrosine kinase.
- *Prognosis and behavior.* Certain genetic alterations are associated with a poor prognosis, and thus the presence of these alterations determines the patient's subsequent therapy. FISH and PCR methods can be used to detect amplification of oncogenes such as *HER2* and *MYCN*, which provide therapeutic and prognostic information for breast cancers and neuroblastomas, respectively. Sequencing of cancer genomes is now routine in many centers, allowing for the identification of point mutations in cancer genes such as *TP53* that predict a poor outcome in many different types of cancer. Although not yet standard of care, efforts are ongoing to develop tests that assess the host immune response to tumors, for example, by quantifying the number of infiltrating cytotoxic T cells, as this too is helpful in gauging prognosis.
- *Detection of minimal residual disease.* Another emerging use of molecular techniques is the detection of minimal residual disease after treatment. For example, detection of *BCR-ABL* transcripts by PCR assay gives a measure of residual disease in patients treated for chronic myeloid leukemia. Recognition that virtually all advanced tumors are associated with both intact circulating tumor cells and products derived from tumors (e.g., cell-free circulating tumor DNA) has led to interest in following tumor burden through sensitive blood tests (so-called *liquid biopsies*) designed to identify circulating tumor-specific nucleic acid sequences.

- *Diagnosis of hereditary predisposition to cancer.* Germline mutation of several tumor suppressor genes, such as *BRCA1*, increases a patient's risk for developing certain types of cancer. Thus, detection of these mutated alleles may allow the patient and the physician to devise an aggressive screening protocol or to opt for prophylactic surgery. In addition, detection through screening allows genetic counseling for relatives who are at risk.
- *Therapeutic decision-making.* There is increasing development of therapies that directly target specific mutations; detection of such mutations in a tumor can guide "personalized" therapy, as discussed later. It is now becoming evident that certain targetable mutations are seen in multiple malignancies. One example involves a valine for glutamate substitution in amino acid 600 (V600E) of the serine/threonine kinase BRAF, which lies downstream of RAS in the growth factor signaling pathway. Melanomas with the V600E *BRAF* mutation respond well to BRAF inhibitors, whereas melanomas without this mutation show no response. Subsequently, this same V600E mutation was also found in a subset of many other cancers, including carcinomas of the colon and thyroid gland, most hairy cell leukemias, and many cases of Langerhans cell histiocytosis (Fig. 6.35). These tumors are morphologically diverse and have distinct cells of origin, but they share identical oncogenic lesions in a common progrowth pathway.

Molecular Profiling of Tumors

Until recently, molecular studies of tumors involved the analysis of individual genes. However, the past few years have seen the introduction of technologies that can rapidly sequence an entire genome; assess epigenetic modifications genome-wide (the epigenome); quantify all of the RNAs expressed in a cell population (the transcriptome); measure many proteins simultaneously (the proteome); and take a snapshot of all of the cell's metabolites (the metabolome).

The most common method for large-scale analysis of RNA expression is now RNA sequencing, which offers a comprehensive and quantitative assessment of RNA expression that has supplanted older methods. However, RNA is prone to degradation and is a more difficult analyte to work with than DNA in clinical practice.

Furthermore, DNA sequencing is technically simpler than RNA sequencing, permitting the development of methods that rely on massively parallel sequencing (so-called "Next-generation [NextGen] sequencing") that can be performed on virtually any tissue specimen. Increases in DNA sequencing capacity and speed over the past decade have been breathtaking and are matched by an equally remarkable decrease in cost. The first reasonably complete draft of the sequence of the human genome, released in 2003, took 12 years of work and cost about $2,700,000,000. The cost of sequencing the whole genome has now decreased to less than $1000. At present, the entire genome of individual tumors can be sequenced in a few weeks, including the time for the extraordinarily complex task of assembling and analyzing the sequencing data.

These advances have enabled the systematic sequencing and cataloging of genomic alterations in various human cancers, an effort sponsored by the National Cancer Institute called The Cancer Genome Atlas (TCGA). The main impact of these systematic efforts has been in the area of research: identification of recurrent mutations in various types of cancer; description of the full panoply of genetic lesions that are found in individual cancers; and a greater appreciation of the genetic heterogeneity that exists in individual cancers from site to site. While whole-genome sequencing can also be used for individual patient care, most efforts in the clinical realm are focused on sequencing methods that permit identification of therapeutically "actionable" genetic lesions in a timely fashion at a reasonable cost. Such approaches are particularly useful when applied to tumors, such as lung and breast carcinomas, that are genetically diverse and require a "personalized" approach if targeted therapy is to succeed (Fig. 6.36). Most molecular diagnostic laboratories rely on "NextGen" methods that sequence the exons of several hundred key cancer genes at sufficient "depth" (fold coverage of the sequence in question) to detect mutations that are present in as few as 5% of tumor cells. In the process of doing this analysis, it is also possible to identify tumors that have exceptionally high mutational burdens, as is seen in cancers caused by carcinogen exposure or by mutations in DNA repair genes. This "hypermutated" phenotype is associated with response to checkpoint inhibitors,

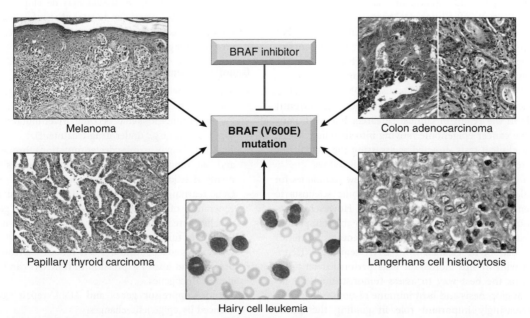

FIG. 6.35 Diverse tumor types sharing a common mutation, *BRAF* (V600E), are candidates for treatment with BRAF inhibitors.

ANATOMY

MOLECULAR TARGET

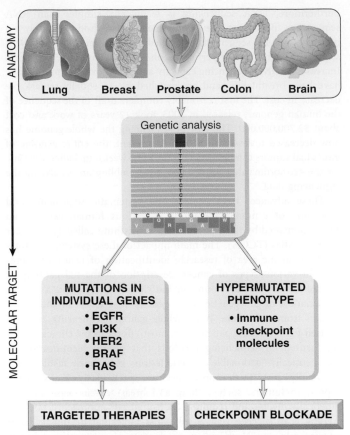

Lung Breast Prostate Colon Brain

Genetic analysis

MUTATIONS IN INDIVIDUAL GENES
- EGFR
- PI3K
- HER2
- BRAF
- RAS

HYPERMUTATED PHENOTYPE
- Immune checkpoint molecules

TARGETED THERAPIES

CHECKPOINT BLOCKADE

FIG. 6.36 Molecularly guided cancer therapy. Genetic analysis of cancers is utilized to identify mutated oncoproteins that can be targeted by specific drugs or, in the case of tumors with a "hypermutated" phenotype, immune checkpoint inhibitors that target molecules such as PD-1, PD-L1, and CTLA-4. *EGFR,* Epidermal growth factor receptor; *HER2,* human epidermal growth factor receptor 2; *PI3K,* phosphatidylinositol 3-kinase.

which unleash the immune response to neoantigens expressed by mutated cancer cells. A second method that is also used clinically involves the hybridization of tumor DNA to arrays containing oligonucleotide probes, a method that identifies changes in DNA copy number such as amplifications and deletions. Arrays containing probes that span the entire genome can detect all but the smallest copy number aberrations, providing information that is complementary to that obtained from focused DNA sequencing. Other "omics," such as proteomics and epigenomics, are currently being used mainly in the realm of clinical research, but with many drugs that target the cancer epigenome moving into the clinic, it can be anticipated that clinical tests directed at assessing the state of the epigenome that predict response to such agents will follow.

The excitement created by the development of new techniques for the global molecular analysis of tumors has led some scientists to predict that the end of histopathology is in sight. However, histopathologic inspection of tumors provides information about important characteristics of cancers, such as anaplasia, invasiveness, and tumor heterogeneity, that cannot be gleaned from DNA sequences. Histopathology coupled with in situ biomarker tests performed on tissue sections also remains the best way to assess tumor:stromal cell interactions, such as angiogenesis and host immune responses; the latter may have an increasingly important role in guiding therapeutic

interventions that are designed to counteract immune evasion by tumors. Thus, for the foreseeable future the most accurate diagnosis and assessment of prognosis in cancer patients will be arrived at by a combination of morphologic and molecular techniques.

Recent advances in imaging, computer technology, machine learning, and artificial intelligence indicate that diagnostic pathology is on the cusp of a revolution, in which qualitative evaluation of tumors (and other pathologic conditions) with the light microscope is replaced by more quantitative approaches that involve computer analysis of digitized images. It is hoped that integrating diverse types of data from computational analyses and "omic" characterization of tumors will further advance "precision oncology," the ability to select the right combination of treatments for each individual patient's tumor.

■ RAPID REVIEW

Benign and Malignant Tumors

- Benign and malignant tumors are distinguished based on differentiation, local invasiveness, and distant spread.
- In general, benign tumors resemble the tissue of origin, are well differentiated, are well circumscribed, have a capsule, and remain localized.
- In general, malignant tumors are poorly or completely undifferentiated (anaplastic), often (but not always) grow rapidly, are poorly circumscribed, invade surrounding normal tissues, and have the ability to metastasize to distant sites.

Epidemiology of Cancer

- Cancer incidence varies with age, geographic factors, and genetic background; it is most frequent in older adults, but certain types characteristically occur in children.
- Geographic variation in cancer incidence results mostly from different environmental exposures, such as infectious agents, smoking, alcohol, diet, obesity, reproductive history, and exposure to carcinogens.
- Cancer risk rises in the setting of chronic inflammation or excessive hormonal stimulation.
- Epithelial cell linings of tissues may develop morphologic changes (dysplasia) that signify an increased risk for developing cancer.
- Cancer risk is modified by interactions between environmental exposures and genetic variants.

Genetic Lesions in Cancer

- Mutations belong to two major classes, *driver (pathogenic)* and *passenger (neutral).*
- Passenger mutations may become driver mutations if selective pressure changes (e.g., under drug treatment).
- Tumor cells may acquire driver mutations through point mutations and nonrandom chromosomal abnormalities (gene rearrangements, deletions, and amplifications).
- Gene rearrangements often lead to overexpression of oncogenes or generation of novel fusion proteins, whereas gene amplifications usually increase the expression of oncogenes and deletions cause the loss of tumor suppressor genes.
- Overexpression of miRNAs can reduce expression of tumor suppressors and loss of expression of miRNAs can lead to overexpression of oncogenes.
- Tumor suppressor genes and DNA repair genes may also be silenced by epigenetic changes.

Self-Sufficiency in Growth Signals

- Proto-oncogenes are normal cellular genes whose products stimulate cell proliferation.
- Oncogenes are mutant or overexpressed versions of proto-oncogenes that produce inappropriate growth-promoting signals.
- Oncoproteins drive uncontrolled cell proliferation by several mechanisms, including autocrine signaling by secreted factors (e.g., PDGF in brain tumors); constitutive activity of proteins involved in progrowth signaling pathways (e.g., HER2 in breast cancer; BCR-ABL in leukemia; and RAS, in many cancers); excessive activity of transcription factors that turn on a program of gene expression that promotes cell growth (e.g., MYC, in many cancers); and constitutive expression of proteins that directly regulate cell cycle progression (e.g., cyclin D, in diverse cancers).

RB: Governor of the Cell Cycle

- Like other tumor suppressors, both copies of *RB* must be dysfunctional for tumorigenesis to occur.
- In *familial retinoblastoma*, one defective copy of the *RB* gene is present in the germline.
- RB inhibits G_1-to-S transition of cells by binding to E2F transcription factors.
- RB is negatively regulated by growth factor signaling, which leads to activation of cyclin D–CDK4/6 complexes, inactivation of RB by phosphorylation, and release of E2F factors.
- Almost all cancers have a disabled G_1 checkpoint due to mutation of *RB* or genes that regulate RB (e.g., genes encoding cyclin D, CDK4, and CDK inhibitors).
- Several oncogenic DNA viruses (e.g., HPV) encode proteins that bind and inhibit RB.

TP53: Guardian of the Genome

- *TP53* encodes p53, a central monitor of stress in the cell.
- DNA damage leads to phosphorylation and activation of p53, which upregulates factors such as p21 that sustain the activity of RB and cause a G_1-S block in the cell cycle.
- If DNA damage cannot be repaired, p53 turns on additional genes that induce cellular senescence or apoptosis.
- The majority of human cancers demonstrate biallelic mutations in *TP53*.
- Patients with *Li-Fraumeni syndrome* inherit one defective copy of *TP53* in the germline and develop a wide variety of tumors.
- p53 is inhibited by proteins encoded by oncogenic DNA viruses (e.g., HPV).

TGF-β, Contact Inhibition, and APC-β-Catenin Pathways

- TGF-β inhibits proliferation by activating growth-inhibiting genes (e.g., genes encoding cyclin-dependent kinase inhibitors) and suppressing growth-promoting genes (e.g., *MYC*).
- TGF-β pathway components are frequently compromised by mutations in many tumors, including pancreatic, colorectal, gastric, and esophageal carcinomas.
- E-cadherin maintains contact inhibition, which is lost in malignant cells.
- APC blocks proliferation of colonic epithelial cells by enhancing the destruction of β-catenin, a transcription factor in the WNT signaling pathway.
- With the loss of APC, β-catenin is stabilized, translocates to the nucleus, and upregulates progrowth genes (e.g., *MYC*).
- Familial adenomatous polyposis syndrome is caused by germline mutations in *APC* and is associated with the development of hundreds of colonic polyps and eventually colon carcinoma.

Altered Cellular Metabolism

- *Warburg metabolism* favors glycolysis over oxidative phosphorylation. It is induced in normal cells by exposure to growth factors and becomes fixed in cancer cells due to the action of certain driver mutations.
- Many oncoproteins (e.g., RAS, MYC, mutated growth factor receptors) induce Warburg metabolism to provide cellular building blocks needed for prolieration, and many tumor suppressors (e.g., PTEN, NF1, p53) oppose it.
- Stress may induce cells to consume their components in a process called autophagy, which is a double-edged sword in cancers, as cancer cells may accumulate mutations to avoid autophagy yet also use autophagy to provide nutrients for growth and survival.
- Some oncoproteins (e.g., mutated IDH) are enzymes that catalyze the formation of "oncometabolites" that alter the epigenome, leading to oncogenic changes in gene expression.

Evasion of Apoptosis

- Evasion of cell death mainly involves acquired abnormalities that interfere with the intrinsic (mitochondrial) pathway of apoptosis.
- Evasion often involves loss of p53 (a proapoptotic transcription factor) or overexpression of p53 inhibitors (e.g., MDM2).
- Other evasion mechanisms involve overexpression of antiapoptotic members of the BCL2 family (e.g., BCL2, BCL-XL).
- In follicular lymphoma, BCL2 is overexpressed because of a (14;18) translocation that fuses *BCL2* with regulatory elements of the immunoglobulin heavy chain gene.
- MDM2 inhibitors (which lead to activation of p53) and BCL2 family member inhibitors stimulate apoptosis through the intrinsic pathway.

Limitless Replicative Potential (Immortality)

- Normal cells lack telomerase, leading to telomere shortening, activation of cell cycle checkpoints, and senescence.
- In cells with disabled checkpoints, DNA repair pathways are activated by shortened telomeres, leading to chromosomal instability and mitotic crisis.
- Tumor cells reactivate telomerase, staving off mitotic catastrophe and achieving immortality.

Sustained Angiogenesis

- Vascularization of tumors is essential for their growth.
- Angiogenesis is controlled by a balance between angiogenic and antiangiogenic factors.
- Hypoxia triggers angiogenesis by stabilizing HIF-1α, leading to upregulation of VEGF, a key growth factor for endothelial cells.
- Many factors regulate angiogenesis, including p53, which induces synthesis of the angiogenesis inhibitor thrombospondin-1, and RAS, MYC, and MAPK, which upregulate VEGF expression.
- VEGF inhibitors slow the growth of advanced cancers but are not curative.

Invasion and Metastasis

- Invasion of tissues, a hallmark of malignancy, occurs in four steps: (1) loosening of cell–cell contacts; (2) degradation of ECM; (3) attachment to ECM components; and (4) migration of tumor cells.
- Cell–cell contacts are weakened due to loss of E-cadherin.
- Basement membrane and interstitial matrix degradation is mediated by proteolytic enzymes secreted by tumor cells and stromal cells (e.g., MMPs and cathepsins).

- Proteolytic enzymes also release growth factors from ECM and generate chemotactic and angiogenic fragments.
- Many tumors arrest in the first capillary bed they encounter (lung and liver, most commonly).
- Other tumors show marked organ tropism that is not explained by anatomy.

Evasion of Immune Surveillance

- Tumor cells can be recognized by the immune system as nonself and destroyed.
- Antitumor activity is mediated by predominantly cell-mediated mechanisms.
- Tumor antigens are presented on the cell surface by MHC class I molecules and are recognized by CD8+ CTLs.
- Tumor antigens include products of mutated genes, overexpressed or aberrantly expressed proteins, and tumor antigens produced by oncogenic viruses.
- Patients who are immunosuppressed have an increased risk for cancer, particularly types caused by oncogenic DNA viruses.
- In immunocompetent patients, tumors may avoid the immune system by several mechanisms, including selective outgrowth of antigen-negative variants, loss or reduced expression of histocompatibility molecules, and immunosuppression due to expression of certain factors (e.g., TGF-β, PD-1 ligands) by the tumor cells.
- Antibodies that block some of these mechanisms are used to treat patients with advanced cancers.

Genomic Instability as an Enabler of Malignancy

- Inherited mutations in DNA repair genes are associated with increased cancer risk.
- Hereditary nonpolyposis colorectal cancer (Lynch syndrome) is caused by defects in the mismatch repair system that lead to instability of short DNA repeat regions called microsatellites and the development of several tumors, particularly colon cancer.
- *Xeroderma pigmentosum* is caused by a defect in nucleotide excision repair that leads to a failure to repair DNA damage caused by UV light and development of skin cancers in sites exposed to sunlight.
- Other syndromes are caused by defects in the homologous recombination DNA repair; these defects variously lead to *Bloom syndrome, ataxia-telangiectasia, Fanconi anemia,* and *hereditary breast/ovarian cancer.*
- Familial breast/ovarian cancer syndrome is most often caused by mutations in the genes encoding the DNA repair factors BRCA1 and BRCA2.
- Intrinsic genomic instability in lymphocytes undergoing antigen receptor gene rearrangement/mutation may lead to mutations that result in lymphoid neoplasms.

Chemical and Radiation Carcinogenesis

- Chemical carcinogens have highly reactive electrophile groups that damage DNA.
- Carcinogens include *direct-acting agents* (e.g., alkylating agents used as chemotherapy) that do not require metabolic conversion to become carcinogenic and *indirect-acting agents* (e.g., benzo[a]-pyrene, azo dyes, aflatoxin) that are not active until converted to an ultimate carcinogen by endogenous metabolic pathways.
- Tumor promoters act by stimulating the proliferation of cells exposed to carcinogens either directly or indirectly, the latter through tissue injury and associated regenerative repair.
- Ionizing radiation causes mutations that may affect cancer genes, thereby driving carcinogenesis.

- UV rays in sunlight induce the formation of pyrimidine dimers within DNA, leading to mutations due to error-prone repair.

Infections Associated With Cancer

- *HTLV-1* causes a T-cell leukemia that is endemic in Japan and the Caribbean.
- *HPV* is associated with benign warts and cervical cancer.
- Oncogenic strains of HPV encode two viral oncoproteins, E6 and E7, that inhibit p53 and RB, respectively.
- *EBV* is implicated in the pathogenesis of diverse lymphomas (e.g., Burkitt lymphoma), nasopharyngeal carcinoma, a subset of gastric carcinoma, and rarely smooth muscle tumors.
- Certain EBV gene products contribute to oncogenesis by stimulating normal B-cell proliferation pathways.
- Compromise of T-cell function often leads to EBV-driven B-cell lymphomas.
- Chronic HBV and HCV infection is associated with 70% to 85% of hepatocellular carcinomas worldwide, which appear to be caused largely by chronic inflammation and ongoing repair of the liver.
- *H. pylori* infection is implicated in both gastric adenocarcinoma and B-cell lymphomas known as extranodal marginal zone lymphomas.
- Development of gastric carcinoma involves chronic inflammation and gastric epithelial cell regeneration.
- Development of B-cell lymphoma involves an initial reactive polyclonal proliferation of B-cells that are susceptible to acquiring mutations that lead to clonal B-cell outgrowth (transformation).

Clinical Aspects of Tumors

- *Cachexia* is a common complication of advanced cancer that is defined by the progressive loss of body fat and lean body mass and accompanied by profound weakness, anorexia, and anemia.
- Cachexia is caused by release of cytokines by the tumor or host.
- *Paraneoplastic syndromes* are defined by the presence of symptoms that are not explained by tumor spread or by release of hormones appropriate to the tissue.
- Paraneoplastic syndromes are caused by the ectopic production and secretion of bioactive substances (e.g., ACTH, PTHrP, or TGF-α) by tumor cells.
- *Tumor grading* is determined by cytologic appearance and is based on the idea that behavior and differentiation are related (poorly differentiated = aggressive behavior).
- *Tumor staging* (extent of tumor) is determined by surgical exploration or imaging and is based on tumor size, local and regional lymph node spread, and distant metastases.
- Staging is of greater clinical value than grading.

Laboratory Diagnosis of Cancer

- Several sampling approaches exist for tumors (e.g., excision, biopsy, fine-needle aspiration, cytologic smears).
- Testing modalities include *immunohistochemistry* and *flow cytometry* (used to identify protein expression patterns that define different entities); *serum markers* (e.g., PSA), used to screen populations for cancer and to monitor for recurrence after treatment; and *molecular profiling* (e.g., DNA or RNA sequencing).
- Molecular profiling is used to determine diagnosis and prognosis; identify therapeutic targets; detect minimal residual disease after therapy; diagnose patients with a hereditary predisposition to cancer; and characterize circulating tumor cells and DNA shed into blood, stool, sputum, and urine (liquid biopsies).

■ Laboratory Tests

These are some samples of laboratory tests used in patients who have various cancers. Additional tumor specific testing is covered in systemic pathology chapters.

Test	Normal Value	Pathophysiology/Clinical Relevance
Alphafetoprotein (AFP), serum	<8.4 ng/mL	AFP is a glycoprotein normally expressed by embryonic hepatocytes and fetal yolk sac cells. Production drops after birth but rises again in patients with certain tumors. Serum AFP levels are increased in 90% of patients with hepatocellular carcinoma and in patients with certain germ cell tumors of the ovary and testis (e.g., yolk sac tumor, embryonal carcinoma). AFP levels are neither specific nor sensitive for the diagnosis of any tumor but they are useful to monitor postoperative course of tumors that produce them such as testicular tumors. AFP is also elevated in maternal serum in the setting of open neural tube defects (e.g., anencephaly, spina bifida).
Cancer antigen 19-9 (Carbohydrate antigen 19-9, CA 19-9), serum	<35 U/mL	CA 19-9 is the sialylated form of the Lewis(a) blood group antigen. It is elevated in the blood of ~70%–90% of patients with pancreatic ductal adenocarcinoma and may be elevated in other malignancies (e.g., cholangiocarcinoma, colon cancer, gastric cancer, ovarian cancer). In patients who are Lewis blood group antigen negative, tumor cells cannot produce CA 19-9, a limitation of this marker. CA 19-9 is not useful in screening due to lack of specificity but can be used to follow therapeutic response/disease recurrence.
Cancer antigen 125 (CA-125), serum	<46 U/mL	CA-125 is a glycoprotein that is normally expressed on cells derived from coelomic epithelium (e.g., fallopian tube, ovary, colon). Serum CA-125 is increased in advanced epithelial ovarian cancer and can be used to assess the presence of residual disease following debulking surgery or to monitor for recurrence.
Carcinoembryonic antigen (CEA), serum	Nonsmokers: ≤3.0 ng/mL Smokers: <5.0 ng/mL	CEA is an oncofetal antigen normally expressed during fetal development. It is also expressed by certain epithelial malignancies (e.g., colorectal, pancreatic, and lung cancer). Serum CEA elevations of >20 ng/mL are usually (but not always) indicative of malignancy. It is a useful marker for monitoring recurrence of colon cancer after resection but is not useful for screening.
Cervical cancer screening: Pap test cytology +/– high-risk HPV (hrHPV) test	Positive Pap test: Squamous cells with morphologic features consistent with HPV infection. Positive hrHPV test: Presence of any of several hrHPV types.	Most invasive cervical cancers are squamous cell carcinoma; persistent infection with hrHPV is usually necessary but not sufficient for the development of squamous cell carcinoma. The goal of cervical cancer screening is to identify precursor lesions and/or HPV types likely to progress to cervical carcinoma. Pap tests assess the morphologic features of cells scraped from the cervix and endocervix and are reported in terms of degree of dysplasia. hrHPV tests are molecular tests that look for the presence of certain HPV types. Pap and hrHPV tests may be used alone or in combination; many countries and professional organizations recommend testing for hrHPV types first, followed by a Pap test if a hrHPV is detected.
PD-L1 expression	Varies depending on tumor type, PD-L1 clone, scoring methods	Expression of PD-L1 on tumor cells allows tumors to evade the host immune response. Immunohistochemistry for PD-L1 is performed in multiple tumor types (e.g., melanoma, non-small cell lung cancer, Hodgkin lymphoma) to predict treatment response to PD-L1 inhibitors ("checkpoint inhibitors").
Prostate specific antigen (PSA), serum	Total PSA 0–4 ng/mL	PSA is a protease secreted by the epithelial cells of the acini and ducts of the prostate gland that is found in the blood in protein-bound and free forms. Total PSA (bound + unbound) is a marker for prostate cancer and is useful in diagnosis and staging and monitoring treatment, though it is not specific for malignancy. Definitive diagnosis of prostate cancer requires biopsy and pathologist examination.

Molecular Tests of Broad Relevance in Cancer		
Mutational burden/ microsatellite instability	Several methods available: (1) immunohistochemical identification of loss of mismatch repair proteins; (2) PCR-based assays that detect microsatellite instability; and (3) Next-Gen sequencing methods that measure mutational load	High mutational load is observed in cancers that are caused by carcinogens (e.g., melanoma and lung cancer) or that have defects in mismatch repair genes or acquired mutations in genes encoding DNA proofreading factors. The presence of a high mutational burden or associated defects is predictive of response to immune checkpoint inhibitors across a spectrum of cancers.
MYC gene amplification	Not amplified	The MYC transcription factor promotes cell growth and is tightly controlled. When deregulated (e.g., by amplification, overexpression) MYC promotes carcinogenesis by affecting cell cycle progression, promoting metabolic reprogramming (the Warburg effect), upregulating telomerase, and increasing protein synthesis. *MYC* amplification is a prognostic marker, associated with aggressive disease and/or poor outcome in several tumor types (e.g., neuroblastomas with *MYCN* are less likely to respond to treatment). *MYC* amplification can also be seen in lymphomas, breast cancer, medulloblastoma, glioblastoma, alveolar rhabdomyosarcoma, small cell lung cancer, and prostate cancer.
TP53 mutation	Several methods available: (1) immunohistochemical detection of p53 staining, which is correlated with mutations that stabilize p53 and render it dysfunctional; (2) Next-Gen sequencing methods that directly detect *TP53* mutation and/or deletion; (3) in those suspected of having germline mutation of *TP53* (Li-Fraumeni syndrome), PCR amplification and sequencing of the *TP53* gene	*TP53* mutation is the most common event in a wide range of cancers. Loss of p53 function is correlated with resistance to therapy and predicts a worse outcome in many cancers. Individuals with germline *TP53* mutations are at high risk for developing diverse cancers, including lymphomas, leukemias, and sarcomas.

References values from https://www.mayocliniclabs.com/ by permission of Mayo Foundation for Medical Education and Research. All rights reserved.

Adapted from Deyrup AT, D'Ambrosio D, Muir J, et al. Essential Laboratory Tests for Medical Education. *Acad Pathol*. 2022;9. doi: 10.1016/j.acpath.2022.100046.

Environmental and Nutritional Diseases

Most diseases are influenced by environmental factors, and some are directly caused by environmental insults. Broadly defined, the *ambient environment* encompasses the various outdoor, indoor, and occupational settings in which humans live and work. In each of these settings, the air people breathe, the food and water they consume, the toxic agents they are exposed to, and the stresses they encounter are major determinants of health. Other environmental factors pertain to the individual ("personal environment") and include tobacco use, alcohol ingestion, therapeutic and nontherapeutic drug consumption, and diet. Many of these personal factors are related to gender, class, and socially defined race.

The term environmental disease refers to disorders caused by exposure to chemical or physical agents in the ambient, workplace, and personal environments, including diseases of nutritional origin. Environmental diseases are very common: the International Labor Organization has estimated that work-related injuries and illnesses kill more people per year globally than do road accidents and wars combined. Most of these work-related problems are caused by illnesses rather than accidents. The burden of disease in the general population created by nonoccupational exposures to toxic agents is more difficult to estimate, mostly because of the diversity of agents and difficulties in measuring the dose and duration of exposures. Whatever the precise numbers, environmental diseases are major causes of disability and suffering and constitute a heavy financial burden, particularly in lower-income countries.

Environmental diseases are sometimes the consequence of major disasters, such as the methyl mercury contamination of Minamata Bay in Japan in the 1960s and lead poisoning resulting from contaminated drinking water in the city of Flint, Michigan, in the United States in 2016. Less dramatic, but much more common, are disease and injury produced by chronic exposure to relatively low levels of contaminants. Disease related to nutrition is even more pervasive. In 2014 it was estimated that globally 462 million adults were underweight and 1.9 billion were either overweight or obese. Children are disproportionately affected by undernutrition: in 2016 an estimated 155 million children worldwide under the age of 5 years showed low height for age (stunting), a finding associated with chronic or recurrent undernutrition.

Health disparities in the United States are increasingly linked to social, cultural, and economic factors that include income, education, and occupation as well as variables that are more challenging to measure such as medical literacy, generational wealth, access to healthcare, food availability, living environment, and racial bias.

In this chapter, we first consider the problem of health disparities. We then discuss the issue of climate change followed by a section on the mechanisms of toxicity of chemical and physical agents and finally address specific environmental disorders, including those of nutritional origin.

HEALTH DISPARITIES

Health disparities are the differences in the incidence, prevalence, and severity of diseases between populations. Disparities may occur between groups based upon various attributes of an individual's identity, including gender, class, and socially defined race. Racism is a deeply rooted and ongoing feature of modern societies, so a clear understanding of the concept of "race" is critical in any discussion of health disparities. In the 19th century, different naturalists argued that there were anywhere from 2 to 63 human biological races, a state of confusion that reflected an inability to agree on the characteristics that should define race. The difficulty of dividing human populations into specific biological races was brought into focus when scientists began using genetics to examine human biological diversity. In the 1960s it was recognized that groups formerly considered distinct races (e.g., Africans, Asians, and Europeans) could not be differentiated based on the frequency of genetic polymorphisms. In recent years, this finding has been reinforced by various international DNA sequencing projects, which have produced data that invalidate the idea that there are distinct human biological races. The modern biological conception of race is defined by two criteria: (1) the amount of genetic variation within such groups compared to that between them and (2) whether any group within a species can be shown to be an evolutionarily distinct population. Studies of human populations have shown greater genetic variation within populations (e.g., African, East Asian, European) than between populations, leading to the conclusion that because of high levels of gene flow between populations, no population is truly genetically distinct. Furthermore, while geographically based genetic variation exists within our species, there is no unambiguous way to partition that genetic variation into groups, because human genetic variation is continuous, not discrete. Based on these considerations, the consensus position of modern population geneticists and biological anthropologists is that **there are no biologically distinct races in modern humans.**

However, throughout history, societies have distinguished certain populations based on arbitrary criteria such as appearance and geographic origin. This resulted in individuals being assigned to *socially defined races,* which continue to serve as the basis for social dominance in nations around the world. Social subordination results in groups being more likely to be exposed to environmental variables that have a negative impact on their health, such as air and water pollution, crowding, poor diet, inadequate education, greater exposure to toxic chemicals, lack of access to health care and infectious disease. When compared to European Americans, African Americans have increased infant mortality (more than 2-fold), prostate cancer mortality (2.5-fold), and COVID-19 mortality (nearly 2-fold). Type 2 diabetes, hypertension, and obesity are also more common in this population. The United States Latin American population also has increased rates of type 2 diabetes and obesity. Rates of health insurance coverage vary by socially defined race, which contributes to these disparities: according to CDC data, U.S. Latin American adults are least likely to have health insurance, whereas Asian Americans and European Americans are most likely.

While population-specific genetic differences do exist, socially defined race does not accurately reflect this genetic variability. Ethnicity, which is defined as group identity based on multiple characteristics including culture, country of origin, language and religion, can also influence health outcomes. In the United States, ethnicity is usually dichotomized as Hispanic or non-Hispanic. The term "Hispanic" in the U.S. census and many research studies refers to Americans of Spanish origin or descent, whereas "Latin American" includes non-Spanish speaking populations (e.g., Brazilians) of Central and South America with varying amounts of African, Amerindian, and European ancestry.

Historically, descriptors of socially defined race have included skin pigmentation (e.g., white, black), references to origin (African American, Asian American), and archaic 18th century anthropological terms such as "Caucasian"; in this textbook, we will use terms related to *geographic origin* for socially defined race: European American, African American, etc. Associations related to genetic disorders that are more prevalent in certain populations (e.g., cystic fibrosis) are best considered within the framework of *geographic ancestry* such as "of European descent." This approach is useful but imperfect due to (1) gene flow between populations (population admixture) and (2) historic associations of diseases with socially defined races or countries (e.g., "African American" or "Indian") that do not fully reflect the distribution of causative genetic variants across population. For example, sickle cell disease is commonly associated with African Americans; however, the basis for this association is positive selection for an allele that offers protection wherever falciparum malaria is found, including equatorial Africa, Southern Europe, the Middle East, and parts of Asia.

Thus, while racial and ethnic associations with disease are commonly stated in the medical literature, care must be taken in interpreting these relationships since they are not the result of inherent biological differences. Furthermore, while there may be statistically significant differences in disease incidence between socially defined races, the clinical relevance of these disparities is not always clear in rare diseases. Health disparities also reflect associations with socioeconomic status, geography, occupation, gender identity, and sexual orientation. Awareness of the issues that contribute to health disparities continues to increase, and an understanding of the social determinants of health and their impact on an individual's health is critical for the future health professional.

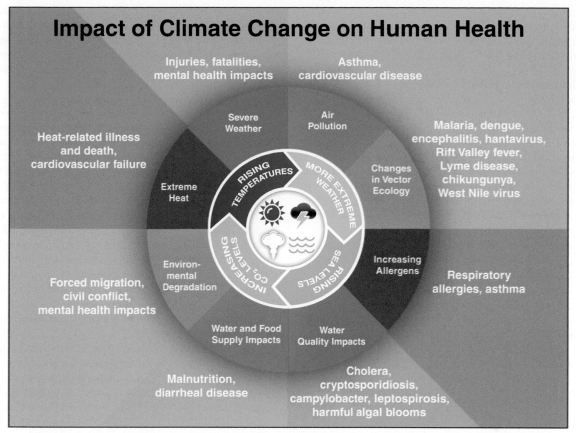

FIG. 7.1 Climate change impacts a wide-range of health outcomes. This slide illustrates the most significant climate change impacts (rising temperatures, more extreme weather, rising sea levels, and increasing carbon dioxide levels), their effect on exposures, and the subsequent health outcomes that can result from these changes in exposures. (From CDC: https://www.cdc.gov/climateandhealth/effects/default.htm.)

HEALTH EFFECTS OF CLIMATE CHANGE

Without immediate action, climate change stands to become the preeminent global cause of environmental disease in the 21st century and beyond (Fig. 7.1). Global temperature measurements show that the Earth has warmed significantly since the early 20th century and especially since the mid-1960s. Record-breaking global temperatures have become common, and the 5 years from 2016 to 2020 were the warmest since record keeping began in 1880. During 2020 the global land temperature was 1.59°C warmer than the 20th century average. Mean global ocean temperatures also continue to rise.

The rising atmospheric and oceanic temperatures have led to a large number of effects that include changes in storm frequency, drought, and flood, as well as large-scale ice losses in glaciated regions and dramatic reduction in the amount of sea ice in the Arctic Ocean. The melting of land-based glacial ice and the thermal expansion of the warming oceans have produced approximately 13 to 20 cm of global average sea level rise since 1900, and the sea level is currently rising at a global average rate of 3.6 mm/year.

Scientists have conclusively demonstrated that climate change is due to human activity through rising atmospheric level of "greenhouse" gases, particularly carbon dioxide (CO_2) released by the burning of fossil fuels (Fig. 7.2), ozone (an important air pollutant, discussed later), and methane. These gases, along with water vapor, produce the so-called greenhouse effect by absorbing energy radiated

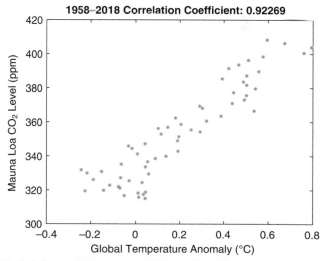

FIG. 7.2 Correlation of carbon dioxide (CO_2) levels measured at the Mauna Loa Observatory in Hawaii with average global temperature trends over the past 60 years. Global temperature in any given year was deduced at the Hadley Center (United Kingdom) from measurements taken at more than 3000 weather stations located around the globe. (Courtesy of Dr. Richard Aster, Department of Geosciences, Colorado State University, Fort Collins, Colorado.)

from Earth's surface that would otherwise be lost into space. Deforestation and the attendant decrease in carbon fixation by plants also increase CO_2 levels. Depending on the computer model used, the global temperature is projected to rise by 2°C to 5°C by the year 2100 (Fig. 7.3).

The health consequences of climate change will depend on its extent and rapidity, the severity of the ensuing consequences, and humankind's ability to mitigate the damaging effects. The World Health Organization (WHO) estimates that approximately 250,000 excess deaths will occur annually between 2030 and 2050 because of climate change, a toll that does not include morbidity and disruption of health services due to extreme changes in weather. Because of residential segregation, those most severely affected will include individuals of low socioeconomic status and those living in racially subordinated communities, as was the case when Hurricane Katrina struck New Orleans in 2005.

Climate change is expected to have a serious negative impact on human health by increasing the incidence and severity of many diseases, including the following:

- *Cardiovascular, cerebrovascular, and respiratory diseases,* all of which will be exacerbated by heat waves and air pollution
- *Gastroenteritis, cholera, and other foodborne and waterborne infectious diseases,* caused by contamination of water supplies and disruption of sewage treatment due to floods and other environmental disasters
- *Vector-borne infectious diseases* such as malaria and dengue fever, worsened by changes in the prevalence and geographic distribution of vectors due to increased temperatures, crop failures, and extreme weather variation
- *Malnutrition,* caused by changes in local climate that disrupt crop production. Such changes are anticipated to be most severe in tropical locations, in which average temperatures may already be near or above crop tolerance levels; it is estimated that by 2080, agricultural productivity may decline by 10% to 25% in some lower-income countries as a consequence of climate change.

Beyond these disease-specific effects, it is estimated that the melting of glacial ice combined with the thermal expansion of warming oceans will raise sea levels by 2 to 6 feet by 2100. Approximately 10% of the world's population—roughly 600 million people—live in low-lying

areas that are at risk for flooding. It is estimated that some countries such as the Maldives will be completely submerged and hence cease to exist. The resulting displacement of people will disrupt lives and commerce, creating conditions ripe for political unrest, war, and poverty—the "vectors" of malnutrition, sickness, and death.

TOXICITY OF CHEMICAL AND PHYSICAL AGENTS

Toxicology **is defined as the science of poisons. It studies the distribution, effects, and mechanisms of action of toxic agents.** More broadly, it also includes the study of the effects of physical agents such as radiation and heat. In general, little is known about the potential health effects of chemicals. Of the approximately 100,000 chemicals in use in the United States, less than 1% have been tested experimentally for health effects. Furthermore, much of the testing to date is scientifically inadequate to determine long-term health effects. This is further complicated by the complex interaction between various pollutants and the age, genetic predisposition, and different tissue sensitivities of exposed persons. Thus, there are wide variations in individual sensitivity to toxic agents, limiting the value of establishing "safe levels" for entire populations.

We now consider general principles regarding the toxicity of exogenous chemicals and drugs.

- The definition of a *poison* is not straightforward. It is a quantitative concept strictly dependent on dosage. The quote from Paracelsus in the 16th century that "all substances are poisons; the right dosage differentiates a poison from a remedy" is perhaps even more valid today, in view of the proliferation of therapeutic drugs with potentially harmful effects.
- *Xenobiotics* are exogenous chemicals in the environment that may be absorbed by the body through inhalation, ingestion, or skin contact (Fig. 7.4).
- Chemicals may act at the site of entry, or they may be transported to other sites. Some agents are not modified on entry in the body, but most solvents and drugs are metabolized to form water-soluble products *(detoxification)* or can be activated to form toxic metabolites. Most solvents and drugs are lipophilic, which facilitates their transport in the blood by lipoproteins and penetration through lipid components of cell membranes.
- The *cytochrome P-450 system* is the most important cellular enzyme system involved in reactions that either detoxify xenobiotics or, less commonly, convert xenobiotics into active compounds that cause cellular injury. Both types of reactions may produce reactive oxygen species (ROS) that can cause cellular damage (Chapter 1). The P-450 system is present in organs throughout the body, but it is most active in the endoplasmic reticulum (ER) of the liver. Examples of metabolic activation of chemicals through the P-450 system include the conversion of carbon tetrachloride to the toxic trichloromethyl free radical and the generation of a carcinogenic DNA-binding metabolite from benzo[a]pyrene, present in cigarette smoke. The cytochrome P-450 system also participates in the metabolism of many common therapeutic drugs such as acetaminophen, barbiturates, and warfarin, and in alcohol metabolism (discussed later).

P-450 enzymes vary widely in activity among different people, due to both polymorphisms in the genes encoding the enzymes and interactions with drugs that are metabolized through the system. Enzyme activity may be decreased by fasting or starvation, and increased by alcohol consumption, smoking, and hormones.

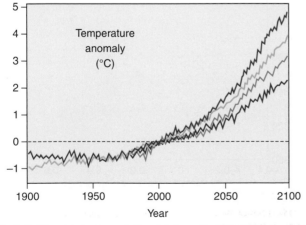

FIG. 7.3 Climate change, past and future. Predicted temperature increases during the 21st century. Different colors represent various computer models that plot anticipated rises in global temperatures of 2°C to 5°C by the year 2100.

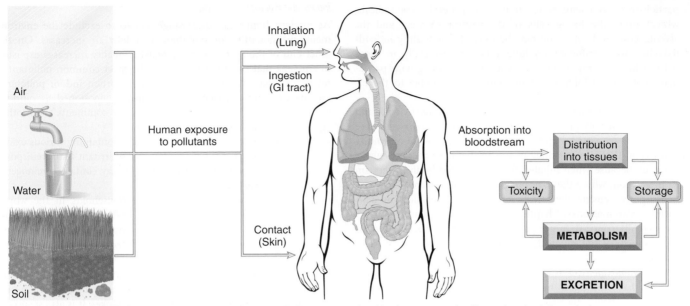

FIG. 7.4 Human exposure to pollutants. Pollutants contained in air, water, and soil are absorbed through the lungs, gastrointestinal (GI) tract, and skin. In the body, they may act at the site of absorption, but they are generally transported through the bloodstream to various organs, where they are stored or metabolized. Metabolism of xenobiotics may result in the formation of water-soluble compounds, which are excreted, or in activation of the agent, creating a toxic metabolite.

ENVIRONMENTAL POLLUTION

Air Pollution

Air pollution is a significant cause of morbidity and mortality worldwide, particularly among individuals with preexisting pulmonary or cardiac disease. In addition, airborne microorganisms have long been major causes of morbidity and death and the causes of two of the modern world's great pandemics, influenza in 1918 to 1919 and COVID-19 beginning in 2019. More widespread are the chemical and particulate pollutants found in the air worldwide. Specific hazards have been recognized for both outdoor and indoor air.

Outdoor Air Pollution

The ambient air is contaminated with a mixture of gaseous and particulate pollutants, more so in cities and in proximity to heavy industry. Exposure to air pollutants is disproportionately greater among marginalized populations of lower socioeconomic status. In the United States, the Environmental Protection Agency (EPA) monitors and sets allowable upper limits for five pollutants: sulfur dioxide, carbon monoxide (CO), nitrogen dioxide, ozone, and particulate matter. Smog (from the words *smoke* and *fog*) is composed of these and other compounds; particulate matter and ground level ozone make the greatest contribution. Levels of these five pollutants are quantified and reported as the air quality index.

The lungs bear the brunt of the adverse consequences of air pollution, but air pollutants, like other environmental toxins (e.g., lead, mercury), affect many organ systems. More detailed discussion of pollutant-caused lung diseases is found in Chapter 11. Here we consider the major health effects of ozone, sulfur dioxide, particulates, and CO (Table 7.1).

- *Ozone is one of the most pervasive air pollutants*; levels in many cities exceed EPA standards. It is a gas formed by sunlight-driven reactions involving nitrogen oxides, which are released mostly by automobile exhaust. Its toxicity stems from its

Table 7.1 Health Effects of Outdoor Air Pollutants

Pollutant	Populations at Risk	Effect(s)
Ozone	Healthy adults and children	Decreased lung function Increased airway reactivity Lung inflammation
	Athletes, outdoor workers	Decreased exercise capacity
	Patients with asthma	Increased hospitalizations
Nitrogen dioxide	Healthy adults Patients with asthma Children	Increased airway reactivity Decreased lung function Increased respiratory infections
Sulfur dioxide	Healthy adults	Increased respiratory symptoms
	Patients with COPD Patients with asthma	Increased mortality Increased hospitalization Decreased lung function
Acid aerosols	Healthy adults	Altered mucociliary clearance
	Children	Increased respiratory infections
	Patients with asthma	Decreased lung function Increased hospitalizations
Particulates	Children	Increased respiratory infections
	Patients with chronic lung or heart disease	Decreased lung function
	Patients with asthma	Increased mortality Increased asthma attacks

COPD, Chronic obstructive pulmonary disease.
Data from Health Effects of Outdoor Air Pollution, Part 2. Committee of the Environmental and Occupational Health Assembly of the American Thoracic Society. *Am J Respir Crit Care Med* 153:477, 1996.

participation in chemical reactions that generate free radicals, which injure the lining cells of the respiratory tract and the alveoli. Low levels of ozone may be tolerated by healthy individuals but are detrimental to lung function, especially in those with asthma or emphysema, or when present along with particulate pollution. Children are particularly susceptible to the effects of ozone.

- *Sulfur dioxide, particles, and acid aerosols* are emitted by coal- and oil-fired power plants and industrial processes burning these fuels. Of these, particles appear to be the main cause of morbidity and death. Particles less than 10 μm in diameter are particularly harmful, because when inhaled they are carried by the airstream to the alveoli, where they are phagocytosed by macrophages and neutrophils, causing the release of mediators (possibly by activating inflammasomes, Chapter 2) and inciting an inflammatory reaction. By contrast, larger particles are removed in the nose or are trapped by the mucociliary barrier and consequently cause less harm.

- *Carbon monoxide (CO)* is a nonirritating, colorless, tasteless, odorless gas that is produced by the incomplete oxidation of carbonaceous materials. Its sources include automotive engines, industries using fossil fuels, home oil burners, and cigarette smoke. The low levels often found in ambient air may contribute to impaired respiratory function but are usually not life threatening. However, workers in confined environments in which fumes accumulate, such as tunnels and underground garages, may develop chronic poisoning. CO is included here as an air pollutant but is also an important cause of accidental and suicidal death. In a small, closed garage, exhaust from a running car engine can induce a lethal coma within 5 minutes. Death is due to lack of O_2 delivery to tissues, as hemoglobin has a 200-fold greater affinity for CO than for O_2 and the carboxyhemoglobin that is formed by binding of CO is incapable of carrying oxygen. Hypoxia leads to central nervous system (CNS) depression, which develops so insidiously that victims are caught unaware. Systemic hypoxia occurs when the hemoglobin is 20% to 30% saturated with CO, and unconsciousness and death are probable with 60% to 70% saturation. The diagnosis of CO poisoning is based on detection of high levels of carboxyhemoglobin in the blood.

MORPHOLOGY

Chronic poisoning by CO develops because carboxyhemoglobin, once formed, is remarkably stable. As a result, with low-level persistent exposure to CO, carboxyhemoglobin may accumulate to life-threatening concentrations in the blood. The slowly developing hypoxia can evoke widespread ischemic changes in the brain, particularly in the basal ganglia and lenticular nuclei. With cessation of exposure to CO, the patient usually recovers, but there may be permanent neurologic damage.

Acute poisoning by CO is generally a consequence of accidental exposure or suicide attempt. The mucous membranes may appear erythematous due to the presence of carboxyhemoglobin. If death occurs rapidly, morphologic changes may not be present; with longer survival, the brain may be slightly edematous and exhibit punctate hemorrhages and hypoxia-induced neuronal changes (Chapter 21). These changes result from systemic hypoxia and are not specific to CO poisoning. In individuals who survive, complete recovery is possible; however, impairment of memory, vision, hearing, and speech sometimes remain.

Indoor Air Pollution

As modern homes are increasingly sealed to exclude the environment, the potential for pollution of indoor air increases. On the other end of the spectrum, poor housing quality increases exposure to antigens that can trigger asthma. The most common pollutant is tobacco smoke (discussed later); other important indoor pollutants include CO and nitrogen dioxide (already mentioned as outdoor pollutants) and asbestos (Chapter 11). A few comments about other agents are presented here.

- *Smoke from burning of organic materials,* containing various oxides of nitrogen and carbon particulates, is an irritant that predisposes exposed persons to lung infections and may contain carcinogenic polycyclic hydrocarbons.

  It is estimated that one-third of households in the world, mainly in lower-income areas, burn carbon-containing material such as wood, dung, or charcoal for cooking, heating, and light and are therefore at risk for disease related to pollutants in indoor smoke.

- *Radon,* a radioactive gas derived from uranium, is widely present in soil and in homes. Radon exposure can cause lung cancer in uranium miners (particularly in those who smoke). It is also suspected that low-level chronic exposures in the home increase lung cancer risk, particularly in those who smoke tobacco.

- *Bioaerosols* may contain pathogenic microbiologic agents, such as those that cause Legionnaires' disease, viral pneumonia, and the common cold, as well as allergens derived from pet dander, dust mites, and fungi and molds, which can cause rhinitis, eye irritation, and asthma. All of these are more common in families of lower socioeconomic status.

Metals as Environmental Pollutants

Lead, mercury, arsenic, and cadmium, the heavy metals most associated with harmful effects in human populations, are considered here.

Lead

Lead is a readily absorbed metal that binds to sulfhydryl groups in proteins and interferes with calcium metabolism, leading to hematologic, skeletal, neurologic, GI, and renal toxicities. Lead exposure occurs through contaminated air, food, and water. For most of the 20th century the major sources of lead in the environment were house paints and gasoline. The use of lead-based paints and leaded gas has greatly diminished in higher-income countries; however, in lower-income areas lead persists in the environment and in older homes, where it remains a significant cause of toxicity. Blood levels of lead in children living in older homes containing lead-based paint or lead-contaminated dust often exceed 5 μg/dL, the level at which the Centers for Disease Control and Prevention (CDC) recommends intervention to limit further exposure. Lead exposure is related to socially defined race: average blood lead levels are higher in African American children than in European American children. From 2014 to 2016 widespread lead contamination of drinking water occurred in the US city of Flint, Michigan, a city in which 57% of the population is African American and about 40% of the population live in poverty. Following a change in the source of the city water supply, higher chloride concentrations leached lead from the century-old lead pipes, raising lead levels in tap water to as high as 13,200 parts per billion (ppb) (acceptable limit, 15 ppb). Six thousand to 12,000 residents developed very high lead levels in their blood.

The clinical features of lead poisoning are shown in Fig. 7.5. Children are disproportionately affected by lead exposure since they absorb more than 50% of ingested lead, in comparison to the 15% absorbed by adults. Furthermore, a more permeable blood—brain barrier in children increases susceptibility to brain damage. The effects of lead poisoning are related to its concentration in the blood (eFig. 7.1). Most absorbed lead (80% to 85%) is taken up into teeth and bone, where it binds phosphates and thus competitively reduces binding of calcium. Once incorporated into bone, lead is fairly stable, with a half-life of 20 to 30 years; however, in conditions in which bone turnover is accelerated (e.g., pregnancy, hyperthyroidism, osteoporosis), lead can be released into the bloodstream. About 5% to 10% of the absorbed lead remains in the blood, and the remainder is distributed throughout soft tissues. Excess lead is toxic to nervous tissues in adults and children; peripheral neuropathies predominate in adults, whereas central effects are more common in children. The

effects of chronic lead exposure in children may be subtle, producing mild dysfunction, or they may be massive and lethal. In young children, sensory, motor, intellectual, and psychologic impairments have been described, including reduced IQ, learning disabilities, retarded psychomotor development, and, in more severe cases, blindness, psychoses, seizures, and coma. Lead-induced peripheral neuropathies in adults generally remit with the elimination of exposure, but both peripheral and CNS abnormalities in children are usually irreversible.

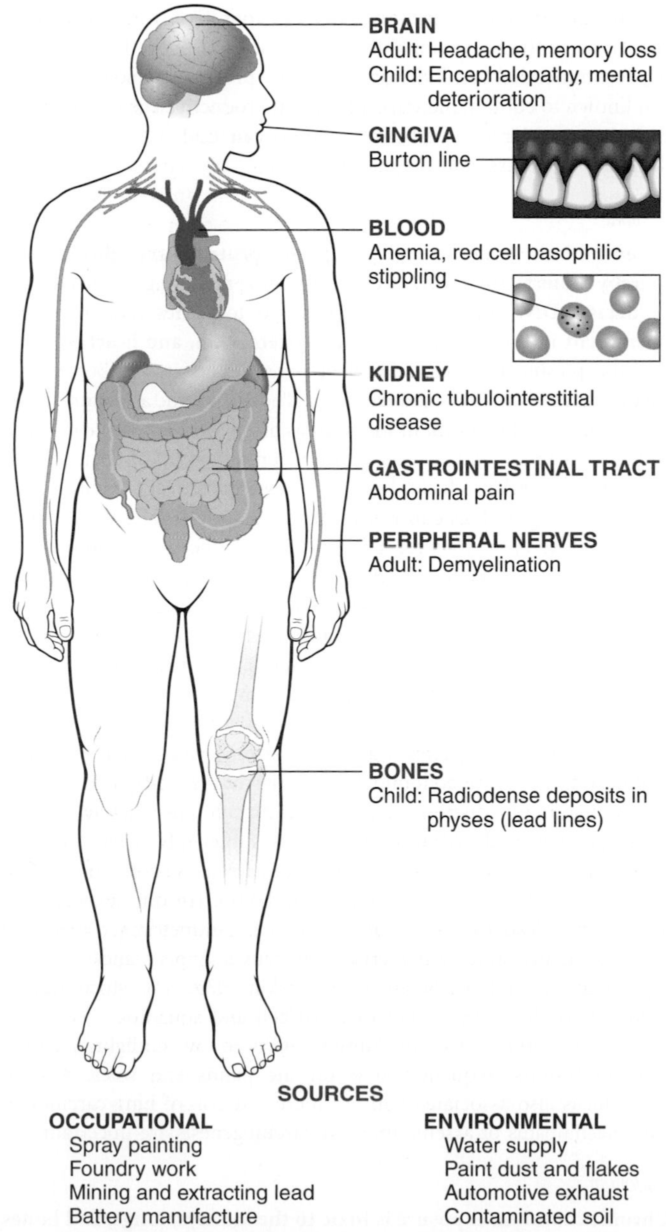

Excess lead interferes with the normal remodeling of the growth plate (physis) in children, causing increased bone density detected as radiodense "lead lines" (Fig. 7.6). Lead inhibits the healing of fractures by increasing chondrogenesis and delaying cartilage mineralization. Linear hyperpigmentation in the gums can also be seen (Burton line). Acute exposures and renal excretion of lead may cause damage to proximal tubules.

Lead has a high affinity for sulfhydryl groups and interferes with two enzymes involved in heme synthesis: delta-aminolevulinic acid dehydratase and ferrochelatase. Zinc-protoporphyrin (ZPP) is formed instead of heme, leading to decreased iron incorporation into heme and subsequent anemia. Lead also inhibits sodium- and potassium-dependent ATPases in cell membranes, an effect that may increase the fragility of red cells, causing *hemolysis.*

Lead poisoning may be suspected based on neurologic changes in children or unexplained anemia with basophilic stippling in red cells in adults and children. Elevated blood lead, red cell free protoporphyrin, or zinc-protoporphyrin levels are required for definitive diagnosis. In milder cases of lead exposure, anemia may be the only obvious finding.

The GI tract is also a site of major clinical manifestations: lead "colic" is characterized by severe, poorly localized abdominal pain that may mimic an acute abdomen. The mechanism is unclear.

BRAIN
Adult: Headache, memory loss
Child: Encephalopathy, mental deterioration

GINGIVA
Burton line

BLOOD
Anemia, red cell basophilic stippling

KIDNEY
Chronic tubulointerstitial disease

GASTROINTESTINAL TRACT
Abdominal pain

PERIPHERAL NERVES
Adult: Demyelination

BONES
Child: Radiodense deposits in physes (lead lines)

SOURCES

OCCUPATIONAL
Spray painting
Foundry work
Mining and extracting lead
Battery manufacture

ENVIRONMENTAL
Water supply
Paint dust and flakes
Automotive exhaust
Contaminated soil

FIG. 7.5 Pathologic features of lead poisoning.

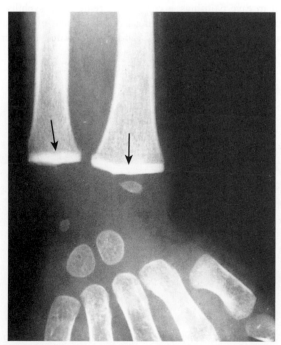

FIG. 7.6 Lead poisoning. Impaired remodeling of calcified cartilage in the physes *(arrows)* of the wrist has caused a marked increase in their radiodensity, so that they are as radiopaque as the cortical bone. (Courtesy of Dr. GW Dietz, Department of Radiology, University of Texas Southwestern Medical School, Dallas, Texas.)

The major anatomic targets of lead toxicity are the blood, bone marrow, nervous system, GI tract, and kidneys (see Fig. 7.5).

Blood changes are one of the earliest signs of lead accumulation and are characteristic, consisting of a microcytic, hypochromic anemia associated with a distinctive punctate **basophilic stippling** of red cells (Fig. 7.7). These changes in the blood are due to reduced heme synthesis in marrow erythroid progenitors.

Brain damage is prone to occur in children. The anatomic changes underlying the more subtle functional deficits are ill defined; at the more severe end of the spectrum, changes include brain edema, demyelination of the cerebral and cerebellar white matter, and necrosis of cortical neurons accompanied by diffuse astrocytic proliferation. In adults, the CNS is less often affected, but **peripheral demyelinating neuropathy** can occur, typically involving motor neurons innervating the muscles that are most used. Thus, the extensor muscles of the wrist and fingers are often the first to be affected, followed by paralysis of the peroneal muscles (**wristdrop and footdrop**).

The **kidneys** may develop proximal tubular damage with intranuclear lead inclusions. Chronic renal damage leads eventually to interstitial fibrosis and sometimes renal failure and findings suggestive of gout. Other features of lead poisoning are shown in Fig. 7.5.

Mercury

Mercury, like lead, binds with high affinity to sulfhydryl groups, thereby inhibiting enzymes such as choline acetyl transferase, which is involved in the production of acetylcholine, and inactivating other proteins, leading to damage in the CNS and several other organs, such as the GI tract and the kidneys. Humans have used mercury in many ways throughout history, including as a pigment in cave paintings, a cosmetic, a remedy for syphilis, and a component of diuretics. Poisoning from inhalation of mercury vapors has long been recognized and is associated with tremor,

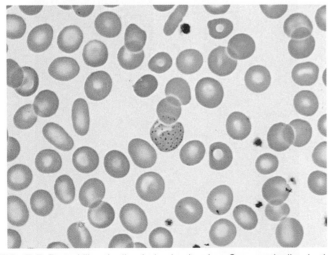

FIG. 7.7 Basophilic stippling in lead poisoning. Coarse stippling in the red cell in the middle of the field is common in lead poisoning and is also seen in other anemias caused by impaired hemoglobin synthesis (e.g., megaloblastic anemia). (From McPherson R et al: *Henry's Clinical Diagnosis and Management by Laboratory Methods,* ed 22, Philadelphia, 2011, Saunders, p 526.)

gingivitis, and bizarre behavior, such as that of the "Mad Hatter" in Lewis Carroll's *Alice in Wonderland* (mercury was formerly used in hat making).

Though no longer used in large-scale gold mining, mercury waste from that process as well as inorganic mercury from the Earth's crust are converted to organic compounds such as methyl mercury by bacteria. Methyl mercury enters the food chain and concentrates in carnivorous fish (e.g., swordfish, shark, tuna), in which mercury levels may be 1 million times higher than in the surrounding water. Today the main sources of mercury exposure are contaminated fish. Almost 90% of ingested mercury is absorbed in the GI tract where it can cause precipitation of proteins in intestinal epithelial cells, leading to vomiting, abdominal pain, and bloody diarrhea. Mercury is cleared by the kidney which can cause renal damage. Acute toxicity is associated with renal tubular injury and oliguria or anuria. Because mercury is lipophilic, it concentrates in the CNS and can cross the placenta.

The developing brain is extremely sensitive to methyl mercury which can affect the motor, sensory, cognitive, and behavioral functions of the brain; for this reason, the CDC in the United States has recommended that individuals who are pregnant avoid consuming fish known to contain mercury and that reproductive age women limit their intake. Mercury exposure in utero can lead to cerebral palsy, deafness, blindness, and major CNS defects.

Arsenic

Arsenic binds to sulfhydryl groups on proteins and glutathione, thereby interfering with numerous enzymes (e.g., glutathione reductase, DNA ligases) and leading to toxicities that are most prominent in the GI tract, nervous system, skin, and heart. Arsenic was the poison of choice of skilled practitioners in the Borgia and Medici families in Renaissance Italy. Today, arsenic exposure is an important health problem in many areas of the world. Arsenic is found in soil and water and is used in wood preservatives, pesticides, and other agricultural products. It may be released into the environment by the mining and smelting industries. Arsenic is present in some traditional herbal medicines, and arsenic trioxide is a component of the treatment for acute promyelocytic leukemia (Chapter 10). High concentrations of inorganic arsenic are present in ground water in several countries, particularly Bangladesh, where arsenic poisoning is a continuing health crisis. In the United States, arsenic contamination of rice has received attention since rice is a component of infant formula and cereals.

When ingested in large quantities, arsenic causes acute toxicity manifesting as severe abdominal pain, diarrhea, cardiac arrhythmias, shock, respiratory distress syndrome, and acute encephalopathy. GI, cardiovascular, and CNS toxicity may be sufficiently severe to cause death. These effects have been attributed to arsenic's ability to interfere with mitochondrial oxidative phosphorylation. Chronic exposure to arsenic may lead to the development of a symmetric sensorimotor polyneuropathy and characteristically causes hyper- and/or hypopigmentation and hyperkeratosis of the skin (eFig. 7.2), which may be followed by the development of basal cell and squamous cell carcinomas. In contrast to skin tumors induced by sunlight, arsenic-induced tumors frequently arise on the palms and soles. Arsenic exposure is also associated with an increased risk of lung carcinoma. The mechanisms of arsenic-induced carcinogenesis are uncertain.

Cadmium

Chronic cadmium exposure is toxic to the kidneys, lungs, and bones through uncertain mechanisms that may involve increased

production of reactive oxygen species. Cadmium (Cd) principally enters the environment through industrial waste, in particular the production of nickel-cadmium batteries that can contaminate ground water and soil when disposed of in household waste. Agricultural crops may concentrate cadmium derived from the soil or from fertilizers and irrigation water. In the 1960s cadmium-contaminated water used to irrigate rice fields in Japan caused a disease known as "itai-itai" ("ouch-ouch"), a combination of osteoporosis and osteomalacia associated with multiple fractures and renal disease.

Cadmium is present in some foods (e.g., cereals, leafy vegetables) and in cigarette smoke, and these are the most important sources of exposure for the general population. Due to its long biologic half-life, cadmium continues to accumulate throughout an individual's lifetime. Chronic cadmium excess can lead to emphysema and renal toxicity through unknown mechanisms, particularly in the setting of occupational exposure (e.g., smelting and refining of metals, recycling of nickel-cadmium batteries). Skeletal abnormalities are associated with increased urinary excretion of calcium and phosphorus, which can also lead to kidney stones.

Industrial and Agricultural Exposures

More than 10 million occupational injuries occur annually in the United States, and approximately 65,000 people die each year as a consequence of occupational injuries and illnesses. Industrial exposures to toxic agents are as varied as the industries themselves, ranging from simple irritation of respiratory airways by formaldehyde or ammonia fumes, to lung cancers arising from exposure to asbestos, arsenic, or uranium. Human diseases associated with occupational exposures are listed in Table 7.2. In addition to toxic metals (already discussed), other important agents that contribute to environmental diseases include the following:

- *Organic solvents*, such as chloroform and toluene, are widely used in vast quantities worldwide, primarily in industry. Acute exposure to high levels of vapors from these agents can cause dizziness, confusion, CNS depression, and even coma. Lower levels may cause liver and kidney toxicity. Occupational exposure and residential proximity to hazardous waste sites containing organic solvents, particularly benzene, are associated with an increased risk of leukemia. Benzene is oxidized to an epoxide through hepatic CYP2E1, a component of the P-450 enzyme system. This and other metabolites disrupt progenitor cell differentiation in the bone marrow and may lead to marrow aplasia and acute myeloid leukemia.
- *Polycyclic hydrocarbons* are released during the combustion of coal and gas, particularly at the high temperatures used in steel foundries, and are also present in tar and soot. When metabolized, polycyclic hydrocarbons form potent carcinogens that can covalently attach to DNA, leading to mutations and changes in gene expression that can cause neoplasia.
- *Organochlorines* (and halogenated organic compounds in general) are synthetic products that resist degradation and are lipophilic. Important organochlorines used as pesticides are DDT (dichlorodiphenyltrichloroethane) and its metabolites, and agents such as lindane, aldrin, and dieldrin, all of which have been banned in the United States due to concerns about toxicity. Although DDT was banned in 1973, its long-lasting metabolite p,p′-DDE is detectable in the serum of much of the American population, including individuals born after the ban went into effect. Acute organochlorine toxicity primarily affects the body through stimulating the central nervous system by interfering with sodium channel activity (DDT) or by inhibiting GABA receptors (lindane, aldrin).
- *Nonpesticide organochlorines* include polychlorinated biphenyls (PCBs) and dioxin (TCDD [2,3,7,8-tetrachlorodibenzo-p-dioxin]).

Table 7.2 Human Diseases Associated With Occupational Exposures

Organ/System	Effect(s)	Environmental Toxins
Cardiovascular system	Heart disease	CO, lead, solvents, cobalt, cadmium
Respiratory system	Nasal cancer	Wood dust, leather dust
	Lung cancer	Radon, asbestos, silica, bis(chloromethyl) ether, nickel, arsenic, chromium, mustard gas
	Chronic obstructive pulmonary disease	Grain dust, coal dust, cadmium
	Hypersensitivity	Beryllium, isocyanates
	Irritation	Ammonia, sulfur oxides, formaldehyde
	Fibrosis	Silica, asbestos, cobalt
Nervous system	Peripheral neuropathies	Solvents, acrylamide, methyl chloride, mercury, lead, arsenic, DDT
	Ataxic gait	Chlordane, toluene, acrylamide, mercury
	CNS depression	Alcohols, ketones, aldehydes, solvents
	Cataracts	Ultraviolet radiation
Urinary system	Renal toxicity	Mercury, lead, glycol ethers, solvents
	Bladder cancer	Naphthylamines, 4-aminobiphenyl, benzidine, rubber products
Reproductive system	Male infertility	Lead, dibromochloropropane, cadmium, mercury
	Female infertility	Cadmium, lead, phthalates
	Teratogenesis	Mercury, polychlorinated biphenyls
Hematopoietic system	Leukemia	Benzene, radon, uranium
Skin	Folliculitis and chloracne	Polychlorinated biphenyls, dioxins, herbicides
	Cancer	Ultraviolet radiation
GI tract	Liver angiosarcoma	Vinyl chloride

CNS, Central nervous system; *CO,* carbon monoxide; *DDT,* dichlorodiphenyltrichloroethane; *GI,* gastrointestinal.
Data from Leigh JP, Markowitz SB, Fahs M, et al: Occupational injury and illness in the United States: estimates of costs, morbidity, and mortality. *Arch Intern Med* 157:1557, 1997; Mitchell FL: Hazardous waste. In Rom WN, editor: *Environmental and Occupational Medicine,* ed 2, Boston, 1992, Little, Brown, p 1275; and Levi PE: Classes of toxic chemicals. In Hodgson E, Levi PE, editors: *A Textbook of Modern Toxicology,* Stamford, CT, 1997, Appleton & Lange, p 229.

High doses of dioxins and PCBs can cause skin disorders such as chloracne, which is characterized by acne, cyst formation, hyperpigmentation, and hyperkeratosis, generally around the face and behind the ears. The mechanism is thought to be related to activation of a signaling pathway mediated by an aryl hydrocarbon receptor in skin stem cell progenitors. Other findings include liver dysfunction, encephalopathy, and transient peripheral neuropathy. Because PCBs induce the P-450 enzyme system, workers exposed to these substances may show altered drug metabolism. Low levels of PCB and TCDD are present in the blood of most of the US population. Most organochlorines are endocrine disruptors (i.e., they may mimic hormones or affect hormone levels) with antiestrogenic or antiandrogenic activity in laboratory animals, but long-term health effects in humans have not been firmly established.

- *Bisphenol A* (BPA) is used in the synthesis of polycarbonate food and water containers and of epoxy resins that line almost all food bottles and cans; as a result, exposure to BPA is virtually ubiquitous in humans. BPA is a proven endocrine disruptor; though its effect is weak, its omnipresence is cause for concern. There is some evidence that early exposure to BPA may increase the risk of chronic diseases such as diabetes, cancer, and hypertension in adulthood due to its hormone-like properties. In 2010 Canada was the first country to list BPA as a toxic substance; in 2012 its use was banned in baby bottles and "sippy" cups in the United States. However, potential replacements for BPA, such as bisphenol S and bisphenol F, have similar structures and research has questioned their safety.
- *Vinyl chloride,* used in the synthesis of polyvinyl resins, can cause angiosarcoma of the liver, a rare type of liver tumor.
- Inhalation of certain mineral dusts, inorganic particulates, and fumes and vapors may cause chronic, nonneoplastic lung diseases called *pneumoconioses.* This group of disorders includes diseases induced by organic and inorganic particulates as well as chemical fume- and vapor-induced nonneoplastic lung diseases. The most common pneumoconioses are caused by exposures to coal dust (in mining of hard coal), silica (in sandblasting and stone cutting), asbestos (in mining, fabrication, and insulation work), and beryllium (in mining and fabrication). Exposure to these agents nearly always occurs in the workplace. Notably, the increased risk of cancer because of asbestos exposure extends to family members of asbestos workers due to residua carried on the workers' clothing. Pneumoconioses and their pathogenesis are discussed in Chapter 11.

EFFECTS OF TOBACCO

Tobacco is the most common exogenous cause of human cancers, being responsible for 80% to 90% of lung cancers. The primary contributor is cigarette smoking, which is causal in cardiovascular disease, various types of cancer, and chronic respiratory diseases. Smokeless tobacco in its various forms (e.g., chewing tobacco) is also harmful to health and is an important cause of oral cancer. Not only does the use of tobacco products create personal risk, but also passive tobacco inhalation from the environment ("second-hand smoke") can cause lung cancer in nonsmokers. The percentage of Americans who smoke cigarettes has decreased from 20.9% in 2005 to 14% in 2019, and about 34 million Americans are current smokers. In the United States, tobacco is responsible for about 480,000 deaths per year. Worldwide, there are 1.3 billion tobacco users, with more than 80%

living in low- and middle-income countries. More than 8 million deaths per year are attributed to tobacco use.

Smoking is the most important cause of preventable human death. It reduces overall survival in a dose-dependent fashion. Whereas 80% of nonsmokers are alive at age 70, only about 50% of smokers survive to this age (Fig. 7.8). Within 5 years, cessation of smoking greatly reduces overall mortality and the risk of death from cardiovascular diseases. Lung cancer mortality decreases by 21% within 5 years, but the excess risk persists for 30 years. Adverse effects of smoking in various organ systems are shown in Fig. 7.9.

The number of potentially harmful chemicals in tobacco smoke is vast; Table 7.3 presents a partial list and includes the type of injury produced by these agents. Nicotine, an alkaloid present in tobacco leaves, is not a direct cause of tobacco-related diseases but is highly addictive. Nicotine binds to receptors in the brain and, through the release of catecholamines, is responsible for the acute effects of smoking, such as increased heart rate and blood pressure and increased cardiac contractility and output.

The most common diseases caused by cigarette smoking involve the lung and include emphysema, chronic bronchitis, and lung cancer, all discussed in Chapter 11. The mechanisms responsible for some tobacco-induced diseases include the following:

- *Direct irritant effect on the tracheobronchial mucosa,* producing inflammation and increased mucus production (bronchitis). Cigarette smoke also causes the recruitment of leukocytes to the lung, increasing local elastase production and subsequent injury to lung tissue that leads to emphysema.
- *Carcinogenesis.* Components of cigarette smoke, particularly polycyclic hydrocarbons and nitrosamines (Table 7.4), are potent

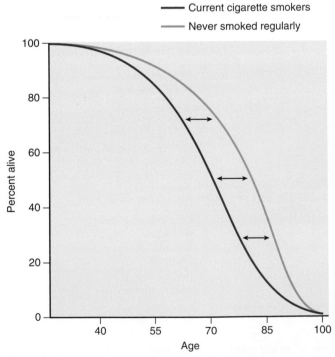

FIG. 7.8 The effects of smoking on survival. The study compared age-specific death rates for current cigarette smokers with those of individuals who never smoked regularly (British Doctors Study). The difference in survival, measured at age 75, between smokers and nonsmokers is 7.5 years. (Modified from Stewart BW, Kleihues P, editors: *World Cancer Report,* Lyon, 2003, IARC Press.)

CANCERS   CHRONIC DISEASES

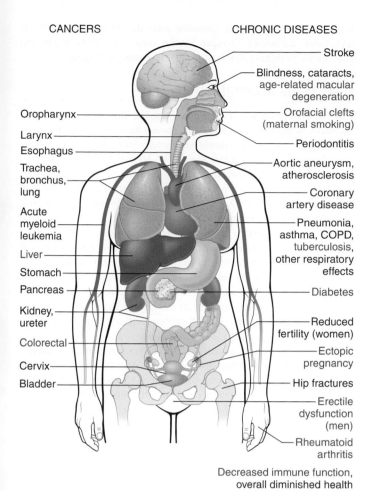

FIG. 7.9 Health consequences causally linked to smoking. Items in red were added relatively recently to the list of ill effects of smoking. *COPD,* Chronic obstructive pulmonary disease. (US Department of Health and Human Services: *The Health Consequences of Smoking—50 Years of Progress: A Report of the Surgeon General,* Atlanta, 2016, US Department of Health and Human Services, Centers for Disease Control and Prevention, National Center for Chronic Disease Prevention and Health Promotion, Office on Smoking and Health.)

Table 7.4 Organ-Specific Carcinogens in Tobacco Smoke

Organ	Carcinogen(s)
Lung, larynx	Polycyclic aromatic hydrocarbons 4-(Methylnitrosoamino)-1-(3-pyridyl)-1-butanone Nicotine-derived nitrosamine ketone (NNK) ^{210}Polonium
Esophagus	N′-Nitrosonornicotine (NNN)
Pancreas	NNK (?)
Bladder	4-Aminobiphenyl, 2-naphthylamine
Oral cavity: smoking	Polycyclic aromatic hydrocarbons, NNK, NNN
Oral cavity: chewing tobacco	NNK, NNN, ^{210}polonium

Data from Szczesny LB, Holbrook JH: Cigarette smoking. In Rom WH, editor: *Environmental and Occupational Medicine,* ed 2, Boston, 1992, Little, Brown, p 1211.

carcinogens in animals and are involved in the pathogenesis of lung carcinomas in humans (see Chapter 11). The risk of developing lung cancer is related to the intensity of exposure, frequently expressed in terms of "pack years" (e.g., one pack daily for 20 years equals 20 pack years) or in cigarettes smoked per day (Fig. 7.10). In addition to lung cancers, tobacco smoke contributes to the development of cancers of the oral cavity, esophagus, pancreas, and bladder (see Table 7.4). Moreover, smoking multiplies the risk associated with other carcinogens; well-recognized examples are the 10-fold increased incidence of lung carcinomas in asbestos workers and uranium miners who smoke compared to those who do not. The combination of tobacco (chewed or smoked) and alcohol consumption has multiplicative effects on the risks of oral, laryngeal, and esophageal cancers. An example of the carcinogenic interaction of these two factors is shown for laryngeal cancer (Fig. 7.11).

- *Atherosclerosis* and its major complication, myocardial infarction, are strongly linked to cigarette smoking. The causal mechanisms probably relate to several factors, including increased platelet aggregation, decreased myocardial oxygen supply (due to lung disease

Table 7.3 Effects of Selected Tobacco Smoke Constituents

Substance	Effect(s)
Tar	Carcinogenesis
Polycyclic aromatic hydrocarbons	Carcinogenesis
Nicotine	Ganglionic stimulation and depression, tumor promotion
Phenol	Tumor promotion; mucosal irritation
Benzopyrene	Carcinogenesis
Carbon monoxide	Impaired oxygen transport and use
Formaldehyde	Toxic to cilia; mucosal irritation
Oxides of nitrogen	Toxic to cilia; mucosal irritation
Nitrosamine	Carcinogenesis

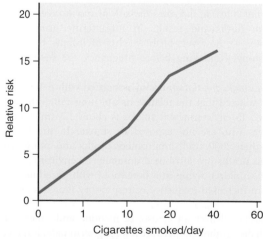

FIG. 7.10 The risk of lung cancer is determined by the number of cigarettes smoked. (Data from Stewart BW, Kleihues P, editors: *World Cancer Report,* Lyon, 2003, IARC Press.)

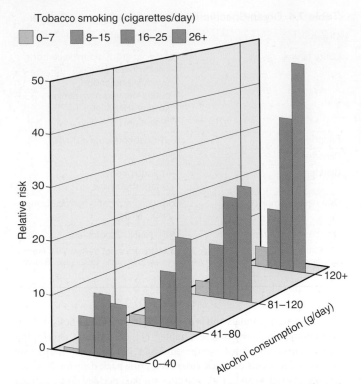

FIG. 7.11 Multiplicative increase in the risk of laryngeal cancer from the interaction between cigarette smoking and alcohol consumption. (Data from Stewart BW, Kleihues P, editors: *World Cancer Report*, Lyon, 2003, IARC Press.)

coupled with hypoxia related to CO in cigarette smoke) accompanied by increased oxygen demand, and a decreased threshold for ventricular fibrillation. According to the CDC, about 20% of all cardiovascular deaths are caused by cigarette smoking. Smoking has a multiplicative effect on risk when combined with hypertension and hypercholesterolemia.

- The 2016 US Surgeon General's report added several additional diseases to the previously known list of smoking-associated diseases (see Fig. 7.9), including type 2 diabetes, rheumatoid arthritis, age-related macular degeneration, ectopic pregnancy, and erectile dysfunction.
- *Maternal smoking increases the risk of spontaneous abortions and preterm births* and results in intrauterine growth retardation (Chapter 4); however, birth weights of infants born to mothers who stopped smoking before pregnancy are within the normal range.
- *Passive smoke inhalation* is also associated with detrimental effects. It is estimated that the relative risk of lung cancer in nonsmokers exposed to environmental smoke is about 1.3 times that in nonsmokers who are not exposed to smoke. In the United States, more than 7000 adult lung cancer deaths and more than 30,000 cardiac deaths are attributed annually to environmental tobacco smoke. Children living in a household with an adult who smokes have an increased frequency of respiratory illnesses and asthma.

E-cigarettes deliver an aerosol of nicotine and other components that is inhaled. Although there are few long-term data, it is thought that risk of cardiopulmonary disease and cancer is lower than with conventional tobacco cigarettes. However, e-cigarette use (vaping) may be associated with a form of acute lung injury related to compounds in the vaping fluid and typically presents with dyspnea, cough, and GI symptoms. Pathologic changes in the lung vary from organizing pneumonia to diffuse alveolar damage (discussed in Chapter 11).

EFFECTS OF ALCOHOL

Despite the attention focused on use of illicit substance use, excessive alcohol use is a more widespread hazard and claims many more lives. A person who drinks excessively does not necessarily meet the *Diagnostic and Statistical Manual of Mental Disorders* (DSM-V) criteria for an alcohol use disorder (AUD). Similarly, individuals who drink what most people would consider a moderate amount may still meet criteria for an AUD, depending on their life situation and consequences of their alcohol consumption.

It is estimated that 1 in 8 Americans meets the criteria for AUD and that excess alcohol consumption is directly responsible for approximately 95,000 deaths annually, about 10,000 of which are due to alcohol-related motor vehicle accidents. The remaining deaths are secondary to alcohol-related homicides and suicides, cirrhosis of the liver, cardiac disease, and cancer. In the United States, approximately 75,000 cancer cases and 19,000 cancer deaths are attributable to alcohol each year.

After consumption, ethanol is absorbed unaltered in the stomach and small intestine and then distributes to the tissues and fluids of the body in direct proportion to the blood level. Less than 10% is excreted unchanged in the urine, sweat, and breath. The amount exhaled is proportional to the blood level and forms the basis for the breath alcohol test. The federal legal driving limit for blood alcohol content is 0.08%, though states may set a lower limit, and lower limits may apply for drivers under the age of 21 years. Many factors determine blood alcohol concentration including sex, age, medications, and rate of consumption. Drowsiness occurs at 200 mg/dL, stupor at 300 mg/dL, and coma, with possible respiratory arrest, at higher levels. Over time, sustained heavy alcohol use increases its rate of metabolism and can lead to the development of tolerance; as a result, when the same amount of alcohol is consumed, lower peak alcohol levels are seen in heavy alcohol drinkers than in seldom drinkers.

Blood alcohol is metabolized to acetaldehyde in the liver by one of three enzyme systems: alcohol dehydrogenase (in the cytosol of hepatocytes), cytochrome P-450 isoenzymes (in the microsomes), and catalase (in the peroxisomes) (Fig. 7.12). Of these, the main enzyme involved in alcohol metabolism is alcohol dehydrogenase. At high blood alcohol levels, the microsomal ethanol-oxidizing system also plays an important role. This system involves cytochrome P-450 enzymes, particularly the CYP2E1 isoform. As alcohol is an inducer of P-450 enzymes, heavy alcohol use can increase an individual's susceptibility to other compounds metabolized by the same enzyme system, which include drugs (e.g., acetaminophen, cocaine), anesthetics, carcinogens, and industrial solvents. When alcohol is present in the blood at high concentrations, it competes with other CYP2E1 substrates such as medications and may delay their catabolism, thereby potentiating their effects. Catalase is of minor importance, being responsible for about 5% of alcohol metabolism. Acetaldehyde produced by these systems is in turn converted by acetaldehyde dehydrogenase to acetate, which is used in the mitochondrial respiratory chain.

Several toxic effects result from ethanol metabolism. Listed here are the most important of these:
- *Alcohol oxidation* by alcohol dehydrogenase causes a decrease in nicotinamide adenine dinucleotide (NAD^+) and an increase in NADH (the reduced form of NAD^+). Since NAD^+ is required

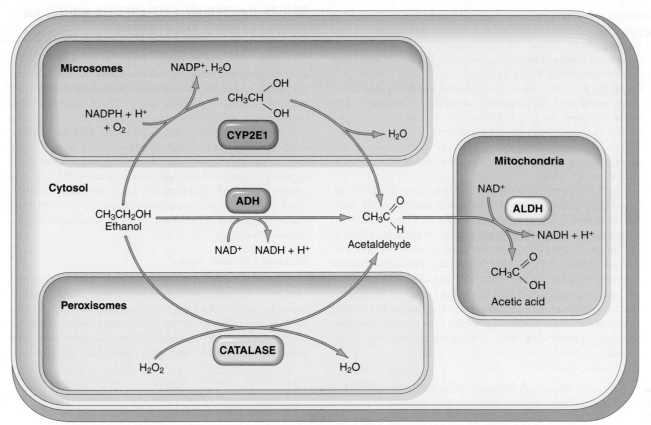

FIG. 7.12 Metabolism of ethanol: oxidation of ethanol to acetaldehyde by three different routes, and the generation of acetic acid. Note that oxidation by alcohol dehydrogenase (ADH) takes place in the cytosol; the cytochrome P-450 system and its CYP2E1 isoform are located in the endoplasmic reticulum (microsomes), and catalase is located in peroxisomes. Oxidation of acetaldehyde by aldehyde dehydrogenase (ALDH) occurs in mitochondria. (Figure from Parkinson A: Biotransformation of xenobiotics. In Klassen CD, editor: *Casarett and Doull's Toxicology: The Basic Science of Poisons*, ed 6, New York, 2001, McGraw-Hill, p 133.)

for hepatic fatty acid oxidation, excess alcohol intake can lead to fat accumulation in the liver over time. In addition, the increase in the NADH/NAD$^+$ ratio can result in lactic acidosis.

- *Acetaldehyde toxicity* may be responsible for some of the acute effects of alcohol. Acetaldehyde metabolism differs between populations due to genetic variation. One polymorphism that originated in China causes acetaldehyde accumulation in individuals of East Asian descent (e.g., China, Korea, Japan). After ingesting alcohol, individuals with this allele experience flushing, tachycardia, and hyperventilation.
- *ROS generation.* Metabolism of ethanol in the liver by CYP2E1 produces ROS and causes lipid peroxidation of cell membranes. However, the precise mechanisms that account for alcohol-induced cellular injury have not been well defined.
- *Endotoxin release.* Alcohol may cause the release of endotoxin (lipopolysaccharide), a product of gram-negative bacteria, from the intestinal flora. Endotoxin stimulates the release of tumor necrosis factor (TNF) and other cytokines from macrophages and from Kupffer cells in the liver, causing cell injury.

Acutely, excess alcohol exerts its effects mainly on the CNS but may also induce reversible hepatic and gastric injuries. Even with moderate alcohol intake, multiple fat droplets accumulate in hepatocytes (*fatty change* or *hepatic steatosis*). Gastric damage occurs in the form of acute *gastritis* and *ulceration*. In the CNS, alcohol is a depressant, first affecting subcortical structures that modulate cerebral cortical activity followed by stimulation and disordered cortical, motor, and intellectual behavior. At progressively higher blood levels, cortical neurons and then lower medullary centers are depressed, including those that regulate respiration. Respiratory arrest may follow.

Sustained excessive alcohol intake has been associated with increased morbidity and shortened life span, related principally to damage to the liver, GI tract, CNS, cardiovascular system, and pancreas.

- The *liver* is the main site of chronic injury. In addition to fatty change, mentioned earlier, chronic excess alcohol intake can lead to steatohepatitis and cirrhosis (Chapter 14). Cirrhosis is associated with portal hypertension and an increased risk of hepatocellular carcinoma.
- In the *GI tract*, chronic excess alcohol intake can cause massive bleeding from gastritis, gastric ulcer, or esophageal varices (associated with cirrhosis), which may prove fatal.
- *Neurologic effects.* Thiamine deficiency is common in the setting of sustained heavy alcohol intake; the principal lesions resulting from this deficiency are peripheral neuropathies and the Wernicke-Korsakoff syndrome (Chapter 21). Cerebral atrophy, cerebellar degeneration, and optic neuropathy may also occur.
- *Cardiovascular effects.* Alcohol has diverse effects on the cardiovascular system. Injury to the myocardium may produce dilated

congestive cardiomyopathy *(alcohol-related cardiomyopathy)* (Chapter 9). Chronic heavy alcohol consumption increases risk for coronary heart disease and hypertension.

- *Pancreatitis.* Excess alcohol intake increases the risk of acute and chronic pancreatitis (Chapter 15).
- *Effects on the fetus.* No safe level for alcohol use during pregnancy has been established; consequently, abstinence is recommended, particularly during the first trimester. The use of alcohol during pregnancy can cause fetal alcohol syndrome, which is marked by microcephaly, growth retardation, and facial dysmorphism in the newborn (Chapter 4). Brain dysfunction may not become apparent until children are older.
- *Carcinogenesis.* Chronic alcohol consumption is associated with an increased incidence of cancer, particularly in heavy drinkers. Cancers of the upper airways and digestive tract (oral cavity, pharynx, esophagus, and larynx) and liver (secondary to cirrhosis) are most closely linked to heavy alcohol use. Low to moderate levels of alcohol use increase the risk of breast cancer. The mechanisms of the carcinogenic effect are uncertain; however, alcohol and cigarette smoke synergize in the causation of various cancers.
- *Malnutrition.* Ethanol is a substantial source of calories but is often consumed at the expense of food. Chronic alcohol use is thus associated with malnutrition and deficiencies, particularly of B vitamins.

INJURY CAUSED BY THERAPEUTIC DRUGS AND NONPRESCRIBED SUBSTANCES

Injury by Therapeutic Drugs: Adverse Drug Reactions

Adverse drug reactions (ADRs) are untoward effects of drugs that are administered in conventional therapeutic settings. ADRs are extremely common, affecting almost 7% of patients admitted to a hospital, and are often serious, accounting for over 100,000 deaths annually. Table 7.5 lists common pathologic findings in ADRs and the drugs most frequently involved. Many of the drugs causing ADRs, such as the antineoplastic agents, are toxic at doses that are predicted to achieve maximal therapeutic effects. Because they are widely used, estrogens and oral contraceptives (OCs) are discussed next in more detail. In addition, acetaminophen and aspirin, nonprescription drugs that are important causes of accidental or intentional overdose, merit consideration.

Menopausal Hormone Therapy

The most common type of menopausal hormone therapy (MHT) consists of the administration of an estrogen together with a progestogen. In women who have had hysterectomies, the carcinogenic risk of progestogen on the uterus is eliminated and they may be treated solely with estrogen. Though MHT was initially used primarily to counteract hot flashes and other symptoms of menopause, early

Table 7.5 Some Common Adverse Drug Reactions and Their Agents

Reaction	Major Offenders
Blood Dyscrasias[a]	
Granulocytopenia, aplastic anemia, pancytopenia	Antineoplastic agents, immunosuppressives, chloramphenicol
Hemolytic anemia, thrombocytopenia	Penicillin, methyldopa, quinidine
Cutaneous	
Urticaria, macules, papules, vesicles, petechiae, exfoliative dermatitis, fixed drug eruptions, abnormal pigmentation	Antineoplastic agents, sulfonamides, hydantoins, some antibiotics, and many other agents
Cardiac	
Arrhythmias	Theophylline, hydantoins
Cardiomyopathy	Doxorubicin, daunorubicin
Renal	
Glomerulonephritis	Penicillamine
Acute tubular injury	Aminoglycoside antibiotics, cyclosporine, amphotericin B
Tubulointerstitial disease with papillary necrosis	Phenacetin, salicylates
Pulmonary	
Asthma	Salicylates
Acute pneumonitis	Nitrofurantoin
Interstitial fibrosis	Busulfan, nitrofurantoin, bleomycin
Hepatic	
Fatty change	Tetracycline
Diffuse hepatocellular damage	Halothane, isoniazid, acetaminophen
Cholestasis	Chlorpromazine, estrogens, contraceptive agents
Systemic	
Anaphylaxis	Penicillin
Lupus erythematosus syndrome (drug-induced lupus)	Hydralazine, procainamide
Central Nervous System	
Tinnitus and dizziness	Salicylates
Acute dystonic reactions and parkinsonian syndrome	Phenothiazine antipsychotics
Respiratory depression	Sedatives

[a]Feature in almost half of all drug-related deaths.

clinical studies suggested that MHT in postmenopausal women could prevent or slow the progression of osteoporosis (Chapter 19) and reduce the likelihood of myocardial infarction. However, subsequent randomized clinical trials revealed several adverse cardiovascular effects of MHT, including increased risk of stroke, congestive heart failure, and venous thromboembolism. Several mechanisms have been proposed for the deleterious effects of MHT, including increased serum triglycerides, reduced levels of antithrombotic factors (e.g., fibrinogen, factor VII, antithrombin), increased production of proinflammatory markers and increased resistance to activated protein C, which results in a prothrombotic state due to dysregulation of factors V and VIII (Chapter 3). An increased risk of breast cancer was also noted. As a result, use of MHT has declined significantly in the United States, despite recent studies that support a more individualized approach to MHT. These newer analyses showed that MHT effects depend on several factors:

- *Type of regimen.* Combination estrogen-progesterone treatment increases the risk of breast cancer. By contrast, estrogen alone in women with hysterectomy is associated with a borderline reduction in risk of breast cancer. There is no increase in ovarian cancer risk.
- *Age.* MHT may have a protective effect on the development of atherosclerosis and coronary disease in women younger than age 60 years, but there is no protection in women who start MHT at an older age.
- *Duration of treatment.* When taken for less than 4 to 5 years, combined estrogen-progestin MHT does not appear to increase breast cancer risk; risk increases with longer durations.
- *Route of administration.* Transdermal estrogen is associated with a lower risk of venous thromboembolism and stroke compared to oral estrogen preparations.
- *Baseline risk for cardiovascular disease, thromboembolism (e.g., factor V Leiden allele), and breast carcinoma.* Depending on risk assessment, nonhormonal therapies may be indicated in individuals at increased risk for these conditions.

Assessment of risks and benefits when considering the use of MHT is complex. Current recommendations indicate that, while these agents have a role in managing the symptoms of early menopause in selected patients, they should not be used long term for disease prevention.

Combined Hormonal Contraception

Combined hormonal (estrogen-progestin) contraception has evolved from high-dose estrogen formulations (100 μg) to much lower doses (less than 35 μg of ethinyl estradiol in monophasic oral preparations) and has expanded from oral contraceptive pills (OCs) to include transvaginal rings and dermal patches. Epidemiologic studies must be interpreted in the context of the changing dosage. Nevertheless, there is reasonable evidence to support the following conclusions:

- *Breast carcinoma:* There is a small ($\sim$1.2-fold) increased risk of breast cancer in women using OCs.
- *Endometrial cancer and ovarian cancers:* OCs have a protective effect against these tumors.
- *Cervical cancer:* OCs may increase the risk of cervical carcinomas in women infected with human papillomavirus.
- *Thromboembolism:* Combined hormone therapy of all types is associated with an increased risk of thromboembolism due to increased hepatic synthesis of coagulation factors. It is therefore contraindicated in women with thrombophilia (e.g., factor V Leiden) who are not receiving anticoagulation therapy.

- *Cardiovascular disease:* There is considerable uncertainty about the risk of atherosclerosis and myocardial infarction associated with OCs. It seems that OCs do not increase the risk of coronary artery disease in women younger than 30 years or in older women who are nonsmokers, but the risk is approximately double in women older than 35 years who smoke.
- *Hepatic adenoma:* There is a well-defined association between the use of OCs and this rare benign hepatic tumor (Chapter 14), especially in older women who have used OCs for prolonged periods.

These hazards must be viewed in the context of the wide availability and relative safety of combined hormone contraception. This is a changing field so therapy must be based on the latest available data.

Acetaminophen

At therapeutic doses, acetaminophen, a widely used nonprescription analgesic and antipyretic, is mostly conjugated in the liver with glucuronide or sulfate. About 5% or less is metabolized to a potentially toxic compound, *NAPQI* (*N*-acetyl-*p*-benzoquinoneimine), through the hepatic cytochrome P-450 system. With very large doses, however, NAPQI accumulates, leading to *centrilobular hepatic necrosis.* The mechanisms of hepatocyte injury produced by NAPQI include (1) covalent binding to hepatic proteins and (2) depletion of reduced glutathione (GSH). The depletion of GSH renders hepatocytes more susceptible to cell death caused by reactive oxygen species. A variety of factors influence acetaminophen toxicity including an individual's baseline glutathione levels (depleted in chronic disease, poor nutrition, exposure to xenobiotics) and cytochrome P450 activity. In adults, toxicity is likely with a single dose of 250 mg/kg or more than 12 g in a 24-hour period; severe liver toxicity is seen in nearly all adults who consume greater than 350 mg/kg. Since the maximal therapeutic dose (up to 4 g/day in adults) is substantially lower than the toxic dose, the drug is ordinarily very safe. However, accidental overdoses occur in children and suicide attempts using acetaminophen are not uncommon. Moreover, since multiple over-the-counter medications include acetaminophen, patients are not always aware of the extent of their exposure.

In the United States, acetaminophen toxicity accounts for about 50% of cases of acute liver failure and is the second most common cause of liver failure requiring transplantation. Toxicity begins with nausea, vomiting, diarrhea, and sometimes shock, followed in a few days by the appearance of jaundice. Overdoses of acetaminophen can be treated in early stages by the administration of *N*-acetylcysteine, which restores glutathione. With significant overdoses, liver failure ensues, and centrilobular necrosis may extend to involve entire lobules; these patients often require liver transplantation. Depending on the amount of acetaminophen ingested, 10% to 50% of patients have concurrent renal damage.

Aspirin (Acetylsalicylic Acid)

Aspirin overdose may result from accidental ingestion in young children or suicide attempts in adults. The major consequences are metabolic, with few morphologic changes. At first, *respiratory alkalosis* develops due to stimulation of the respiratory center in the medulla; this is followed by *metabolic acidosis* and accumulation of pyruvate and lactate caused by uncoupling of oxidative phosphorylation and inhibition of the Krebs cycle. Fatal doses may be as low as 3 g in children and 10 to 30 g in adults, but survival has been reported after doses five times larger.

Chronic aspirin toxicity (salicylism) may develop in persons who take 100 mg/kg/day to treat chronic pain or inflammatory conditions. Symptoms include headache, dizziness, ringing in the ears (tinnitus), difficulty in hearing, mental confusion, drowsiness, nausea, vomiting, and diarrhea. The neurologic abnormalities may progress to convulsions and coma. The morphologic consequences of chronic salicylism are varied; most often, there is an acute erosive gastritis (Chapter 13), which may produce overt or covert GI bleeding and lead to gastric ulceration. A bleeding tendency may manifest concurrently with chronic toxicity because aspirin irreversibly inhibits platelet cyclooxygenase and blocks the ability to make thromboxane A_2 (Chapter 3), an activator of platelet aggregation (this effect is the basis of low-dose aspirin intake to reduce the risk of acute coronary events). Petechial hemorrhages may appear in the skin and internal viscera, and bleeding from gastric ulcerations may increase.

When taken for several years, proprietary analgesic mixtures of aspirin and phenacetin or its active metabolite, acetaminophen, can cause tubulointerstitial nephritis with renal papillary necrosis (Chapter 12). This clinical entity is referred to as *analgesic nephropathy*.

Injury Due to Nontherapeutic Use of Substances

Substance use disorder and overdose are serious public health problems. Commonly misused substances are listed in Table 7.6. Considered here are psychostimulants, opiates, and marijuana, with a brief mention of a few other drugs.

Psychostimulants

In the United States, cocaine is the nonprescribed substance most often implicated in visits to hospital emergency departments. Overdose deaths attributed to cocaine and other psychostimulants continue to increase in number, perhaps due to surges in concomitant use of opioids contaminated with fentanyl (see later). Cocaine is extracted from the leaves of the coca plant to form a water-soluble powder that may be liberally diluted with talcum powder, lactose, or other look-alikes. Crystallization of the pure alkaloid from cocaine hydrochloride yields nuggets of crack cocaine, so called because of the sound it makes when heated.

Cocaine produces a sense of intense euphoria and mental alertness, making it one of the most psychologically addictive of all drugs. Experimental animals will press a lever more than 1000 times and will forgo food and drink to obtain cocaine. Although physical dependence does not seem to occur in individuals who use cocaine, psychologic dependence is profound. Intense cravings are particularly severe in the first several months after abstinence and can recur for years. Stimulant withdrawal can also manifest as depression, anhedonia, anxiety, and suicidal tendencies. Stimulant toxicity exists on a spectrum and can include anxiety, restlessness, repetitive behaviors (e.g., skin picking), agitation, and psychotic symptoms. Risk of stimulant toxicity can rise with increasing dose, sleep deprivation, and sensitization from prior episodes of toxicity. Cocaine toxicity, for example, has been associated with risk of seizures, cardiac arrythmias, cardiac ischemia, and respiratory arrest. The following are the important manifestations of cocaine toxicity:

- *Cardiovascular effects.* Cocaine acutely affects the cardiovascular system through its sympathomimetic effects (Fig. 7.13) both in the CNS, where it blocks the reuptake of dopamine, and at adrenergic nerve endings, where it blocks the reuptake of both epinephrine and norepinephrine while stimulating the presynaptic release of norepinephrine. The net effect is the accumulation of these neurotransmitters in synapses and excessive stimulation, manifested by tachycardia, hypertension, and peripheral vasoconstriction. Cocaine also induces myocardial ischemia, the basis for which is multifactorial, including coronary artery vasoconstriction and promotion of thrombus formation by facilitating platelet aggregation. Cigarette smoking potentiates cocaine-induced coronary vasospasm. By increasing myocardial oxygen demand by its sympathomimetic action and, at the same time, reducing coronary blood flow, cocaine induced myocardial ischemia may lead to myocardial infarction. Cocaine can also precipitate lethal arrhythmias by enhanced sympathetic activity as well as disruption of normal ion (K^+, Ca^{2+}, Na^+) transport in the myocardium. Ischemic and hemorrhagic stroke are also associated with cocaine use.
- *CNS effects.* Hyperthermia can be seen and is thought to be caused by aberrations of the dopaminergic pathways that control body

Table 7.6 Commonly Misused Substances

Class	Molecular Target	Examples
Opioid narcotics	Mu opioid receptor (agonist)	Heroin, fentanyl Oxycodone Methadone (Dolophine)
Sedative-hypnotics	GABA receptor (agonist)	Barbiturates Ethanol Benzodiazepines
Psychomotor stimulants	Biogenic amine transporter (antagonist)	Cocaine Amphetamine 3,4-methylenedioxymethamphetamine (MDMA) (i.e., "ecstasy")
Phencyclidine-like drugs	NMDA glutamate receptor channel (antagonist)	Phencyclidine (PCP) (i.e., "angel dust") Ketamine
Cannabinoids	CB1 cannabinoid receptors (agonist)	Marijuana Hashish
Nicotine	Nicotine acetylcholine receptor (agonist)	Tobacco products
Hallucinogens	Serotonin 5-HT2 receptors (agonist)	Lysergic acid diethylamide (LSD) Mescaline Psilocybin

CB1, Cannabinoid receptor type 1; *GABA*, γ-aminobutyric acid; *5-HT2*, 5-hydroxytryptamine; *NMDA*, N-methyl-D-aspartate; *PCP*, 1-(1-phenylcyclohexyl)piperidine.
Data from Hyman SE: A 28-year-old man addicted to cocaine. *JAMA* 286:2586, 2001.

CENTRAL NERVOUS SYSTEM SYNAPSE

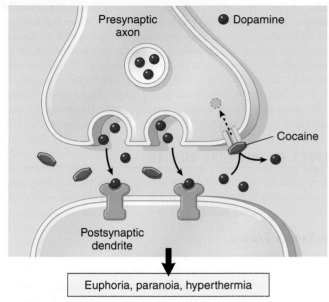

SYMPATHETIC NEURON–TARGET CELL INTERFACE

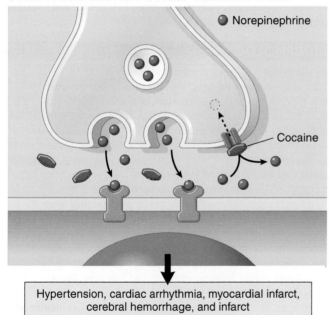

FIG. 7.13 The effect of cocaine on neurotransmission. The drug inhibits reuptake of the neurotransmitters dopamine and norepinephrine in the central and peripheral nervous systems.

temperature. With chronic cocaine use, imaging studies demonstrate gray matter atrophy in the frontal and temporal lobes.
- *Effects on the fetus.* In pregnant women, cocaine may cause decreased placental blood flow, resulting in fetal hypoxia, increased risk of spontaneous abortion, and potential for impaired fetal neurologic development.
- *Chronic cocaine use.* Chronic use may cause (1) perforation of the nasal septum in intranasal users; (2) wheezing, dyspnea, and hemoptysis in users who inhale the smoke; and (3) the development of dilated cardiomyopathy (Chapter 9).

Other psychostimulants include methamphetamine, amphetamine, "ecstasy" (3,4-methylenedioxymethamphetamine [MDMA]), ketamine (and related anesthetic agents), and "bath salts," synthetic cathinones that are chemically related to khat, a stimulant used in East Africa. Chronic use of ecstasy may deplete the CNS of serotonin, potentially leading to sleep disorders, depression, and anxiety. Ketamine has recently been approved by the FDA for treatment-resistant depression.

Opioids

Opioids include *opiates* (e.g., heroin, morphine, codeine) that are derived from the poppy plant and synthetic *opioids* such as fentanyl, oxycodone, hydrocodone, methadone, and buprenorphine. Some opioids have a medical use in pain control; however heroin has no approved medical use. Opioids bind receptors in the peripheral and central nervous system; stimulation of G proteins coupled to the receptor initiates signal transduction pathways that involve secondary messengers such as cAMP. Central effects include respiratory depression, analgesia, constriction of the pupils (miosis), and euphoria, while peripheral effects result in cough suppression and constipation. Opioids are highly addictive, and their misuse has taken a tremendous toll in the United States, particularly over the past several decades. Opioid-related deaths first began rising in the 1990s with increased prescribing of opioids. A second increase in deaths began in 2010 and was related to rapid increases in overdoses due to heroin. Most recently, the third and largest increase in deaths began in 2013 as synthetic opioids, particularly highly potent agents such as fentanyl and carfentanyl, became more available. Altogether, nonprescribed opioid use and opioid use disorders nearly doubled in prevalence from 2002 to 2018 and have resulted in nearly 500,000 deaths since 1999 and close to 100,000 deaths in the year ending in March of 2021.

Misuse often begins with prescribed or nonprescribed oral opioid pills, but most users eventually switch to heroin, which is substantially less expensive but also frequently admixed with highly potent synthetic opioids. Current efforts to reverse the ongoing opioid epidemic are focused on increasing the availability of treatments for opioid overdose to first responders (e.g., naloxone); promoting harm reduction (e.g., distribution of safe injection kits and medications to prevent HIV infection, needle exchange programs, better access to treatment programs using agents such as methadone and buprenorphine that reduce the craving for more dangerous opioids); and decreasing the medical use of prescription opioids.

Heroin and other opioids may be diluted (cut) with agents such as talc or quinine or mixed with fentanyl; thus, the size of the dose is not only variable but usually unknown to the user. The high potency of fentanyl and its increasing use are a main driver in overdose deaths. Heroin may be injected intravenously or subcutaneously or taken intranasally, while other opioids are often taken orally, intranasally, or mixed with water and injected. Effects are varied and include euphoria, hallucinations, somnolence, and sedation. Adverse physical effects can be ascribed to (1) the pharmacologic action of the agent; (2) reactions to the cutting agents or contaminants; (3) hypersensitivity reactions to the drug or its adulterants; and (4) infectious complications related to risky injection practices. Some of the most important adverse effects of opioids are the following:
- *Sudden death.* Sudden death, usually related to overdose, is an ever-present risk because drug purity is generally unknown and may range from 2% to 90%. Sudden death may be due to a loss of tolerance for the drug, such as after a period of incarceration. The mechanisms of death include profound respiratory depression, arrhythmia and cardiac arrest, and pulmonary edema.

- *Pulmonary disease.* Pulmonary complications include edema, septic embolism, lung abscess, opportunistic infections, and foreign body granulomas caused by inflammatory reactions to talc and other adulterants. Although granulomas occur principally in the lung, they are also sometimes found in the spleen, liver, and lymph nodes that drain the upper extremities. Examination under polarized light often highlights trapped talc crystals, sometimes enclosed within foreign body giant cells.
- *Infections.* Infectious complications are common. The sites most often affected are the skin and subcutaneous tissue, heart valves, liver, and lungs. Endocarditis is a common sequela and often involves right-sided heart valves, particularly the tricuspid valve. Most cases are caused by *Staphylococcus aureus,* but fungi and a multitude of other organisms have also been implicated. Unsafe injection practices can result in transmission of hepatitis B (HBV), hepatitis C (HCV), and human immunodeficiency virus.
- *Skin lesions.* Cutaneous lesions include abscesses, cellulitis, and ulcerations resulting from injections. Scarring at injection sites, hyperpigmentation over commonly used veins, and thrombosed veins are the usual sequelae of repeated intravenous inoculations.
- *Renal disease.* Kidney disease is a relatively common hazard when opioids are injected and includes secondary amyloidosis (due to skin infections), focal segmental glomerulosclerosis (Chapter 12), membranous nephropathy (due to HBV infection), and membranoproliferative glomerulonephritis (due to HCV infection).
- *Effects on the fetus.* Opioid exposure in utero can result in withdrawal symptoms after delivery; however, neonatal abstinence syndrome can be safely treated with methadone or buprenorphine.

Cannabis

Cannabis (marijuana) is a commonly used psychoactive drug derived from the leaves of the *Cannabis sativa* and *Cannabis indica* plants. In 2019, 48.2 million people (18% of the population) used cannabis at least once. As of 2022, 38 states and the District of Columbia legalized cannabis for medical use, and 18 states and the District of Columbia legalized cannabis for nonmedical use. Cannabis remains illegal under federal law.

The psychoactive substance in cannabis is Δ^9-tetrahydrocannabinol (THC). When cannabis is smoked, about 5% to 10% of the THC content is absorbed. Cannabis acutely distorts sensory perception and impairs motor coordination, attention, and concentration, but these effects generally clear in 4 to 5 hours. Evidence of long-term neurocognitive deficits due to chronic cannabis use is mixed, and it appears that effects resolve with abstinence. Beneficial effects of THC include its capacity to decrease intraocular pressure in glaucoma and to combat intractable nausea secondary to cancer chemotherapy. Although not supported by scientific studies, individuals may use cannabis for relaxation, as a sleep aid, for pain relief, and for pleasure.

Cannabis has many of the same carcinogens and lung irritants as tobacco; however, chronic cannabis use has not been shown to impair pulmonary function, and epidemiologic studies have not shown an increase in the incidence of lung cancer, though there are potentially confounding methodologic factors (e.g., small sample size, inaccuracies of self-reporting). Consequences of marijuana smoking on the lungs include cough, chest tightness, bronchitis, airway inflammation, and bronchodilation. Acutely, cannabis increases sympathetic activity while decreasing parasympathetic activity, thereby increasing cardiac output without a rise in blood pressure, which may result in orthostatic hypotension. There is no strong evidence linking cannabis use to myocardial infarction or stroke.

Hallucinogens

Hallucinogens are substances that alter sensory perception, thought patterns, and mood. They include PCP (1-[1-phenylcyclohexyl] piperidine, also known as phencyclidine), lysergic acid diethylamide (LSD), and psilocybin. Acutely, LSD has unpredictable effects on mood, affect, and thought, sometimes leading to bizarre and dangerous behaviors. Conversely, there is substantial current interest in using these substances in the treatment of posttraumatic stress disorder, cancer-related anxiety, and treatment-resistant depression.

INJURY BY PHYSICAL AGENTS

Injury induced by physical agents is divided into the following categories: mechanical trauma, thermal injury, electrical injury, and injury produced by ionizing radiation. Each type is considered separately.

Mechanical Trauma

Mechanical forces may inflict a variety of forms of damage. The type of injury depends on the shape of the colliding object, the amount of energy discharged at impact, and the tissues or organs that bear the impact. Bone and head injuries result in unique damage and are discussed elsewhere (Chapters 19 and 21). All soft tissues react similarly to mechanical forces, and the patterns of injury can be divided into abrasions, contusions, lacerations, incised wounds, and puncture wounds.

> **MORPHOLOGY**
>
> An **abrasion** is a wound produced by scraping or rubbing the skin surface, which damages the superficial layer. Typical skin abrasions remove only the epidermal layer. A **contusion,** or bruise, is usually produced by blunt trauma and is characterized by damage to a vessel and extravasation of blood into tissues. A **laceration** is a tear or disruptive stretching of tissue caused by the application of force by a blunt object. In contrast to an incision, most lacerations have intact bridging blood vessels and jagged, irregular edges. An **incised wound** is one inflicted by a sharp instrument that severs blood vessels. A **puncture wound** is typically caused by a long, narrow instrument and is termed **penetrating** when the instrument pierces the tissue and **perforating** when it traverses a tissue to also create an exit wound. Gunshot wounds are special forms of puncture wounds that demonstrate distinctive features important to the forensic pathologist. For example, a wound from a bullet fired at close range leaves powder burns, whereas one fired from more than 4 or 5 feet away does not.
>
> One of the most common causes of mechanical injury is **vehicular accident.** Typically, injuries are sustained as a result of (1) hitting part of the interior of the vehicle or being hit by objects that enter the passenger compartment during the crash, such as engine parts; (2) being thrown from the vehicle; or (3) being trapped in a burning vehicle. The pattern of injury relates to whether one or more of these mechanisms are operative. For example, in a head-on collision, a common pattern of injury sustained by a driver who is not wearing a seat belt includes trauma to the head (windshield impact), chest (steering column impact), and knees (dashboard impact). Common chest injuries stemming from such accidents include sternal and rib fractures, heart contusions, aortic lacerations, and (less commonly) lacerations of the spleen and liver. Thus, in caring for an automobile injury victim, it is essential to recognize that internal wounds often accompany superficial abrasions, contusions, and lacerations. Indeed, in many cases, external evidence of serious internal damage is completely absent.

Thermal Injury

Both excess heat and excess cold are important causes of injury. Burns are the most common type of thermal injury and are discussed first; a brief discussion of hyperthermia and hypothermia follows.

Thermal Burns

In the United States, burns cause approximately 3500 deaths per year and result in the hospitalization of more than 10 times that many persons. Many victims are children, in whom the cause of injury is often scalding by hot liquids. Since the 1970s, marked decreases have been seen in both mortality rates and the length of hospitalizations following burns. These improvements have been achieved through better understanding of the systemic effects of massive burns and more effective strategies for preventing and treating wound infection and facilitating the healing of skin surfaces.

The clinical severity of burns depends on the following important variables:

- *Depth* of the burns
- *Percentage* of body surface involved
- *Internal injuries* caused by inhalation of hot and toxic fumes
- *Promptness and efficacy of therapy,* especially fluid and electrolyte management and prevention or control of wound infections

A *full-thickness* burn totally destroys the epidermis and dermis, including the dermal appendages that harbor cells needed for epithelial regeneration; it results in anesthesia due to the destruction of nerve endings. In *partial-thickness* burns, at least the deeper portions of the dermal appendages are spared, so regeneration of the epidermis is possible; these are painful. Partial-thickness burns include first-degree burns (epithelial involvement only) and second-degree burns (involving both the epidermis and the superficial dermis); depending on the depth, they are erythematous or mottled and blistered. Histologic examination of devitalized tissue shows coagulative necrosis associated with acute inflammation and edema.

Shock, sepsis, and respiratory insufficiency are the greatest threats to life in burn patients. Any burn exceeding 50% of the total body surface, whether superficial or deep, is potentially fatal. With burns of more than 20% of the body surface, there is a rapid shift of body fluids into the interstitial compartments, both at the burn site and systemically, which can result in hypovolemic shock (Chapter 3). Due to widespread vascular leakiness, generalized edema (including pulmonary edema) can be severe. An important pathophysiologic effect of burns is the development of a hypermetabolic state associated with excess heat loss and an increased need for nutritional support. It is estimated that when more than 40% of the body surface is burned, the resting metabolic rate doubles.

Another important consideration is the degree of injury to the airways and lungs. *Inhalation injury* is frequent in persons trapped in burning buildings and may result from the direct effect of heat on tissues or from the inhalation of heated air and gases in the smoke. Water-soluble gases, such as chlorine, sulfur oxides, and ammonia, may react with water to form acids or alkalis, particularly in the upper airways, resulting in inflammation and swelling, which may lead to partial or complete airway obstruction. Lipid-soluble gases, such as nitrous oxide and products of burning plastics, are more likely to reach deeper airways, producing pneumonitis. Pulmonary manifestations may not develop for 24 to 48 hours.

Organ system failure resulting from sepsis continues to be the leading cause of death in burn patients. The burn site is a nidus for the growth of microorganisms; the serum and debris provide nutrients, and the burn injury compromises blood flow, blocking effective inflammatory responses. The most common offender is the opportunist *Pseudomonas aeruginosa,* but antibiotic-resistant strains of other common hospital-acquired bacteria, such as *S. aureus* and fungi, particularly *Candida* spp., also may be involved. Furthermore, systemic inflammatory response syndrome (Chapter 3) may impair or dysregulate both innate and adaptive immune responses. Direct bacteremic spread and release of toxic substances such as endotoxin from the local site have serious consequences. Pneumonia or septic shock, accompanied by renal failure and/or acute respiratory distress syndrome (ARDS) (Chapter 11), are the most common serious sequelae.

Hyperthermia

Prolonged exposure to elevated ambient temperatures can result in heat cramps, heat exhaustion, or heat stroke.

- *Heat cramps* result from loss of electrolytes through sweating. Cramping of voluntary muscles, usually in association with vigorous exercise, is the hallmark sign. Heat-dissipating mechanisms are intact, allowing affected individuals to maintain a normal core body temperature.
- *Heat exhaustion* is probably the most common hyperthermic syndrome. Its onset is sudden, with prostration and collapse, and it results from a failure of the cardiovascular system to compensate for hypovolemia secondary to water depletion. Equilibrium is spontaneously reestablished if the victim can rehydrate.
- *Heat stroke* is associated with high ambient temperatures and high humidity. Elderly people, persons with cardiovascular disease, and otherwise healthy people undergoing physical stress (such as young athletes and military recruits) are prime candidates for heat stroke. Thermoregulatory mechanisms fail, sweating ceases, and the core body temperature rises to more than 104°F, leading to multiorgan dysfunction that can be rapidly fatal.

Malignant hyperthermia, although similar in name, is not caused by exposure to high temperatures. It is a genetic condition resulting from mutations in genes such as ryanodine receptor 1 *(RYR1)* that control calcium levels in skeletal muscles. In affected individuals, exposure to certain anesthetics during surgery triggers a rapid rise in calcium levels in skeletal muscle, which in turn leads to muscle rigidity and increased heat production. The resulting hyperthermia has a mortality rate of approximately 80% if untreated, but this falls to less than 5% if the condition is recognized and muscle relaxants are administered promptly.

Hypothermia

Prolonged exposure to low ambient temperature leads to hypothermia. The condition is seen all too frequently in individuals who are unsheltered in whom wet or inadequate clothing and lack of housing hasten the lowering of body temperature. At a body temperature of about 90°F, loss of consciousness occurs, followed by bradycardia and atrial fibrillation at lower core temperatures.

Chilling or freezing of cells and tissues causes injury by two mechanisms:

- *Direct effects* of frostbite are due to crystallization of intra- and extracellular water, which lead to physical disruption of plasma membranes and intracellular organelles.
- *Indirect effects* result from circulatory changes, which vary depending on the rate and the duration of the temperature drop. Slow chilling may induce vasoconstriction and increased permeability, leading to edema. Over a long period of time, this can lead to nerve damage and gangrene, necessitating amputation. Alternatively,

with sudden, persistent chilling, the vasoconstriction and increased viscosity of the blood in the local area may cause ischemic injury and degenerative changes in peripheral nerves. Vascular injury and edema become evident only after the temperature begins to return to normal. If the period of ischemia is prolonged, hypoxic changes and infarction of the affected tissues (e.g., gangrene of toes or feet) may result.

Electrical Injury

Electrical injuries may be caused by low-voltage currents (i.e., in the home and workplace) or high-voltage currents carried in power lines or by lightning. The resulting injuries may include burns, ventricular fibrillation, and respiratory center failure resulting from disruption of normal electrical impulses, all of which may be fatal. The type of injury and the severity and extent of burning depend on the amperage of the electric current and its path within the body.

Voltage in the household and the workplace (120 or 220 V) is high enough that with low resistance at the site of contact (as when the skin is wet), sufficient current can pass through the body to cause serious injury, including ventricular fibrillation. If current flow continues long enough, it generates sufficient heat to produce burns at the site of entry and exit as well as in internal organs. An important characteristic of alternating current, the type available in most homes, is that it induces tetanic muscle spasm, so that when a live wire or switch is grasped, irreversible clutching is likely to occur, prolonging the period of current flow. This results in a greater likelihood of extensive electrical burns and, in some cases, spasm of the chest wall muscles, producing death from asphyxia. Currents generated from high-voltage sources cause similar damage; however, because of the large current flows generated, these injuries are more likely to produce paralysis of medullary centers and extensive burns. Lightning is a classic cause of high-voltage electrical injury.

Injury Caused by Ionizing Radiation

Radiation is energy that travels in the form of waves or high-speed particles. It has a wide range of energies that spans the electromagnetic spectrum and can be divided into nonionizing and ionizing radiation. The energy of nonionizing radiation, such as ultraviolet (UV) and infrared light, microwaves, and sound waves, can move atoms in a molecule or cause them to vibrate but is not sufficient to displace electrons from atoms. By contrast, ionizing radiation has sufficient energy to remove tightly bound electrons. Collision of these free electrons with other atoms releases additional electrons, in a reaction cascade referred to as ionization. The main types of ionizing radiation are x-rays and gamma rays (electromagnetic waves of very high frequencies), high-energy neutrons, alpha particles (composed of two protons and two neutrons), and beta particles, which are essentially electrons. At equivalent energies, alpha particles induce significant damage in a restricted area, whereas x-rays and gamma rays dissipate energy over a longer, deeper course and produce considerably less damage per unit of tissue. About 50% of the dose of ionizing radiation received by the US population is human made, mostly originating from medical devices and radioisotopes. The exposure of patients to ionizing radiation during radiologic imaging tests roughly doubled between the early 1980s and 2006 because of increased use of computed tomography (CT) scans but has since leveled off, in part because of a conscious effort by radiologists to change practices so as to limit exposures.

Ionizing radiation is a double-edged sword. It is indispensable in medical practice, being used in the treatment of cancer, in diagnostic imaging, and in therapeutic or diagnostic radioisotopes, but it also produces adverse short-term and long-term effects such as fibrosis, mutagenesis, carcinogenesis, and teratogenesis.

There are many terms used to express the dose of radiation. Of these Gray (Gy) is most commonly employed.

- *Gray* (Gy) is a unit that expresses the energy absorbed by a target tissue. It corresponds to the absorption of 10^4 ergs per gram of tissue. A centigray (cGy), which is the absorption of 100 ergs per gram of tissue, is equivalent to the exposure of tissue to 100 Rads (R) ("radiation absorbed dose"). The cGy nomenclature has now replaced the Rad in medical parlance.
- *Sievert* (Sv) is a unit of equivalent dose that depends on the biologic effects rather than the physical effects of radiation, replacing a unit called the Rem. For the same absorbed dose, various types of radiation differ in the extent of damage they produce. The equivalent dose controls for this variation, providing a uniform unit of measure.

Main Determinants of the Biologic Effects of Ionizing Radiation

In addition to the physical properties of the radiation, its biologic effects depend heavily on the following variables:

- *Rate of delivery* significantly modifies the biologic effect. Although the effect of radiant energy is cumulative, delivery in divided doses may allow cells to repair some of the damage in the intervals. Thus, fractional doses of radiant energy have a cumulative effect only to the extent that repair during the intervals is incomplete. Radiotherapy of tumors exploits the capability of normal cells to repair themselves and to recover more rapidly than tumor cells.
- *Field size* has a great influence on the consequences of radiation exposure. The body can withstand relatively high doses of radiation when they are delivered to small, carefully shielded fields, whereas smaller doses delivered to larger fields may be lethal.
- *Rate of cell division.* Dividing cells are more vulnerable to injury than quiescent cells because ionizing radiation damages DNA. Except at extremely high doses that impair DNA transcription, DNA damage is compatible with survival in nondividing cells, such as neurons and muscle cells. However, as discussed in Chapter 6, in dividing cells DNA damage is detected by sensors that produce signals leading to the upregulation of p53, the "guardian of the genome." p53 in turn upregulates the expression of genes that initially lead to cell-cycle arrest and, if the DNA damage is too great to repair, cause cell death through apoptosis. Therefore, tissues with a high rate of cell turnover, such as the gonads, bone marrow, lymphoid tissue, and the mucosa of the GI tract, are extremely vulnerable to radiation, and the injury is manifested early after exposure.
- *Oxygen levels* influence the rate of production of free radicals generated by radiolysis of water, which is the major mechanism by which DNA is damaged by ionizing radiation. As a result, poorly vascularized hypoxic tissues, such as the center of rapidly growing tumors, are generally less sensitive to radiation therapy than nonhypoxic tissues.
- *Damage to endothelial cells*, which are moderately sensitive to radiation. This may cause narrowing or occlusion of blood vessels, leading to impaired healing, fibrosis, and chronic ischemic atrophy, changes that typically appear months or years after exposure. Despite the low sensitivity of brain cells to radiation, vascular damage after irradiation can lead to late manifestations of radiation injury in the brain.

DNA Damage and Carcinogenesis

The most important cellular target of ionizing radiation is DNA (Fig. 7.14). If the damaged DNA is not precisely repaired, mutations result that can manifest years or decades later as cancer. Ionizing radiation can cause many types of DNA damage, including single-base damage, single- and double-strand breaks, and crosslinks between

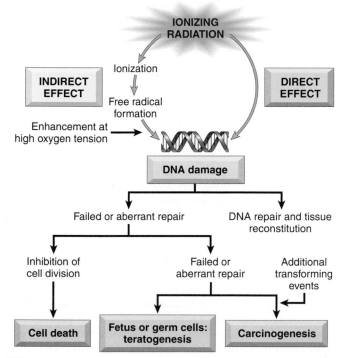

FIG. 7.14 Effects of ionizing radiation on DNA and their consequences. The effects on DNA can be direct or, most importantly, indirect, through free radical formation.

DNA and protein. In surviving cells, simple defects may be corrected by various enzyme repair systems (Chapter 6). These repair systems are linked to cell-cycle regulation through "sensor" proteins such as ATM (ataxia-telangiectasia mutated) that detect the damage, and p53, an effector molecule that can transiently arrest the cell cycle to allow DNA repair or to trigger apoptosis of cells that are irreparably damaged. However, double-strand breaks may persist without repair or repair may be imprecise, creating mutations. When cell-cycle checkpoints are impaired (for instance, because of *TP53* mutations), cells with abnormal and unstable genomes survive and may expand as abnormal clones that eventually transform into cancers.

Fibrosis

A common consequence of cancer radiotherapy is the development of fibrosis in the irradiated field (Fig. 7.15). Fibrosis may occur weeks or months after irradiation, as dead parenchymal cells are replaced by connective tissue and scars and adhesions form (Chapter 2). Vascular damage and the killing of tissue stem cells by ionizing radiation combined with the release of inflammatory cytokines and chemokines contribute to fibroblast activation and the development of radiation-induced fibrosis.

Effects on Organ Systems

Fig. 7.16 depicts the main consequences of radiation injury. As already mentioned, the most sensitive organs and tissues are the gonads, the hematopoietic and lymphoid systems, and the lining of the GI tract. Estimated threshold doses for the effects of acute exposure to radiation in various organs are shown in Table 7.7. The changes in the hematopoietic and lymphoid systems, along with the carcinogenic effects of environmental or occupational exposure to ionizing radiation, are summarized as follows:

- *The hematopoietic and lymphoid systems are extremely susceptible to radiation injury.* Radiation directly destroys lymphocytes in the blood and in tissues (e.g., in lymph nodes, spleen, thymus, gastrointestinal tract). With high dose levels and large exposure fields, severe lymphopenia and shrinkage of lymphoid tissues appear

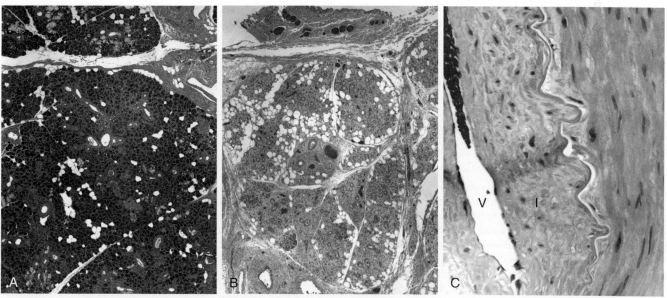

FIG. 7.15 Vascular changes and fibrosis of salivary glands produced by radiation therapy of the neck region. (A) Healthy salivary gland; (B) fibrosis caused by radiation; (C) vascular changes consisting of fibrointimal thickening and arteriolar sclerosis. *I*, Thickened intima; *V*, vessel lumen. (A–C, Courtesy of Dr. Melissa Upton, Department of Pathology, University of Washington, Seattle, Washington.)

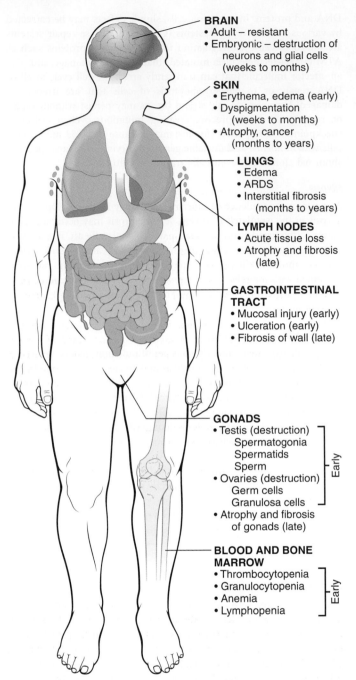

BRAIN
- Adult – resistant
- Embryonic – destruction of neurons and glial cells (weeks to months)

SKIN
- Erythema, edema (early)
- Dyspigmentation (weeks to months)
- Atrophy, cancer (months to years)

LUNGS
- Edema
- ARDS
- Interstitial fibrosis (months to years)

LYMPH NODES
- Acute tissue loss
- Atrophy and fibrosis (late)

GASTROINTESTINAL TRACT
- Mucosal injury (early)
- Ulceration (early)
- Fibrosis of wall (late)

GONADS
- Testis (destruction) Spermatogonia Spermatids Sperm — Early
- Ovaries (destruction) Germ cells Granulosa cells
- Atrophy and fibrosis of gonads (late)

BLOOD AND BONE MARROW
- Thrombocytopenia
- Granulocytopenia
- Anemia
- Lymphopenia — Early

FIG. 7.16 Overview of the major morphologic consequences of radiation injury. Early changes occur in hours to weeks; late changes occur in months to years. *ARDS,* Acute respiratory distress syndrome.

Table 7.7 Estimated Threshold Doses for Acute Radiation Effects on Specific Organs

Organ/ Structure	Injurious Dose (Sv)	Health Effect
Testes	0.15	Temporary sterility
Bone marrow	0.50	Depression of hematopoiesis
Skin	1.0–2.0	Reversible skin effects (e.g., erythema)
Ovaries	2.5–6.0	Permanent sterility
Skin	3.0–5.0	Temporary hair loss
Testis	3.5	Permanent sterility
Lens of eye	5.0	Cataract

require 2 to 3 months. *Thrombocytopenia* appears by the end of the first week, with the platelet count nadir occurring somewhat later than that of granulocytes; recovery is similarly delayed. *Anemia* appears after 2 to 3 weeks and may persist for months. Higher doses of radiation produce more severe cytopenias and more prolonged periods of recovery. Very high doses kill marrow stem cells and induce permanent aplasia *(aplastic anemia)* marked by a failure of blood count recovery, whereas aplasia is transient at lower doses.

- *Radiation exposure and cancer development.* Any cell capable of division that has sustained mutations has the potential to become cancerous. Thus, an increased incidence of neoplasms may occur in any organ after exposure to ionizing radiation. The minimal level of radiation required to increase the risk of cancer is difficult to determine, but there is little doubt that acute or prolonged exposures that result in doses of 100 mSv are carcinogenic. This is documented by the increased incidence of leukemias and tumors at various sites (e.g., thyroid, breast, and lung) in survivors of the atomic bombings of Hiroshima and Nagasaki, the increase in thyroid cancers in survivors of the Chernobyl accident, and the development of "second cancers," such as acute myeloid leukemia and various solid tumors in individuals who received radiation therapy for cancers such as Hodgkin lymphoma. It is believed that the risk of secondary cancers following irradiation is greatest in the young. This is based on a large-scale epidemiologic study showing that children who receive at least two CT scans have very small but measurable increased risks for leukemia and malignant brain tumors, and older studies showing that radiation therapy to the chest is particularly likely to produce breast cancers when administered to adolescent females. A well-documented example of an environmental radiation exposure that is carcinogenic involves radon gas, a ubiquitous product of the spontaneous decay of uranium. The carcinogenic agents are two radon decay byproducts (polonium-214 and polonium-218), which emit alpha particles and have a short half-life. These particulates are deposited in the lung, and chronic exposure in uranium miners may give rise to lung carcinomas. Risks are also present in those homes in which radon levels are very high, comparable to those found in mines. It is suspected that lower levels of household radon may contribute to lung cancer development, particularly in individuals who also smoke tobacco.

Total-Body Irradiation

Exposure of large areas of the body to even small doses of radiation may have devastating effects. Dosages less than 1 Sv produce minimal

within hours of irradiation. With sublethal doses of radiation, regeneration from viable progenitors is prompt, leading to restoration of a normal lymphocyte count. Hematopoietic precursors in the bone marrow are also quite sensitive to radiant energy, which produces a dose-dependent *marrow aplasia.* The acute effects of marrow irradiation on peripheral blood counts reflect the kinetics of turnover of the formed elements—the granulocytes, platelets, and red cells, which have half-lives of less than 1 day, 10 days, and 120 days, respectively. *Neutropenia* appears within several days and falls to a nadir, often at counts near zero, during the second week. If the patient survives, full recovery of granulocytes may

Table 7.8 Effects of Whole-Body Ionizing Radiation

	0–1 Sv	1–2 Sv	2–10 Sv	10–20 Sv	>50 Sv
Main site of injury	None	Lymphocytes	Bone marrow	Small bowel	Brain
Main signs and symptoms	—	Moderate leukopenia	Leukopenia, hemorrhage, epilation, vomiting	Diarrhea, fever, electrolyte imbalance, vomiting	Ataxia, coma, convulsions, vomiting
Timing	—	1 day–1 week	2–6 weeks	5–14 days	1–4 hours
Lethality	—	None	Variable (0–80%)	100%	100%

or no symptoms. Greater exposures, however, cause health effects known as acute radiation syndromes, which at progressively higher doses involve the hematopoietic system, GI system, and CNS. The syndromes associated with total-body exposure to ionizing radiation are summarized in Table 7.8.

NUTRITIONAL DISEASES

Millions of people in all parts of the world are affected by starvation, food insecurity, and obesity; while these represent a spectrum of food access, they all contribute to malnutrition.

Malnutrition

A healthy diet provides sufficient carbohydrates, fats, and proteins to support the body's daily metabolic needs and adequate amounts of vitamins and minerals, which function as coenzymes or hormones in vital metabolic pathways or as important structural components (e.g., calcium, phosphate). A high-quality diet is also rich in complex foods, including different fruits and vegetables, which contain phytochemicals and plant pigments that provide protective health benefits. In *primary malnutrition,* one or all these components are missing from the diet. By contrast, in *secondary,* or *conditional, malnutrition,* the dietary intake of nutrients is adequate, and malnutrition results from nutrient malabsorption, impaired use or storage, excess losses, or increased requirements. The causes of secondary malnutrition can be grouped into three general but overlapping categories: gastrointestinal diseases, chronic wasting diseases, and acute critical illness.

Malnutrition is widespread and may be obvious or subtle. Some common causes of dietary insufficiencies are listed here.

- *Poverty.* Unsheltered persons, elderly persons, marginalized communities, and children of lower socioeconomic status often experience severe malnutrition as well as trace nutrient deficiencies. In lower-resource countries, poverty, crop failures, livestock deaths, and drought, often in times of war and political upheaval, create the setting for the malnourishment of children and adults.
- *Ignorance.* Even well-educated individuals may not recognize that infants, adolescents, pregnant women, and elderly persons have increased nutritional needs. Ignorance about the nutritional content of various foods also contributes to malnutrition; for example, iodine is often lacking in food and water in regions removed from the oceans, leading to deficiencies unless supplementation is provided through iodized salt.
- *Chronic excess alcohol use.* Individuals who chronically drink excess alcohol may be malnourished but are more frequently lacking in several vitamins, especially thiamine, pyridoxine, folate, and vitamin A, as a result of poor diet, defective gastrointestinal absorption, abnormal nutrient utilization and storage, increased metabolic needs, and an increased rate of loss. A failure to recognize thiamine

deficiency in these patients may result in irreversible brain damage (e.g., Korsakoff psychosis, discussed in Chapter 21).

- *Acute and chronic illnesses.* The basal metabolic rate (BMR) rises in many conditions (e.g., severe burns, in which the BMR may double), resulting in increased daily requirements for nutrients. If these needs are unmet, recovery may be delayed. Malnutrition is often present in patients with wasting diseases, such as advanced cancers, disseminated tuberculosis, and AIDS, that are complicated by cachexia.
- *Self-imposed dietary restriction.* Anorexia nervosa, bulimia nervosa, and less overt eating disorders affect a large population of persons who struggle with underlying mental health challenges, in particular anxiety and depression. These may result in a hypervigilant focus on body image, calorie counting, or excessive exercise.
- *Other causes.* Additional causes of malnutrition include GI diseases, acquired and inherited malabsorption syndromes, specific drug therapies (which interfere with the uptake or function of particular nutrients), and total parenteral nutrition.

The remainder of this section presents a general overview of nutritional disorders. Particular attention is devoted to severe acute malnutrition, anorexia nervosa and bulimia nervosa, deficiencies of vitamins and trace minerals, and obesity, with a brief consideration of the relationships of diet to atherosclerosis and cancer. Other nutrients and nutritional issues are discussed in the context of specific diseases throughout the text.

Severe Acute Malnutrition

The World Health Organization (WHO) defines severe acute malnutrition (SAM) as a state characterized by weight-to-height ratio that is 3 standard deviations below the median growth standard, visible wasting, or the presence of nutritional edema. Worldwide about 50 million children are affected by SAM. Malnutrition is most common in low-resource countries, where about 45% of deaths in children under 5 years are due to undernutrition, and in the setting of war due to the abject poverty of many refugees. In camps set up for refugees from Syria, for example, as many as 20% of the children are severely or moderately malnourished, and widespread famine is currently afflicting the people of Afghanistan.

SAM, previously called protein energy malnutrition (PEM), manifests as a range of clinical syndromes, all resulting from an inadequate intake of dietary protein and calories to meet the body's needs. The two ends of the spectrum of SAM are known as *marasmus* and *kwashiorkor.* From a functional standpoint, there are two protein compartments in the body: the somatic compartment, represented by proteins in skeletal muscles, and the visceral compartment, represented by protein stores in visceral organs, primarily the liver. These two compartments are regulated differently, as detailed later. The somatic compartment is affected more severely in marasmus and the visceral compartment is depleted more severely in kwashiorkor.

The diagnosis of SAM is obvious when severe. In mild to moderate forms, the diagnosis is made by comparing body weight for a given height against standard tables; other helpful parameters are fat stores, muscle mass, and levels of certain serum proteins. With loss of body fat, measured skinfold thickness (which includes skin and subcutaneous tissue) is reduced. When the somatic protein compartment is catabolized, the reduction in muscle mass is reflected by reduced circumference of the midarm. Measurement of serum proteins (e.g., albumin, transferrin) provides an estimate of the adequacy of the visceral protein compartment. Recent studies suggest a role for the gut microbiome in the pathogenesis of SAM: there is a substantial difference in the microbial flora of children with SAM when compared with the gut microbiome of properly nourished children. It appears that the alterations in the microbiome are not merely the consequences of SAM but play a role in their causation.

Marasmus

Marasmus develops when the diet is severely lacking in calories (Fig. 7.17A). A child with marasmus experiences growth retardation and loss of muscle mass due to catabolism and depletion of the somatic protein compartment. This seems to be an adaptive response that provides the body with amino acids as a source of energy. The visceral protein compartment, which presumably is more critical for survival, is depleted only marginally; therefore, *serum albumin levels are normal or only slightly reduced*. In addition to muscle proteins, subcutaneous fat is also mobilized and used as fuel. Leptin (discussed later) production is low, which may stimulate the hypothalamic-pituitary-adrenal axis to produce the high levels of cortisol that contribute to lipolysis. Due to losses of muscle and subcutaneous fat, the extremities are emaciated; by comparison, the head appears too large for the body. Anemia and manifestations of multivitamin deficiencies are present, and there is evidence of *immune deficiency*, particularly of T cell–mediated immunity. Hence, concurrent infections are usually present, which impose an additional stress on a weakened body.

Kwashiorkor

Kwashiorkor occurs when protein deprivation is relatively greater than the reduction in total calories (Fig. 7.17B). This is the most common form of SAM in children who have been weaned early and subsequently fed, almost exclusively, a carbohydrate diet (the name kwashiorkor, from the Ga language in Ghana, describes the illness in a child who is weaned when another baby is born). The prevalence of kwashiorkor is high in impoverished areas of Africa, Southeast Asia, and Central America. Less severe forms may occur in persons with chronic diarrheal states, in which protein is not absorbed, or in those with chronic protein loss (e.g., protein-losing enteropathies, the nephrotic syndrome, or the aftermath of extensive burns). Rare cases of kwashiorkor resulting from fad diets or replacement of milk by rice-based beverages have been reported in the United States.

In kwashiorkor, unlike in marasmus, marked protein deprivation is associated with severe loss of the visceral protein compartment, and the resultant hypoalbuminemia gives rise to *generalized* or *dependent edema*. The weight of children with severe kwashiorkor is typically 60% to 80% of normal. However, true weight loss is masked by increased fluid retention (edema). In further contrast with marasmus, there is relative sparing of subcutaneous fat and muscle mass. The modest loss of these compartments may also be masked by edema.

Children with kwashiorkor have characteristic *skin lesions* with alternating zones of hyperpigmentation, desquamation, and hypopigmentation (eFig. 7.3). *Hair changes* include loss of color or alternating bands of pale and darker color, straightening, fine texture, and loss of firm attachment to the scalp. Other features that distinguish kwashiorkor from marasmus include an enlarged, *fatty liver* (due to reduced synthesis of the carrier protein component of lipoproteins) and the development of apathy, listlessness, and loss of appetite. As in marasmus, vitamin deficiencies are likely to be present, as are *defects in immunity* and *secondary infections*, which produce a catabolic state

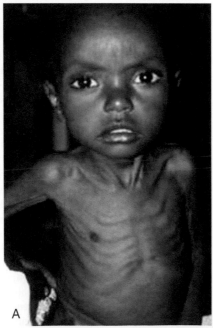
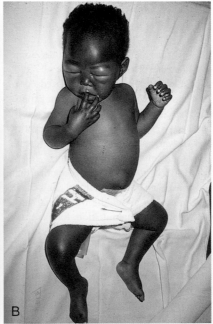

FIG. 7.17 Childhood malnutrition. (A) Marasmus. Note the loss of muscle mass and subcutaneous fat; the head appears to be too large for the emaciated body. (B) Kwashiorkor. The infant shows generalized edema, seen as ascites and puffiness of the face, hands, and legs. (A, From Clinic Barak, Reisebericht Kenya.)

that aggravates the malnutrition. As already mentioned, marasmus and kwashiorkor represent two ends of a spectrum, and considerable overlap exists.

Secondary Malnutrition

Secondary malnutrition is more commonly seen in higher-income countries in individuals who are chronically ill, elderly, or bedridden. It is estimated that more than 50% of residents in US nursing homes are malnourished; weight loss of more than 5% due to malnutrition increases the risk of mortality in these individuals by almost 5-fold.

MORPHOLOGY

The characteristic anatomic changes in SAM are (1) growth failure; (2) peripheral edema in kwashiorkor; and (3) muscle atrophy and loss of body fat, more marked in marasmus. The **liver** in kwashiorkor, but not in marasmus, is enlarged and fatty; superimposed cirrhosis is rare. In kwashiorkor (rarely in marasmus) the **small bowel** shows a decreased mitotic index in the crypts of the glands, associated with mucosal atrophy and loss of villi and microvilli. In such cases, concurrent loss of small intestinal enzymes occurs, most often manifested as disaccharidase deficiency. Hence, infants with kwashiorkor are lactose intolerant initially and may not respond well to full-strength, milk-based diets. With treatment, the mucosal changes are reversible. The **bone marrow** in both kwashiorkor and marasmus may be hypoplastic, mainly due to a decrease in red cell precursors. Thus, anemia is usually present. It is most often hypochromic and microcytic due to iron deficiency, but a concurrent deficiency of folate may lead to a mixed microcytic-macrocytic anemia (Chapter 10). The **brain** in infants who are born to mothers who are malnourished and who experience SAM during the first 1 or 2 years of life has been reported to show cerebral atrophy, a reduced number of neurons and impaired myelination of white matter. Many other abnormalities may be present, including (1) thymic and lymphoid atrophy (more marked in kwashiorkor than in marasmus); (2) anatomic alterations induced by intercurrent infections, particularly with endemic helminths and other parasites; and (3) deficiencies of other required nutrients such as iodine and vitamins.

The most obvious signs of secondary malnutrition include (1) depletion of subcutaneous fat in the arms, chest wall, shoulders, or metacarpal regions; (2) wasting of the quadriceps and deltoid muscles; and (3) ankle or sacral edema.

Anorexia Nervosa and Bulimia Nervosa

Anorexia nervosa is a state of self-induced starvation resulting in marked weight loss, whereas bulimia nervosa is a condition in which the patient binges on food and then seeks to use some compensatory mechanism such as vomiting. Bulimia nervosa is more common than anorexia nervosa and carries a better prognosis. It is estimated to occur in 1% to 2% of women and 0.1% of men, with an average age at onset of 20 years. However, any eating disorder, including other subtypes such as *binge eating disorder* and *avoidant restrictive food intake disorder*, can begin as early as childhood or present much later in life.

The clinical findings in anorexia nervosa are generally similar to those in SAM. In addition, effects on the endocrine system are prominent. In women, *amenorrhea*, resulting from decreased secretion of gonadotropin-releasing hormone (and consequent decreased secretion of luteinizing and follicle-stimulating hormones), is so common that its presence is almost a diagnostic feature. Other common findings in males and females are related to *decreased thyroid hormone* release and include cold intolerance, bradycardia, constipation, and changes in the skin and hair. Dehydration and electrolyte abnormalities are frequently seen. Body hair may be increased but is usually fine and pale (lanugo). *Bone density can be decreased* in men and women, most likely due to lower testosterone and estrogen, respectively, as well as reduced body weight. As expected with severe malnutrition, anemia, lymphopenia, and hypoalbuminemia may be present. A major complication of anorexia nervosa is an increased susceptibility to *cardiac arrhythmia* and *sudden death,* both resulting from hypokalemia.

Binge eating is part of the Diagnostic and Statistical Manual of Mental Disorders - V (DSM-V) criteria for bulimia nervosa. Huge amounts of food, principally carbohydrates, are ingested, only to be followed by induced vomiting or some other compensatory mechanism such as laxatives and/or diuretics, food restriction for several days, and overexercising to burn off calories. Although menstrual irregularities are common, amenorrhea occurs in less than 50% of patients with bulimia, probably because weight and gonadotropin levels are typically nearly normal. The major medical complications are related to continual induced vomiting and/or chronic use of laxatives and diuretics. These include (1) electrolyte imbalances (hypokalemia), which predispose the patient to cardiac arrhythmias; (2) pulmonary aspiration of gastric contents; and (3) rupture of the esophagus or stomach. Nevertheless, there are no specific signs and symptoms for this syndrome, and the diagnosis must rely on a comprehensive assessment of the patient.

Vitamin Deficiencies and Toxicity

Thirteen vitamins are necessary for health; vitamins A, D, E, and K are fat soluble, and all others are water soluble. The distinction between fat-soluble and water-soluble vitamins is important: fat-soluble vitamins are more readily stored in the body, but they may be poorly absorbed in fat malabsorption disorders caused by disturbances of digestive functions (Chapter 13). Certain vitamins can be synthesized endogenously—vitamin D from precursor steroids; vitamin K and biotin by the intestinal microflora; and niacin from tryptophan, an essential amino acid. Notwithstanding this endogenous synthesis, a dietary supply of all vitamins is essential for health.

In the following sections, vitamins A, D, and C are presented in some detail because their functions are wide ranging and their deficiency states have characteristic morphologic changes. This is followed by a summary in tabular form of the main consequences of deficiencies of the remaining vitamins—E, K, and B complex—and some essential minerals. However, it should be emphasized that deficiency of a single vitamin is uncommon, and that single or multiple vitamin deficiencies may be associated with SAM.

Vitamin A

The major functions of vitamin A are maintenance of normal vision, regulation of cell growth and differentiation, and regulation of lipid metabolism. Vitamin A is a generic name for a group of related fat-soluble compounds that include *retinol, retinal,* and *retinoic acid,* which have similar biologic activities. Retinol is the transport form and, as retinol ester, the storage form of vitamin A. A widely used term, *retinoids,* refers to both natural and synthetic chemicals that are structurally related to vitamin A but that may not necessarily have vitamin A activity. Animal-derived foods such as liver, fish, eggs, milk, and butter are important dietary sources of vitamin A. Yellow and leafy green vegetables such as carrots, squash, and spinach supply large amounts of carotenoids, many of which are provitamins that are metabolized to vitamin A in the body. Carotenoids contribute approximately 30% of the vitamin A in human diets; the most important of these is β-carotene, which is efficiently converted to vitamin A. The recommended dietary allowance for vitamin A is expressed in retinol equivalents, which reflects the contributions of both preformed vitamin A and β-carotene.

Metabolism. As with all fat soluble vitamins, vitamin A is hydrophobic and its absorption requires bile as well as pancreatic enzymes and some level of antioxidant activity in the food. Retinol (generally ingested as retinol ester) and β-carotene are absorbed through the intestinal wall, where β-carotene is converted to retinol (Fig. 7.18). Retinol is then transported through the blood in chylomicrons to the liver, where it is taken up through the apolipoprotein E receptor. More than 90% of the body's vitamin A reserves are found in the liver, predominantly as retinol ester in the perisinusoidal stellate (Ito) cells. In healthy persons who consume an adequate diet, these reserves are sufficient to support the body's needs for at least 6 months. For transport from the liver, retinol is bound to retinol-binding protein (RBP), which is synthesized in the liver. The uptake of retinol/RBP in peripheral tissues depends on cell surface RBP receptors. After uptake by cells, retinol is released, and RBP is recycled back into the blood. Retinol may be stored in peripheral tissues as retinyl ester or may be oxidized to form retinoic acid.

Function. In humans, the best-defined functions of vitamin A are the following:

- *Maintaining normal vision in reduced light.* Vision involves four forms of vitamin A–containing pigments: rhodopsin, located in rod cells, the most light-sensitive pigment and therefore important in reduced light, and three iodopsins, located in cone cells, each responsive to a specific color in bright light. Synthesis of all four pigments is reduced when vitamin A is deficient.
- *Potentiating the differentiation of specialized epithelial cells.* Vitamin A and retinoids play an important role in the orderly differentiation of mucus-secreting columnar epithelium; when a deficiency state exists, the epithelium undergoes *squamous metaplasia,* differentiating into keratinizing epithelium. Activation of retinoic acid receptors (RARs) by their ligands causes the formation of heterodimers with another retinoid receptor known as the *retinoic X receptor (RXR).* RAR/RXR heterodimers bind to retinoic acid response elements located in the regulatory regions of various genes, including some that encode receptors for growth factors, tumor suppressor genes, and secreted proteins. Through these effects, retinoids regulate cell growth and differentiation, cell-cycle control, and other biologic responses.
- *Metabolic effects of retinoids.* Retinoids inhibit adipogenesis and stimulate lipid breakdown. RXR is activated by 9-*cis* retinoic acid and can form heterodimers with nuclear receptors other than RAR, such as the peroxisome proliferator-activated receptors (PPARs) and vitamin D receptors. PPARs are key regulators of fatty acid metabolism, including fatty acid oxidation in fat and muscle, adipogenesis, and lipoprotein metabolism. The metabolic effects of retinoids on adipogenesis are thought to be mediated through the activities of RXR-PPAR heterodimers.
- *Enhancing resistance to infections.* Vitamin A supplementation can reduce morbidity and mortality rates from diarrhea by approximately 15% and 30%, respectively. Vitamin A may promote the regeneration of damaged epithelia and, through uncertain mechanisms, may also be required for optimal immune function.

Deficiency States. Vitamin A deficiency may occur as a consequence of either poor nutrition or fat malabsorption. In adults,

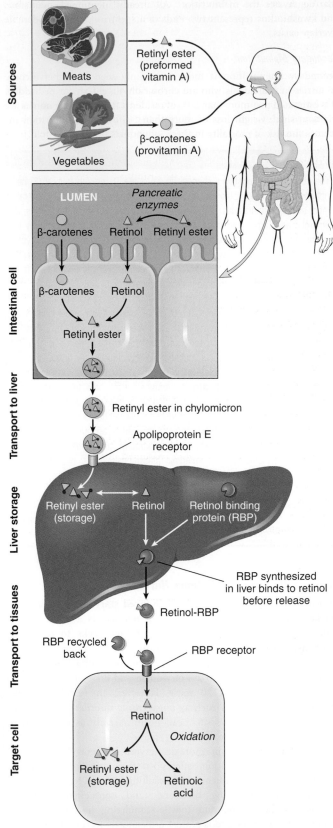

FIG. 7.18 Vitamin A metabolism.

vitamin A deficiency, in conjunction with depletion of other fat-soluble vitamins, may develop in patients with malabsorption syndromes such as celiac disease, Crohn disease, and colitis. Bariatric surgery and the continuous use of mineral oil laxatives may also lead to deficiency. The pathologic effects of vitamin A deficiency are summarized in Fig. 7.19.

As already discussed, vitamin A is a component of rhodopsin and other visual pigments; therefore, one of the earliest manifestations of vitamin A deficiency is impaired vision, particularly in reduced light (night blindness). Other effects of deficiency are related to the role of vitamin A in regulating the differentiation of epithelial cells. Persistent deficiency gives rise to epithelial metaplasia and keratinization. The most clinically significant changes occur in the eyes and are referred to as xerophthalmia (dry eye). First, there is dryness of the conjunctiva *(xerosis conjunctivae)* as the normal lacrimal and mucus-secreting epithelium is replaced by keratinized epithelium, followed by a buildup of keratin debris in small opaque plaques *(Bitot spots)* that progresses to erosion of the roughened corneal surface, softening and destruction of the cornea (keratomalacia), and blindness.

The epithelium lining the upper respiratory passage and urinary tract may also undergo squamous metaplasia. Loss of the mucociliary epithelium of the airways predisposes to secondary pulmonary infections, and desquamation of keratin debris in the urinary tract can result in renal and urinary bladder stones. Hyperplasia and hyperkeratinization of the epidermis and plugging of the ducts of the adnexal glands may produce follicular or papular dermatosis. In parts of the world where deficiency of vitamin A is prevalent, dietary supplements reduce mortality by 20% to 30% by improving immune function.

Toxicity. Both short-term and long-term excesses of vitamin A may produce toxic manifestations. The consequences of acute hypervitaminosis A were first described by Gerrit de Veer in 1597, a ship's carpenter stranded in the Arctic, who recounted in his diary the serious symptoms that he and other members of the crew developed after eating polar bear liver. With this cautionary tale in mind, the adventurous eater should be aware that acute vitamin A toxicity has also been described in individuals who ingested the livers of whales, sharks, and even tuna.

The symptoms of acute vitamin A toxicity include headache, dizziness, vomiting, stupor, and blurred vision, symptoms that may be confused with those of a brain tumor (pseudotumor cerebri). Chronic toxicity is associated with weight loss, anorexia, nausea, vomiting, and bone and joint pain. Retinoic acid stimulates osteoclast production and activity, leading to increased bone resorption and high risk of fractures. Although synthetic retinoids used for the treatment of acne are not associated with these types of conditions, their use in pregnancy should be avoided because of the well-established teratogenic effects of retinoids.

Vitamin D

The major function of vitamin D is the maintenance of adequate plasma levels of calcium and phosphorus to support metabolic functions, bone mineralization, and neuromuscular transmission. Vitamin D is required for the prevention of bone diseases known as *rickets* (in children whose epiphyses have not already closed) and *osteomalacia* (in adults), as well as *hypocalcemic tetany*. With respect to tetany, vitamin D maintains the correct concentration of ionized calcium in the extracellular fluid compartment. When deficiency develops, the drop in ionized calcium in the extracellular fluid results in continuous excitation of muscle (tetany). Any reduction in the level of serum calcium is usually corrected by increased secretion of parathyroid hormone followed by bone resorption; hence, bone changes dominate the clinical picture and tetany is quite uncommon. Our attention here is focused on the function of vitamin D in the regulation of serum calcium levels.

Metabolism. The major source of vitamin D in humans is its endogenous synthesis in the skin through a reaction that requires solar or artificial UV light. Irradiation of the precursor compound, 7-dehydrocholesterol forms cholecalciferol, known as vitamin D_3; in the following discussion, for the sake of simplicity, the term vitamin D is used to refer to this compound. Under usual conditions of sun exposure, approximately 90% of the needed vitamin D is endogenously derived. However, individuals with dark skin tones may have a lower level of vitamin D production in the skin because of absorption of UV light by melanin. The small remainder comes from dietary sources, such as deep-sea fish, plants and grains, and supplemented milk. In plant sources, vitamin D is present in a precursor form, ergosterol, which is converted to vitamin D in the body.

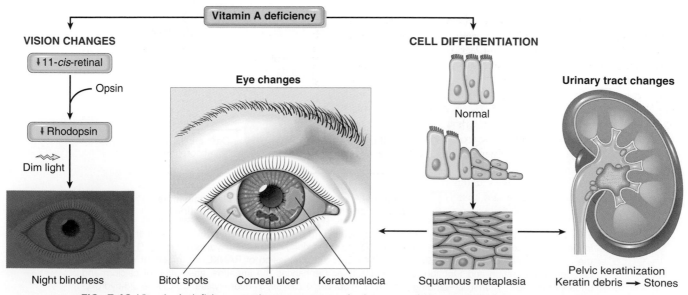

FIG. 7.19 Vitamin A deficiency: major consequences in the eye and due to squamous metaplasia. Not depicted is immune deficiency.

The metabolism of vitamin D can be outlined as follows (Fig. 7.20):

- Absorption of vitamin D along with other fats in the gut or synthesis from precursors in the skin
- Binding to plasma α_1-globulin (vitamin D—binding protein) and transport to liver
- Conversion to 25-hydroxyvitamin D (25-OH-D) by 25-hydroxylase in the liver

- Conversion of 25-OH-D to 1,25-dihydroxyvitamin D [1,25-(OH)$_2$-D] (the most active form of vitamin D) by α1-hydroxylase in the kidney

Renal production of 1,25-(OH)$_2$-D is regulated by three mechanisms:
- *Hypocalcemia stimulates secretion of parathyroid hormone (PTH), which in turn augments the conversion of 25-OH-D to 1,25-(OH)$_2$-D by activating α1-hydroxylase.*

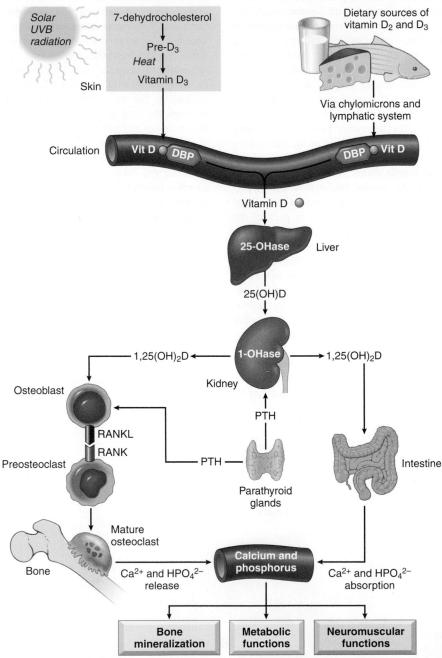

FIG. 7.20 Vitamin D metabolism. Vitamin D is produced from 7-dehydrocholesterol in the skin or is ingested in the diet. It is converted in the liver into 25(OH)D and in the kidney into 1,25-dihydroxyvitamin D (1,25[OH]$_2$D), the active form of the vitamin. 1,25(OH)$_2$D stimulates the expression of RANKL, an important regulator of osteoclast maturation and function, on osteoblasts and enhances the intestinal absorption of calcium and phosphorus. *DBP,* Vitamin D—binding protein (α_1-globulin); *1-OHase,* α_1-hydroxylase; *25-OHase,* 25-hydroxylase; *PTH,* parathyroid hormone; *RANK,* receptor activator of nuclear factor kappa-β; *RANKL,* receptor activator of nuclear factor kappa-β ligand.

- *Hypophosphatemia directly activates α1-hydroxylase,* thereby increasing the formation of 1,25(OH)$_2$-D.
- Through a feedback mechanism, increased levels of 1,25-(OH)$_2$-D downregulate its own synthesis through inhibition of 1α-hydroxylase activity.

Functions. Like retinoids and steroid hormones, 1,25-(OH)$_2$-D acts by binding to a high-affinity nuclear receptor that in turn binds to regulatory DNA sequences, thereby inducing transcription of specific target genes. The receptors for 1,25-(OH)$_2$-D are present in most nucleated cells of the body and, when activated, they induce the expression of genes that regulate various biologic activities. The best-understood of these functions relate to the maintenance of normal plasma levels of calcium and phosphorus through actions on the intestines, bones, and kidneys (Fig. 7.21).

The main functions of 1,25-dihydroxyvitamin D on calcium and phosphorus homeostasis are the following:

- *Stimulation of intestinal absorption of calcium* through upregulation of calcium transport in enterocytes
- *Stimulation of calcium resorption in renal distal tubules* through upregulation of proteins involved in calcium uptake (e.g., plasma membrane calcium pump, epithelial calcium channel), intracellular trafficking (e.g., calbindin), and basolateral transport
- *Regulation of PTH synthesis by chief cells.* Increased serum concentrations of 1,25-(OH)$_2$-D decrease transcription of the PTH gene.
- *Bone mineralization and resorption.* Vitamin D is needed for the mineralization of osteoid matrix and epiphyseal cartilage during the formation of flat and long bones. Vitamin D also upregulates expression of RANK ligand on osteoblasts, which activates RANK receptors on osteoclast precursors. RANK activation produces signals that increase osteoclast differentiation and bone resorptive activities (Chapter 19).

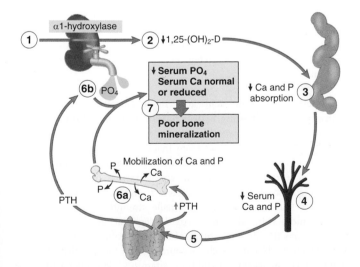

FIG. 7.21 Vitamin D deficiency. Inadequate substrate (1) for renal hydroxylase leads to a deficiency of 1,25(OH)$_2$-D (2) and decreased absorption of calcium (Ca) and phosphorus (P) from the gut (3), with consequent depressed serum levels of both (4). The hypocalcemia activates the parathyroid glands (5), causing mobilization of calcium and phosphorus from bone (6a). Simultaneously, parathyroid hormone (PTH) induces wasting of phosphate in the urine (6b) and calcium retention. Consequently, the serum levels of calcium are normal or nearly normal, but the phosphate is low; hence, mineralization is impaired (7).

Of note, effects of vitamin D on bone depend on the plasma levels of calcium. In hypocalcemic states 1,25-(OH)$_2$-D together with PTH increases the resorption of calcium and phosphorus from bone to support blood levels. In normocalcemic states, vitamin D is required for calcium deposition in epiphyseal cartilage and osteoid matrix.

Deficiency States. Vitamin D deficiency causes rickets in growing children and osteomalacia in adults. These skeletal diseases occur worldwide and may result from diets deficient in calcium and vitamin D, but limited exposure to sunlight is probably a more important factor in their etiology. Insufficient sun exposure is most frequent in inhabitants of northern latitudes but may also be seen in other regions in individuals whose skin is nearly completely protected by clothing or sunscreen and in children born to mothers who have frequent pregnancies followed by lactation due to deficient vitamin D in milk. In these situations, vitamin D deficiency can be prevented by a diet high in fish oils or by supplementation. Other, less common causes of rickets and osteomalacia include renal disorders leading to decreased synthesis of 1,25-(OH)$_2$-D or phosphate depletion and malabsorption disorders. Although rickets and osteomalacia rarely occur outside high-risk groups, milder forms of vitamin D deficiency that lead to bone loss and hip fractures are common among elderly persons. Studies also suggest that vitamin D may be important for preventing demineralization of bones, as certain genetic variants of the vitamin D receptor are associated with accelerated loss of bone minerals with aging and certain familial forms of osteoporosis (Chapter 19).

Vitamin D deficiency tends to cause hypocalcemia, which stimulates PTH production. This results in (1) activation of renal α$_1$-hydroxylase, which increases levels of active vitamin D and calcium absorption; (2) mobilization of calcium from bone; (3) a decrease in renal calcium excretion; and (4) an increase in renal excretion of phosphate. The serum level of calcium is restored to near normal, but hypophosphatemia persists, resulting in impaired bone mineralization or high bone turnover.

The basic derangement in both rickets and osteomalacia is an excess of unmineralized bone matrix. An understanding of the morphologic changes in rickets and osteomalacia is facilitated by a brief summary of normal bone development and maintenance. The development of flat bones in the skeleton involves intramembranous ossification, whereas the formation of long tubular bones proceeds by endochondral ossification. With intramembranous bone formation, mesenchymal cells differentiate directly into osteoblasts, which synthesize the collagenous osteoid matrix on which calcium is deposited. By contrast, with endochondral ossification, growing cartilage at the epiphyseal plates is provisionally mineralized and then progressively resorbed and replaced by osteoid matrix, which undergoes mineralization to create bone (Fig. 7.22A).

In the growing bones of children with rickets, hypocalcemia results in inadequate provisional calcification of epiphyseal cartilage and consequent derangements of enchondral bone growth. The following sequence ensues in rickets:

- Overgrowth of epiphyseal cartilage caused by inadequate provisional calcification and failure of the cartilage cells to mature and disintegrate
- Persistence of distorted, irregular masses of cartilage, many of which project into the marrow cavity
- Deposition of osteoid matrix on inadequately mineralized cartilaginous remnants
- Disruption of the orderly replacement of cartilage by osteoid matrix, with enlargement and lateral expansion of the osteochondral junction (Fig. 7.22B)

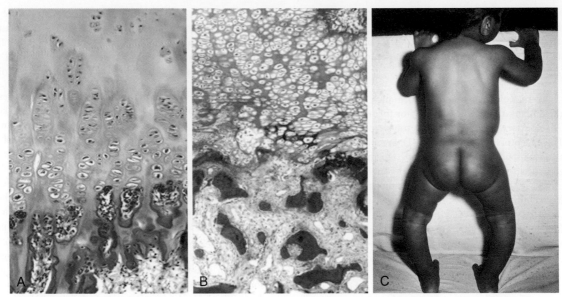

FIG. 7.22 Rickets. (A) Normal costochondral junction of a young child. Note cartilage palisade formation and orderly transition from cartilage to new bone. (B) Rachitic costochondral junction in which the palisade of cartilage is absent. Darker trabeculae are well-formed bone; paler trabeculae consist of uncalcified osteoid. (C) Note bowing of legs as a consequence of the formation of poorly mineralized bone in a child with rickets. (B, Courtesy of Dr. Andrew E. Rosenberg, Massachusetts General Hospital, Boston, Massachusetts.)

- Abnormal overgrowth of capillaries and fibroblasts in the disorganized bone resulting from microfractures and weak, poorly formed bone
- Deformation of the skeleton resulting from the loss of structural rigidity of the developing bones

MORPHOLOGY

The gross skeletal changes depend on the severity of the rachitic (related to rickets) process; its duration; and (in particular) the stresses to which individual bones are subjected. During the nonambulatory stage of infancy, the head and chest sustain the greatest stresses. The softened occipital bones may become flattened and the parietal bones can be buckled inward by pressure; with the release of the pressure, elastic recoil snaps the bones back into their original positions **(craniotabes).** An excess of osteoid produces **frontal bossing** and a squared appearance to the head. Deformation of the chest results from overgrowth of cartilage or osteoid tissue at the costochondral junction, producing characteristic nodularity of the junctions. The weakened metaphyseal areas of the ribs are subject to the pull of the respiratory muscles, causing them to bend inward, creating anterior protrusion of the sternum. The inward pull at the margin of the diaphragm creates the **Harrison groove,** girdling the thoracic cavity at the lower margin of the rib cage. The pelvis may become deformed. When an ambulating child develops rickets, deformities are likely to affect the spine, pelvis, and lower extremity long bones, causing, most notably, **lumbar lordosis** and **bowing of the legs** (Fig. 7.22C).

In adults with **osteomalacia,** the lack of vitamin D deranges the normal bone remodeling that occurs throughout life. Newly formed osteoid matrix laid down by osteoblasts is inadequately mineralized, producing the excess persistent osteoid that characterizes osteomalacia. Although the contours of the bone are not affected, the bone is weak and vulnerable to gross fractures or microfractures, which most often affect vertebral bodies and femoral necks. On histologic examination, the unmineralized osteoid can be visualized as a thickened layer of eosinophilic matrix arranged about the more basophilic, normally mineralized trabeculae.

Vitamin C (Ascorbic Acid)

A deficiency of water-soluble vitamin C leads to the development of scurvy, characterized principally by bone disease in growing children and by hemorrhages and healing defects in both children and adults. Sailors of the British Royal Navy were nicknamed "limeys" because at the end of the 18th century the Navy began to provide lime and lemon juice, rich sources of vitamin C, to prevent scurvy during their long sojourns at sea. It was not until 1932 that ascorbic acid was identified and synthesized. Unlike vitamin D, ascorbic acid is not synthesized endogenously in humans, who are entirely dependent on the diet for this nutrient. Vitamin C is abundant in a variety of fruits and vegetables and is present in milk and some animal products (liver, fish). All but the most restricted diets provide adequate amounts of vitamin C.

Function. Ascorbic acid acts in a variety of biosynthetic pathways by accelerating hydroxylation and amidation reactions. The most clearly established function of vitamin C is the activation of prolyl and lysyl hydroxylases from inactive precursors, allowing for hydroxylation of procollagen. Inadequately hydroxylated procollagen cannot acquire a stable helical configuration or be adequately crosslinked, so it is poorly secreted from the fibroblasts. Those molecules that are secreted lack tensile strength, are more soluble, and are more vulnerable to enzymatic degradation. Collagen, which normally has the highest content of hydroxyproline, is most affected, particularly in blood vessels, accounting for the predisposition to hemorrhages in scurvy. In addition, vitamin C deficiency suppresses the synthesis of collagen polypeptides, independent of effects on proline hydroxylation. Vitamin C also has *antioxidant properties.* These include an ability to scavenge free radicals directly and the participation in metabolic reactions that regenerate the antioxidant form of vitamin E.

Deficiency States. Consequences of vitamin C deficiency are illustrated in Fig. 7.23. Because of the abundance of ascorbic acid in foods, scurvy has ceased to be a global problem. It is sometimes

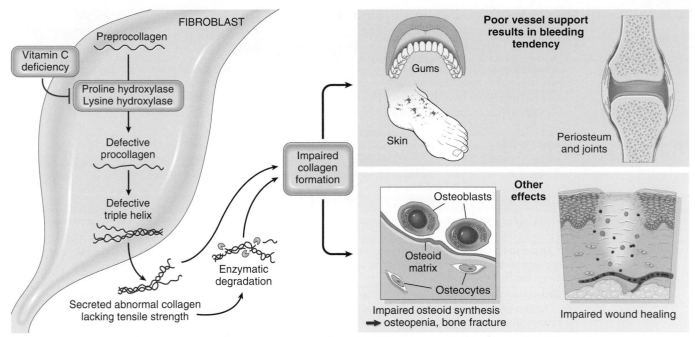

FIG. 7.23 Major consequences of impaired formation of collagen caused by vitamin C deficiency.

encountered in affluent populations as a secondary deficiency, particularly among elderly persons, people who live alone, and individuals who chronically overuse alcohol—groups often characterized by erratic and inadequate eating patterns. Occasionally, scurvy appears in patients undergoing peritoneal dialysis or hemodialysis and among food faddists.

Toxicity. The popular notion that megadoses of vitamin C protect against the common cold or at least allay the symptoms has not been borne out by controlled clinical studies. Such slight relief as may be experienced is probably a result of the mild antihistamine action of ascorbic acid. All excess vitamin C is promptly excreted in the urine but may cause uricosuria and increased absorption of iron, with the potential for iron overload.

Other vitamins and some essential minerals are listed and briefly described in Tables 7.9 and 7.10. Folic acid and vitamin B_{12} are discussed in Chapter 10.

Obesity

Obesity and excess body weight are associated with increased incidence of several of the most important human diseases, including type 2 diabetes, dyslipidemias, cardiovascular disease, hypertension, and cancer. The strength of this association is related not only to the extent of excess fat but also to its distribution: central, or visceral, obesity, in which excess fat accumulates preferentially in the trunk and in the abdominal cavity (in the mesentery and around viscera), is associated with a much higher risk for several diseases than is excess accumulation of subcutaneous fat.

Since weight covaries with height, a metric called the body mass index (BMI), which is calculated as (weight in kilograms)/(height in meters)^2 or kg/m^2, is used for initial health assessment. Healthy BMI ranges from 18.5 to 25 kg/m^2, with some variation by country and population. Individuals with BMI greater than 30 kg/m^2 are classified as obese; individuals with BMI between 25 kg/m^2 and 30 kg/m^2 are considered overweight. It is generally agreed that a BMI greater than 30 kg/m^2 imparts a health risk. However, since body weight includes all weight (e.g., muscle, bone, fat), it does not account for body composition: an athlete with a low body fat percentage may have a high BMI and an individual with minimal muscle mass may present with a "healthy" BMI. Other metrics, such as circumference measures, should ideally supplement the BMI to validate a diagnosis of obesity. Unless otherwise noted, the term obesity herein applies to both truly obese and overweight individuals.

Obesity is a major public health problem in higher income countries and an emerging health problem in lower-income nations. In the United States, obesity has reached epidemic proportions. The prevalence of obesity increased from 13% to 34% between 1960 and 2008, and as of 2018 42.4% of Americans between 20 and 75 years of age were obese as were 19.3% of children and adolescents. Globally, the World Health Organization (WHO) estimates that in 2016, 650 million adults were obese. The causes of this epidemic are complex but are undoubtedly related to societal changes in diet and levels of physical activity.

The etiology of obesity is complex and incompletely understood. Genetic, environmental, and psychologic factors are involved. However, simply put, obesity is a disorder of energy balance. The two sides of the energy equation, intake and expenditure, are finely regulated by neural and hormonal mechanisms so that body weight is maintained within a narrow range for many years. Apparently, this fine balance is controlled by an internal setpoint, or "lipostat," that senses the quantity of energy stores (adipose tissue) and appropriately regulates food intake as well as energy expenditure. Several "obesity genes" have been identified that encode molecular components of the physiologic system that regulates energy balance. A key player in energy homeostasis is the *LEP* gene and its product, *leptin*. This unique member of the cytokine family, secreted by adipocytes, regulates both sides of the energy equation—intake of food and expenditure of energy. As discussed later, the net effect of leptin is to reduce food intake and to enhance the expenditure of energy.

Table 7.9 Vitamins: Major Functions and Deficiency Syndromes

Vitamin	Functions	Deficiency Syndromes
Fat-Soluble		
Vitamin A	A component of visual pigment Maintenance of specialized epithelia Maintenance of resistance to infection	Night blindness, xerophthalmia, blindness Squamous metaplasia Vulnerability to infection, particularly measles
Vitamin D	Facilitates intestinal absorption of calcium and phosphorus and mineralization of bone	Rickets in children Osteomalacia in adults
Vitamin E	Major antioxidant; scavenges free radicals	Spinocerebellar degeneration; hemolytic anemia in premature infants
Vitamin K	Cofactor in hepatic carboxylation of procoagulants—factors II (prothrombin), VII, IX, and X; and protein C and protein S	Bleeding diathesis
Water-Soluble		
Vitamin B_1 (thiamine)	As pyrophosphate, is coenzyme in decarboxylation reactions	Dry and wet beriberi, Wernicke syndrome, Korsakoff syndrome
Vitamin B_2 (riboflavin)	Converted to coenzymes flavin mononucleotide and flavin adenine dinucleotide, cofactors for many enzymes in intermediary metabolism	Cheilosis, stomatitis, glossitis, dermatitis, corneal vascularization
Niacin	Incorporated into nicotinamide adenine dinucleotide (NAD) and NAD phosphate; involved in a variety of oxidation-reduction (redox) reactions	Pellagra—"three Ds": dementia, dermatitis, diarrhea
Vitamin B_6 (pyridoxine)	Derivatives serve as coenzymes in many intermediary reactions	Cheilosis, glossitis, dermatitis, peripheral neuropathy
Vitamin B_{12}[a]	Required for normal folate metabolism and DNA synthesis Maintenance of myelinization of spinal cord tracts	Combined system disease (megaloblastic anemia and degeneration of posterolateral spinal cord tracts)
Vitamin C	Serves in many redox reactions and hydroxylation of collagen	Scurvy
Folate[a]	Essential for transfer and use of one-carbon units in DNA synthesis	Megaloblastic anemia, neural tube defects
Pantothenic acid	Incorporated in coenzyme A	No nonexperimental syndrome recognized
Biotin	Cofactor in carboxylation reactions	No clearly defined clinical syndrome

[a]See also Chapter 10.

Table 7.10 Selected Trace Elements and Deficiency Syndromes

Element	Function	Basis of Deficiency	Clinical Features
Zinc	Component of enzymes, principally oxidases	Inadequate supplementation in artificial diets Interference with absorption by other dietary constituents Inborn error of metabolism	Anorexia and diarrhea Growth retardation in children Depressed mental function Depressed wound healing and immune response Impaired night vision Infertility Rash around eyes, mouth, nose, and anus called *acrodermatitis enteropathica*
Iron	Essential component of hemoglobin as well as several iron-containing metalloenzymes	Inadequate diet Chronic blood loss	Hypochromic, microcytic anemia
Iodine	Component of thyroid hormone	Inadequate supply in food and water	Goiter and hypothyroidism
Copper	Component of cytochrome c oxidase, dopamine β-hydroxylase, tyrosinase, and lysyl oxidase (involved in crosslinking collagen)	Inadequate supplementation in artificial diet Interference with absorption	Muscle weakness Neurologic defects Abnormal collagen crosslinking
Fluoride	Replaces calcium during remineralization of teeth, producing fluorapatite, which is more resistant to acids	Inadequate supply in soil and water Inadequate supplementation	Dental caries
Selenium	Component of GSH peroxidase Antioxidant with vitamin E	Inadequate amounts in soil and water	Myopathy Cardiomyopathy (Keshan disease)

In a simplified way, the neurohumoral mechanisms that regulate energy balance and body weight may be divided into three components—a peripheral or afferent system, a central processing system, and an efferent system (Fig. 7.24):

- The *peripheral* or *afferent system* generates signals from various sites. Its main components are leptin produced by fat cells, ghrelin from the stomach, peptide YY (PYY) and glucagon-like peptide 1 (GLP-1) from the ileum and colon, and insulin from the pancreas.

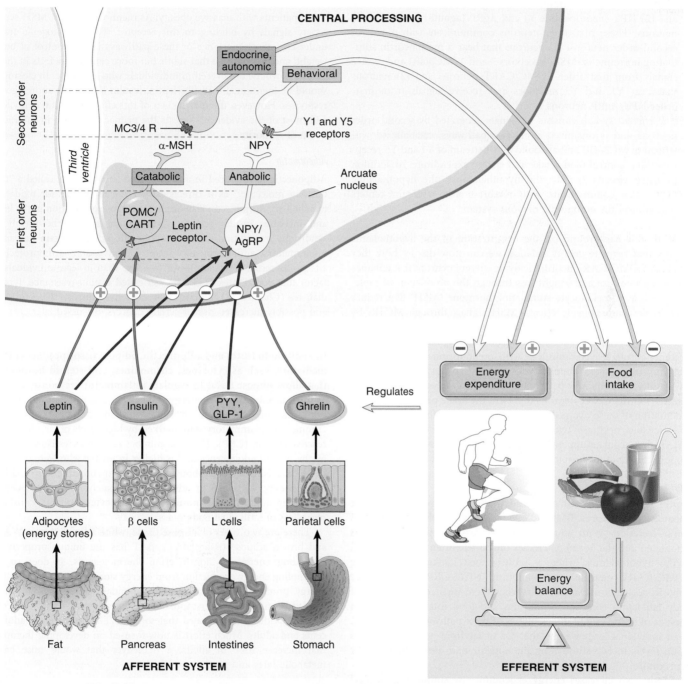

FIG. 7.24 Energy balance regulatory circuitry. When sufficient energy is stored in adipose tissue and the individual is well fed, afferent adiposity signals (insulin, leptin, ghrelin, peptide YY) are delivered to the central neuronal processing units, in the hypothalamus. Here the adiposity signals inhibit anabolic circuits and activate catabolic circuits. The effector arms of these central circuits then influence energy balance by inhibiting food intake and promoting energy expenditure. This in turn reduces the energy stores, and proadiposity signals are blunted. Conversely, when energy stores are low, the available anabolic circuits take over, at the expense of catabolic circuits, to generate energy stores in the form of adipose tissue. *AgRP,* Agouti-related peptide; *α-MSH,* α-melanocyte stimulating hormone; *CART,* cocaine- and amphetamine-regulated transcript; *GLP-1,* glucagon-like peptide-1; *MC3/4 R,* melanocortin receptors 3 and 4; *NPY,* neuropeptide Y; *POMC,* proopio-melanocortin; *PYY,* peptide YY.

The afferent systems provide signals to the central processing system in the brain.

- The *central processing system* resides in the arcuate nucleus of the hypothalamus, where neurohumoral peripheral signals are integrated to generate efferent signals that are transmitted by a pair of first-order neurons: (1) POMC (proopiomelanocortin) and CART (cocaine- and amphetamine-regulated transcript) neurons; and (2) NPY (neuropeptide Y) and AgRP (agouti-related peptide) neurons. These first-order neurons communicate with a pair of second-order neurons: (1) neurons that bear α melanocortin stimulating hormone (α-MSH) receptors 3 and 4 (MC3/4R) and receive signals from first-order POMC/CART neurons and (2) neurons that bear Y1 and Y5 receptors and receive signals from first-order NPY/AgRP neurons.

- The *efferent system* consists of signals generated by second-order neurons and is organized along two pathways, catabolic (downstream of MC3/4R) and anabolic (downstream of Y1 and Y5 receptors), that control food intake and energy expenditure. In addition to these circuits (within the hypothalamus), the hypothalamic nuclei also communicate with forebrain and midbrain centers that control the autonomic nervous system.

With this background on the organization of the hypothalamic centers that regulate energy balance, we can now discuss how they function. POMC/CART neurons activate efferent neurons that enhance energy expenditure and weight loss through the production of molecules such as α-melanocyte stimulating hormone (MSH) that reduce food intake (anorexigenic effect). MSH signals through MC4R. By contrast, NPY/AgRP neurons activate efferent neurons that promote food intake (orexigenic effect) and weight gain. Signals transmitted by efferent neurons also communicate with forebrain and midbrain centers that control the autonomic nervous system. To put it more simply, NPY/AgRP neurons may be thought of as the gas pedals for appetite, whereas POMC/CART neurons represent the brake pedal. The orderly functioning of these two pedals maintains energy homeostasis.

Discussed next are two important components of the afferent system that regulate appetite and satiety: leptin, gut hormones, and adiponectin, another hormone produced by fat cells.

Leptin

Leptin is secreted by fat cells, and its output is regulated by the adequacy of fat stores. BMI and body fat stores are directly related to leptin secretion. With abundant adipose tissue, leptin secretion is stimulated and the hormone crosses the blood–brain barrier to travel to the hypothalamus, where it reduces food intake by stimulating POMC/CART neurons and inhibiting NPY/AgRP neurons. The opposite sequence of events occurs when there are inadequate stores of body fat; leptin secretion diminishes and food intake increases. In persons of stable weight, the activities of these pathways are balanced. If an individual loses weight, the loss of fat from adipocytes causes leptin levels to fall, stimulating the appetite and diminishing energy expenditure.

Leptin also increases energy expenditure by stimulating physical activity, energy expenditure, and thermogenesis. Although the effects of leptin on food intake and energy expenditure can be readily demonstrated in nonobese mice and humans, the anorexigenic response of leptin is blunted in states of obesity despite high levels of circulating leptin. Leptin resistance in obese mice can be bypassed by intraventricular injection of leptin. However, injections of leptin in humans who are obese do not affect food intake and energy expenditure, dashing initial hopes surrounding leptin therapy for obesity.

In rodents and humans, loss-of-function mutations affecting components of the leptin pathway give rise to massive obesity. Mice with mutations that disable the leptin gene or its receptor fail to sense the adequacy of fat stores, so they behave as if they are undernourished, eating ravenously. As in mice, rare mutations of the leptin gene or receptor in humans cause massive obesity. More common are mutations in the *melanocortin receptor-4 gene (MC4R)*, found in 4% to 5% of patients with massive obesity. As mentioned earlier, MSH sends satiety signals by binding to this receptor. These monogenic traits underscore the importance of these pathways in the control of body weight, and it is possible that subtle but more common defects in these pathways will be discovered in individuals who are obese. In closing it should be mentioned that, like leptin, insulin also exerts anorexigenic responses. However, the mechanism of this effect of insulin is unclear and most of the evidence suggests the primacy of leptin in the regulation of adiposity.

Adiponectin

Adiponectin is produced in adipose tissue and has been called a "fat-burning molecule," as it directs fatty acids to muscle for oxidative metabolism. Adiponectin also decreases glucose production in the liver and increases insulin sensitivity, protecting against the metabolic syndrome. In addition to its metabolic effects, adiponectin has anti-inflammatory, antiatherogenic, antiproliferative, and cardioprotective effects. Its serum levels are lower in obese than in lean individuals, a factor that contributes to obesity-associated insulin resistance, type 2 diabetes (Chapter 18), nonalcoholic fatty liver disease (Chapter 14), and possibly increased risk of certain cancers, discussed later.

Other Mediators

In addition to leptin and adiponectin, adipose tissue produces other mediators, such as cytokines, chemokines, and steroid hormones, that allow adipose tissue to regulate inflammatory responses as well as lipid metabolism and energy intake. The increased production of cytokines and chemokines by adipose tissue in obesity creates a chronic proinflammatory state marked by high levels of circulating C-reactive protein (CRP). The total number of adipocytes is established by the time of adolescence and is higher in people who were obese as children, raising concern about the long-term consequences of childhood obesity. Although in adults approximately 10% of adipocytes turn over annually, the number of adipocytes remains constant, regardless of individual body mass.

There are two types of adipose tissue, white adipose tissue (WAT) and brown adipose tissue (BAT). BAT has the unique property of expending energy by nonshivering thermogenesis. It does so by uncoupling energy production from energy storage and converting the energy produced into heat. BAT is abundant in newborns and is located primarily in interscapular and supraclavicular areas. Recent imaging studies have revealed that some BAT is preserved in adolescents and adults. Much effort is now focused on developing therapies that increase BAT in adults, a maneuver that would raise basal metabolic rates and produce weight loss.

Gut Hormones

Gut hormones are rapidly acting initiators and terminators of volitional eating. Prototypical examples are ghrelin, peptide YY (PYY), and GLP-1 (glucagon-like peptide-1). *Ghrelin* is produced in the stomach and the arcuate nucleus of the hypothalamus. It increases food intake, most likely by stimulating the NPY/AgRP neurons in the hypothalamus. Ghrelin levels normally rise before meals and fall 1 to 2 hours afterward, but this drop is attenuated in obesity. Ghrelin levels are lower in individuals who are obese as compared to lean people, and they increase with a reduction in obesity.

PYY and GLP-1 are secreted from endocrine cells in the ileum and colon. Plasma levels of PYY and GLP-1 are low during fasting and increase shortly after food intake. Both PYY and GLP-1 act centrally by inhibiting NPY/AgRP neurons in the hypothalamus to decrease food intake. Agonists of GLP-1 receptor have recently been approved for treatment of selected patients with obesity and type 2 diabetes since, in addition to reducing food intake, GLP-1 receptor signaling enhances glucose-dependent insulin secretion.

The Role of the Gut Microbiome

An interesting series of observations in mice suggest that the gut microbiome may be involved in the development of obesity. The profiles of gut microbiota differ between genetically obese mice and their lean littermates, as the microbiome of the former can harvest much more energy from food than the latter. Colonization of the gut of germ-free mice by microbiota from obese mice (but not microbiota from lean mice) is associated with increased body weight. The relevance of the mouse models to human obesity remains to be proven. Differences between the gut microbiome of obese and lean humans have also been reported, but it is not clear if this is causal or merely correlative.

Clinical Consequences of Obesity

Obesity, particularly central obesity, is associated with an increase in all-cause mortality and is a known risk factor for type 2 diabetes, cardiovascular disease, and cancer. Central obesity is also linked to alterations collectively known as *metabolic syndrome*, characterized by abnormalities of glucose and lipid metabolism, hypertension, and systemic inflammation. Inflammation appears to stem from activation of the inflammasome by free fatty acids and excess levels of lipids in cells and tissue. This is turn stimulates secretion of IL-1, which induces systemic inflammation and insulin resistance. The following associations are worthy of note:

- *Obesity is associated with insulin resistance and hyperinsulinemia,* important features of type 2 diabetes (Chapter 18).
- *Insulin resistance and hyperinsulinemia may contribute to obesity-related hypertension* by increasing sympathetic activity and renal sodium absorption and by causing endothelial dysfunction.
- *Individuals who are obese generally have hypertriglyceridemia and low HDL cholesterol levels,* factors that increase the risk of coronary artery disease. The association between obesity and heart disease is not straightforward, however, and may be more directly related to the associated diabetes and hypertension than to weight *per se.*
- *Nonalcoholic fatty liver disease* is commonly associated with obesity and type 2 diabetes. It can progress to fibrosis and cirrhosis, and imparts an increased risk of liver cancer (Chapter 14).
- *Cholelithiasis (gallstones)* is six times more common in obese than in lean subjects. The elevated risk stems from an increase in total body cholesterol, increased cholesterol turnover, and augmented biliary excretion of cholesterol in the bile, which predisposes affected persons to the formation of cholesterol-rich gallstones (Chapter 14).
- *Obstructive sleep apnea* and consequent right-sided heart failure is strongly associated with obesity. Hypoventilation syndrome is a constellation of respiratory abnormalities in persons who are very obese.
- *Marked adiposity is a predisposing factor for the development of degenerative joint disease* (osteoarthritis) (Chapter 19). This form of arthritis, which typically appears in older persons, is attributed

in large part to the cumulative effects of wear and tear on joints. The greater the body burden, the greater the trauma to joints with the passage of time.

- *Markers of inflammation, such as CRP and proinflammatory cytokines like TNF, are often elevated in persons who are obese, in particular people with central obesity.* It is thought that chronic inflammation may contribute to many of the complications of obesity including insulin resistance, metabolic abnormalities, thrombosis, cardiovascular disease, and cancer.

Obesity and Cancer. **There is an increased incidence of certain cancers in the overweight, including cancers of the esophagus, thyroid, colon, and kidney in men and cancers of the esophagus, endometrium, gallbladder, and kidney in women.** Though the risk associated with obesity is modest, because of the prevalence of obesity in the population, it is associated with approximately 40% of all cancers in the United States, somewhat more in women than in men. The underlying mechanisms are unknown and are likely to be multiple:

- *Elevated insulin levels.* Insulin resistance leads to hyperinsulinemia, which induces multiple effects that may directly or indirectly contribute to cancer. For example, hyperinsulinemia causes a rise in levels of free insulin-like growth factor-1 (IGF-1). IGF-1 is a mitogen, and its receptor, IGFR-1, is highly expressed in many human cancers. IGFR-1 activates the RAS and PI3K/AKT pathways, which promote the growth of normal and neoplastic cells (Chapter 6).
- Obesity has effects on *steroid hormones,* which regulate cell growth and differentiation in the breast, uterus, and other tissues. Specifically, obesity increases the synthesis of estrogen from androgen precursors, increases androgen synthesis in ovaries and adrenals, and enhances estrogen availability in persons who are obese by inhibiting the production of sex-hormone—binding globulin (SHBG) in the liver.
- As discussed earlier, *adiponectin* secretion from adipose tissue is reduced in obese individuals. Adiponectin suppresses cell proliferation and promotes apoptosis. In individuals who are obese, these antineoplastic actions of adiponectin may be compromised.
- The *proinflammatory state* that is associated with obesity may itself be carcinogenic, through mechanisms discussed in Chapter 6.

Diet and Systemic Diseases

Currently, one of the most important and controversial issues is the contribution of diet to atherogenesis. The central question is whether dietary modification—specifically, reduction in the consumption of foods high in cholesterol and saturated animal fats (e.g., eggs, butter, beef)—can reduce serum cholesterol levels and prevent or retard the development of atherosclerosis (and coronary heart disease) in those without a history of cardiovascular disease. This is called "primary prevention." We know some but not all the answers. The average adult in the United States consumes a large amount of fat and cholesterol daily, with a ratio of saturated fatty acids to polyunsaturated fatty acids of about 3:1. Lowering the level of saturated fats to the level of polyunsaturated fats causes a 10% to 15% reduction in serum cholesterol within a few weeks. Vegetable oils (e.g., corn and safflower oils) and fish oils contain polyunsaturated fatty acids and are good sources of cholesterol-lowering lipids. Fish oil fatty acids belonging to the omega-3 family have more double bonds than do the omega-6 fatty acids found in vegetable oils. A corollary of this idea is that supplementation of diet with fish oils might protect against atherosclerosis. However, a recent large metaanalysis of 79 randomized controlled trials showed that dietary supplements of omega-3 fatty acids or consumption of oily fish had little or no effect on cardiovascular disease (ischemic heart disease, stroke).

Other specific effects of diet on disease have been recognized:

- Restricting sodium intake reduces hypertension.
- *High dietary fiber (roughage)* results in increased fecal bulk and is thought by some investigators to protect against diverticulosis of the colon and reduce the risk of colorectal cancers.
- Caloric restriction has been convincingly demonstrated to increase life span in experimental animals, including monkeys. However, the degree of calorie restriction required to produce this effect is substantial, leading some to question whether such a prolonged life is worth living. Furthermore, while caloric restriction may be successful in short-term weight loss, it can create a lifelong struggle with diet, body image, and weight management.

Diet and Cancer

With respect to carcinogenesis, three aspects of the diet are potentially contributory: (1) the content of exogenous carcinogens; (2) the endogenous synthesis of carcinogens from dietary components; and (3) the lack of protective factors.

- *Aflatoxin* is an example of an exogenous carcinogen. It is an important factor in the development of hepatocellular carcinoma in parts of Asia and Africa, generally in cooperation with hepatitis B virus. Exposure to aflatoxin causes a specific mutation in codon 249 of the *TP53* gene. This mutation can thus be used as a molecular signature of aflatoxin exposure in epidemiologic studies.
- *Endogenous synthesis* of carcinogens or tumor promoters from components of the diet relates most clearly to gastric carcinomas. Exposure to *nitrosamines* and *nitrosamides* are suspected of causing these tumors in humans, as they induce gastric cancer in animals. These compounds are formed in the body from nitrites and amines or amides derived from digested proteins. Sources of nitrites include sodium nitrite, added to foods as a preservative, and nitrates, present in common vegetables, which are reduced in the gut by bacterial flora. There is, then, the potential for endogenous production of carcinogenic agents from dietary components.
- *High animal fat intake combined with low fiber intake has been implicated in the causation of colon cancer.* The most plausible explanation for this association is that high fat intake increases the level of bile acids in the gut, which in turn modifies intestinal flora, favoring the growth of microaerophilic bacteria. Bile acid metabolites produced by these bacteria may function as carcinogens. The protective effect of a high-fiber diet might relate to (1) increased stool bulk and more rapid transit time, which decreases the exposure of mucosa to putative offenders and (2) the capacity of certain fibers to bind carcinogens and thereby protect the mucosa. However, attempts to document these theories in clinical and experimental studies have not generated consistent results.
- Vitamins C and E, β-carotenes, and selenium have been assumed to have anticarcinogenic effects because of their antioxidant properties. To date, however, no convincing evidence has emerged to show that these antioxidants prevent cancer. As already mentioned, retinoic acid promotes epithelial differentiation and may reverse squamous metaplasia. Associations between low levels of vitamin D and cancer of the colon, prostate, and breast have been reported, but studies have yet to show that vitamin D supplementation can decrease cancer risk.

■ RAPID REVIEW

Environmental Diseases and Environmental Pollution

- Environmental diseases are conditions caused by exposure to chemical or physical agents in the ambient, workplace, and personal environments.
- Health disparities are the differences in disease incidence, prevalence, morbidity, and mortality between populations.
- Biological race does not exist in modern humans; socially defined race and ethnicity have a significant impact on health and well-being.
- Exogenous chemicals, known as xenobiotics, enter the body through inhalation, ingestion, and skin contact and can either be eliminated or accumulate in fat, bone, brain, and other tissues.
- Xenobiotics can be converted into nontoxic products or toxic compounds through a two-phase reaction process that involves the cytochrome P-450 system.
- The most common air pollutants are ozone (which in combination with oxides and particulate matter forms smog), sulfur dioxide, acid aerosols, and particles less than 10 μm in diameter.
- CO is an air pollutant and an important cause of death from accidents and suicide; it binds hemoglobin with high affinity, leading to systemic hypoxia and CNS depression.

Toxic Effects of Heavy Metals

- Lead, mercury, arsenic, and cadmium are the heavy metals most commonly associated with toxic effects in humans.
- Children absorb more ingested lead than adults; the main source of exposure for children is lead-containing paint.
- Excess lead causes CNS defects in children and peripheral neuropathy in adults. Excess lead competes with calcium in bones and interferes with the remodeling of cartilage; it also causes anemia.
- The major source of mercury is contaminated fish. The developing brain is highly sensitive to methyl mercury, which accumulates in the brain and blocks ion channels.
- Exposure of the fetus to high levels of mercury in utero may lead to cerebral palsy, deafness, and blindness.
- Arsenic is naturally found in soil and water and is a component of some wood preservatives and herbicides. Excess arsenic interferes with mitochondrial oxidative phosphorylation and causes toxic effects in the GI tract, CNS, and cardiovascular system; long-term exposure causes polyneuropathy, skin lesions, and carcinomas.
- Cadmium from nickel-cadmium batteries and chemical fertilizers can contaminate soil. Excess cadmium causes obstructive lung disease and kidney damage.

Health Effects of Tobacco

- Smoking is the most preventable cause of human death.
- Tobacco smoke contains more than 2000 compounds, including nicotine, which is responsible for tobacco addiction, and strong carcinogens—mainly, polycyclic aromatic hydrocarbons, nitrosamines, and aromatic amines.
- Approximately 90% of lung cancers occur in smokers. Smoking is also associated with an increased risk of cancers of the oral cavity, larynx, esophagus, stomach, bladder, and kidney, as well as some forms of leukemia. Cessation of smoking reduces the risk of lung cancer.
- Smokeless tobacco use is an important cause of oral cancers.

- Tobacco interacts with alcohol in multiplying the risk of oral, laryngeal, and esophageal cancer and increases the risk of lung cancers from occupational exposures to asbestos, uranium, and other agents.
- Tobacco consumption is an important risk factor for development of atherosclerosis and myocardial infarction, peripheral vascular disease, and cerebrovascular disease. In the lungs, in addition to cancer, it predisposes to emphysema, chronic bronchitis, and chronic obstructive disease.
- Maternal smoking increases the risk of abortion, premature birth, and intrauterine growth retardation.

Alcohol—Metabolism and Health Effects

- Acute alcohol excess causes drowsiness at blood levels of approximately 200 mg/dL. Stupor and coma develop at higher levels.
- Alcohol is oxidized to acetaldehyde in the liver primarily by alcohol dehydrogenase, and to a lesser extent by the cytochrome P-450 system, and by catalase. Acetaldehyde is converted to acetate in mitochondria and is used in the respiratory chain.
- Alcohol oxidation by alcohol dehydrogenase depletes NAD, leading to accumulation of fat in the liver and to metabolic acidosis.
- The main effects of chronic excess alcohol use are fatty liver, alcohol-related hepatitis, and cirrhosis, which leads to portal hypertension and increases the risk for development of hepatocellular carcinoma.
- Chronic excess alcohol use can cause bleeding from gastritis and gastric ulcers and alcohol-related cardiomyopathy, and it increases the risk for development of acute and chronic pancreatitis.
- Chronic alcohol use is often associated with poor diet, leading to deficiencies of B vitamins such as folate and thiamine.
- Chronic excess alcohol use is a major risk factor for cancers of the oral cavity, larynx, and esophagus. The risk is greatly increased by concurrent smoking or the use of smokeless tobacco.

Injury by Therapeutic Drugs and Nontherapeutic Agents

- Both therapeutic drugs and nontherapeutic agents commonly cause injury.
- Antineoplastic agents, long-acting tetracyclines, and other antibiotics, menopausal hormone therapy (MHT) oral contraceptives (OCs), acetaminophen, and aspirin are the drugs most frequently involved in adverse drug reactions (ADRs).
- MHT increases the risk of endometrial and breast cancer and thromboembolism and does not appear to protect against ischemic heart disease. OCs have a protective effect against endometrial and ovarian cancers but increase the risk of thromboembolism and hepatic adenoma.
- Overdose of acetaminophen may cause centrilobular liver necrosis, leading to liver failure. Early treatment with agents that restore GSH levels may limit toxicity. Aspirin blocks the production of prostaglandins, which may produce gastric ulceration and bleeding.
- Substance use disorder and overdose are serious public health problems. Substances that are commonly misused include sedative-hypnotics (barbiturates, ethanol), psychomotor stimulants (cocaine, amphetamine, ecstasy), opioid narcotics (heroin, methadone, oxycodone), hallucinogens (LSD, mescaline), and cannabinoids (marijuana, hashish). They have diverse effects on various organs.

Radiation Injury

- Ionizing radiation may injure cells directly or indirectly by generating free radicals from water or molecular oxygen.
- Ionizing radiation damages DNA; therefore, rapidly dividing cells such as germ cells and those in the bone marrow and GI tract, are very sensitive to radiation injury.
- DNA damage that is not adequately repaired may result in mutations that predispose affected cells to neoplastic transformation.
- Ionizing radiation may cause vascular damage and sclerosis, resulting in ischemic necrosis of parenchymal cells and their replacement by fibrous tissue.

Nutritional Diseases

- Primary severe acute malnutrition (SAM) is a common cause of childhood deaths in lower-income countries. The two main primary SAM syndromes are marasmus and kwashiorkor. Secondary SAM occurs in the chronically ill and in patients with advanced cancer (as a result of cachexia).
- Kwashiorkor is characterized by hypoalbuminemia, generalized edema, fatty liver, skin changes, and defects in immunity. It is caused by diets low in protein but sufficient in calories.
- Marasmus is characterized by emaciation resulting from loss of muscle mass and fat with relative preservation of serum albumin. It is caused by diets severely lacking in calories—both protein and nonprotein.
- Anorexia nervosa is self-induced starvation; it is characterized by amenorrhea and multiple manifestations of low thyroid hormone levels. Bulimia nervosa is a condition in which food binges alternate with induced vomiting or excess exercise.
- Vitamins A and D are fat-soluble vitamins with a wide range of activities. Vitamin C and members of the vitamin B family are water soluble (Table 7.9 lists vitamin functions and deficiency syndromes).

Obesity

- Obesity is a disorder of energy regulation. It increases the risk for a number of important conditions such as insulin resistance, type 2 diabetes, hypertension, and hypertriglyceridemia, which are associated with the development of coronary artery disease.
- The regulation of energy balance has three main components: (1) afferent signals, provided mostly by insulin, leptin, ghrelin, and peptide YY; (2) the central hypothalamic system, which integrates afferent signals and triggers the efferent signals; and (3) efferent signals, which control energy balance.
- Leptin plays a key role in energy balance. Its output from adipose tissues is regulated by the abundance of fat stores. Leptin binding to its receptors in the hypothalamus reduces food intake by stimulating POMC/CART neurons and inhibiting NPY/AgRP neurons.
- In addition to diabetes and cardiovascular disease, obesity is also associated with increased risk for certain cancers, nonalcoholic fatty liver disease, and gallstones.

■ **Laboratory Tests**

Test	Reference Values	Pathophysiology/Clinical Relevance
25-Hydroxyvitamin D2 and D3, serum	20–50 ng/mL (optimal)	When UVB strikes the epidermis, 7-dehydrocholesterol is converted into previtamin D_3, which is next converted into vitamin D_3 (cholecalciferol). In the liver, vitamin D_3 is hydroxylated to form 25-hydroxyvitamin-D_3. In the kidney, it is finally converted into the biologically active form: 1,25-dihydroxyvitamin-D_3. Initial laboratory assessment for vitamin D status analyzes levels of 25-hydroxyvitamin-D_3, not the biologically active form; testing for 1,25-dihydroxyvitamin D may be indicated in the setting of renal disease. In children, vitamin D deficiency is associated with rickets and muscle pain/weakness and tetany (due to hypocalcemia). In adults with vitamin D deficiency, risk of osteoporosis and fracture is increased.
Acetaminophen, plasma	10–25 μg/mL[a]	Acetaminophen is processed in the liver to the reactive, toxic metabolite N-acetyl-p-benzoquinoneimine (NAPQI), which is then conjugated to glutathione and excreted in urine. When supratherapeutic doses are ingested, glutathione is depleted; high levels of NAPQI cause mitochondrial dysfunction and hepatocellular damage. N-acetylcysteine is used to treat acetaminophen overdose; it functions as a glutathione substitute, binding directly to NAPQI. In the United States, acetaminophen toxicity accounts for about 50% of cases of acute liver failure.
Arsenic, blood/hair	Blood: <13 ng/mL Hair: <1.0 μg/g	Arsenic is rapidly cleared from the circulation; therefore, blood levels are only useful for acute toxicity. In chronic exposure, arsenic accumulates in hair, which can be assessed. Acute arsenic toxicity presents as arrhythmias and nonspecific gastrointestinal symptoms (e.g., diarrhea, nausea). Chronic exposure results in hyperkeratosis, peripheral neuropathies, renal failure, anemia, liver dysfunction, or cardiac arrhythmias and is associated with an increased risk of cancers of the urinary bladder, liver, skin, and lung.
Cadmium, urine/blood	Urine: <3 μg/g creatinine Blood: <4.9 μg/L	Cadmium binds serum proteins and is concentrated primarily in the liver and the proximal tubule of the kidneys. Excess cadmium exposure can result in (1) obstructive lung disease secondary to alveolar epithelial cell necrosis; (2) renal tubular damage; and (3) skeletal abnormalities (e.g., osteoporosis, osteomalacia) due to calcium loss. The mechanism of cadmium toxicity is unknown but is thought to involve reactive oxygen species. Common sources of cadmium exposure include tobacco smoke, occupations (e.g., smelting, nickel-cadmium battery manufacture), and some foods.
Ethanol, blood	Legal limit of intoxication in most of the United States: >80 mg/dL (0.08%) Potentially lethal: ≥400 mg/dL (0.4%)	Ethanol is metabolized in the liver, primarily through an oxidative pathway in which alcohol dehydrogenase converts ethanol into acetaldehyde, which is further metabolized to acetic acid by aldehyde dehydrogenase. With increasing blood alcohol levels or chronic ethanol consumption, microsomal cytochrome P450 metabolism of ethanol becomes increasingly significant, particularly the CYP2E1 isoform. CYP2E1 levels increase with chronic alcohol consumption, which contributes to increased tolerance; relatively unimpaired behavior in the context of high blood alcohol levels suggests chronic alcohol intake.
Lead, blood (venous)	Children <3.5 μg/dL (see explanation) Adults: ≤70 μg/dL (occupational)	Most lead is absorbed via the gastrointestinal tract and is distributed throughout the body, predominantly in developing teeth and bone. Adults absorb about 15% of ingested lead while children absorb up to 50%, particularly if they have coexistent nutritional deficiencies. Lead forms covalent bonds with protein cysteine sulfhydryl groups, which contributes to renal toxicity. Lead decreases heme biosynthesis and acts as a mitochondrial toxin. No safe blood lead level has been established for children. At levels above 3.5 μg/dL, the CDC provides a series of recommendations; chelation therapy may be indicated in children with blood levels >45 μg/dL. Blood lead levels are monitored to ensure occupational exposures meet established federal standards.

Mercury, blood	Blood: <10 ng/mL	Mercury is primarily absorbed in the GI tract. It can bind to sulfhydryl groups on proteins. It is lipophilic, which enables it to cross the placenta and to concentrate in lipid-rich tissues such as the central nervous system. Because it is cleared by the kidney, renal damage may result. Mercury affects the motor, sensory, cognitive, and behavioral functions of the brain. Acute toxicity is associated with renal tubular necrosis and oliguria or anuria. Mercury exposure in utero can cause major CNS pathology, cerebral palsy, and blindness. Vomiting and abdominal pain may develop upon acute ingestion. Severe symptoms and high blood mercury levels may require chelation therapy.
Salicylate, serum	Therapeutic: <30 mg/dL	Aspirin has a short half-life (15 minutes) and is rapidly metabolized to salicylate. In aspirin overdose, stimulation of the medulla results in early hyperventilation, respiratory alkalosis, nausea and vomiting, followed by disruption of cellular metabolism (oxidative phosphorylation) and metabolic acidosis. Serum salicylate levels of 50 mg/dL or higher are toxic.

[a]Duke University Health Systems Clinical Laboratories reference values.

References values from https://www.mayocliniclabs.com/ by permission of Mayo Foundation for Medical Education and Research. All rights reserved.

Adapted from Deyrup AT, D'Ambrosio D, Muir J, et al. Essential Laboratory Tests for Medical Education. *Acad Pathol.* 2022;9. doi: 10.1016/j.acpath.2022.100046.

8

Blood Vessels

Vascular diseases are responsible for some of the most common and lethal conditions afflicting humans. Although most clinically significant disorders involve arterial lesions, venous pathologies can also wreak havoc. Two types of vascular lesions cause disease:

- *Narrowing* or *complete obstruction of* vessel lumina, occurring either progressively (e.g., by atherosclerosis) or acutely (e.g., by thrombosis or embolism)
- *Weakening* of vessel walls, causing dilation and/or rupture

We start with an overview of vascular structure and function, as background for the diseases of blood vessels discussed in the chapter.

STRUCTURE AND FUNCTION OF BLOOD VESSELS

Blood vessels are essentially tubular structures composed of smooth muscle cells (SMCs) and extracellular matrix (ECM), with an inner luminal surface covered by a lining of continuous endothelial cells (ECs). The relative amounts of SMCs and ECM and the properties of the ECs vary throughout the vasculature according to functional need (Fig. 8.1). To accommodate pulsatile flow and higher blood

The contributions to this chapter by Dr. Richard Mitchell, Department of Pathology, Brigham and Women's Hospital, Harvard Medical School, Boston, Massachusetts, in several previous editions of this book are gratefully acknowledged.

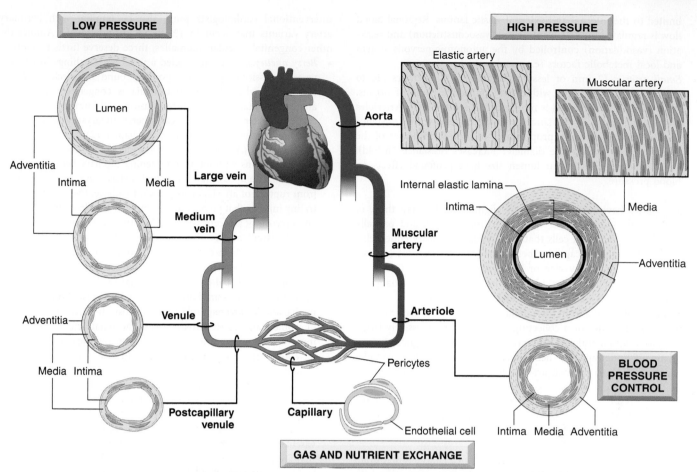

FIG. 8.1 Regional specializations of the vasculature. Although the basic organization of the vasculature is constant, the thickness and composition of the various layers differ according to hemodynamic forces and tissue requirements. Thus, the aorta and other elastic arteries have substantial elastic tissue to accommodate high pulsatile forces, with the capacity to recoil and transmit energy into forward blood flow. These vessels have lamellar units that comprise repetitions of a layer of elastic fibers, a smooth muscle cell, and intervening extracellular matrix. Purely muscular arteries have elastic fibers only at the intersection of the intima and media or media and adventitia. In comparison, the venous system has relatively poorly developed thinner medial layers that permit greater capacitance, and the capillary wall permits ready diffusion of oxygen and nutrients because it comprises only an endothelial cell and sparse encircling pericytes. The different structure and functional attributes also influence the disorders that can affect the various parts of the vascular tree. Thus, loss of aortic elastic tissue will result in aneurysm, while stasis in a dilated venous bed can result in thrombosis.

pressures, *arterial* walls are thicker than veins and invested with several reinforcing layers of SMCs. As arteries narrow to *arterioles*, the ratio of wall thickness to lumen diameter increases to allow more precise regulation of intravascular pressure. *Veins*, by contrast, are distensible thin-walled vessels with high capacitance. To facilitate maximal diffusion, *capillaries* are lined by a single layer of ECs apposed to a basement membrane. Notably, certain disorders characteristically involve only specific types of vessels. For example, atherosclerosis occurs mainly in larger, muscular arteries, while hypertension affects small arterioles, and specific forms of vasculitis preferentially involve vessels of a particular caliber.

Vessel walls are organized into three concentric layers: *intima, media,* and *adventitia* (see Fig. 8.1). The intima consists of an EC monolayer resting on a basement membrane with minimal underlying ECM; it is separated from the media by a dense elastic membrane called the *internal elastic lamina*. The media is composed predominantly of SMCs and ECM, surrounded by the loose connective tissue and nerve fibers of the adventitia. An *external elastic lamina* is present in some arteries and defines the transition between media and adventitia. Diffusion of oxygen and nutrients from the lumen is adequate to sustain thin-walled vessels and the innermost SMCs of all vessels. In large and medium-sized vessels, however, small arterioles within the adventitia (called *vasa vasorum*—literally, "vessels of the vessels") perfuse the outer half to two-thirds of the media.

Organization of Blood Vessels

Arteries are divided into three types based on their size and structure:
- *Large elastic arteries* (e.g., aorta, aortic arch vessels, iliac and pulmonary arteries). In these vessels, elastic fibers alternate with SMCs throughout the media, which expands during systole and recoils during diastole to propel blood forward.
- *Medium-sized muscular arteries* (e.g., coronary and renal arteries). Here, the media is composed primarily of SMCs, with elastin

limited to the internal and external elastic lamina. Regional blood flow is regulated by SMC contraction (vasoconstriction) and relaxation (vasodilation) controlled by the autonomic nervous system and local metabolic factors (e.g., acidosis).

- *Small arteries* (2 mm or less in diameter) *and arterioles* (20 to 100 μm in diameter) lie within the connective tissue of organs. The media in these vessels is mostly composed of SMCs. Arterioles are where blood flow resistance is regulated. Because the resistance to fluid flow is inversely proportional to the fourth power of the diameter (i.e., halving the diameter increases resistance 16-fold), small changes in arteriolar lumen size have profound effects on blood pressure.

Capillaries have luminal diameters slightly smaller than those of red cells (7 to 8 μm). These vessels are lined by ECs and partially surrounded by pericytes, cells that may regulate capillary endothelial function. Collectively, capillary beds have a very large total cross-sectional area and a low rate of blood flow. With their thin walls and slow flow, capillaries are ideally suited to the rapid exchange of diffusible substances between blood and tissue.

Veins receive blood from the capillary beds as postcapillary venules, which anastomose to form collecting venules and progressively larger veins. The vascular leakage (edema) and leukocyte emigration characteristic of inflammation occur mainly in postcapillary venules (Chapter 2). Compared with arteries at the same level of branching, veins have larger diameters, larger lumina, and thinner walls with less distinct layers, all adaptations to the low pressures found on the venous side of the circulation. Collectively, the venous system has a huge capacity and normally contains approximately two-thirds of the blood.

Lymphatics are thin-walled, endothelium-lined channels that drain lymph from the interstitium of tissues, eventually reconnecting with the bloodstream via the *thoracic duct*. Lymphatics transport fluid and cells from epithelia and parenchymal tissues to lymph nodes, thereby facilitating antigen presentation and lymphocyte activation in the lymph nodes, and enabling continuous monitoring of peripheral tissues for infection.

CONGENITAL ANOMALIES

Although rarely symptomatic, unusual anatomic variants of blood vessels can cause complications during surgery, such as injury of a vessel in an unexpected location. Cardiac surgeons and interventional cardiologists must also be familiar with coronary artery variants that occur in 1% to 5% of individuals. Among the other congenital vascular anomalies, three deserve further mention:

- *Berry aneurysms* are thin-walled arterial outpouchings in cerebral vessels, classically at branch points around the circle of Willis; they occur where the arterial media is congenitally attenuated and can spontaneously rupture, causing fatal intracerebral hemorrhage (Chapter 21). In some cases berry aneurysms are associated with adult polycystic renal disease (Chapter 12).
- *Arteriovenous (AV) fistulas* are abnormal connections between arteries and veins without an intervening capillary bed. They occur most commonly as developmental defects but can also result from rupture of arterial aneurysms into adjacent veins, from penetrating injuries that pierce arteries and veins, or from inflammation and necrosis of adjacent vessels. AV fistulas are created surgically to provide vascular access for hemodialysis. Large or multiple AV fistulas can cause high-output cardiac failure by shunting large volumes of blood from the arterial to venous circulation.
- *Fibromuscular dysplasia* is focal irregular thickening of the walls of medium- and large-sized muscular arteries due to a combination of medial and intimal hyperplasia and fibrosis. It is primarily a disease of women and preferentially affects the renal arteries, which are involved in 75% to 90% of cases. The median age at diagnosis is 52 years. The cause is unknown. The focal wall thickening results in luminal stenosis or can be associated with vessel spasm that reduces vascular flow; in the renal arteries, this decrease in flow may lead to renovascular hypertension due to activation of the renin-angiotensin-aldosterone axis. Between the focal segments of the thickened wall, the artery often exhibits medial attenuation; vascular outpouchings may develop in these portions of the vessel that are prone to rupture.

BLOOD PRESSURE REGULATION

Systemic and local blood pressure must be held within a narrow range to maintain health. Low blood pressure *(hypotension)* leads to inadequate organ perfusion, organ dysfunction, and sometimes tissue necrosis. Conversely, high blood pressure *(hypertension)* causes vessel and end-organ damage and is one of the major risk factors for atherosclerosis (see later).

Blood pressure is determined by cardiac output and peripheral vascular resistance, both of which are influenced by multiple genetic and environmental factors (Fig. 8.2).

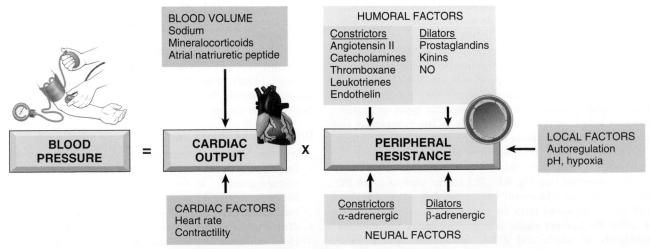

FIG. 8.2 Blood pressure regulation. *NO,* Nitric oxide.

- *Cardiac output is a function of stroke volume and heart rate.* The most important determinant of stroke volume is filling pressure, which is regulated through sodium homeostasis (described later) and its effect on blood volume. Heart rate and myocardial contractility (a second factor affecting stroke volume) are controlled by the α- and β-adrenergic systems (which also have significant effects on vascular tone).

- *Peripheral resistance is regulated predominantly at the level of the arterioles* by neural and humoral inputs. Vascular tone reflects a balance between the actions of vasoconstrictors (including angiotensin II, catecholamines, and endothelin) and vasodilators (including kinins, prostaglandins, and nitric oxide [NO]). Resistance vessels also exhibit autoregulation, whereby increased blood flow induces vasoconstriction to protect tissues against hyperperfusion. Finally, blood pressure is fine-tuned by tissue pH and hypoxia to accommodate local metabolic demands.

Factors released from the kidneys, adrenal glands, and myocardium interact to influence vascular tone and to regulate blood volume by adjusting sodium balance. The forces that regulate blood pressure are depicted in Fig. 8.3 and described next.

- *Sodium homeostasis.* Each day, the kidneys filter on average 170 liters of plasma containing 23 moles of salt. With a typical diet containing 100 mEq of sodium, 99.5% of the filtered salt must be reabsorbed to maintain total body sodium levels. About 98% of the filtered sodium is reabsorbed by several constitutively active transporters. Recovery of the remaining 2% of sodium occurs by way of the epithelial sodium channel (ENaC), which is tightly regulated by aldosterone, a downstream effector of the renin-angiotensin system; it is this pathway that determines net sodium balance.

- The kidneys and heart contain cells that sense changes in blood pressure and/or blood volume. In response, these cells release several important regulators that act in concert to maintain normal blood pressure. The kidneys influence peripheral resistance and sodium excretion/retention primarily through the renin-angiotensin system.
  - *Renin* is a proteolytic enzyme produced by renal juxtaglomerular cells—myoepithelial cells that surround the glomerular afferent arterioles. It is released in response to low blood pressure in afferent arterioles or low sodium levels in the distal convoluted renal tubules. The latter occurs when the glomerular

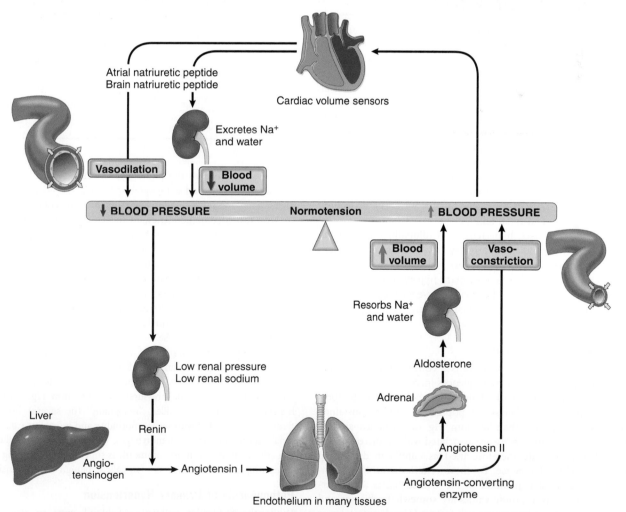

FIG. 8.3 Interplay of renin, angiotensin, aldosterone, and atrial natriuretic peptide in blood pressure regulation. Low blood pressure caused either by vasodilation and/or a reduction in blood volume triggers the release of renin from the kidney, which raises the blood pressure through angiotensin-aldosterone systems. In the reverse situation, high blood pressure triggers the secretion of "cardiac volume sensors"—atrial natriuretic peptide (ANP) and brain natriuretic peptide (BNP), which in turn normalize the blood pressure.

filtration rate falls (e.g., when cardiac output is low), leading to increased sodium resorption by the proximal tubules.

- *Angiotensin.* Renin cleaves plasma angiotensinogen to angiotensin I, which in turn is converted to *angiotensin II* by angiotensin-converting enzyme (ACE), which is mainly expressed by vascular endothelium. Angiotensin II raises blood pressure by (1) inducing vascular SMC contraction; (2) stimulating aldosterone secretion by the adrenal gland; and (3) increasing tubular sodium resorption.
- *Aldosterone.* Adrenal aldosterone increases blood pressure by its effect on blood volume; it increases sodium resorption (and thus water resorption) in the distal convoluted and collecting tubules while also increasing potassium excretion into the urine.
- *Vasodilators.* The kidney produces a variety of vascular relaxing substances (including prostaglandins and NO) that counterbalance the vasopressor effects of angiotensin.
- *Natriuretic peptides.* Myocardial natriuretic peptides are released from atrial and ventricular myocardium in response to volume expansion; these inhibit sodium resorption in the distal renal tubules, thus leading to sodium excretion and diuresis. They also induce systemic vasodilation.

HYPERTENSIVE VASCULAR DISEASE

Hypertension is a major health problem in higher-income countries. Although it occasionally manifests in an acute aggressive form, high blood pressure is typically asymptomatic for many years. This insidious condition is referred to as benign or essential hypertension, so called because the gradual age-associated rise in blood pressure was considered "essential" for normal perfusion of end organs such as the brain. However, such increases are neither essential nor benign; it is best called primary hypertension because it is typically without any identifiable cause (idiopathic). The terms idiopathic, essential, and benign all continue to be used for this form of hypertension. Primary hypertension increases the risk for stroke and atherosclerotic coronary heart disease, and can also lead to cardiac hypertrophy and heart failure (hypertensive heart disease; see Chapter 9), aortic dissection, multiinfarct dementia, and renal failure.

In close to 95% of cases, hypertension is idiopathic. Most of the remaining cases are secondary to primary renal disease, renal artery narrowing (renovascular hypertension), adrenal disorders, or obstructive sleep apnea (Table 8.1). Primary hypertension is compatible with long life unless a complication supervenes (e.g., myocardial infarction, stroke). Prognosis of secondary hypertension depends on adequate treatment of the underlying cause.

Epidemiology of Hypertension

Like height and weight, blood pressure is a continuously distributed variable; moreover, detrimental consequences increase progressively as the pressure rises, with no rigidly defined threshold dependably predicting total safety. Nevertheless, in population studies, sustained diastolic pressures greater than 80 mm Hg or sustained systolic pressures in excess of 120 mm Hg are associated with an increased risk for atherosclerosis and are therefore used as cutoffs in diagnosing hypertension in clinical practice. By these criteria, over 40% of individuals in the general population in the United States are hypertensive. As noted, however, these values are somewhat arbitrary, and in patients with other cardiovascular risk factors (e.g., diabetes), lower thresholds may be applicable.

Table 8.1 Types and Causes of Hypertension

Primary Hypertension
Accounts for 90% to 95% of all cases
Secondary Hypertension
Renal
Acute glomerulonephritis
Chronic renal disease
Polycystic kidney disease
Renal artery stenosis
Renal vasculitis
Renin-producing tumors
Endocrine
Adrenocortical hyperfunction (Cushing syndrome, primary aldosteronism, congenital adrenal hyperplasia)
Exogenous hormones (glucocorticoids, estrogen [including pregnancy-induced and oral contraceptives], sympathomimetics, and monoamine oxidase inhibitors)
Pheochromocytoma
Acromegaly
Hypothyroidism (myxedema)
Hyperthyroidism (thyrotoxicosis)
Pregnancy-induced (preeclampsia)
Cardiovascular
Coarctation of the aorta
Polyarteritis nodosa
Increased intravascular volume
Increased cardiac output
Neurologic
Psychogenic
Increased intracranial pressure
Obstructive sleep apnea
Acute stress, including surgery

The prevalence of the pathologic effects of high blood pressure increases with age and is higher in particular populations. Generally, high-income countries suffer less from hypertension-related diseases than do low-income countries. In the United States, African Americans have the highest rate of hypertension when compared to European Americans, Asian Americans, and Latin Americans, due to a combination of environmental and genetic factors. Without appropriate treatment, about half of patients with hypertension die of ischemic heart disease (IHD) or congestive heart failure, and another third succumb to stroke. Reduction of blood pressure reduces the incidence and clinical sequelae (including death) of all forms of hypertension-related disease.

A small percentage of patients with hypertension (approximately 5%) present with a rapidly rising blood pressure that, if untreated, leads to death within 1 to 2 years. Such patients have systolic pressures over 180 mm Hg or diastolic pressures over 120 mm Hg. This form of hypertension has been called "malignant" (or severe) because it is frequently associated with severe morbidity and mortality, e.g., caused by renal failure and retinal hemorrhages, with or without papilledema. It can arise de novo but most commonly is superimposed on long-standing preexisting primary, less severe (so-called "benign") hypertension.

Pathogenesis of Primary Hypertension

While the molecular pathways of blood pressure regulation are reasonably well understood, the mechanisms leading to hypertension in the vast majority of affected individuals remain unknown. The accepted wisdom is that primary hypertension results from the interplay of genetic polymorphisms and environmental factors, which synergize to increase blood volume and/or peripheral resistance.

Although the specific triggers are unknown, it appears that both altered renal sodium handling and increased vascular resistance contribute to primary hypertension.

- *Reduced renal sodium excretion* in the presence of normal arterial pressure is probably a key pathogenic feature; indeed, this is a common etiologic factor in most forms of hypertension. Decreased sodium excretion causes an obligatory increase in fluid volume and increased cardiac output, thereby elevating blood pressure (see Fig. 8.3). At the new higher blood pressure, the kidneys excrete additional sodium. Thus, a new steady state of sodium excretion is achieved, but at the expense of an elevated blood pressure.
- *Increased vascular resistance may stem from vasoconstriction or structural changes in vessel walls.* These are not necessarily independent factors, as chronic vasoconstriction may result in permanent thickening of the walls of affected vessels.
- *Genetic factors* play an important role in determining blood pressure, as shown by familial clustering of hypertension and by studies of monozygotic and dizygotic twins. Susceptibility genes for primary hypertension in the vast majority of cases are unknown but probably include those that influence renal sodium resorption, the production of endogenous pressors, and SMC growth. In a small proportion of cases there is linkage to specific angiotensinogen polymorphisms and angiotensin II receptor variants; polymorphisms affecting the renin-angiotensin system may also contribute to the differences in blood pressure regulation seen in different populations.
- *Environmental factors,* such as stress, obesity, smoking, physical inactivity, high levels of salt consumption, and lack of access to health care, modify the impact of genetic determinants. Evidence linking dietary sodium intake with hypertension is particularly strong.

MORPHOLOGY

Hypertension accelerates atherogenesis and causes degenerative changes in the walls of large and medium-sized arteries that can lead to aortic dissection and cerebrovascular hemorrhage. Two related forms of small blood vessel disease are recognized (Fig. 8.4):

- **Hyaline arteriolosclerosis** is associated with primary hypertension. It is marked by thickening of arteriolar walls, with deposition of homogeneous, pink hyaline material and loss of underlying structural detail, and luminal narrowing (Fig. 8.4A). The lesions stem from leakage of plasma components across injured ECs into vessel walls and increased ECM production by SMCs in response to chronic hemodynamic stress. In the kidneys, the arteriolar narrowing caused by hyaline arteriosclerosis leads to diffuse vascular compromise and **nephrosclerosis** (glomerular scarring) (Chapter 12). Although the vessels of even normotensive older adult individuals may show the same changes, hyaline arteriolosclerosis is more generalized and severe in patients with hypertension. The same lesions are also seen in diabetic microangiopathy; in this disorder, the underlying etiology is hyperglycemia-associated EC dysfunction.
- **Hyperplastic arteriolosclerosis** is more typical of severe hypertension. Vessels exhibit "onion skin," concentric, laminated thickening of arteriolar walls and luminal narrowing (see Fig. 8.4B). The laminations consist of SMCs and thickened, reduplicated basement membrane. In severe ("malignant") hypertension, these changes are accompanied by **fibrinoid necrosis** which are particularly prominent in the kidney.

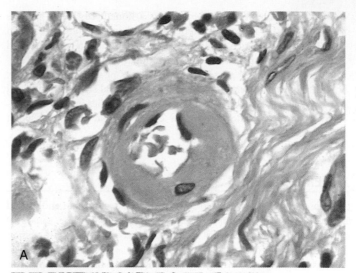

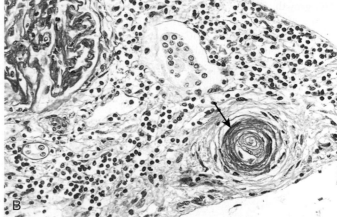

FIG. 8.4 Hypertensive vascular disease. (A) Hyaline arteriolosclerosis. The arteriolar wall is thickened with the deposition of amorphous proteinaceous material (hyalinized), and the lumen is markedly narrowed. (B) Hyperplastic arteriolosclerosis ("onion-skinning") *(arrow)* causing luminal obliteration (periodic acid–Schiff stain). (B, Courtesy of Helmut Rennke, MD, Brigham and Women's Hospital, Boston, Massachusetts.)

ARTERIOSCLEROSIS

Arteriosclerosis literally means "hardening of the arteries"; it is a generic term reflecting arterial wall thickening and loss of elasticity. Four types are recognized, each with different causes and consequences:

- *Arteriolosclerosis* affects small arteries and arterioles and may cause downstream ischemic injury. The two variants, hyaline and hyperplastic arteriolosclerosis, were discussed earlier in relation to hypertension.
- *Atherosclerosis,* from Greek root words for "gruel" and "hardening," is the most common and clinically important vascular disease and is discussed in the next section.
- *Mönckeberg medial sclerosis* is characterized by the presence of calcific deposits in muscular arteries, usually centered on the internal elastic lamina, typically in individuals older than 50 years of age. The lesions do not encroach on the vessel lumen and usually are not clinically significant (eFig. 8.1). In breast tissue, they may be identified on mammography.

- *Fibromuscular intimal hyperplasia* is a nonatherosclerotic process that occurs in muscular arteries larger than arterioles. This is an SMC- and ECM-rich lesion caused by inflammation (as in a healed arteritis or transplant-associated arteriopathy; Chapter 9) or by mechanical injury (e.g., associated with stents or balloon angioplasty. The resulting hyperplasia can cause substantial stenosis of affected vessels; indeed, such intimal hyperplasia underlies in-stent restenosis and is the major long-term cause of solid organ transplant failure.

ATHEROSCLEROSIS

Atherosclerosis is best viewed as the vascular response to endothelial injury. Since the response of the vessel wall to diverse causes of endothelial injury is quite stereotypic, we begin our discussion describing this process.

Vascular injury leading to EC loss or dysfunction stimulates SMC growth, ECM synthesis, and thickening of the vascular wall. Healing of injured vessels involves the migration of SMCs from the media or from circulating SMC precursor cells into the intima. These cells then proliferate and synthesize ECM in much the same way that fibroblasts fill wounds elsewhere in the body (Fig. 8.5A), forming a neointima that is typically covered by an intact EC layer. The migratory, proliferative, and synthetic activities of the intimal SMCs are regulated by growth factors and cytokines produced by platelets, ECs, and macrophages, as well as by activated coagulation and complement proteins. This neointimal response occurs with any form of vascular damage or dysfunction, including infection, inflammation, immune injury, physical trauma (e.g., from a balloon catheter or hypertension), or toxic exposure (e.g. oxidized lipids or cigarette smoke). With persistent or recurrent insults, further thickening can occur that leads to the stenosis of small- and medium-sized blood vessels.

Atherosclerosis is characterized by intimal lesions called *atheromas* (or *atherosclerotic plaques*) that impinge on the vascular lumen. It underlies the pathogenesis of coronary, cerebral, and peripheral vascular disease, and causes more morbidity and mortality (roughly half of all deaths) in the Western world than any other disorder. Atheromatous plaques are raised lesions composed of soft friable (grumous) lipid cores (mainly cholesterol and cholesterol esters, with necrotic debris) covered by fibrous caps (Fig. 8.5B). As they enlarge, atherosclerotic plaques may mechanically obstruct vascular lumina, leading to stenosis. Of greater concern, however, is that atherosclerotic plaques are prone to rupture, an event that may result in thrombosis and sudden occlusion of the vessel. The thickness of the intimal lesions also may be sufficient to impede the perfusion of the underlying media, which may then be compromised by ischemia and by changes in the ECM caused by subsequent inflammation. Together, these two factors weaken the media, setting the stage for the formation of aneurysms.

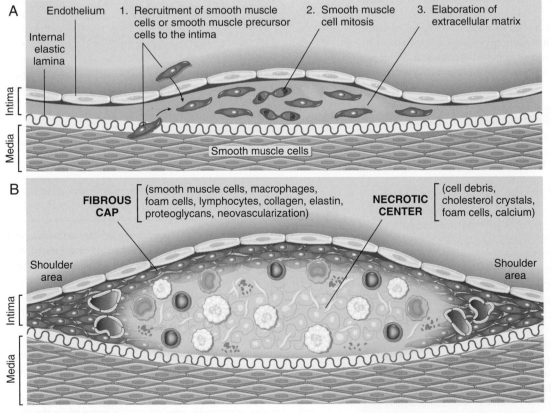

FIG. 8.5 (A) Vascular response to endothelial injury. Healing of injured vessels involves the migration of SMCs from the media or from circulating SMC precursor cells into the intima. These cells then proliferate and synthesize ECM in much the same way that fibroblasts fill in a wound elsewhere in the body, forming a neointima that typically is covered by an intact EC layer. Intimal smooth muscle cells are depicted in a color different from that of the medial smooth muscle cells, to emphasize their distinct phenotype. (B) Atheromatous plaque. With persistence of vascular injury in the presence of risk factors such as hypercholesterolemia, atheromatous plaques develop at the site of injury. Atheromatous plaques are raised lesions composed of soft friable (grumous) lipid cores (mainly cholesterol and cholesterol esters, with necrotic debris) covered by fibrous caps. Shoulder areas may be more cellular due to the presence of smooth muscle cells, macrophages, and T cells.

Epidemiology

Atherosclerosis is virtually ubiquitous among higher-income nations, with prevalence increasing at an alarming pace in lower-income countries. This is thought to be associated with increasing urbanization and the globalization of Western diets. As a result, the death rate for coronary artery disease in Africa, India, and Southeast Asia now exceeds that in the United States; eastern European countries have rates 3 to 5 times higher than the United States and 7 to 12 times higher than Japan. Because coronary artery disease is an important manifestation of atherosclerosis, epidemiologic data related to atherosclerosis-related mortality typically reflect deaths caused by ischemic heart disease (IHD) (Chapter 9); indeed, myocardial infarction is responsible for roughly one-quarter of all deaths in the United States.

The prevalence and severity of atherosclerosis and IHD have been correlated with a number of risk factors in several prospective analyses including the landmark Framingham Heart Study; some of these risk factors are constitutional (and therefore less controllable), but others are acquired or related to modifiable behaviors (Table 8.2). These risk factors are roughly multiplicative in effect. Thus, two factors increase the risk for myocardial infarction approximately 4-fold, and three (i.e., hyperlipidemia, hypertension, and smoking) increase the rate by a factor of 7 (Fig. 8.6).

Constitutional Risk Factors

- *Genetics. Family history is the most important independent risk factor for atherosclerosis.* Certain mendelian disorders are strongly associated with atherosclerosis (e.g., familial hypercholesterolemia) (Chapter 4), but these account for only a small percentage of cases. Most familial risk is related to multifactorial traits that go hand in hand with atherosclerosis, including hypertension and diabetes.
- *Age.* Atherosclerosis usually is clinically silent until lesions reach a critical threshold in middle age or later. Thus, the incidence of myocardial infarction increases 5-fold between 40 and 60 years of age. Death rates from IHD continue to rise with each successive decade. It is now evident that with aging, there is a tendency for the outgrowth of hematopoietic clones (so-called *clonal hematopoiesis of indeterminate potential [CHIP]*) carrying mutations that alter the functions of monocytes and macrophages, and that this too may play an important role in atherogenesis (discussed later).
- *Gender.* All other factors being equal, premenopausal women are relatively protected against atherosclerosis compared with age-matched men. Thus, myocardial infarction and other complications

Table 8.2 Major Risk Factors for Atherosclerosis

Nonmodifiable (Constitutional)
Inherited causes (e.g., familial hypercholesterolemia)
Family history
Increasing age
Male sex

Modifiable
Hyperlipidemia
Hypertension
Cigarette smoking
Diabetes
Inflammation

of atherosclerosis are uncommon in premenopausal women in the absence of other predisposing factors such as diabetes, hyperlipidemia, or severe hypertension. After menopause, however, the incidence of atherosclerosis-related disease increases and can even exceed that in men. Although a salutary effect of estrogen has long been proposed to explain this gender difference, clinical trials have shown that hormone replacement therapy does not prevent vascular disease. Indeed, estrogen replacement after 65 years of age appears to result in a small increase of cardiovascular risk. In addition to atherosclerosis, gender also influences other factors that can affect outcome in patients with IHD, such as hemostasis, infarct healing, and myocardial remodeling.

Modifiable Major Risk Factors

- **Hyperlipidemia—and, in particular, hypercholesterolemia—is a major risk factor for development of atherosclerosis and is sufficient to induce lesions in the absence of other risk factors.** The main cholesterol component associated with increased risk is low-density lipoprotein (LDL) cholesterol ("bad cholesterol"), which distributes cholesterol to peripheral tissues. By contrast, high-density lipoprotein (HDL) cholesterol ("good cholesterol") mobilizes cholesterol from developing and existing vascular plaques and transports it to the liver for biliary excretion. Consequently, higher levels of HDL correlate with reduced risk. Recognition of these relationships has spurred the development of dietary and pharmacologic interventions that lower total serum cholesterol or LDL and/or raise serum HDL, as follows:
  - *High dietary intake of cholesterol* and saturated fats (e.g., present in egg yolks, animal fats, and butter) raises plasma cholesterol levels. Conversely, diets low in cholesterol and/or containing higher ratios of polyunsaturated fats lower plasma cholesterol levels.
  - The *type of lipid consumed* has a significant impact. Omega-3 fatty acids (abundant in fish oils) are beneficial, whereas (trans)-unsaturated fats produced by artificial hydrogenation of polyunsaturated oils (used in baked goods and margarine) adversely affect cholesterol profiles.
  - *Exercise* and moderate consumption of ethanol raise HDL levels, whereas obesity and smoking lower them.
  - *Statins* are a widely used class of drugs that lower circulating cholesterol levels by inhibiting hydroxymethylglutaryl coenzyme A (HMG-CoA) reductase, the rate-limiting enzyme in hepatic cholesterol biosynthesis (Chapter 4).
- *Hypertension* (see earlier discussion) is another major risk factor for development of atherosclerosis. On its own, hypertension can increase the risk for IHD by approximately 60% (see Fig. 8.6). Hypertension is also the major cause of left ventricular hypertrophy (LVH) by increasing oxygen demand, thereby contributing to myocardial ischemia (see Fig. 8.6).
- *Cigarette smoking* is a well-established risk factor and changes in smoking habits probably account for the increasing incidence and severity of atherosclerosis in women. Prolonged smoking (for years) doubles the rate of IHD-related mortality, while smoking cessation reduces the risk.
- *Diabetes* is associated with increased levels of serum cholesterol and markedly increases the risk for atherosclerosis. Other factors being equal, the incidence of myocardial infarction is twice as high in people with diabetes as in those without. In addition,

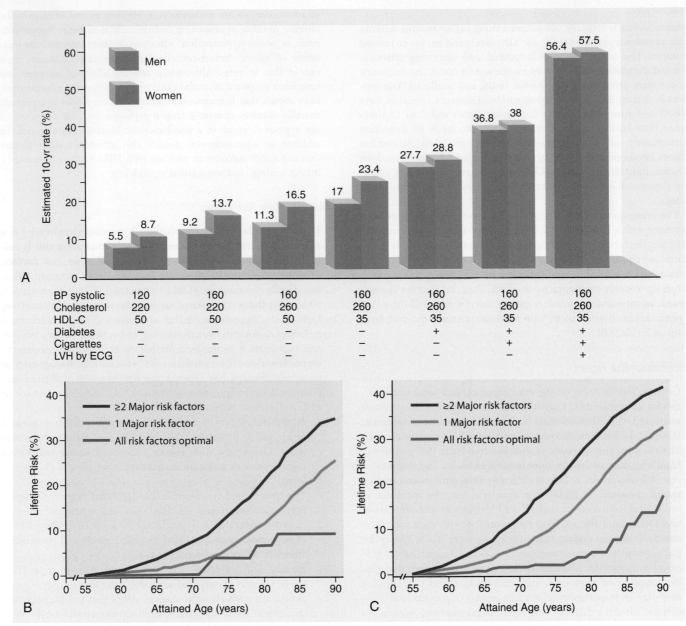

FIG. 8.6 Lifetime risk of death from cardiovascular disease. (A) Estimated 10-year risk of coronary artery disease in hypothetical 55-year-old men and women as a function of well-established risk factors (hyperlipidemia, hypertension, smoking, and diabetes). *BP*, Blood pressure; *ECG*, electrocardiogram; *HDL-C*, high-density lipoprotein cholesterol; *LVH*, left ventricular hypertrophy. In women (B) and men (C), one or more risk factors (blood pressure, cholesterol, diabetes, and cigarette smoking) significantly increase the lifetime risk of a cardiovascular event. (A, From O'Donnell CJ, Kannel WB: Cardiovascular risks of hypertension: lessons from observational studies. *J Hypertens Suppl* 16[6]:S3–S7, 1998, with permission from Lippincott Williams & Wilkins; B and C, Modified from Berry JD, Dyer A, Cai X, et al: Lifetime risks of cardiovascular disease. *N Eng J Med* 366:321–329, 2012.)

this disorder is associated with an increased risk for stroke and a 100-fold increase in atherosclerosis-induced gangrene of the lower extremities.

Additional Risk Factors

Other factors that contribute to risk include the following:
- *Inflammation.* Inflammatory cells are present during all stages of atheromatous plaque formation and are intimately linked with

plaque progression and rupture (see the following discussion). There is some evidence that a systemic proinflammatory state is associated with the development of atherosclerosis. Of various systemic markers of inflammation, determination of C-reactive protein (CRP) has emerged as one of the simplest and most sensitive. CRP is an acute-phase reactant synthesized primarily by the liver in response to a variety of inflammatory cytokines (Chapter 2). In some studies, CRP levels independently predict the risk for myocardial infarction, stroke, peripheral arterial disease, and sudden cardiac death, even among apparently healthy individuals (Fig. 8.7). Accordingly, CRP levels are now incorporated into risk stratification algorithms. However, whether CRP is a marker of the inflammatory state that accompanies atherosclerosis or a causative factor remains unknown. Quite tantalizingly, inhibition of interleukin-1 beta lowered the inflammatory biomarkers CRP and IL-6 and decreased the risk of nonfatal myocardial infarction in individuals with a previous myocardial infarct.

- *Homocystinuria,* due to rare inborn errors of metabolism, causes elevated circulating homocysteine (greater than 100 μmol/L) and is associated with early-onset vascular disease. Although low folate and vitamin B_{12} levels can increase homocysteine levels, supplemental vitamin ingestion does not affect the incidence of cardiovascular disease.

- *Metabolic syndrome.* This clinical entity is associated with central obesity and is characterized by insulin resistance, hypertension, dyslipidemia (elevated triglycerides and depressed HDL), hypercoagulability, and a proinflammatory state, which may be triggered by cytokines released from adipocytes. The dyslipidemia, hyperglycemia, and hypertension are all cardiac risk factors, while the systemic hypercoagulable and proinflammatory state may contribute to endothelial dysfunction and/or thrombosis.

- *Lipoprotein(a) levels.* Lipoprotein(a) is an LDL-like particle that contains apolipoprotein B-100 linked to apolipoprotein(a). It shares many proatherogenic properties of LDL, and lipoprotein(a) levels are correlated with risk of coronary and cerebrovascular disease, independent of total cholesterol or LDL levels. Lipoprotein(a) promotes endothelial cell dysfunction; impairs plasminogen activation, plasmin generation, and fibrinolysis; and promotes thrombogenesis, which in turn promotes atherogenesis.

- *Clonal hematopoiesis.* It is now recognized that a high fraction of older individuals have clonal hematopoiesis (Chapter 10), defined by the presence of a major clone of cells in the bone marrow that have acquired somatic driver mutations in one or more well-characterized oncogenes or tumor suppressor genes. Despite the presence of these mutations, such patients typically have normal blood counts. Unexpectedly, epidemiologic studies have found that clonal hematopoiesis is strongly associated with an increased risk of death from cardiovascular disease, possibly because of alterations in the function of innate immune cells derived from clones of hematopoietic stem cells.

- *Other factors* associated with difficult-to-quantify risks include lack of exercise and living a competitive, stressful lifestyle ("type A personality").

It should be kept in mind that roughly 20% of cardiovascular events occur in the absence of identifiable risk factors.

Pathogenesis

The currently held view of pathogenesis is that atherosclerosis is a chronic inflammatory response of the arterial wall to endothelial injury (the *response to injury hypothesis*). Lesion progression involves interaction of modified lipoproteins, monocyte-derived macrophages, T lymphocytes, and the cellular constituents of the arterial wall (Fig. 8.8). According to this model, atherosclerosis results from the following pathogenic events:

- *EC injury*—and resultant endothelial dysfunction—leading to increased permeability, leukocyte adhesion, and thrombosis
- *Accumulation of lipoproteins* (mainly oxidized LDL and cholesterol crystals) in the vessel wall
- *Accumulation and activation of macrophages* in the intima
- *Platelet adhesion*
- *Factor release from activated platelets, macrophages, and vascular wall cells* inducing *SMC* recruitment, either from resident SMCs in the media or from circulating precursors
- *Lipid accumulation both extracellularly and within macrophages and SMC*
- *SMC proliferation, ECM production, and recruitment of T cells*

Each of the steps is described next.

Endothelial Injury. **EC injury is the cornerstone of the response to injury hypothesis.** Early human atherosclerotic lesions begin at sites of intact, but dysfunctional, endothelium. Dysfunction implies defective ability of endothelium to perform or maintain blood vessel (vascular) tone, regulate hemostasis, act as barrier to potentially toxic materials, and control inflammation. Suspected triggers of endothelial dysfunction and early atheromatous lesions include hypertension, hyperlipidemia, and toxins from cigarette smoke (Fig. 8.8). Inflammatory cytokines (e.g., tumor necrosis factor [TNF]) can also stimulate proatherogenic patterns of EC gene expression. Nevertheless, the two most important causes of endothelial dysfunction are hemodynamic disturbances and hypercholesterolemia. Dysfunctional ECs exhibit increased permeability, increased tendency for thrombus formation, and enhanced leukocyte adhesion, all of which may contribute to the development of atherosclerosis.

Hemodynamic Disturbances. The importance of hemodynamic factors in atherogenesis is illustrated by the observation that plaques tend to occur where there is turbulent blood flow: at ostia of exiting vessels, at branch points, and along the posterior wall of the abdominal aorta. In vitro studies further demonstrate that nonturbulent laminar flow leads to the induction of endothelial genes whose products protect against atherosclerosis. Such "atheroprotective" genes may explain the nonrandom localization of early atherosclerotic lesions.

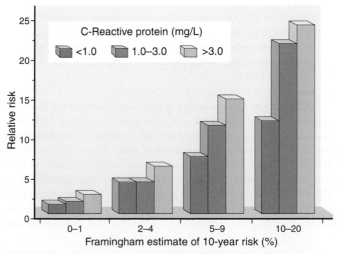

FIG. 8.7 Prognostic value of C-reactive protein (CRP) in coronary artery disease. Relative risk (y-axis) reflects the risk for a cardiovascular event (e.g., myocardial infarction). The x-axis shows the 10-year risk for a cardiovascular event calculated from the traditional risk factors identified in the Framingham Study. In each risk group, CRP levels further stratify the patients. (Data from Ridker PM, et al: Comparison of C-reactive protein and low-density lipoprotein cholesterol levels in the prediction of first cardiovascular events. *N Engl J Med* 347:1557, 2002.)

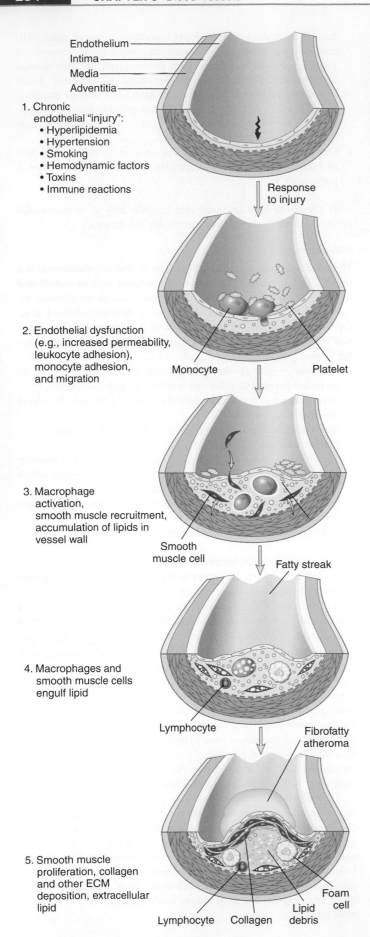

1. Chronic
   endothelial "injury":
   • Hyperlipidemia
   • Hypertension
   • Smoking
   • Hemodynamic factors
   • Toxins
   • Immune reactions

Response to injury

2. Endothelial dysfunction
   (e.g., increased permeability,
   leukocyte adhesion),
   monocyte adhesion,
   and migration

Monocyte   Platelet

3. Macrophage
   activation,
   smooth muscle recruitment,
   accumulation of lipids in
   vessel wall

Smooth
muscle cell

Fatty streak

4. Macrophages and
   smooth muscle cells
   engulf lipid

Lymphocyte

Fibrofatty
atheroma

5. Smooth muscle
   proliferation, collagen
   and other ECM
   deposition, extracellular
   lipid

Lymphocyte   Collagen   Lipid
debris

Foam
cell

FIG. 8.8 Response to injury in atherogenesis: *1,* Endothelial injury. *2,* Endothelial dysfunction with monocyte and platelet adhesion. *3,* Monocyte and smooth muscle cell migration into the intima, with macrophage activation. *4,* Macrophage and smooth muscle cell uptake of modified lipids and further activation. *5,* Intimal smooth muscle cell proliferation and extracellular matrix elaboration, forming a well-developed plaque.

Lipids. Common lipoprotein abnormalities in the general population (and indeed, present in many myocardial infarction survivors) include (1) increased LDL cholesterol levels; (2) decreased HDL cholesterol levels; and (3) increased levels of lipoprotein(a). Lipids are transported in the bloodstream bound to specific apoproteins (forming lipoprotein complexes) (Chapter 4). *Dyslipoproteinemias* result from mutations in genes that encode apoproteins or lipoprotein receptors or from disorders that derange lipid metabolism, (e.g., nephrotic syndrome, alcoholism, hypothyroidism, or diabetes).

Several lines of evidence implicate hypercholesterolemia in atherogenesis:

• *The dominant lipids in atheromatous plaques are cholesterol and cholesterol esters.*
• *Genetic defects in lipoprotein uptake and metabolism that cause hyperlipoproteinemia are associated with accelerated atherosclerosis.* Thus, homozygous familial hypercholesterolemia, caused by defective LDL receptors and inadequate hepatic LDL uptake, can lead to myocardial infarction by 20 years of age (Chapter 4). Other genetic or acquired disorders (e.g., diabetes, hypothyroidism) that cause hypercholesterolemia lead to premature atherosclerosis.
• *Epidemiologic analyses* (e.g., the Framingham study) demonstrate a significant correlation between the levels of total plasma cholesterol or LDL and the severity of atherosclerosis.
• *Lowering serum cholesterol* by diet or drugs slows the rate of progression of atherosclerosis, causes regression of some plaques, and reduces the risk for cardiovascular events.

The mechanisms by which dyslipidemia contributes to atherogenesis include the following:

• *Chronic hyperlipidemia, particularly hypercholesterolemia, can directly impair EC function* by increasing local oxygen free radical production; one effect of oxygen free radicals is to accelerate NO decay, damping its vasodilator activity.
• *With chronic hyperlipidemia, lipoproteins accumulate within the intima,* where they are thought to generate two pathogenic derivatives, oxidized LDL and cholesterol crystals. LDL is oxidized through the action of oxygen free radicals generated locally by macrophages or ECs and ingested by macrophages through the scavenger receptor, resulting in foam cell formation. Oxidized LDL stimulates the local release of growth factors, cytokines, and chemokines, increasing monocyte recruitment, and is also cytotoxic to ECs and SMCs.

Inflammation. Chronic inflammation contributes to the initiation, progression, and complications of atherosclerotic lesions. Inflammation is triggered by the accumulation of cholesterol crystals and free fatty acids in macrophages and other cells. These cells sense the presence of abnormal materials such as cholesterol crystals via cytosolic innate immune receptors that activate the inflammasome (Chapter 5). This leads to the production of the proinflammatory cytokine interleukin (IL-1), which promotes the recruitment of leukocytes, including macrophages and T lymphocytes. Activated T cells

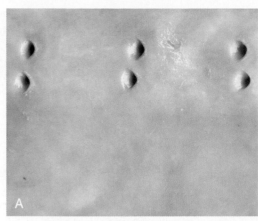
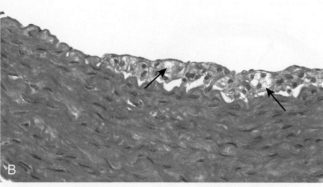

FIG. 8.9 Fatty streaks. (A) Aorta with yellowish fatty streaks mainly near the ostia of branch vessels. (B) Fatty streak in an experimental hypercholesterolemic rabbit, demonstrating intimal, macrophage-derived foam cells *(arrows)*. (A, Image courtesy of Dr. Joseph J. Maleszewski, Mayo Clinic, Rochester, Minnesota; B, Courtesy of Myron I. Cybulsky, MD, University of Toronto, Toronto, Ontario, Canada.)

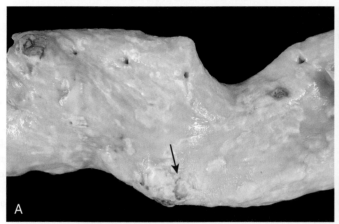
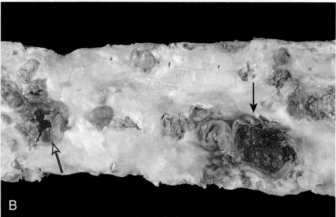

FIG. 8.10 Atherosclerotic lesions. (A) Aorta with mild atherosclerosis composed of fibrous plaques, one denoted by the *arrow*. (B) Aorta with severe diffuse complicated lesions, including an ulcerated plaque *(open arrow)*, and a lesion with overlying thrombus *(closed arrow)*.

in the growing intimal lesions elaborate inflammatory cytokines (e.g., IFN-γ), which activate macrophages, ECs, and SMCs.

SMC Proliferation and Matrix Synthesis. Intimal SMC proliferation and ECM deposition lead to conversion of the earliest lesion, a fatty streak, into a mature atheroma, thus contributing to the progressive growth of atherosclerotic lesions (see Fig. 8.8). Several growth factors are implicated in SMC proliferation and matrix synthesis, including platelet-derived growth factor (released by locally adherent platelets, macrophages, ECs, and SMCs), and fibroblast growth factor. The recruited SMCs synthesize ECM (most notably collagen), which stabilizes atherosclerotic plaques. However, activated inflammatory cells in atheromas can also cause intimal SMC apoptosis and breakdown of matrix, leading to the development of unstable plaques (see later).

MORPHOLOGY

The development of atherosclerosis tends to follow a sequence of morphologic changes, as follows:

Fatty Streaks. Fatty streaks begin as minute yellow, flat macules that coalesce into elongated lesions, 1 cm or more in length (Fig. 8.9). They are composed of lipid-filled foamy macrophages but are only minimally raised and do not cause any significant flow disturbance. Fatty streaks can appear in the aortas of infants younger than 1 year of age and are present in virtually all children older than 10 years of age, regardless of genetic, clinical, or dietary risk factors. Not all fatty streaks are destined to progress to atherosclerotic plaques. Nevertheless, it is notable that coronary fatty streaks form during adolescence at the same anatomic sites that are prone to plaques later in life.

Atherosclerotic Plaque. The key features of these lesions are intimal thickening and lipid accumulation (see Fig. 8.5B). Atheromatous plaques are white to yellow raised lesions; they range from 0.3 to 1.5 cm in diameter but can coalesce to form larger masses. Thrombus superimposed on ulcerated plaques imparts a red-brown color (Fig. 8.10).

Atherosclerotic plaques are patchy, usually involving only a portion of any given arterial wall; on cross-section, therefore, the lesions appear "eccentric" (Fig. 8.11A). The focal nature of atherosclerotic lesions may be related to the vagaries of vascular hemodynamics. Local flow disturbances, such as turbulence at branch points, make certain parts of a vessel wall especially susceptible to plaque formation.

In descending order of severity, atherosclerosis involves the infrarenal abdominal aorta, the coronary arteries, the popliteal arteries, the internal carotid arteries, and the vessels of the circle of Willis. In a given individual, atherosclerosis is typically more severe in the abdominal aorta than in the

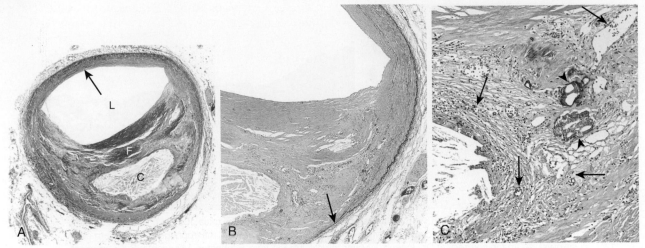

FIG. 8.11 Atherosclerotic plaque, coronary artery. (A) Overall architecture demonstrating fibrous cap *(F)* and a central necrotic (largely lipid) core *(C)*; collagen *(blue)* is stained with Masson trichrome. The lumen *(L)* is moderately narrowed by this eccentric lesion, which leaves part of the vessel wall unaffected *(arrow)*. (B) Medium-power view of the plaque shown in *A*, stained for elastin *(black)*; the internal and external elastic membranes are attenuated, and the media of the artery is thinned under the most advanced plaque *(arrow)*. (C) High-power view of the junction of the fibrous cap and core, showing scattered inflammatory cells, calcification *(arrowheads)*, and neovascularization *(small arrows)*.

thoracic aorta. Vessels of the upper extremities are usually spared, as are the mesenteric and renal arteries, except at their ostia.

Atherosclerotic plaques have three principal components: (1) cells, including SMCs, macrophages, and T cells; (2) ECM, including collagen, elastic fibers, and proteoglycans; and (3) intracellular and extracellular lipids (see Fig. 8.11A and B). The proportion and configuration of each component vary from lesion to lesion. Most commonly, plaques have a superficial fibrous cap composed of SMCs and relatively dense collagen. Where the cap meets the vessel wall (the "shoulder") is a more cellular area containing macrophages, T cells, and SMCs. Deep to the fibrous cap is a necrotic core, containing lipid (primarily cholesterol and cholesterol esters), necrotic debris, lipid-laden macrophages and SMCs **(foam cells),** fibrin, variably organized thrombus, and other plasma proteins. The extracellular cholesterol frequently takes the form of crystalline aggregates that are washed out during routine tissue processing, leaving behind empty "cholesterol clefts." The periphery of the lesions shows **neovascularization** (proliferating small blood vessels) (see Fig. 8.11C). The media deep to the plaque may be attenuated and exhibit fibrosis secondary to smooth muscle atrophy and loss.

Plaques generally enlarge over time through cell death and degeneration, synthesis and degradation of ECM (remodeling), and thrombus organization. The necrotic material in atheromas also often undergoes dystrophic calcification (see Fig. 8.11C).

Consequences of Atherosclerosis

The natural history, morphologic features, and main pathogenic events are schematized in Fig. 8.12. The principal pathophysiologic outcome stemming from atherosclerotic lesions varies depending on the size of the affected vessel, the size and stability of the plaques, and the degree to which plaques disrupt the vessel wall.

Large elastic arteries (e.g., aorta, carotid, and iliac arteries) and large and medium-sized muscular arteries (e.g., coronary, renal, and popliteal arteries) are the vessels most commonly involved by atherosclerosis. Accordingly, atherosclerosis is most likely to present with signs and symptoms related to ischemia of the heart, brain, kidneys, and lower extremities. **Myocardial infarction (heart attack), cerebral infarction (stroke), aortic aneurysm, and peripheral vascular disease (gangrene of extremities) are the major clinical consequences of atherosclerosis.**

We next describe the features of atherosclerotic lesions that are typically responsible for the clinical manifestations.

Atherosclerotic Stenosis

At early stages, remodeling of the media tends to preserve the luminal diameter by increasing the overall vessel circumference. Due to limits on remodeling, however, eventually the expanding atheroma may impinge on blood flow. Although this most commonly happens as a consequence of acute plaque change (described next), it can also occur gradually, with *critical stenosis* being the tipping point at which chronic occlusion limits flow so severely that tissue demand exceeds supply. In the coronary artery (and other) circulations, this typically occurs when the vessel is approximately 70% occluded. At rest, affected patients have adequate cardiac perfusion; but with even modest exertion, demand exceeds supply, and chest pain develops because of cardiac ischemia (stable angina) (Chapter 9). The toll of chronic arterial hypoperfusion due to atherosclerosis in various vascular beds includes bowel ischemia, sudden cardiac death, chronic IHD, ischemic encephalopathy, and intermittent claudication (ischemic leg pain).

Acute Plaque Change

Plaque changes fall into three general categories:

- *Rupture, ulceration, or erosion* of the luminal surface of atheromatous plaques exposes highly thrombogenic substances and induces thrombus formation (Fig. 8.13, eFig. 8.2, and eFig. 8.3).
- *Hemorrhage* into a plaque. Rupture of the overlying fibrous cap or of the thin-walled vessels in the areas of neovascularization can

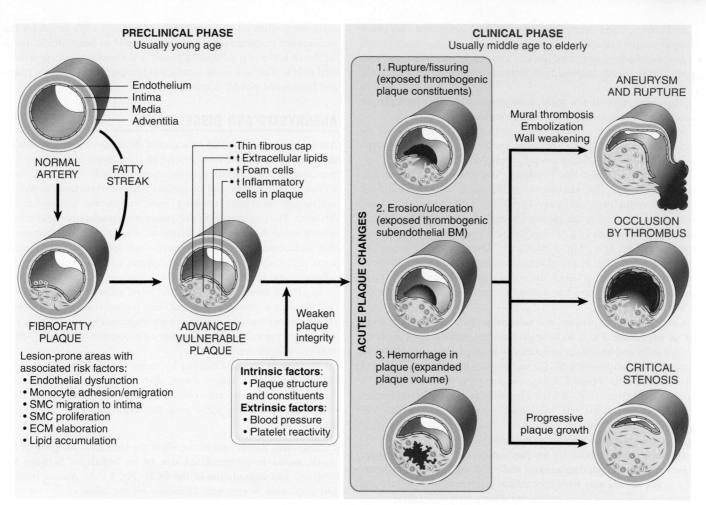

PRECLINICAL PHASE
Usually young age

- Endothelium
- Intima
- Media
- Adventitia

NORMAL
ARTERY

FATTY
STREAK

FIBROFATTY
PLAQUE

- Thin fibrous cap
- ↑ Extracellular lipids
- ↑ Foam cells
- ↑ Inflammatory cells in plaque

ADVANCED/
VULNERABLE
PLAQUE

Lesion-prone areas with associated risk factors:
- Endothelial dysfunction
- Monocyte adhesion/emigration
- SMC migration to intima
- SMC proliferation
- ECM elaboration
- Lipid accumulation

Weaken plaque integrity

Intrinsic factors:
- Plaque structure and constituents

Extrinsic factors:
- Blood pressure
- Platelet reactivity

CLINICAL PHASE
Usually middle age to elderly

ACUTE PLAQUE CHANGES

1. Rupture/fissuring (exposed thrombogenic plaque constituents)

2. Erosion/ulceration (exposed thrombogenic subendothelial BM)

3. Hemorrhage in plaque (expanded plaque volume)

Mural thrombosis
Embolization
Wall weakening

ANEURYSM
AND RUPTURE

OCCLUSION
BY THROMBUS

Progressive plaque growth

CRITICAL
STENOSIS

FIG. 8.12 Summary of the natural history, morphologic features, main pathogenic events, and clinical complications of atherosclerosis—critical stenosis, complete thrombotic occlusion, aneurysm, and vascular rupture. *BM,* Basement membrane; *ECM,* extracellular matrix; *SMC,* smooth muscle cell.

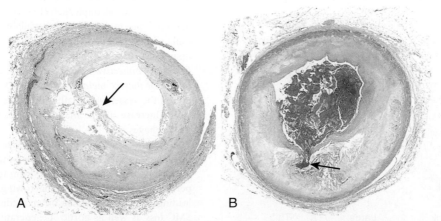

FIG. 8.13 Atherosclerotic plaque rupture. (A) Plaque rupture without superimposed thrombus in a patient who died suddenly. (B) Acute coronary thrombosis superimposed on an atherosclerotic plaque with focal disruption of the fibrous cap, triggering fatal myocardial infarction. In both A and B, an arrow points to the site of plaque rupture. (B, Reproduced from Schoen FJ: *Interventional and Surgical Cardiovascular Pathology: Clinical Correlations and Basic Principles,* Philadelphia, 1989, Saunders, p 61.)

cause intraplaque hemorrhage; the resulting hematoma may cause rapid plaque expansion or plaque rupture.

- *Atheroembolism.* Ruptured plaque can discharge debris into the blood, producing microemboli composed of plaque contents.

Thrombosis, partial or total, associated with a disrupted plaque is a central factor in acute coronary syndromes.

It is now recognized that plaques responsible for myocardial infarctions and other acute coronary syndromes are often asymptomatic before the acute event; symptoms are triggered by thrombosis on a lesion that previously did not produce significant luminal occlusion. The worrisome conclusion is that large numbers of asymptomatic individuals are at risk for a catastrophic coronary event. The causes of acute plaque change are complex and include both intrinsic factors (e.g., plaque structure and composition) and extrinsic factors (e.g., blood pressure). These factors combine to weaken the integrity of the plaque, making it unable to withstand vascular shear forces. It should be noted that while thrombosis most often occurs on a ruptured or disrupted plaque, it may also occur on an intact plaque.

Certain types of plaques are believed to be at particularly high risk of rupturing. These include plaques that contain large numbers of foam cells and abundant extracellular lipid, plaques that have thin fibrous caps containing few SMCs, and plaques that contain clusters of inflammatory cells. Plaques at high risk for rupture are referred to as *vulnerable plaques* (Fig. 8.14). The fibrous cap also undergoes continuous remodeling; its mechanical strength and stability are proportional to its collagen content, so the balance of collagen synthesis and degradation affects cap integrity.

Inflammation destabilizes the mechanical integrity of the plaque by increasing collagen degradation and reducing collagen synthesis. Of interest, statins may have a beneficial effect not only by reducing circulating cholesterol levels but also by other poorly understood effects on atherogenesis. These include reversal of endothelial dysfunctions and stabilizing plaques through a reduction in plaque inflammation.

Factors extrinsic to plaques are also important. Adrenergic stimulation (as with intense emotions) can increase systemic blood pressure or induce local vasoconstriction, thereby increasing the

mechanical stress on a given plaque. Indeed, one explanation for the pronounced circadian periodicity in the onset of heart attacks (peak incidence between 6 AM and 12 noon) is the adrenergic surge associated with waking and rising—sufficient to cause blood pressure spikes and heightened platelet reactivity.

ANEURYSMS AND DISSECTIONS

Aneurysms are congenital or acquired dilations of blood vessels or the heart. "True" aneurysms involve all three layers of the artery (intima, media, and adventitia) or the attenuated wall of the heart; these include atherosclerotic and congenital vascular aneurysms, as well as ventricular aneurysms resulting from transmural myocardial infarctions. By comparison, a false aneurysm (pseudoaneurysm) results when a wall defect leads to the formation of an extravascular hematoma that communicates with the intravascular space ("pulsating hematoma"). Examples are ventricular ruptures contained by pericardial adhesions and leaks at the junction of a vascular graft with an artery.

In arterial dissections, pressurized blood gains entry to the arterial wall through a surface defect and then pushes apart the underlying layers. Aneurysms and dissections are important causes of stasis and subsequent thrombosis; they also have a propensity to rupture—often with catastrophic results.

Aneurysms can be classified by shape (Fig. 8.15B). *Saccular aneurysms* are discrete outpouchings often with a contained thrombus. *Fusiform aneurysms* are circumferential dilations; these most commonly involve the aortic arch, the abdominal aorta, or the iliac arteries.

Pathogenesis. **Aneurysms occur when the structural integrity of the aortic media is compromised due to an imbalance between the synthesis and degradation of the ECM** (Fig. 8.15A). Among the factors implicated in aneurysm formation are the following:

- *Inadequate or abnormal connective tissue synthesis.* Several rare inherited diseases provide insight into the types of abnormalities that can lead to aneurysm formation. As discussed earlier, TGF-β regulates SMC proliferation and matrix synthesis. Thus, mutations in TGF-β receptors or downstream signaling pathways result in defective elastin and collagen synthesis. In *Marfan syndrome* (Chapter 4), for example, defective synthesis of the scaffold protein *fibrillin* leads to increased bioavailability of TGF-β in the aortic wall, with subsequent dilation due to progressive loss of elastic tissue.
- *Excessive connective tissue degradation by inflammation-associated release of matrix metalloproteases* (MMP). Transmural inflammation of the vessel wall in atherosclerotic aneurysms is characterized by an increase in the amounts of elastolytic MMPs produced by macrophages.
- *Loss of SMCs or change in SMC synthetic phenotype.* Atherosclerotic thickening of the intima can cause ischemia of the inner media by increasing the diffusion distance from the lumen, and systemic hypertension can cause luminal narrowing of the aortic vasa vasorum, leading to ischemia of the outer media. Such ischemia results in SMC loss as well as aortic "degenerative changes," which include fibrosis (replacing distensible elastic tissue), inadequate ECM synthesis by SMCs, and accumulation of increasing amounts of amorphous proteoglycans. Histologically, these changes are collectively called *cystic medial degeneration* (Fig. 8.16), although no true cysts are formed. Such changes are nonspecific; they can occur whenever ECM synthesis is defective, including in inherited disorders such as Marfan syndrome and acquired conditions such as scurvy.

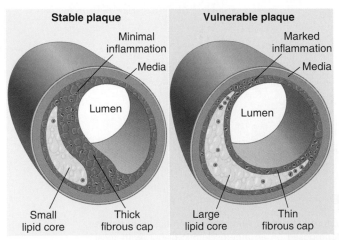

FIG. 8.14 Stable and vulnerable atherosclerotic plaques. Stable plaques have densely collagenized and thickened fibrous caps with minimal inflammation and negligible underlying atheromatous cores, whereas vulnerable plaques have thin fibrous caps, large lipid cores, and more inflammation. (Adapted from Libby P: Molecular bases of the acute coronary syndromes. *Circulation* 91:2844, 1995.)

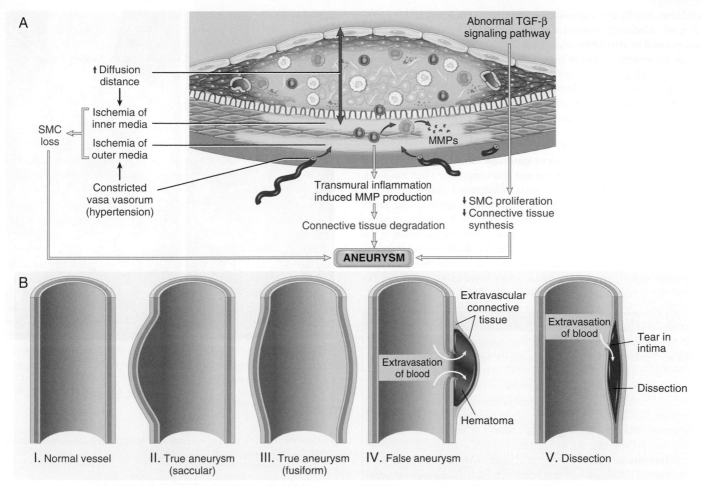

FIG. 8.15 Aneurysms. (A) Pathogenesis of aneurysms. (B) Different type of aneurysms. *MMP*, Membrane metalloproteinase; *SMC*, smooth muscle cell; *TGF-β*, transforming growth factor beta.

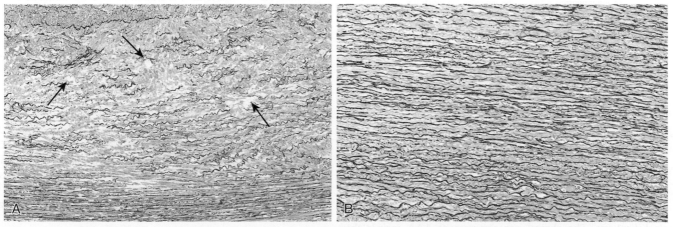

FIG. 8.16 Cystic medial degeneration. (A) Cross-section of aortic media from a patient with Marfan syndrome, showing marked elastin fragmentation and areas devoid of elastin that resemble cystic spaces *(arrows)*. (B) Healthy media for comparison, showing the regular layered pattern of elastic tissue. In both (A) and (B), elastin is stained black.

The three most important predisposing conditions for aortic aneurysms are atherosclerosis, hypertension, and smoking. Atherosclerosis and tobacco smoking are the dominant factors in abdominal aortic aneurysms, while hypertension is associated with ascending aortic aneurysms. Other conditions that weaken vessel walls and lead to aneurysms include trauma, vasculitis (see later), congenital anomalies, and infections, which give rise to so-called "mycotic aneurysms." Mycotic aneurysms may result from (1) embolization of a septic embolus, usually as a complication of infective endocarditis; (2) extension of an adjacent suppurative process; or (3) direct infection of an arterial wall by circulating organisms. Tertiary syphilis is a rare cause of aortic aneurysms. A predilection of the spirochetes for the vasa vasorum of the ascending thoracic aorta—and the subsequent immune response to them—results in an *obliterative endarteritis* that compromises blood flow to the media; the ensuing ischemic injury leads to aneurysmal dilation that occasionally also involves the aortic valve annulus.

Abdominal Aortic Aneurysm

Atherosclerotic aneurysms occur most commonly in the abdominal aorta and common iliac arteries and less commonly affect the aortic arch and descending thoracic aorta. Abdominal aortic aneurysms (AAAs) occur more frequently in men and in smokers and rarely develop before 50 years of age. Atherosclerosis is a major cause of AAA, but other factors clearly contribute, since the incidence is less than 5% in men older than 60 years of age despite the almost universal presence of abdominal aortic atherosclerosis in this population. As discussed earlier, aneurysms occur when there is an imbalance between the synthesis and degradation of the ECM.

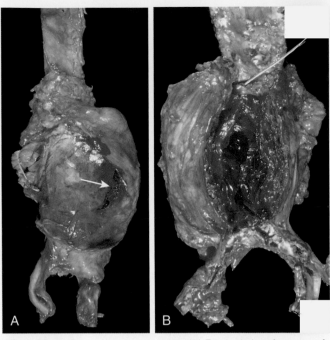

FIG. 8.17 Abdominal aortic aneurysm. (A) External site of rupture of a large aortic aneurysm is indicated by the *arrow*. (B) Opened aorta, with the location of the rupture tract indicated by a *probe*. The wall of the aneurysm is attenuated, and the lumen is filled by a large, layered thrombus.

MORPHOLOGY

Abdominal aortic aneurysms typically occur between the renal arteries and the aortic bifurcation; they can be saccular or fusiform and up to 15 cm in diameter and 25 cm in length (Fig. 8.17). In the vast majority of cases, extensive atherosclerosis is present, with thinning and focal destruction of the underlying media. The aneurysm sac usually contains bland, laminated, poorly organized mural thrombus, which can fill much of the dilated segment. Not infrequently, AAAs are accompanied by smaller iliac artery aneurysms. Next, we describe some other forms of aortic aneurysms:

- **Inflammatory AAAs** are a distinct subtype characterized by dense periaortic fibrosis containing abundant chronic inflammatory cells with lymphocytes, plasma cells, and many macrophages and giant cells. They account for 5% to 10% of all AAAs and typically occur in individuals younger than those who have atherosclerotic AAA.
- A subset of inflammatory AAAs is the vascular manifestation of **immunoglobulin G4-related disease.** This disorder is marked by tissue fibrosis associated with infiltrates rich in IgG4-expressing plasma cells. As discussed in Chapter 5, IgG4-related chronic disease can also affect a variety of other tissues, including the pancreas, biliary system, thyroid gland, and salivary gland. There may be retroperitoneal fibrosis and bilateral hydronephrosis. Affected individuals have aortitis and periaortitis that weaken the wall sufficiently to give rise to aneurysms. IgG4-related chronic disease responds well to steroids and anti—B-cell therapies.
- **Mycotic AAAs** occur when circulating microorganisms (as in bacteremia from infective endocarditis) seed the aneurysm wall or the associated thrombus; the resulting suppuration accelerates the medial destruction and may lead to rapid dilation and rupture.

Clinical Features. The clinical consequences of AAA include the following:

- *Obstruction* of a vessel branching off the aorta (e.g., the renal, iliac, vertebral, or mesenteric arteries), resulting in ischemic injury of the kidneys, legs, spinal cord, or gastrointestinal tract, respectively
- *Embolism* of atheromatous material or mural thrombus
- *Impingement on adjacent structures* (e.g., compression of a ureter or erosion of vertebrae by the expanding aneurysm)
- *An abdominal mass* (often palpably pulsating) that simulates a tumor

- *Rupture* into the peritoneal cavity or retroperitoneal tissues, leading to massive, often fatal, hemorrhage

The risk for rupture is related to the size. AAAs 4 cm or less in diameter almost never burst, while those larger than 5.5 cm are at a high risk. Thus, aneurysms 5.5 cm in diameter or larger are surgically repaired. Timely intervention is critical, because the mortality rate for elective procedures is much lower than the rate for emergency surgery after rupture.

A point worthy of emphasis is that because atherosclerosis is a systemic disease, a patient with AAA is also likely to have atherosclerosis in other vascular beds and is at a significantly increased risk for ischemic heart disease and stroke.

Thoracic Aortic Aneurysm

Thoracic aortic aneurysms are most commonly associated with hypertension, bicuspid aortic valves, and Marfan syndrome. Less commonly, tertiary syphilis and mutations in the TGF-β signaling pathway (e.g., *Loeys-Dietz syndrome*) are causative. These aneurysms manifest with the following signs and symptoms:

- *Respiratory or feeding difficulties* due to airway or esophageal compression, respectively
- *Persistent cough* from irritation of the recurrent laryngeal nerves
- *Pain* caused by erosion of bone (i.e., ribs and vertebral bodies)
- *Cardiac disease* due to valvular insufficiency or narrowing of the coronary ostia, or heart failure induced by aortic valvular incompetence
- *Aortic dissection* or rupture

Aortic Dissection

Aortic dissection occurs when the laminar planes of the media split apart and form a blood-filled channel within the aortic wall

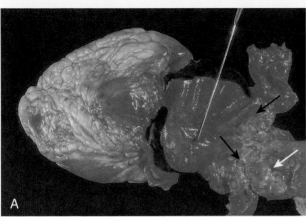
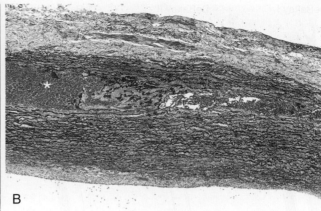

FIG. 8.18 Aortic dissection. (A) An opened aorta with a proximal dissection originating from a small, oblique intimal tear *(identified by the probe)* associated with an intramural hematoma. Note that the intimal tear occurred in a region largely free of atherosclerotic plaque. The distal edge of the intramural hematoma *(black arrows)* lies at the edge of a large area of atherosclerosis *(white arrow)*, which arrested the propagation of the dissection. The heart is on the left. (B) Histologic preparation showing the dissection and intramural hematoma *(asterisk)*. Aortic elastic layers are *black*, and blood is *red* in this section, stained with Movat stain.

(Fig. 8.18; eFig. 8.4). This development can be catastrophic if the dissecting blood ruptures through the adventitia and escapes into adjacent spaces. Aortic dissection occurs mainly in two age groups: (1) men 40 to 60 years of age with antecedent hypertension (more than 90% of cases); and (2) younger patients with connective tissue abnormalities that affect the aorta (e.g., Marfan syndrome). Dissections can also be iatrogenic (e.g., complicating arterial cannulation during diagnostic catheterization or cardiopulmonary bypass).

Rarely, pregnancy is associated with aortic (or other vessel) dissection (roughly 10 to 20 cases per 1 million births). This event typically occurs during or after the third trimester and may be related to hormone-induced vascular remodeling and the hemodynamic stresses of the perinatal period. Dissection is unusual in the presence of substantial atherosclerosis or other causes of medial scarring, presumably because the medial fibrosis inhibits propagation of the dissecting hematoma (see Fig. 8.18).

Pathogenesis. **Hypertension is the major risk factor for aortic dissection.** Aortas in patients with hypertension show narrowing of the vasa vasora associated with degenerative changes in ECM and variable loss of medial SMCs, suggesting that diminished flow through the vasa vasora is contributory. Abrupt, transient increases in blood pressure, as may occur with cocaine use, is also known to cause aortic dissection. Most other dissections are related to inherited or acquired connective tissue disorders that give rise to abnormal aortic ECM, including Marfan syndrome, Ehlers-Danlos syndrome type IV, and defects in copper metabolism.

The trigger for the intimal tear and subsequent intramural hemorrhage is not known in most cases. Nevertheless, once the tear has occurred, blood under systemic pressure dissects through the media along laminar planes. Accordingly, aggressive antihypertensive treatment may be effective in limiting an evolving dissection. In rare cases, disruption of the vasa vasora can give rise to an intramural hematoma without an intimal tear.

MORPHOLOGY

In most dissections, the intimal tear marking the point of origin is found in the ascending aorta within 10 cm of the aortic valve (see Fig. 8.18A). Such tears are usually transverse or oblique in orientation and 1 to 5 cm long, with sharp, jagged edges. The dissection plane can extend retrograde toward the heart or distally, occasionally as far as the iliac and femoral arteries, and usually lies between the middle and outer thirds of the media (see Fig. 8.18B).

External rupture causes massive hemorrhage or cardiac tamponade if it occurs into the pericardial sac. In some instances, the dissecting hematoma reenters the lumen of the aorta through a second distal intimal tear, creating a second vascular channel within the media (so-called "double-barreled aorta"). Over time, such a false channel becomes endothelialized, forming a chronic dissection.

The most frequent histologically detectable lesion is **cystic medial degeneration** (discussed earlier); this is characterized by SMC dropout and necrosis, elastic tissue fragmentation, and accumulations of amorphous proteoglycan-rich ECM (see Fig. 8.16). Inflammation is characteristically absent. However, recognizable medial damage is not a prerequisite for dissection as in most instances no specific underlying defect is identified in the aortic wall.

Clinical Features. The clinical manifestations of dissection depend primarily on the portion of the aorta affected; the most serious complications occur with dissections involving the proximal aorta and arch. Thus, aortic dissections generally are classified into two types (Fig. 8.19):

- *Proximal (type A) dissections*, involving the ascending aorta, with or without involvement of the descending aorta (DeBakey type I or II, respectively)
- *Distal (type B) dissections*, usually beginning beyond the subclavian artery (DeBakey type III)

The classic clinical symptom of aortic dissection is the sudden onset of excruciating tearing or stabbing pain, usually beginning in the anterior chest, radiating to the back between the scapulae, and moving downward as the dissection progresses. The most common cause of death is rupture of the dissection into the pericardial, pleural, or peritoneal cavity. Retrograde dissection into the aortic root also can cause fatal disruption of the aortic valvular apparatus or compression of the coronary arteries. Common clinical presentations

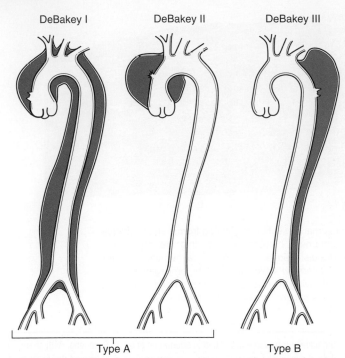

FIG. 8.19 Classification of dissections. Type A dissections (proximal) involve the ascending aorta, either as part of a more extensive dissection (DeBakey type I), or in isolation (DeBakey type II). Type B dissections (distal, or DeBakey type III) arise after the takeoff of the great vessels. Type A dissections typically have the most serious complications and the greatest associated mortality.

stemming from cardiac involvement include tamponade, aortic insufficiency, and myocardial infarction. Other complications are related to extension of the dissection to the great arteries of the neck and the renal, mesenteric, or iliac arteries, any of which may become obstructed. Similarly, compression of spinal arteries can cause transverse myelitis.

Type A dissections are medical emergencies requiring rapid diagnosis and institution of intensive antihypertensive therapy coupled with surgical intervention. Most type B dissections are managed conservatively with antihypertensive therapy.

VASCULITIS

Vasculitis is a general term for vessel wall inflammation. The two most common pathogenic mechanisms of vasculitis are immune-mediated inflammation and direct vascular invasion by infectious pathogens. Infections can also indirectly precipitate immune-mediated vasculitis (e.g., by generating immune complexes or triggering cross-reactivity). In any given patient, it is critical to distinguish between infectious and immunologic mechanisms because immunosuppressive therapy is appropriate for immune-mediated vasculitis but could exacerbate infectious vasculitis. Physical and chemical injury caused by various insults (e.g., radiation, mechanical trauma, toxins) also can cause vasculitis.

Some 20 primary forms of vasculitis are recognized, and classification schemes attempt (with variable success) to group them according to vessel diameter, role of immune complexes, presence of specific autoantibodies, granuloma formation, organ specificity, and population demographics (Table 8.3 and Fig. 8.20).

The possible clinical manifestations are protean but largely depend on the specific vascular bed that is affected. In addition to findings referable to the affected tissue(s), there are also usually signs and symptoms of systemic inflammation, such as fever, myalgia, arthralgias, and malaise. There is considerable clinical and pathologic overlap among these entities, as will be evident from the following discussion of individual forms. We begin our discussion with pathogenic mechanisms and then describe selected types.

Noninfectious Vasculitis

The main immunologic alterations associated with noninfectious vasculitis are as follows:

- Immune complex deposition
- Antineutrophil cytoplasmic antibodies
- Antiendothelial cell antibodies
- Autoreactive T cells

Immune Complex—Associated Vasculitis

This form of vasculitis is seen in immunologic disorders such as systemic lupus erythematosus (Chapter 5) that are associated with autoantibody production. The vascular lesions resemble those found in experimental immune complex—mediated disorders, such as the Arthus reaction and serum sickness, and in some cases contain readily identifiable antibody and complement. Only rarely is the specific antigen responsible for immune complex formation known, and in some suspected cases, the antigen-antibody deposits are scarce, perhaps because the immune complexes have been degraded by the time of biopsy.

Immune complex deposition is also implicated in the following vasculitides:

- *Drug hypersensitivity vasculitis.* In some cases, drugs (e.g., penicillin) may bind to host proteins and elicit immune responses; other agents are themselves foreign proteins (e.g., streptokinase). In either case, antibodies directed against the drug-modified proteins or foreign molecules result in immune complex formation. The clinical manifestations can be mild and self-limiting, or severe and even fatal; skin lesions are most common. It is always important to consider drug hypersensitivity as a cause of vasculitis, since discontinuation of the offending agent usually leads to resolution.
- *Vasculitis secondary to infections.* Antibodies to microbial constituents can form immune complexes that deposit in vascular lesions. For example, in up to 30% of patients with *polyarteritis nodosa* (discussed later), the vasculitis can be ascribed to immune complexes composed of hepatitis B surface antigen (HBsAg) and anti-HBsAg antibody.

Antineutrophil Cytoplasmic Antibodies

Many patients with vasculitis have circulating antibodies that react with neutrophil cytoplasmic antigens, so-called "antineutrophil cytoplasmic antibodies" (ANCAs). ANCAs are a heterogeneous group of autoantibodies directed against constituents (mainly enzymes) of neutrophil primary granules, monocyte lysosomes, and ECs. ANCAs are very useful diagnostic markers; their titers generally mirror clinical severity, and a rise in titers after periods of quiescence is predictive of disease recurrence.

Although a number of ANCAs have been described, two are most important. These are classified according to their antigen specificity:

- *Antiproteinase-3 (PR3-ANCA),* previously called c-ANCA. PR3 is a neutrophil azurophilic granule constituent that shares homology with numerous microbial peptides, possibly explaining the

Table 8.3 Classification and Characteristic Pathologic Features of Vasculitides

Name	Characteristic Pathologic Features
Large-vessel vasculitis	Predominantly affects large arteries
Takayasu arteritis	Arteritis, often granulomatous; patients usually younger than 50 years
Giant cell arteritis	Arteritis, often granulomatous; usually affecting the aorta and/or its major branches (carotid, vertebral, temporal); patients usually older than 50 years
Medium-vessel vasculitis	Predominantly affects medium arteries (main visceral arteries and their branches); inflammatory aneurysms and stenoses are common
Polyarteritis nodosa	Necrotizing arteritis of medium or small arteries (not affecting pulmonary circulation, glomeruli, arterioles, capillaries, or venules) not associated with antineutrophil cytoplasmic antibodies (ANCAs)
Kawasaki disease	Arteritis associated with mucocutaneous lymph node syndrome; predominantly affects medium and small arteries (especially coronary arteries); most common in infants and young children
Small-vessel vasculitis	Vasculitis predominantly affecting small vessels (small intraparenchymal arteries, arterioles, capillaries, and venules)
ANCA-associated vasculitis	Necrotizing vasculitis, with few or no immune deposits; associated with myeloperoxidase (MPO) ANCA or proteinase 3 (PR3) ANCA
Microscopic polyangiitis	Necrotizing vasculitis, with few or no immune deposits; necrotizing glomerulonephritis is very common and pulmonary capillaritis often occurs; associated with MPO-ANCA
Granulomatosis with polyangiitis (Wegener)	Necrotizing granulomatous inflammation of upper and lower respiratory tract, and necrotizing vasculitis affecting predominantly small to medium vessels; necrotizing glomerulonephritis is common. PR3-ANCAs are present in 95% of cases
Eosinophilic granulomatosis with polyangiitis (Churg-Strauss)	Eosinophil-rich and necrotizing granulomatous inflammation of respiratory tract, and necrotizing vasculitis of small to medium vessels; associated with asthma and eosinophilia; MPO-ANCAs in over 50% of cases; ANCA is more frequent when glomerulonephritis is present
Immune complex vasculitis Antiglomerular basement membrane disease (Goodpasture); Cryoglobulinemic vasculitis; Immunoglobulin A (IgA) vasculitis (Henoch-Schönlein purpura); Vasculitis associated with systemic disease (SLE, rheumatoid arthritis)	Moderate to marked vessel-wall deposits of immunoglobulin and/or complement components predominantly affecting small vessels; glomerulonephritis is frequent.

SLE, Systemic lupus erythematosus.

[a]Adapted from Jennette JC, Falk RJ, Bacon PA, et al.: 2012 Revised International Chapel Hill Consensus Conference Nomenclature of Vasculitides, *Arthritis Rheum* 65:1, 2013.

generation of PR3-ANCAs. They are associated with *granulomatosis with polyangiitis* (see later).

- *Antimyeloperoxidase (MPO-ANCA)*, previously called *p-ANCA.* MPO is a lysosomal granule constituent involved in oxygen free radical generation (Chapter 2). MPO-ANCAs are induced by several therapeutic agents, particularly propylthiouracil (used to treat hyperthyroidism). MPO-ANCAs are associated with *microscopic polyangiitis* and eosinophilic granulomatosis with polyangiitis (also called *Churg-Strauss syndrome*) (see later).

The close association between ANCA titers and disease activity suggests a pathogenic role for these antibodies. Of note, ANCAs can directly activate neutrophils, stimulating the release of reactive oxygen species and proteolytic enzymes; in vascular beds, this may lead to EC injury. While the antigenic targets of ANCA are primarily intracellular, ANCA antigens (especially PR3) are either constitutively expressed at low levels on the plasma membrane or are translocated to the cell surface in activated and apoptotic leukocytes, allowing them to be accessible to circulating antibodies.

A plausible pathogenic sequence for the development of ANCA vasculitis is the following:

- Drugs or cross-reactive microbial antigens induce ANCA formation; alternatively, leukocyte surface expression or release of PR3 and MPO (in the setting of infection) incites ANCA development in a susceptible individual.
- Subsequent inflammatory stimuli elicit the release of cytokines such as TNF that upregulate the surface expression of PR3 and MPO on neutrophils and other cell types.
- ANCAs bind to these cytokine-activated cells, causing further neutrophil activation.
- ANCA-activated neutrophils cause EC injury by releasing granule contents and elaborating reactive oxygen species.

The ANCA autoantibodies are directed against cellular constituents and do not form circulating immune complexes, nor do the vascular lesions typically contain demonstrable antibody and complement; therefore, ANCA-associated vasculitides often are described as "pauci-immune."

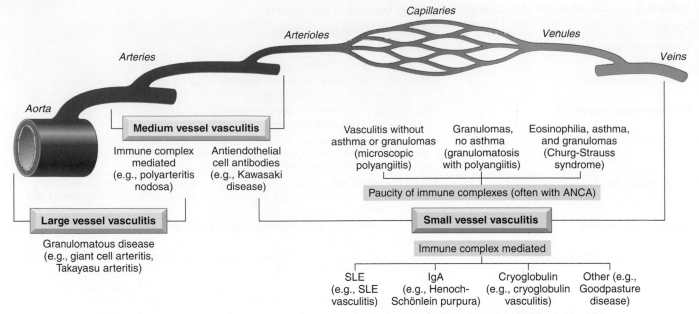

FIG. 8.20 Vascular sites involved in the more common vasculitides and their presumptive etiology. Note the considerable overlap in distributions. *ANCA,* Antineutrophil cytoplasmic antibody; *IgA,* immunoglobulin A; *SLE,* systemic lupus erythematosus. (Data from Jennette JC, Falk RJ: Nosology of primary vasculitis. *Curr Opin Rheumatol* 19:17, 2007.)

Antiendothelial Cell Antibodies and Autoreactive T Cells

Antibodies to ECs underlie certain vasculitides, such as Kawasaki disease (discussed later). Autoreactive T cells cause injury in some forms of vasculitis characterized by formation of granulomas.

Presented next is a brief overview of several of the best-characterized vasculitides (Table 8.3). Although each is presented as a distinct entity, many cases of vasculitis lack a classic constellation of findings and have overlapping features that may render classification difficult.

Large Vessel Vasculitis

There are two major forms of large vessel vasculitis: giant cell arteritis and Takayasu arteritis (see Table 8.3).

Giant Cell (Temporal) Arteritis

Giant cell (temporal) arteritis is a chronic inflammatory disorder, typically with granulomatous inflammation, that principally affects large to medium-sized arteries in the head. The temporal arteries are not more vulnerable than other arteries but have given their name to the disorder because the diagnosis is typically established by biopsy of these vessels. Vertebral and ophthalmic arteries, as well as the aorta *(giant cell aortitis),* are other common sites of involvement. Because ophthalmic artery vasculitis can lead to sudden and permanent blindness, affected individuals must be promptly diagnosed and treated. It is the most common form of vasculitis in the US. Older age and North European descent are risk factors.

Pathogenesis. **Giant cell arteritis likely occurs as a result of a T cell–mediated immune response to an as-yet uncharacterized vessel wall antigen.** The characteristic granulomatous inflammation, an association with certain MHC class II alleles, and the excellent therapeutic response to steroids, all strongly support a T cell–mediated

injury. Both Th1 and Th17 pathways are involved; in keeping with this, high levels of IFN-γ and IL-17 can be detected in the walls of affected vessels. The predilection for vessels of the head remains unexplained.

> ## MORPHOLOGY
>
> In giant cell arteritis, the pathologic changes are notoriously patchy along the length of affected vessels. Involved arterial segments exhibit nodular intimal thickening (and occasional thromboses) that reduce the vessel diameter and cause distal ischemia. The majority of lesions exhibit **granulomatous inflammation** within the inner media; there is an infiltrate of T lymphocytes and macrophages, with multinucleate giant cells. Inflammation of the vascular wall causes **loss of vascular smooth muscle cells and fragmentation of the internal elastic lamina** (Fig. 8.21). In up to 25% of cases, granulomas and giant cells are absent, and lesions exhibit only nonspecific panarteritis with acute and chronic inflammation. Healing is marked by intimal thickening, medial thinning and scarring, and adventitial fibrosis. Characteristically, lesions at different stages of development are seen within the same artery.

Clinical Features. Temporal arteritis is rare before 50 years of age. Signs and symptoms may be vague and constitutional (e.g., fever, fatigue, weight loss) or take the form of facial pain or headache, most intense along the course of the superficial temporal artery, which is painful to palpation. Ocular symptoms (associated with involvement of the ophthalmic artery) appear abruptly in about 50% of patients; these range from diplopia to complete vision loss. Diagnosis depends on biopsy and histology; however, because the vascular inflammation is patchy, a negative biopsy result does not exclude the diagnosis. Corticosteroids are the mainstay of treatment. Anti-IL-6 therapy is useful in those who are resistant to steroids.

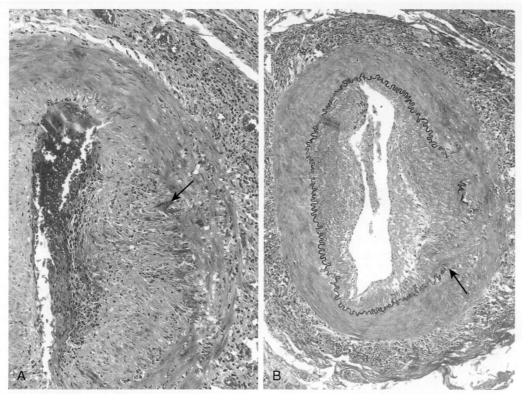

FIG. 8.21 Giant cell arteritis. (A) Hematoxylin-eosin-stained section of a temporal artery showing giant cells near the fragmented internal elastic membrane *(arrow)*, along with medial and adventitial inflammation. (B) Elastic tissue stain demonstrating focal destruction of the internal elastic membrane *(arrow)* and medial attenuation and scarring.

Takayasu Arteritis

Takayasu arteritis is a granulomatous vasculitis of medium- and large-sized arteries characterized principally by ocular disturbances and marked weakening of the pulses in the upper extremities (hence the alternate name, *pulseless disease*). This disorder manifests with transmural scarring and thickening of the aorta—particularly the aortic arch and great vessels—with severe luminal narrowing of the major branch vessels (Fig. 8.22). Aortic lesions share many of the clinical and histologic features of giant cell aortitis. Indeed, the distinction between the two entities is made largely on the basis of the patient's age: those older than 50 years of age are said to have *giant cell arteritis* while lesions that occur in those younger than 50 years of age are designated *Takayasu arteritis*. Although historically associated with Japanese ethnicity and certain HLA alleles, Takayasu arteritis has a global distribution. An autoimmune etiology is likely. As with giant cell arteritis, it is a T cell–mediated disease.

MORPHOLOGY

Takayasu arteritis classically affects the aortic arch and arch vessels; one-third of cases also involve the remainder of the aorta and its branches. The abdominal aorta and pulmonary arteries are involved in 50% of patients; renal and coronary arteries can also be affected. The origins of the great vessels can be markedly narrowed and even obliterated (see Fig. 8.22A and B), explaining the upper-extremity weakness and faint carotid pulses. The histologic picture (see Fig. 8.22C) encompasses a spectrum ranging from adventitial mononuclear infiltrates and perivascular cuffing of the vasa vasorum, to intense transmural mononuclear inflammation, to granulomatous inflammation, replete with giant cells and patchy medial necrosis. The inflammation is associated with irregular thickening of the vessel wall, intimal hyperplasia, and adventitial fibrosis.

Clinical Features. Initial signs and symptoms are usually nonspecific, including fatigue, weight loss, and fever. With progression, vascular signs and symptoms appear and dominate the clinical picture. These include reduced upper-extremity blood pressure and pulse strength; neurologic deficits; and ocular disturbances, including visual field defects, retinal hemorrhages, and blindness. Involvement of the distal aorta can manifest as leg claudication, and pulmonary artery involvement can cause pulmonary hypertension. Narrowing of the coronary ostia can lead to myocardial infarction, and involvement of the renal arteries causes systemic hypertension in roughly one-half of patients. The course of the disease is variable. Some cases rapidly progress, while others become quiescent after 1 to 2 years. In the latter scenario, long-term survival, albeit with visual or neurologic deficits, is possible.

Medium Vessel Vasculitis

Polyarteritis Nodosa

Polyarteritis nodosa (PAN) is a systemic vasculitis of small or medium-sized muscular arteries; it typically involves the renal and visceral vessels and spares the pulmonary circulation. There is no association with ANCAs, but up to one-third of patients have chronic hepatitis B infection, which leads to the formation of immune

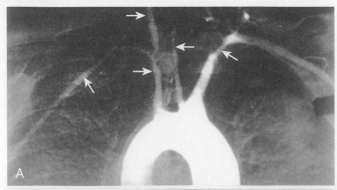

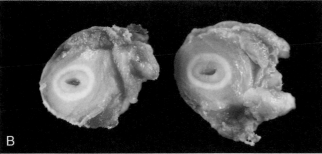

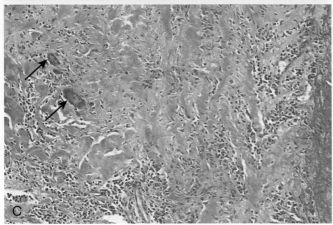

FIG. 8.22 Takayasu arteritis. (A) Aortic arch angiogram showing reduced flow of contrast material into the great vessels and narrowing of the brachiocephalic, carotid, and subclavian arteries *(arrows)*. (B) Cross-sections of the right carotid artery from the patient shown in A demonstrating marked intimal thickening and luminal narrowing. The *white circles* correspond to the original vessel wall; the inner core of tan tissue is the area of intimal hyperplasia. (C) Histologic appearance in active Takayasu aortitis illustrating destruction and fibrosis of the arterial media associated with mononuclear infiltrates and giant cells *(arrows)*.

complexes containing hepatitis B antigens that deposit in affected vessels. Hepatitis C is also an antecedent in some cases but less commonly than is hepatitis B. The cause is unknown in the remaining cases.

MORPHOLOGY

Classic PAN is a **segmental transmural necrotizing inflammation** of small to medium-sized arteries, often with superimposed thrombosis. Kidney, heart, liver, and gastrointestinal tract vessels are affected in descending order of frequency. Lesions usually involve only part of the vessel wall and have a predilection for branch points. Of note, glomeruli are spared. Impaired perfusion may lead to ulcerations, infarcts, ischemic atrophy, or

hemorrhages in the distribution of affected vessels. The inflammatory process also weakens the arterial wall, leading to aneurysms and rupture.

In the acute phase, there is a transmural mixed inflammatory infiltrate composed of neutrophils and mononuclear cells, frequently accompanied by **fibrinoid necrosis** and luminal thrombosis (Fig. 8.23). Older lesions show fibrous thickening of the vessel wall extending into the adventitia. Characteristically, all stages of activity (from early to late) coexist in different vessels or even within the same vessel, suggesting ongoing and recurrent immunologically mediated insults.

Clinical Features. PAN is primarily a disease of young adults but also occurs in middle or older adults. The clinical course is typically episodic, with long symptom-free intervals. The systemic findings—malaise, fever, and weight loss—are nonspecific, and the vascular involvement is widely scattered, so the clinical manifestations can be varied and puzzling. The "classic" presentation manifests itself with some combination of rapidly accelerating hypertension due to renal artery involvement; abdominal pain and bloody stools caused by gastrointestinal lesions; diffuse muscular aches and pains; and peripheral neuritis, predominantly affecting motor nerves. Renal involvement is often prominent and is a major cause of death. Untreated, PAN is typically fatal; however, with immunosuppression, 5-year survival is close to 80%. Relapse occurs in up to 25% of cases, more often in non—HBV-associated cases than those that follow HBV infection. The latter have a better long-term prognosis.

Kawasaki Disease

Kawasaki disease is an acute, febrile, usually self-limited illness of infancy and childhood associated with an arteritis of mainly large to medium-sized vessels. Less commonly, aorta and large arteries may be involved. The vast majority of patients are younger than 5 years of age. Its clinical significance stems from the involvement of coronary arteries. Coronary arteritis can result in aneurysms that rupture or thrombose, causing myocardial infarction. Originally described in Japan, Kawasaki disease has a global distribution but is more common

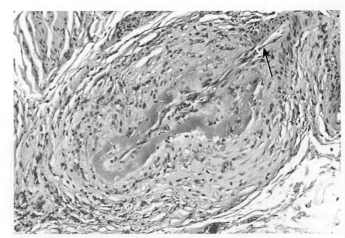

FIG. 8.23 Polyarteritis nodosa, associated with segmental fibrinoid necrosis and thrombotic occlusion of a small artery. Note that part of the vessel *(upper-right, arrow)* is uninvolved. (Courtesy of Sidney Murphree, MD, Department of Pathology, University of Texas Southwestern Medical School, Dallas, Texas.)

in children of east Asian descent. Although genetic factors are suspected, no clear genetic mechanism has been identified.

In genetically susceptible individuals, a variety of infectious agents (mostly viral) have been postulated to trigger the disease. Most recently, a Kawasaki-like disease has been documented in children infected with SARS-CoV-2. The precise pathogenesis of Kawasaki disease remains unknown. It is suspected that the vasculitis results from a delayed-type hypersensitivity response directed against cross-reactive or newly uncovered vascular antigen(s). Subsequent cytokine production and B-cell activation result in autoantibodies to ECs and SMCs that precipitate the vasculitis.

MORPHOLOGY

The vasculitis resembles that seen in polyarteritis nodosa. There is a **dense transmural inflammatory infiltrate,** although fibrinoid necrosis is usually less prominent than in PAN. The vasculitis usually subsides spontaneously or in response to treatment, but aneurysm formation due to wall damage may supervene. As with other arteritides, healing may be accompanied by the development of obstructive intimal thickening. Pathologic changes outside the cardiovascular system are rarely significant except when it occurs in association with SARS-CoV-2 infection. In the latter, many organs are involved.

Clinical Features. Kawasaki disease typically manifests with conjunctival and oral erythema and blistering, edema of the hands and feet, erythema of the palms and soles, a desquamative rash, and cervical lymph node enlargement (hence its other name, *mucocutaneous lymph node syndrome*). Approximately 20% of untreated patients develop cardiovascular sequelae, ranging from asymptomatic coronary arteritis, to coronary artery ectasia, to coronary artery aneurysms (7 to 8 mm in diameter); the latter may be associated with rupture, thrombosis, myocardial infarction, and/or sudden death. Treatment consists of intravenous immunoglobulin infusions (which suppress inflammation through unclear mechanisms) and aspirin, which when given with the former markedly decrease the incidence of symptomatic coronary artery disease.

Small Vessel Vasculitis

This group includes two pathogenetically distinct subgroups: ANCA-associated vasculitis and immune complex—associated vasculitis (see Table 8.3). Only some of the more common entities are described in this section.

Microscopic Polyangiitis

Microscopic polyangiitis is a necrotizing vasculitis that generally affects capillaries, small arterioles, and venules. It is also called *hypersensitivity vasculitis* or *leukocytoclastic vasculitis*. Unlike in PAN, all lesions of microscopic polyangiitis tend to be of the same age in any given patient. The skin, mucous membranes, lungs, brain, heart, gastrointestinal tract, kidneys, and muscle can all be involved; *necrotizing glomerulonephritis* (seen in 90% of patients) and *pulmonary capillaritis* are particularly common.

Most cases of microscopic polyangiitis are associated with MPO-ANCA. Recruitment and activation of neutrophils within affected vascular beds are probably responsible for the disease manifestations. Immune complexes are absent. Pathogenesis is unknown. In some cases drugs such as hydralazine and microbes (*S. aureus*) are suspected to trigger the disease.

MORPHOLOGY

Microscopic polyangiitis is characterized by segmental fibrinoid necrosis of the media with **focal transmural necrotizing lesions;** granulomatous inflammation is absent. These lesions resemble those of polyarteritis nodosa but spare medium- and large-sized arteries, so macroscopic infarcts are uncommon. In some areas (typically postcapillary venules), only infiltrating neutrophils undergoing nuclear fragmentation (karyorrhexis) are seen, giving rise to the term *leukocytoclastic vasculitis* (Fig. 8.24A). Although immunoglobulins and complement components can be demonstrated in early skin lesions, most lesions are "pauci-immune" (i.e., show little or no antibody).

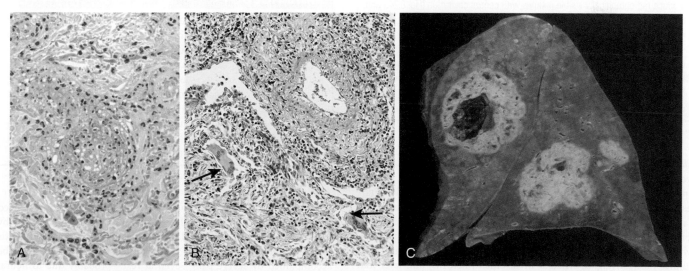

FIG. 8.24 ANCA-associated small vessel vasculitis. (A) Microscopic polyangiitis (leukocytoclastic vasculitis) with fragmented neutrophils in the thickened vessel wall. (B and C) Granulomatosis with polyangiitis. (B) Vasculitis of a small artery with adjacent granulomatous inflammation including giant cells *(arrows)*. (C) Lung from a patient with granulomatosis with polyangiitis, demonstrating large nodular cavitating lesions. (A, Courtesy of Scott Granter, MD, Brigham and Women's Hospital, Boston, Massachusetts. C, Courtesy of Sidney Murphree, MD, Department of Pathology, University of Texas Southwestern Medical School, Dallas, Texas.)

Clinical Features. This disease typically occurs in older adults, although children can also be affected. Depending on the vascular bed involved, major features include hemoptysis, hematuria, proteinuria, abdominal pain or bleeding, muscle pain or weakness, and palpable cutaneous purpura. With the exception of patients with widespread renal or CNS involvement, immunosuppression and removal of the offending agent (most often a drug) induce durable remissions.

Granulomatosis With Polyangiitis

Previously called *Wegener granulomatosis,* granulomatosis with polyangiitis is an ANCA-positive necrotizing vasculitis characterized by the following triad:

- *Necrotizing granulomas* of the upper respiratory tract (ear, nose, sinuses, throat), the lower respiratory tract (lung), or both
- *Necrotizing or granulomatous vasculitis* affecting small to medium-sized vessels (e.g., capillaries, venules, arterioles, and arteries), most prominently the lungs and upper airways but other sites as well
- *Focal necrotizing, often crescentic, glomerulonephritis*

"Limited" forms of disease can be restricted to the respiratory tract. Conversely, when widespread the disease may affect the eyes, skin, and other organs, most notably the heart; clinically, widespread vasculitis resembles PAN with the additional feature of respiratory involvement.

Granulomatosis polyangiitis is likely initiated as a cell-mediated hypersensitivity response to inhaled infectious or environmental antigens. PR3-ANCAs are present in almost 95% of cases and probably drive the tissue injury. The ANCA level is also a useful marker of disease activity, as antibody titers fall dramatically with effective immunosuppressive therapy and rise prior to disease relapse.

MORPHOLOGY

Upper respiratory tract lesions include **granulomatous sinusitis** and **ulcerated lesions** of the nose, palate, or pharynx; lung findings also vary, ranging from diffuse parenchymal infiltrates to granulomatous nodules. There is multifocal necrotizing **granulomatous vasculitis** with a surrounding fibroblastic proliferation (Fig. 8.24B). Multiple granulomas can coalesce to produce radiographically visible nodules with central cavitation (Fig. 8.24B and C). Destruction of vessels can lead to hemorrhage and hemoptysis. Lesions can ultimately undergo progressive fibrosis and organization.

The **renal lesions** range from mild, focal glomerular necrosis associated with thrombosis of isolated glomerular capillary loops **(focal and segmental necrotizing glomerulonephritis)** to more advanced glomerular lesions with diffuse necrosis and parietal cell proliferation forming epithelial crescents **(crescentic glomerulonephritis)** (Chapter 12).

Clinical Features. The typical patient is a middle-aged man, although women and individuals of other ages can be affected. Classic presentations include bilateral pneumonitis with nodules and cavitary lesions (95%), chronic sinusitis (90%), mucosal ulcerations of the nasopharynx (75%), and renal disease (80%). Patients with mild renal involvement may demonstrate only hematuria and proteinuria, whereas more severe disease may portend rapidly progressive renal failure. Rash, myalgias, articular involvement, neuritis, and fever may also occur. If untreated, the mortality rate at 1 year is 80%. Treatment with steroids, cyclophosphamide, TNF inhibitors, and anti–B-cell antibodies (rituximab) has improved this picture considerably. Most patients with GPA now survive but remain at high risk for relapses that may ultimately lead to renal failure.

Eosinophilic Granulomatosis With Polyangiitis (Churg-Strauss Syndrome)

Eosinophilic granulomatosis with polyangiitis is a small-vessel necrotizing vasculitis associated with asthma, allergic rhinitis, lung infiltrates, peripheral eosinophilia, extravascular necrotizing granulomas, and a striking infiltration of vessels and perivascular tissues by eosinophils. It is a rare disorder, affecting 1 in 1 million individuals. Cutaneous involvement (with palpable purpura), gastrointestinal bleeding, and renal disease (primarily as focal and segmental glomerulosclerosis) are the major findings. Cytotoxicity secondary to myocardial eosinophilic infiltrates often leads to cardiomyopathy; cardiac involvement is seen in 60% of patients and is a major cause of morbidity and death.

This form of vasculitis may stem from "hyperresponsiveness" to some usually innocuous allergic stimulus. MPO-ANCAs are present in close to half of the cases and hence are classified as an ANCA-associated vasculitis. ANCA-positive cases more commonly have glomerulonephritis. The vascular lesions differ from those of PAN or microscopic polyangiitis by virtue of the presence of granulomas and eosinophils.

Thromboangiitis Obliterans (Buerger Disease)

Thromboangiitis obliterans is characterized by segmental, thrombosing, acute and chronic inflammation of medium- and small-sized arteries, principally the tibial and radial arteries, with occasional secondary extension into the veins and nerves of the extremities. Visceral vessels are rarely involved. Thromboangiitis obliterans occurs almost exclusively in heavy tobacco smokers and usually develops before 35 years of age. Endothelial dysfunction including reduced endothelium-dependent vasodilation and release of prothrombotic substances has been found. Direct EC toxicity caused by some component of tobacco is suspected; alternatively, a reactive compound in tobacco may modify vessel wall components and induce an immune response. Indeed, most patients are hypersensitive to tobacco extracts. An association has been seen with certain HLA haplotypes suggesting a genetic predisposition.

MORPHOLOGY

Thromboangiitis obliterans is characterized by a **sharply segmental acute and chronic vasculitis of medium- and small-sized arteries accompanied by luminal thrombosis** affecting predominantly vessels of the extremities. In the early stages, mixed inflammatory infiltrates are accompanied by luminal thrombosis; small microabscesses, occasionally rimmed by granulomatous inflammation, also may be present (Fig. 8.25). The inflammation then extends outward, sometimes into contiguous veins and nerves (a feature that is rare in other forms of vasculitis). With time, thrombi can organize and recanalize, and eventually the artery and adjacent structures become encased in fibrous tissue.

Clinical Features. Early manifestations include cold-induced Raynaud phenomenon (see later), instep foot pain induced by exercise *(instep claudication),* and superficial nodular phlebitis (venous inflammation). The vascular insufficiency tends to be accompanied by severe pain—even at rest—probably due to neural involvement. Chronic extremity ulcerations may develop, progressing over time to gangrene. Smoking abstinence in the early stages of the disease often ameliorates further attacks; however, once established, the vascular lesions do not respond to smoking abstinence.

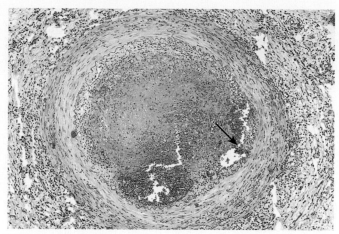

FIG. 8.25 Thromboangiitis obliterans (Buerger disease). The lumen is occluded by thrombus containing a sterile abscess *(arrow)*, and the vessel wall is infiltrated with leukocytes.

Infectious Vasculitis

Localized arteritis may be caused by the direct invasion of arteries by infectious agents, usually bacteria or fungi, and in particular *Aspergillus* and *Mucor* spp. Vascular invasion may be part of a nearby local tissue infection (e.g., bacterial pneumonia or an adjacent abscess), or—less commonly—may arise from hematogenous spread of bacteria or embolization from infective endocarditis.

Vascular infections may weaken arterial walls and give rise to *mycotic aneurysms* described earlier or may induce thrombosis and infarction. Thus, inflammation of vessels in bacterial meningitis can cause thrombosis and infarction, ultimately leading to extension of a subarachnoid infection into the brain parenchyma.

DISORDERS OF BLOOD VESSEL HYPERREACTIVITY

Several disorders are characterized by inappropriate or exaggerated vasoconstriction of blood vessels.

Raynaud Phenomenon

Raynaud phenomenon is an exaggerated vasoconstrictive response to cold temperature and emotional stress. It affects arteries and arterioles in the extremities, particularly the fingers and toes, but also sometimes the nose, earlobes, or lips. The involved digits change color according to a temporal sequence reflecting initial vasoconstriction, subsequent tissue anoxia, and eventual return of oxygenated blood due to warming. While in fair skin types the accompanying color changes may transition from white (due to vasoconstriction), to blue (anoxia), and then red (reperfusion), in individuals of darker skin types color change may appear as pallor (vasoconstriction), to purple (anoxia), and finally pink to dull red (reperfusion). Raynaud phenomenon can be a primary entity or may be secondary to other disorders.

Primary Raynaud phenomenon occurs in the absence of any associated disorders; it affects 3% to 5% of the general population and has a predilection for young women. The course usually is benign, but in chronic cases, atrophy of the skin, subcutaneous tissues, and muscles may occur. Ulceration and ischemic gangrene are rare.

Secondary Raynaud phenomenon refers to vascular insufficiency due to arterial disease caused by other entities including systemic lupus erythematosus, scleroderma, thromboangiitis obliterans, or even atherosclerosis. Indeed, since Raynaud phenomenon may be the first manifestation of such conditions, every patient with Raynaud phenomenon should be evaluated for these secondary causes.

VEINS AND LYMPHATICS

Varicose veins and phlebothrombosis/thrombophlebitis account for over 90% of cases of clinically relevant venous disease.

Varicose Veins of the Extremities

Varicose veins are abnormally dilated, tortuous veins caused by chronically increased intraluminal pressures and weakened vessel wall support. The superficial veins of the upper and lower leg typically are involved. Up to one-fifth of men and one-third of women develop lower-extremity varicose veins. Obesity increases the risk as does pregnancy due to compression of the inferior vena cava by the gravid uterus. There is also a familial tendency toward premature varicosities.

Clinical Features. Varicose dilation renders the venous valves incompetent and leads to lower-extremity stasis, congestion, edema, pain, and thrombosis. The most disabling sequelae include persistent edema in the extremity and secondary ischemic skin changes, including stasis dermatitis and ulcerations. The latter can become chronic varicose ulcers as a consequence of poor wound healing and superimposed infections. Of note, embolism from these superficial veins is very rare, in contrast with the relatively frequent emboli that arise from thrombosed deep veins (Chapter 3).

Varicosities of Other Sites

Venous dilations in two other sites merit special attention:

- *Esophageal varices.* Liver cirrhosis (and, less frequently, portal vein obstruction or hepatic vein thrombosis) causes portal venous hypertension (Chapter 14). This, in turn, leads to the opening of portosystemic shunts and increased blood flow into veins in several locations: (1) the gastroesophageal junction (forming esophageal varices); (2) the rectum (forming hemorrhoids); and (3) the periumbilical veins of the abdominal wall (forming a caput medusae). Esophageal varices are the most important clinically since they are prone to ruptures that can lead to massive (even fatal) upper gastrointestinal hemorrhage.
- *Hemorrhoids* are varicose dilations of the venous plexus at the anorectal junction that result from prolonged pelvic vascular congestion associated with pregnancy or straining to defecate. Hemorrhoids are a source of bleeding and are prone to thrombosis and painful ulceration.

Thrombophlebitis and Phlebothrombosis

Thrombosis of deep leg veins accounts for more than 90% of cases of thrombophlebitis and phlebothrombosis. These two terms are largely interchangeable designations for venous thrombosis accompanied by inflammation. Pulmonary embolism is a common and serious clinical complication of deep vein thrombosis of the legs. The pathogenesis and clinical features of deep vein thrombosis have been discussed in detail in Chapters 3 and 11.

Superior and Inferior Vena Cava Syndromes

Superior vena cava syndrome is usually caused by neoplasms that compress or invade the superior vena cava, such as bronchial carcinoma or mediastinal lymphoma. The resulting obstruction produces a characteristic clinical complex consisting of marked dilation of the veins of the head, neck, and arms associated with cyanosis. Findings are typically more pronounced in the morning due to overnight pooling of blood during rest. Pulmonary vessels can also be compressed, causing respiratory distress.

Inferior vena cava syndrome can be caused by neoplasms that compress or invade the inferior vena cava or by a thrombus that has propagated from the hepatic, renal, or lower-extremity veins. Certain neoplasms—particularly hepatocellular carcinoma and renal cell carcinoma—show a striking tendency to grow within veins, and these tumors may ultimately occlude the inferior vena cava. Obstruction of the inferior vena cava induces marked lower-extremity edema, distention of the superficial collateral veins of the lower abdomen, and—with renal vein involvement—marked proteinuria.

Lymphangitis and Lymphedema

Primary disorders of lymphatic vessels are extremely uncommon. Much more commonly, lymphatic vessels are secondarily involved by inflammatory, infectious, or malignant processes.

Lymphangitis refers to acute inflammation caused by bacterial entry in the lymphatic vessels (Chapter 2). Clinically, the inflamed lymphatics appear as red, painful subcutaneous streaks, usually associated with tender enlargement of draining lymph nodes (acute lymphadenitis). If the bacteria are not trapped within the lymph nodes, they can pass into the venous circulation and cause bacteremia or sepsis.

Primary *lymphedema* may occur as an isolated congenital anomaly (simple congenital lymphedema or as the familial *Milroy disease* [heredofamilial congenital lymphedema]), resulting from agenesis or hypoplasia of lymphatics. Secondary or obstructive lymphedema is caused by the accumulation of interstitial fluid in an obstructed, previously normal lymphatic; such obstruction can result from the following disorders or conditions:

- *Tumors* involving either the lymphatic channels or the regional lymph nodes
- *Surgical procedures* that sever lymphatic connections (e.g., axillary lymph nodes in mastectomy)
- *Postradiation fibrosis*
- *Filariasis*
- *Postinflammatory thrombosis* and scarring

Regardless of the cause, lymphedema increases the hydrostatic pressure in the lymphatics distal to the obstruction and causes edema. Chronic edema in turn may lead to deposition of ECM and fibrosis, producing brawny induration or a *peau d'orange* appearance of the overlying skin (as may occur in the skin overlying a breast carcinoma that extensively involves lymphatic channels). Eventually, inadequate tissue perfusion may lead to skin ulceration. Rupture of dilated lymphatics, typically following obstruction by an infiltrating tumor mass, can lead to milky accumulations of lymph in various spaces designated *chylous ascites* (abdomen), *chylothorax,* and *chylopericardium.*

TUMORS

Tumors of blood vessels and lymphatics include benign hemangiomas (common), locally aggressive neoplasms that metastasize infrequently, and rare, highly malignant angiosarcomas (Table 8.4).

Vascular neoplasms arise either from endothelium (e.g., hemangioma, lymphangioma, angiosarcoma) or cells that support or surround blood vessels (e.g., glomus tumor). Primary tumors of large vessels (e.g., aorta, pulmonary artery, and vena cava) occur infrequently and are mostly sarcomas. Although a benign hemangioma

Table 8.4 Classification of Vascular Tumors and Tumorlike Conditions

Benign Neoplasms: Developmental and Acquired Conditions
Hemangioma
Capillary hemangioma
Cavernous hemangioma
Pyogenic granuloma
Lymphangioma
Simple (capillary) lymphangioma
Cavernous lymphangioma (cystic hygroma)
Glomus tumor
Reactive vascular proliferations
Bacillary angiomatosis
Intermediate-Grade Neoplasms
Kaposi sarcoma
Hemangioendothelioma
Malignant Neoplasms
Angiosarcoma

cannot be confused with an anaplastic angiosarcoma, lesions of uncertain malignancy are sometimes observed. Congenital or developmental malformations and nonneoplastic reactive vascular proliferations (e.g., *bacillary angiomatosis*) can also manifest as tumorlike lesions that may present diagnostic challenges. In general, benign and malignant vascular neoplasms are distinguished by the following features:

- Benign tumors are usually composed of well-formed vascular channels filled with blood cells or lymph that are lined by a monolayer of bland ECs.
- Malignant tumors are more cellular, show cytologic atypia, are proliferative, and usually do not form well-organized vessels; confirmation of the endothelial derivation of such proliferations may require immunohistochemical detection of EC-specific markers.

Benign Tumors and Tumorlike Conditions

Vascular Ectasias

Ectasia is a generic term for any local dilation of a structure, while *telangiectasia* is used to describe a permanent dilation of preexisting small vessels (e.g., capillaries, venules, and arterioles, usually in the skin or mucous membranes) that forms a discrete red lesion. These lesions can be congenital or acquired and are not true neoplasms.

- *Nevus flammeus* (a "birthmark"), the most common form of vascular ectasia, is a light pink to deep purple, flat lesion on the head or neck composed of dilated vessels. Most regress spontaneously over time.
- The so-called "port wine stain" is a particular form of nevus flammeus. These lesions tend to grow during childhood and thicken the skin surface; they do not regress. Such lesions occurring in the distribution of the trigeminal nerve are associated with the *Sturge-Weber syndrome* (also called encephalotrigeminal angiomatosis). This uncommon congenital disorder is associated with facial port wine nevi, ipsilateral venous angiomas in the cortical leptomeninges, mental disability, seizures, hemiplegia, and radiologic opacities of the skull. Thus, a large facial telangiectasia in a child with mental disability may indicate the presence of additional vascular malformations.

- *Spider telangiectasias* are nonneoplastic vascular lesions. These lesions manifest as radial, often pulsatile arrays of dilated subcutaneous arteries or arterioles (the "legs" of the spider) about a central core (the spider's "body") that blanch with pressure. Spider telangiectasias commonly occur on the face, neck, or upper chest and are most frequently associated with hyperestrogenic states (e.g., in pregnant women or patients with cirrhosis).

- *Hereditary hemorrhagic telangiectasia (Osler-Weber-Rendu disease)* is an autosomal dominant disorder caused by mutations in genes that encode components of the TGF-β signaling pathway in ECs. The telangiectasias are malformations composed of dilated capillaries and veins that are present at birth. They are widely distributed over the skin and oral mucous membranes, as well as in the respiratory, gastrointestinal, and urinary tracts. The lesions can spontaneously rupture, causing serious epistaxis (nosebleed), gastrointestinal bleeding, or hematuria.

Hemangiomas

Hemangiomas are common tumors composed of blood-filled vessels (see also Chapter 4). They constitute 7% of all benign tumors of infancy and childhood; most are present from birth and, after an initial increase in size, regress spontaneously. While hemangiomas are typically localized lesions confined to the head and neck, they occasionally are more extensive *(angiomatosis)* or arise internally. Nearly one-third of the internal lesions are found in the liver. Malignant transformation is extremely rare. Several histologic and clinical variants have been described:

- *Capillary hemangiomas* are the most common type; these occur in the skin, subcutaneous tissues, and mucous membranes of the oral cavities and lips, as well as in the liver, spleen, and kidneys (Fig. 8.26A). Histologically, they are composed of thin-walled capillaries with scant stroma (Fig. 8.26B).

- *Infantile hemangiomas* of the skin are extremely common and can be multiple. They grow rapidly for a few months but then begin to involute by 1 to 3 years of age, and completely regress by 7 years of age in the vast majority of cases.

- *Pyogenic granulomas* are capillary proliferations of uncertain etiology that manifest as rapidly growing red pedunculated lesions on the skin, or gingiva or oral mucosa. Microscopically they resemble exuberant granulation tissue. They bleed easily and often ulcerate (Fig. 8.26C). Roughly one-fourth of the lesions develop after trauma, reaching a size of 1 to 2 cm within a few weeks. Curettage and cautery are usually curative. They are seen at all ages, most commonly in the second and third decades. Pyogenic granulomas of the gingiva occasionally occur in women who are pregnant. These lesions may spontaneously regress (especially after pregnancy) or undergo fibrosis but occasionally require surgical excision.

- *Cavernous hemangiomas* are composed of large, dilated vascular channels. Compared with capillary hemangiomas, cavernous hemangiomas are more infiltrative, frequently involve deep structures, and do not spontaneously regress. Although they may affect any tissue, the liver is a common site. Most are asymptomatic and are found by imaging studies performed for other reasons. On

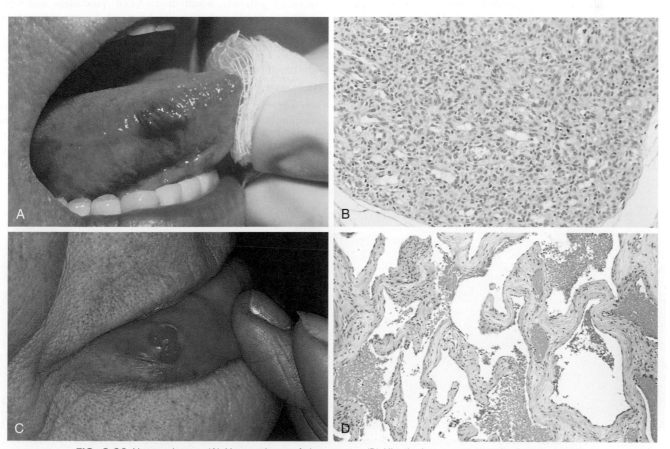

FIG. 8.26 Hemangiomas. (A) Hemangioma of the tongue. (B) Histologic appearance of infantile capillary hemangioma. (C) Pyogenic granuloma of the lip. (D) Histologic appearance of cavernous hemangioma. (A and D, Courtesy of John Sexton, MD, Beth Israel Hospital, Boston, Massachusetts. B, Courtesy of Christopher D.M. Fletcher, MD, Brigham and Women's Hospital, Boston, Massachusetts. C, Courtesy of Thomas Rogers, MD, University of Texas Southwestern Medical School, Dallas, Texas.)

histologic examination, the mass is sharply defined but unencapsulated and is composed of large blood-filled vascular spaces separated by connective tissue stroma (Fig. 8.26D). Intravascular thrombosis and dystrophic calcification are common. Brain hemangiomas are problematic because of symptoms related to compression of adjacent tissue and the possibility of rupture. Cavernous hemangiomas constitute one component of *von Hippel-Lindau disease* (Chapter 21), in which vascular lesions are commonly found in the cerebellum, brain stem, retina, pancreas, and liver. In some cases, cerebral cavernous hemangiomas are familial, caused by mutations in one of three tumor suppressor genes called *CCM1, CCM2,* and *CCM3.* Genetic testing should be performed if there are multiple lesions.

Lymphangiomas

Lymphangiomas are the benign lymphatic counterpart of hemangiomas and are much less frequent than hemangiomas.

- *Simple (capillary) lymphangiomas* are slightly elevated or sometimes pedunculated lesions up to 1 to 2 cm in diameter that occur predominantly in the head, neck, and axillary subcutaneous tissues. Histologically, lymphangiomas are composed of networks of endothelium-lined spaces that are distinguished from capillary channels only by the absence of blood cells.
- *Cavernous lymphangiomas (cystic hygromas)* are typically found in the neck or axilla of children, and more rarely in the retroperitoneum. Cavernous lymphangiomas of the neck are common in Turner syndrome. They can be large (up to 15 cm), filling the axilla or producing gross deformities of the neck. Cavernous lymphangiomas are composed of massively dilated lymphatic spaces lined by ECs and separated by intervening connective tissue stroma containing lymphoid aggregates. The tumor margins are indistinct and unencapsulated, making definitive resection difficult.

Glomus Tumors (Glomangiomas)

Glomus tumors are benign, exquisitely painful tumors arising from specialized SMCs of glomus bodies, arteriovenous structures involved in thermoregulation. Distinction from hemangiomas is based on clinical features and immunohistochemical staining for smooth muscle markers. They are most commonly found in the distal portion of the digits, especially under the fingernails. Excision is curative. Malignant glomus tumors are very rare; they are more deeply situated and locally invasive.

Bacillary Angiomatosis

Bacillary angiomatosis is a rare vascular proliferation in patients who are immunocompromised (e.g., patients with AIDS or solid organ transplants and a CD4 count <100); it is caused by opportunistic gram-negative bacilli of the *Bartonella* family. The lesions can involve the skin, bone, brain, and other organs. Two bacterial species have been implicated:

- *Bartonella henselae,* whose principal reservoir is the domestic cat; this organism causes cat-scratch disease (a necrotizing granulomatous inflammation of lymph nodes) in immunocompetent hosts.
- *Bartonella quintana,* which is transmitted by human body lice; this microbe was the cause of "trench fever" in World War I.

Skin lesions bleed easily and take the form of red papules and nodules or rounded subcutaneous masses. Clinically, the lesions can mimic Kaposi sarcoma (see later). Histologically, there is a proliferation of capillaries lined by prominent epithelioid ECs, which exhibit nuclear atypia and mitoses (Fig. 8.27). Other features include infiltrating neutrophils, nuclear debris, and purplish granular collections of the causative bacteria.

The bacteria induce host tissues to produce hypoxia-inducible factor-1α (HIF-1α), which drives VEGF production and vascular proliferation. The infections (and lesions) are cured by antibiotic treatment.

Intermediate-Grade (Borderline) Tumors

Kaposi Sarcoma

Kaposi sarcoma (KS) is a vascular neoplasm caused by Kaposi sarcoma herpesvirus (KSHV, also known as human herpesvirus 8 [HHV8]). Although it occurs in a number of contexts, it is most common in patients with AIDS; indeed, its presence is used as a criterion for the diagnosis. While it occurs in patients with AIDS, it is not

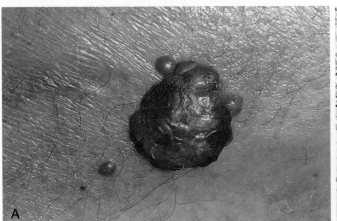
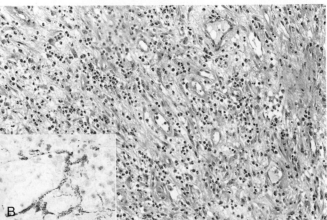

FIG. 8.27 Bacillary angiomatosis. (A) Characteristic cutaneous lesion. (B) Histologic features are those of acute inflammation and capillary proliferation. *Inset,* Modified silver (Warthin-Starry) stain demonstrates clusters of tangled bacilli *(black).* (A, Courtesy of Richard Johnson, MD, Beth Israel Deaconess Medical Center, Boston, Massachusetts. B and inset, courtesy of Scott Granter, MD, Brigham and Women's Hospital, Boston, Massachusetts.)

caused by HIV. Four forms of KS, based on population demographics and risks, are recognized:

- *Classic KS* has a worldwide distribution but is most common in individuals of Central and Eastern European and Mediterranean ancestry. It is a disease of older men and is uncommon in the United States. It can be associated with other malignancies or altered immunity. Classic KS manifests as multiple red-purple skin plaques or nodules, usually on the distal lower extremities; these progressively increase in size and number and spread proximally. Although persistent, the tumors are typically asymptomatic and remain localized to the skin and subcutaneous tissue.

- *Endemic African KS* occurs in equatorial, particularly sub-Saharan, Africa in younger (under 40 years of age) HIV-seronegative individuals and can follow an indolent or aggressive course; it involves lymph nodes much more frequently than the classic variant. A particularly severe form, with prominent lymph node and visceral involvement, occurs in prepubertal children; the prognosis is poor, with an almost 100% mortality within 3 years.

- *Transplantation-associated KS* occurs in solid organ transplant recipients in the setting of T-cell immunosuppression. In these patients, the risk for KS is increased 100-fold. The disease pursues an aggressive course and often involves lymph nodes, mucosa, and viscera; cutaneous lesions may be absent. Lesions often regress with attenuation of immunosuppression, but at the risk for organ rejection.

- *AIDS-associated (epidemic) KS* is an AIDS-defining illness; worldwide it represents the most common HIV-related malignancy (Chapter 5). Although the incidence of KS has fallen greatly with the advent of highly active antiretroviral therapy, it still occurs far more commonly in individuals infected with HIV than in the general population. AIDS-associated KS often involves lymph nodes and disseminates widely to viscera early in its course. Most patients eventually die of opportunistic infections rather than from KS.

Pathogenesis. **Virtually all KS lesions are infected by KSHV (HHV8), but not all individuals who are infected develop KS.** Like Epstein-Barr virus, KSHV is a γ-herpesvirus. It is transmitted both through sexual contact and potentially via oral secretions and cutaneous exposures. Altered T-cell immunity is probably required for KS development; in older adults, diminished T-cell immunity may be related to aging. Inherited variations in genes that modulate cytokine expression such as interleukin 8 receptor-beta (IL8Rβ) and interleukin 13 (IL-13) genes have been noted in some individuals.

KSHV causes lytic and latent infections in ECs, both of which are probably important in KS pathogenesis. A virally encoded G protein induces VEGF production, stimulating endothelial growth, and cytokines produced by inflammatory cells recruited to sites of lytic infection also create a local proliferative milieu. In latently infected cells, KSHV-encoded proteins disrupt normal cellular proliferation controls (e.g., through synthesis of a viral homologue of cyclin D) and prevent apoptosis by inhibiting p53. Thus, the local inflammatory environment favors cellular proliferation, and latently infected cells have a growth advantage. In its early stages, only a few cells are KSHV infected, but with time, virtually all the proliferating cells carry the virus. The proliferating spindle cells are initially polyclonal or oligoclonal, but most advanced lesions become monoclonal.

MORPHOLOGY

In classic Kaposi sarcoma (and sometimes in the other variants), the cutaneous lesions progress through three stages: patch, plaque, and nodule.

- **Patches** are pink, red, or purple macules, typically affecting the distal lower extremities (Fig. 8.28A). Microscopic examination reveals dilated, irregular, and angulated blood vessels lined by ECs and an interspersed infiltrate of chronic inflammatory cells, sometimes containing hemosiderin. These lesions can be difficult to distinguish from granulation tissue.

- With time, lesions spread proximally and become larger, **violaceous, raised plaques** (Fig. 8.28A) composed of dilated, jagged dermal vascular channels lined and surrounded by plump spindle cells. Other prominent features include extravasated red cells, hemosiderin-laden macrophages, and other mononuclear cells.

- Eventually, **nodular lesions** appear. They are composed of plump, proliferating spindle cells, mostly located in the dermis or subcutaneous tissues (Fig. 8.28B), often with interspersed slitlike spaces. Hemorrhage and hemosiderin deposition are more pronounced, and mitotic figures are common. The nodular stage is often accompanied by nodal and visceral involvement, particularly in the African and AIDS-associated variants.

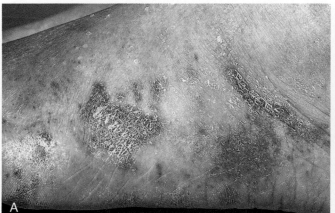
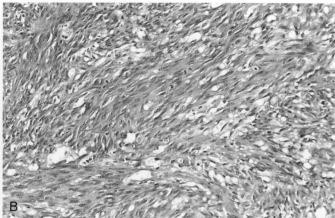

FIG. 8.28 Kaposi sarcoma. (A) Characteristic coalescent cutaneous red-purple macules and plaques. (B) Histologic view of the nodular stage, demonstrating sheets of plump, proliferating spindle cells and slitlike vascular spaces. (Courtesy of Christopher D.M. Fletcher, MD, Brigham and Women's Hospital, Boston, Massachusetts.)

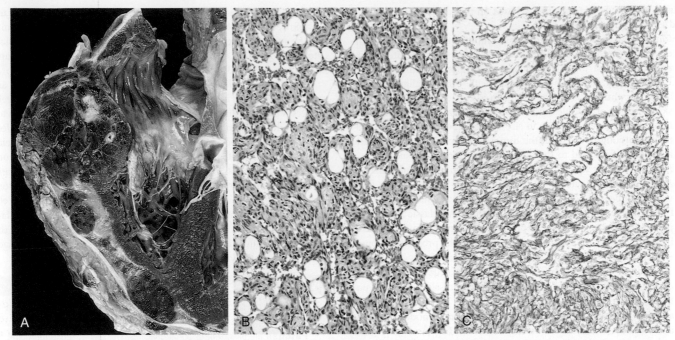

FIG. 8.29 Angiosarcoma. (A) Angiosarcoma of the right ventricle. (B) Moderately differentiated angiosarcoma with dense clumps of atypical cells lining distinct vascular lumina. (C) Immunohistochemical staining of angiosarcoma for the endothelial cell marker CD31.

Clinical Features. The course of disease varies widely according to the clinical setting. Most primary KSHV infections are asymptomatic. Classic KS is—at least initially—largely restricted to the surface of the body, and surgical resection is usually adequate for an excellent prognosis. Radiation therapy can be used for multiple lesions in a restricted area, and chemotherapy yields satisfactory results for more disseminated disease, including nodal involvement. In KS associated with iatrogenic immunosuppression, withdrawal of immunosuppressive agents (with or without adjunct chemotherapy or radiotherapy) is often effective. For AIDS-associated KS, HIV antiretroviral therapy is generally beneficial, with or without additional chemotherapy depending on the extent of the disease.

Malignant Tumors

Angiosarcomas

Angiosarcomas are malignant endothelial neoplasms ranging from highly differentiated tumors resembling hemangiomas to wildly anaplastic lesions. Older adults are more commonly affected, without gender predilection; lesions can occur at any site, but most often involve the skin, soft tissue, breast, and liver. Clinically, angiosarcomas are aggressive tumors that invade locally and metastasize, with a poor survival.

Angiosarcomas can arise in the setting of lymphedema, classically in the ipsilateral upper extremity several years after lymph node resection for breast cancer *(Steward-Treves syndrome)*. In such instances, the tumor presumably arises from lymphatic vessels *(lymphangiosarcoma)*. Angiosarcomas affecting the breast and/or overlying skin may also occur following radiation therapy for breast cancers in the absence of lymphedema.

Hepatic angiosarcomas are associated with certain carcinogens, including arsenical pesticides and polyvinyl chloride (one of the best-known examples of human chemical carcinogenesis). Multiple years typically transpire between exposure and subsequent tumor development.

■ RAPID REVIEW

Structure and Function of Blood Vessels

- All vessels are lined by endothelium; although all endothelial cells (ECs) share certain homeostatic properties, ECs in specific vascular beds have special features that allow for tissue-specific functions (e.g., fenestrated ECs in renal glomeruli).
- The relative smooth muscle cell (SMC) and extracellular matrix (ECM) content of vessel walls (e.g., in arteries, veins, and capillaries) varies according to hemodynamic demands (e.g., pressure, pulsatility) and functional requirements.
- EC function is tightly regulated in both the basal and activated states. Various physiologic and pathophysiologic stimuli induce endothelial activation and dysfunction that alter the EC phenotype (e.g., procoagulative versus anticoagulative, proinflammatory versus antiinflammatory, nonadhesive versus adhesive).

Blood Pressure Regulation

- Blood pressure is determined by vascular resistance and cardiac output.

- Vascular resistance is regulated at the level of the arterioles, influenced by neural and hormonal inputs.
- Cardiac output is determined by heart rate and stroke volume, the latter of which is strongly influenced by blood volume. Blood volume in turn is regulated mainly by renal sodium excretion or resorption.
- Renin, a major regulator of blood pressure, is secreted by the kidneys in response to decreased blood pressure in afferent arterioles. Renin cleaves angiotensinogen to angiotensin I; subsequent peripheral catabolism produces angiotensin II, which regulates blood pressure by increasing vascular SMC tone and by increasing adrenal aldosterone secretion, which stimulates renal sodium resorption.

Hypertension

- Hypertension is a common disorder affecting 40% of the population; it is a major risk factor for atherosclerosis, congestive heart failure, and renal failure.
- Hypertension may be primary (idiopathic) or less commonly secondary to an identifiable underlying condition. In close to 95% of cases hypertension is idiopathic or "essential."
- Idiopathic hypertension is a complex, multifactorial disorder, involving both environmental influences and genetic polymorphisms that may influence sodium resorption, aldosterone pathways, the adrenergic nervous system, and the renin-angiotensin system.
- Secondary hypertension is occasionally caused by single-gene disorders but is more commonly related to diseases of the renal arteries, kidneys, adrenal glands, or other endocrine organs.

Atherosclerosis

- Atherosclerosis is an intima-based lesion composed of a fibrous cap and an atheromatous (literally, "gruel-like") core; the constituents of the atherosclerotic plaque include SMCs, ECM, inflammatory cells, lipids, and necrotic debris.
- Atherogenesis is driven by an interplay of vessel wall injury and inflammation. The multiple risk factors for atherosclerosis all cause EC dysfunction and influence SMC recruitment and stimulation.
- Major modifiable risk factors for atherosclerosis are hypercholesterolemia, hypertension, cigarette smoking, and diabetes.
- Atherosclerotic plaques develop and grow slowly over decades. Stable plaques can produce symptoms related to narrowing of vessels and chronic ischemia, whereas unstable plaques can cause dramatic and potentially fatal ischemic complications related to acute plaque rupture, thrombosis, or embolization.
- Stable plaques tend to have a dense fibrous cap, minimal lipid accumulation, and little inflammation, whereas "vulnerable" unstable plaques have thin caps, large lipid cores, and relatively dense inflammatory infiltrates.

Aneurysms and Dissections

- Aneurysms are congenital or acquired dilations of the heart or blood vessels that involve the entire wall thickness. Complications are related to rupture, thrombosis, and embolization.
- Dissections occur when blood enters the wall of a vessel and separates the various layers. Complications arise as a result of rupture or obstruction of vessels branching off the aorta.
- Aneurysms and dissections result from structural weakness of the vessel wall caused by loss of SMCs or weakening of the ECM, which can be a consequence of ischemia, genetic defects, or defective matrix remodeling.

Vasculitis

- Vasculitis is defined as inflammation of vessel walls; it is frequently associated with systemic manifestations (including fever, malaise, myalgias, and arthralgias) and organ dysfunction that depends on the pattern of vascular involvement.
- Vasculitis can result from infections but more commonly have an immunologic basis such as immune complex deposition, antineutrophil antibodies (ANCAs), or anti-EC antibodies.
- Different forms of vasculitis tend to specifically affect vessels of a particular caliber and location.

Vascular Tumors

- Vascular ectasias are not neoplasms, but rather dilations of existing vessels.
- Vascular neoplasms can derive from either blood vessels or lymphatics, and can be composed of ECs (e.g., hemangioma, lymphangioma, angiosarcoma) or other cells of the vascular wall (e.g., glomus tumor).
- Most vascular tumors are benign (e.g., hemangioma); some have an intermediate, locally aggressive behavior (e.g., Kaposi sarcoma); and others are highly malignant (e.g., angiosarcoma).
- Benign tumors typically form obvious vascular channels lined by normal-appearing ECs. Malignant tumors are more often solid and cellular, exhibit cytologic atypia, and lack well-defined vessels.

■ **Laboratory Tests**

Test	Reference Values	Pathophysiology/Clinical Relevance
Antineutrophil cytoplasmic antibody (ANCA), serum	Negative	Antineutrophil cytoplasmic antibodies (ANCAs) are sensitive and specific markers for ANCA-associated systemic vasculitis. They are identified using indirect immunofluorescence; the two main patterns are diffuse cytoplasmic staining and perinuclear staining. Cytoplasmic staining is typically due to autoantibodies against proteinase 3 (PR3-ANCA), while perinuclear staining is associated with autoantibodies against myeloperoxidase (MPO-ANCA).
Antineutrophil cytoplasmic antibody (ANCA)—myeloperoxidase (MPO), serum	Negative	MPO is found in the granules of neutrophils and the lysosomes of monocytes; MPO-ANCAs are predominantly of IgG isotype and activate both cell types. MPO-ANCA was formerly known as p-ANCA (perinuclear-ANCA) based on indirect immunofluorescent staining. Eosinophilic granulomatosis with polyangiitis is typically associated with MPO-ANCA, which is also the ANCA most commonly associated with microscopic polyangiitis.
Antineutrophil cytoplasmic antibody (ANCA)—proteinase 3 (PR3), serum	Negative	PR3-ANCA was formerly known as c-ANCA (cytoplasmic-ANCA) based on indirect immunofluorescent staining. The primary target of these antibodies is proteinase 3 (PR3) in the cytoplasm of neutrophils. PR3-ANCA is positive in the majority of cases of granulomatosis with polyangiitis.
High-density lipoprotein (HDL), serum	Males: ≥40 mg/dL Females: ≥50 mg/dL	Of the lipoproteins (HDL, LDL, VLDL), HDL is the smallest and has the highest ratio of proteins to lipids (about 50% protein). HDL transports cholesterol from the periphery to the liver where it is catabolized and excreted. Low levels of HDL are a risk factor for atherosclerosis. HDL is increased by exercise, alcohol consumption, and some medications (e.g., hormone replacement therapy).
Human herpesvirus 8 (HHV8)	Quantitative real-time PCR: <1000 copies/mL	HHV8 (also known as Kaposi sarcoma-associated herpesvirus, KSHV) is a DNA virus that is associated with Kaposi sarcoma (KS), primary effusion lymphoma, and Castleman disease. HHV8 is associated with all four types of KS (i.e., classic, endemic, organ transplant-associated, epidemic/AIDS related). In the latter two categories, KS often regresses with reduction in immunosuppression. Primary effusion lymphoma arises in the pericardial, pleural, and peritoneal cavities. HHV8 positivity is most often observed in multicentric Castleman disease, which frequently arises in the context of HIV infection.
Lipoprotein(a) (Lp[a]), serum	<5 mg/dL	Lp(a) is composed of apolipoprotein(a) bound to the apo-B100 moiety of LDL via a disulfide bridge. Lp(a) is atherogenic and prothrombotic. Proposed mechanisms include interference with fibrinolysis, macrophage binding and recruitment to atherosclerotic plaques, and disruption of normal endothelial function. Increased Lp(a) is an independent risk factor for atherosclerotic cardiovascular disease.
Low-density lipoprotein (LDL), serum	Adults: <100 mg/dL, desirable	LDL is a product of VLDL metabolism. It is composed primarily of cholesterol (50%), protein (25%), phospholipid (20%), and a trace amount of triglycerides. LDL delivers cholesterol to peripheral tissues. LDL is a major component of atheromatous plaques, and elevated LDL is a risk factor in cardiovascular disease. Serum levels are affected by lifestyle factors (e.g., diet, exercise) and some diseases. Conditions in which LDL levels are elevated include familial hypercholesterolemia, hypothyroidism, uncontrolled diabetes, nephrotic syndrome, Cushing syndrome, and corticosteroid use. LDL levels are typically decreased in severe liver disease, hyperthyroidism, and, in the setting of severe acute or chronic illness, malnutrition, malabsorption, or extensive burns.
Total cholesterol, serum	Desirable: <200 mg/dL Borderline high: 200–239 mg/dL High risk: ≥240 mg/dL	Total cholesterol includes high-density lipoprotein (20%–30%), low-density lipoprotein (60%–70%), and very-low-density lipoprotein (10%–15%). Low-density lipoprotein (LDL) is usually calculated from total cholesterol, high-density lipoprotein (HDL), and triglycerides. Tests for direct measurement are also available and are useful if triglyceride level is very high. Total cholesterol is elevated in a number of conditions including familial hypercholesterolemia (deficiency of LDL receptors), uncontrolled diabetes, hypothyroidism, nephrotic syndrome, and biliary obstruction. Corticosteroids also increase total cholesterol. Total cholesterol may be decreased in severe liver disease, hyperthyroidism, severe acute or chronic illness, malnutrition, malabsorption, and extensive burns.

| Triglycerides, serum | Normal: <150 mg/dL
Borderline high:
  150–199 mg/dL
High: 200–499 mg/dL
Very high: ≥500 mg/dL | Triglycerides, LDL, and HDL are the primary lipids found in plasma. Triglycerides are transported from the small bowel inside chylomicrons and as VLDL particles. Triglycerides are directly measured in the laboratory. This value, along with total cholesterol and HDL, is used to calculate LDL. Elevated triglycerides are a risk factor for coronary artery disease and acute pancreatitis. Triglycerides are increased by some medications (e.g., β-blockers, corticosteroids) and in a wide range of conditions including diabetes, nephrotic syndrome, biliary tract obstruction, obesity, cirrhosis, and some glycogen storage diseases (I, III, and VI). |

[a]Assistance of Dr. Pankti D. Reid and Dr. Bauer Ventura, Department of Medicine, University of Chicago, is gratefully acknowledged for their help in reviewing this table.

References values from https://www.mayocliniclabs.com/ by permission of Mayo Foundation for Medical Education and Research. All rights reserved.

Adapted from Deyrup AT, D'Ambrosio D, Muir J, et al. Essential Laboratory Tests for Medical Education. *Acad Pathol.* 2022;9. doi: 10.1016/j.acpath.2022.100046.

9

Heart

OUTLINE

The heart is a truly remarkable organ, beating more than 40 million times per year and pumping over 7500 liters of blood a day; in a typical life span, its cumulative output would fill three supertankers. The cardiovascular system is the first organ system to become functional in utero (at approximately 8 weeks of gestation); without a beating heart and vascular supply, development cannot proceed, and the embryo dies. When the heart fails during postnatal life, the results are equally catastrophic. Indeed, cardiovascular disease is the leading cause of mortality worldwide and accounts for one in four of all deaths in the United States.

OVERVIEW OF HEART DISEASE

Although a wide range of diseases can affect the cardiovascular system, the pathophysiologic pathways that result in a "broken" heart can be distilled down to six principal mechanisms:
- *Failure of the pump.* In the most common situation, the cardiac muscle contracts weakly and the chambers cannot empty properly—so-called *systolic dysfunction*. In some cases, the muscle

The contributions to this chapter by Dr. Richard Mitchell, Department of Pathology, Brigham and Women's Hospital, Harvard Medical School, Boston, Massachusetts, in several previous editions of this book are gratefully acknowledged.

cannot relax sufficiently to permit ventricular filling, resulting in *diastolic dysfunction.*

- *Obstruction to flow.* Lesions that prevent valve opening (e.g., calcific aortic valve stenosis) or cause increased ventricular chamber pressures (e.g., systemic hypertension or aortic stenosis) can overwork the myocardium, which has to pump against the increased obstruction (as in valvular stenosis) or resistance (as in hypertension).
- *Regurgitant flow.* Valve pathology that allows backward flow of blood results in increased volume workload and may overwhelm the pumping capacity of the affected chambers.
- *Shunted flow.* Defects (congenital or acquired) that divert blood inappropriately from one chamber to another, or from one vessel to another, lead to pressure and volume overloads.
- *Disorders of cardiac conduction.* Uncoordinated cardiac impulses or blocked conduction pathways can cause arrhythmias that slow contractions or prevent effective pumping altogether.
- *Rupture of the heart or major vessel.* Loss of circulatory continuity (e.g., a gunshot wound through the thoracic aorta) may lead to massive blood loss, shock, and death.

HEART FAILURE

Heart failure, often referred to as *congestive heart failure (CHF),* is the common end point for many forms of cardiac disease and is typically a progressive condition with a poor prognosis.

CHF occurs when the heart cannot generate sufficient output to meet the metabolic demands of the tissues or can only do so at higher-than-normal filling pressures. In a minority of cases, heart failure is a consequence of greatly increased tissue demands, as in hyperthyroidism, or decreased oxygen-carrying capacity, as in anemia *(high-output failure).* The onset of CHF is sometimes abrupt, as in the setting of a large myocardial infarct or acute valve dysfunction. In most cases, however, CHF develops gradually and insidiously owing to the cumulative effects of chronic work overload or progressive loss of myocardial function.

Heart failure may result from any cause that impairs the ability of the ventricle to fill with or eject blood. The inability to eject blood (systolic failure) results from inadequate myocardial contractile function, usually as a consequence of ischemic heart disease or hypertension. Diastolic failure refers to an inability of the heart to adequately relax and fill. This form of heart failure is called heart failure with preserved ejection fraction. It is said to exist when symptoms of heart failure are associated with left ventricular ejection fraction $\geq 50\%$. Approximately one-half of CHF cases are attributable to diastolic dysfunction, with a greater frequency seen in older adults, patients with diabetes, and women. When the failing heart can no longer efficiently pump blood, there is an increase in end-diastolic ventricular volumes, increased end-diastolic pressures, and elevated venous pressures. Thus, inadequate cardiac output—called *forward failure*—is almost always accompanied by increased congestion of the venous circulation—that is, *backward failure.* Although the root problem in CHF is typically deficient cardiac function, virtually every other organ is eventually affected by some combination of forward and backward failure.

Several homeostatic mechanisms are employed by the cardiovascular system to compensate for reduced myocardial contractility or increased hemodynamic burden:

- *The Frank-Starling mechanism.* Increased filling volumes dilate the heart, thereby increasing actin-myosin cross-bridge formation and enhancing contractility and stroke volume. As long as the dilated ventricle is able to maintain cardiac output by this means, the patient is said to be in *compensated heart failure.* However, ventricular dilation comes at the expense of increased wall tension and also

increases the oxygen requirements of an already-compromised myocardium. With time, the failing muscle is no longer able to propel sufficient blood to meet the needs of the body, and the patient develops *decompensated heart failure.*

- Activation of neurohumoral systems:
  - Release of the neurotransmitter norepinephrine by the autonomic nervous system increases heart rate and augments myocardial contractility and vascular resistance.
  - Activation of the renin-angiotensin-aldosterone system spurs water and salt retention (augmenting circulatory volume) and increases vascular tone.
  - Release of atrial natriuretic peptide acts to balance the renin-angiotensin-aldosterone system through diuresis and vascular smooth muscle relaxation.
- *Myocardial structural changes, including increased muscle mass.* Cardiac myocytes adapt to increased workload by assembling new sarcomeres, a change that is accompanied by myocyte enlargement (hypertrophy) (Fig. 9.1).
  - In *pressure overload states* (e.g., hypertension or valvular stenosis), new sarcomeres tend to be added parallel to the long axis of the myocytes, adjacent to existing sarcomeres. The growing muscle fiber diameter thus results in *concentric hypertrophy,* and the ventricular wall thickness increases without an increase in the size of the chamber.
  - In *volume overload states* (e.g., valvular regurgitation or shunts), the new sarcomeres are added in series with existing sarcomeres so that the muscle fiber length increases. Consequently, the ventricle tends to dilate, and the resulting wall thickness can be increased, normal, or decreased; thus, heart weight—rather than wall thickness—is the best measure of hypertrophy in volume-overloaded hearts.

Compensatory hypertrophy comes at a cost. The oxygen requirements of hypertrophic myocardium are greater due to increased myocardial cell mass. Because the myocardial capillary bed does not expand sufficiently to meet the increased myocardial oxygen demands, the myocardium becomes vulnerable to ischemic injury.

Pathologic compensatory cardiac hypertrophy is correlated with increased mortality; indeed, cardiac hypertrophy is an independent risk factor for sudden cardiac death. By contrast, the volume-loaded hypertrophy induced by regular aerobic exercise (physiologic hypertrophy) is typically accompanied by an increase in capillary density and decreased resting heart rate and blood pressure. These physiologic adaptations reduce overall cardiovascular morbidity and mortality. On the other hand, anaerobic exercise (e.g., weightlifting) is associated with pressure hypertrophy and may not have the same beneficial effects.

Left-Sided Heart Failure

Heart failure can affect predominantly the left or right side of the heart or may involve both sides. The most common causes of left-sided cardiac failure are ischemic heart disease (IHD), systemic hypertension, mitral or aortic valve disease, and primary diseases of the myocardium (e.g., amyloidosis). The morphologic and clinical effects of left-sided CHF stem from diminished systemic perfusion and elevated back-pressures within the pulmonary circulation.

MORPHOLOGY

Heart. The gross cardiac findings depend on the underlying disease process; for example, myocardial infarction or valvular deformities may be present. With the exception of failure due to mitral valve stenosis or restrictive cardiomyopathies (described later), the left ventricle is usually **hypertrophied** and can be **dilated**, sometimes massively. Left ventricular dilation can result in mitral insufficiency and left atrial enlargement, which is associated with an increased incidence of atrial fibrillation. The microscopic changes in heart failure are nonspecific, consisting primarily of **myocyte hypertrophy with interstitial fibrosis** of variable severity. Superimposed on this background may be other lesions that contribute to the development of heart failure (e.g., recent or old myocardial infarction).

Lungs. In acute left-sided heart failure, rising pressure in the pulmonary veins is ultimately transmitted back to the capillaries and arteries of the lungs, resulting in congestion and edema as well as pleural effusion due to increased hydrostatic pressure in the venules of the visceral pleura. The lungs are heavy and wet and microscopically show perivascular and interstitial transudates, alveolar septal edema, and **accumulation of edema fluid in the alveolar spaces.** In chronic heart failure, variable numbers of red cells extravasate from the leaky capillaries into alveolar spaces, where they are phagocytosed by macrophages. The subsequent breakdown of red cells and hemoglobin leads to the appearance of hemosiderin-laden alveolar macrophages — so-called **heart failure cells** — that reflect previous episodes of pulmonary edema.

Clinical Features. **Dyspnea (shortness of breath) on exertion is usually the earliest and most significant symptom of left-sided heart failure;** cough is also common as a consequence of fluid transudation into air spaces. As failure progresses, patients experience dyspnea when recumbent *(orthopnea)* because the supine position increases venous return from the lower extremities and also elevates the diaphragm. Orthopnea is typically relieved by sitting or standing, so patients usually sleep in a semiseated position. *Paroxysmal nocturnal dyspnea* is a particularly dramatic form of breathlessness, awakening patients from sleep with extreme dyspnea bordering on feelings of suffocation.

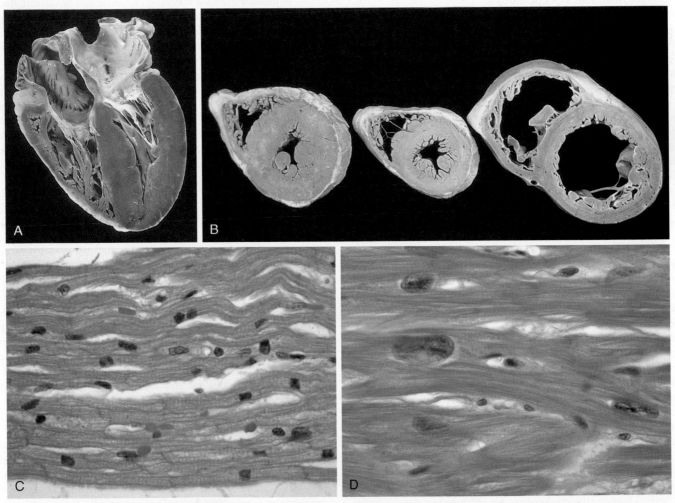

FIG. 9.1 Left ventricular hypertrophy. (A) Pressure hypertrophy due to left ventricular outflow obstruction. The left ventricle is on the *lower right* in this apical four-chamber view of the heart. (B) Left ventricular hypertrophy with and without dilation, viewed in transverse heart sections. Compared with a normal heart *(center),* the pressure-hypertrophied hearts *(left and in A)* have increased mass and a thick left ventricular wall, while the hypertrophied, dilated heart *(right)* has increased mass and a normal wall thickness. (C) Normal myocardium. (D) Hypertrophied myocardium (panels *C* and *D* are photomicrographs at the same magnification). Note the increases in both cell size and nuclear size in the hypertrophied myocytes. (A and B, Reproduced with permission from Edwards WD: Cardiac anatomy and examination of cardiac specimens. In Emmanouilides GC, et al, editors: *Moss and Adams Heart Disease in Infants, Children, and Adolescents: Including the Fetus and Young Adults,* ed 5, Philadelphia, 1995, Williams & Wilkins, p 86.)

Other manifestations of left ventricular failure include an enlarged heart (cardiomegaly), tachycardia, a third heart sound (S_3), which represents rapid passive ventricular filling, and fine rales at the lung bases, caused by the opening of edematous pulmonary alveoli by inspired air. With progressive ventricular dilation, the papillary muscles are displaced outward, resulting in mitral regurgitation and a systolic murmur. Subsequent chronic dilation of the left atrium can cause atrial fibrillation due to firing from stretch sensitive ion channels. It is manifested by an "irregularly irregular" heartbeat. Such uncoordinated, chaotic atrial contractions reduce the atrial contribution to ventricular filling, thus reducing the ventricular stroke volume. Atrial fibrillation also causes stasis of the blood (particularly in the atrial appendage), frequently leading to the formation of thrombi that can shed emboli, causing infarction in other organs (e.g., stroke).

Diminished cardiac output leads to decreased renal perfusion that in turn triggers the renin-angiotensin-aldosterone axis, increasing intravascular volume and pressures (Chapters 3 and 8). However, with a failing heart, these compensatory effects exacerbate the pulmonary edema. With further progression of CHF, prerenal failure may supervene, with impaired excretion of wastes and increasing metabolic derangement. In severe CHF, diminished cerebral perfusion may manifest as hypoxic encephalopathy marked by irritability, diminished cognition, and restlessness that can progress to stupor and coma.

Treatment for CHF is typically focused—at least initially—on correcting the underlying cause, for example, a valvular defect or inadequate cardiac perfusion. In lieu of such options, the clinical approach includes salt restriction or pharmacologic agents that variously reduce volume overload (e.g., diuretics), increase myocardial contractility (so-called "positive inotropes"), or reduce afterload (adrenergic blockade or inhibitors of angiotensin-converting enzymes). Angiotensin-converting enzyme inhibitors appear to benefit patients not only by opposing aldosterone-mediated salt and water retention but also by limiting cardiomyocyte hypertrophy and remodeling.

Right-Sided Heart Failure

Right-sided heart failure is usually the consequence of left-sided heart failure, since any pressure increase in the pulmonary circulation inevitably produces an increased burden on the right side of the heart. Consequently, the causes of right-sided heart failure include all those that induce left-sided heart failure. Isolated right-sided heart failure is infrequent and typically occurs in patients with one of a variety of disorders affecting the lungs; hence, it is often referred to as *cor pulmonale*. In addition to parenchymal lung diseases, cor pulmonale may also arise secondary to disorders that affect the pulmonary vasculature, for example, primary pulmonary hypertension (Chapter 11), recurrent pulmonary thromboembolism, or conditions that cause pulmonary vasoconstriction (obstructive sleep apnea). The common feature of these disorders is pulmonary hypertension (discussed later), which results in hypertrophy and dilation of the right side of the heart. In cor pulmonale, myocardial hypertrophy and dilation are generally confined to the right ventricle and atrium, although bulging of the ventricular septum to the left can reduce cardiac output by causing outflow tract obstruction.

The major morphologic and clinical effects of pure right-sided heart failure differ from those of left-sided heart failure in that engorgement of the systemic and portal venous systems is typically pronounced, and pulmonary congestion is minimal.

MORPHOLOGY

Liver and Portal System. The liver is usually increased in size and weight **(congestive hepatomegaly).** A cut section displays prominent **passive congestion** characterized by congested centrilobular areas surrounded by peripheral paler, noncongested parenchyma, a pattern referred to as **nutmeg liver** (Chapter 3). When left-sided heart failure is also present, severe central hypoxia produces **centrilobular necrosis** in addition to the sinusoidal congestion. With long-standing severe right-sided heart failure, the central areas can become fibrotic, creating so-called **cardiac cirrhosis.**

Right-sided heart failure can also lead to elevated pressure in the portal vein and its tributaries **(portal hypertension),** with vascular congestion producing a tense, enlarged spleen **(congestive splenomegaly).** When severe, chronic passive congestion and attendant edema of the bowel wall may interfere with absorption of nutrients and medications.

Pleural, Pericardial, and Peritoneal Spaces. Systemic venous congestion due to right-sided heart failure can lead to transudates **(effusions)** in the pleural and pericardial spaces but usually does not cause pulmonary parenchymal edema. Pleural effusions are most pronounced when there is combined right-sided and left-sided heart failure, leading to elevated pulmonary and systemic venous pressures. A combination of hepatic congestion (with or without diminished albumin synthesis) and portal hypertension can lead to peritoneal transudates (ascites). When uncomplicated, effusions associated with right-sided CHF are transudates with a low protein content and lack of inflammatory cells.

Subcutaneous Tissues. Pitting edema of dependent portions of the body, especially the feet and lower legs, is a hallmark of right-sided CHF. In chronically bedridden patients, the edema may be primarily presacral.

Clinical Features. Unlike left-sided heart failure, pure right-sided heart failure is not typically associated with respiratory symptoms. Instead, the clinical manifestations are related to systemic and portal venous congestion and include hepatic and splenic enlargement, peripheral edema, pleural effusion, and ascites. Venous congestion and hypoxia of the kidneys and brain due to right-sided heart failure can produce deficits comparable to those caused by the hypoperfusion of left-sided heart failure.

Of note, cardiac decompensation is often marked by the appearance of biventricular CHF, encompassing features of both right-sided and left-sided heart failure. As CHF progresses, patients may become cyanotic and acidotic, as a consequence of decreased tissue perfusion resulting from both diminished cardiac output and increasing congestion.

CONGENITAL HEART DISEASE

Congenital heart diseases are abnormalities of the heart or great vessels that are present at birth. They account for 20% to 30% of all birth defects and include a broad spectrum of malformations, ranging from severe anomalies incompatible with intrauterine or perinatal survival, to lesions that produce few or no symptoms, such that they may go unrecognized during life. Congenital heart disease affects nearly 1% of newborns (or roughly 40,000 infants per year in the United States). The incidence is higher in premature infants and in stillborns, approximately one-fourth of whom have significant cardiac malformations. Defects that permit live birth usually involve only single chambers or regions of the heart. Twelve entities account for 85% of congenital heart disease; their frequencies are shown in Table 9.1.

Table 9.1 Frequency of Congenital Cardiac Malformations

Malformation	Incidence per 1 Million Live Births	%
Ventricular septal defect	4482	42
Atrial septal defect	1043	10
Pulmonary stenosis	836	8
Patent ductus arteriosus	781	7
Tetralogy of Fallot	577	5
Coarctation of aorta	492	5
Atrioventricular septal defect	396	4
Aortic stenosis	388	4
Transposition of great arteries	388	4
Truncus arteriosus	136	1
Total anomalous pulmonary venous connection	120	1
Tricuspid atresia	118	1
TOTAL	9757	

aSummary of 44 published studies. Percentages do not add to 100% because of rounding.
Data from Hoffman JI, Kaplan S: The incidence of congenital heart disease, *J Am Coll Cardiol* 39:1890, 2002.

Thanks to advances in surgical techniques, the number of patients surviving with congenital heart disease is increasing rapidly and is currently estimated at 1.5 million individuals in the United States alone. In 25% of cases, surgical intervention is required for survival in the first year of life.

Pathogenesis. **Congenital heart disease most commonly arises from faulty embryogenesis during gestational weeks 3 through 8, when major cardiovascular structures develop.** The cause is unknown in almost 90% of cases. The mechanisms specific for congenital heart disease are also not known. Most likely they are similar to those responsible for other congenital malformations discussed in Chapter 4. The following risk factors have been identified:

- *Prematurity*
- *Family history*
- *Maternal conditions* such as diabetes, hypertension, obesity, phenylketonuria, thyroid disorders, and systemic connective tissue disorders; maternal exposure to therapeutic drugs taken during pregnancy such as phenytoin and retinoic acid as well as smoking and alcohol ingestion
- *Assisted reproductive technology* such as in vitro fertilization
- *Genetic disorders and extra cardiac abnormalities* are common in patients with congenital heart diseases. Examples include trisomy 21, 18, 13, and Turner syndrome.
- *In utero infections* caused by rubella, cytomegalovirus, coxsackie virus, human herpesvirus 6, parvovirus B19, herpes simplex, and toxoplasmosis

Clinical Features. **The various structural anomalies in congenital heart disease can be assigned to three major groups based on their hemodynamic and clinical consequences: (1) malformations causing a left-to-right shunt; (2) malformations causing a right-to-left shunt (cyanotic congenital heart diseases); and (3) malformations causing obstruction.**

A *shunt* is an abnormal communication between chambers or blood vessels. Depending on pressure relationships, shunts permit the flow of blood from the left to the right side of the heart or vice versa.

- A *right-to-left shunt* causes a dusky blueness of the skin *(cyanosis)* because the pulmonary circulation is bypassed, and poorly oxygenated blood collected from the venous system enters the systemic arterial circulation.
- By contrast, *left-to-right shunts* increase blood flow into the pulmonary circulation and are not associated (at least initially) with cyanosis. However, they expose the low-pressure, low-resistance pulmonary circulation to high pressures and increased volumes, leading to adaptive changes that increase lung vascular resistance to protect the pulmonary bed. The result is right ventricular hypertrophy and eventually right-sided failure. With time, increased pulmonary resistance can also cause shunt reversal (right to left) and late-onset cyanosis.
- Some congenital anomalies *obstruct vascular flow* by narrowing the chambers, valves, or major blood vessels. In some disorders (e.g., tetralogy of Fallot), an obstruction (pulmonary stenosis) is also associated with a shunt (right-to-left, through a VSD).

Malformations Associated With Left-to-Right Shunts

Disorders associated with left-to-right shunts are the most common types of congenital cardiac malformations. They include **atrial septal defects (ASDs), ventricular septal defects (VSDs),** and **patent ductus arteriosus (PDA)** (Fig. 9.2). ASDs typically increase only right

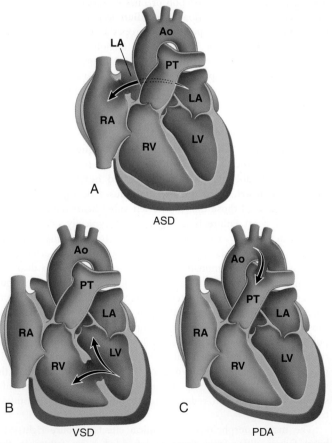

FIG. 9.2 Common congenital causes of left-to-right shunts (*arrows* indicate direction of blood flow). (A) Atrial septal defect (ASD). (B) Ventricular septal defect (VSD). (C) Patent ductus arteriosus (PDA). *Ao,* Aorta; *LA,* left atrium; *LV,* left ventricle; *PT,* pulmonary trunk; *RA,* right atrium; *RV,* right ventricle.

ventricular and pulmonary outflow volumes, while VSDs and PDAs cause both increased pulmonary blood flow and pressure. Manifestations of these shunts range from completely asymptomatic to fulminant heart failure.

Cyanosis is not an early feature of these defects. However, as discussed earlier, prolonged left-to-right shunting may eventually give rise to pulmonary hypertension and right-to-left shunting of unoxygenated blood into the systemic circulation, a change marked by the appearance of cyanosis *(Eisenmenger syndrome)*. Once significant pulmonary hypertension develops, the structural defects of congenital heart disease are considered irreversible. This is the rationale in most cases for early intervention, which is usually surgical.

Atrial Septal Defect and Patent Foramen Ovale

ASD and patent foramen ovale (PFO) are distinct defects that result from incomplete separation of the two atria, thus allowing communication between right and left atria. During normal cardiac development, patency is maintained between the right and left atria by a series of fenestrations *(ostium primum* and *ostium secundum)* that eventually become the *foramen ovale.* The patent foramen ovale allows oxygenated blood from the maternal circulation to flow from the right to the left atrium, thereby sustaining fetal development. At later stages of intrauterine development, tissue flaps between the right and left atrium called *septum primum* and *septum secundum* grow to occlude the foramen ovale. In 80% of individuals the higher left-sided pressures in the heart that occur at birth permanently fuse the septa, thereby closing the foramen ovale; in the remaining 20% of cases, a PFO results. While the flaps are of adequate size to cover the foramen, the unsealed septa can allow transient right-to-left blood flow, as may occur during sneezing or straining during bowel movements. Although this typically has little significance, it can cause *paradoxical embolism,* defined as venous emboli (e.g., from deep leg veins) that enter the systemic arterial circulation via a foramen ovale defect.

In contrast to patent foramen ovale, an ASD is an abnormal fixed opening in the atrial septum that allows unrestricted blood flow between the atrial chambers. A majority of ASDs are so-called "ostium secundum" defects in which growth of the septum secundum is insufficient to occlude the second ostium.

> ## MORPHOLOGY
>
> **Ostium secundum** ASDs (90% of ASDs) are smooth-walled defects near the foramen ovale, typically without other associated cardiac abnormalities. Hemodynamically significant lesions are accompanied by right atrial and ventricular dilation, right ventricular hypertrophy, and dilation of the pulmonary artery, reflecting the effects of a chronically increased volume load.
>
> **Ostium primum** ASDs (5% of these defects) occur at the lowest part of the atrial septum and can be associated with mitral and tricuspid valve abnormalities, reflecting the close relationship between development of the septum primum and the endocardial cushions. In more severe cases, additional defects may include a VSD and a **common atrioventricular canal.**
>
> **Sinus venosus ASDs** (5% of cases) are located high in the atrial septum and are often accompanied by anomalous drainage of the pulmonary veins into the right atrium or superior vena cava.

Clinical Features. ASDs are usually asymptomatic until adulthood. Although VSDs are more common, many close spontaneously. Consequently, **ASDs—which are less likely to spontaneously close— are the most common defects with initial diagnosis in adulthood.**

ASDs initially cause left-to-right shunts due to lower pressures in the pulmonary circulation and the right side of the heart. In general, these defects are well tolerated, especially if they are less than 1 cm in diameter; even larger lesions do not usually produce any symptoms in childhood. Over time, however, chronic volume and pressure overloads can cause pulmonary hypertension. Surgical or intravascular ASD closure is performed to prevent the development of heart failure, paradoxical embolization, and irreversible pulmonary vascular disease. Mortality is low, and postoperative survival is comparable to that of the unaffected population.

Ventricular Septal Defect

Defects in the ventricular septum allow left-to-right shunting and constitute the most common congenital cardiac anomaly diagnosed at birth (see Table 9.1 and Fig. 9.3). The ventricular septum is normally formed by a muscular ridge that grows upward from the heart apex and fuses with a thinner membranous partition that grows downward from the endocardial cushions. The basal (membranous) region is the last part of the septum to develop and is the site of approximately 90% of VSDs. Most VSDs close spontaneously in childhood; only 20% to 30% of VSDs occur in isolation; the remainder are associated with other cardiac malformations.

> ## MORPHOLOGY
>
> The size and location of VSDs are variable (see Fig. 9.3), ranging from minute defects in the membranous septum to large defects involving virtually the entire interventricular wall. In defects associated with a significant left-to-right shunt, the right ventricle is hypertrophied and often dilated. The diameter of the pulmonary artery is increased due to the increased right ventricular output and higher right-sided pressures. Vascular changes typical of pulmonary hypertension are common (Chapter 11).

Clinical Features. Small VSDs may be asymptomatic; half of those in the muscular portion of the septum close spontaneously during infancy or childhood. Larger defects, however, result in chronic left-to-right shunting, often complicated by pulmonary hypertension and CHF.

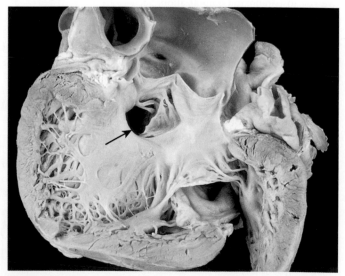

FIG. 9.3 Ventricular septal defect of the membranous type *(arrow).* (Courtesy of William D. Edwards, MD, Mayo Clinic, Rochester, Minnesota.)

Progressive pulmonary hypertension, with resultant reversal of the shunt and cyanosis, occurs earlier and more frequently with VSDs than with ASDs due to the higher flow volumes and pressures experienced by the pulmonary circulation in the former. Therefore, early surgical correction is indicated for such lesions. Small- or medium-sized defects that produce jet lesions in the right ventricle cause endothelial damage and increase the risk for infective endocarditis.

Patent Ductus Arteriosus

The *ductus arteriosus* arises from the left pulmonary artery and joins the aorta just distal to the origin of the left subclavian artery (see Fig. 9.2). During intrauterine life, it permits blood to flow from the pulmonary artery to the aorta, bypassing the unoxygenated lungs. Within 1 to 2 days of birth in healthy term infants, the ductus constricts and closes; these changes occur in response to increased arterial oxygenation, decreased pulmonary vascular resistance, and declining local levels of prostaglandin E_2. Complete obliteration occurs within the first few months of extrauterine life, leaving only a strand of residual fibrous tissue known as the *ligamentum arteriosum*. Ductal closure can be delayed (or even absent) in infants with hypoxia (related to respiratory distress or heart disease). PDAs account for about 7% of congenital heart lesions (see Table 9.1); the great majority of these (90%) are isolated defects.

Clinical Features. **PDAs are high-pressure left-to-right shunts that produce harsh, "machinery-like" murmurs.** A small PDA generally causes no symptoms, but larger defects can eventually lead to Eisenmenger syndrome with cyanosis and congestive heart failure. High-pressure shunts also predispose patients to developing infective endocarditis. Isolated PDAs should be closed as early in life as is feasible.

Malformations Associated With Right-to-Left Shunts

Cardiac malformations associated with right-to-left shunts are distinguished by early cyanosis, which occurs because poorly oxygenated blood from the right side of the heart flows directly into the arterial circulation. Two of the most important conditions associated with cyanotic congenital heart disease are tetralogy of Fallot and transposition of the great vessels (Fig. 9.4). Clinical consequences of severe, systemic cyanosis include clubbing of the tips of the fingers and toes (hypertrophic osteoarthropathy) and polycythemia. They can also give rise to paradoxical embolization.

Tetralogy of Fallot

Tetralogy of Fallot is the most common cause of cyanotic congenital heart disease. It accounts for about 5% of all congenital cardiac malformations (see Table 9.1). The four cardinal features are (Fig. 9.4A):
- VSD
- Right ventricular outflow tract obstruction (subpulmonic stenosis)
- Overriding of the VSD by the aorta
- Right ventricular hypertrophy

Developmentally, all the features of tetralogy of Fallot result from anterosuperior displacement of the infundibular septum leading to abnormal septation between the pulmonary trunk and the aortic root.

MORPHOLOGY

The heart is enlarged and "boot-shaped" as a consequence of **right ventricular hypertrophy;** the proximal aorta is dilated, while the pulmonary trunk is hypoplastic. The left-sided cardiac chambers are of normal size, while the right ventricular wall is markedly hypertrophied, sometimes even

exceeding the thickness of the left ventricle. The **VSD** is usually large and lies in the vicinity of the membranous portion of the interventricular septum; the aortic valve lies immediately over the VSD **(overriding aorta)** and is the major site of egress for blood flow from both ventricles. The obstruction of the right ventricular outflow is most often due to narrowing of the infundibulum **(subpulmonic stenosis)** but can also be caused by pulmonary valve stenosis or complete atresia of the valve and the proximal pulmonary arteries. In such cases, a persistent PDA or dilated bronchial arteries are the only route for blood to reach the lungs.

Clinical Features. **The hemodynamic consequences of tetralogy of Fallot are right-to-left shunting, decreased pulmonary blood flow, and increased aortic volumes.** The clinical severity largely depends on the degree of the pulmonary outflow obstruction; even untreated, some patients survive into adult life. Thus, if the pulmonic obstruction is mild, the condition resembles an isolated VSD because the high left-sided pressure causes only a left-to-right shunt with no cyanosis. More commonly, severe degrees of pulmonic stenosis cause early cyanosis. Moreover, as the child grows and the heart increases in size, the

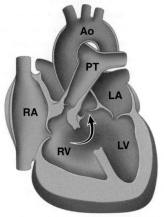

A Classic tetralogy of Fallot

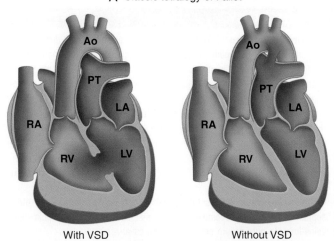

With VSD   Without VSD

B Complete transposition

FIG. 9.4 Common congenital right-to-left shunts (cyanotic congenital heart disease). (A) Tetralogy of Fallot (*arrow* indicates direction of blood flow). (B) Transposition of the great vessels with and without VSD. *Ao,* Aorta; *LA,* left atrium; *LV,* left ventricle; *PT,* pulmonary trunk; *RA,* right atrium; *RV,* right ventricle.

pulmonic orifice does not expand proportionately, leading to progressive worsening of the stenosis. Fortuitously, the pulmonic outflow stenosis protects the pulmonary vasculature from pressure and volume overloads, so pulmonary hypertension does not develop, and right ventricular failure is rare. Nevertheless, patients develop the typical sequelae of cyanotic heart disease, such as hypertrophic osteoarthropathy and polycythemia (due to hypoxia) with attendant hyperviscosity; right-to-left shunting also increases the risk for infective endocarditis and systemic embolization. Complete surgical repair is possible with classic tetralogy of Fallot but is more complicated in the setting of pulmonary atresia.

Transposition of the Great Arteries

Transposition of the great arteries is a discordant connection of the ventricles to their vascular outflow. The embryologic defect is an abnormal formation of the truncal and aortopulmonary septa so that the aorta arises from the right ventricle and the pulmonary artery emanates from the left ventricle (Fig. 9.4B). The atrium-to-ventricle connections, however, are normal (concordant), with the right atrium joining the right ventricle and the left atrium emptying into the left ventricle.

The functional outcome is separation of the systemic and pulmonary circulations, a condition incompatible with postnatal life unless a shunt (such as a VSD) allows delivery of oxygenated blood to the aorta. Indeed, VSDs occur in one-third of cases (see Fig. 9.4B). There is marked right ventricular hypertrophy since that chamber functions as the systemic ventricle; the left ventricle is hypoplastic since it pumps only to the low-resistance pulmonary circulation. Some newborns with transposition of the great arteries have a patent foramen ovale or PDA that allows oxygenated blood to reach the aorta, but these tend to close; such infants typically require emergent surgical intervention within the first few days of life.

Clinical Features. The dominant manifestation is cyanosis, with the prognosis depending on the magnitude of shunting, the degree of tissue hypoxia, and the ability of the right ventricle to maintain systemic pressures. Without surgery (even with stable shunting), most patients with uncorrected transposition of the great arteries die within the first months of life. However, improved surgical techniques now permit definitive repair, and such patients typically survive into adulthood.

Malformations Associated With Obstructive Lesions

Congenital obstruction of blood flow can occur at the level of the heart valves or more distally within a great vessel. Obstruction can also occur proximal to the valve, as with subpulmonic stenosis in tetralogy of Fallot. Relatively common examples of congenital obstructions are pulmonic valve stenosis, aortic valve stenosis or atresia, and coarctation of the aorta (described next).

Aortic Coarctation

Coarctation (narrowing, or constriction) of the aorta is a common form of obstructive congenital heart disease (see Table 9.1). Males are affected twice as often as females, although females with Turner syndrome frequently have coarctation. There are two classic forms (Fig. 9.5):
- A *preductal* ("infantile") form featuring hypoplasia of the aortic arch proximal to a patent ductus arteriosus (PDA)
- A *postductal* ("adult") form consisting of a discrete ridge-like infolding of the aorta, adjacent to the ligamentum arteriosum, without an associated PDA)

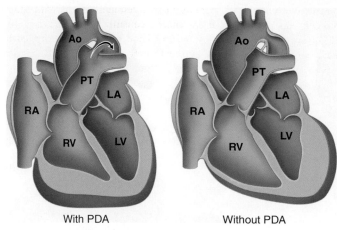

With PDA   Without PDA

Coarctation of aorta

FIG. 9.5 Coarctation of the aorta. A patent ductus arteriosus may be present ("infantile" or preductal form) or absent ("adult" or postductal form); *arrow* indicates direction of blood flow. *Ao,* Aorta; *LA,* left atrium; *LV,* left ventricle; *PT,* pulmonary trunk; *RA,* right atrium; *RV,* right ventricle.

Coarctation can occur as a solitary defect, but in more than half of cases is accompanied by a bicuspid aortic valve. Aortic valve stenosis, ASD, VSD, or mitral regurgitation can also be present.

MORPHOLOGY

Preductal coarctation is characterized by circumferential narrowing of the aortic segment between the left subclavian artery and the ductus arteriosus; the ductus is typically patent and is the main source of (unoxygenated) blood delivered to the distal aorta. The pulmonary trunk is dilated to accommodate the increased blood flow; because the right side of the heart now perfuses the body distal to the narrowed segment ("coarct"), the right ventricle is typically hypertrophied.

In the more common **postductal coarctation,** the aorta is sharply constricted by a tissue ridge adjacent to the nonpatent ligamentum arteriosum (Fig. 9.6). The constricted segment is made up of smooth muscle and elastic fibers derived from the aortic media. Proximal to the coarctation, the aortic arch and its branch vessels are dilated, and the left ventricle is hypertrophied.

Clinical Features. Clinical manifestations depend on the severity of the narrowing and the patency of the ductus arteriosus.
- *Preductal coarctation with a PDA* usually presents early in life, classically as cyanosis localized to the lower half of the body; without intervention, most affected infants die in the neonatal period.
- *Postductal coarctation without a PDA* is usually asymptomatic, and the disease may remain unrecognized well into adult life. Classically, there is upper-extremity hypertension paired with weak pulses and relative hypotension in the lower extremities, associated with symptoms of claudication and coldness. Exuberant collateral circulation often develops through markedly enlarged intercostal and internal mammary arteries; expansion of the flow through these vessels can lead to radiographically visible "notching" of the ribs.

In most cases, significant coarctations are associated with systolic murmurs and occasionally palpable thrills. Balloon dilation and stent placement or surgical resection with end-to-end anastomosis

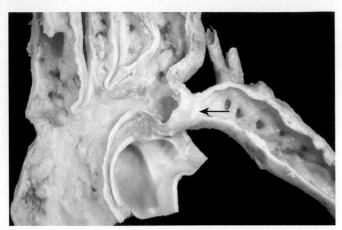

FIG. 9.6 Coarctation of the aorta, postductal type. The coarctation is a segmental narrowing of the aorta *(arrow)*. Such lesions typically manifest later in life than preductal coarctations. The dilated ascending aorta and major branch vessels are to the left of the coarctation. The lower extremities are perfused predominantly by way of dilated, tortuous collateral channels. (Courtesy of Sid Murphree, MD, Department of Pathology, University of Texas Southwestern Medical School, Dallas, Texas.)

(or replacement of the affected aortic segment by a prosthetic graft) yields excellent results.

ISCHEMIC HEART DISEASE

Ischemic heart disease (IHD) is a broad term encompassing several closely related syndromes caused by an imbalance between cardiac blood supply (perfusion) and myocardial oxygen and nutritional demands. Despite dramatic improvements in therapy in the past quarter century, IHD in its various forms remains the leading cause of mortality in the United States and other higher income nations, accounting for 7.5 million deaths worldwide each year.

In more than 90% of cases, IHD is a consequence of reduced coronary blood flow secondary to obstructive atherosclerotic vascular disease (Chapter 8). Thus, unless otherwise specified, IHD is usually synonymous with coronary artery disease (CAD). In most cases, the various syndromes of IHD are consequences of coronary atherosclerosis that has been gradually progressing for decades. In the remaining cases, cardiac ischemia may be the result of *increased demand* (e.g., with increased heart rate or hypertension); *diminished blood volume* (e.g., with hypotension or shock); *diminished blood oxygenation* (e.g., due to pneumonia or CHF); or *diminished blood oxygen-carrying capacity* (e.g., due to anemia or carbon monoxide poisoning).

Cardiac myocytes generate energy almost exclusively through mitochondrial oxidative phosphorylation, and their function and survival are strictly dependent upon the continuous flow of oxygenated blood through the coronary arteries. The manifestations of IHD are a direct consequence of the insufficient delivery of oxygen to the heart. The clinical presentation may include one or more of the following *cardiac syndromes:*

- *Angina pectoris* (literally, "chest pain"). Ischemia induces pain but is insufficient to cause myocyte death. Angina can be *stable* (occurring predictably at certain levels of exertion), can be caused by vessel spasm *(vasospatic angina, Prinzmetal angina),* or can be *unstable* (occurring with progressively less exertion or even at rest).

- *Myocardial infarction (MI).* This occurs when the severity or duration of ischemia is sufficient to cause cardiomyocyte death.
- *Chronic IHD with CHF.* This progressive cardiac decompensation, which occurs after acute MI or secondary to the accumulated effect of multiple ischemic insults, eventually precipitates mechanical pump failure.
- *Sudden cardiac death (SCD).* This occurs as a consequence of myocardial ischemia that induces a lethal ventricular fibrillation. Typically, there is underlying coronary artery disease.

The term *acute coronary syndrome* is applied to any of the three catastrophic manifestations of IHD: unstable angina, MI, and SCD.

Epidemiology

About 800,000 Americans experience an MI each year, and roughly half of those affected die. As troubling as this toll is, it represents spectacular progress: since peaking in 1963, the mortality related to IHD in the United States has declined by 50%. The improvement is largely attributed to interventions that have diminished *cardiac risk factors* (behaviors or conditions that promote atherosclerosis; Chapter 8), in particular smoking cessation programs, hypertension and diabetes treatment, and use of cholesterol-lowering agents. To a lesser extent, diagnostic and therapeutic advances have also contributed; these include aspirin prophylaxis, better arrhythmia control, establishment of coronary care units, thrombolysis for MI, angioplasty and endovascular stenting, use of ventricular assist devices, and coronary artery bypass graft surgery. Maintaining this downward trend in mortality will be particularly challenging given the predicted longevity of "baby boomers," as well as the epidemic of obesity that is sweeping the United States and other parts of the world.

Pathogenesis of Ischemic Heart Disease

IHD is a consequence of inadequate coronary perfusion relative to myocardial demand. In the vast majority of cases this is due to either or both of the following:

- Preexisting ("fixed") atherosclerotic occlusion of the coronary arteries
- Acute plaque change with superimposed thrombosis and/or vasospasm

Next we will discuss each of these two factors in greater detail.

Chronic Vascular Occlusion

Fixed obstructions that occlude less than 70% of a coronary vessel lumen are typically asymptomatic, even with exertion. In comparison, lesions that occlude more than 70% of a vessel lumen—resulting in so-called "critical stenosis"—generally cause symptoms in the setting of increased demand; with critical stenosis, certain levels of exertion predictably cause chest pain, and the patient is said to have stable angina. A fixed stenosis that occludes 90% or more of a vascular lumen can lead to inadequate coronary blood flow with symptoms even at rest—one of the forms of unstable angina (discussed later in the chapter). Atherosclerotic narrowing can affect any of the coronary arteries—left anterior descending (LAD), left circumflex (LCX), and right coronary artery (RCA)—singly or in combination. Clinically significant plaques tend to occur within the first several centimeters of the LAD and LCX takeoff from the aorta, and along the entire length of the RCA. Sometimes, secondary branches are also involved (i.e., diagonal branches of the LAD, obtuse marginal branches of the LCX, or posterior descending branch of the RCA). Of note, if an atherosclerotic lesion progressively occludes a coronary artery at a slow rate over years, other coronary vessels may undergo remodeling and provide compensatory blood flow to the area at risk; such *collateral perfusion* can protect against MI, even if the original vessel becomes completely occluded. Unfortunately, with acute coronary blockage, there is no time for collateral flow to develop, and infarction results.

Vasoconstriction directly compromises lumen diameter; moreover, by increasing local mechanical shear forces, vessel spasm can cause plaque disruption. Vasoconstriction in atherosclerotic plaques can be stimulated by the following:

- Circulating adrenergic agonists
- Locally released platelet contents
- Imbalance between endothelial cell—relaxing factors (e.g., nitric oxide) and endothelial cell—contracting factors (e.g., endothelin) due to endothelial dysfunction
- Mediators released from perivascular inflammatory cells

Acute Plaque Change

In most patients, unstable angina, infarction, and sudden cardiac death occur because of abrupt plaque change followed by thrombosis—hence the term *acute coronary syndrome* (Fig. 9.7).

The initiating event is typically a sudden disruption (rupture or erosion) of a partially occlusive plaque. Rupture, fissuring, ulceration, or erosion of plaques exposes highly thrombogenic constituents or underlying subendothelial basement membrane, leading to rapid thrombosis. In addition, hemorrhage into the core of plaques can expand plaque volume, thereby acutely exacerbating the degree of luminal occlusion. Even partial luminal occlusion by a thrombus can compromise blood flow sufficiently to cause an infarction of the innermost zone of the myocardium *(subendocardial infarct)*. Mural thrombi in a coronary artery can also embolize; indeed, small emboli may be found in the distal intramyocardial circulation (along with associated microinfarcts) at autopsy of patients with unstable angina.

Most seriously, completely obstructive thrombus over a disrupted plaque typically results in MI.

Factors that trigger loss of endothelial cells without plaque rupture *(plaque erosion)* include endothelial injury and apoptosis, likely attributable to some combination of inflammatory and toxic exposures. Acute *plaque rupture*, on the other hand, involves factors that influence plaque susceptibility to disruption by mechanical stress. These include intrinsic aspects of plaque composition and structure (Chapter 8) and extrinsic factors, such as blood pressure and platelet reactivity:

Plaques that contain large atheromatous cores or have thin overlying fibrous caps are more likely to rupture and are therefore termed vulnerable. Fissures frequently occur at the junction of the fibrous cap and the adjacent normal (plaque-free) arterial segment, where the mechanical stresses are highest and the fibrous cap is thinnest. Fibrous caps are also continuously remodeling; the overall balance of collagen synthesis and degradation within the plaque determines its mechanical strength and stability. Collagen is produced by smooth muscle cells and degraded by the action of metalloproteases elaborated by macrophages. Consequently, atherosclerotic lesions with a paucity of smooth muscle cells or large numbers of inflammatory cells are vulnerable to rupture. Of interest, statins may have a beneficial effect not only by reducing circulating cholesterol levels but also by multiple poorly understood effects on atherogenesis. These include reversal of endothelial dysfunctions and stabilizing plaques through a reduction in plaque inflammation.

In a majority of cases, the "culprit lesion" in patients who experience an MI was not critically stenotic or even symptomatic before its rupture. As noted previously, anginal symptoms typically occur with fixed lesions exhibiting greater than 70% chronic occlusion. Pathologic and clinical studies show that two-thirds of ruptured plaques are less than or equal to 50% stenotic before plaque rupture, and 85% exhibit

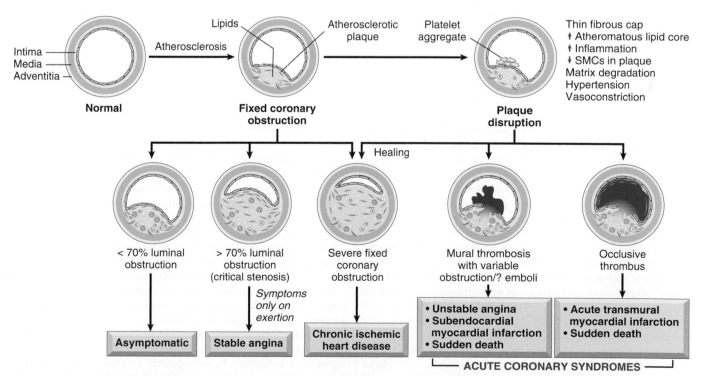

FIG. 9.7 Diagram of sequential progression of coronary artery lesions leading to various acute coronary syndromes. (Modified from Schoen FJ: *Interventional and Surgical Cardiovascular Pathology: Clinical Correlations and Basic Principles*, Philadelphia, 1989, Saunders, p 63.)

initial stenotic occlusion of less than or equal to 70%. Thus, it is sobering to note that a large number of asymptomatic adults are at significant risk for a catastrophic coronary event. At present, it is impossible to predict plaque rupture in any given patient.

Plaque disruption and ensuing nonocclusive thrombosis are additional common, repetitive, and often clinically silent complications of atheromas. The healing of subclinical disrupted plaques is an important mechanism by which atherosclerotic lesions progressively enlarge (see Fig. 9.7).

Angina Pectoris

Angina pectoris is intermittent chest discomfort or pain caused by transient, reversible myocardial ischemia that is insufficient to cause myocyte necrosis. It is a consequence of the ischemia-induced release of adenosine, bradykinin, and other molecules that stimulate autonomic nerves. Three variants are recognized:

- *Typical* or *stable angina* is predictable episodic chest discomfort associated with exertion or some other cause of increased demand (e.g., tachycardia). The discomfort is described as a crushing or squeezing substernal sensation radiating down the left arm or to the left jaw (referred pain). The discomfort is usually relieved by rest (reducing demand) or by medications such as nitroglycerin, a vasodilator that increases coronary perfusion.
- *Prinzmetal* or *variant angina* occurs at rest and is caused by coronary artery spasm. Although vasospasm typically involves atherosclerotic vessels, a completely healthy vessel can be affected. Prinzmetal angina typically responds promptly to vasodilators such as nitroglycerin and calcium channel blockers.
- *Unstable angina* is characterized by increasingly frequent chest pain, precipitated by progressively less exertion or occurring at rest. Unstable angina is associated with plaque disruption and superimposed thrombosis, distal embolization of the thrombus, and/or vasospasm. Recent studies have shown that the majority of cases of unstable angina are associated with evidence of myocyte injury, and such patients are treated aggressively to limit irreversible myocardial damage.

Myocardial Infarction

Myocardial infarction (MI), also commonly referred to as "heart attack," is necrosis of the heart muscle resulting from ischemia. The 2018 joint task force of U.S. and European Cardiology groups defines MI "as the presence of acute myocardial injury detected by abnormal cardiac biomarkers in the setting of evidence of acute myocardial ischemia." The major underlying cause of IHD is atherosclerosis; while MIs can occur at virtually any age, the frequency rises progressively with aging and with increasing risk factors for atherosclerosis (Chapter 8). Nevertheless, approximately 10% of MIs occur before 40 years of age, and 45% occur before 65 years of age. Men are at greater risk than women, but the gap progressively narrows with age. In general, women tend to be protected against MI during their reproductive years. However, menopause—with declining estrogen production—is associated with exacerbation of coronary artery disease, and IHD is the most common cause of death in older adult women.

Pathogenesis. **The vast majority of MIs are caused by acute thrombosis within coronary arteries** (see Fig. 9.7). In most instances, disruption or erosion of preexisting atherosclerotic plaque serves as the nidus for thrombus generation and consequent vascular occlusion. In 10% of MIs, however, transmural infarction occurs in the absence of occlusive atherosclerotic vascular disease; such

infarcts are mostly ascribed to coronary artery vasospasm or to embolization from mural thrombi (e.g., in the setting of atrial fibrillation) or from valve vegetations. Occasionally, especially with infarcts limited to the innermost (subendocardial) myocardium, thrombi or emboli are absent. In such cases, severe fixed coronary atherosclerosis leads to marginal perfusion of the heart (eFig. 9.1). In this setting, a prolonged period of increased demand (e.g., due to tachycardia or hypertension) can lead to ischemic necrosis of endomyocardium, the portion of the heart that is most distal to the epicardial vessels. Finally, ischemia without detectable atherosclerosis or thromboembolic disease can be caused by disorders of small intramyocardial arterioles, including vasculitis, amyloid deposition, or stasis, as in sickle cell disease.

Coronary Artery Occlusion

In a typical MI, the following sequence of events takes place:

1. *An atheromatous plaque is eroded* or suddenly disrupted by endothelial injury, intraplaque hemorrhage, or mechanical forces, exposing subendothelial collagen and necrotic plaque contents to the blood.
2. *Platelets adhere, aggregate, and are activated*, releasing thromboxane A_2, adenosine diphosphate (ADP), and serotonin, all of which cause further platelet aggregation and vasospasm (Chapter 3).
3. *Activation of coagulation* by exposure of tissue factor adds to the growing thrombus.
4. Within minutes, the enlarging thrombus may completely occlude the coronary artery lumen.

The evidence for this scenario derives from autopsy studies of patients dying of acute MI, as well as imaging studies demonstrating a high frequency of thrombotic occlusion early after MI. Angiography performed within 4 hours of the onset of MI demonstrates coronary thrombosis (eFig. 9.2) in almost 90% of cases. When angiography is performed 12 to 24 hours after onset of symptoms, however, evidence of thrombosis is seen in only 60% of patients, even without intervention. Thus, at least some occlusions clear spontaneously through lysis of the thrombus or relaxation of spasm. This sequence of events in a typical MI also has therapeutic implications: early thrombolysis and/or angioplasty can be highly successful in limiting the extent of myocardial necrosis.

Myocardial Response to Ischemia

Loss of blood supply has profound functional, biochemical, and morphologic consequences for the myocardium. Within seconds of vascular obstruction, aerobic metabolism ceases, leading to a drop in adenosine triphosphate (ATP) and accumulation of potentially noxious metabolites (e.g., lactic acid) in cardiac myocytes. The functional consequence is a rapid loss of contractility, occurring within minutes of the onset of ischemia. These early changes are reversible, but if ischemia persists for 20 to 40 minutes, it leads to irreversible damage and coagulative necrosis of myocytes.

The earliest detectable feature of myocyte necrosis is disruption of the integrity of the sarcolemmal membrane, allowing intracellular macromolecules to leak out of necrotic cells into the cardiac interstitium and the vasculature (Chapter 1).

If blood flow is restored before irreversible injury occurs, myocardium can be preserved; this is the goal of early diagnosis and prompt intervention by thrombolysis or angioplasty. However, as discussed later, reperfusion can have deleterious effects. Even when reperfusion is timely, postischemic myocardium can be profoundly dysfunctional for a number of days due to persistent abnormalities in cellular biochemistry that result in a noncontractile state (stunned myocardium) which may be sufficiently severe to produce transient but reversible cardiac failure.

Myocardial ischemia also contributes to arrhythmias, probably by causing electrical instability (irritability) of ischemic regions of the heart. Although massive myocardial damage can cause fatal mechanical failure, in 80% to 90% of cases cardiac death in the setting of myocardial ischemia is due to ventricular fibrillation caused by myocardial irritability.

Irreversible injury of ischemic myocytes first occurs in the subendocardial zone (Fig. 9.8). As mentioned, this region is especially susceptible to ischemia, as it is the last area to receive blood delivered by the epicardial vessels and is exposed to relatively high intramural pressures, which impede the inflow of blood. With more prolonged ischemia, a wavefront of cell death moves through other regions of the myocardium, driven by progressive tissue edema and myocardial-derived reactive oxygen species and inflammatory mediators. In the

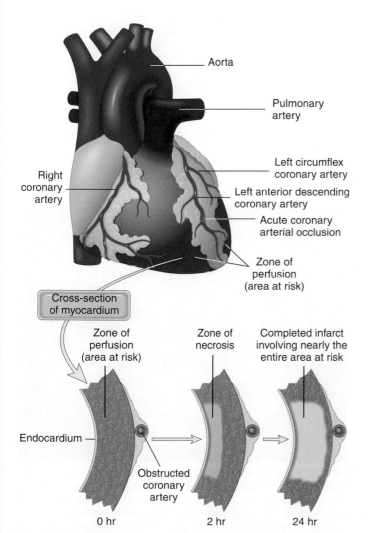

FIG. 9.8 Progression of myocardial necrosis after coronary artery occlusion. A transmural segment of myocardium that is dependent on the occluded vessel for perfusion constitutes the area at risk (dotted line). Necrosis begins in the subendocardial region in the center of the ischemic zone and with time expands to involve the entire wall thickness. Note that a very narrow zone of myocardium immediately beneath the endocardium is spared from necrosis because it can be oxygenated by diffusion from the ventricle.

absence of intervention, an infarct caused by occlusion of an epicardial vessel can involve the entire wall thickness (transmural infarct). An infarct achieves its full extent in 3 to 6 hours. Clinical intervention within this critical window of time can lessen the size of the infarct.

Patterns of Infarction

The location, size, and morphologic features of an acute myocardial infarct depend on multiple factors:

- *Size and distribution* of the involved vessel (Fig. 9.9)
- *Rate of development* and duration of the occlusion
- *Metabolic demands* of the myocardium (affected, for example, by blood pressure and heart rate)
- *Extent of collateral supply*

Acute occlusion of the proximal left anterior descending (LAD) artery is the cause of 40% to 50% of all MIs and typically results in infarction of the anterior wall of the left ventricle, the anterior two-thirds of the ventricular septum, and most of the heart apex; acute proximal obstructions are often fatal while more distal occlusion of the same vessel may affect only the apex. Similarly, acute occlusion of the proximal left circumflex (LCX) artery (seen in 15% to 20% of MIs) causes necrosis of the lateral left ventricle, and proximal right coronary artery (RCA) occlusion (30% to 40% of MIs) affects much of the right ventricle.

The posterior third of the septum and the posterior left ventricle are perfused by the posterior descending artery. The posterior descending artery can arise from either the RCA (in 90% of individuals) or the LCX. By convention, the coronary artery—either RCA or LCX—that gives rise to the posterior descending artery and thereby perfuses portions of the inferior/posterior left ventricle and the posterior third of the septum is considered the dominant vessel. Thus, in a right dominant heart, occlusion of the RCA leads to posterior septal and posterior wall ischemic injury. In comparison, in a left dominant heart, where the posterior descending artery arises from the circumflex artery, occlusion of the LCX generally affects the left lateral wall as well as the posterior third of the septum, and the inferior and posterior wall of the left ventricle.

Occlusions can also occur within secondary branches, such as the diagonal branches of the LAD artery or marginal branches of the LCX artery. Atherosclerosis is primarily a disease of epicardial vessels; significant atherosclerosis or thrombosis of penetrating intramyocardial branches of coronary arteries is rare—although these can be affected by vasculitis, vasospasm, or embolization.

Even though the three major coronary arteries are end arteries, they are interconnected by numerous anastomoses (collateral circulation). Gradual narrowing of one artery allows blood to flow from high- to low-pressure areas through the collateral channels. In this manner, gradual collateral dilation can provide adequate perfusion to areas of the myocardium despite occlusion of an epicardial vessel.

Based on the size of the involved vessel and the degree of collateral circulation, myocardial infarcts may take one of the following patterns:

- *Transmural infarctions* involve the full thickness of the ventricle and are caused by epicardial vessel occlusion resulting from atherosclerosis and acute plaque change with occlusive thrombosis.
- *Subendocardial infarctions* are MIs limited to the inner third of the myocardium. They occur as a result of plaque disruption followed by a coronary thrombus that is lysed spontaneously or therapeutically before the necrosis becomes transmural. As mentioned earlier, the subendocardial region is most vulnerable to hypoperfusion and hypoxia. Thus, in the setting of severe coronary artery disease, transient

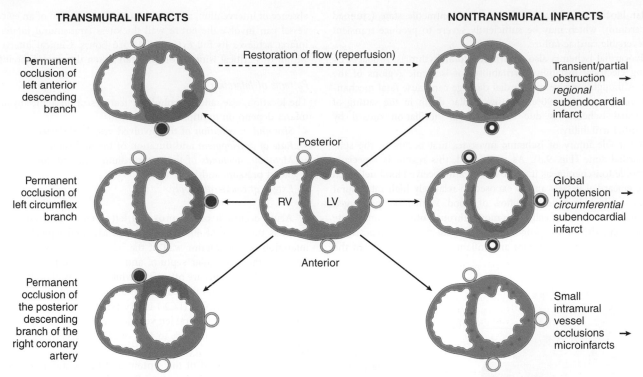

TRANSMURAL INFARCTS

Permanent occlusion of left anterior descending branch

Permanent occlusion of left circumflex branch

Permanent occlusion of the posterior descending branch of the right coronary artery

Restoration of flow (reperfusion)

Posterior

RV   LV

Anterior

NONTRANSMURAL INFARCTS

Transient/partial obstruction → *regional* subendocardial infarct

Global hypotension → *circumferential* subendocardial infarct

Small intramural vessel occlusions → microinfarcts

FIG. 9.9 Dependence of myocardial infarction on the location and nature of the diminished perfusion. *Left,* Patterns of transmural infarction resulting from major coronary artery occlusion. The right ventricle may be involved with occlusion of the right main coronary artery *(not depicted). Right,* Patterns of infarction resulting from partial or transient occlusion *(top),* global hypotension superimposed on fixed three-vessel disease *(middle),* or occlusion of small intramyocardial vessels *(bottom).*

decreases in oxygen delivery (as from hypotension, anemia, or pneumonia) or increases in oxygen demand (as with tachycardia or hypertension) can cause subendocardial ischemic injury.

- *Microscopic infarcts* occur in the setting of small-vessel occlusions and may not show any diagnostic ECG changes. These can occur in the setting of vasculitis, embolization of valve vegetations or mural thrombi, or vessel spasm due to elevated catecholamines, as may occur in extreme emotional stress, with certain tumors (e.g., pheochromocytoma), or as a consequence of cocaine use.

MORPHOLOGY

Nearly all transmural infarcts (involving 50% or more of the ventricle thickness) affect at least a portion of the left ventricle and/or interventricular septum. Roughly 15% to 30% of MIs that involve the posterior or posteroseptal wall also extend into the right ventricle. Isolated right ventricle infarcts occur in only 1% to 3% of cases of IHD.

The gross and microscopic appearance of an MI depends on the age of the injury. Areas of damage progress through a highly characteristic sequence of morphologic changes from coagulative necrosis, to acute and then chronic inflammation, to fibrosis (Table 9.2). Myocardial necrosis proceeds invariably to scar formation without any significant regeneration.

Gross and/or microscopic recognition of very recent myocardial infarcts can be challenging, particularly when death occurs within a few hours. **Myocardial infarcts less than 12 hours old are usually not grossly apparent.** However, infarcts more than 3 hours old can be visualized by exposing myocardium to vital stains, such as triphenyl tetrazolium chloride, a substrate for lactate dehydrogenase. Because this enzyme leaks out of damaged cells in the area of ischemic necrosis, the infarcted area

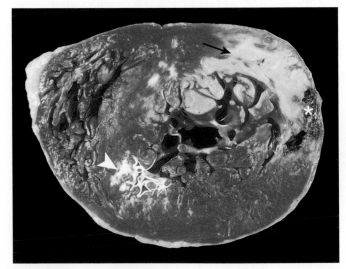

FIG. 9.10 Acute myocardial infarct of the posterolateral left ventricle demonstrated by a lack of triphenyl tetrazolium chloride staining in areas of necrosis *(arrow);* the absence of staining is due to enzyme leakage after cell death. Note the anterior scar *(arrowhead),* indicative of remote infarction. The myocardial hemorrhage at the right edge of the infarct *(asterisk)* is due to ventricular rupture that was the acute cause of death in this patient (specimen is oriented with the posterior wall at the *top).*

is unstained (pale) in contrast to healthy myocardium, while old scars appear white and glistening (Fig. 9.10). **By 12 to 24 hours after MI, an infarct can usually be grossly identified by a red-blue**

Table 9.2 Evolution of Morphologic Changes in Myocardial Infarction

Time Frame	Gross Features	Light Microscopic Findings	Electron Microscopic Findings
Reversible Injury			
0–½ hour	None	None	Relaxation of myofibrils; glycogen loss; mitochondrial swelling
Irreversible Injury			
½–4 hours	None	Usually none; variable waviness of fibers at border	Sarcolemmal disruption; mitochondrial amorphous densities
4–12 hours	Occasionally dark mottling	Onset coagulation necrosis; edema; hemorrhage	
12–24 hours	Dark mottling	Ongoing coagulation necrosis; pyknosis of nuclei; hypereosinophilic appearance of myocytes; marginal contraction band necrosis; early neutrophilic infiltrate	
1–3 days	Mottling with yellow-tan infarct center	Coagulation necrosis with loss of nuclei and striations; increased infiltrate of neutrophils	
3–7 days	Hyperemic border; central yellow-tan softening	Initial disintegration of dead myofibers, with dying neutrophils; early phagocytosis of dead cells by macrophages at infarct border	
7–10 days	Maximally yellow-tan and soft, with depressed red-tan margins	Well-developed phagocytosis of dead cells; early formation of granulation tissue at margins	
10–14 days	Red-gray depressed infarct borders	Well-established granulation tissue with new blood vessels and collagen deposition	
2–8 weeks	Gray-white scar, progressing from border toward core of infarct	Increased collagen deposition, with decreased cellularity	
>2 months	Scarring complete	Dense collagenous scar	

discoloration due to stagnant, trapped blood. Thereafter, infarcts become progressively better delineated as soft, yellow-tan areas; by 10 to 14 days, infarcts are rimmed by hyperemic (highly vascularized) granulation tissue. Over the succeeding weeks, the infarcted tissue evolves to a fibrous scar.

The microscopic appearance also undergoes a characteristic sequence of changes (see Table 9.2 and Fig. 9.11). Typical features of coagulative necrosis (Chapter 1) become detectable within 4 to 12 hours of infarction. "Wavy fibers," which reflect the stretching and buckling of noncontractile dead fibers, may be present at the edges of an infarct. Sublethal ischemia may induce intracellular **myocyte vacuolization;** such myocytes are viable but frequently contract poorly.

Necrotic myocardium elicits acute inflammation (typically 1 to 3 days after MI), followed by a wave of macrophages that remove necrotic myocytes and neutrophil fragments (most pronounced 5 to 10 days after MI). The infarcted zone is progressively replaced by granulation tissue by 1 to 2 weeks after MI, which in turn forms the provisional scaffolding upon which dense collagenous scar forms. In most instances, scarring is well advanced by the end of the sixth week, but the extent of repair depends on the size of the original lesion and the ability of the host tissues to heal. Healing requires the migration of inflammatory cells and ingrowth of new vessels from the infarct margins. Thus, an MI heals from its borders toward the center, and a large infarct may not heal as quickly nor as completely as a small one. Moreover, malnutrition, poor vasculature, or exogenous corticosteroids can impede infarct scarring (Chapter 2). Once an MI is completely healed, it is impossible to distinguish its age: whether present for 8 weeks or 10 years, fibrous scars look the same.

Infarct Modification by Reperfusion

The therapeutic goal in acute MI is restoration of tissue perfusion as quickly as possible (hence the adage "time is myocardium"). Such reperfusion is achieved by thrombolysis (dissolution of thrombus by tissue plasminogen activator), angioplasty, or coronary arterial bypass graft. While preservation of a viable (but at-risk) heart can improve short- and long-term outcomes, reperfusion is not an unalloyed blessing because of a phenomenon called reperfusion injury (Chapter 1). The factors that contribute to reperfusion injury include the following:

- *Mitochondrial dysfunction.* Ischemia alters mitochondrial membrane permeability, which leads to swelling and rupture of the outer membrane, releasing mitochondrial contents that promote apoptosis.
- *Myocyte hypercontracture.* During periods of ischemia, the intracellular levels of calcium increase due to increased influx through the damaged plasma membrane and release from intracellular stores. The increased intracellular calcium leads to cytoskeletal contraction, causing enhanced and uncontrolled myofibril contractions and culminating in cell death.
- *Free radicals,* including superoxide anion $(O_2^{\cdot})$, hydrogen peroxide (H_2O_2), hypochlorous acid $(HOCl)$, nitric oxide—derived peroxynitrite, and hydroxyl radicals ($\cdot OH$) are produced within minutes of reperfusion and cause damage to the myocytes by altering membrane proteins and phospholipids. ROS generated by infiltrating leukocytes may also contribute to the damaged vulnerable cells.
- *Leukocyte aggregation* within the reperfused vessels may occlude the microvasculature and contribute to the impairment of blood flow, the so-called "no-reflow" phenomenon. This is mediated in part by activation of phospholipase A2, which gives rise to

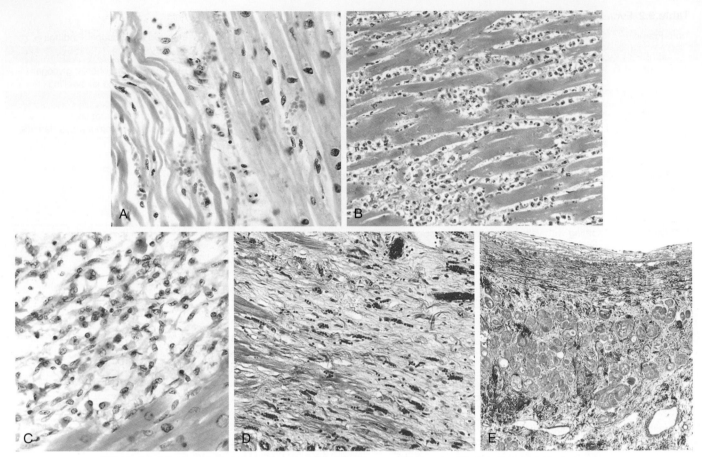

FIG. 9.11 Microscopic features of myocardial infarction and its repair. (A) One-day-old infarct showing coagulative necrosis and wavy fibers *(left)*, compared with adjacent healthy fibers *(right)*. Necrotic cells are separated by edema fluid. (B) Dense neutrophilic infiltrate in the area of a 2- to 3-day-old infarct. (C) Nearly complete removal of necrotic myocytes by phagocytic macrophages (7 to 10 days). (D) Granulation tissue characterized by loose connective tissue and abundant capillaries. (E) Healed myocardial infarct consisting of a dense collagenous scar. A few residual cardiac muscle cells are present. (D) and (E) are Masson trichrome stain, which stains collagen blue.

arachidonic acid metabolites such as prostaglandins that trigger acute inflammation.

- *Platelet and complement activation* also contribute to microvascular injury. Complement activation is thought to play a role in the "no-reflow" phenomenon by causing injury and swelling of the endothelium.

The typical appearance of reperfused myocardium in the setting of an acute MI is shown in Fig. 9.12. Such infarcts are hemorrhagic because of vascular injury and leakiness. Microscopically, myocytes that are irreversibly damaged after reperfusion develop *contraction band necrosis*, characterized by the presence of intense eosinophilic bands of hypercontracted sarcomeres created by an influx of calcium. In the absence of ATP, the sarcomeres cannot relax and are fixed in an agonal tetanic state. Thus, while reperfusion can salvage reversibly injured cells, it also alters the morphology of irreversibly injured cells.

Clinical Features. **The classic MI is heralded by severe, crushing substernal chest pain (or pressure) that radiates to the neck, jaw, epigastrium, or left arm.** In contrast to angina pectoris, the associated pain typically lasts several minutes to hours and is not relieved by nitroglycerin or rest. However, in a substantial minority of patients (as

many as 25%), MIs are entirely asymptomatic. Such "silent" infarcts are particularly common in patients with underlying diabetes (in whom autonomic neuropathy may prevent perception of pain) and in older adults.

The pulse is generally rapid and weak, and patients are often diaphoretic (sweating) and nauseated (particularly with posterior wall MIs). Dyspnea is common, resulting from impaired myocardial contractility and dysfunction of the mitral valve apparatus, with resultant acute pulmonary congestion and edema. With massive MIs (involving more than 40% of the left ventricle), cardiogenic shock develops. Arrhythmias caused by electrical abnormalities in the ischemic myocardium and conduction system are common; indeed, sudden cardiac death from a lethal arrhythmia accounts for most MI-related deaths occurring before hospitalization.

Electrocardiographic abnormalities are important for the diagnosis of MI; these include Q waves, ST segment changes, and T wave inversions (the latter two representing abnormalities in myocardial repolarization). MIs are classified into two categories based on ECG changes, ST-elevated MI *(STEMI)* and non-ST-elevated MI *(NSTEMI)*.

- *STEMI* is invariably due to complete occlusion of a coronary artery and indicates the presence of a transmural infarct. Typically, patients need urgent coronary artery thrombolysis or stent placement.

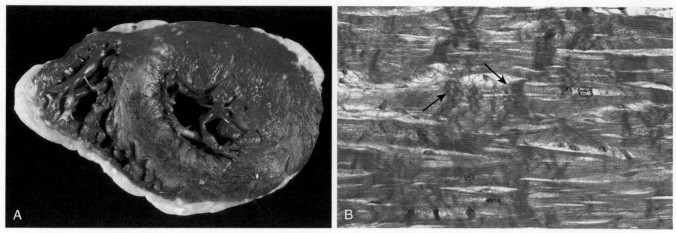

FIG. 9.12 Reperfused myocardial infarction. (A) The transverse heart slice (stained with triphenyl tetrazolium chloride) exhibits a large anterior wall myocardial infarction that is hemorrhagic because of bleeding from damaged vessels. The posterior wall is at the *top*. (B) Contraction bands, visible as prominent hypereosinophilic cross-striations spanning myofibers *(arrow)*, are seen microscopically. (B, Courtesy of Dr. Joseph J. Maleszewski, Mayo Clinic, Rochester, Minnesota USA.)

- *NSTEMI* is not associated with complete coronary artery occlusion or full-thickness infarction and can often be managed conservatively.

  The laboratory evaluation of MI is based on measuring blood levels of normally intracellular proteins that leak out of injured myocardial cells through damaged cell membranes (Fig. 9.13). These molecules include myoglobin, cardiac troponins T and I (TnT, TnI), creatine kinase (CK; specifically, the myocardial isoform, CK-MB), and lactate dehydrogenase. Troponins (and to a lesser extent CK-MB) have high specificity and sensitivity for myocardial damage.
- *CK-MB* has long been used as the biomarker of myocardial injury but is now tested for less frequently in favor of the more sensitive cardiac-specific troponins. CK-MB activity begins to rise within 2 to 4 hours of MI, peaks at 24 to 48 hours, and returns to normal within approximately 72 hours.
- *TnI* and *TnT* are normally not found in the circulation; however, after acute MI, both are detectable within 2 to 4 hours, with levels peaking at 48 hours and remaining elevated for 7 to 10 days. Persistence of elevated troponin levels allows the diagnosis of an acute MI to be made long after CK-MB levels have returned to normal. With reperfusion, both troponin and CK-MB levels may peak earlier owing to more rapid washout of the enzyme from the necrotic tissue.

Consequences and Complications of Myocardial Infarction

Extraordinary progress has been made in improving patient outcomes after acute MI; the overall in-hospital death rate for MI is approximately 7% to 8%. Patients with STEMI experience higher mortality rates (10%) than those with NSTEMI (approximately 6%). With better and earlier in-hospital care such differences are narrowing. Out-of-hospital mortality is substantially poorer: one-third of individuals with STEMIs die, usually of an arrhythmia within 1 hour of symptom onset, before they receive appropriate medical attention. Such statistics make the rising rate of coronary artery disease in lower-income countries with scarce hospital facilities all the more worrisome.

There may be multiple complications of acute MI, of which three are potentially lethal: rupture of the left ventricular free wall, rupture of the interventricular septum, and acute mitral regurgitation due to papillary muscle necrosis. Nearly three-fourths of patients experience one or more of these complications (Fig. 9.14):

- *Myocardial rupture.* Rupture complicates 1% to 5% of MIs and is frequently fatal. Ventricular septal rupture is the most common (Fig. 9.14B), creating a VSD, followed in frequency by papillary muscle rupture (Fig. 9.14C), often producing severe mitral regurgitation. Ventricular free wall rupture is the least common but the most serious, resulting in fatal hemopericardium and cardiac tamponade (Fig. 9.14A). Rupture occurs most often 3 to 7 days after MI—the time in the healing process when lysis of necrotic myocardium is maximal and when much of the infarct has been converted to soft, friable granulation tissue.

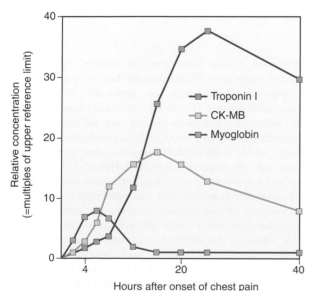

FIG. 9.13 Acute increases in myocardium-derived troponin I, myocardial creatine kinase (CK-MB), and myoglobin following myocardial infarction. The kinetics of enzyme elevations can be used to estimate the timing of the MI. Myoglobin can also be measured but is substantially less sensitive and specific for myocardial injury.

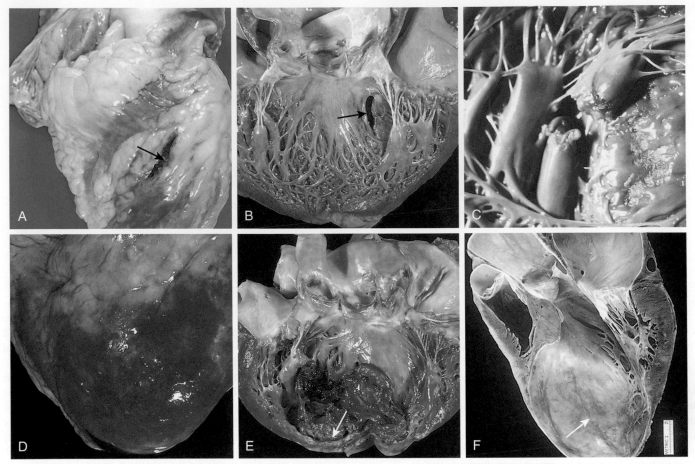

FIG. 9.14 Complications of myocardial infarction. (A to C) Cardiac rupture. (A) Anterior free wall myocardial rupture *(arrow)*. (B) Ventricular septal rupture *(arrow)*. (C) Papillary muscle rupture. (D) Fibrinous pericarditis, with a hemorrhagic, roughened epicardial surface overlying an acute infarct. (E) Recent expansion of an anteroapical infarct with wall stretching and thinning *(arrow)* and mural thrombus. (F) Large apical left ventricular aneurysm *(arrow)*. (A to E, Reproduced by permission from Schoen FJ: *Interventional and Surgical Cardiovascular Pathology: Clinical Correlations and Basic Principles*, Philadelphia, 1989, Saunders. F, Courtesy of William D. Edwards, MD, Mayo Clinic, Rochester, Minnesota.)

- *Contractile dysfunction.* In general, MIs impair left ventricular pump function in proportion to the extent of damage. In most cases, there is some degree of left ventricular failure manifested as hypotension, pulmonary congestion, and pulmonary edema. Severe "pump failure" *(cardiogenic shock)* occurs in roughly 10% of patients with transmural MIs and is typically associated with infarcts that damage 40% or more of the left ventricle.
- *Papillary muscle dysfunction.* Papillary muscles may be poorly contractile as a result of ischemia, leading to postinfarct mitral regurgitation. Later, papillary muscle fibrosis and shortening or global ventricular dilation can also cause mitral valve insufficiency.
- *Right ventricular infarction.* Isolated right ventricular infarction occurs in only 1% to 3% of MIs, but right ventricle is vulnerable to RCA occlusions, which also produce left ventricular damage. In either case, right-sided heart failure is a common outcome, leading to pooling of blood in the venous circulation and systemic hypotension.
- *Arrhythmias.* MIs lead to myocardial irritability and conduction disturbances that can cause sudden death. Approximately 90% of patients develop some form of rhythm disturbance, with the incidence being higher in STEMIs versus NSTEMIs. MI-associated arrhythmias include heart block of variable degree (including asystole), bradycardia, supraventricular tachyarrhythmias, ventricular premature contractions or ventricular tachycardia, and ventricular fibrillation. The risk for serious arrhythmias (e.g., ventricular fibrillation) is greatest in the first hour and declines thereafter.
- *Pericarditis.* Transmural MIs can elicit a fibrinohemorrhagic pericarditis, which is an epicardial manifestation of the underlying myocardial inflammation (Fig. 9.14D). Heralded by anterior chest pain and a pericardial friction rub, pericarditis typically appears 2 to 3 days after infarction and then gradually resolves over the next few days. Extensive infarcts or severe pericardial inflammation can occasionally lead to large effusions or can organize to form dense adhesions that eventually manifest as a constrictive lesion. Rarely, pericarditis may develop weeks later *(Dressler syndrome)* due to development of antibodies against injured myocardium.
- *Chamber dilation.* Because of the weakening of necrotic muscle, there may be disproportionate stretching, thinning, and dilation of the infarcted region (especially with anteroseptal infarcts).
- *Mural thrombus.* With any infarct, the combination of attenuated myocardial contractility (causing stasis), chamber dilation, and endocardial damage (exposing a thrombogenic surface) can foster

mural thrombosis (Fig. 9.14E), which may lead to left-sided thromboembolism.

- *Ventricular aneurysm.* A late complication, aneurysm of the ventricle most commonly results from a large transmural anteroseptal infarct that heals with the formation of a thinned wall of scar tissue (Fig. 9.14F). Although ventricular aneurysms frequently give rise to mural thrombi, arrhythmias, and heart failure, they do not rupture.
- *Progressive heart failure.* This is discussed under "Chronic Ischemic Heart Disease" next.

The long-term prognosis after MI depends on many factors, the most important of which are the quality of left ventricular function and the severity of atherosclerotic narrowing of vessels perfusing the remaining viable myocardium.

Chronic Ischemic Heart Disease

Chronic IHD, also called ischemic cardiomyopathy, is progressive heart failure secondary to ischemic myocardial damage. In most instances, there is a known clinical history of previous MI. After prior infarction(s), chronic IHD appears when the compensatory mechanisms (e.g., hypertrophy) of residual myocardium begin to fail. In other cases, severe CAD can cause diffuse myocardial dysfunction, micro-infarction and replacement fibrosis, without a clinically evident episode of infarction.

The heart failure of chronic IHD is typically severe and is occasionally punctuated by new episodes of angina or infarction. Arrhythmias, CHF, and intercurrent MI account for most of the associated morbidity and mortality.

ARRHYTHMIAS

Aberrant rhythms can be initiated anywhere in the conduction system, from the sinoatrial (SA) node down to the level of an individual myocyte; they are typically designated as originating from the atrium (*supraventricular*) or within the ventricular myocardium. Abnormalities in myocardial conduction can be sustained or sporadic (*paroxysmal*). They can manifest as *tachycardia* (fast heart rate); *bradycardia* (slow heart rate); an irregular rhythm with normal ventricular contraction; chaotic depolarization without functional ventricular contraction (*ventricular fibrillation*); or no electrical activity at all (*asystole*). Patients may be unaware of a rhythm disorder or may note a "racing heart" or *palpitations* (irregular rhythm); loss of adequate cardiac output due to sustained arrhythmia can produce lightheadedness (near syncope), loss of consciousness (*syncope*), or *sudden cardiac death* (see later).

Ischemic injury is the most common cause of rhythm disorders, either causing direct damage of the conduction system or altered conduction of signals resulting from dilation of heart chambers.

- When the SA node is damaged (e.g., *sick sinus syndrome*), other fibers or even the atrioventricular (AV) node can take over pacemaker function, albeit at a much slower intrinsic rate (causing bradycardia).
- When the atrial myocytes become "irritable" as occurs with atrial dilation, firing from stretch sensitive ion channels, gives rise to the random "irregularly irregular" heart rate of *atrial fibrillation*.
- When the AV node is dysfunctional, varying degrees of *heart block* occur, ranging from asymptomatic prolongation of the P-R interval on ECG (*first-degree heart block*), to intermittent transmission of

the signal (*second-degree heart block*), to complete failure (*third-degree heart block*).

Certain rare heritable conditions can also cause arrhythmias. They are important to recognize because they may alert physicians to the need for intervention to prevent sudden cardiac death (discussed later) in the proband and their family members. Some of these disorders are associated with recognizable anatomic findings (e.g., congenital anomalies, hypertrophic cardiomyopathy, mitral valve prolapse). However, other heritable disorders precipitate arrythmias and sudden death in the absence of other cardiac pathology (so-called "primary electrical disorders"). These syndromes are diagnosed by genetic testing, which is performed in those with a positive family history or an unexplained nonlethal arrhythmia. The most important of these are the *channelopathies*, which are caused by mutations in genes that encode various ion channels or ion channel regulators. Since ion channels are responsible for conducting the electrical currents that mediate contraction of the heart, defects in these channels may provoke arrythmias. The prototype is the *long QT syndrome*, characterized by prolongation of the QT segment in ECGs and susceptibility to ventricular arrhythmias. Mutations in several different genes cause long QT syndrome; the most frequently culpable gene, *KCNQ1*, encodes a K^+ channel that controls levels of potassium ions in myocardial cells, which regulate electrical activity.

Sudden Cardiac Death

Sudden cardiac death (SCD) is defined as unexpected death due to cessation of normal cardiac electrical activity with hemodynamic collapse. SCD results most commonly from lethal arrhythmias such as ventricular tachycardia, ventricular fibrillation, and asystole. If the individual is successfully resuscitated (e.g., by timely defibrillation), the event is called sudden cardiac arrest (SCA). Roughly 450,000 individuals succumb to SCD each year in the United States. The majority (65% to 70%) have underlying coronary atherosclerosis and ischemic heart disease; approximately 10% have structural heart disease (listed below); 5% to 10% are due to arrhythmias in the absence of structural heart disease, and the rest stem from noncardiac causes. SCD may be the first manifestation of IHD. Of interest, coronary angiography shows thrombotic occlusion of a coronary artery in approximately 50% of cases. Thus, in many cases, there is no associated myocardial infarction, and 80% to 90% of patients who suffer SCA do not show any enzymatic or ECG evidence of myocardial necrosis—even if the cause is IHD. Healed remote MIs are present in about 40% of cases.

In younger patients with SCD, nonatherosclerotic causes are more common, including the following:

- *Hereditary (channelopathies)* or acquired abnormalities of the cardiac conduction system
- *Congenital coronary artery abnormalities*
- *Mitral valve prolapse*
- *Myocarditis or sarcoidosis*
- *Dilated or hypertrophic cardiomyopathy*
- *Pulmonary hypertension*
- *Myocardial hypertrophy.* Increased cardiac mass is an independent risk factor for SCD; thus, in some young individuals who die suddenly, including athletes, hypertensive hypertrophy or unexplained increased cardiac mass is the only pathologic finding.

The prognosis of many patients at risk for SCD, including those with chronic IHD, is markedly improved by implantation of a pacemaker or an automatic cardioverter defibrillator, which senses and electrically counteracts episodes of ventricular fibrillation.

The relationship of coronary artery disease to the various clinical end points discussed earlier is depicted in Fig. 9.15.

HYPERTENSIVE HEART DISEASE

Hypertensive heart disease is a consequence of the increased demands placed on the heart by hypertension. As discussed in Chapter 8, hypertension is a common disorder associated with considerable morbidity that affects many organs, including the heart, brain, and kidneys. The discussion here will focus specifically on the major cardiac complications of hypertension, which result from pressure overload and ventricular hypertrophy. Myocyte hypertrophy is an adaptive response to pressure overload; there are limits to myocardial adaptive capacity, however, and persistent hypertension can eventually culminate in dysfunction, cardiac dilation, CHF, and sudden death. Although hypertensive heart disease most commonly affects the left side of the heart because hypertension is

usually systemic, pulmonary hypertension can also cause right-sided hypertensive changes (cor pulmonale).

Systemic (Left-Sided) Hypertensive Heart Disease

The criteria for the diagnosis of systemic hypertensive heart disease are (1) left ventricular hypertrophy in the absence of other cardiovascular pathology (e.g., valvular stenosis) and (2) a history or pathologic evidence of hypertension in other organs (e.g., kidneys). With the recent revision of criteria for hypertension to pressures above 120 mm systolic and 80 mm diastolic, approximately 50% of the general population in the United States has hypertension.

MORPHOLOGY

As discussed earlier, systemic hypertension imposes pressure overload on the heart and is associated with gross and microscopic changes somewhat distinct from those caused by volume overload. The essential feature of hypertensive heart disease is **left ventricular hypertrophy,** typically without ventricular dilation until very late in the process (Fig. 9.16A). The heart weight can exceed 500 g (typical for a 60- to 70-kg individual is 320 to 360 g), and the left ventricular wall thickness can exceed 2.0 cm (usually 1.2 to 1.4 cm). With time, the increased left ventricular wall thickness imparts a stiffness that impairs diastolic filling and can result in left atrial dilation. In long-standing systemic hypertensive heart disease leading to congestive failure, the hypertrophic left ventricle is typically dilated.

Microscopically, the transverse diameter of myocytes is increased and there are prominent nuclear enlargement and hyperchromasia ("boxcar nuclei"), as well as intercellular fibrosis (see also Fig. 9.1D).

Clinical Features. Compensated hypertensive heart disease is typically asymptomatic and is suspected only from discovery of elevated blood pressure on routine physical examination, or from ECG or echocardiographic findings of left ventricular hypertrophy. In some patients, the disease comes to attention with the onset of atrial fibrillation (secondary to left atrial enlargement) and/or CHF. The mechanisms by which hypertension leads to heart failure are incompletely understood; presumably the hypertrophic myocytes fail to contract efficiently, possibly due to structural abnormalities in newly assembled sarcomeres and because the vascular supply is inadequate to meet the demands of the increased muscle mass. Patients with left ventricular hypertrophy have a higher incidence of heart failure, ventricular arrhythmias, death following myocardial infarction, sudden cardiac death, and cerebrovascular accident. Effective hypertension control can prevent or lead to the regression of cardiac hypertrophy and its attendant risks.

Pulmonary Hypertensive Heart Disease: Cor Pulmonale

Cor pulmonale consists of right ventricular hypertrophy and dilation—frequently accompanied by right-sided heart failure—caused by pulmonary hypertension attributable to primary disorders of the lung parenchyma, such as chronic obstructive pulmonary disease and interstitial fibrosis, or the pulmonary vasculature (Table 9.3). Right ventricular dilation and hypertrophy caused by left ventricular failure (or by congenital heart disease) is substantially more common but is excluded by this definition.

Cor pulmonale can be acute in onset, as with pulmonary embolism, or can have a slow and insidious onset when due to prolonged pressure overload in the setting of chronic lung and pulmonary vascular disease (see Table 9.3).

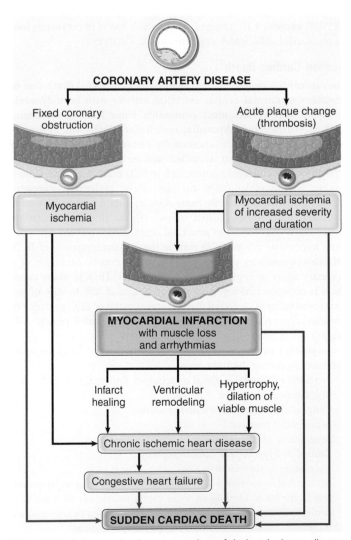

FIG. 9.15 Pathways in the progression of ischemic heart disease showing the relationships among coronary artery disease and its major sequelae.

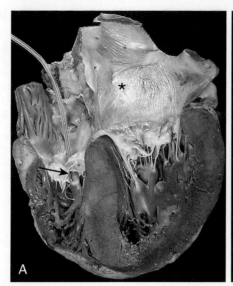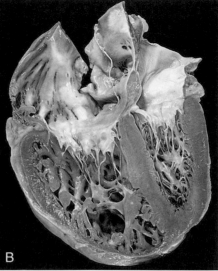

FIG. 9.16 Hypertensive heart disease. (A) Systemic (left-sided) hypertensive heart disease. There is marked concentric thickening of the left ventricular wall causing reduction in lumen size. The left ventricle and left atrium are shown on the *right* in this four-chamber view of the heart. A pacemaker is present in the right ventricle *(arrow)*. Note also the left atrial dilation *(asterisk)* due to stiffening of the left ventricle and impaired diastolic relaxation, leading to atrial volume overload. (B) Chronic cor pulmonale. The right ventricle *(shown on the left)* is markedly dilated and hypertrophied with a thickened free wall and hypertrophied trabeculae. The shape and volume of the left ventricle have been distorted by the enlarged right ventricle.

MORPHOLOGY

In **acute cor pulmonale,** the right ventricle usually shows only dilation; if an embolism causes sudden death, the heart may even be of normal size. **Chronic cor pulmonale** is characterized by right ventricular (and often right atrial) hypertrophy. In extreme cases, the thickness of the right ventricular wall may be comparable to or even exceed that of the left ventricle (Fig. 9.16B). When ventricular failure develops, the right ventricle and atrium are often dilated. Because chronic cor pulmonale occurs in the setting of pulmonary hypertension, the pulmonary arteries may show abnormal intimal thickening.

VALVULAR HEART DISEASE

Valvular disease may result in stenosis, insufficiency (regurgitation or incompetence), or both.
- *Stenosis* is the failure of a valve to open completely, obstructing forward flow. Valvular stenosis is almost always due to a primary cuspal abnormality stemming from a chronic process (e.g., calcification or valve scarring).
- *Insufficiency* results from failure of a valve to close completely, thereby allowing regurgitation (backflow) of blood. Valvular insufficiency can result from either intrinsic disease of the valve cusps (e.g., endocarditis) or disruption of the support structures (e.g., the aorta, mitral annulus, tendinous cords, papillary muscles, or ventricular free wall) without primary cuspal injury. It can appear abruptly, as with chordal rupture, or insidiously as a consequence of leaflet scarring and retraction.

Valvular disease can involve only one valve (typically the mitral valve) or multiple valves. Turbulent flow through diseased valves produces abnormal heart sounds called *murmurs*; severe lesions can be externally palpated as *thrills*. Depending on the valve involved, murmurs are best heard at different locations on the chest wall; moreover, the nature (regurgitation versus stenosis) and severity of the valvular disease determines the quality and timing of the murmur (e.g., harsh systolic or soft diastolic murmurs).

The outcome of valvular disease depends on the valve involved, the degree of impairment, the tempo of its development, and the effectiveness of compensatory mechanisms. For example, rapid destruction

Table 9.3 Disorders Predisposing to Cor Pulmonale

Diseases of the Pulmonary Parenchyma
Chronic obstructive pulmonary disease
Diffuse pulmonary interstitial fibrosis
Pneumoconiosis
Cystic fibrosis
Bronchiectasis
Diseases of the Pulmonary Vessels
Recurrent pulmonary thromboembolism
Primary pulmonary hypertension
Extensive pulmonary arteritis (e.g., granulomatosis with polyangiitis)
Drug-, toxin-, or radiation-induced vascular obstruction
Extensive pulmonary tumor microembolism
Disorders Affecting Chest Movement
Kyphoscoliosis
Marked obesity
Neuromuscular diseases
Disorders Inducing Pulmonary Arterial Constriction
Metabolic acidosis
Hypoxemia
Obstructive sleep apnea
Idiopathic alveolar hypoventilation

of an aortic valve cusp by infection can cause massive regurgitation and the abrupt onset of cardiac failure. By contrast, rheumatic mitral stenosis usually progresses over years, and its clinical effects are well tolerated until late in the course.

Valvular abnormalities can be congenital or acquired. By far the most common congenital valvular lesion is a *bicuspid aortic valve*, composed of only two functional cusps instead of the usual three; this malformation occurs with a frequency of 1% to 2% of all live births and has been associated with mutations in several genes. The two cusps are of unequal size, with the larger cusp exhibiting a midline *raphe* resulting from incomplete cuspal separation (see Fig. 9.17B). The function of bicuspid aortic valves is generally normal early in life; however, with aging they are abnormally susceptible to progressive degenerative calcification, resulting in stenosis (see later).

The most important causes of acquired valvular diseases are summarized in Table 9.4; acquired stenoses of the aortic and mitral valves account for approximately two-thirds of all valve disease.

Degenerative Valve Disease

Degenerative valve disease is a term used to describe changes that affect the integrity of valvular extracellular matrix (ECM). These diseases are probably an inevitable aspect of aging, related to the repetitive mechanical stresses to which valves are subjected—40 million beats per year, with each normal opening and closing requiring substantial valve deformation.

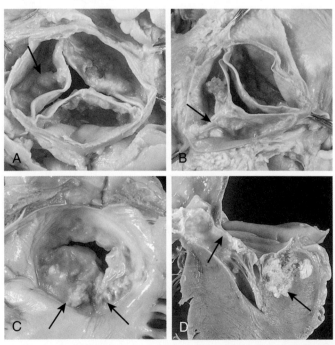

FIG. 9.17 Calcific valvular degeneration. (A) Calcific aortic stenosis of a previously normal valve (viewed from above the valve). Nodular masses of calcium are heaped up within the sinuses of Valsalva *(arrow)*. Note that the commissures are not fused, as in rheumatic aortic valve stenosis (see Fig. 9.19C). (B) Calcific aortic stenosis occurring on a congenitally bicuspid valve. One cusp has a partial fusion at its center, called a raphe *(arrow)*. (C and D) Mitral calcification, with calcific nodules within the annulus (attachment margin) of the mitral leaflets *(arrows)*. (C) Left atrial view. (D) Section demonstrating the extension of calcification *(arrow)* into the underlying myocardium. Such involvement of adjacent structures near the interventricular septum can impinge on the conduction system.

Table 9.4 Etiology of Acquired Heart Valve Disease

Mitral Valve Disease	Aortic Valve Disease
Mitral Stenosis	**Aortic Stenosis**
Postinflammatory scarring (rheumatic heart disease)	Postinflammatory scarring (rheumatic heart disease)
	Senile calcific aortic stenosis
	Calcification of congenitally deformed valve
Mitral Regurgitation	**Aortic Regurgitation**
Abnormalities of leaflets and commissures	Intrinsic valvular disease
Postinflammatory scarring	Postinflammatory scarring (rheumatic heart disease)
Infective endocarditis	Infective endocarditis
Mitral valve prolapse	
"Fen-phen"—induced valvular fibrosis	Aortic disease
	Degenerative aortic dilation
Abnormalities of tensor apparatus	Syphilitic aortitis
Rupture of papillary muscle	Ankylosing spondylitis
Papillary muscle dysfunction (fibrosis)	Rheumatoid arthritis
Rupture of chordae tendineae	Marfan syndrome
Abnormalities of left ventricular cavity and/or annulus	
Left ventricular enlargement (myocarditis, dilated cardiomyopathy)	
Calcification of mitral ring	

Fen-phen, Fenfluramine-phentermine.
Data from Schoen FJ: Surgical pathology of removed natural and prosthetic valves, *Hum Pathol* 18:558, 1987.

Degenerative changes include the following:
- *Calcifications,* which can be cuspal (typically in the aortic valve) (Fig. 9.17A and B) or annular (in the mitral valve) (Fig. 9.17C and D). Mitral annular calcification is usually asymptomatic unless it encroaches on the adjacent conduction system.
- *Alterations in the ECM.* In some cases, changes consist of increased proteoglycan and diminished fibrillar collagen and elastin *(myxomatous degeneration)*; in other cases, the valve becomes fibrotic and scarred.

Calcific Aortic Stenosis

Calcific aortic degeneration is the most common cause of aortic stenosis. In most cases, calcific degeneration is asymptomatic and is discovered only incidentally on chest radiograph or at autopsy. In other patients, valvular sclerosis and/or calcification can be sufficiently severe to cause stenosis, necessitating surgical intervention. The incidence of calcific aortic stenosis is increasing in pace with longevity. In anatomically normal valves, it typically begins to manifest when patients reach their 70s and 80s; onset with bicuspid aortic valves is at a much earlier age (often 40 to 50 years of age).

Although simple progressive age-associated "wear and tear" is often invoked to explain the process, cuspal fibrosis and calcification also can be viewed as the valvular counterparts to age-related arteriosclerosis. Risk factors for aortic valve degeneration and calcification include male sex, high low-density lipoprotein cholesterol, hypertension, and smoking, all of which are also associated with atherosclerosis.

The accumulation of lipoproteins induces local inflammation, which may be exacerbated by flow abnormalities (e.g., bicuspid valve, hypertension) that alter endothelial cell function. The resulting injury predisposes the valve for calcification.

Clinical Features. In severe disease, valve orifices can be compromised by as much as 70% to 80%. Cardiac output is maintained only by virtue of concentric left ventricular hypertrophy; the chronic outflow obstruction can drive left ventricular pressures to 200 mm Hg or more. The hypertrophied myocardium is prone to ischemia, and angina may develop. Systolic and diastolic dysfunction combine to cause CHF, and cardiac decompensation eventually ensues. The development of angina, CHF, or syncope in aortic stenosis heralds the exhaustion of compensatory cardiac hyperfunction and carries a poor prognosis; without surgical intervention, 50% to 80% of patients die within 2 to 3 years.

Mitral Valve Prolapse (Myxomatous Mitral Valve)

In mitral valve prolapse, one or both mitral leaflets are "floppy" and balloon back into the left atrium during systole. It can be primary or secondary:

- *Primary mitral valve prolapse* is idiopathic. It is associated with myxomatous mitral valve degeneration affecting some 0.5% to 2.4% of adults. It can be sporadic or familial and is one of the most common forms of valvular heart disease.
- *Secondary mitral valve prolapse* is associated with an identifiable genetic disorder such as Marfan syndrome (Chapter 4).

Clinical Features. Most patients are asymptomatic, and the valvular abnormality is discovered incidentally. In a minority of cases, patients present with palpitations, dyspnea, or atypical chest pain. Auscultation discloses a midsystolic click, caused by abrupt tension on the redundant valve leaflets and chordae tendineae as the valve attempts to close; sometimes there is an associated regurgitant murmur. Although in

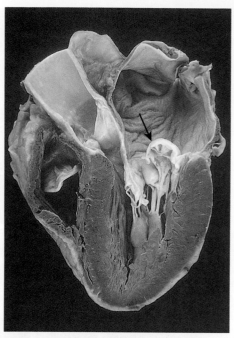

FIG. 9.18 Myxomatous degeneration of the mitral valve. There is prominent hooding with prolapse of the posterior mitral leaflet *(arrow)* into the left atrium; the atrium also is dilated, reflecting long-standing valvular insufficiency and volume overload. The hypertrophic left ventricle is shown on the *right* in this four-chamber view. (Courtesy of William D. Edwards, MD, Mayo Clinic, Rochester, Minnesota.)

most instances the natural history and clinical course are benign, approximately 3% of patients develop complications such as hemodynamically significant mitral regurgitation and CHF, particularly if the chordae or valve leaflets rupture. Patients with primary myxomatous degeneration are also at increased risk for the development of infective endocarditis (see later), as well as sudden cardiac death due to ventricular arrhythmias. Stroke or other systemic infarctions may rarely occur from embolism of thrombi formed in the left atrium.

Rheumatic Valvular Disease

Rheumatic fever is an acute, immunologically mediated, multisystem inflammatory disease that occurs after group A β-hemolytic streptococcal infections (usually pharyngitis, but also occasionally infections at other sites, such as skin). Rheumatic heart disease is the cardiac manifestation of rheumatic fever. It is associated with inflammation of all parts of the heart, but valvular inflammation and scarring produce the most important clinical features.

The valvular disease principally takes the form of deforming fibrotic mitral stenosis; indeed, rheumatic heart disease is essentially the *only* cause of acquired mitral stenosis. The incidence of rheumatic fever (and thus rheumatic heart disease) has declined greatly in many parts of higher-income countries over the past several decades due to a combination of improved socioeconomic conditions, rapid diagnosis and treatment of streptococcal pharyngitis, and an unexplained decline in the virulence of many strains of group A streptococci. *Nevertheless, in lower-income countries rheumatic heart disease remains the most important form of acquired heart disease in children and young adults.*

Pathogenesis. **Acute rheumatic fever results from host immune responses to group A streptococcal antigens that cross-react with**

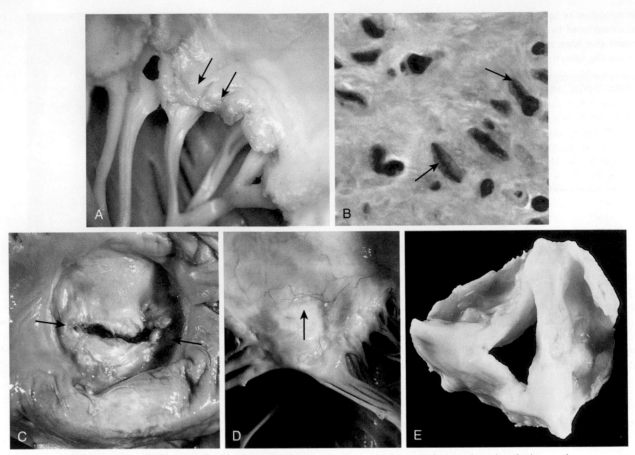

FIG. 9.19 Rheumatic heart disease. (A) Acute rheumatic mitral valvulitis superimposed on chronic rheumatic heart disease. Small vegetations (verrucae) are visible along the line of closure of the mitral valve leaflet *(arrows)*. Previous episodes of rheumatic valvulitis have caused fibrous thickening and fusion of the chordae tendineae. (B) Microscopic appearance of an Aschoff body in acute rheumatic carditis showing activated macrophages with prominent nucleoli and central wavy (caterpillar) chromatin (Anitschkow cells) *(arrows)*. (C and D) Mitral stenosis with diffuse fibrous thickening and distortion of the valve leaflets, commissural fusion *(arrows)*, and thickening and shortening of the chordae tendineae. There is marked left atrial dilation as seen from above the valve (C). (D) Anterior leaflet of an opened rheumatic mitral valve; note the neovascularization *(arrow)*. (E) Surgically removed specimen of rheumatic aortic stenosis, demonstrating thickening and distortion of the cusps with commissural fusion. (B, From Diagnostic Pathology: Cardiovascular. Copyright Elsevier. E, From Schoen FJ, St John-Sutton M: Contemporary issues in the pathology of valvular heart disease. *Hum Pathol* 18:568, 1967.)

host proteins present in the myocardium and valves. Both T cells and antibodies against M proteins of certain streptococcal strains can recognize the proteins in the myocardium and cardiac valves. Antibodies cause injury through the activation of complement and Fc receptor–bearing cells (including macrophages). Cytokine production by the stimulated T cells leads to macrophage activation (e.g., within Aschoff bodies). The characteristic 2- to 3-week delay in symptom onset after infection is explained by the time needed to generate an immune response; by this time streptococci are completely absent from the lesions. Since only a small minority of infected patients develop rheumatic fever (estimated at 1% to 3%), genetic susceptibility to the development of the cross-reactive immune responses is likely in those affected. The deforming fibrotic lesions are the consequence of healing and scarring associated with the resolution of the acute inflammation.

MORPHOLOGY

Acute rheumatic fever is characterized by discrete inflammatory foci within a variety of tissues. The myocardial inflammatory lesions—called **Aschoff bodies**—are pathognomonic for rheumatic fever (see Fig. 9.19B); these are collections of lymphocytes (primarily T cells), scattered plasma cells, and plump activated macrophages called **Anitschkow cells** associated with zones of fibrinoid necrosis. The Anitschkow cells have abundant cytoplasm and nuclei with chromatin that is centrally condensed into a slender, wavy ribbon (so-called "caterpillar cells"). During acute rheumatic fever, Aschoff bodies can be found in any of the three layers of the heart—pericardium, myocardium, or endocardium (including valves). Hence, rheumatic fever is said to cause pancarditis, with the following salient features:

• The pericardium may exhibit a fibrinous exudate, which generally resolves without sequelae.

- The myocardial involvement—myocarditis—takes the form of scattered Aschoff bodies within the interstitial connective tissue.
- Valve involvement results in fibrinoid necrosis and fibrin deposition along the lines of closure (Fig. 9.19A) forming 1- to 2-mm vegetations—verrucae—that cause little disturbance in cardiac function.

Chronic rheumatic heart disease is characterized by organization of acute inflammation and subsequent scarring. Aschoff bodies are replaced by fibrous scar so that these lesions are rarely seen in chronic disease. Characteristically, valve cusps and leaflets become permanently thickened and retracted. Classically, the mitral valves exhibit **leaflet thickening, commissural fusion and shortening, and thickening and fusion of the chordae tendineae** (Fig. 9.19 C to E). Fibrous bridging across the valvular commissures and calcification create "fishmouth" or "buttonhole" stenoses (Fig. 9.19C). Microscopic examination shows neovascularization (grossly evident in Fig. 9.19D) and diffuse fibrosis that obliterates the normal leaflet architecture.

The most important functional consequence of rheumatic heart disease is **valvular stenosis and regurgitation;** stenosis tends to predominate. The mitral valve alone is involved in 70% of cases, and combined mitral and aortic disease is seen in another 25%. The tricuspid valve is less frequently (and less severely) involved, and the pulmonic valve almost always escapes injury. With tight mitral stenosis, the left atrium progressively dilates owing to pressure overload, precipitating atrial fibrillation. The combination of dilation and fibrillation is a fertile substrate for thrombosis, and formation of large mural thrombi is common. Long-standing passive venous congestion of the lungs gives rise to pulmonary vascular and parenchymal changes typical of left-sided heart failure. In time, this leads to right ventricular hypertrophy and failure. With pure mitral stenosis, the left ventricle is generally normal.

Clinical Features. Acute rheumatic fever occurs most often in children between the ages of 5 to 15 years; the principal clinical manifestation is carditis. The clinical signs of carditis include pericardial friction rubs and arrhythmias; myocarditis may be sufficiently severe to cause cardiac dilation and resultant functional mitral insufficiency and CHF. Nevertheless, fewer than 1% of patients die of acute rheumatic fever. About 20% of first attacks occur in adults, and in this age group arthritis is the predominant feature. Symptoms in all age groups typically begin 2 to 3 weeks after streptococcal infection and are heralded by fever and migratory polyarthritis: one large joint after another becomes painful and swollen for a period of days, followed by spontaneous resolution with no residual disability. Although cultures are negative for streptococci at the time of symptom onset, serum titers of antibodies against one or more streptococcal antigens (e.g., streptolysin O or DNAase) are usually elevated.

The diagnosis of acute rheumatic fever is made based on serologic evidence of previous streptococcal infection in conjunction with two or more of the *Jones criteria:* (1) carditis; (2) migratory polyarthritis of large joints; (3) subcutaneous nodules; (4) erythematous annular rash (erythema marginatum); and (5) Sydenham chorea, a neurologic disorder characterized by involuntary purposeless, rapid movements. Minor criteria such as fever, arthralgias, ECG changes, or elevated acute phase reactants can help support the diagnosis.

After an initial attack and the generation of immunologic memory, patients are increasingly vulnerable to disease reactivation with subsequent streptococcal infections. Carditis is likely to worsen with each recurrence, and the damage is cumulative. However, chronic rheumatic carditis is usually not clinically evident until years or even decades after the initial episode of rheumatic fever. The signs and symptoms depend on the extent and degree of valvular involvement. In addition to various cardiac murmurs, cardiac hypertrophy and dilation, and CHF, patients with chronic rheumatic heart disease often have arrhythmias (particularly atrial fibrillation in the setting of mitral stenosis), and thromboembolic complications due to atrial mural thrombi. In addition, scarred and deformed valves are more susceptible to infective endocarditis. The long-term prognosis is highly variable. Surgical repair or replacement of diseased valves—mitral valvuloplasty—has greatly improved the outlook for patients with rheumatic heart disease.

Infective Endocarditis

Infective endocarditis (IE) is a microbial infection of the heart valves or endocardium that leads to the formation of *vegetations* composed of thrombotic debris and organisms, often associated with destruction of the underlying cardiac tissue. The aorta, aneurysmal sacs, other blood vessels, and prosthetic devices may also become infected. Although fungi, rickettsiae (agents of Q fever), and chlamydial species can cause endocarditis, the vast majority of cases are caused by bacteria.

Infective endocarditis is classified as *acute* and *subacute* based on the tempo and severity of the clinical course; the distinctions are related to the virulence of the responsible microbe and whether underlying cardiac disease is present. Of note, a clear delineation between acute and subacute endocarditis is not always possible, and many cases fall somewhere along the spectrum between the two forms.

- *Acute endocarditis* refers to rapidly progressing, destructive infections. It is associated with substantial morbidity and mortality, even with appropriate antibiotic therapy and/or surgery.
- *Subacute endocarditis* refers to infections that appear insidiously and even if untreated follow a protracted course of weeks to months; most patients recover after appropriate antibiotic therapy.

Pathogenesis. Infective endocarditis can develop on previously normal valves, but cardiac abnormalities predispose to such infections; rheumatic heart disease, mitral valve prolapse, bicuspid aortic valves, and calcific valvular stenosis are all common substrates. As rheumatic valvular heart disease has become much less common, mitral valve prolapse has become the leading preexistent risk factor. Prosthetic heart valves are also at risk for IE and account for 10% to 20% of all cases of IE. Sterile platelet-fibrin deposits at sites of pacemaker lines, indwelling vascular catheters, or endocardium damage by flow "jets" stemming from preexisting cardiac disease are other potential foci for bacterial seeding and development of endocarditis. Host factors such as neutropenia, immunodeficiency, malignancy, diabetes, and alcohol or intravenous drug use also increase the risk for IE and adversely affect outcomes.

The three most common causes of IE worldwide are staphylococci, streptococci, and enterococci. The frequency of each is dependent on the clinical setting. In community-acquired IE, 50% to 60% of cases are caused by *Streptococcus viridans,* a relatively benign group of normal oral flora. Typically, such infections occur on damaged or deformed valves and present as subacute IE. By contrast, the more virulent *S. aureus* (common to skin) is the most common cause of IE arising in healthcare settings and in intravenous drug users. It can attack healthy as well as deformed valves and often presents as acute IE. Because medical interventions are the major risk factor for bloodstream infections, *S. aureus* has emerged as the most common cause of infective endocarditis in most higher-income countries. Additional bacterial agents include enterococci and the so-called "HACEK group" (*Haemophilus, Actinobacillus, Cardiobacterium, Eikenella,* and *Kingella*), all commensals in the oral cavity. More rarely, gram-negative bacilli and fungi are involved. In about 10% of all cases of endocarditis, no organism is isolated from the blood ("culture-negative" endocarditis) because of previous antibiotic therapy or difficulty in isolating the offending agent from the blood.

Foremost among the factors predisposing to endocarditis is seeding of the blood with microbes. The mechanism or portal of entry of the agent into the bloodstream may be an obvious infection elsewhere, a dental or surgical procedure that causes a transient bacteremia, injection of contaminated material directly into the bloodstream by intravenous substance users, an occult source from the gut or oral cavity, or trivial injuries. Recognition of predisposing anatomic sites and clinical conditions causing bacteremia allows appropriate antibiotic prophylaxis.

MORPHOLOGY

In both acute and subacute forms of the disease, friable, bulky, and potentially destructive vegetations containing fibrin, inflammatory cells, and microorganisms are present on the heart valves (Figs. 9.20 and 9.21). **The aortic and mitral valves are the most common sites of infection, although the tricuspid valve is a frequent target in the setting of intravenous substance use.** Vegetations may be single or multiple and may involve more than one valve; they can sometimes erode into the underlying myocardium to produce an abscess cavity **(ring abscess)** (Fig. 9.21B). Shedding of **emboli** is common because of the friable nature of the vegetations. Since the fragmented vegetations contain large numbers of organisms, abscesses often develop at the sites where emboli lodge, leading to development of **septic infarcts** and aneurysms resulting from bacterial infection of the arterial wall **(mycotic aneurysms).**

Clinical Features. **Fever is the most consistent sign of infective endocarditis.** However, in subacute disease (particularly in older adults), fever may be absent, and the only manifestations may be nonspecific fatigue, weight loss, and a flulike syndrome; splenomegaly is also common in subacute cases. By contrast, acute endocarditis typically manifests with rapidly developing fever, chills, and lassitude (lack of energy). Murmurs are present in 90% of patients with left-sided lesions. In those who are not treated promptly, microemboli are formed, which can give rise to petechiae; nail bed *(splinter)* hemorrhages; retinal hemorrhages *(Roth spots)*; painless, erythematous lesions of the palm or sole *(Janeway lesions)*; or painful fingertip nodules *(Osler nodes)*; diagnosis is confirmed by positive blood cultures and echocardiographic findings.

Prognosis depends on the infecting organism and the development of complications. Adverse sequelae generally begin within the first weeks after onset of the infectious process and can include glomerulonephritis due to glomerular trapping of antigen-antibody complexes, with hematuria, albuminuria, or renal failure (Chapter 12). Clinical features of septicemia, arrhythmias (suggesting extension to underlying myocardium and conduction system), and systemic embolization are associated with a worse prognosis. Left untreated, IE is generally fatal. However, with appropriate antibiotic therapy and/or valve replacement, mortality is reduced.

Noninfected Vegetations

Nonbacterial Thrombotic Endocarditis

Nonbacterial thrombotic endocarditis (NBTE) is characterized by the deposition of sterile thrombi on cardiac valves, typically in patients with an underlying hypercoagulable state. Although NBTE can occur in otherwise healthy individuals, a wide variety of diseases associated with general debility or wasting are associated with an increased risk for NBTE. In contrast to infective endocarditis, the sterile valvular lesions of NBTE are nondestructive (Fig. 9.22).

The vegetations in NBTE are typically small (1 to 5 mm in diameter) and usually occur on previously normal valves. Hypercoagulable states are the usual precursor to NBTE; underlying malignancy is the most common cause, particularly mucinous adenocarcinomas, probably related to the effect of circulating mucin and/or other procoagulants elaborated by these tumors. Other predisposing conditions include chronic disseminated intravascular coagulation, hyperestrogenic states, and endocardial trauma (e.g., from an indwelling catheter).

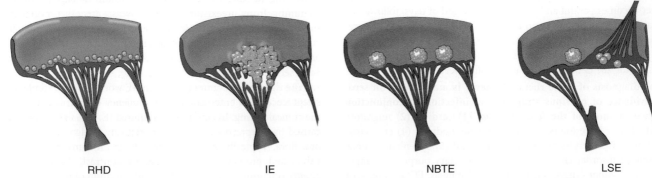

RHD   IE   NBTE   LSE

FIG. 9.20 Major forms of vegetative endocarditis. The acute phase of rheumatic heart disease (RHD) is marked by the appearance of small, warty, inflammatory vegetations along the lines of valve closure; as the inflammation resolves, substantial scarring can result. Infective endocarditis (IE) is characterized by large, irregular, often destructive masses that can extend from valve leaflets onto adjacent structures (e.g., chordae or myocardium). Nonbacterial thrombotic endocarditis (NBTE) typically manifests with small- to medium-sized, bland, nondestructive vegetations at the line of valve closure. Libman-Sacks endocarditis (LSE) is characterized by small- to medium-sized inflammatory vegetations that can be attached on either side of the valve leaflets; these heal with scarring.

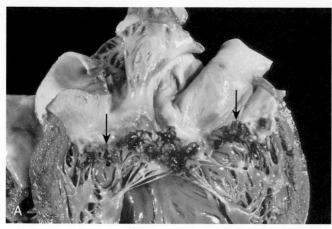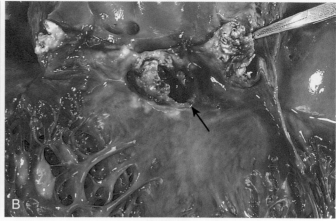

FIG. 9.21 Infective endocarditis. (A) Subacute endocarditis caused by *Streptococcus viridans* on a previously myxomatous mitral valve. The large, friable vegetations are denoted by *arrows*. (B) Acute endocarditis caused by *Staphylococcus aureus* on a congenitally bicuspid aortic valve with extensive cuspal destruction and ring abscess *(arrow)*.

Although the local effect on the valve is usually trivial, NBTE lesions are easily dislodged due to the lack of underlying inflammation and can give rise to emboli that cause infarcts in the brain, heart, and other organs. NBTE can also serve as a nidus for bacterial colonization and the consequent development of infective endocarditis.

Endocarditis in Systemic Lupus Erythematosus: Libman-Sacks Endocarditis

Libman-Sacks endocarditis is a form of NBTE characterized by the presence of sterile vegetations on the valves of patients with systemic lupus erythematosus. The lesions probably develop as a consequence of immune complex deposition and exhibit associated inflammation, often with fibrinoid necrosis of the valve adjacent to the vegetation; subsequent fibrosis and serious deformity can result in lesions that resemble chronic rheumatic heart disease. These can occur anywhere on the valve surface, on the cords, or even on the atrial or ventricular endocardium (see Fig. 9.20). Similar lesions can occur in the setting of antiphospholipid antibody syndrome (Chapter 3).

CARDIOMYOPATHIES

Cardiac diseases due to intrinsic myocardial dysfunction are termed *cardiomyopathies* (literally, "heart muscle diseases"); these can be primary—that is, principally confined to the myocardium—or secondary, presenting as the cardiac manifestation of a systemic disorder. This definition excludes myocardial dysfunction secondary to coronary artery disease, hypertension, valvular disease, and congenital heart diseases. Cardiomyopathies are a diverse group that includes inflammatory disorders (e.g., myocarditis), immunologic diseases (e.g., sarcoidosis), systemic metabolic disorders (e.g., hemochromatosis), muscular dystrophies, and genetic disorders of myocardial fibers. In many cases, the cardiomyopathy is of unknown etiology and has been termed idiopathic; however, a number of previously "idiopathic" cardiomyopathies have been shown to be the consequence of specific genetic abnormalities in cardiac energy metabolism or in structural and contractile proteins.

Cardiomyopathies can be classified according to a variety of criteria, including the underlying genetic basis of dysfunction; some of the arrhythmia-inducing channelopathies that are included in classifications of cardiomyopathy were alluded to earlier. For purposes of general diagnosis and therapy, however, three time-honored clinical, functional, and pathologic patterns are recognized (Fig. 9.23 and Table 9.5):

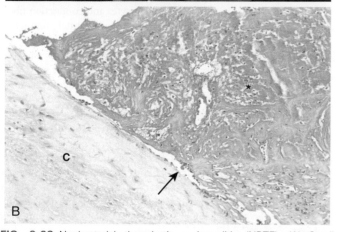

FIG. 9.22 Nonbacterial thrombotic endocarditis (NBTE). (A) Small thrombotic vegetations along the line of closure of the mitral valve leaflets *(arrows)*. (B) Photomicrograph of NBTE lesion, showing bland thrombus, with virtually no inflammation in the valve cusp *(C)* or the thrombotic deposit *(*)*. The thrombus is only loosely attached to the cusp *(arrow)*.

- Dilated cardiomyopathy (DCM) (including arrhythmogenic right ventricular cardiomyopathy)
- Hypertrophic cardiomyopathy (HCM)
- Restrictive cardiomyopathy

Of the three major patterns, DCM is the most common (90% of cases), and restrictive cardiomyopathy is the least frequent. Within each pattern, there is a spectrum of clinical severity, and in some cases clinical features overlap among the groups. In addition, each of these patterns can be caused by a specific identifiable etiology or can be idiopathic (see Table 9.5).

Dilated Cardiomyopathy

Dilated cardiomyopathy (DCM) is characterized by progressive cardiac dilation and contractile (systolic) dysfunction, usually with concurrent hypertrophy; regardless of the cause, the clinicopathologic patterns are similar.

Pathogenesis. At diagnosis, dilated cardiomyopathy has usually progressed to end-stage disease marked by heart failure secondary to poor myocardial contractility and does not reveal any specific pathologic features. The damage that culminates in end-stage dilated cardiomyopathy can be initiated by inherited abnormalities or by environmental exposures, as follows:

- *Genetic causes.* DCM has a hereditary basis in 20% to 50% of cases. Over 50 genes are known to be mutated in this form of cardiomyopathy, with autosomal dominant inheritance being the predominant pattern. It is most often caused by loss of function mutations affecting cytoskeletal proteins or proteins that link the sarcomere to the cytoskeleton (Fig. 9.24). Examples include mutations affecting the genes for β-myosin heavy chain, α-myosin heavy chain, cardiac troponin T, and titin. Of these, mutations affecting titin, which is a key component of sarcomeric force generation, are the most common. It should be noted that gain-of-function mutations in some of the same sarcomere genes cause hypertrophic cardiomyopathy. X-linked DCM is most frequently associated with mutations in dystrophin, a cell membrane protein that physically couples the intracellular cytoskeleton to the ECM (Chapter 20). Other genetic forms of DCM include those with mutations in cytoskeletal proteins such as desmin (the principal intermediate filament protein in cardiac myocytes) and nuclear lamins A and C. Since contractile myocytes and conduction fibers share a common developmental pathway, congenital conduction abnormalities also can be a feature of inherited forms of DCM.
- *Infection.* In earlier studies, adenovirus and enterovirus were the most commonly implicated organisms. More recently, parvovirus B-19 and human herpesvirus 6 have been identified more frequently. The nucleic acid "footprints" of coxsackievirus B and other enteroviruses can occasionally be detected in the myocardium from patients with late-stage DCM. Moreover, sequential endomyocardial biopsies have documented instances in which infectious myocarditis progressed to DCM. Simply identifying viral transcripts or demonstrating elevated antiviral antibody titers may be sufficient to invoke a myocarditis that was "missed" in its early stages. Consequently, many cases of DCM are attributed to viral infections, even though inflammation is absent from the end-stage heart.
- *Alcohol or other toxic exposure.* Excess alcohol use is strongly associated with the development of DCM. Alcohol and its metabolites (especially acetaldehyde) have a direct toxic effect on the myocardium. Moreover, chronic alcohol use disorder can be associated

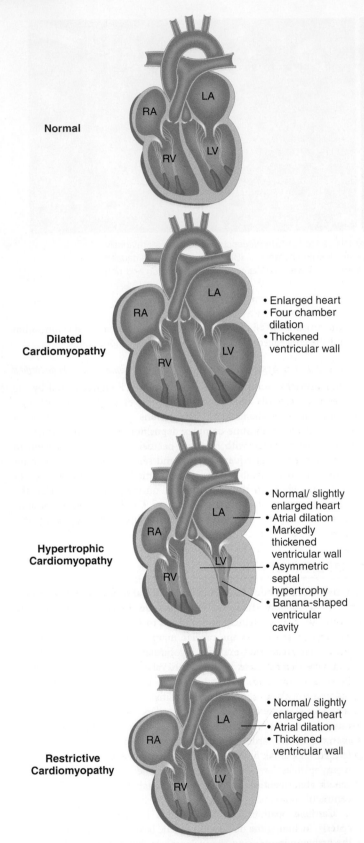

FIG. 9.23 The three major forms of cardiomyopathy. Dilated cardiomyopathy leads primarily to systolic dysfunction, whereas restrictive and hypertrophic cardiomyopathies result in diastolic dysfunction. Note the changes in atrial and/or ventricular dilation and in ventricular wall thickness. In DCM the ventricular wall may be thickened (as shown) or thinner or normal. *LA,* Left atrium; *LV,* left ventricle; *RA,* right atrium; *RV,* right ventricle.

Labels within figure:

Normal

Dilated Cardiomyopathy
- Enlarged heart
- Four chamber dilation
- Thickened ventricular wall

Hypertrophic Cardiomyopathy
- Normal/ slightly enlarged heart
- Atrial dilation
- Markedly thickened ventricular wall
- Asymmetric septal hypertrophy
- Banana-shaped ventricular cavity

Restrictive Cardiomyopathy
- Normal/ slightly enlarged heart
- Atrial dilation
- Thickened ventricular wall

Table 9.5 Cardiomyopathies: Functional Patterns, Causes

Functional Pattern	Left Ventricular Ejection Fraction[a]	Mechanisms of Heart Failure	Causes	Secondary Myocardial Dysfunction (Mimicking Cardiomyopathy)
Dilated	<40%	Impairment of contractility (systolic dysfunction)	Genetic; alcohol; peripartum; myocarditis; hemochromatosis; chronic anemia; doxorubicin; sarcoidosis; idiopathic	Ischemic heart disease; valvular heart disease; hypertensive heart disease; congenital heart disease
Hypertrophic	50%–80%	Impairment of compliance (diastolic dysfunction)	Genetic; Friedreich ataxia; storage diseases; infants of mothers with diabetes	Hypertensive heart disease; aortic stenosis
Restrictive	25%–50%	Impairment of compliance (diastolic dysfunction)	Amyloidosis; radiation-induced fibrosis; idiopathic	Pericardial constriction

[a]Range of normal values is approximately 50% to 65%.

with thiamine deficiency, introducing an element of beriberi heart disease (Chapter 7). DCM can also develop after exposure to other toxic agents, such as cobalt, and particularly doxorubicin, a chemotherapeutic drug.

- *Peripartum cardiomyopathy* occurs late in gestation or several weeks to months postpartum. The etiology is unknown; pregnancy-associated hypertension, volume overload, nutritional deficiency, metabolic derangements (e.g., gestational diabetes), and impaired angiogenic signaling have all been invoked as potential contributing factors. Approximately one-half of these patients spontaneously recover normal function.

- *Iron overload* in the heart can result from hereditary hemochromatosis (Chapter 14) or from multiple transfusions (in those with chronic anemia). Iron overload can cause restrictive cardiomyopathy due to interstitial fibrosis, but DCM is the most common manifestation. It is thought to be due to interference with metal-dependent enzyme systems or to injury caused by iron-mediated production of reactive oxygen species.

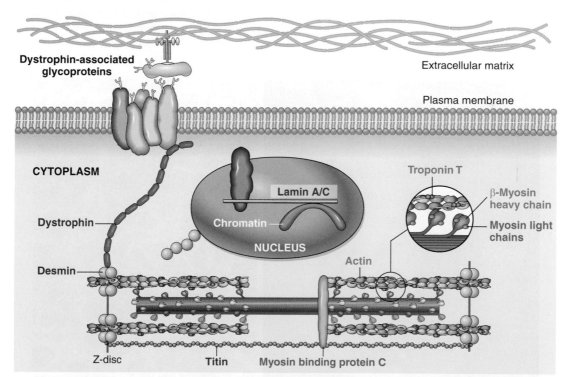

FIG. 9.24 Schematic of a myocyte, showing key proteins mutated in dilated cardiomyopathy *(red labels)*, hypertrophic cardiomyopathy *(blue labels)*, or both *(green labels)*. Mutations in titin (the largest known human protein at approximately 30,000 amino acids) account for approximately 20% of all dilated cardiomyopathy. Titin spans the sarcomere and connects the Z and M bands, thereby limiting the passive range of motion of the sarcomere as it is stretched. M band is not illustrated.

The heart in DCM is characteristically enlarged (up to two to three times the normal weight) and **flabby,** with dilation of all chambers (Fig. 9.25). Because of the wall thinning that accompanies dilation, the ventricular thickness may be less than, equal to, or greater than normal. **Mural thrombi** are often present and may be a source of thromboemboli. By definition, valvular and vascular lesions (e.g., atherosclerotic coronary artery disease) that can cause secondary cardiac dilation are absent.

The histologic abnormalities in DCM are nonspecific. Most myocytes exhibit **hypertrophy** with enlarged nuclei, but many are attenuated, stretched, and irregular. There is also variable interstitial and endocardial fibrosis, with scattered areas of replacement fibrosis; the latter may mark previous areas of myocyte ischemic necrosis caused by hypoperfusion or may be the "fingerprints" of a previous missed myocarditis.

In DCM secondary to iron overload, there is a marked accumulation of intramyocardial hemosiderin, which is demonstrable by staining with Prussian blue.

Clinical Features. **The fundamental defect in DCM is ineffective contraction.** Thus, in end-stage DCM, the cardiac ejection fraction typically is less than 25% (normal is 50% to 65%). Secondary mitral regurgitation and abnormal cardiac rhythms are common, and embolism from intracardiac (mural) thrombi can occur. DCM is most commonly diagnosed between 20 and 50 years of age. It typically manifests with signs of slowly progressive CHF, including dyspnea, easy fatigability, and poor exertional capacity. Median survival to transplant or death is 4 to 6 years. Death is usually due to progressive cardiac failure or arrhythmia. Cardiac transplantation is the only definitive treatment, although implantation of long-term ventricular assist devices is increasingly utilized; in some patients, a course of mechanical assistance can produce durable regression of cardiac dysfunction.

Arrhythmogenic Right Ventricular Cardiomyopathy

Arrhythmogenic right ventricular cardiomyopathy is an autosomal dominant disorder that manifests with right-sided heart failure and rhythm disturbances, which can cause sudden cardiac death. Its prevalence in the general adult population is 1 in 2000 to 1 in 5000. Almost 10% of cases of sudden deaths in athletes have been ascribed to this entity. Morphologically, the right ventricular wall is severely thinned because of myocyte replacement by fatty infiltration and lesser amounts of fibrosis (Fig. 9.26). Many of the causative mutations involve genes encoding desmosomal junctional proteins at the intercalated disk (e.g., plakoglobin), as well as proteins that interact with the desmosome (e.g., the intermediate filament desmin). It is thought that myocyte death is caused by desmosomal detachment, particularly during strenuous exercise.

Hypertrophic Cardiomyopathy

Hypertrophic cardiomyopathy (HCM) is characterized by myocardial hypertrophy, defective diastolic filling, and—in one-third of cases—ventricular outflow obstruction. The heart is thick-walled, heavy, and hypercontractile, in striking contrast to the flabby, poorly contractile heart in DCM. Systolic function is usually preserved in HCM, but the myocardium does not relax and the result is a form of diastolic dysfunction. HCM must be distinguished clinically from disorders causing ventricular stiffness (e.g., amyloid deposition) and ventricular hypertrophy (e.g., aortic stenosis and hypertension).

Pathogenesis. **Most cases of HCM are caused by missense mutations in one of several genes encoding proteins that form the contractile apparatus.** The usual pattern of transmission is autosomal dominant, with variable expression. Although more than 400 causative mutations

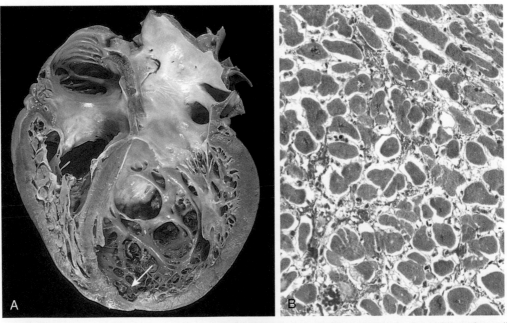

FIG. 9.25 Dilated cardiomyopathy (DCM). (A) Four-chamber dilation and hypertrophy are evident. A small mural thrombus can be seen at the apex of the left ventricle *(arrow).* (B) The nonspecific histologic picture in typical DCM, with myocyte hypertrophy and interstitial fibrosis. (Collagen is *blue* in this Masson trichrome–stained preparation.)

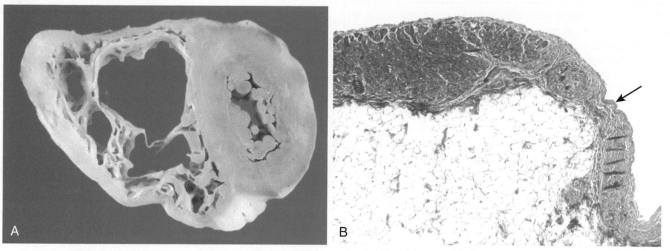

FIG. 9.26 Arrhythmogenic right ventricular cardiomyopathy. (A) The right ventricle is markedly dilated with focal, almost transmural replacement of the free wall by adipose tissue and fibrosis. The left ventricle has a grossly normal appearance in this heart; it can be involved (albeit to a lesser extent) in some instances. (B) The right ventricular myocardium *(red)* is focally replaced by fibrous connective tissue *(blue, arrow)* and fat (Masson trichrome stain).

in nine different genes have been identified, they have one unifying feature: they are all gain-of-function mutations that affect sarcomeric proteins and thus enhance myofilament function. This results in myocyte hypercontractility, increased energy use, and a net negative energy balance. Of the various sarcomeric proteins, β-myosin heavy chain is most frequently involved, followed by myosin-binding protein C and troponin T. Mutations in these three genes account for 70% to 80% of all cases of HCM.

Some of the genes mutated in HCM are also mutated in DCM (e.g., β-myosin), but in DCM the mutations cause loss of function as opposed to the gain of function mutations in HCM.

MORPHOLOGY

Hypertrophic cardiomyopathy is marked by massive myocardial hypertrophy without ventricular dilation (Fig. 9.27A). In 90% of cases, there is disproportionate thickening of the ventricular septum relative to the left ventricle free wall (so-called **asymmetric septal hypertrophy**); in the remaining 10% of cases, concentric hypertrophy is seen. On longitudinal sectioning, the ventricular cavity loses its usual round-to-ovoid shape and is compressed into a "banana-like" configuration. The anterior mitral leaflet contacts the septum during ventricular systole, producing a plaque in the left ventricular outflow tract and thickening of the mitral leaflet; these changes

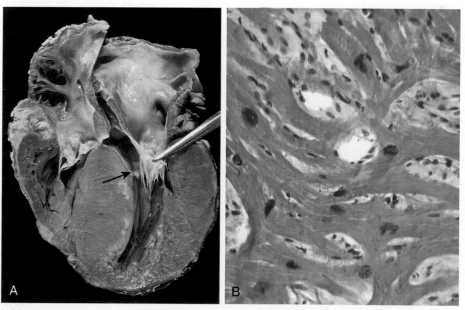

FIG. 9.27 Hypertrophic cardiomyopathy with asymmetric septal hypertrophy. (A) The septal muscle bulges into the left ventricular outflow tract, giving rise to a "banana-shaped" ventricular lumen, and the left atrium is enlarged. The anterior mitral leaflet has been moved away from the septum to reveal a fibrous endocardial plaque *(arrow)* (see text). (B) Histologic appearance demonstrating disarray, extreme hypertrophy, and characteristic branching of myocytes, as well as interstitial fibrosis.

produce variable degrees of left ventricular outflow tract obstruction due to systolic anterior motion of the mitral valve.

The characteristic histologic features in HCM are marked myocyte hypertrophy, haphazard **myocyte** (and **myofiber**) **disarray,** and interstitial fibrosis (Fig. 9.27B).

Clinical Features. Although HCM can present at any age, it typically manifests during the postpubertal growth spurt. The clinical symptoms can be best understood in the context of the functional abnormalities. Following systole, the myocardium does not fully relax, which limits ventricular filling during diastole. This, combined with functional obstruction of the ventricular outflow tract, decreases the effectiveness of cardiac pumping. Reduced cardiac output and a secondary increase in pulmonary venous pressure cause exertional dyspnea, with a harsh systolic ejection murmur. A combination of massive hypertrophy, high left ventricular pressures, and compromised intramural arterial blood flow frequently leads to myocardial ischemia (with angina), even in the absence of concomitant coronary artery disease. Major clinical problems include atrial fibrillation with mural thrombus formation, ventricular fibrillation leading to sudden cardiac death, infectious endocarditis of the mitral valve, and CHF. Most patients' symptoms are improved by therapy that promotes ventricular relaxation; partial surgical excision or controlled therapeutic infarction of septal muscle (by local injection of alcohol) can also relieve the outflow tract obstruction. As mentioned earlier, HCM is an important cause of sudden cardiac death. In almost one-third of cases of sudden cardiac death in athletes younger than 35 years of age, the underlying cause is HCM.

Restrictive Cardiomyopathy

Restrictive cardiomyopathy is characterized by a decrease in ventricular compliance, resulting in impaired ventricular filling during diastole; simply put, the wall is stiffer. This form of cardiomyopathy may be idiopathic or may be associated with a variety of conditions that affect the myocardium such as radiation fibrosis, amyloidosis, sarcoidosis, or products of inborn errors of metabolism such as mucopolysaccharides and sphingolipids.

Three forms of restrictive cardiomyopathy merit brief mention:
- *Amyloidosis* is caused by the deposition of extracellular proteins with a predilection for forming insoluble β-pleated sheets (Chapter 5). Cardiac amyloidosis can occur in the setting of systemic amyloidosis (e.g., multiple myeloma) or can be restricted to the heart. In the latter case, deposition of normal (or mutant) forms of transthyretin (a liver-synthesized circulating protein that transports thyroxine and retinol) in the hearts of older adult patients results in a restrictive cardiomyopathy. Four percent of African Americans carry a specific mutation of transthyretin that increases the risk of cardiac amyloidosis in that population over fourfold. Immunoglobulin light chains in AL-type amyloid not only deposit as amyloid but also have the potential to be cardiotoxic and may contribute to myocardial dysfunction.
- *Endomyocardial fibrosis* is principally a disease of children and young adults in Africa and other tropical areas; on a worldwide basis it is believed to be the most common form of restrictive cardiomyopathy. It is characterized by diffuse fibrosis of the ventricular endocardium and subendocardium, often involving the tricuspid and mitral valves. The fibrous tissue markedly diminishes the volume and compliance of affected chambers, resulting in a restrictive physiology.

Endomyocardial fibrosis has been linked to nutritional deficiencies and/or inflammation related to helminthic infections.
- *Loeffler endomyocarditis* also exhibits endocardial fibrosis, typically associated with formation of large mural thrombi. It has no geographic or population predilection. It is characterized by peripheral hypereosinophilia and eosinophilic tissue infiltrates. Release of eosinophil granule contents, especially major basic protein, probably causes endocardial and myocardial necrosis, followed by scarring, layering of the endocardium by thrombus, and finally thrombus organization.

MORPHOLOGY

In restrictive cardiomyopathy, the ventricles are of approximately normal size or only slightly enlarged, the cavities are not dilated, and the myocardium is firm. However, both atria are typically dilated as a consequence of restricted ventricular filling and pressure overloads. Microscopic examination reveals variable degrees of interstitial fibrosis. Although gross morphologic findings are similar for restrictive cardiomyopathy of disparate causes, endomyocardial biopsy often reveals a specific etiology (e.g., amyloid, endomyocardial fibrosis).

MYOCARDITIS

Myocarditis encompasses a diverse group of clinical entities in which infectious agents and/or inflammatory processes target the myocardium. It is important to distinguish myocarditis from conditions such as IHD, where the inflammatory process is secondary to some other cause of myocardial injury.

Pathogenesis. **In the United States, viral infections are the most common cause of myocarditis, with coxsackieviruses A and B and other enteroviruses accounting for the majority of cases.** Increasingly, human herpesvirus 6 and parvovirus B19 are detected in viral myocarditis. Less commonly, cytomegalovirus (CMV), human immunodeficiency virus (HIV), and influenza virus are involved. Etiologic agents can be identified by serologic studies that show rising antibody titers or through molecular diagnostic techniques using infected tissues. While some viruses cause direct cell death, in most cases the injury results from an immune response directed against virally infected cells; this is analogous to the damage inflicted by virus-specific T cells on hepatitis virus–infected liver cells (Chapter 14). In some cases, viruses trigger an immune reaction that cross-reacts with myocardial proteins such as myosin heavy chain.

The nonviral infectious causes of myocarditis run the entire spectrum of the microbial world. Some of the most important causes are described next.
- The protozoan *Trypanosoma cruzi* is the agent of Chagas disease. Chagas disease is common in parts of South America, Central America, and Mexico, and about 300,000 individuals who are infected with *T. cruzi* live in the United States. Myocardial involvement is seen in the vast majority of patients: about 10% of the patients die during an acute attack while others can enter a chronic immune-mediated phase with development of progressive signs of CHF and arrhythmia 10 to 20 years later.
- *Toxoplasma gondii* can also cause myocarditis, particularly in immunocompromised individuals. Household cats are the most common vector.
- *Trichinosis*, also known as Trichinellosis, is the most common helminthic disease associated with cardiac involvement. Trichinosis is

contracted by eating raw or undercooked meat from an animal containing *Trichinella* larvae.

- *Lyme disease.* Myocarditis occurs in approximately 5% of patients with *Lyme disease,* a systemic illness caused by the bacterial spirochete *Borrelia burgdorferi.* Lyme myocarditis manifests primarily as self-limited conduction system disease, frequently requiring temporary pacemaker insertion.
- *mRNA COVID-19 vaccination.* Rare cases of postvaccination myocarditis occur especially in male adolescents and young adults, more often after the second dose, and usually within a week of vaccination. Most cases recover uneventfully.

Noninfectious causes of myocarditis include systemic diseases of immune origin, such as systemic lupus erythematosus and polymyositis. Drug hypersensitivity reactions affecting the heart (hypersensitivity myocarditis) may occur with exposure to a wide range of agents; such reactions are typically mild and only in rare circumstances lead to CHF or sudden death.

MORPHOLOGY

In acute myocarditis, the heart may appear normal or dilated; in advanced stages, the myocardium is typically flabby and often mottled with pale and hemorrhagic areas. Mural thrombi may be present.

Microscopically, viral myocarditis is characterized by edema, interstitial inflammatory infiltrates, and myocyte injury (Fig. 9.28). A diffuse lymphocytic infiltrate is most common (see Fig. 9.28A), although the inflammatory involvement is often patchy and may not be sampled on endomyocardial biopsy. If the patient survives the acute phase of myocarditis, lesions may resolve without significant sequelae or heal by fibrosis.

In **hypersensitivity myocarditis,** interstitial and perivascular infiltrates are composed of lymphocytes, macrophages, and a high proportion of eosinophils (Fig. 9.28B). **Giant cell myocarditis** is a morphologically distinctive entity thought to be caused by autoreactive T cells. It is characterized by widespread inflammatory cell infiltrates containing multinucleate giant cells (formed by macrophage fusion). It is an aggressive disease with focal—and frequently extensive—necrosis (Fig. 9.28C). This variant carries a poor prognosis.

Chagas myocarditis is characterized by the parasitization of scattered myofibers by trypanosomes accompanied by an inflammatory infiltrate of neutrophils, lymphocytes, macrophages, and occasional eosinophils (Fig. 9.28D).

Clinical Features. The clinical spectrum of myocarditis is broad; at one end, the disease is asymptomatic and patients recover without sequelae. At the other extreme is the precipitous onset of heart failure or arrhythmias, occasionally resulting in sudden death. Between these

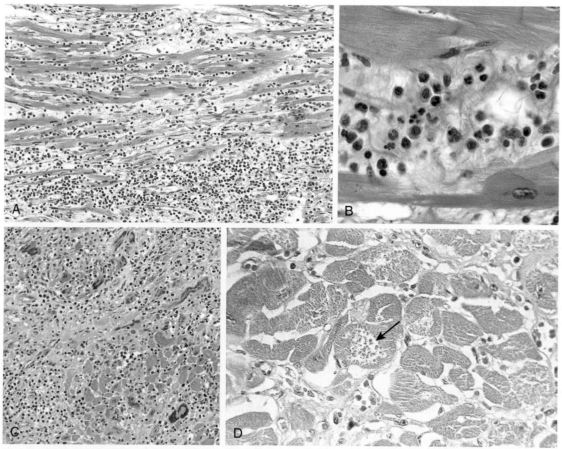

FIG. 9.28 Myocarditis. (A) Lymphocytic myocarditis, with edema and associated myocyte injury. (B) Hypersensitivity myocarditis characterized by eosinophil-rich inflammatory infiltrates. (C) Giant cell myocarditis, with lymphocyte and macrophage infiltrates, myocyte damage, and multinucleate giant cells. (D) Chagas myocarditis. A myofiber distended with trypanosomes *(arrow)* is present, along with mononuclear inflammation and myofiber necrosis. (B and C, From Diagnostic Pathology: Cardiovascular. Copyright Elsevier.)

extremes are many levels of involvement associated with a variety of signs and symptoms, including fatigue, dyspnea, palpitations, pain, and fever. The clinical features of myocarditis can mimic those of acute MI. Clinical progression from myocarditis to DCM is occasionally seen.

Other Causes of Myocardial Disease

Cardiotoxic Drugs

Cardiac complications of cancer therapy are important clinical problems. Cardiotoxicity can be associated with conventional chemotherapeutic agents, targeted drugs such as tyrosine kinase inhibitors, and certain forms of immunotherapy (e.g., immune checkpoint blockade for cancer). **The anthracyclines doxorubicin and daunorubicin are the chemotherapeutic agents that are most frequently associated with myocardial toxicity,** which often takes the form of a dilated cardiomyopathy and heart failure. Anthracycline toxicity is dose dependent (cardiotoxicity becomes progressively more frequent above a total dose of 500 mg/m^2) and is attributed primarily to peroxidation of lipids in myocyte membranes.

A variety of nonanthracycline agents, such as antimetabolites (fluorouracil), microtubule targeting agents (vinca alkaloids), and alkylating agents (cyclophosphamide), can also damage the heart. Common findings in hearts injured by many of these chemicals and drugs are myofiber swelling, cytoplasmic vacuolization, and fatty change. Discontinuing such agents leads to complete resolution, with no apparent sequelae. Sometimes, however, more extensive damage produces myocyte necrosis and leads to a dilated cardiomyopathy.

Catecholamines

Foci of myocardial necrosis with contraction bands, often associated with a sparse mononuclear inflammatory infiltrate (mostly macrophages), can occur in individuals with pheochromocytoma, a tumor that elaborates catecholamines (Chapter 18). Similar changes can occur with a variety of agents—endogenous or exogenous—under the rubric of "catecholamine effect." These include cocaine, high doses of ephedrine (an adrenergic agent in many cold and allergy formulations), intense autonomic stimulation secondary to intracranial lesions, or vasopressor agents such as dopamine. The mechanism of catecholamine cardiotoxicity is uncertain but seems to relate either to a direct toxicity of catecholamines on cardiac myocytes via calcium overload or to vasoconstriction in the face of an increased heart rate. The mononuclear cell infiltrate is probably a reaction to microscopic foci of myocyte cell death.

PERICARDIAL DISEASE

Pericardial lesions are typically associated with a pathologic process elsewhere in the heart or surrounding structures or are secondary to a systemic disorder. Pericardial disorders include effusions and inflammatory conditions, sometimes resulting in fibrous constriction.

Pericardial Effusion and Hemopericardium

Ordinarily, the pericardial sac contains less than 50 mL of thin, clear, straw-colored fluid. Under various circumstances, the pericardial sac may be distended by accumulations of serous fluid (*pericardial effusion*), blood (*hemopericardium*), or lymph (*chylous pericarditis*), as follows:
- *Serous:* Congestive heart failure, hypoalbuminemia of any cause

- *Serosanguineous:* Blunt chest trauma, malignancy, ruptured MI, or aortic dissection
- *Chylous:* Mediastinal lymphatic obstruction

With slowly accumulating fluid, the pericardium has time to stretch, allowing chronic pericardial effusions to become quite large without interfering with cardiac function. Thus, with chronic effusions of less than 500 mL in volume, the only clinical finding is a characteristic globular enlargement of the heart shadow on chest radiograph. By contrast, rapidly developing fluid collections of as little as 200 to 300 mL (e.g., due to hemopericardium caused by a ruptured MI or aortic dissection) can compress the thin-walled atria and venae cavae, or the ventricles themselves; cardiac filling is thereby restricted, producing potentially fatal cardiac tamponade.

Pericarditis

Primary pericarditis is uncommon. It is typically due to viral infection (often with concurrent myocarditis), although bacteria, fungi, or parasites may also be involved. Secondary pericarditis is more common and may be seen in the setting of acute MI or develop weeks later (*Dressler syndrome*) due to development of antibodies against injured myocardium, radiation to the mediastinum, or processes involving other thoracic structures (e.g., pneumonia or pleuritis). *Uremia* is the most common systemic disorder associated with pericarditis. Less common secondary causes include rheumatic fever, systemic lupus erythematosus, and metastatic malignancies. Pericarditis can (1) cause immediate hemodynamic complications if it elicits a large effusion (resulting in cardiac tamponade); (2) resolve without significant sequelae; or (3) progress to a chronic fibrosing process.

MORPHOLOGY

In patients with acute viral pericarditis or uremia, the exudate is typically fibrinous, imparting an irregular, shaggy appearance to the pericardial surface. In acute bacterial pericarditis, the exudate is fibrinopurulent (suppurative), often with areas of pus (Fig. 9.29); tuberculous pericarditis can exhibit areas of caseation. Pericarditis due to malignancy is often associated with an exuberant, shaggy fibrinous exudate and a bloody effusion; metastases can be grossly evident as irregular excrescences or may be grossly inapparent, especially in the case of leukemia. In most cases, acute fibrinous or fibrinopurulent pericarditis resolves without any sequelae. With extensive suppuration or caseation, however, healing can result in fibrosis (chronic pericarditis).

Chronic pericarditis may be associated with delicate adhesions or dense, fibrotic scars that obliterate the pericardial space. In extreme cases, the heart is so completely encased by dense fibrosis that it cannot expand normally during diastole—resulting in the condition known as **constrictive pericarditis.**

Clinical Features. Pericarditis classically manifests with atypical chest pain (not related to exertion and worse in recumbency) and a prominent friction rub. When associated with significant fluid accumulation, acute pericarditis can cause cardiac tamponade, which leads to declining cardiac output and consequent shock. Chronic constrictive pericarditis produces a combination of right-sided venous distention and low cardiac output, similar to the clinical picture in restrictive cardiomyopathy.

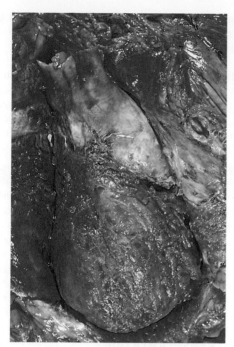

FIG. 9.29 Acute suppurative (purulent, exudative) pericarditis, caused by extension from pneumonia.

CARDIAC TUMORS

Primary Neoplasms

Primary cardiac tumors are uncommon; moreover, most are benign. The five most common have no malignant potential and account for 80% to 90% of all primary heart tumors. In descending order of frequency, these are myxoma, fibroma, lipoma, papillary fibroelastoma, and rhabdomyoma. Angiosarcoma is the most common primary malignant tumor of the heart. Only myxoma and rhabdomyoma merit further mention here.

Myxoma is the most common primary tumor of the adult heart. Roughly 90% are atrial, with the left atrium accounting for 80% of those.

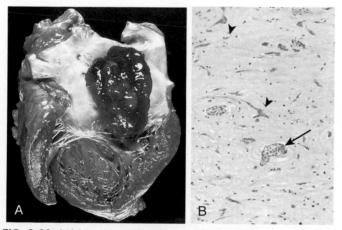

FIG. 9.30 Atrial myxoma. (A) A large pedunculated lesion arises from the region of the fossa ovalis and extends into the mitral valve orifice. (B) Abundant amorphous extracellular matrix contains scattered multinucleate myxoma cells *(arrowheads)* in various groupings, including abnormal vascular formations *(arrow)*.

Cardiac rhabdomyomas occur with high frequency in patients with tuberous sclerosis caused by mutations in the *TSC1* or *TSC2* tumor suppressor genes (Chapter 21); loss of TSC-1 and TSC-2 activity leads to myocyte overgrowth. Because they often regress spontaneously, rhabdomyomas are sometimes considered to be hamartomas rather than true neoplasms. In keeping with this, not all cardiac rhabdomyomas that occur in patients with tuberous sclerosis are clonal.

MORPHOLOGY

Myxomas are almost always single, classically arising in the region of the fossa ovalis (atrial septum). They can be small (less than 1 cm in diameter) or massive (up to 10 cm across), sessile or pedunculated masses (Fig. 9.30A), most often manifesting as soft, translucent, villous lesions with a gelatinous appearance. Pedunculated forms are often sufficiently mobile to swing into the mitral or tricuspid valve during systole, causing intermittent obstruction or exerting a "wrecking ball" effect that damages the valve leaflets.

Histologically, myxomas are composed of stellate, frequently multinucleate cells (typically with hyperchromatic nuclei), admixed with cells showing endothelial, smooth muscle, and/or fibroblastic differentiation, all of which are part of the neoplastic clone. The cells are embedded in an abundant acid mucopolysaccharide ground substance (Fig. 9.30B). Vessel-like and glandlike structures are characteristic. Hemorrhage, poorly organizing thrombus, and mononuclear inflammation are also usually present.

Rhabdomyomas are gray-white masses up to several centimeters in diameter that protrude into the ventricular chambers. They are usually multiple. Histologic examination shows a mixed population of cells; most characteristic, however, are large, rounded, or polygonal cells containing numerous glycogen-laden vacuoles separated by strands of cytoplasm running from the plasma membrane to the centrally located nucleus, so-called "spider cells."

Clinical Features. The major clinical manifestations of myxomas are due to valvular obstruction, embolization, or a syndrome of constitutional signs and symptoms including fever and malaise. This syndrome is caused by elaboration of the cytokine IL-6 by the tumor cells, a mediator of the acute-phase response. Echocardiography is the diagnostic modality of choice, and surgical resection is almost uniformly curative.

Rhabdomyomas demonstrate skeletal muscle differentiation and are the most frequent primary tumors of the heart in infants and children; they are frequently discovered due to valvular or outflow obstruction.

Cardiac Effects of Noncardiac Neoplasms

With increased patient survival due to diagnostic and therapeutic advances, diverse cardiovascular effects of noncardiac neoplasms and their therapy are increasingly encountered (Table 9.6). These effects may be mediated by metastatic spread to the pleura or heart but are more commonly caused by substances released from tumors. Examples include nonbacterial thrombotic endocarditis, carcinoid heart disease, pheochromocytoma-associated myocardial damage, and myeloma-associated AL-type amyloidosis. Many of these conditions are discussed elsewhere in this book. Only carcinoid heart disease is discussed here.

Carcinoid Heart Disease

The carcinoid syndrome results from bioactive compounds such as serotonin released by carcinoid tumors (Chapter 13); systemic

Table 9.6 Cardiovascular Effects of Noncardiac Neoplasms

Direct Consequences of Tumor
Pericardial and myocardial metastases
Large vessel obstruction
Pulmonary tumor emboli
Indirect Consequences of Tumor (Complications of Circulating Mediators)
Nonbacterial thrombotic endocarditis
Carcinoid heart disease
Pheochromocytoma-associated heart disease
Myeloma-associated amyloidosis
Effects of Tumor Therapy
Chemotherapy
Radiation therapy

Modified from Schoen FJ, et al: Cardiac effects of non-cardiac neoplasms, *Cardiol Clin* 2:657, 1984.

manifestations include flushing, diarrhea, dermatitis, and bronchoconstriction. Carcinoid heart disease refers to cardiac manifestation caused by bioactive compounds and occurs in one-half of patients in whom the systemic syndrome develops. Cardiac lesions typically do not occur until there is a large hepatic metastatic burden, since the liver efficiently inactivates circulating mediators before they can affect the heart. Classically, endocardium and valves of the right heart are primarily affected since they are the first cardiac tissues bathed by the mediators released by gastrointestinal carcinoid tumors. The left side of the heart is afforded some measure of protection because the pulmonary vascular bed degrades the mediators. However, left-sided heart carcinoid lesions can occur in the setting of atrial or ventricular septal defects and right-to-left flow, or they can arise in association with primary pulmonary carcinoid tumors.

Pathogenesis. The mediators elaborated by carcinoid tumors include serotonin (5-hydroxytryptamine), kallikrein, bradykinin, histamine, prostaglandins, and tachykinins. Of these, serotonin seems to be the culprit. This is supported by the following:

- Plasma levels of serotonin and urinary excretion of the serotonin metabolite 5-hydroxyindoleacetic acid correlate with the severity of right-sided heart lesions.

- In patients with the carcinoid syndrome, 70% of dietary tryptophan is converted to serotonin as compared to 1% in unaffected individuals.

The valvular plaques in carcinoid syndrome are also similar to lesions that occur with the administration of fenfluramine (an appetite suppressant) or ergot alkaloids (previously used for migraine headaches); of interest, these agents affect either systemic serotonin metabolism or directly bind to hydroxytryptamine receptors on heart valves.

MORPHOLOGY

The cardiovascular lesions associated with the carcinoid syndrome are distinctive, glistening white, plaque-like thickenings on the endocardial surfaces of the cardiac chambers and valve leaflets (Fig. 9.31). The lesions are composed of smooth muscle cells and sparse collagen fibers embedded in an acid mucopolysaccharide—rich matrix. Underlying structures are intact. With right-sided involvement, typical findings are tricuspid insufficiency and pulmonic stenosis.

CARDIAC TRANSPLANTATION

Although permanent ventricular assist devices are increasingly being used for management of end-stage heart disease, cardiac transplantation remains the treatment of choice for patients with intractable heart failure. Without transplantation, medically managed end-stage heart failure carries a 50% 1-year mortality rate, and fewer than 10% of patients survive 5 years. Over 3,500 heart transplantation procedures are performed annually worldwide, mostly for DCM and IHD.

The major complications of cardiac transplantation are acute graft rejection and allograft arteriopathy. The immunosuppression required for allograft survival also increases the risk for opportunistic infections and certain malignancies (e.g., Epstein-Barr virus—associated lymphoma).

- *Rejection* is characterized by interstitial lymphocytic inflammation, myocyte damage, and a histologic pattern similar to that seen in viral myocarditis. Both T-cell and antibody responses to the allograft are involved in the rejection reaction.

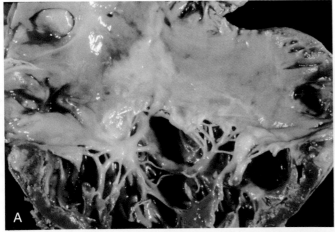
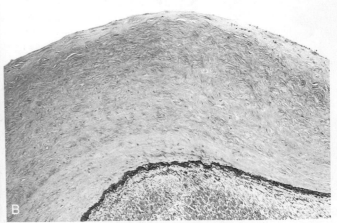

FIG. 9.31 Carcinoid heart disease. (A) Characteristic endocardial fibrotic *(light gray)* lesion "coating" the right ventricle and tricuspid valve, and extending onto the chordae tendineae. (B) Microscopic appearance of the thickened endocardium, which contains smooth muscle cells and abundant acid mucopolysaccharides (blue-green in this Movat stain, which colors the underlying endocardial elastic tissue black).

- *Allograft arteriopathy* is the most important lesion of chronic rejection in transplanted hearts, and the major cause of graft loss. It is marked by progressive, diffusely stenosing intimal proliferation in the coronary arteries, leading to ischemic injury.

Despite these problems, the outlook for transplant recipients generally is good, with a 1-year survival rate of 90% and a 5-year survival rate of more than 70%.

■ RAPID REVIEW

Heart Failure

- CHF occurs when the heart is unable to provide adequate perfusion to meet the metabolic demands of peripheral tissues; inadequate cardiac output is usually accompanied by congestion of the venous circulation.
- Left-sided heart failure is most commonly secondary to ischemic heart disease, systemic hypertension, mitral or aortic valve disease, or primary diseases of the myocardium; symptoms are mainly a consequence of pulmonary congestion and edema, although systemic hypoperfusion can cause renal and cerebral dysfunction.
- Right-sided heart failure is due most often to left-sided heart failure and, less commonly, to primary pulmonary disorders; signs and symptoms are related chiefly to peripheral edema and visceral congestion.

Congenital Heart Disease

- Congenital heart disease represents defects of cardiac chambers or the great vessels; these either result in shunting of blood between the right- and left-sided circulation or cause outflow obstructions.
- Malformations associated with left-to-right shunts are the most common and include ASDs, VSDs, and PDA. Shunting results in right-sided volume overload that eventually causes pulmonary hypertension and, with reversal of flow and right-to-left shunting, cyanosis (*Eisenmenger syndrome*).
- Malformations associated with right-to-left shunts include tetralogy of Fallot and transposition of the great arteries. These lesions cause early-onset cyanosis and are associated with polycythemia, hypertrophic osteoarthropathy, and paradoxical embolization.
- Obstructive lesions include forms of aortic coarctation; the clinical severity of these lesions depends on the degree of stenosis and the patency of the ductus arteriosus.

Ischemic Heart Disease

- In the vast majority of cases, cardiac ischemia is due to coronary artery atherosclerosis; vasospasm, vasculitis, and embolism are less common causes.
- Cardiac ischemia results from a mismatch between coronary supply and myocardial demand and manifests as different, albeit overlapping syndromes:
  - *Angina pectoris* is exertional chest pain due to inadequate perfusion and is typically due to atherosclerotic disease causing greater than 70% fixed stenosis (so-called "critical stenosis").
  - *Unstable angina* is characterized by increasingly frequent pain, precipitated by progressively less exertion or even occurring at rest. It results from an erosion or rupture of atherosclerotic plaque triggering platelet aggregation, vasoconstriction, and formation of a thrombus that need not be occlusive.
  - *Acute myocardial infarction* typically results from acute thrombosis after plaque disruption; a majority occur in plaques that did not previously exhibit critical stenosis.
  - *Sudden cardiac death* usually results from a fatal arrhythmia, typically without significant acute myocardial damage.
  - *Ischemic cardiomyopathy* is progressive heart failure due to ischemic injury, either from previous infarction(s) or chronic ischemia.
- Myocardial ischemia leads to loss of myocyte function within 1 to 2 minutes and myocyte death after 20 to 40 minutes. Myocardial infarction is diagnosed on the basis of symptoms, electrocardiographic changes, and measurement of serum levels of cardiac-specific troponins. Gross and histologic changes of infarction require hours to days to develop.
- Infarction can be modified by therapeutic intervention (e.g., thrombolysis or stenting), which salvages myocardium at risk but may also induce reperfusion-related injury.
- Complications of infarction include arrhythmia, ventricular rupture, papillary muscle rupture, aneurysm formation, mural thrombus, pericarditis, and CHF.

Arrhythmias

- Arrhythmias can be caused by ischemic or structural changes in the conduction system or by myocyte electrical instability. In structurally normal hearts, arrhythmias may be due to mutations in ion channels that cause aberrant repolarization or depolarization.
- Sudden cardiac death (SCD) most frequently is due to coronary artery disease leading to ischemia. Myocardial irritability typically results from nonlethal ischemia or from preexisting fibrosis from previous myocardial injury. In younger patients acquired or hereditary defects in conduction defects are present.

Hypertensive Heart Disease

- Hypertensive heart disease can affect either the left ventricle or the right ventricle; in the latter case, the disorder is due to primary pulmonary disease and is called *cor pulmonale*. Elevated pressures induce myocyte hypertrophy and interstitial fibrosis that increase wall thickness and stiffness.
- The chronic pressure overload of systemic hypertension causes left ventricular concentric hypertrophy, often associated with left atrial dilation due to impaired diastolic filling of the ventricle. Persistently elevated pressure overload can cause ventricular failure with dilation.
- Cor pulmonale results from pulmonary hypertension due to primary lung parenchymal (e.g., COPD) or vascular disorders (e.g., pulmonary hypertension). Hypertrophy of both the right ventricle and the right atrium is characteristic; dilation also may be seen when failure supervenes.

Valvular Heart Disease

- Valve pathology can lead to occlusion (*stenosis*) and/or regurgitation (*insufficiency*); acquired aortic or mitral valve stenosis accounts for approximately two-thirds of all valve disease.
- Stenosis typically results from valve calcification, as in aortic stenosis; abnormal matrix synthesis and turnover leads to myxomatous degeneration and insufficiency (as in floppy mitral valve).
- Inflammatory valve diseases cause postinflammatory scarring. Rheumatic heart disease results from antistreptococcal antibodies that cross-react with cardiac tissues; it most commonly affects the mitral valve and is responsible for almost all cases of acquired mitral stenosis.

- Acute infective endocarditis (IE), caused most often by *S. aureus,* can rapidly destroy normal valves; subacute IE, caused often by *Streptococcus viridans,* is indolent and usually occurs on previously abnormal valves. Systemic embolization can produce septic infarcts.
- Nonbacterial thrombotic endocarditis occurs on previously normal valves as a result of hypercoagulable states; embolization is an important complication.

Cardiomyopathies and Myocarditis

- *Cardiomyopathy* refers to intrinsic cardiac muscle disease; there may be specific causes, or it may be idiopathic.
- The three general pathophysiologic categories of cardiomyopathy are *dilated (DCM)* (accounting for 90% of the cases), *hypertrophic (HCM),* and *restrictive* (least common).
- DCM results in systolic (contractile) dysfunction. In 20% to 50% of cases, mutations affecting cytoskeletal proteins are responsible. Acquired causes include myocarditis, toxic exposures (e.g., alcohol), and pregnancy. The heart is enlarged with four chamber dilation.
- HCM results in diastolic (relaxation) dysfunction. Virtually all cases are due to autosomal dominant mutations in the proteins that make up the contractile apparatus, in particular β-myosin heavy chain. There is massive cardiac hypertrophy with asymmetric septal hypertrophy.
- Restrictive cardiomyopathy results in a stiff, noncompliant myocardium and can be due to depositions (e.g., amyloid), or endomyocardial scarring.
- Arrhythmogenic right ventricular cardiomyopathy is an autosomal dominant disorder of cardiac muscle that manifests with right-sided heart failure and rhythm disturbances that can cause sudden cardiac death in athletes; fibrosis and fat infiltration are characteristic.
- Myocarditis is an inflammatory disorder caused by infections or immune reactions. Coxsackieviruses A and B are the most common pathogens in the United States. Clinically, myocarditis may be asymptomatic, give rise to acute heart failure, or evolve to DCM.

■ Laboratory Tests

Test	Reference Values	Pathophysiology/Clinical Relevance
Brain natriuretic peptide or B-type natriuretic peptide (BNP), plasma/ N-terminal (NT)-prohormone BNP (NT-proBNP), serum	Varies with sex and age	In response to ventricular wall stretch and volume overload, cardiac myocytes cleave an N-terminal section from the BNP prohormone (NT-proBNP) to release active BNP. BNP downregulates the renin-angiotensin-aldosterone system, decreases sympathetic tone in the heart and kidney, and increases renal blood flow and sodium excretion. NT-proBNP has a longer half-life than BNP and is more commonly used clinically. It is useful in distinguishing acute onset dyspnea secondary to congestive heart failure versus lung disease since it is elevated in the former, but not the latter. However, NT-proBNP should not be used in isolation to establish the diagnosis of CHF.
C-reactive protein (CRP), serum	≤8.0 mg/L	CRP is an acute phase protein that is made by the liver and released in response to inflammatory cytokines. It is a very sensitive test for inflammation. Since inflammation is a risk factor for atherosclerosis and consequent atherosclerotic cardiovascular disease, CRP levels can be useful in cardiovascular risk stratification.
High-sensitivity troponin T (hs-cTnT), plasma	Males: ≤20 ng/L Females: ≤15 ng/L	Troponin is a regulatory protein of striated muscle composed of three subunits: T, C, and I. The T, or tropomyosin-binding subunit, binds to muscle fibers. cTnT is specific for cardiac muscle and is released into the circulation after myocardial cell death. Its level begins to rise 2 to 3 hours after acute myocardial infarction and peaks at 48 hours. The blood level remains elevated for 2 weeks or longer. In addition to myocardial infarction, elevated cTnT can be seen in cardiac contusion, congestive heart failure, renal failure, pulmonary embolism, and myocarditis.

Adapted from Deyrup AT, D'Ambrosio D, Muir J, et al. Essential Laboratory Tests for Medical Education. *Acad Pathol.* 2022;9. doi: 10.1016/j.acpath.2022.100046.

Hematopoietic and Lymphoid Systems

The hematopoietic and lymphoid systems are affected by a wide spectrum of diseases. One useful way to organize these disorders is based on whether they primarily affect red cells, white cells, or the coagulation system, which includes platelets and clotting factors. The most common red cell disorders are those that lead to *anemia*, a state of red cell deficiency. Clinically significant white cell disorders, by contrast, are most often associated with excessive proliferation resulting from malignant transformation. Derangements in blood coagulation may result in hemorrhagic diatheses (bleeding disorders). Blood products are frequently lifesaving when given to patients but may also produce serious complications, which are reviewed in brief. Finally, splenomegaly, a feature of numerous diseases, is discussed at the end of the chapter, as are tumors of the thymus.

Although these divisions are useful, in reality the production, function, and destruction of red cells, white cells, and components of the hemostatic system are closely linked, and derangements primarily affecting one cell type or component of the system often lead to alterations in others. Other levels of interplay and complexity stem from the anatomically dispersed nature of the hematolymphoid system and the capacity of both normal and malignant white cells to "traffic" between various compartments. Hence, a patient who is diagnosed with lymphoma by lymph node biopsy may also be found to have neoplastic lymphoid cells in the bone marrow and blood. The malignant clone of lymphoid cells in the marrow may suppress hematopoiesis, giving rise to low blood cell counts (cytopenias), and the dissemination of tumor cells to the liver and spleen may lead to organomegaly. Thus, in both benign and malignant hematolymphoid disorders, a single underlying abnormality can result in diverse systemic manifestations. Keeping these complexities in mind, we will use the time-honored classification of hematolymphoid disorders based on predominant involvement of red cells, white cells, and the hemostatic system.

RED CELL DISORDERS

Disorders of red cells can result in anemia or, less commonly, *polycythemia* (an increase in red cells, also known as *erythrocytosis*). *Anemia* is defined as a decrease in the red cell mass to subnormal levels and results in a reduction of the oxygen-transporting capacity of blood.

Anemia can stem from bleeding, increased red cell destruction (hemolysis), or decreased red cell production. These mechanisms serve as one basis for classifying anemia (Table 10.1). In some entities both mechanisms may occur; for example, in thalassemia, both reduced red cell production and increased destruction contribute to anemia. With the exception of anemia caused by chronic renal failure or chronic inflammation (described later), the decrease in tissue oxygen tension that accompanies anemia triggers increased production of the growth factor *erythropoietin* from specialized cells in the kidney. Erythropoietin in turn drives a compensatory hyperplasia of erythroid precursors in the bone marrow and, in severe anemia, the induction of *extramedullary hematopoiesis* within the secondary hematopoietic organs (the liver, spleen, and lymph nodes). In well-nourished persons who become anemic because of acute bleeding or increased red cell destruction (hemolysis), the compensatory response can increase the production of red cells 5- to 8-fold. The marrow response is signaled by the appearance of increased numbers of newly formed red cells *(reticulocytes)* in the peripheral blood. By contrast, anemia caused by decreased red cell production (aregenerative anemia) is associated with subnormal reticulocyte counts (reticulocytopenia).

Table 10.1 Classification of Anemia According to Underlying Mechanism

Blood Loss
Acute: trauma
Chronic: gastrointestinal tract lesions, gynecologic disturbances

Increased Destruction (Hemolytic Anemias)

Intrinsic (Intracorpuscular) Abnormalities

Hereditary
Membrane abnormalities
  Membrane skeleton proteins: spherocytosis, elliptocytosis
  Membrane lipids: abetalipoproteinemia
Enzyme deficiencies
  Enzymes of hexose monophosphate shunt: glucose-6-phosphate dehydrogenase, glutathione synthetase
  Glycolytic enzymes: pyruvate kinase, hexokinase
Disorders of hemoglobin synthesis
  Structurally abnormal globin synthesis (hemoglobinopathies): sickle cell anemia, unstable hemoglobins
  Deficient globin synthesis: thalassemia syndromes
Acquired
Membrane defect: paroxysmal nocturnal hemoglobinuria

Extrinsic (Extracorpuscular) Abnormalities

Antibody-mediated
  Isohemagglutinins: transfusion reactions, immune hydrops (Rh disease of the newborn)
  Autoantibodies: idiopathic (primary), drug-associated, autoimmune diseases, e.g., systemic lupus erythematosus
Mechanical trauma to red cells
  Microangiopathic hemolytic anemias: thrombotic thrombocytopenic purpura, disseminated intravascular coagulation
  Dysfunctional cardiac valves
Infections: malaria

Impaired Red Cell Production

Disturbed proliferation and differentiation of stem cells: aplastic anemia, pure red cell aplasia
Disturbed proliferation and maturation of erythroblasts
  Defective DNA synthesis: deficiency or impaired use of vitamin B_{12} and folic acid (megaloblastic anemias)
  Anemia of renal failure (erythropoietin deficiency)
  Anemia of chronic disease (iron sequestration, relative erythropoietin deficiency)
  Anemia of endocrine disorders
  Defective hemoglobin synthesis
    Deficient heme synthesis: iron deficiency, sideroblastic anemias
    Deficient globin synthesis: thalassemias
Marrow replacement: primary hematopoietic neoplasms (acute leukemia, myelodysplastic syndromes)
Marrow infiltration (myelophthisic anemia): metastatic neoplasms, granulomatous disease

Anemia can also be classified on the basis of red cell morphology, which often points to particular causes. Features that provide etiologic clues include the size, color, and shape of the red cells. These are judged subjectively by visual inspection of peripheral smears and also are expressed quantitatively using the following indices:

- *Mean cell volume* (MCV): the average volume of each red cell, expressed in femtoliters (cubic microns)
- *Mean corpuscular hemoglobin* (MCH): the average mass of hemoglobin per red cell, expressed in picograms
- *Mean corpuscular hemoglobin concentration* (MCHC): the average concentration of hemoglobin in a given volume of packed red cells, expressed in grams per deciliter

- *Red cell distribution width* (RDW): the coefficient of variation of red cell volume

Red cell indices are quantified by specialized instruments in clinical laboratories. The same instruments also determine the *reticulocyte count,* a simple measure that distinguishes between hemolytic anemia and anemia due to reduced production (see later). Adult reference ranges for these tests are shown in Table 10.2. Depending on the differential diagnosis, a number of other blood tests may also be performed to evaluate anemia, including (1) *serum iron indices* (iron levels, iron-binding capacity, transferrin saturation, and ferritin concentrations), which help distinguish among microcytic anemia caused by iron deficiency, chronic inflammation, or thalassemia; (2) *plasma unconjugated bilirubin, haptoglobin, and lactate dehydrogenase levels,* which are abnormal in hemolytic anemia; (3) *serum and red cell folate and vitamin B_{12} concentrations,* which are low in megaloblastic anemia; (4) *hemoglobin electrophoresis,* which is used to detect abnormal hemoglobins; and (5) the *Coombs test,* which is used to detect antibodies or complement bound to red cells in suspected cases of antibody-mediated hemolytic anemia. In isolated anemia, tests performed on the peripheral blood usually suffice to establish the cause. By contrast, when anemia occurs along with thrombocytopenia and/or granulocytopenia, it is much more likely to be associated with marrow aplasia or infiltration; in such instances a marrow examination is usually warranted.

As discussed later, the clinical consequences of anemia are determined by its severity, rapidity of onset, and underlying pathogenic mechanism. If the onset is slow, the deficit in O_2-carrying capacity is compensated for by increases in cardiac output, respiratory rate, and red cell 2,3-diphosphoglycerate (DPG), a glycolytic pathway intermediate that enhances the release of O_2 from hemoglobin. These adaptive changes mitigate the effects of mild to moderate anemia in otherwise healthy persons but are less effective in those with compromised pulmonary or cardiac function. Pallor, fatigue, and lassitude are common to all forms of anemia. Features that are specific to various subtypes are discussed in the following sections.

ANEMIA OF BLOOD LOSS: HEMORRHAGE

Anemia of blood loss can be divided into anemia caused by acute bleeding (hemorrhage) and anemia caused by chronic blood loss (described later). **The effects of acute bleeding are mainly due to the loss of intravascular volume, which if greater than 20%, can lead to cardiovascular collapse, shock, and death.** If the patient survives and is resuscitated with oral or intravenous fluids, hemodilution begins at once and achieves its full effect within 2 to 3 days; only then is the full extent of the red cell loss revealed. The anemia is normocytic and normochromic. Recovery from blood loss is enhanced by a compensatory rise in erythropoietin, which stimulates increased red cell production and reticulocytosis following a lag of 5 to 7 days.

With chronic blood loss, iron stores are gradually depleted. Iron is essential for hemoglobin synthesis and erythropoiesis, and its deficiency leads to a chronic anemia of underproduction. Iron deficiency anemia can occur in other clinical settings as well; it is described later along with other forms of anemia caused by decreased red cell production.

HEMOLYTIC ANEMIA

Hemolytic anemias are a diverse group of disorders that have as a common feature accelerated red cell destruction. The red cell life span is shortened to less than its normal 120 days, often markedly so. The resulting anemia and low tissue O_2 levels stimulate erythropoietin release from the kidney, leading to increased production of reticulocytes by the bone marrow. Thus, marrow erythroid hyperplasia and peripheral blood reticulocytosis are hallmarks of hemolytic anemias. In severe hemolytic anemias, the erythropoietic drive may be so pronounced that extramedullary hematopoiesis appears in the liver, spleen, and lymph nodes.

There are several ways to organize hemolytic anemias. One approach groups them according to whether the pathogenic red cell defect is *intrinsic (intracorpuscular)* or *extrinsic (extracorpuscular)* (see Table 10.1). A second more clinically useful approach groups hemolytic anemias according to whether hemolysis is primarily extravascular or intravascular. **Extravascular hemolysis is caused by defects that increase the destruction of red cells by phagocytes, particularly in the spleen.** The spleen contains large numbers of macrophages, the principal cells responsible for the removal of damaged or antibody-coated red cells from the circulation. Because marked alterations of shape are necessary for red cells to navigate the splenic sinusoids, any reduction in red cell deformability makes this passage difficult, and red cells that become "stuck" are phagocytosed by resident splenic macrophages. As described later in the chapter, diminished deformability is a major cause of red cell destruction in several hemolytic anemias. Findings that are relatively specific for extravascular hemolysis (as compared to intravascular hemolysis) include the following:

- *Hyperbilirubinemia* and *jaundice,* stemming from degradation of hemoglobin in macrophages
- Varying degrees of *splenomegaly* due to "work hyperplasia" of phagocytes in the spleen
- If long-standing, increased risk of *cholelithiasis* with formation of *bilirubin-rich gallstones* (pigment stones)

Intravascular hemolysis, **by contrast, is characterized by injuries so severe that red cells burst within the circulation.** Intravascular hemolysis may result from mechanical forces (e.g., turbulence created by a defective heart valve) or biochemical or physical agents that severely damage the red cell membrane (e.g., fixation of complement or exposure to clostridial toxins or heat). Findings that distinguish intravascular hemolysis from extravascular hemolysis include the following:

- *Hemoglobinemia, hemoglobinuria,* and *hemosiderinuria.* Hemoglobin released into the circulation is small enough to pass into the

Table 10.2 Adult Reference Ranges for Red Blood Cells[a]

	Units	Men	Women
Hemoglobin (Hb)	g/dL	13.2–16.6	11.6–15.0
Hematocrit (Hct)	%	38–49	35–45
Red cell count	$\times 10^6/\mu L$	4.4–5.6	3.9–5.1
Reticulocyte count	%	0.6–2.7	0.6–2.7
Mean cell volume (MCV)	fL	78–98	78–98
Mean cell Hb (MCH)	pg	26–34	26–34
Mean cell Hb concentration (MCHC)	g/dL	32–36	31–36
Red cell distribution width (RDW)		11.8–14.5	12.2–16.1

[a]Reference ranges vary among laboratories. The reference ranges for the laboratory providing the result should always be used in interpreting a laboratory test. Reference values from https://mayocliniclabs.com/ by permission of Mayo Foundation for Medical Education and Research. All rights reserved.

urinary space. Here, it is partially resorbed by renal tubular cells and processed into hemosiderin, which is then lost in the urine when renal tubular cells are sloughed.

- *Loss of iron,* which may lead to iron deficiency if hemolysis is persistent. By contrast, iron recycling by phagocytes is very efficient, and so iron deficiency is not a feature of extravascular hemolytic anemias.

A feature of both intravascular and extravascular hemolysis is decreased serum levels of *haptoglobin,* a plasma protein that binds free hemoglobin and is then removed from the circulation. Apparently, macrophages "regurgitate" sufficient hemoglobin during consumption of red cells to cause haptoglobin levels to fall, even when hemolysis is entirely extravascular.

We now turn to some of the relatively common hemolytic anemias.

Hereditary Spherocytosis

This disorder stems from inherited (intrinsic) defects in the red cell membrane that lead to the formation of spherocytes, non-deformable cells that are highly vulnerable to sequestration and destruction in the spleen. Hereditary spherocytosis is usually transmitted as an autosomal dominant trait; a more severe, autosomal recessive form of the disease affects a small minority of patients.

Pathogenesis. **Hereditary spherocytosis is caused by inherited defects in the membrane skeleton, a network of proteins that stabilizes the lipid bilayer of the red cell** (Fig. 10.1). The major membrane skeleton protein is spectrin, a long, flexible heterodimer that self-associates at one end and binds short actin filaments at its other end. These contacts create a two-dimensional meshwork that is connected to the intrinsic membrane proteins band 3 and glycophorin via linker proteins like ankyrin and band 4.1. The common feature of the mutations that cause hereditary spherocytosis is that they weaken interactions between the membrane skeleton and intrinsic red cell membrane proteins. This results in the destabilization of the lipid bilayer of red cells, which shed membrane vesicles into the circulation as they age. Little cytoplasm is lost in the process and as a result the surface area-to-volume ratio decreases progressively with time until the cells become spherical (Fig. 10.1).

The floppy discoid shape of normal red cells allows considerable latitude for shape changes. By contrast, spherocytes have limited deformability and are sequestered in the splenic cords, where they are destroyed by the plentiful resident macrophages (Fig. 10.1). **The critical role of the spleen in hereditary spherocytosis is illustrated by the beneficial effect of splenectomy; although the red cell defect and spherocytes persist, the anemia is corrected.**

MORPHOLOGY

On peripheral blood smears, **spherocytes** are dark red and lack central pallor (Fig. 10.2). The excessive red cell destruction and resultant anemia lead to a compensatory hyperplasia of red cell progenitors in the marrow and an increase in red cell production marked by reticulocytosis. **Splenomegaly** is more common and prominent in hereditary spherocytosis than in other forms of hemolytic anemia. The splenic weight is usually between 500 g and 1000 g (normal, 150 g to 200 g). The enlargement results from marked congestion of the splenic cords and increased numbers of macrophages. Phagocytosed red cells are seen within macrophages lining the sinusoids and within the cords. Other general features of hemolytic anemia may also be seen, including **cholelithiasis,** which occurs in 40% to 50% of patients with hereditary spherocytosis.

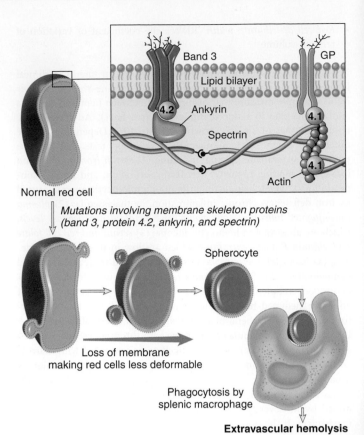

FIG. 10.1 Pathogenesis of hereditary spherocytosis. *(Top)* Normal organization of the major red cell membrane skeleton proteins. Mutations in spectrin, ankyrin, band 4.2, and band 3 that weaken the association of the membrane skeleton with the overlying plasma membrane cause red cells to shed membrane vesicles and transform into spherocytes *(bottom).* The nondeformable spherocytes are trapped in the splenic cords and phagocytosed by macrophages. *GP,* Glycophorin.

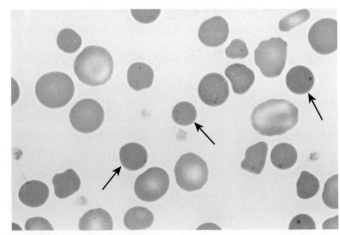

FIG. 10.2 Hereditary spherocytosis—peripheral blood smear. Note the anisocytosis and several hyperchromic spherocytes *(arrows).* Howell-Jolly bodies (small nuclear remnants, which appear as small dark inclusions) are also present in the red cells of this asplenic patient. (Courtesy of Dr. Robert W. McKenna, Department of Pathology, University of Texas Southwestern Medical School, Dallas, Texas.)

Clinical Features. **The characteristic features are anemia, spleno-megaly, and jaundice.** The anemia is variable in severity, ranging from subclinical to profound; most commonly it is moderate in degree. Because of their spherical shape, red cells in hereditary spherocytosis show increased osmotic fragility when placed in hypotonic salt solutions, a characteristic that can help establish the diagnosis.

The course is generally stable but may be punctuated by *aplastic crises*, the most severe of which are triggered by *parvovirus B19 infection*. This virus has a marked tropism for erythroblasts, which undergo apoptosis during viral replication. Until the immune response controls the infection (usually in 10 to 14 days), the marrow may be virtually devoid of red cell progenitors. Because of the shortened life span of red cells in hereditary spherocytosis, a lack of red cell production, even for a few days, results in rapid worsening of the anemia. Blood transfusions may be needed to support patients until the infection is cleared.

There is no specific treatment. Splenectomy improves the anemia by removing the major site of red cell destruction. The benefits of splenectomy must be weighed against the increased risk of serious infections by encapsulated bacteria, particularly in children. Partial splenectomy is gaining favor in young children because this approach produces hematologic improvement while maintaining protection against sepsis. The downside is that because the partially resected spleen eventually regains its size, many patients will need a second resection. The hope is that this can be delayed until later in childhood, when the risk of serious infection is lower.

Sickle Cell Anemia

Hemoglobinopathies **are a group of hereditary disorders caused by inherited mutations that lead to structural abnormalities in hemoglobin.** Sickle cell anemia, the prototypic hemoglobinopathy, is caused by a mutation in β-globin that creates sickle hemoglobin (HbS). Numerous other hemoglobinopathies have been described, but these are less common and beyond the scope of this discussion.

Sickle cell anemia is the most common familial hemolytic anemia. The presence of HbS is protective against falciparum malaria and because of this selective pressure the HbS allele is prevalent in areas where malaria was (and, in some instances, still is) endemic, including equatorial Africa and parts of India, southern Europe, and the Middle East. In the United States, approximately 8% of people of African descent are heterozygous HbS carriers, and about 1 in 600 have sickle cell anemia.

Pathogenesis. **Sickle cell anemia is caused by a single amino acid substitution in β-globin that results in a tendency for deoxygenated HbS to self-associate into polymers.** Normal hemoglobins are tetramers composed of two pairs of similar chains. On average, the normal adult red cell contains 96% HbA ($\alpha_2\beta_2$), 3% HbA2 ($\alpha_2\delta_2$), and 1% fetal Hb (HbF, $\alpha_2\gamma_2$). In patients with sickle cell anemia, HbA is completely replaced by HbS, whereas in heterozygous carriers, only about half is replaced. HbS differs from HbA by having a valine residue instead of a glutamate residue at the 6th amino acid position in β-globin. On deoxygenation HbS molecules undergo a conformational change that allows polymers to form via intermolecular contacts involving the abnormal valine residue. These polymers distort the red cell, which assumes an elongated crescentic or sickle shape (Fig. 10.3).

The sickling of red cells is initially reversible on reoxygenation. However, membrane distortion produced by each sickling episode leads to an influx of calcium, which causes the loss of potassium and water and also damages the membrane skeleton. With time, this cumulative damage creates *irreversibly sickled cells* that are prone to hemolysis.

Three factors are particularly important in determining whether clinically significant polymerization of HbS occurs in patients:

- *The intracellular levels of hemoglobins other than HbS.* In heterozygotes approximately 40% of Hb is HbS and the remainder is HbA, which interacts only weakly with deoxygenated HbS. Because HbA greatly retards HbS polymerization, the red cells of HbS heterozygotes have little tendency to sickle in vivo. Such persons are said to have *sickle cell trait.* Similarly, because fetal hemoglobin (HbF) interacts weakly with HbS, newborns with sickle cell anemia do not manifest the disease until HbF falls to adult levels, generally around the age of 5 to 6 months. Hemoglobin C (HbC), another mutant β-globin, has a lysine residue instead of the normal glutamic acid residue at position 6. Like HbS, HbC confers protection to falciparum malaria and is prevalent in similar populations (sub-Saharan Africa, parts of India, etc.). Due to equatorial African ancestry, about 2.3% of Americans of

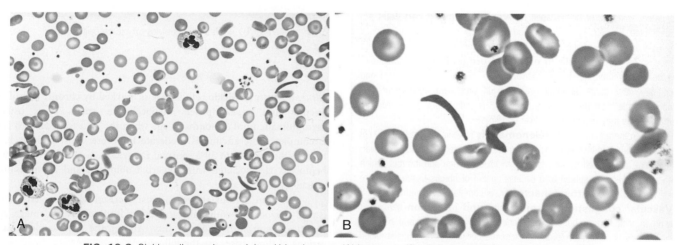

FIG. 10.3 Sickle cell anemia—peripheral blood smear. (A) Low magnification shows sickle cells, anisocytosis, poikilocytosis, and target cells. (B) Higher magnification shows two irreversibly sickled cells in the center. (Courtesy of Dr. Robert W. McKenna, Department of Pathology, University of Texas Southwestern Medical School, Dallas, Texas.)

African descent are heterozygous carriers of HbC, and about 1 in 1250 are compound HbC/HbS heterozygotes.

- *The intracellular concentration of HbS.* The polymerization of deoxygenated HbS is strongly concentration dependent. Thus, red cell dehydration, which increases the Hb concentration, facilitates sickling. Conversely, the coexistence of α-thalassemia (described later), which decreases the Hb concentration, reduces sickling.

- *The time required for red cells to pass through the microvasculature.* The normal transit times of red cells through capillary beds are too short for significant polymerization of deoxygenated HbS to occur. Hence, the tissues that are most susceptible to obstruction by sickle cells are those in which blood flow is sluggish, such as the spleen and the bone marrow. However, sickling may occur in other microvascular beds in the presence of factors that retard the passage of red cells, particularly inflammation. Recall that inflammation slows blood flow by increasing the adhesion of leukocytes and red cells to endothelium and by inducing the exudation of fluid through leaky vessels (Chapter 2). In addition, sickle red cells have a greater tendency than normal red cells to adhere to endothelial cells, as repeated bouts of sickling cause membrane damage that makes the red cells abnormally "sticky." These factors conspire to prolong the transit times of sickle red cells, increasing the probability of clinically significant vascular obstruction.

The sickling of red cells has two major pathologic consequences: **chronic moderately severe hemolytic anemia, due to red cell membrane damage; and vascular obstructions, which result in ischemic tissue damage and pain crises** (Fig. 10.4). The mean life span of red cells in sickle cell anemia averages only 20 days (one-sixth of normal) and the severity of the hemolysis correlates with the fraction of irreversibly sickled cells that are present in the blood. Vasoocclusion, by contrast, is not related to the number of irreversibly sickled cells and instead appears to be triggered by superimposed factors such as infection, inflammation, dehydration, and acidosis, all of which enhance the tendency of red cells to arrest and sickle within the microvasculature.

MORPHOLOGY

The abnormalities in sickle cell anemia stem from (1) chronic hemolytic anemia, (2) increased breakdown of heme to bilirubin, and (3) microvascular obstructions, which provoke tissue ischemia and infarction. In peripheral smears, elongated, spindled, or boat-shaped **irreversibly sickled red cells** are evident (see Fig. 10.3). Both the anemia and the vascular stasis produce hypoxia-induced fatty changes in the heart, liver, and renal tubules. There is a compensatory **hyperplasia of erythroid progenitors** in the marrow. The cellular proliferation in the marrow often causes bone resorption and secondary new bone formation, resulting in prominent cheekbones and changes in the skull resembling a "crewcut" in radiographs. Extramedullary hematopoiesis may appear in the liver and spleen.

In children there is moderate **splenomegaly** (splenic weight up to 500 g) due to red pulp congestion caused by entrapped sickled red cells. However, chronic splenic red cell stasis produces hypoxic damage and infarcts, which with time reduce the spleen to a useless nubbin of fibrous tissue. This process, referred to as **autosplenectomy**, is complete by adulthood.

Vascular congestion, thrombosis, and infarction can affect any organ, including the bones, liver, kidney, retina, brain, lung, and skin. The bone marrow is particularly prone to ischemia because of its sluggish blood flow and high rate of metabolism. Priapism, another frequent problem, can lead to penile fibrosis and erectile dysfunction. As with the other hemolytic anemias, **pigment gallstones** are common.

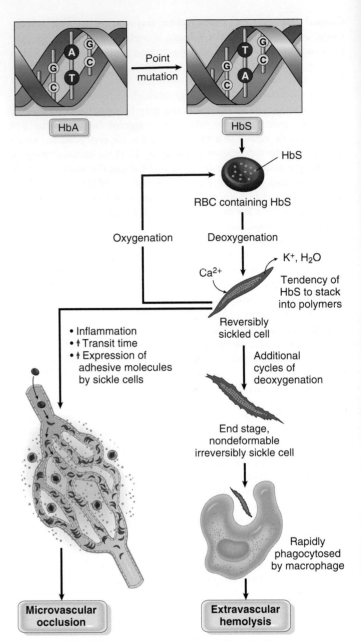

FIG. 10.4 Pathophysiology of sickle cell disease.

Clinical Features. **Sickle cell disease is marked by chronic hemolytic anemia and superimposed vasoocclusive crises.** It is usually asymptomatic until 6 months of age when the shift from HbF to HbS is complete. The anemia is moderate to severe; most patients have hematocrits of 18% to 30% (normal range, 38% to 48%). The chronic hemolysis is associated with hyperbilirubinemia and compensatory reticulocytosis.

Much more serious are vasoocclusive crises, which are characteristically associated with pain and often lead to tissue damage and significant morbidity and mortality. Among the most common and serious of these crises are the following:

- *Hand-foot syndrome,* resulting from infarction of bones in the hands and feet, is the most common presenting symptom in young children.

- *Acute chest syndrome,* in which sluggish blood flow in an inflamed lung (e.g., an area of pneumonia) leads to sickling within hypoxemic pulmonary beds. This exacerbates pulmonary dysfunction, creating a vicious circle of worsening pulmonary and systemic hypoxemia, sickling, and vasoocclusion. Acute chest syndrome may also be triggered by fat emboli emanating from infarcted bone.
- *Stroke,* which sometimes occurs in the setting of the acute chest syndrome. Stroke and the acute chest syndrome are the two leading causes of ischemia-related death.
- *Proliferative retinopathy,* a consequence of vasoocclusions in the eye that can lead to loss of visual acuity and blindness.

Another acute event, *aplastic crisis,* is caused by a sudden decrease in red cell production. As in hereditary spherocytosis, this is usually triggered by infection of erythroblasts by parvovirus B19 and, although severe, is self-limited.

In addition to these crises, patients with sickle cell disease are prone to infections. Both children and adults with sickle cell disease are functionally asplenic, making them susceptible to infections caused by encapsulated bacteria, such as pneumococci. In adults the basis for "hyposplenism" is autoinfarction. In the earlier childhood phase of splenic enlargement, congestion caused by trapped sickled red cells apparently interferes with bacterial sequestration and killing; hence, even children with enlarged spleens are at risk for developing fatal septicemia. Patients with sickle cell disease are also predisposed to bacterial osteomyelitis, which may result from bacterial seeding of infarcted bone. The most common causative organisms are encapsulated bacterial species and gram-negative organisms, particularly *E. coli* and *Salmonella.*

In homozygous sickle cell disease, irreversibly sickled red cells are seen in routine peripheral blood smears. In sickle cell trait, sickling can be induced in vitro by exposing cells to hypoxia. In the United States, newborn screening for sickle cell disease is now mandated; HbS and other hemoglobins are identified by methods such as gel electrophoresis in blood obtained by heel-stick. Prenatal diagnosis of sickle cell anemia is performed by analyzing fetal DNA obtained by amniocentesis or biopsy of chorionic villi.

The clinical course of sickle cell disease is highly variable. As a result of improvements in supportive care, approximately 50% of patients now survive beyond the fifth decade. Of particular importance is vaccination and prophylactic treatment with penicillin to prevent pneumococcal infections, especially in children younger than age 5. A mainstay of therapy is hydroxyurea, a "gentle" inhibitor of DNA synthesis. Hydroxyurea reduces pain crises and lessens the anemia through several effects, including (1) an increase in levels of HbF; (2) an anti-inflammatory effect because of the inhibition of white cell production; (3) an increase in red cell size, which lowers the intracellular hemoglobin concentration; and (4) its metabolism to NO, a potent vasodilator and inhibitor of platelet aggregation. More recently, encouraging results have been obtained with allogeneic bone marrow transplantation and corrective gene therapy, both of which are potentially curative.

Thalassemia

Thalassemias are inherited disorders caused by mutations in globin genes that decrease the synthesis of α- or β-globin. Decreased synthesis of one globin chain results not only in a deficiency of Hb but also in the formation of intracellular precipitates from the excess of unpaired normal globin chain that cause red cell damage and hemolysis. The mutations that cause thalassemia are particularly common in Mediterranean, African, and Asian regions in which malaria is endemic. As with HbS, it is hypothesized that globin mutations associated with thalassemia protect against falciparum malaria.

Pathogenesis. A diverse collection of α-globin and β-globin mutations underlie the thalassemias, which are autosomal codominant conditions. As described previously, adult hemoglobin, or HbA, is a tetramer composed of two α chains and two β chains. The α chains are encoded by two α-globin genes lying in tandem on chromosome 16, whereas the β chains are encoded by a single β-globin gene located on chromosome 11. The clinical features vary widely depending on the specific combination of mutated alleles that are inherited by the patient (Table 10.3).

Table 10.3 Clinical and Genetic Classification of Thalassemias

Clinical Syndrome	Genotype	Clinical Features	Molecular Genetics
β-Thalassemias			Mainly point mutations that lead to defects in the transcription, splicing, or translation of β-globin mRNA
β-Thalassemia major	Homozygous β-thalassemia (β^0/β^0, β^+/β^+, β^0/β^+)	Severe anemia; regular blood transfusions required	
β-Thalassemia intermedia	Variable (β^0/β^+, β^+/β^+, β^0/β, β^+/β)	Moderately severe anemia; regular blood transfusions not required	
β-Thalassemia minor	Heterozygous β-thalassemia (β^0/β, β^+/β)	Asymptomatic with mild or absent anemia; red cell abnormalities seen	
α-Thalassemias			Mainly gene deletions
Silent carrier	$-/\alpha$, α/α	Asymptomatic; no red cell abnormality	
α-Thalassemia trait	$-/-$, α/α (Asian) $-/\alpha$, $-/\alpha$ (black African, Asian)	Asymptomatic, resembles β-thalassemia minor	
HbH disease	$-/-$, $-/\alpha$	Moderately severe; resembles β-thalassemia intermedia	
Hydrops fetalis	$-/-$, $-/-$	Lethal in utero without transfusions	

HbH, Hemoglobin H; *mRNA,* messenger ribonucleic acid.

β-Thalassemia

Mutations associated with β-thalassemia fall into two categories: (1) β^0, in which no β-globin chains are produced; and (2) β^+, in which there is reduced (but detectable) β-globin synthesis. Sequencing of β-thalassemia genes has shown more than 100 different causative mutations, a majority consisting of single-base changes. Persons inheriting one abnormal allele have *β-thalassemia minor* (also known as *β-thalassemia trait*), which is asymptomatic or mildly symptomatic. Most people inheriting any two β^0 and β^+ alleles have *β-thalassemia major*; occasionally, persons inheriting at least one β^+ allele have a milder disease termed *β-thalassemia intermedia*. In contrast with α-thalassemia (described later), gene deletions rarely underlie β-thalassemia (Table 10.3).

The mutations responsible for β-thalassemia are diverse and disrupt β-globin synthesis in several ways. The most common lead to abnormal RNA splicing, whereas others lie in the β-globin gene promoter (leading to decreased transcription) or in coding regions (leading to decreased translation). The specific nature of the mutation determines whether the outcome is a β^+ or β^0 allele.

Defective synthesis of β-globin in β-thalassemia contributes to anemia through two mechanisms: (1) inadequate HbA formation, resulting in small (microcytic), poorly hemoglobinized (hypochromic) red cells; and (2) accumulation of unpaired α-globin chains, which form toxic precipitates that severely damage the membranes of red cells and erythroid precursors. A large fraction of erythroid precursors is so badly damaged that they die by apoptosis in the bone marrow (Fig. 10.5), a phenomenon termed *ineffective erythropoiesis*, and the few red cells that are produced have a shortened life span. Ineffective hematopoiesis is also associated with an inappropriate increase in the absorption of dietary iron, which without medical intervention inevitably leads to *iron overload*. The increased iron absorption is caused by low plasma levels of hepcidin, a critical negative regulator of iron absorption that is discussed later.

α-Thalassemia

Unlike β-thalassemia, **α-thalassemia is caused mainly by deletions involving one or more of the α-globin genes.** The severity of the disease is proportional to the number of α-globin genes that are

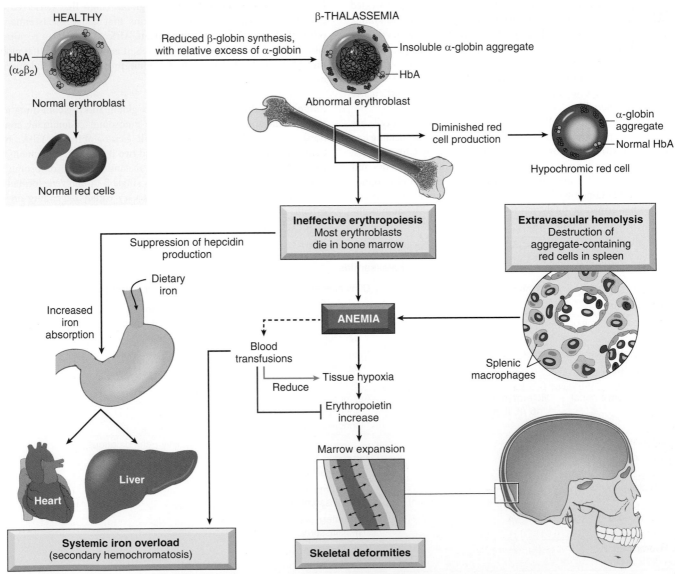

FIG. 10.5 Pathophysiology of β-thalassemia major. See text for details.

deleted (see Table 10.3). For example, loss of a single α-globin gene produces a silent-carrier state, whereas deletion of all four α-globin genes is lethal in utero because the red cells have virtually no oxygen-delivering capacity. With loss of three α-globin genes there is a relative excess of β-globin or (early in life) γ-globin chains. Excess β-globin and γ-globin chains form relatively stable β4 and γ4 tetramers known as *HbH* and *Hb Bart*, respectively, which cause less membrane damage than the free α-globin chains that are found in β-thalassemia; as a result, ineffective erythropoiesis is less pronounced in α-thalassemia. Unfortunately, both HbH and Hb Bart have an abnormally high affinity for oxygen, which prevents release of oxygen in tissues and thus renders them ineffective at delivering oxygen.

MORPHOLOGY

A range of morphologies is seen, depending on the specific underlying molecular lesion. On one end of the spectrum is β-thalassemia minor and α-thalassemia trait, in which abnormalities are confined to the peripheral blood. In smears, the red cells are small (microcytic) and pale (hypochromic), but regular in shape. Often seen are **target cells,** cells with an increased surface area-to-volume ratio that allows the cytoplasm to collect in a central dark red "puddle." On the other end of the spectrum, in β-thalassemia major peripheral blood smears show marked **microcytosis, hypochromia, poikilocytosis** (variation in cell shape), and **anisocytosis** (variation in cell size). Nucleated red cells (normoblasts) are also seen that reflect the underlying erythropoietic drive. β-Thalassemia intermedia and HbH disease are associated with peripheral smear findings that lie between these two extremes.

The anatomic changes in β-thalassemia major are similar to those seen in other hemolytic anemias but profound in degree. Ineffective erythropoiesis and hemolysis result in a striking hyperplasia of erythroid progenitors, with a shift toward early forms. The expanded erythropoietic marrow may completely fill the intramedullary space of the skeleton, invade the bony cortex, impair bone growth, and produce **skeletal deformities.** Extramedullary hematopoiesis and hyperplasia of mononuclear phagocytes result in prominent **splenomegaly,** hepatomegaly, and lymphadenopathy. The ineffective erythropoietic precursors consume nutrients and produce growth retardation and a degree of **cachexia** reminiscent of that seen in cancer patients. Unless steps are taken to prevent iron overload, during the span of years severe **hemosiderosis** develops (see Fig. 10.5). HbH disease and β-thalassemia intermedia are also associated with splenomegaly, erythroid hyperplasia, and growth retardation related to anemia, but these are less severe than in β-thalassemia major.

Clinical Features. β-Thalassemia trait and α-thalassemia trait are typically asymptomatic. There is usually only a mild microcytic hypochromic anemia; these patients have a normal life expectancy. Iron deficiency anemia is associated with a similar red cell appearance and must be excluded by appropriate laboratory tests (described later).

β-Thalassemia major manifests postnatally as HbF synthesis diminishes. Affected children have growth retardation that commences in infancy. They are sustained by blood transfusions, which improve the anemia and reduce the skeletal deformities associated with excessive erythropoiesis. With transfusions alone, survival into the second or third decade is possible, but systemic iron overload gradually develops owing to inappropriate uptake of iron from the gut and the iron load in transfused red cells. The excessive uptake of iron from the gut occurs because the expanded pool of erythroblasts secrete a hormone called *erythroferrone*, which circulates to the liver and suppresses the release of hepcidin (described later). Unless

patients are treated aggressively with iron chelators, cardiac dysfunction from *secondary hemochromatosis* inevitably develops and often is fatal in the second or third decade of life. When feasible, hematopoietic stem cell transplantation at an early age is the treatment of choice.

HbH disease and β-thalassemia intermedia are not as severe as β-thalassemia major because the imbalance in globin chain synthesis is not as profound and hematopoiesis is more effective. Anemia is of moderate severity, patients usually do not require transfusions, and iron overload is rarely seen.

The diagnosis of β-thalassemia major can be strongly suspected on clinical grounds. Hb electrophoresis shows a profound reduction or absence of HbA and increased levels of HbF. The HbA_2 level may be normal or increased. Similar but less severe changes are noted in patients affected by β-thalassemia intermedia. Prenatal diagnosis of β-thalassemia is challenging but can be made in specialized centers by DNA analysis. In fact, thalassemia was the first disease diagnosed by DNA-based tests, opening the way for the field of molecular diagnostics. The diagnosis of β-thalassemia minor is made by Hb electrophoresis, which typically shows a reduced level of HbA ($α_2β_2$) and an increased level of HbA_2 ($α_2δ_2$). HbH disease can be diagnosed by detection of β4 tetramers by electrophoresis.

Glucose-6-Phosphate Dehydrogenase Deficiency

Red cells are constantly exposed to both endogenous and exogenous oxidants, which are normally inactivated by reduced glutathione (GSH). Abnormalities affecting enzymes responsible for the synthesis of GSH leave red cells vulnerable to oxidative injury and hemolysis. By far the most common of these conditions is glucose-6-phosphate dehydrogenase (G6PD) deficiency. The G6PD gene is on the X chromosome. More than 400 G6PD variants have been identified, but only a few are associated with disease.

Pathogenesis. **G6PD deficiency is typically associated with transient episodes of intravascular hemolysis caused by exposure to an environmental factor (usually infectious agents or drugs) that produces oxidant stress.** Incriminated drugs include antimalarials (e.g., primaquine), sulfonamides, nitrofurantoin, phenacetin, aspirin (in large doses), and vitamin K derivatives. Consumption of certain foods, such as fava beans, may also lead to hemolysis. More commonly, episodes of hemolysis are triggered by infection, which induce phagocytes to generate oxidants as part of the host response. These oxidants, such as hydrogen peroxide, are normally sopped up by GSH, which is converted to oxidized GSH in the process. Because regeneration of GSH is impaired in G6PD-deficient cells, oxidants are free to "attack" other red cell components, including globin chains. Oxidized hemoglobin denatures and precipitates, forming intracellular inclusions called *Heinz bodies,* which can damage the red cell membrane so severely that intravascular hemolysis results. Other cells with less damage lose their deformability and suffer further injury when splenic phagocytes attempt to "pluck out" the Heinz bodies, creating *bite cells* (Fig. 10.6). Such cells become trapped on recirculation to the spleen and are destroyed by phagocytes.

Clinical Features. Hemolysis typically develops 2 or 3 days after drug exposure and is of variable severity. Because G6PD is X-linked, the red cells of affected males are uniformly deficient and vulnerable to oxidant injury. By contrast, random inactivation of one X chromosome in heterozygous females (Chapter 4) creates two populations of red cells, one normal and the other G6PD deficient. Most carrier females are unaffected except for those with a large proportion of deficient red

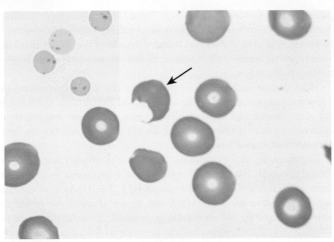

FIG. 10.6 Glucose-6-phosphate dehydrogenase deficiency after oxidant drug exposure—peripheral blood smear. *(Inset)* Red cells with precipitates of denatured globin (Heinz bodies) shown by supravital staining. As the splenic macrophages pluck out these inclusions, "bite cells" *(arrow)* similar to the one in this smear are produced. (Courtesy of Dr. Robert W. McKenna, Department of Pathology, University of Texas Southwestern Medical School, Dallas, Texas.)

cells (a chance situation known as unfavorable lyonization). Susceptibility to hemolysis among different mutated forms of G6PD varies according to the degree of G6PD deficiency. In the case of the G6PD A⁻ variant, which is common in areas of Africa where malaria is endemic, the half-life of the variant is only modestly decreased. As a result, only older red cells are susceptible to lysis. Because the marrow compensates for the anemia by increasing its production of new red cells with adequate levels of G6PD, the hemolysis abates even if the drug exposure continues. Other variants such as G6PD Mediterranean, found mainly in the Middle East, produce more marked enzyme deficiency and as a result the hemolysis that occurs on exposure to oxidants is more severe.

Paroxysmal Nocturnal Hemoglobinuria

Paroxysmal nocturnal hemoglobinuria (PNH) is a hemolytic anemia that stems from acquired mutations in *PIGA*, a gene required for the synthesis of phosphatidylinositol glycan (PIG), which serves as a membrane anchor for many proteins. Because *PIGA* is X-linked, normal cells have only one active *PIGA* gene, mutation of which is sufficient to cause PIGA deficiency. The pathogenic mutations in PNH occur in an early hematopoietic progenitor that is capable of giving rise to red cells, leukocytes, and platelets. Progeny of the *PIGA*-mutated clone lack the ability to make "PIG-tailed" proteins, including several that limit the activity of complement; as a result, red cells derived from *PIGA*-deficient precursors are inordinately sensitive to lysis by the complement C5b-C9 membrane attack complex. Leukocytes share the same deficiency but are less sensitive to complement than are red cells, and so red cells take the brunt of the attack. The nocturnal hemolysis that gives PNH its name occurs because complement fixation is enhanced by the decrease in blood pH that accompanies sleep (owing to CO_2 retention). However, most patients present less dramatically with anemia and iron deficiency resulting from chronic intravascular hemolysis. Interestingly, PNH is sometimes associated with aplastic anemia, which may precede or follow the onset of PNH. The basis for this association is uncertain.

The most feared complication of PNH is thrombosis, which often occurs within abdominal vessels such as the portal vein and the hepatic vein. The prothrombotic state also is somehow related to excessive complement activity, as eculizumab, a therapeutic antibody that binds C5 and inhibits the assembly of the C5b—C9 membrane attack complex, greatly lessens the incidence of thrombosis as well as the degree of intravascular hemolysis. Eculizumab has no effect on early stages of complement fixation, and treated patients continue to have varying degrees of extravascular hemolysis because of the deposition of C3b on red cell surfaces. Loss of C5b-C9 activity in patients receiving eculizumab poses a risk for *Neisseria* infections, particularly meningococcal sepsis; thus, all treated patients must be vaccinated against *N. meningococcus*.

Immunohemolytic Anemia

Immunohemolytic anemia is caused by antibodies that bind to antigens on red cell membranes. These antibodies may arise spontaneously or be induced by exogenous agents such as drugs or chemicals. Immunohemolytic anemia is uncommon and is classified based on (1) the nature of the antibody and (2) the presence of predisposing conditions, summarized in Table 10.4.

The diagnosis depends on the detection of antibodies and/or complement on red cells. This is done with the *direct Coombs test*, in which the patient's red cells are incubated with antibodies against human immunoglobulin or complement. These antibodies cause the patient's red cells to clump (agglutinate), indicating that the patient's red cells are coated with immunoglobulin and/or complement. The *indirect Coombs test*, which assesses the ability of the patient's serum to agglutinate test red cells bearing defined surface determinants, can then be used to characterize the target of the antibody.

Warm Antibody Immunohemolytic Anemia

In this entity, hemolysis results from the binding of high-affinity autoantibodies to red cells, which are then removed from the circulation by phagocytes in the spleen and elsewhere. In addition to erythrophagocytosis, incomplete consumption ("nibbling") of antibody-coated red cells by macrophages removes membrane and transforms red cells into spherocytes, which are rapidly destroyed in the spleen, just as in hereditary spherocytosis (described earlier). Warm antibody immunohemolytic anemia is caused by immunoglobulin G (IgG) or (rarely) IgA antibodies that are active at 37°C. More than 60% of cases are idiopathic (primary), while 25% occur in the setting of an immunologic disorder (e.g., systemic lupus erythematosus) or are induced by drugs. The clinical severity is variable, but most patients have chronic mild anemia and moderate splenomegaly and require no treatment.

The mechanisms of hemolysis induced by drugs are varied and, in some instances, poorly understood. Drugs such as α-methyldopa induce autoantibodies against intrinsic red cell constituents, in particular Rh blood group antigens. Presumably, the drug somehow alters the immunogenicity of native epitopes and thereby circumvents

Table 10.4 Classification of Immunohemolytic Anemias

Warm Antibody Type
Primary (idiopathic)
Secondary: B-cell neoplasms (e.g., chronic lymphocytic leukemia), autoimmune disorders (e.g., systemic lupus erythematosus), drugs (e.g., α-methyldopa, penicillin, quinidine)

Cold Antibody Type
Acute: Mycoplasma infection, infectious mononucleosis
Chronic: idiopathic, B-cell lymphoid neoplasms (e.g., lymphoplasmacytic lymphoma)

T-cell tolerance (Chapter 5). Other drugs, such as penicillin, induce an antibody response by binding covalently to red cell membrane proteins and thereby produce neoantigens. Sometimes antibodies recognize a drug in the circulation and form immune complexes that are deposited on red cells. Here they may fix complement or act as opsonins, either of which can lead to hemolysis.

Cold Antibody Immunohemolytic Anemia

Cold antibody immunohemolytic anemia is usually caused by low-affinity IgM antibodies that bind to red cell membranes only at temperatures below 30°C, such as may occur in distal parts of the body (e.g., ears, hands, and toes) in cold weather. Cold agglutinins sometimes appear transiently during recovery from pneumonia caused by *Mycoplasma* spp. and infectious mononucleosis, producing a mild anemia of little clinical importance. More significant chronic forms of cold agglutinin hemolytic anemia occur in association with certain B-cell neoplasms or as an idiopathic condition.

Pathogenesis. IgM binding to red cells initiates the fixation of complement, but later steps of the complement cascade occur inefficiently at temperatures lower than 37°C. As a result, red cells with bound IgM are coated with complement C3 fragments C3b and C3d but are not lysed intravascularly. When these cells travel to warmer areas, the weakly bound IgM is released, but the coating of C3b and C3d fragments remains. Because C3b and C3d fragments are opsonins (Chapter 2), the cells are phagocytosed by macrophages, mainly in the spleen and liver; hence, in most cases the hemolysis is mainly extravascular. Because IgM is pentavalent, each molecule can bind to more than one red cell, crosslinking red cells and causing them to clump *(agglutinate)*. Sludging of blood in capillaries because of agglutination of red cells often produces *Raynaud phenomenon* in the extremities of affected individuals.

Mechanical Hemolysis

Hemolysis of red cells due to their exposure to abnormal mechanical forces occurs in two major settings. Clinically significant *traumatic hemolysis* is sometimes produced by dysfunctional cardiac valve prostheses, which may create sufficient turbulence to shear red cells (the blender effect). More commonly, traumatic hemolysis occurs incidentally during an activity producing repeated physical pounding of one or more body parts (e.g., marathon racing, karate chopping, bongo drumming). *Microangiopathic hemolytic anemia* is observed in pathologic states in which small vessels become partially obstructed or narrowed by lesions that predispose passing red cells to mechanical damage. The most frequent of these conditions is disseminated intravascular coagulation (DIC) (see later), in which vessels are narrowed by the intravascular deposition of fibrin. Other causes of microangiopathic hemolytic anemia include severe hypertension, thrombotic thrombocytopenic purpura (TTP), hemolytic uremic syndrome (HUS), and disseminated intravascular cancer, in which tumor cells occlude small vessels. Mechanical fragmentation of red cells *(schistocytosis)* leads to the appearance of characteristic "burr cells," "helmet cells," and "triangle cells" in peripheral blood smears (Fig. 10.7). Although microangiopathic hemolysis is not usually a major clinical problem in and of itself, it often points to a serious underlying condition. TTP and HUS are discussed later in this chapter.

Malaria

In 2020 the World Health Organization estimated that there were more than 200 million cases of malaria worldwide that resulted in over 600,000 deaths, making it one of the most serious afflictions of

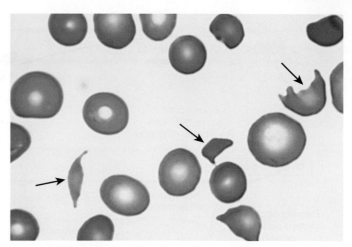

FIG. 10.7 Microangiopathic hemolytic anemia—peripheral blood smear. This specimen from a patient with hemolytic uremic syndrome contains several fragmented red cells *(arrows)*. (Courtesy of Dr. Robert W. McKenna, Department of Pathology, University of Texas Southwestern Medical School, Dallas, Texas.)

humans. Malaria is endemic in Asia and Africa, but with widespread jet travel, cases are now seen all over the world. It is caused by five species of plasmodia. Of these, the most important is *Plasmodium falciparum*, which is responsible for tertian malaria (falciparum malaria), a disorder with a high fatality rate. The other four species of *Plasmodium* that infect humans—*Plasmodium malariae, Plasmodium vivax, Plasmodium knowlesi*, and *Plasmodium ovale*—cause relatively mild disease. All forms are transmitted by the bite of female *Anopheles* mosquitoes and humans are the only natural reservoir.

Pathogenesis. The life cycle of plasmodia is complex and varies among species; Fig. 10.8 shows the life cycle of *P. falciparum*. As *Anopheles* mosquitoes feed on human blood, *sporozoites* are introduced into the circulation and travel through the blood to the liver, where two sporozoite surface proteins, thrombospondin-related adhesive protein and circumsporozoite protein, bind to factors such as proteoglycans on the surface of hepatocytes. The sporozoites then enter the liver and differentiate into *merozoites*. After an incubation period of 1 to 4 weeks, the infected hepatocytes rupture and release the merozoites. Next, a lectinlike molecule on the surface of the merozoite binds to sialidated glycophorin, a red cell transmembrane protein, allowing the merozoite to invaginate into red cells within a "digestive" vacuole. Intraerythrocytic organisms then differentiate into *trophozoites*, which follow two paths. Some trophozoites differentiate into *gametocytes*, which restart the life cycle in mosquitoes when the infected human is again bitten by another *Anopheles* mosquito. Most trophozoites differentiate into *schizonts*, which express an adhesion molecule called PfEMP1 (*Plasmodium falciparum* erythrocyte membrane protein 1) that concentrates in knoblike extensions on the red cell surface. Normally, red cells bear negatively charged surfaces that interact poorly with endothelial cells, but PfEMP1 binds to adhesion molecules on the surface of endothelium such as intercellular adhesion molecule-1 (ICAM-1), vascular cell adhesion molecule-1 (VCAM-1), and CD36, causing the parasitized red cells to arrest in capillary beds. After a period of several days, schizonts differentiate into merozoites, leading to lysis of the infected red cell and another cycle of red cell infection.

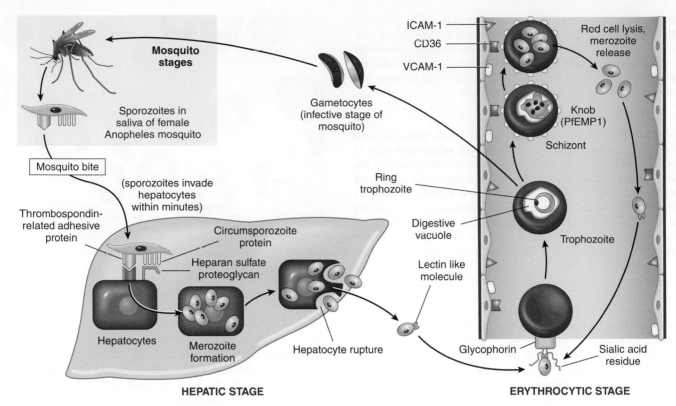

FIG. 10.8 Life cycle of *Plasmodium falciparum*. See text for details. *ICAM-1,* Intercellular adhesion molecule-1; *PfEMP1, Plasmodium falciparum* erythrocyte membrane protein 1; *VCAM-1,* vascular cell adhesion molecule-1.

Fatal falciparum malaria often involves the small vessels of the brain, a complication known as cerebral malaria. In an unfortunate minority of patients, mainly children, this process involves cerebral vessels, which become engorged and occluded.

MORPHOLOGY

Red cell trophozoites from each *Plasmodium* species have a somewhat distinctive appearance, allowing expert observers to determine which species is responsible for an infection from examination of appropriately stained thick smears of peripheral blood. The destruction of red cells leads to **hemolytic anemia,** with its attendant features and laboratory findings. A characteristic brown malarial pigment derived from hemoglobin called **hematin** is released from the ruptured red cells and produces discoloration of the spleen, liver, lymph nodes, and bone marrow. Activation of defense mechanisms in the host leads to a marked hyperplasia of mononuclear phagocytes, producing **massive splenomegaly** and occasional hepatomegaly.

Clinical Features. Malaria is associated with episodic shaking chills and fever that coincide with the release of "showers" of merozoites from infected red cells at intervals of approximately 24 hours for *P. knowlesi;* 48 hours for *P. vivax, P. ovale,* and *P. falciparum;* and 72 hours for *P. malariae.* Hemolytic anemia of varying severity is a constant feature. Cerebral malaria associated with *P. falciparum* is rapidly progressive; convulsions, coma, and death usually occur within days to weeks. Falciparum malaria more often pursues a chronic course that may be punctuated by *blackwater fever,* a poorly understood complication marked by massive intravascular hemolysis, hemoglobinemia, hemoglobinuria, jaundice, and renal failure.

With appropriate drug therapy, the prognosis for patients with most forms of malaria is good; however, falciparum malaria is becoming more difficult to treat due to the emergence of drug-resistant strains. Because of the potentially serious consequences of the disease, early diagnosis and treatment are important. An encouraging advance is the recent development of a vaccine containing sporozoite antigens; although the protection afforded by the vaccine is partial, when fully deployed it is expected to prevent thousands of cases of fatal cerebral malaria in children. Currently, the best method of preventing malaria is by public health measures such as removal of stagnant bodies of water (mosquitoes breeding sites) close to living areas, use of insecticide-treated bed nets, and prophylactic intake of antimalarial drugs.

ANEMIA OF DIMINISHED ERYTHROPOIESIS

Anemias of diminished erythropoiesis include those caused by an inadequate dietary supply of nutrients, particularly iron, folic acid, and vitamin B$_{12}$. Other anemias of this type are associated with bone marrow failure (aplastic anemia), systemic inflammation (anemia of chronic inflammation), or bone marrow infiltration by tumor or inflammatory cells (myelophthisic anemia). In this section, some common examples of anemias of these types are discussed individually.

Iron Deficiency Anemia

Iron deficiency is the most common nutritional deficiency in the world and results in clinical signs and symptoms that are mostly related to anemia. About 10% of people living in higher-resource countries and 25% to 50% of those in lower-resource countries are anemic, and in both settings the most frequent cause is iron deficiency.

The factors responsible for iron deficiency differ in various populations and are best understood in the context of iron metabolism.

The normal total body iron mass is about 2.5 g for women and 3.5 g for men. Approximately 80% of this iron is present in hemoglobin, myoglobin, and iron-containing enzymes (e.g., catalase, cytochromes). The remaining 15% to 20% of body iron is in a storage pool consisting of hemosiderin and ferritin-bound iron, which is mainly found in macrophages in the liver, spleen, and bone marrow and in skeletal muscle cells. Because serum ferritin is largely derived from the storage pool, the serum ferritin level is usually a good surrogate measure of iron stores. Bone marrow aspiration to assess iron stores is another reliable but more invasive method for estimating iron stores. Iron is transported in the plasma bound to the protein transferrin. Normally, transferrin is about 33% saturated with iron, yielding serum iron levels that average 120 μg/dL in men and 100 μg/dL in women. Thus, the normal total iron-binding capacity of serum is 300 to 350 μg/dL.

In keeping with the high prevalence of iron deficiency, evolutionary pressures have produced metabolic pathways that are strongly biased toward iron retention. Iron is lost at a rate of 1 to 2 mg/day through the shedding of mucosal and skin epithelial cells. This loss must be balanced by the absorption of dietary iron, which is tightly regulated (described later). The normal daily Western diet contains 10 to 20 mg of iron. Most is found in heme within meat and poultry, with the remainder present as inorganic iron in vegetables. About 20% of heme and 1% to 2% of nonheme iron are absorbable; hence, the average Western diet contains sufficient iron to balance fixed daily losses.

Regulation of iron absorption occurs within the duodenum (Fig. 10.9). After reduction by duodenal cytochrome B, a ferric reductase, ferrous iron (Fe^{2+}) is transported across the apical membrane of enterocytes by divalent metal transporter-1 (DMT1). A second transporter, ferroportin, then moves iron from the cytoplasm to the plasma across the basolateral membrane. The newly absorbed iron is oxidized by hephaestin and ceruloplasmin to ferric iron (Fe^{3+}), the form that binds to transferrin. Both DMT1 and ferroportin are widely distributed in the body and are involved in iron transport in many tissues. As depicted in Fig. 10.9 (middle panel), part of the iron that enters enterocytes is delivered to transferrin by ferroportin, whereas the remainder is incorporated into cytoplasmic ferritin and is lost through the exfoliation of epithelial cells.

The fraction of dietary iron that is absorbed from the duodenum is determined by the plasma level of hepcidin, a small peptide secreted by the liver in an iron-dependent fashion that negatively regulates ferroportin. Plasma iron levels are "sensed" by a protein called HFE that is expressed on the surface of hepatocytes, and as iron levels rise, HFE and associated proteins send signals that upregulate hepcidin production, creating a feedback loop that maintains iron stores within a physiologic range. In addition, hepatic hepcidin production is positively regulated by inflammatory mediators (e.g., IL-6) and negatively regulated by *erythroferrone*, which is secreted from erythroblasts in the bone marrow.

Alterations in hepcidin production are a common feature of disorders of iron metabolism. Thus, disorders associated with sustained high levels of erythroferrone (e.g., β-thalassemia major) or inherited defects in HFE (hereditary hemochromatosis, Chapter 14) suppress hepcidin production (Fig. 10.9, *left panel*), leading to iron overload, whereas chronic inflammation stimulates hepcidin production (Fig. 10.9, *right panel*), leading to the anemia of chronic inflammation (discussed later).

Pathogenesis. Iron deficiency arises in a variety of settings:
- *Chronic blood loss is the most important cause of iron deficiency anemia in higher-resource countries.* The most common sources

of bleeding are the gastrointestinal tract (e.g., peptic ulcers, colon cancer, hemorrhoids) and the female genital tract (e.g., menorrhagia, metrorrhagia, endometrial cancer).
- *In lower-resource countries, low intake and poor bioavailability of iron because of predominantly vegetarian diets are the most common causes of iron deficiency.* In the United States, low dietary intake is infrequent but is sometimes seen in infants fed exclusively milk, in individuals with food insecurity, and the elderly.
- *Increased iron demands not met by normal dietary intake occur worldwide during pregnancy and infancy.*
- *Malabsorption of iron may occur with celiac disease, various forms of gastritis, or after gastrectomy* (Chapter 13).

Regardless of cause, iron deficiency develops insidiously. Iron stores are depleted first, marked by a decline in serum ferritin and the absence of stainable iron in bone marrow macrophages. These changes are followed by a decrease in serum iron and a rise in serum transferrin. Ultimately, the capacity to synthesize hemoglobin, myoglobin, and other iron-containing proteins is diminished, leading to microcytic anemia, impaired work and cognitive performance, and even reduced immunocompetence.

Clinical Features. In most instances iron deficiency anemia is mild and asymptomatic. Nonspecific manifestations, such as weakness, listlessness, and pallor, may be present in severe cases. With long-standing anemia, abnormalities of the fingernails, including thinning, flattening, and "spooning," may appear. A curious but characteristic neurobehavioral complication is pica, the compunction to consume nonfoodstuffs such as dirt or clay.

In peripheral smears, red cells are microcytic and hypochromic (Fig. 10.10). Characteristic findings include decreased hematocrit; hypochromic, microcytic red cell indices; low serum ferritin and iron levels; low transferrin saturation; increased total iron-binding capacity; and, ultimately, response to iron therapy. For unclear reasons, the platelet count is often high. Erythropoietin levels are elevated, but the marrow response is blunted by the iron deficiency; thus, marrow cellularity is usually only slightly increased.

Persons often die with iron deficiency anemia but virtually never of it. An important point to remember is that in well-nourished persons, microcytic hypochromic anemia is not a disease but rather a symptom of another underlying disorder (e.g., colon cancer leading to chronic blood loss).

Anemia of Chronic Inflammation

Often referred to as the anemia of chronic disease, anemia associated with chronic inflammation is the most common form of anemia in hospitalized patients. It superficially resembles the anemia of iron deficiency but arises instead from the suppression of erythropoiesis by systemic inflammation. It occurs in a variety of disorders associated with sustained inflammation, including the following:
- *Chronic microbial infections* such as osteomyelitis, bacterial endocarditis, and lung abscess
- *Chronic immune disorders* such as rheumatoid arthritis and Crohn disease
- *Cancers* such as Hodgkin lymphoma and carcinomas of the lung and breast

Pathogenesis. **The anemia of chronic inflammation stems from high levels of plasma hepcidin,** which blocks the transfer of iron to erythroid precursors by downregulating ferroportin in marrow macrophages. The elevated hepcidin levels are caused by pro-inflammatory cytokines such

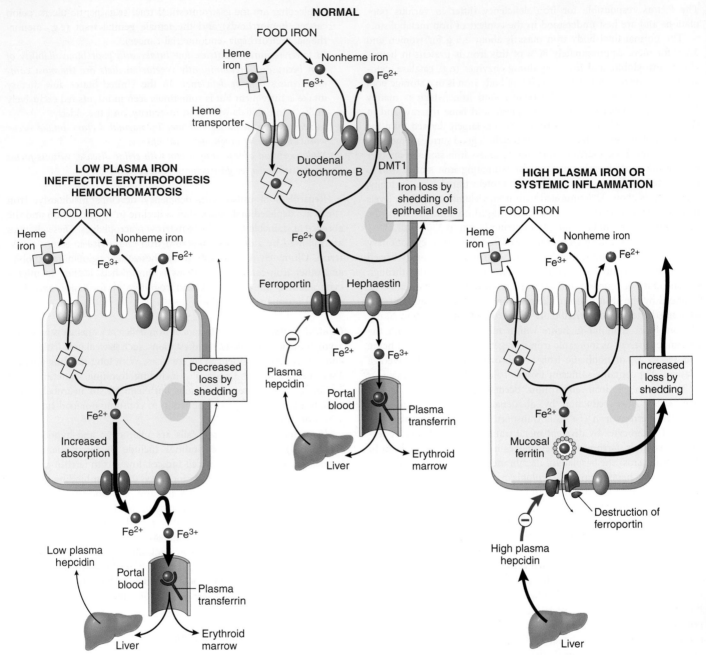

FIG. 10.9 Regulation of iron absorption. Duodenal epithelial cell uptake of heme and nonheme iron is depicted. When the storage sites of the body are replete with iron and erythropoietic activity is normal, plasma hepcidin balances iron uptake and loss to maintain iron hemostasis by downregulating ferroportin and limiting iron uptake *(middle panel)*. Hepcidin rises in the setting of systemic inflammation or when iron levels are high, decreasing iron uptake and increasing iron loss by the shedding of duodenocytes *(right panel)*, whereas it falls in the setting of low plasma iron or primary hemochromatosis, resulting in increased iron uptake *(left panel)*. *DMT1,* Divalent metal transporter-1.

as IL-6, which increase hepatic hepcidin synthesis. In addition, chronic inflammation blunts erythropoietin synthesis by the kidney, lowering red cell production by the marrow. The functional advantages of these adaptations in the face of systemic inflammation are unclear; they may serve to inhibit the growth of iron-dependent microorganisms.

Clinical Features. Serum iron levels usually are low in the anemia of chronic disease, and the red cells may be slightly hypochromic and microcytic. In contrast to iron deficiency anemia, however, storage iron in the bone marrow and serum ferritin are increased and the total iron-binding capacity is reduced. Administration of erythropoietin and iron can improve the anemia but only effective treatment of the underlying condition is curative.

Megaloblastic Anemias

The two principal causes of megaloblastic anemia are folate deficiency and vitamin B$_{12}$ deficiency. Both vitamins are required for DNA synthesis and the effects of their deficiency on hematopoiesis are

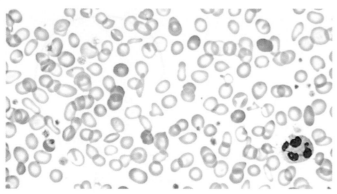

FIG. 10.10 Iron deficiency anemia—peripheral blood smear. Note the increased central pallor of most of the red cells. Scattered fully hemoglobinized cells, from a recent blood transfusion, stand out in contrast. (Courtesy of Dr. Robert W. McKenna, Department of Pathology, University of Texas Southwestern Medical School, Dallas, Texas.)

identical. However, the causes and consequences of folate and vitamin B_{12} deficiency differ in important ways. We will first review some of the common features and then touch on those that are specific to folate and vitamin B_{12} deficiency.

Pathogenesis. **Megaloblastic anemia stems from metabolic defects that lead to inadequate biosynthesis of thymidine, one of the building blocks of DNA.** Folate and vitamin B_{12} are both essential for thymidine synthesis, which is required for DNA replication. Thymidine deficiency causes abnormalities in rapidly dividing cells throughout the body, but the hematopoietic marrow is most severely affected. Because the synthesis of RNA and cytoplasmic elements proceeds in parallel at a relatively normal rate and thus outpaces that of DNA, the hematopoietic precursors show *nuclear-cytoplasmic asynchrony* (described later). This maturational derangement contributes to the anemia in several ways. DNA synthesis is so defective in many red cell progenitors that a DNA damage response is triggered, leading to apoptosis *(ineffective hematopoiesis)*. Other progenitors mature into red cells but do so after fewer cell divisions, further diminishing the output of red cells. Granulocyte and platelet precursors are also affected (although not as severely), and most patients present with pancytopenia (anemia, thrombocytopenia, and granulocytopenia).

MORPHOLOGY

Certain morphologic features are common to all megaloblastic anemias. The bone marrow is markedly hypercellular and contains numerous megaloblastic erythroid progenitors. **Megaloblasts** are larger than normal erythroid progenitors (normoblasts) and have delicate, finely reticulated nuclear chromatin (indicative of nuclear immaturity). As megaloblasts differentiate and acquire hemoglobin, the nucleus retains its finely distributed chromatin and fails to undergo the chromatin clumping typical of normoblasts, a classic example of nuclear-cytoplasmic asynchrony. Granulocytic precursors also demonstrate nuclear-cytoplasmic asynchrony, yielding **giant metamyelocytes.** Megakaryocytes may also be abnormally large and contain bizarre multilobed nuclei.

In the peripheral blood the earliest change is the appearance of **hypersegmented neutrophils** (Fig. 10.11), which appear before the onset of anemia. Normal neutrophils have three or four nuclear lobes, but in megaloblastic anemias they often have five or more. The red cells typically include large **egg-shaped macroovalocytes;** the MCV is often greater than 110 fL (normal, 78–98 fL). Although macroovalocytes appear hyperchromic, in reality

their hemoglobin concentration is normal. Large, misshapen platelets also may be seen. Morphologic changes in other systems, especially the gastrointestinal tract, also occur, giving rise to some of the clinical manifestations.

Folate (Folic Acid) Deficiency Anemia

Folate deficiency is usually the result of inadequate dietary intake, sometimes complicated by increased metabolic demands. Folate is present in nearly all foods but is destroyed by 10 to 15 minutes of cooking; as a result, folate stores are marginal in a surprising number of healthy persons. The risk of folate deficiency is highest in those with a poor diet (individuals with food insecurity and the elderly) or those with increased metabolic needs (pregnant women and patients with chronic hemolytic anemias such as sickle cell disease). Deficiency may also stem from problems with absorption or metabolism. Food folates are predominantly in polyglutamate form and must be split into monoglutamates for absorption, a conversion that is inhibited by acidic foods and substances found in beans and other legumes. Some drugs such as phenytoin also interfere with folate absorption, while others such as methotrexate inhibit folate metabolism. Malabsorptive disorders such as *celiac disease* and *environmental enteropathy* (Chapter 13) that affect the upper third of the small intestine, where folate is absorbed, may also impair folate uptake.

Pathogenesis. **Tetrahydrofolate acts as an acceptor and donor of one-carbon units in several reactions that are required for the synthesis of deoxythymidine monophosphate (dTMP), which is used in DNA synthesis.** Although the metabolism and functions of folate are complex, here it is sufficient to note that its conversion within cells from dihydrofolate to tetrahydrofolate by dihydrofolate reductase (the target of the drug methotrexate) is particularly important for dTMP synthesis. If intracellular stores of folate fall, insufficient dTMP is synthesized and DNA replication is blocked, leading to megaloblastic anemia.

Clinical Features. The onset of the anemia of folate deficiency is insidious, associated with nonspecific symptoms such as weakness and easy fatigability. The clinical picture may be complicated by coexistent deficiency of other vitamins, especially in those with alcohol use disorder. Because the cells lining the gastrointestinal tract, like the

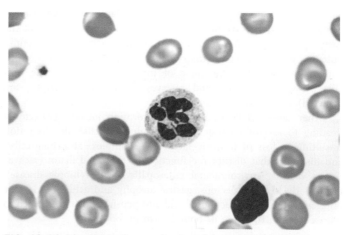

FIG. 10.11 Megaloblastic anemia. A peripheral blood smear shows a hypersegmented neutrophil with a six-lobed nucleus. (Courtesy of Dr. Robert W. McKenna, Department of Pathology, University of Texas Southwestern Medical School, Dallas, Texas.)

hematopoietic system, turn over rapidly, symptoms referable to the alimentary tract, such as sore tongue, are common. Unlike in vitamin B_{12} deficiency, neurologic abnormalities do not occur.

The diagnosis of a megaloblastic anemia is readily made from the examination of smears of peripheral blood and bone marrow. The anemia of folate deficiency is best distinguished from that of vitamin B_{12} deficiency by measuring serum and red cell folate and vitamin B_{12} levels.

Vitamin B_{12} (Cobalamin) Deficiency Anemia

Vitamin B_{12} is widely present in foods, is resistant to cooking and boiling, and is even synthesized by gut flora. Thus, unlike folate, vitamin B_{12} deficiency is virtually never caused by inadequate intake except in vegetarians who scrupulously avoid milk and eggs. Instead, deficiencies typically arise from some abnormality that interferes with vitamin B_{12} absorption. **Absorption of vitamin B_{12} requires intrinsic factor, which is secreted by the parietal cells of the fundic mucosa** (Fig. 10.12). Vitamin B_{12} is freed from binding proteins in food through the action of pepsin in the stomach and it then binds to a salivary protein called *haptocorrin*. In the duodenum, bound vitamin B_{12} is released from haptocorrin by the action of pancreatic proteases and associates with intrinsic factor. This complex is transported to the ileum, where it is endocytosed by ileal enterocytes that express a receptor for intrinsic factor called *cubilin* on their surfaces. Within ileal cells, vitamin B_{12} associates with transcobalamin II and is secreted into the plasma. Transcobalamin II in turn delivers vitamin B_{12} to the liver and other cells of the body, including rapidly proliferating cells in the bone marrow and the gastrointestinal tract.

After absorption, the body handles vitamin B_{12} efficiently. It is stored in the liver, which normally contains reserves sufficient to support bodily needs for 5 to 20 years. Because of the large storage capacity of the liver, clinical presentations of vitamin B_{12} deficiency typically follow years of unrecognized malabsorption.

Pathogenesis. **The most frequent cause vitamin B_{12} deficiency is *pernicious anemia,* which results from an autoimmune attack on the gastric mucosa that suppresses the production of intrinsic factor** (Chapter 13). Histologically, there is a *chronic atrophic gastritis* marked by a loss of parietal cells, a prominent infiltrate of lymphocytes and plasma cells, and megaloblastic changes in mucosal cells similar to those found in erythroid precursors. The serum of most affected patients contains several types of autoantibodies that block the binding of vitamin B_{12} to intrinsic factor or prevent binding of the intrinsic factor—vitamin B_{12} complex to cubilin. Autoantibodies are of diagnostic use, but they are not thought to be the primary cause of the gastric pathology; rather, it seems that an autoreactive T-cell response initiates gastric mucosal injury and triggers the formation of autoantibodies. When the mass of intrinsic factor—secreting cells falls below a threshold (and reserves of stored vitamin B_{12} are depleted), anemia develops.

Other causes of vitamin B_{12} malabsorption include gastrectomy (leading to loss of intrinsic factor—producing cells), ileal resection (resulting in loss of intrinsic factor—B_{12} complex—absorbing cells), and disorders that disrupt the function of the distal ileum (such as Crohn disease, environmental enteropathy, and Whipple disease). Particularly in older persons, gastric atrophy and achlorhydria may interfere with the production of acid and pepsin, which are needed to release vitamin B_{12} from its bound form in food.

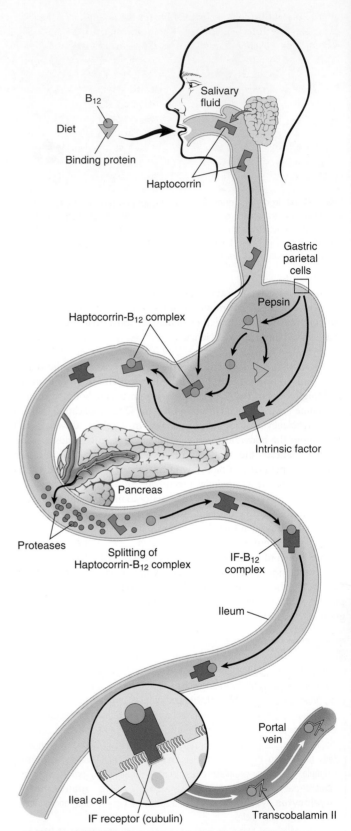

FIG. 10.12 Schematic illustration of vitamin B_{12} absorption. See text for details. *IF,* Intrinsic factor.

The metabolic defects responsible for the anemia of vitamin B_{12} deficiency are intertwined with folate metabolism. Vitamin B_{12} is required for recycling tetrahydrofolate, the form of folate needed for DNA synthesis. In keeping with this relationship, the anemia of vitamin B_{12} deficiency is reversed by administration of folate. Importantly, however, folate administration does not prevent and may worsen neurologic symptoms that are specific to vitamin B_{12} deficiency. The main neurologic lesions associated with vitamin B_{12} deficiency are demyelination of the posterior and lateral columns of the spinal cord, sometimes beginning in the peripheral nerves. In time, axonal degeneration may supervene. The severity of the neurologic manifestations is not related to the degree of anemia and neurologic disease may even occur in the absence of overt megaloblastic anemia.

Clinical Features. The manifestations of vitamin B_{12} deficiency are nonspecific. As with all anemias, findings include pallor, easy fatigability, and (in severe cases) dyspnea and congestive heart failure. The increased destruction of erythroid progenitors because of ineffective erythropoiesis may give rise to mild jaundice. Megaloblastic changes in the oropharyngeal epithelium may produce a beefy red tongue. The spinal cord disease *(subacute combined degeneration)* begins with symmetric numbness, tingling, and burning in the feet or hands, followed by unsteadiness of gait and loss of position sense, particularly in the toes. Although the anemia responds dramatically to parenteral vitamin B_{12}, the neurologic manifestations often fail to resolve. As discussed in Chapter 13, patients with pernicious anemia have an increased risk for the development of gastric carcinoma.

Findings supporting the diagnosis of vitamin B_{12} deficiency are (1) low serum vitamin B_{12} levels, (2) normal or elevated serum folate levels, (3) moderate to severe macrocytic anemia, (4) leukopenia with hypersegmented granulocytes, and (5) a dramatic increase in reticulocytes 2 to 3 days after treatment with vitamin B_{12}. Pernicious anemia is associated with all of these findings plus the presence of serum antibodies to intrinsic factor.

Aplastic Anemia

Aplastic anemia is a disorder in which multipotent myeloid stem cells are suppressed, leading to bone marrow failure and pancytopenia. The marrow is often virtually devoid of recognizable hematopoietic elements. It must be distinguished from pure red cell aplasia, in which only erythroid progenitors are affected and anemia is the only manifestation.

Pathogenesis. The pathogenesis of aplastic anemia is not fully understood, but two major etiologies have been invoked: an extrinsic, immune-mediated suppression of marrow progenitors and an intrinsic abnormality of stem cells. Experimental studies have focused on a model in which activated T cells suppress hematopoietic stem cells. It is hypothesized that stem cells are first antigenically altered by exposure to drugs, infectious agents, or other unidentified environmental insults. This provokes a cellular immune response, during which activated Th1 cells produce cytokines that suppress hematopoietic progenitors. In keeping with this scenario, immunosuppressive therapy directed against T cells restores hematopoiesis in 60% to 70% of patients.

Alternatively, the notion that aplastic anemia results from an intrinsic stem cell abnormality is supported by observations showing that from 5% to 10% of patients have inherited defects in telomerase, which is needed for the maintenance and stability of chromosomes. It is hypothesized that telomerase defects lead to premature senescence of hematopoietic stem cells. Of further interest, the bone marrow cells in an additional 50% of cases have unusually short telomeres, possibly stemming from as-yet undiscovered defects in telomerase or excessive replication of hematopoietic stem cells. These two mechanisms are not mutually exclusive, because genetically altered stem cells (e.g., those with abnormal telomeres) also might express "neoantigens" that serve as targets for a T-cell attack.

Clinical Features. Aplastic anemia affects persons of all ages and both sexes. The slowly progressive anemia causes the insidious development of weakness, pallor, and dyspnea. Thrombocytopenia often manifests with petechiae and ecchymoses. Neutropenia may set the stage for serious infections.

It is important to separate aplastic anemia from anemia caused by marrow infiltration (myelophthisic anemia), "aleukemic leukemia," and granulomatous diseases, which may have similar clinical presentations but are easily distinguished by examination of the bone marrow. Aplastic anemia does not cause splenomegaly; if present, another diagnosis should be sought.

The prognosis is unpredictable. Withdrawal of an inciting drug sometimes leads to recovery, but this is the exception. Hematopoietic stem cell transplantation is often curative, particularly in patients younger than 40 years of age. Transfusion necessary to correct anemia sensitizes patients to alloantigens, producing a high rate of engraftment failure; thus, it must be minimized in persons eligible for transplantation. Successful transplantation requires "conditioning" with immunosuppressive radiation or chemotherapy, reinforcing the notion that autoimmunity has an important role in the disease. As mentioned earlier, patients who are not transplant candidates often benefit from immunosuppressive therapy.

Myelophthisic Anemia

Myelophthisic anemia is caused by extensive infiltration of the marrow by tumors or other lesions. It is most commonly associated with metastatic breast, lung, or prostate cancer. Other tumors, advanced tuberculosis, lipid storage disorders, and osteosclerosis may produce a similar clinical picture. The principal manifestations include anemia and thrombocytopenia; in general, the white cell series is less affected. Characteristic misshapen red cells, some resembling teardrops, are seen in the peripheral blood. Immature granulocytic and erythrocytic precursors may also be present *(leukoerythroblastosis)* along with mild leukocytosis. Treatment is directed at the underlying condition.

POLYCYTHEMIA

Polycythemia (erythrocytosis) denotes an increase in red cells per unit volume of peripheral blood. It may be absolute (defined as an increase in total red cell mass) or relative. Relative polycythemia results from dehydration, such as occurs with water deprivation, prolonged vomiting, diarrhea, or excessive use of diuretics. Absolute polycythemia is described as primary when the increased red cell mass results from an autonomous proliferation of erythroid progenitors, and secondary when the excessive proliferation stems from elevated levels of erythropoietin. Primary polycythemia is usually caused by a myeloid neoplasm, *polycythemia vera*, considered later in this chapter. The increases in erythropoietin that lead to secondary forms of absolute polycythemia stem from diverse causes (Table 10.5).

Table 10.5 Pathophysiologic Classification of Polycythemia

Relative
Reduced plasma volume (hemoconcentration)
Absolute
Primary
Abnormal proliferation of myeloid stem cells, normal or low erythropoietin levels (polycythemia vera)
Inherited activating mutations in the erythropoietin receptor (rare)
Secondary
Increased erythropoietin levels
Adaptive: Lung disease, high-altitude living, cyanotic heart disease
Paraneoplastic: Erythropoietin-secreting tumors (e.g., renal cell carcinoma, hepatocellular carcinoma, cerebellar hemangioblastoma)
"Blood doping": Endurance athletes

WHITE CELL DISORDERS

Disorders of white cells include deficiencies (leukopenias) and proliferations, which may be reactive or neoplastic. Reactive proliferation in response to diseases such as microbial infections is common. Neoplastic disorders, although less common, are more ominous. They cause approximately 9% of all cancer deaths in adults and approximately 30% in people younger than 20 years of age.

Presented next are brief descriptions of some nonneoplastic conditions, followed by more detailed considerations of the malignant proliferations of white cells.

NONNEOPLASTIC DISORDERS OF WHITE CELLS

Leukopenia

Leukopenia results most commonly from a decrease in granulocytes, the most numerous circulating white cells. Lymphopenia is less common; it is associated with rare congenital immunodeficiency diseases, advanced human immunodeficiency virus (HIV) infection, and treatment with high doses of corticosteroids. Only the more common leukopenias of granulocytes are discussed here.

Neutropenia/Agranulocytosis

A reduction in the number of granulocytes in blood is known as *neutropenia* or, when severe, *agranulocytosis*. People who are neutropenic are susceptible to severe, potentially fatal bacterial and fungal infections. The risk of infection rises sharply as the neutrophil count falls below 500 cells/μL.

Pathogenesis. The mechanisms underlying neutropenia can be divided into two broad categories:

- *Decreased granulocyte production.* Clinically important reductions in granulopoiesis are most often caused by marrow hypoplasia (as occurs transiently with cancer chemotherapy and chronically with aplastic anemia) or extensive replacement of the marrow by tumor (such as with leukemia). Alternatively, neutrophil production may be selectively suppressed while other blood lineages are unaffected. This is most often caused by certain drugs or by neoplastic proliferations of cytotoxic T cells and natural killer (NK) cells (so-called "large granular lymphocytic leukemia"),

both of which suppress myelopoiesis through uncertain mechanisms.

- *Increased granulocyte destruction.* This can be encountered with immune-mediated injury (triggered in some cases by drugs) or in overwhelming bacterial, fungal, or rickettsial infections resulting from increased peripheral "use." Splenomegaly can also lead to the sequestration and accelerated removal of neutrophils.

> ### MORPHOLOGY
>
> The morphologic changes in the bone marrow depend on the underlying cause. Compensatory marrow hypercellularity is seen when there is excessive neutrophil destruction or ineffective granulopoiesis, such as occurs in megaloblastic anemia. Drugs that selectively suppress granulocytopoiesis are associated with decreased numbers of granulocytic precursors and preservation of erythroid elements and megakaryocytes, while myelotoxic chemotherapy drugs reduce the number of elements from all lineages.

Clinical Features. Infections constitute the major clinical problem. They commonly take the form of ulcerating, necrotizing lesions of the gingiva, floor of the mouth, buccal mucosa, pharynx, or other sites within the oral cavity. Owing to the lack of leukocytes, such lesions often contain large masses or sheets of microorganisms. In addition to local inflammation, systemic symptoms are usually present, consisting of malaise, chills, and fever. Because of the danger of sepsis, patients with neutropenia are started on broad-spectrum antibiotics at the first sign of infection. Depending on the clinical context, patients may also be treated with granulocyte colony-stimulating factor (G-CSF), a growth factor that speeds recovery of neutrophil counts.

Reactive Leukocytosis

An increase in the number of white cells in the blood is common in a variety of inflammatory states caused by microbial and nonmicrobial stimuli. Leukocytoses are relatively nonspecific and are classified according to the particular white cell series that is affected (Table 10.6). As discussed later, in some cases reactive leukocytosis may lead to white cell counts that are high enough to mimic leukemia. Such *leukemoid reactions* must be distinguished from true white cell malignancies. Infectious mononucleosis merits separate consideration because it gives rise to a distinctive syndrome associated with lymphocytosis.

Infectious Mononucleosis

Infectious mononucleosis is an acute self-limited disease of adolescents and young adults that is caused by Epstein-Barr virus (EBV), a member of the herpesvirus family. The infection is characterized by (1) fever, sore throat, and generalized lymphadenitis and (2) a lymphocytosis of activated CD8+ T cells. Of note, cytomegalovirus infection induces a similar syndrome that can be distinguished only by serologic assays.

EBV is ubiquitous in human populations. In lower-income parts of the world, EBV infection in early childhood is nearly universal. Even though infected children mount an immune response, most remain asymptomatic and more than half continue to shed virus, usually for life. By contrast, in higher-income areas with better hygiene, infection is typically delayed until adolescence or young adulthood and symptomatic infection is much more common. For unclear reasons, only about 20% of healthy seropositive persons in higher-income countries

Table 10.6 Causes of Leukocytosis

Neutrophilic Leukocytosis

Acute bacterial infections (especially those caused by pyogenic organisms); sterile inflammation caused by, e.g., tissue necrosis (myocardial infarction, burns)

Eosinophilic Leukocytosis (Eosinophilia)

Allergic disorders such as asthma, hay fever, allergic skin diseases (e.g., pemphigus, dermatitis herpetiformis); parasitic infestations; drug reactions; certain malignancies (e.g., Hodgkin lymphoma and some non-Hodgkin lymphomas); collagen-vascular disorders and some vasculitides; atheroembolic disease (transient)

Basophilic Leukocytosis (Basophilia)

Rare, often indicative of a myeloproliferative neoplasm (e.g., chronic myeloid leukemia)

Monocytosis

Chronic infections (e.g., tuberculosis), bacterial endocarditis, rickettsiosis, and malaria; collagen-vascular disorders (e.g., systemic lupus erythematosus); and inflammatory bowel diseases (e.g., ulcerative colitis)

Lymphocytosis

Accompanies monocytosis in many disorders associated with chronic immunologic stimulation (e.g., tuberculosis, brucellosis); viral infections (e.g., hepatitis A, cytomegalovirus, Epstein-Barr virus); *Bordetella pertussis* infection

shed the virus, and only about 50% of those exposed to the virus acquire the infection.

Pathogenesis. Transmission to a seronegative individual usually involves direct oral contact. It is hypothesized that the virus initially infects oropharyngeal epithelial cells and then spreads to underlying lymphoid tissue (tonsils and adenoids), where mature B cells are infected. An EBV envelop glycoprotein binds to CD21, expressed on all B cells, thus explaining the B cell tropism of EBV. The infection of B cells takes one of two forms. In most infected B cells the virus is latent, persisting as an extrachromosomal episome. In the remaining cells, the infection shifts to a lytic phase marked by viral replication and the release of virions.

B cells that are latently infected with EBV may become activated and proliferate as a result of the action of several viral proteins (Chapter 6). These cells disseminate in the circulation and secrete antibodies with unusual specificities, including those recognizing sheep red cells, which are detected in diagnostic tests for mononucleosis. During acute infections, EBV is shed in the saliva; it is not known whether the source of these virions is oropharyngeal epithelial cells or B cells.

The host T-cell response controls the proliferation of EBV-infected B cells and the spread of the virus. Early in the course of the infection, IgM antibodies are formed against viral capsid antigens. Later the serologic response shifts to IgG antibodies, which persist for life. More important in the control of the EBV-positive B-cell proliferation are cytotoxic CD8+ T cells. Virus-specific CD8+ T cells appear in the circulation as large, so-called atypical lymphocytes, a finding that is characteristic of mononucleosis. In otherwise healthy persons, the fully developed immune responses to EBV act as brakes on viral shedding. In most cases, however, a small number of latently infected EBV-positive B cells escape the immune response and persist for the life of the patient. As described later, **impaired T-cell immunity places patients at high risk for EBV-driven B-cell proliferations.**

MORPHOLOGY

The major alterations involve the blood, lymph nodes, spleen, liver, and occasionally other organs. There is peripheral blood **leukocytosis;** the white cell count is usually between 12,000 and 18,000 cells/μL. Typically more than half of these cells are large **atypical lymphocytes,** 12 to 16 μm in diameter, with an oval, indented, or folded nucleus and abundant cytoplasm with a few azurophilic granules (Fig. 10.13). These atypical lymphocytes, which are sufficiently distinctive to suggest the diagnosis, are mainly CD8+ T cells.

Lymphadenopathy is common and is most prominent in the posterior cervical, axillary, and groin regions. On histologic examination, the enlarged nodes are flooded by atypical lymphocytes, which occupy the paracortical (T-cell) areas. A few cells resembling Reed-Sternberg (RS) cells, the hallmark of Hodgkin lymphoma, are often seen. Because of these atypical features, special tests are sometimes needed to distinguish the reactive changes of mononucleosis from lymphoma.

The **spleen** is enlarged in most cases, weighing between 300 and 500 g, and exhibits a heavy infiltrate of atypical lymphocytes. As a result of the rapid increase in splenic size and the infiltration of the trabeculae and capsule by the lymphocytes, such spleens are fragile and are prone to rupture after even minor trauma.

Atypical lymphocytes usually also infiltrate the portal areas and sinusoids of the liver. Scattered apoptotic cells or foci of parenchymal necrosis associated with a lymphocytic infiltrate may also be present—a picture that can be difficult to distinguish from other forms of viral hepatitis.

Clinical Features. Infectious mononucleosis classically manifests with fever, sore throat, and lymphadenitis, but atypical presentations are not unusual. Sometimes there is little or no fever and only fatigue and lymphadenopathy, raising the specter of lymphoma; fever of unknown origin, unassociated with lymphadenopathy or other localized findings; hepatitis that is difficult to differentiate from other hepatotropic viral syndromes (Chapter 14); or a febrile rash resembling rubella. Ultimately, the diagnosis depends on the following, in increasing order of specificity: (1) the presence of atypical lymphocytes in the peripheral blood; (2) a positive heterophil reaction (Monospot test); and (3) a rising titer of antibodies specific for EBV antigens. In most patients, mononucleosis resolves within 4 to 6 weeks, but sometimes the fatigue lasts longer. Occasionally one or

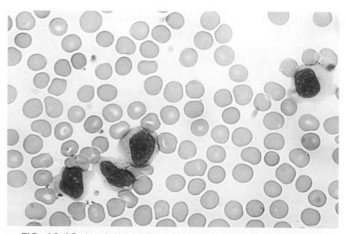

FIG. 10.13 Atypical lymphocytes in infectious mononucleosis.

more complications supervene. Perhaps the most common of these is hepatitis associated with jaundice, elevated liver enzyme levels, loss of appetite, and, rarely, liver failure. Other complications involve the nervous system, kidneys, bone marrow, lungs, eyes, heart, and spleen (including fatal splenic rupture).

EBV is a potent transforming virus that plays a role in the pathogenesis of several human malignancies, including certain B-cell lymphomas (Chapter 6). A serious complication in those lacking T-cell immunity is unimpeded EBV-driven B-cell proliferation. This process can be initiated by an acute infection or by the reactivation of a latent infection and generally begins as a polyclonal proliferation that transforms to overt monoclonal B-cell lymphoma over time. Reconstitution of immunity (e.g., by cessation of immunosuppressive drugs) is sometimes sufficient to cause complete regression of the B-cell proliferation, which is uniformly fatal if left untreated.

The importance of the cellular immune response in controlling EBV infection is also driven home by *X-linked lymphoproliferative syndrome (XLP)*, a rare inherited EBV-specific immunodeficiency characterized by an ineffective response to EBV. Most affected boys have mutations in the *SH2D1A* gene, which encodes a signaling protein that participates in the activation of T and NK cells. In more than 50% of cases, EBV causes an acute overwhelming infection, often complicated by hemophagocytic lymphohistiocytosis (HLH, described later), whereas other patients succumb to EBV-driven lymphoma or secondary infections related to hypogammaglobulinemia, the basis of which is not understood.

Reactive Lymphadenitis

Infections and nonmicrobial inflammatory stimuli often activate immune cells residing in lymph nodes, which act as defensive barriers. Any immune response against foreign antigens can lead to lymph node enlargement (lymphadenopathy). Infections causing lymphadenitis are varied and numerous and may be acute or chronic. In most instances the histologic appearance of the lymph node reaction is nonspecific. A somewhat distinctive form of lymphadenitis that occurs with cat-scratch disease is described separately later.

Acute Nonspecific Lymphadenitis

This form of lymphadenitis may be isolated to a group of nodes draining a local infection or may be generalized, as in systemic infectious and inflammatory conditions.

MORPHOLOGY

Inflamed nodes in acute nonspecific lymphadenitis are swollen, gray-red, and engorged. Histologically, there are **large germinal centers** containing numerous mitotic figures. When the cause is a pyogenic organism, a neutrophilic infiltrate is seen around the follicles and within the lymphoid sinuses. With severe infections, the centers of follicles can undergo necrosis, leading to the formation of an abscess.

Affected nodes are tender and may become fluctuant if abscess formation is extensive. The overlying skin is frequently red and may develop draining sinuses. With control of the infection the lymph nodes may revert to a normal "resting" appearance or, if damaged, undergo scarring.

Chronic Nonspecific Lymphadenitis

Depending on the causative agent, chronic nonspecific lymphadenitis can assume one of three patterns: follicular hyperplasia, paracortical hyperplasia, or sinus histiocytosis.

MORPHOLOGY

Follicular Hyperplasia. This pattern occurs with infections or inflammatory processes that activate B cells, which migrate into follicles and create the **follicular (or germinal center) reaction.** Reactive follicles contain numerous activated B cells, scattered T cells, phagocytic macrophages containing nuclear debris (tingible body macrophages), and a meshwork of antigen-presenting follicular dendritic cells. Causes of follicular hyperplasia include **rheumatoid arthritis, toxoplasmosis,** and early **HIV infection.** This form of lymphadenitis must be distinguished from follicular lymphoma (discussed later). Findings that favor follicular hyperplasia are (1) the preservation of the lymph node architecture; (2) variation in the shape and size of the germinal centers; (3) the presence of a mixture of germinal center lymphocytes of varying shapes and sizes; and (4) prominent phagocytic and mitotic activity in germinal centers.

Paracortical Hyperplasia. This pattern is caused by immune reactions involving the **T-cell regions** of the lymph node. When activated, parafollicular T cells transform into large proliferating immunoblasts that can efface the B-cell follicles. Paracortical hyperplasia is encountered in viral infections (such as EBV), after certain vaccinations, and in immune reactions induced by drugs (especially phenytoin).

Sinus Histiocytosis. This reactive pattern is characterized by distention and prominence of the lymphatic sinusoids, owing to a marked **hypertrophy of lining endothelial cells** and an **infiltrate of macrophages (histiocytes).** It is often encountered in lymph nodes draining cancers and may represent an immune response to the tumor or its products.

Cat-Scratch Disease

Cat-scratch disease is a self-limited lymphadenitis caused by the bacterium *Bartonella henselae.* It is primarily a disease of childhood; 90% of the patients are younger than 18 years of age. It manifests with regional lymphadenopathy, most frequently in the axilla and neck. The nodal enlargement appears approximately 2 weeks after a feline scratch or, less commonly, after a splinter or thorn injury. An inflammatory nodule, vesicle, or eschar is sometimes visible at the site of the skin injury. In most patients the lymph node enlargement regresses during a period of 2 to 4 months. Rarely, encephalitis, osteomyelitis, or thrombocytopenia may develop.

MORPHOLOGY

The nodal changes in cat-scratch disease are quite characteristic. Initially sarcoidlike granulomas form, but these then undergo central necrosis associated with an infiltrate of neutrophils. These **irregular stellate necrotizing granulomas** are similar in appearance to those seen in a limited number of other infections, such as lymphogranuloma venereum. The microbe is extracellular and can be visualized with silver stains. The diagnosis is based on a history of exposure to cats, the characteristic clinical findings, a positive result on serologic testing for antibodies to *Bartonella*, and the distinctive morphologic changes in the lymph nodes.

Hemophagocytic Lymphohistiocytosis (HLH)

HLH is an uncommon disorder in which a viral infection or other proinflammatory exposures trigger activation of macrophages throughout the body, leading to phagocytosis of blood cells and their precursors, cytopenias, and symptoms related to systemic inflammation and organ dysfunction. Because of the widespread activation of macrophages in HLH it is sometimes referred to as *macrophage activation syndrome.* Inherited defects in several genes that regulate the cytotoxic function of immune cells are associated with a greatly elevated risk of HLH. The involved genes and proteins are diverse, but they share a common feature in that they are required for the cytolytic function of CD8+ T cells and NK cells. Owing to this defect in "killer lymphocytes," cytotoxic lymphocytes are unable to kill their targets (e.g., virus-infected cells) and remain engaged with targeted cells for longer than normal periods of time, leading to excessive release of cytokines such as IFN-γ. This in turn results in unbridled macrophage activation and the release of toxic levels of other proinflammatory cytokines, such as TNF and IL-6, producing signs and symptoms that closely resemble those associated with sepsis and other conditions that lead to the systemic inflammatory response syndrome (SIRS) (Chapter 2).

HLH occurs in several distinct settings.

- *HLH is most common in infants and young children with homozygous defects in genes that are required for cytotoxic lymphocyte function* such as *PRF1*, which encodes perforin, an essential component of cytotoxic granules. In this setting the trigger for uncontrolled macrophage activation may be some normally trivial childhood viral infection.
- *HLH may arise in older male children and adolescents with X-linked lymphoproliferative disorder,* in which the trigger is EBV infection. In those affected, inherited defects in T cell activation lead to inefficient killing of EBV-infected B cells and sustained inflammation.
- *HLH may complicate other systemic inflammatory disorders, such as rheumatologic conditions.* At least a subset of those affected have heterozygous defects in genes required for cytotoxic lymphocyte function, creating a genetic background that increases the likelihood of HLH.
- *HLH may appear as a secondary phenomenon in patients with peripheral T-cell lymphomas.* The precise mechanism in this context is uncertain; aberrant cytokine production by malignant T cells leading to dysregulation of nonneoplastic cytotoxic lymphocytes and macrophages is suspected.

Regardless of cause, patients with HLH present with fever, splenomegaly, and pancytopenia. In severe cases, DIC and organ failure may supervene. An examination of the bone marrow shows macrophages phagocytosing red cells, platelets, and nucleated marrow cells. Laboratory abnormalities typically include a very high ferritin level (>10,000 μg/L), hypertriglyceridemia, high serum levels of soluble IL-2 receptor, and low levels of circulating NK cells and CD8+ T lymphocytes. Treatment varies depending on the cause but is usually ineffective. In those with HLH stemming from inherited defects, hematopoietic stem cell transplantation offers a chance for cure.

NEOPLASTIC PROLIFERATIONS OF WHITE CELLS

The most important disorders of white cells are neoplasms. Virtually all of these tumors are considered to be malignant, but they demonstrate a wide range of behaviors, ranging from some of the most aggressive cancers to tumors that are so indolent that they were only recognized relatively recently as true neoplasms. Hematologic malignancies occur at all ages and include disorders that preferentially affect infants, children, and young adults as well as the very old. As a group they are quite common; in aggregate, about 185,000 new hematologic malignancies are diagnosed each year in the United States.

Classification systems for white cell neoplasms rely on morphologic and molecular criteria, including lineage-specific protein markers and genetic findings. The number of specific entities in the most recent World Health Classification of hematologic malignancies is numerous (over 70 at last count), reflecting the diversity of the normal hematopoietic and immune cells from which these tumors are derived. Here, we focus on the most common or clinicopathologically distinctive entities. We will first consider malignancies that originate in hematopoietic stem cells or early marrow progenitors, the acute leukemias and myeloid neoplasms. We will then discuss lymphomas and lymphocytic leukemias, plasma cell neoplasms and related entities, and finally relatively rare but distinctive neoplasms of dendritic cells.

Acute Leukemias

Acute leukemias are a diverse group of neoplastic proliferations of immature hematopoietic cells that often replace normal marrow elements, leading to symptoms related to marrow failure. Most can be readily subclassified by immunophenotype into B-cell (B-cell lymphoblastic leukemia, or B-ALL), T-cell (T-cell acute lymphoblastic leukemia, or T-ALL), or myeloid subtypes (acute myeloid leukemia, or AML). The immature neoplastic cells are referred to as blasts. Typically, in ALL there is a complete maturation arrest at early stages of B- or T-cell differentiation, and blasts are the major tumor cell population in involved tissues. By contrast, in AML the block in differentiation is often incomplete and diagnosis is based on the presence of at least 20% blasts in the marrow or blood.

Beyond their immunophenotypic differences, B, T, and myeloid acute leukemias also have somewhat distinct clinicopathologic features, as follows:

- *B-ALL* is the most common childhood leukemia, with a peak incidence between the ages of 2 and 10 years. It almost always arises within the marrow and replaces normal marrow elements, resulting in symptoms related to anemia (weakness, fatigue), thrombocytopenia (petechiae [small bleeds into the skin and mucosal membranes]), and neutropenia (infection).
- *T-ALL* most commonly presents during adolescence and often involves the thymus as well as the bone marrow. In addition to marrow failure, more than half of T-ALLs present with mediastinal masses due to thymic involvement.
- *AML* occurs throughout life but is most common in individuals older than 60 years of age. Unlike ALL, AML often arises from a preexisting myeloid neoplasm (either a myeloproliferative neoplasm or a myelodysplastic syndrome, described later), sometimes after a prodrome lasting for years. Like ALL, most symptoms are related to marrow failure. In addition, specific subtypes of AML are composed of cells that release thromboplastic substances into the blood and induce disseminated intravascular coagulation (DIC), which can lead to serious, sometimes fatal, bleeding complications (discussed later).

Pathogenesis. **Among the most common driver mutations in all types of acute leukemia are gene rearrangements and point substitutions that interfere with the function of transcription factors that regulate normal hematopoietic stem cell differentiation.** These mutations typically affect gene products that regulate the lineage to which the leukemia belongs. For example, B-ALL often contains mutations affecting the transcription factor PAX5, which is specifically required for the differentiation of early B cell progenitors. Many other such examples have now been described in various subtypes of acute leukemia.

Transcription factor mutations are not sufficient for the development of acute leukemia, and diverse complementary recurrent driver mutations have been described. Many of these mutations affect signaling molecules like tyrosine kinases and RAS and serve to promote increased tumor cell proliferation and survival. Other mutations affect factors that regulate chromatin-associated proteins such as histones, suggesting that epigenetic alterations are important in the genesis of acute leukemias.

Certain driver mutations are worthy of further mention, as they not only are important in the pathogenesis of these diseases but also serve as targets for highly effective therapies.

- *BCR-ABL in B-ALL*: Approximately 5% of childhood B-ALL and 25% of adult B-ALL are associated with rearrangements of the *ABL* gene on chromosome 9 and the *BCR* gene on chromosome 22 that are usually created by a balanced (9;22) translocation that creates the Philadelphia chromosome (or Ph chromosome, named for the city where it was discovered). This rearrangement forms a *BCR-ABL* fusion gene that encodes a constitutively active tyrosine kinase that activates essentially all the pathways that lie downstream of growth factor receptors (Chapter 6). *BCR-ABL* fusion genes are also found in chronic myeloid leukemia (described later). Proof of the importance of BCR-ABL is seen in the response of *BCR-ABL+* B-ALLs to tyrosine kinase inhibitors, which have greatly improved the outcome in this type of acute leukemia, particularly in adults.

- *PML-RARA in acute promyelocytic leukemia.* Acute promyelocytic leukemia is a subtype of AML that is virtually always associated with the presence of rearrangements involving the *PML* gene on chromosome 15 and the *RARA* gene on chromosome 17 that are usually created by a balanced (15;17) translocation. *RARA* encodes the retinoic acid receptor, whereas the chimeric *PML-RARA* gene encodes a fusion protein that blocks myeloid differentiation at the promyelocytic stage, probably in part by inhibiting the function of normal retinoic acid receptors. Remarkably, pharmacologic doses of all-*trans* retinoic acid (ATRA), an analogue of vitamin A (Chapter 7), overcome this block and induce the neoplastic promyelocytes to differentiate rapidly into neutrophils. Because neutrophils die after an average life span of a day or so, ATRA treatment results in "death by differentiation." The effect is very specific; AMLs without translocations involving *RARA* do not respond to ATRA. It was subsequently shown that the combination of ATRA and arsenic trioxide, a salt that induces the degradation of the PML/RARA fusion protein, is even more effective than ATRA alone, producing cures in more than 90% of patients.

- *IDH1 and IDH2 mutations in AML*: Approximately 10% of AMLs have mutations in either *IDH1* or *IDH2*, genes that encode isoforms of isocitrate dehydrogenase (IDH), a metabolic enzyme. As you may recall, mutant forms of IDH contribute to transformation by creating the oncometabolite 2-hydroxyglutarate (Chapter 6). Importantly, inhibitors of mutated IDH1 and IDH2 can induce the differentiation of IDH-mutated AMLs. Although not as effective as PML-RARA targeting agents, IDH inhibitors often induce complete remissions in IDH-mutated AMLs, even in patients who have failed conventional chemotherapy.

MORPHOLOGY AND ANCILLARY STUDIES

The diagnosis and subtyping of acute leukemia cannot be done on the basis of morphology alone and requires a combination of complementary test modalities.

Morphology. In leukemic presentations, **the marrow is hypercellular and packed with blasts and other immature elements,** which replace normal marrow elements. **Mediastinal masses** occur in 50% to 70% of T-ALLs, which are also more likely to be associated

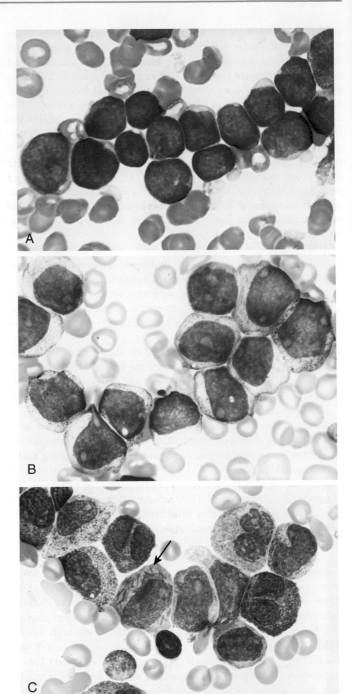

FIG. 10.14 Morphology of acute leukemias. (A) Acute lymphoblastic leukemia. Lymphoblasts are shown with condensed nuclear chromatin, small nucleoli, and scant agranular cytoplasm. (B) Acute myeloid leukemia. Myeloblasts with delicate nuclear chromatin, prominent nucleoli, and fine azurophilic cytoplasmic granules. (C) Acute promyelocytic leukemia. The neoplastic promyelocytes have abnormally coarse and numerous azurophilic granules. Other characteristic findings include a cell in the center of the field with multiple needlelike Auer rods *(arrow)*. (Courtesy of Dr. Robert W. McKenna, Department of Pathology, University of Texas Southwestern Medical School, Dallas, Texas.)

with lymphadenopathy and splenomegaly. The blasts of B-ALL and T-ALL are similar morphologically. Most commonly, lymphoblasts have scant basophilic cytoplasm and nuclei with delicate, finely stippled chromatin and small nucleoli (Fig. 10.14A). By definition, in AML, myeloid blasts or promyelocytes make up more than 20% of the bone marrow cellularity. **Myeloblasts tend to be larger than lymphoid blasts and have fine chromatin, distinct nucleoli, and moderate amounts of cytoplasm with variable numbers of granules** (Fig. 10.14B). In a subset of cases these granules take the form of **Auer rods,** needlelike inclusions that are pathognomonic for AML (Fig. 10.14C). In other instances, blasts with evidence of monocytic, erythroid, and megakaryocytic differentiation may predominate, or the blasts may be so immature that they can only be distinguished from lymphoblasts by immunophenotyping. Blasts can usually be seen in the peripheral blood and bone marrow, although biopsy of a tissue mass may be required for diagnosis, particularly in T-ALL.

Immunophenotyping. Definitive diagnosis relies on stains performed with antibodies specific for B, T, and myeloid lineage-specific markers, usually by flow cytometry (Fig. 10.15). Terminal deoxynucleotidyl transferase (TdT), an enzyme specifically expressed in pre—B and pre—T cells, is a sensitive but not entirely specific marker of ALL. Histochemical stains may also be used, including stains that are specific for myeloperoxidase, which is only expressed by myeloid blasts.

Cytogenetics and Molecular Genetics. Approximately 90% of acute leukemias have nonrandom karyotypic abnormalities. Most common in childhood B-ALL are hyperdiploidy (more than 50 chromosomes/cell) and a (12;21) translocation involving the *ETV6* and *RUNX1* genes, creating a fusion gene encoding an aberrant transcription factor. About 25% of adult pre—B-cell tumors have a (9;22) translocation involving the *ABL* and *BCR* genes. Pre—T-cell tumors are associated with diverse chromosomal aberrations, including frequent translocations involving the T-cell receptor loci and certain transcription factor genes, as well as mutations that inactivate tumor suppressor genes such as *PTEN* (leading to increased progrowth signaling) and *CDKN2A*, which encodes a negative regulator of the cell cycle and a positive regulator of p53. Specific translocations are associated with particular subtypes of acute leukemia, have prognostic importance, and may identify therapeutic targets; included among these are the t(9;22) and the t(15;17) (already discussed). The presence of these fusion genes is typically confirmed by fluorescence in situ hybridization (FISH) studies or by molecular studies.

Certain forms of acute leukemia are now defined by the presence of driver mutations in specific cancer genes and, as already mentioned, therapy and prognosis may be dictated by the results of these analyses. Mutation detection at many centers is now carried out by targeted DNA sequencing.

Clinical Features. Acute leukemia is an aggressive disease. Onset of symptoms is rapid and the natural history of the disease is measured in weeks to months. Peripheral blood findings are highly variable. The white cell count may be markedly elevated (>100,000 cells/μL) but is sometimes normal. Blasts are sometimes absent from the peripheral blood (aleukemic leukemia). Anemia is almost always present, and the platelet count is usually below 100,000/μL. Neutropenia is common. Due to low blood counts, fatigue, lassitude, easy bleeding, and fever are common. Beyond symptoms related to marrow replacement and the attendant pancytopenia, there may also be the following:

- *Bone pain* resulting from marrow expansion and infiltration of the subperiosteum
- *Lymphadenopathy, splenomegaly, and hepatomegaly,* more common and more pronounced in ALL than AML
- *Testicular enlargement* due to leukemic infiltration
- *Infiltration of skin and gums,* most characteristic of AML with monocytic differentiation
- In T-ALL with thymic involvement, *compression of large vessels and airways in the mediastinum*
- *Central nervous system manifestations* resulting from meningeal spread, such as headache, vomiting, and nerve palsies, complications that are more common in ALL

Treatment of acute leukemia varies according to subtype. Most are treated with combination chemotherapy using regimens that differ for ALL and AML. More than 80% of children with B-ALL and T-ALL are cured, one of the great success stories of oncology. Several factors are associated with a worse prognosis in childhood ALL: (1) age younger than 2 years, largely because these tumors are genetically distinct, often being associated with translocations involving the *KMT2A* gene; (2) presentation in adulthood; and (3) peripheral blood blast counts greater than 100,000. Favorable prognostic markers include (1) age between 2 and 10 years, (2) a low white cell count, and (3) hyperdiploidy. The molecular detection of residual disease after therapy is also predictive of a worse outcome in all forms of acute leukemia and is being used to guide therapy.

As already mentioned, highly effective targeted therapies are now available for adults with BCR-ABL-positive B-ALL and acute promyelocytic leukemia. A relatively recent development is treatment of B-ALL with cytotoxic T cells bearing chimeric antigen receptors

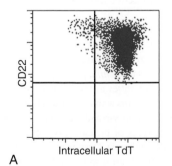 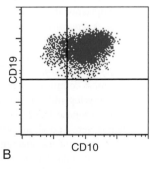 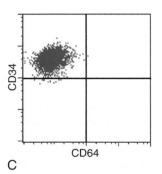 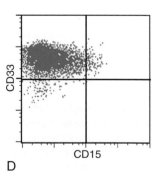

A   Intracellular TdT   B   CD10   C   CD64   D   CD15

FIG. 10.15 Flow cytometric findings in acute leukemia. (A) and (B) show flow cytometry results for a typical B-ALL. The tumor cells are positive for the B-cell markers CD19 and CD22, CD10 (a marker expressed on a subset of ALLs), and TdT (a specialized DNA polymerase that is expressed in pre-B and pre-T cells). (C) and (D) show flow cytometry results for a typical AML. The tumor cells are positive for the stem cell marker CD34 and the myeloid lineage specific markers CD33 and CD15 (subset), and negative for the marker CD64, which is preferentially expressed in monocytic cells. (Courtesy of Dr. Louis Picker, Oregon Health Science Center, Portland, Oregon.)

(CAR) engineered to specifically recognize and kill cells expressing a B-cell surface protein such as CD19, CD20, or CD22. This therapy has produced dramatic responses in relapsed/refractory B-ALL in children and adults, but at the cost of permanent loss of normal B cells (since they also express the target proteins) and sometimes severe or even fatal toxicity caused by production of cytokines by the tumor-specific CAR-T cells.

Challenges remain. For example, infantile acute leukemias associated with rearrangements of the gene *KMT2A* and AML subtypes other than acute promyelocytic leukemia are difficult to treat, and the small subset of acute leukemias with *TP53* mutations have dismal outcomes even with hematopoietic stem cell transplantation.

Myelodysplastic Syndromes

The term *myelodysplastic syndrome* (MDS) refers to a group of clonal stem cell disorders characterized by maturation defects that are associated with ineffective hematopoiesis and a high risk of transformation to AML. In MDS, the bone marrow is partly or wholly replaced by the clonal progeny of a transformed multipotent stem cell that retains the capacity to differentiate into red cells, granulocytes, and platelets, but in a manner that is both ineffective and disordered. As a result, the marrow is usually hypercellular or normocellular, but the peripheral blood shows one or more cytopenias. The abnormal stem cell clone in the bone marrow is genetically unstable and prone to the acquisition of additional mutations and transformation to AML. Most cases are idiopathic, but some develop after exposure to carcinogens, previous cancer therapy, or ionizing radiation therapy.

Pathogenesis. New insights have come from sequencing of MDS genomes, which has identified a number of recurrently mutated genes. These genes can be grouped into three major functional categories, as follows:

- *Epigenetic factors.* Frequent mutations are seen involving many of the same epigenetic factors that are mutated in AML, including factors that regulate DNA methylation and histone modifications; thus, like AML, dysregulation of the epigenome appears to be important in the genesis of MDS, attesting to the relatedness of these two conditions.
- *RNA splicing factors.* A subset of tumors has mutations involving the RNA splicing machinery that are proposed to drive transformation by altering RNA processing so as to alter the function of oncogenes and tumor suppressor genes. These mutations are commonly associated with *ring sideroblasts,* a classic form of dysplasia that is seen in a subset of MDS.
- *Transcription factors.* These mutations affect transcription factors that are required for normal myelopoiesis and may contribute to the deranged differentiation that characterizes MDS.

In addition, roughly **10% of MDS cases have loss-of-function mutations in the tumor suppressor gene *TP53*,** which correlate with the presence of a complex karyotype and particularly poor clinical outcomes. Both primary MDS and therapy-related MDS are associated with similar recurrent chromosomal abnormalities, including monosomies 5 and 7; deletions of 5q, 7q, and 20q; and trisomy 8.

It is now recognized that **MDS often arises from an asymptomatic precursor referred to as clonal hematopoiesis of indeterminant prognosis (CHIP).** CHIP is characterized by normal blood counts despite the presence of one of more clonal acquired "driver" mutations that are identical to those that are found in MDS. CHIP progresses to

an overt white cell neoplasm at a frequency of about 1% per year and may be a risk factor for cardiovascular disease (Chapter 8).

MORPHOLOGY

In MDS, the marrow is populated by abnormal-appearing hematopoietic precursors (eFig. 10.1). Some of the more common abnormalities include **megaloblastoid erythroid precursors** resembling those seen in the megaloblastic anemias, erythroid forms with iron deposits within their mitochondria (**ring sideroblasts**), granulocyte precursors with **abnormal granules** or abnormal nuclear maturation, and small megakaryocytes with single small nuclei or large megakaryocytes with separate nuclei. Myeloblasts may be increased and by definition make up less than 20% of the marrow cellularity.

Clinical Features. MDS is often described as rare but is actually about as common as AML, affecting up to 15,000 people per year in the United States. Most patients present between the ages of 50 and 70. As a result of cytopenias, many suffer from infections, symptoms related to anemia, and abnormal bleeding. The response to conventional chemotherapy is usually poor, perhaps because MDS arises in a background of stem cell damage. Many patients are now treated with DNA hypomethylating agents in an attempt to "reprogram" the aberrant MDS stem cells and improve differentiation, with some sustained responses. Transformation to AML occurs in 10% to 40% of patients. The prognosis is variable; the median survival time ranges from 9 to 29 months and is worse in cases associated with increased marrow blasts, multiple cytogenetic abnormalities, or *TP53* mutations.

Myeloproliferative Neoplasms

Myeloproliferative neoplasms are characterized by the presence of mutated, constitutively activated tyrosine kinases or other acquired aberrations in signaling factors that lead to growth factor independence. This insight provides a satisfying explanation for the observed overproduction of blood cells and is important therapeutically because of the availability of tyrosine kinase inhibitors. The neoplastic progenitors tend to seed secondary hematopoietic organs (the spleen, liver, and lymph nodes), resulting in hepatosplenomegaly (caused by neoplastic extramedullary hematopoiesis).

Four major diagnostic entities are recognized: chronic myeloid leukemia (CML), polycythemia vera, primary myelofibrosis, and essential thrombocythemia. The distinctive features of myeloproliferative neoplasms are as follows:

- *CML is separated from the others by its association with a characteristic abnormality, the BCR-ABL fusion gene,* which produces a constitutively active BCR-ABL tyrosine kinase.
- *Polycythemia vera, essential thrombocythemia, primary myelofibrosis.* The most common genetic abnormalities in these "BCR-ABL negative" myeloproliferative neoplasms are activating mutations in the tyrosine kinase JAK2, which occur in virtually all cases of polycythemia vera and about 50% of cases of primary myelofibrosis and 50% of cases of essential thrombocythemia. Despite their genetic similarity, the clinical features of each of these disorders differs at the time of diagnosis. In polycythemia vera, there is excessive production of red cells, granulocytes, and platelets, whereas in essential thrombocythemia the proliferative drive is confined to platelet precursors (megakaryocytes). In primary myelofibrosis, the leukocyte count may be elevated early in the course, but because of reactive marrow fibrosis, patients tend to develop cytopenias, particularly anemia.

- *Some rare myeloproliferative neoplasms are associated with activating mutations in other tyrosine kinases, such as platelet-derived growth factor receptor-α and platelet-derived growth factor receptor-β.*
- *All myeloproliferative neoplasms have variable propensities to transform to a "spent phase" resembling primary myelofibrosis or to a "blast crisis" identical to acute leukemia, both triggered by the acquisition of additional somatic mutations.*

Only CML, polycythemia vera, and primary myelofibrosis are considered here, as other myeloproliferative neoplasms are too infrequent to merit discussion.

Chronic Myeloid Leukemia

CML principally affects adults between 25 and 60 years of age. The peak incidence is in the fourth and fifth decades of life. About 4500 new cases are diagnosed per year in the United States.

Pathogenesis. **CML is distinguished from other myeloproliferative neoplasms by the presence of a chimeric *BCR-ABL* gene derived from portions of the *BCR* gene on chromosome 22 and the *ABL* gene on chromosome 9.** In about 95% of cases, the *BCR-ABL* gene is the product of a balanced (9;22) translocation that moves *ABL* from chromosome 9 to a position on chromosome 22 adjacent to *BCR*. In the remaining 5% of cases, a *BCR-ABL* fusion gene is created by cytogenetically cryptic or complex rearrangements involving more than two chromosomes. The *BCR-ABL* fusion gene is present in granulocytic, erythroid, megakaryocytic, and B-cell precursors, and in some cases T-cell precursors as well, indicating that CML arises from a transformed hematopoietic stem cell.

As described in Chapter 6, the *BCR-ABL* gene encodes a fusion protein consisting of portions of BCR and the tyrosine kinase domain of ABL. Normal myeloid progenitors depend on signals generated by growth factors and their receptors for growth and survival. **The growth factor dependence of CML progenitors is greatly decreased by constitutive signals generated by BCR-ABL that mimic the effects of growth factor receptor activation, such as activation of RAS.** Importantly, because BCR-ABL does not inhibit differentiation, the early disease course is marked by excessive production of relatively normal blood cells, particularly granulocytes and platelets.

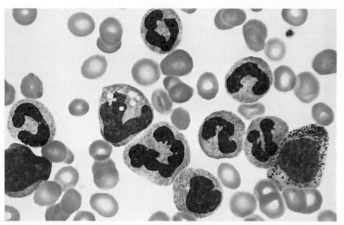

FIG. 10.16 CML—peripheral blood smear. Granulocytic forms at various stages of differentiation are present. (Courtesy of Dr. Robert W. McKenna, Department of Pathology, University of Texas Southwestern Medical School, Dallas, Texas.)

> ### MORPHOLOGY
>
> The peripheral blood findings are highly characteristic. The leukocyte count is elevated, often exceeding 100,000 cells/μL. **The circulating cells are predominantly neutrophils and immature granulocytic progenitors** (Fig. 10.16), but **basophils** and **eosinophils** are also usually increased in number, as are platelets. The bone marrow is hypercellular owing to increased numbers of maturing granulocytic and megakaryocytic precursors. The red pulp of the enlarged spleen resembles bone marrow because of the presence of extensive **extramedullary hematopoiesis**. This burgeoning proliferation often compromises the local blood supply, leading to **splenic infarcts**.

Clinical Features. The onset of CML is insidious, as the initial symptoms are usually nonspecific (e.g., easy fatigability, weakness, weight loss). Sometimes the first symptom is a dragging sensation in the abdomen caused by splenomegaly. On occasion it may be necessary to distinguish CML from a leukemoid reaction, a dramatic elevation of the granulocyte count in response to infection, stress,

chronic inflammation, and certain neoplasms. This distinction can be achieved definitively by testing for the presence of the *BCR-ABL* fusion gene, which can be done by karyotyping, fluorescence in situ hybridization (FISH), or PCR assay.

The natural history of CML is initially one of slow progression. Even without treatment, the median survival is 3 years. After a variable (and unpredictable) period, approximately half of CML cases enter an accelerated phase marked by increasing anemia and new thrombocytopenia, the appearance of additional cytogenetic abnormalities, and finally transformation into a picture resembling acute leukemia (blast crisis). In the remaining 50% of cases, blast crisis occurs abruptly, without an accelerated phase. Of note, in 30% of cases the blast crisis resembles B-cell ALL, further attesting to the origin of CML from hematopoietic stem cells. In the remaining 70% of cases, the blast crisis resembles AML. Less commonly, CML progresses to a spent phase of extensive bone marrow fibrosis resembling primary myelofibrosis.

Fortunately for those affected, the natural history of CML has been altered dramatically by the emergence of targeted therapy. Treatment with tyrosine kinase inhibitors, particularly in patients with early disease, induces sustained remissions with manageable toxicity and prevents progression to blast crisis, apparently by suppressing the proliferative drive that leads to the acquisition of additional mutations. When patients on tyrosine kinase inhibitors relapse, their tumors are often found to have acquired mutations in BCR-ABL that prevent the drugs from binding. The selective outgrowth of these cells is explained by the powerful antitumor effects of BCR-ABL inhibitors and indicates that many resistant tumors are still "addicted" to the progrowth signals created by BCR-ABL. In some instances, resistant tumors can be treated with different inhibitors capable of targeting mutated forms of BCR-ABL. For others, hematopoietic stem cell transplantation offers a chance of cure but carries with it substantial risks, particularly in the elderly.

Polycythemia Vera

Polycythemia vera is strongly associated with activating mutations in the tyrosine kinase JAK2 (Janus kinase 2). JAK2 normally acts in the signaling pathways downstream of the erythropoietin receptor and other growth factor and cytokine receptors. The most common JAK2 mutation sharply lowers the dependence of hematopoietic cells on growth factors for growth and survival. This produces excessive proliferation of erythroid, granulocytic, and megakaryocytic elements (panmyelosis), but most clinical signs and symptoms are related to an absolute increase in red cell mass. Polycythemia vera must be distinguished from relative polycythemia, which results from hemoconcentration. Unlike reactive forms of absolute polycythemia, polycythemia vera is associated with low levels of serum erythropoietin, which is a reflection of the growth factor—independent proliferation of the neoplastic clone.

MORPHOLOGY

The major anatomic changes in polycythemia vera stem from increases in blood volume and viscosity brought about by the polycythemia. **Congestion** of many tissues is characteristic. The liver is enlarged and often contains small foci of extramedullary hematopoiesis. The spleen is usually slightly enlarged (250 to 300 g) because of vascular congestion. As a result of the increased viscosity and vascular stasis, **thromboses and infarctions are common,** particularly in the heart, spleen, and kidneys. Hemorrhages also occur in about a third of the patients. These most often affect the gastrointestinal tract, oropharynx, or brain and may occur spontaneously or following some minor trauma or surgical procedure. Platelets produced from the neoplastic clone are often dysfunctional, a derangement that contributes to the elevated risk of thrombosis and bleeding. As in CML, the peripheral blood often shows **basophilia.**

The bone marrow is hypercellular owing to increased numbers of erythroid, myeloid, and megakaryocytic forms. In addition, some degree of marrow fibrosis is present in 10% of patients at the time of diagnosis. In a subset of patients, this progresses to a spent phase where the marrow is largely replaced by fibroblasts and collagen.

Clinical Features. Polycythemia vera appears insidiously, usually in late middle age. Patients are plethoric and often somewhat cyanotic. Histamine released from the neoplastic basophils may contribute to pruritus and may also account for an increased incidence of peptic ulcers. Other symptoms are related to thrombotic and hemorrhagic tendencies and to hypertension. Headache, dizziness, gastrointestinal symptoms, hematemesis, and melena are common. Because of the high rate of cell turnover, symptomatic gout is seen in 5% to 10% of cases.

The diagnosis is usually made in the laboratory. Red cell counts range from 6 to 10 million/μL, and the hematocrit is often 60% or greater. The granulocyte count can be as high as 50,000 cells/μL, and the platelet count is often more than 400,000/μL. Basophilia is common. The platelets are functionally abnormal in most cases, and giant platelets and megakaryocyte fragments are often seen in the blood. About 30% of patients develop thrombotic complications, usually affecting the brain or heart. Hepatic vein thrombosis giving rise to *Budd-Chiari syndrome* (Chapter 14) is an uncommon but grave complication. Minor hemorrhages (e.g., epistaxis and bleeding from gums) are common, and life-threatening hemorrhages occur in 5% to 10% of patients. In those receiving no treatment, death occurs from vascular complications within months; however, the median survival is increased to about 10 years by lowering the red cell count to near normal through repeated phlebotomy.

Unfortunately, prolonged survival has shown a propensity for polycythemia vera to evolve to a "spent phase" resembling primary myelofibrosis. After an average interval of 10 years, 15% to 20% of cases undergo such a transformation. Owing to the extensive marrow fibrosis, hematopoiesis shifts to the spleen, which enlarges markedly. Inhibitors that target JAK2 have been approved for treatment of the spent phase of polycythemia vera and lead to some improvement in most patients. Transformation to a "blast crisis" identical to AML also occurs, but much less frequently than in CML.

Primary Myelofibrosis

The hallmark of primary myelofibrosis is the development of obliterative marrow fibrosis, which reduces bone marrow hematopoiesis and leads to cytopenias and extensive extramedullary hematopoiesis. Histologically, the appearance is identical to the spent phase that occurs occasionally late in the course of other myeloproliferative disorders.

The molecular pathogenesis of myelofibrosis involves increased JAK-STAT signaling in almost all cases. Many receptors for growth factors and cytokines use a signaling pathway involving JAK kinases and transcription factors called STATs (signal transducers and activators of transcription), and constitutive activation of this pathway seems to be the underlying driver in almost all cases of myelofibrosis. Activating *JAK2* mutations are present in 50% to 60% of cases and activating mutations in *MPL*, the gene encoding the thrombopoietin receptor, are seen in an additional 1% to 5% of cases. Most of the remaining cases have mutations in the *CALR* gene that lead to secretion of a factor called calreticulin that binds and activates MPL. Why *JAK2* mutations are associated with polycythemia vera in some patients and primary myelofibrosis in others is not understood; differences in the cell of origin and the genetic backgrounds that give rise to these two disorders are suspected.

The characteristic marrow fibrosis is caused by the inappropriate release of fibrogenic factors from neoplastic megakaryocytes. Two factors synthesized by megakaryocytes have been implicated: *platelet-derived growth factor* and *TGF-β.* As you recall, platelet-derived growth factor and TGF-β are fibroblast mitogens. In addition, TGF-β promotes collagen deposition and causes angiogenesis, both of which are observed in myelofibrosis. Recall that excessive TGF-β signaling is also responsible for connective tissue defects in Marfan syndrome (Chapter 4).

As marrow fibrosis progresses, displaced hematopoietic stem cells take up residence in niches in secondary hematopoietic organs, such as the spleen, the liver, and the lymph nodes, leading to the appearance of extramedullary hematopoiesis. For incompletely understood reasons, red cell production at extramedullary sites is disordered. This factor and the concomitant suppression of marrow function result in moderate to severe anemia.

MORPHOLOGY

The peripheral blood smear is markedly abnormal (Fig. 10.17). Red cells often exhibit bizarre shapes **(poikilocytes, teardrop cells),** and nucleated erythroid precursors are commonly seen along with immature white cells (myelocytes and metamyelocytes), a combination of findings referred to as **leukoerythroblastosis.** Abnormally large platelets are often present as well. Early in the course, the bone marrow is hypercellular and contains clusters of abnormal megakaryocytes, sometimes within dilated marrow sinusoids, with characteristic hyperchromatic "cloudlike" nuclei (eFig. 10.2). In advanced cases the marrow becomes hypocellular and diffusely fibrotic, and the bone trabeculae become thickened and sclerotic. Marked **splenomegaly** resulting from extensive extramedullary hematopoiesis, often associated with **subcapsular infarcts,** is also typical. The spleen may weigh as much as 4000 g, roughly twenty times its normal weight. Moderate **hepatomegaly,** also due to extramedullary hematopoiesis, is commonplace. Lymph nodes are also involved by extramedullary hematopoiesis, but not to a degree sufficient to cause appreciable enlargement.

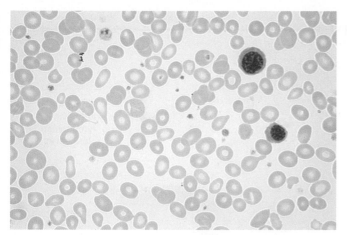

FIG. 10.17 Primary myelofibrosis—peripheral blood smear. Two nucleated erythroid precursors and several teardrop-shaped red cells (dacryocytes) are evident. Immature myeloid cells were present in other fields. An identical histologic picture can be seen in other diseases producing marrow distortion and fibrosis.

Clinical Features. Primary myelofibrosis usually occurs in individuals older than 60 years who come to attention because of progressive anemia and splenomegaly. Nonspecific symptoms such as fatigue, weight loss, and night sweats are common. Hyperuricemia and secondary gout resulting from a high rate of cell turnover are also frequently seen.

Laboratory studies typically show a moderate to severe normochromic normocytic anemia accompanied by leukoerythroblastosis. The white cell count is usually normal or mildly reduced but can be elevated early in the course. The platelet count is usually normal or elevated at diagnosis, but thrombocytopenia often supervenes as the disease progresses. These blood findings are not specific, and bone marrow biopsy is essential for diagnosis.

Primary myelofibrosis is more difficult to treat than polycythemia vera and CML. The median survival is approximately 6 years. Threats to life include infection, thrombosis and bleeding related to platelet abnormalities, and transformation to AML, which occurs in 5% to 20% of cases. JAK2 inhibitors are effective at decreasing the splenomegaly and constitutional symptoms, even in those without *JAK2* mutations, presumably because increased JAK/STAT signaling is common to all molecular subtypes. Hematopoietic stem cell transplantation may be curative in those young and fit enough to withstand the procedure.

Non-Hodgkin Lymphomas and Chronic Lymphoid Leukemias

The non-Hodgkin lymphomas (NHLs) and chronic lymphoid leukemias are composed of tumor cells resembling stages of mature lymphocytic differentiation and vary widely in their clinical presentation and behavior, thus presenting challenges to students and clinicians alike. Some characteristically manifest as *leukemias,* with involvement of the bone marrow and the peripheral blood. Others tend to present as *lymphomas,* tumors that produce masses in lymph nodes or other tissues. Although these tendencies are reflected in the names given to particular entities, in reality all have the potential to spread to lymph nodes and other tissues, especially the liver, spleen, and bone marrow, as well as peripheral blood. Because of their overlapping clinical behavior, the diagnosis of mature lymphoid neoplasms is based on the morphologic and molecular characteristics of the tumor cells. Stated another way, for purposes of diagnosis and prognostication, it is most important to focus on what kind of cells the tumor is made up of, not where the tumor cells reside in the patient.

Two broad groups of lymphoid neoplasms are recognized: Hodgkin lymphomas (discussed later), and non-Hodgkin lymphomas and lymphoid leukemias. An international group of pathologists, molecular biologists, and clinicians working on behalf of the World Health Organization (WHO) has formulated a widely accepted classification scheme for lymphoid neoplasms that relies on a combination of morphologic, phenotypic, genotypic, and clinical features. As background for the subsequent discussion, certain important principles warrant consideration:

- **Tumors of mature B and T cells often resemble a specific stage of normal lymphocyte differentiation** (Fig. 10.18), and (as with acute leukemias) the diagnosis and classification of these tumors rely on tests (either immunohistochemistry or flow cytometry) that detect lineage-specific markers. By convention, many such markers are identified by their cluster of differentiation (CD) number.
- **Class switching and somatic hypermutation are regulated forms of genomic instability that occur in germinal center reactions. They are mistake prone and hence place germinal center B cells at high risk for potentially transforming mutations.** These molecular events in the lives of B cells occur mainly in the germinal centers during B cell activation, involve DNA breaks, and are not seen in T lymphocytes (Chapter 5). Many of the recurrent chromosomal translocations found in mature B-cell malignancies involve the immunoglobulin loci and appear to stem from "accidents" during attempted rearrangement of the immunoglobulin genes. By contrast, mature T cells give rise to neoplasms infrequently and only very rarely have chromosomal translocations involving the T-cell receptor loci.
- **Antigen receptor gene rearrangements in mature lymphoid neoplasms serve as unique markers of the malignant clone.** As described in Chapter 5, precursor B and T cells rearrange their antigen receptor genes through a mechanism that ensures that each lymphocyte makes a single, unique antigen receptor. Because antigen receptor gene rearrangement virtually always precedes transformation, the daughter cells derived from a given malignant progenitor share the same antigen receptor gene configuration and synthesize identical antigen receptor proteins (either immunoglobulins or T-cell receptors). Thus, analyses of antigen receptor genes and their protein products can be used to differentiate lymphoid neoplasms (which are monoclonal and thus have the same rearrangement in all the cells) from immune reactions (which are polyclonal).
- **Lymphoid neoplasms often disrupt normal immune function.** Both immunodeficiency (made evident by increased susceptibility to infection) and autoimmunity may be seen, sometimes in the same patient. Ironically, patients with inherited or acquired immunodeficiencies are at high risk for the development of certain lymphoid neoplasms, particularly those associated with EBV infection.
- **Although non-Hodgkin lymphomas often manifest at a particular tissue site, sensitive molecular assays usually show that the tumor is widely disseminated at diagnosis.** As a result, with few exceptions, only systemic therapies are curative for those with NHL.

The salient features of the more common non-Hodgkin lymphomas, chronic lymphoid leukemias, and plasma cell tumors (discussed later) are summarized in Table 10.7 and are described in the following sections.

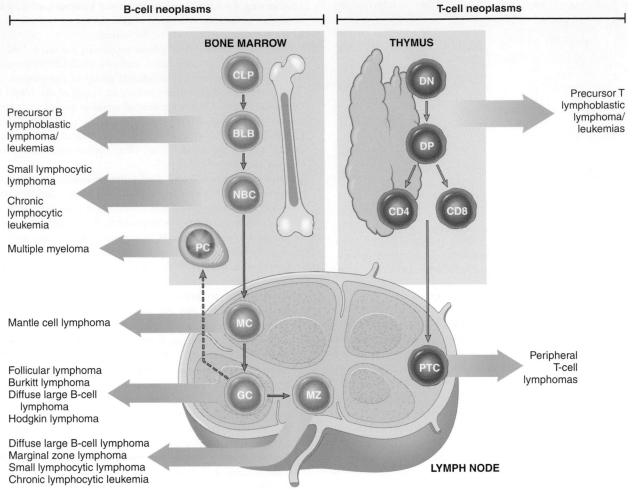

FIG. 10.18 Origin of lymphoid neoplasms. Stages of B- and T-cell differentiation from which specific lymphoid and tumors emerge are shown. *BLB,* Pre-B lymphoblast; *CLP,* common lymphoid progenitor; *DN,* CD4⁻/CD8⁻ (double-negative) pro-T cell; *DP,* CD4+/CD8+ (double-positive) pre-T cell; *GC,* germinal center B cell; *MC,* mantle zone B cell; *MZ,* marginal zone B cell; *NBC,* naïve B cell; *PC,* plasma cell; *PTC,* peripheral T cell.

Chronic Lymphocytic Leukemia/Small Lymphocytic Lymphoma

Chronic lymphocytic leukemia (CLL) and small lymphocytic lymphoma (SLL) are essentially identical, differing only in the extent of peripheral blood involvement. Somewhat arbitrarily, if the peripheral blood lymphocyte count exceeds 5000 cells/μL, the patient is diagnosed with CLL. Most cases fit the diagnostic criteria for CLL, which is the most common leukemia of adults in the Western world. By contrast, SLL (which has predominantly lymph node involvement) constitutes only 4% of NHLs. For unclear reasons, CLL/SLL is less common in Asia.

***Pathogenesis.* CLL/SLL is an indolent, slowly growing tumor in which increased tumor cell survival appears to be more important than tumor cell proliferation per se.** In line with this idea, CLL/SLL cells contain high levels of BCL2, a protein that inhibits apoptosis (Chapters 1 and 6). One mechanism of *BCL2* overexpression appears to be deletion of chromosome 13q that lead to the loss of genes encoding microRNAs that are negative regulators of *BCL2*. Also of critical importance are signals generated by surface immunoglobulin (the so-called B-cell receptor, or BCR). BCR signals flow through an intermediary called *Bruton tyrosine kinase (BTK)* that upregulates the expression of genes that promote the growth and survival of CLL/SLL cells.

CLL/SLL also causes immune dysregulation, particularly of normal B cells. Through unclear mechanisms, the accumulation of CLL/SLL cells suppresses normal B-cell function, often resulting in *hypogammaglobulinemia.* Paradoxically, approximately 15% of patients develop warm autoantibodies against their own red cells or platelets. When present, the autoantibodies are made by nonmalignant bystander B cells, indicating that CLL/SLL cells somehow impair immune tolerance.

MORPHOLOGY AND ANCILLARY STUDIES

Morphology. Involved lymph nodes are effaced by sheets of small lymphocytes. The predominant cells are small, resting lymphocytes with dark, round nuclei, and scanty cytoplasm (Fig. 10.19A). Scattered within are ill-defined foci of larger, actively dividing cells (Fig. 10.19B). The foci of mitotically active cells are called **proliferation centers,** which are pathognomonic for CLL/SLL. The bone marrow, spleen, and liver are also

Table 10.7 Characteristics of the More Common Non-Hodgkin Lymphomas, Lymphoid Leukemias, and Plasma Cell Tumors

Clinical Entity	Frequency	Salient Morphology	Cell of Origin	Comments
Small lymphocytic lymphoma/chronic lymphocytic leukemia	3%–4% of adult lymphomas; 30% of all leukemias	Small resting lymphocytes mixed with loose clusters of large activated cells; lymph nodes diffusely effaced	CD5+ B cell	Occurs in older adults; usually involves nodes, marrow, spleen; and peripheral blood; indolent
Follicular lymphoma	40% of adult lymphomas	Frequent small "cleaved" cells mixed with large cells; nodular (follicular) growth pattern	Germinal center B cell	Associated with t(14;18); indolent
Mantle cell lymphoma	6% of adult lymphomas	Small to intermediate-sized irregular lymphocytes; diffuse or vaguely nodular pattern	CD5+ B cell overexpressing cyclin D1	Associated with t(11;14); moderately aggressive
Diffuse large B-cell lymphoma	40%–50% of adult lymphomas	Variable; most resemble large germinal center B cells; diffuse growth pattern	Germinal center or postgerminal center B cell	Heterogeneous, may arise at extranodal sites; aggressive
Burkitt lymphoma	<1% of lymphomas in the United States; endemic in Africa	Intermediate-sized cells with several nucleoli; diffuse growth pattern; frequent apoptotic cells ("starry sky" appearance)	Germinal center B cell	Associated with t(8;14) and EBV (subset); highly aggressive
Plasmacytoma/multiple myeloma	Most common lymphoid neoplasm in older adults	Plasma cells in sheets, sometimes with prominent nucleoli or inclusions containing immunoglobulin	Postgerminal center B cell	CRAB (hypercalcemia, renal failure, anemia, bone fractures)

EBV, Epstein-Barr virus.

involved in almost all cases. In most patients there is an absolute **lymphocytosis** featuring small, mature-looking lymphocytes. These circulating cells are fragile and during the preparation of smears many are disrupted, producing characteristic **smudge cells.** Variable numbers of larger activated lymphocytes are also usually present in blood smears.

Immunophenotype and Cytogenetics. CLL/SLL is a neoplasm of mature B cells expressing the B-cell marker CD20 and surface immunoglobulins. The tumor cells also express CD5. This is a helpful diagnostic clue, since among B-cell lymphomas only CLL/SLL and mantle cell lymphoma (discussed later) commonly express CD5. Approximately 50% of tumors have karyotypic abnormalities, the most common of which are trisomy 12 and deletions involving portions of chromosomes 11, 13, and 17. Unlike in other B-cell neoplasms, chromosomal translocations are rare.

Clinical Features. When first detected, CLL/SLL is often asymptomatic. The most common signs and symptoms are nonspecific and include fatigue, weight loss, and anorexia. Generalized lymphadenopathy and hepatosplenomegaly are present in 50% to 60% of patients. The leukocyte count may be increased only slightly (in SLL) or may exceed 200,000 cells/μL. Hypogammaglobulinemia develops in more than 50% of the patients, usually late in the course, and leads to an increased susceptibility to bacterial infections. Less commonly, autoimmune hemolytic anemia (warm antibody type) and autoimmune thrombocytopenia are seen.

The course and prognosis are highly variable and depend on the disease stage and genetic findings. For example, the presence of abnormalities in the *TP53* tumor suppressor gene is associated with an overall survival of less than 30% at 10 years, whereas isolated abnormalities of chromosome 13q are associated with an overall

survival that is not significantly different from that of the matched general population. Insights into the molecular pathogenesis of CLL/SLL has led to development of effective new drugs that variously inhibit BCR signaling (e.g., by targeting BTK) or BCL2 function. However, cure may only be achieved with hematopoietic stem cell transplantation, which is reserved for relatively young patients who fail conventional therapies. A small fraction of tumors transforms to aggressive tumors resembling diffuse large B-cell lymphoma *(Richter transformation)*; after transformation occurs, the median survival is less than 1 year.

Follicular Lymphoma

This relatively common tumor constitutes approximately 30% of NHLs in adults in the United States. Like CLL/SLL, it occurs less frequently in Asian populations.

Pathogenesis. **Greater than 85% of follicular lymphomas have a characteristic (14;18) translocation that fuses the *BCL2* gene on chromosome 18 to the *IgH* locus on chromosome 14.** This chromosomal rearrangement results in the inappropriate overexpression of BCL2 protein, which you will recall is an inhibitor of apoptosis (Chapters 1 and 6). Whole-genome sequencing of follicular lymphomas has identified additional mutations in genes encoding histone-modifying proteins, suggesting that epigenetic changes also contribute to the genesis of these tumors.

MORPHOLOGY AND ANCILLARY STUDIES

Morphology. Lymph nodes are usually effaced by a distinctly **nodular proliferation** (Fig. 10.20A). Most commonly, the predominant neoplastic cells are so-called **centrocytes,** cells slightly larger than resting

lymphocytes that have angular "cleaved" nuclei with prominent indentations and linear infoldings (Fig. 10.20B). The nuclear chromatin is coarse and condensed, and nucleoli are indistinct. These centrocytes are mixed with variable numbers of **centroblasts,** larger cells with vesicular chromatin, several nucleoli, and modest amounts of cytoplasm. In most tumors, centroblasts are a minor component of the overall cellularity, mitoses are infrequent, and single dead cells (cells undergoing apoptosis) are not seen. These features help to distinguish follicular lymphoma from follicular hyperplasia, in which mitoses and apoptosis are prominent. Uncommonly, large cells predominate, a histologic pattern that correlates with a more aggressive clinical behavior.

Immunophenotype. These tumors express B-cell markers such as CD20 and the germinal center B-cell markers CD10 and BCL6; of note, BCL6 is a transcription factor that is required for the generation of germinal center B cells.

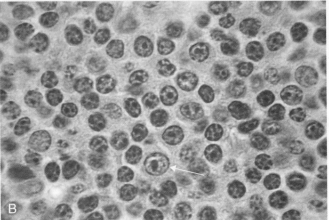

FIG. 10.19 Small lymphocytic lymphoma/chronic lymphocytic leukemia—lymph node. (A) Low-power view shows diffuse effacement of nodal architecture. (B) At high power, a majority of the tumor cells have the appearance of small, round lymphocytes. A "prolymphocyte," a larger cell with a centrally placed nucleolus, is also present in this field *(arrow).* (A, Courtesy of Dr. José Hernandez, Department of Pathology, University of Texas Southwestern Medical School, Dallas, Texas.)

Clinical Features. Follicular lymphoma mainly occurs in adults older than 50 years of age and affects males and females equally. It usually manifests as painless, generalized lymphadenopathy. The bone marrow is involved at diagnosis in approximately 80% of cases. Although the natural history is prolonged (overall median survival approximately 10 years), follicular lymphoma is not curable, a feature shared with most other relatively indolent lymphoid malignancies. As a result, therapy with cytotoxic drugs and agents such as rituximab (anti-CD20 antibody) is reserved for those with bulky, symptomatic disease. In about 30% to 40% of patients, follicular lymphoma progresses to diffuse large B-cell lymphoma. This transformation is an ominous event, since additional mutations that underlie such conversions render these tumors less curable than de novo diffuse large B-cell lymphomas, described later.

Mantle Cell Lymphoma

Mantle cell lymphoma is composed of cells resembling the naïve B cells found in the mantle zones of normal lymphoid follicles. It constitutes approximately 6% of all NHLs and occurs mainly in men older than 50 years of age.

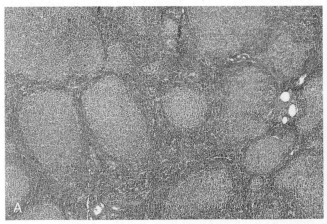
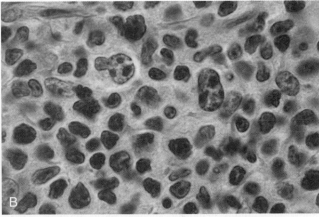

FIG. 10.20 Follicular lymphoma—lymph node. (A) Nodular aggregates of lymphoma cells are present throughout. (B) At high magnification, small lymphoid cells with condensed chromatin and irregular or cleaved nuclear outlines (centrocytes) are mixed with a population of larger cells with nucleoli (centroblasts). (A, Courtesy of Dr. Robert W. McKenna, Department of Pathology, University of Texas Southwestern Medical School, Dallas, Texas.)

Pathogenesis. **These tumors have an (11;14) translocation that fuses the cyclin D1 gene to the IgH locus.** This translocation leads to overexpression of cyclin D1, which you will recall stimulates growth by promoting the progression of cells from the G_1 phase to the S phase of the cell cycle by stimulating hyperphosphorylation of Rb (Chapter 6).

MORPHOLOGY AND ANCILLARY STUDIES

Morphology. Mantle cell lymphoma may involve lymph nodes in a diffuse or vaguely nodular pattern (eFig. 10.3). Proliferation centers are absent, a feature that distinguishes mantle cell lymphoma from CLL/SLL. The tumor cells are usually slightly larger than normal lymphocytes and have an irregular nucleus, inconspicuous nucleoli, and scant cytoplasm. Less commonly, the cells are larger and morphologically resemble lymphoblasts. The bone marrow is involved in most cases and the peripheral blood in about 20% of cases. The tumor sometimes involves the gastrointestinal tract, often manifesting as multifocal submucosal nodules that grossly resemble polyps **(lymphomatoid polyposis).**

Immunophenotype. The tumor cells express surface IgM and IgD, the B-cell antigen CD20, CD5 (as with CLL/SLL), and cyclin D1 protein.

Clinical Features. Most patients present with fatigue and lymphadenopathy and are found to have generalized disease involving the bone marrow, spleen, liver, and often the gastrointestinal tract. These tumors are moderately aggressive and incurable. The median survival is 6 to 7 years. Effective (but noncurative) treatments include BTK inhibitors as, like CLL/SLL cells, mantle cell lymphoma cells depend on signals generated through the B-cell receptor for survival.

Extranodal Marginal Zone Lymphoma

This indolent B-cell tumor arises most commonly in epithelial tissues such as the stomach, salivary glands, small and large bowel, lungs, orbit, and breast. It is also referred to as lymphoma of mucosa-associated lymphoid tissue (so-called MALToma).

Pathogenesis. **Extranodal marginal zone lymphoma is an example of a cancer that arises within and is sustained by chronic inflammation.** It tends to develop within tissues that are involved by chronic inflammation triggered by autoimmune disorders (such as the salivary gland in Sjögren syndrome and the thyroid gland in Hashimoto thyroiditis) or that are the sites of chronic infection (such as *H. pylori* gastritis). In the case of *H. pylori*—associated gastric marginal zone lymphoma, eradication of *H. pylori* with antibiotic therapy often leads to regression of the tumor, because the tumor cells depend on inflammatory cytokines secreted by *H. pylori*—specific T cells for their growth and survival. Based on these observations, it is thought that the disease is initiated within the context of an immune reaction against the bacteria. With the acquisition of driver mutations, a B-cell clone emerges that depends on antigen-stimulated T-helper cells for signals that drive growth and survival. At this stage, withdrawal of the responsible antigen causes tumor involution. As further clonal evolution leads to greater tumor cell autonomy, spread to distant sites or transformation to large B cell lymphoma may occur. This theme of polyclonal to monoclonal transition during lymphomagenesis is also applicable to the pathogenesis of EBV-induced lymphoma (discussed in Chapter 6).

MORPHOLOGY AND ANCILLARY STUDIES

Morphology. The clonal B cells characteristically infiltrate the epithelium of involved tissues, often collecting in small aggregates that are called **lymphoepithelial lesions** (eFig. 10.4). In some cases the tumor cells accumulate abundant pale cytoplasm or exhibit plasma cell differentiation, features that are characteristic but not pathognomonic.

Immunophenotype. This is a tumor of mature B cells expressing CD20 and surface immunoglobulin, usually IgM.

Clinical Features. These tumors often present as swelling of the salivary gland, thyroid, or orbit or are discovered incidentally in the setting of *H. pylori*—induced gastritis or an imaging procedure. When localized, they are often cured by simple excision followed by radiotherapy.

Diffuse Large B-Cell Lymphoma

Diffuse large B-cell lymphoma is the most common type of lymphoma in adults, accounting for approximately 35% of adult NHLs. It includes several subtypes that share an aggressive natural history.

Pathogenesis. About one-third of diffuse large B-cell lymphomas have rearrangements of the *BCL6* gene, located on 3q27, and an even higher fraction have activating point mutations in the *BCL6* promoter. Both aberrations result in increased levels of BCL6 protein, an important transcriptional regulator of gene expression in germinal center B cells. Another 30% of tumors have a (14;18) translocation involving the *BCL2* gene that results in overexpression of BCL2 protein. Some of these tumors may represent "transformed" follicular lymphomas. The remaining tumors have other diverse driver mutations, such as translocations involving the *MYC* gene.

MORPHOLOGY, ANCILLARY STUDIES, AND SPECIAL SUBTYPES

Morphology. The neoplastic B cells are large (at least three to four times the size of resting lymphocytes) and vary in appearance from tumor to tumor. Often, the tumor cells have round or oval nuclear contours, dispersed chromatin, several distinct nucleoli, and modest amounts of pale cytoplasm (Fig. 10.21). Other tumors have a round or multilobate vesicular nucleus, one or two prominent centrally placed nucleoli, and abundant pale or basophilic cytoplasm. Occasionally, the tumor cells are highly anaplastic and include tumor giant cells resembling Reed-Sternberg cells, the malignant cells of Hodgkin lymphoma.

Immunophenotype. These tumors express the B-cell marker CD20. Many also express surface IgM and/or IgG. Other markers (e.g., CD10, MYC, BCL2) are variably expressed.

Special subtypes. Several distinctive clinicopathologic subtypes are included in the category of diffuse large B-cell lymphoma.
- *EBV-associated diffuse large B-cell lymphomas* arise in the setting of AIDS, iatrogenic immunosuppression (e.g., in transplant recipients), and the elderly. In the posttransplant setting, these tumors often begin as EBV-driven polyclonal B-cell proliferations that may regress if immune function is restored.
- *Human herpesvirus type 8* (HHV8), also called *Kaposi sarcoma herpesvirus* (KSHV), is associated with rare *primary effusion lymphomas*, which may arise within the pleural cavity, pericardium, or peritoneum. These tumors

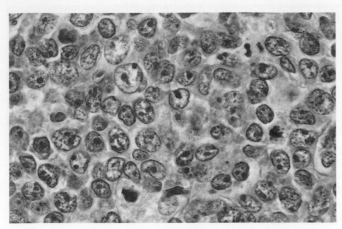

FIG. 10.21 Diffuse large B-cell lymphoma—lymph node. The tumor cells have large nuclei with open chromatin and prominent nucleoli. (Courtesy of Dr. Robert W. McKenna, Department of Pathology, University of Texas Southwestern Medical School, Dallas, Texas.)

are latently infected with HHV8, which encodes proteins homologous to several known oncoproteins, including cyclin D1. As with EBV-related lymphomas, most affected patients are immunosuppressed.
- *Mediastinal large B-cell lymphoma* frequently involves the thymus, occurs most often in young women, and shows a predilection for spread to abdominal viscera and the central nervous system. It is often associated with gene amplifications that lead to overexpression of the checkpoint molecule PD-L1, which is an important mechanism of immunoevasion in this tumor (Chapter 6).

Clinical Features. Although the median age at presentation is about 60 years, diffuse large B-cell lymphoma can occur at any age; it constitutes about 15% of childhood lymphomas. Patients typically present with a rapidly enlarging, often symptomatic mass at one or several sites. Extranodal presentations are common. The gastrointestinal tract is the most common extranodal site, but tumors can appear in virtually any organ or tissue. Unlike the more indolent lymphomas (e.g., follicular lymphoma), involvement of the liver, spleen, and bone marrow is not common at diagnosis.

Without treatment, diffuse large cell B-cell lymphomas are aggressive and rapidly fatal. With intensive combination chemotherapy and anti-CD20 immunotherapy, complete remissions are achieved in 60% to 80% of patients; of these, approximately 50% remain free of disease and appear to be cured. For those not so fortunate, other aggressive treatments (e.g., high-dose chemotherapy and hematopoietic stem cell transplantation) offer hope. As with B-ALL, CAR-T cell therapy directed against B-cell antigens such as CD19 can be curative but is expensive and may be associated with significant toxicity.

Burkitt Lymphoma

Burkitt lymphoma is endemic in parts of Africa and occurs sporadically in other geographic areas, including the United States. Histologically, the African and nonendemic diseases are identical, although there are clinical and virologic differences.

Pathogenesis. **Burkitt lymphoma is highly associated with translocations involving the *MYC* gene on chromosome 8 that result in overexpression of the MYC transcription factor.** As mentioned in Chapter 6, MYC is a master regulator of Warburg metabolism (aerobic glycolysis), a cancer hallmark that is associated with rapid cell growth. In keeping with this association, Burkitt lymphoma is among the fastest growing human tumors. Most translocations fuse *MYC* with the IgH gene on chromosome 14, but variant translocations involving the κ or λ light chain loci on chromosomes 2 and 22, respectively, are also observed. The net result of each is the same—the dysregulation and overexpression of *MYC*. In most endemic cases and about 20% of sporadic cases, the tumor cells are latently infected with EBV, a relationship also discussed in Chapter 6.

MORPHOLOGY AND ANCILLARY STUDIES

Morphology. The tumor cells are intermediate in size and typically have round or oval nuclei and two to five distinct nucleoli (Fig. 10.22). There is a moderate amount of basophilic or amphophilic cytoplasm that often contains small, lipid-filled vacuoles (a feature appreciated on smears). Very high rates of proliferation and apoptosis are characteristic, the latter accounting for the presence of numerous tissue macrophages containing ingested nuclear debris. These benign macrophages often are surrounded by a clear space, creating a **"starry sky" pattern.**

Immunophenotype. These tumors express surface IgM, the B-cell marker CD20, and the germinal center B-cell markers CD10 and BCL6.

Clinical Features. Both the endemic and nonendemic sporadic forms affect mainly children and young adults. Burkitt lymphoma accounts for approximately 30% of childhood NHLs in the United States. The disease usually arises at extranodal sites. Endemic tumors often manifest as maxillary or mandibular masses, whereas abdominal tumors involving the bowel, retroperitoneum, and ovaries are more common in North America. Leukemic presentations sometimes occur and must be distinguished from B-ALL, which is treated with different drug regimens. Burkitt lymphoma is highly aggressive; however, with very intensive chemotherapy regimens, the majority of patients are cured.

Miscellaneous Lymphoid Neoplasms

Among the many other forms of lymphoid neoplasms, several with distinctive or clinically important features merit brief discussion.

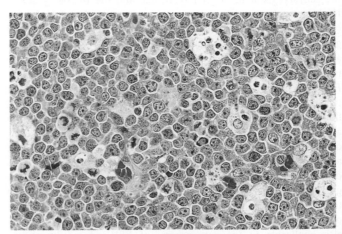

FIG. 10.22 Burkitt lymphoma—lymph node. The tumor cells and their nuclei are fairly uniform, giving a monotonous appearance. Note the high level of mitotic activity and "starry sky" pattern produced by interspersed, lightly staining, macrophages.

Hairy Cell Leukemia. **Hairy cell leukemia is an uncommon, indolent B-cell neoplasm that in virtually all cases is associated with activating mutations in the serine/threonine kinase BRAF, which is also mutated in diverse other cancers** (Chapter 6). It is morphologically distinctive, being characterized by the presence of fine, hairlike cytoplasmic projections (eFig. 10.5). The tumor cells express B-cell markers (CD20), surface immunoglobulin, and CD11c and CD103; the latter two antigens are not present on most other B-cell tumors, making them diagnostically useful.

Hairy cell leukemia occurs mainly in older males, and its manifestations result from infiltration of bone marrow and spleen. Splenomegaly, often massive, is the most common and sometimes only physical finding. Pancytopenia, resulting from marrow infiltration and splenic sequestration, is seen in more than half of cases. Lymph node involvement is rare. Leukocytosis is uncommon, being present in only 15% to 20% of patients, but scattered "hairy cells" can be identified in the peripheral blood smear in most cases.

The disease is indolent but progressive if untreated; pancytopenia and infections are the major clinical problems. Unlike most other indolent lymphoid neoplasms, hairy cell leukemia is extremely sensitive to particular "low dose" chemotherapeutic regimens. Complete, durable responses are the rule, and the overall prognosis is excellent. Tumors that fail conventional therapy respond well to BRAF inhibitors, which ultimately may become the treatment of choice.

Mycosis Fungoides and Sézary Syndrome. **These are tumors of neoplastic CD4+ T cells that home to the skin; as a result, they are often referred to as cutaneous T-cell lymphoma.** Mycosis fungoides usually manifests as a nonspecific erythrodermic rash that progresses with time to a plaque phase and then to a tumor phase. Histologically, neoplastic T cells, often with a cerebriform appearance produced by infolding of the nuclear membrane, infiltrate the epidermis and upper dermis (eFig. 10.6). With disease progression, both nodal and visceral dissemination appear. Sézary syndrome is a clinical variant characterized by (1) generalized exfoliative erythroderma and (2) tumor cells (Sézary cells) in the peripheral blood. Circulating tumor cells are also present in as many as 25% of cases of plaque- or tumor-phase mycosis fungoides. Patients diagnosed with early-phase mycosis fungoides often live with their disease for many years, whereas patients with tumor-phase disease, visceral disease, or Sézary syndrome survive on average for 3 years.

Adult T-Cell Leukemia/Lymphoma. **This neoplasm of CD4+ T cells is caused by a retrovirus, human T-cell leukemia virus type 1 (HTLV-1).** HTLV-1 infection is endemic in southern Japan, the Caribbean basin, and West Africa and occurs sporadically elsewhere, including in the southeastern United States. The pathogenesis of this tumor is discussed in Chapter 6. In addition to lymphoid malignancies, HTLV-1 infection can also cause tropical spastic paraparesis, a progressive demyelinating disease affecting the central nervous system and the spinal cord.

Adult T-cell leukemia/lymphoma is commonly associated with skin lesions, lymphadenopathy, hepatosplenomegaly, hypercalcemia, and variable lymphocytosis, often including cells with markedly irregular nuclear contours (eFig. 10.7). In addition to CD4, the leukemic cells express high levels of CD25, the IL-2 receptor α chain. In most cases the tumor is very aggressive and responds poorly to treatment. The median survival time is about 8 months.

Peripheral T-Cell Lymphoma. This heterogeneous group of tumors makes up about 10% of adult NHLs. Several distinctive subtypes are recognized but most peripheral T cell lymphomas lack defining genetic or immunophenotypic features and are lumped together into a "not otherwise specified" category. In general, these are aggressive tumors that respond poorly to therapy. Moreover, because these are tumors of functional T cells, patients often experience symptoms related to tumor-derived proinflammatory factors, even when the tumor burden is relatively low.

Hodgkin Lymphoma

Although both non-Hodgkin and Hodgkin lymphomas arise most commonly in lymphoid tissues, Hodgkin lymphoma is set apart by several features:

- The presence of distinctive neoplastic *Reed-Sternberg giant cells*
- *A robust, but ineffective, host immune response* to the Reed-Sternberg cells, such that tumor cells typically make up only a small fraction of the tumor mass
- It arises in a single lymph node or chain of lymph nodes and typically *spreads in a stepwise fashion* to anatomically contiguous nodes, a difference in behavior that has therapeutic implications

Classification. Five subtypes of Hodgkin lymphoma are recognized: (1) nodular sclerosis, (2) mixed cellularity, (3) lymphocyte rich, (4) lymphocyte depletion, and (5) nodular lymphocyte predominant. In the first four subtypes the RS cells share certain morphologic and immunophenotypic features (described later), allowing these entities to be lumped together under the rubric *classic Hodgkin lymphoma.* The nodular lymphocyte predominant type is set apart by the expression of germinal center B-cell markers in the Reed-Sternberg cells.

Pathogenesis. The origin of RS cells remained mysterious through most of the 20th century but was finally solved by elegant studies performed on single microdissected RS cells. These showed that every RS cell and variant from any given case possesses the same immunoglobulin gene rearrangements and that these rearranged immunoglobulin genes have undergone somatic hypermutation. As a result, it is now agreed that **Hodgkin lymphoma is a neoplasm that arises from germinal center B cells.**

Another clue into the etiology of Hodgkin lymphoma stems from the frequent involvement of EBV. EBV is present in the RS cells in as many as 70% of cases of the mixed-cellularity subtype and a smaller fraction of other classic forms of Hodgkin lymphoma. The integration site of the EBV genome is identical in all RS cells in a given case, indicating that infection precedes (and therefore may be related to) transformation and clonal expansion. Thus, EBV infection is probably one of several steps contributing to tumor development, particularly of the mixed-cellularity subtype.

The characteristic inflammatory cell infiltrate is generated by a number of cytokines. Some of these are secreted by RS cells, including IL-5, a chemoattractant for eosinophils; transforming growth factor-β, a fibrogenic factor; and IL-13, which may stimulate RS cell growth through an autocrine mechanism. Conversely, the responding inflammatory cells, rather than being innocent bystanders, produce additional factors that aid the growth and survival of RS cells and contribute further to the tissue reaction.

Hodgkin lymphoma is a cardinal example of a tumor that escapes from the host immune response by expressing proteins that inhibit T-cell activation. The RS cells of classic Hodgkin lymphoma often have mutations that lead to loss of β2-microglobulin function and a failure to express class I major histocompatibility complex (MHC) molecules. In addition, RS cells typically express high levels of PD-1 ligands, immune checkpoint factors that antagonize T-cell responses. In many tumors the region on chromosome 9 containing the genes encoding the two PD-1 ligands, PD-L1 and PD-L2, is amplified, an alteration that contributes to their overexpression. The importance of PD-1 ligand expression has been proven in clinical trials of antibodies that block PD-1, which is the T-cell receptor for the ligands (Chapter 6). Most tumors, even those that are resistant to all other therapies, are responsive to anti-PD-1 antibodies, presumably because it reactivates a latent host response that was stifled by the PD-1 ligand/PD-1 signaling axis.

MORPHOLOGY

The *sine qua non* of Hodgkin lymphoma is the **Reed-Sternberg (RS) cell** (Fig. 10.23), a very large cell (15 to 45 μm in diameter) with an enormous multilobate nucleus, exceptionally prominent nucleoli, and abundant, usually slightly eosinophilic, cytoplasm. Particularly characteristic are cells with **two mirror-image nuclei or nuclear lobes, each containing a large (inclusion-like) acidophilic nucleolus surrounded by a clear zone,** features that impart an "owl-eye" appearance. Typical RS cells and variants have a characteristic immunophenotype; they express CD15 and CD30 and fail to express CD45 (leukocyte common antigen) and B-cell and T-cell markers. As we shall see, "classic" RS cells are common in the mixed-cellularity subtype, uncommon in the nodular sclerosis subtype, and rare in the lymphocyte-predominance subtype; in these latter two subtypes, other characteristic RS cell variants predominate.

Nodular sclerosis Hodgkin lymphoma is the most common form. It is equally frequent in men and women and has a striking propensity to involve the lower cervical, supraclavicular, and mediastinal lymph nodes. Most patients are adolescents or young adults, and the overall prognosis is excellent. It is characterized morphologically by the following:

- **Lacunar cells** (Fig. 10.24), an RS cell variant with a single multilobate nucleus, multiple small nucleoli, and abundant, pale-staining cytoplasm. In sections of formalin-fixed tissue, the cytoplasm is often torn away, leaving the nucleus lying in an empty space (a lacune). The immunophenotype of lacunar variants is identical to that of other RS cells found in classic subtypes. As in other forms of classic Hodgkin lymphoma, the RS cells are surrounded by numerous reactive lymphocytes, eosinophils, and macrophages.
- **Collagen bands,** which divide the involved lymphoid tissue into circumscribed cellular nodules (Fig. 10.25). The fibrosis may be scant or abundant.

Mixed-cellularity Hodgkin lymphoma is the most common form of Hodgkin lymphoma in patients older than 50 years of age and comprises about 25% of cases overall. There is a male predominance. **Classic RS cells are plentiful** within a heterogeneous inflammatory infiltrate containing small lymphocytes, eosinophils, plasma cells, and macrophages (Fig. 10.26). This subtype is more likely to be disseminated and to be associated with systemic manifestations than the nodular sclerosis subtype, but the overall prognosis is still very good.

Lymphocyte-rich and lymphocyte depleted Hodgkin lymphoma are uncommon subtypes defined by the tissue reaction to the RS cells and variants. Diagnostic RS cells are found in both with immunophenotypic features identical to other more common forms of "classic" Hodgkin lymphoma.

Nodular lymphocyte-predominant Hodgkin lymphoma, accounting for about 5% of cases, is characterized by the presence of **lymphohistiocytic (L&H) variant RS cells** that have a delicate multilobed nucleus resembling popped corn ("popcorn cell"). L&H variants are usually found within large nodules containing mainly small B cells admixed with variable numbers of macrophages (Fig. 10.27). Other reactive cells, such as eosinophils, are scanty or absent, and typical RS cells are rare. Unlike the RS variants in classic Hodgkin lymphoma, L&H variants express B-cell markers (e.g., CD20) and usually fail to express CD15 and CD30. Most patients present with isolated cervical or axillary lymphadenopathy, and the prognosis typically is excellent.

It is apparent that Hodgkin lymphoma spans a wide range of histologic patterns that often simulate a reactive inflammatory process. Regardless of subtype, **the diagnosis rests on the definitive identification of RS cells or variants in the appropriate background of reactive cells.** Immunophenotyping plays an important role in distinguishing Hodgkin lymphoma from reactive conditions and other forms of lymphoma. In all subtypes, involvement of the spleen, liver, bone marrow, and other organs may appear in due course and takes the form of irregular nodules composed of a mixture of RS cells and reactive cells, similar to what is observed in lymph nodes.

Clinical Features. Hodgkin lymphoma, like NHL, usually manifests as painless lymphadenopathy. Although a definitive distinction from NHL can be made only by examination of a tissue biopsy, several clinical features favor the diagnosis of Hodgkin lymphoma

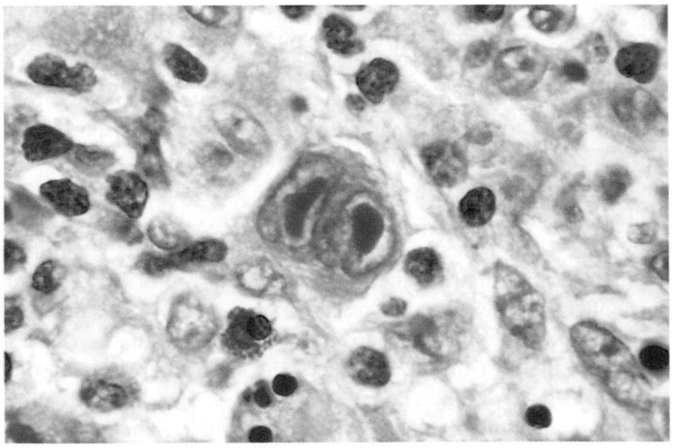

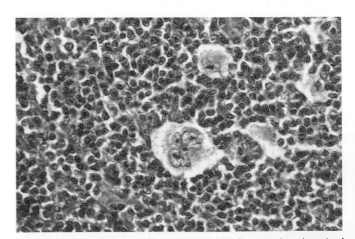

FIG. 10.23 Hodgkin lymphoma—lymph node. A binucleate Reed-Sternberg cell with large, inclusion-like nucleoli and abundant cytoplasm is surrounded by lymphocytes, macrophages, and an eosinophil. (Courtesy of Dr. Robert W. McKenna, Department of Pathology, University of Texas Southwestern Medical School, Dallas, Texas.)

FIG. 10.24 Hodgkin lymphoma, nodular sclerosis type—lymph node. A distinctive "lacunar cell" with a multilobed nucleus containing many small nucleoli is seen lying within a clear space created by retraction of its cytoplasm. It is surrounded by lymphocytes. (Courtesy of Dr. Robert W. McKenna, Department of Pathology, University of Texas Southwestern Medical School, Dallas, Texas.)

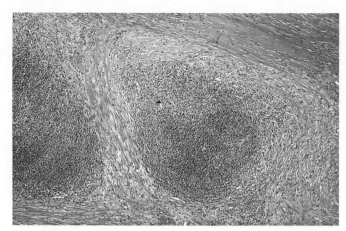

FIG. 10.25 Hodgkin lymphoma, nodular sclerosis type—lymph node. A low-power view shows well-defined bands of pink, acellular collagen that have subdivided the tumor cells into nodules. (Courtesy of Dr. Robert W. McKenna, Department of Pathology, University of Texas Southwestern Medical School, Dallas, Texas.)

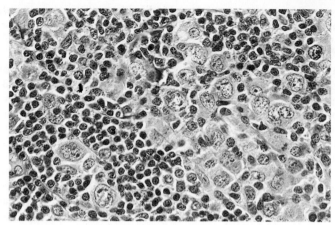

FIG. 10.27 Hodgkin lymphoma, nodular lymphocyte-predominant type—lymph node. Numerous mature-looking lymphocytes surround scattered, large, pale-staining lymphocytic and histiocytic variants ("popcorn" cells).

(Table 10.8). After the diagnosis is established, staging is used to guide therapy and determine prognosis (Table 10.9). Younger patients with more favorable subtypes tend to present with stage I or stage II disease and usually are free of so-called "B symptoms" (fever, weight loss, night sweats). Patients with advanced disease (stages III and IV) are more likely to exhibit B symptoms as well as pruritus and anemia. Because of the long-term complications of radiotherapy, even patients with stage I disease are now treated with systemic chemotherapy. More advanced disease is generally also treated with chemotherapy, and in selected cases with involved field radiotherapy.

The outlook, even for those with advanced disease, is very good. The 5-year survival rate for patients with stage I-A or II-A disease is more than 90%. Even with advanced disease (stage IV-A or IV-B), the overall 5-year disease-free survival rate is around 50%. Among long-term survivors treated with radiotherapy, a higher risk of certain malignancies, including lung cancer and breast cancer, as well as cardiovascular disease, has been reported. These sobering results have spurred development of new regimens that minimize the use of radiotherapy and use less toxic chemotherapy. As already mentioned, anti–PD-1 antibodies produce excellent responses in patients with

Table 10.8 Clinical Differences Between Hodgkin and Non-Hodgkin Lymphomas

Hodgkin Lymphoma	Non-Hodgkin Lymphoma
More often localized to a single axial group of nodes (cervical, mediastinal, paraaortic)	More frequent involvement of multiple lymph node groups
Orderly spread by contiguity	Noncontiguous spread
Mesenteric nodes and Waldeyer ring rarely involved	Mesenteric nodes and Waldeyer ring commonly involved
Extranodal involvement uncommon	Extranodal involvement common

Table 10.9 Clinical Staging of Hodgkin and Non-Hodgkin Lymphomas (Ann Arbor Classification)[a]

Stage	Distribution of Disease
I	Involvement of a single lymph node region (I) or involvement of a single extralymphatic organ or tissue (I_E)
II	Involvement of two or more lymph node regions on the same side of the diaphragm alone (II) or with involvement of limited contiguous extralymphatic organs or tissue (II_E)
III	Involvement of lymph node regions on both sides of the diaphragm (III), which may include the spleen (III_S), limited contiguous extralymphatic organ or site (III_E), or both (III_{ES})
IV	Multiple or disseminated foci of involvement of one or more extralymphatic organs or tissues with or without lymphatic involvement

[a]All stages are further divided based on the absence (A) or presence (B) of the following systemic symptoms and signs: significant fever, night sweats, unexplained loss of more than 10% of normal body weight.
From Carbone PT, et al: Symposium (Ann Arbor): staging in Hodgkin disease, *Cancer Res* 31:1707, 1971.

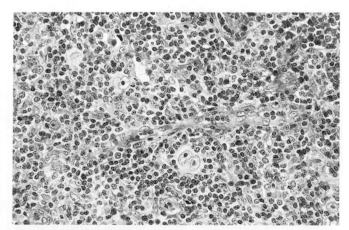

FIG. 10.26 Hodgkin lymphoma, mixed-cellularity type—lymph node. A diagnostic, binucleate Reed-Sternberg cell is surrounded by eosinophils, lymphocytes, and histiocytes. (Courtesy of Dr. Robert W. McKenna, Department of Pathology, University of Texas Southwestern Medical School, Dallas, Texas.)

relapsed, refractory classic Hodgkin lymphoma and is a promising immunotherapy.

Plasma Cell Neoplasms and Related Entities

These B-cell proliferations contain neoplastic plasma cells that virtually always secrete a monoclonal immunoglobulin or immunoglobulin fragments, which serve as tumor markers and often have pathologic effects. Collectively, plasma cell neoplasms and related disorders account for about 10% of hematologic malignancies and about 15% of the deaths caused by lymphoid neoplasms, with most of these deaths being caused by multiple myeloma (discussed later).

The monoclonal immunoglobulins secreted into the blood by these tumors is referred to as an *M protein* (or M component, originally called myeloma protein). Because complete M proteins have molecular weights of 160 kilodaltons or higher, they are restricted to the plasma and extracellular fluid and excluded from the urine in the absence of glomerular damage. However, neoplastic plasma cells often synthesize excess immunoglobulin light chains along with complete immunoglobulins; the free light chains have a molecular weight of approximately 25 kilodaltons and pass through glomerular slit diaphragms into the urinary space. They are referred to as *Bence Jones proteins*. In unusual cases, tumors may produce only light chains, which are detected and quantified in the blood and the urine by highly sensitive tests.

Terms used to describe the abnormal immunoglobulins associated with plasma cell neoplasms include *monoclonal gammopathy, dysproteinemia,* and *paraproteinemia*. These abnormal proteins are associated with several clinicopathologic entities:

- *Multiple myeloma*, the most important plasma cell neoplasm, usually presents as tumor masses scattered throughout the skeletal system. *Solitary plasmacytoma* is an infrequent variant that presents as a single mass in bone or soft tissue. *Smoldering myeloma* is another uncommon variant defined by a lack of symptoms and a high plasma M component.
- *Monoclonal gammopathy of undetermined significance (MGUS)* is applied to patients without signs or symptoms who have small to moderately large M components in their blood. MGUS is very common in older adults and has a low but constant rate of transformation to a symptomatic monoclonal gammopathy, most often multiple myeloma.
- *Primary or immunocyte-associated amyloidosis* results from a monoclonal proliferation of plasma cells secreting light chains that are deposited as amyloid. Some patients have overt multiple myeloma, but others have only a minor clonal population of plasma cells in the marrow.
- *Waldenström macroglobulinemia* is a syndrome in which high levels of IgM lead to symptoms related to hyperviscosity of the blood. It occurs in older adults, most commonly in association with lymphoplasmacytic lymphoma (described later).

With this background, we now turn to specific clinicopathologic entities. Primary amyloidosis was discussed along with other disorders of the immune system in Chapter 5.

Multiple Myeloma

Multiple myeloma is one of the most common lymphoid malignancies; approximately 30,000 new cases are diagnosed in the United States each year. The median age at diagnosis is 70 years, and it is more common in males and, for unknown reasons, occurs more frequently in the United States in people of African descent. It principally involves the bone marrow and is usually associated with lytic lesions throughout the skeletal system.

The most frequent M protein produced by myeloma cells is IgG (60%), followed by IgA (20%—25%); only rarely are IgM, IgD, or IgE M proteins observed. In the remaining cases, the plasma cells produce only κ or λ light chains.

Pathogenesis. As with most other B-cell malignancies, **myeloma often has chromosomal translocations that fuse the IgH locus on chromosome 14 to oncogenes such as the cyclin D1 and cyclin D3 genes.** As might be surmised from this, dysregulation of D cyclins is common in multiple myeloma and is believed to contribute to increases in cell proliferation. Proliferation of myeloma cells is also supported by the cytokine interleukin-6 (IL-6), which is mainly produced by fibroblasts and macrophages in the bone marrow stroma. Late in the course, translocations involving *MYC* are sometimes observed, particularly in patients with aggressive disease.

Multiple myeloma has a number of untoward effects on the skeleton, the immune system, and the kidney, all of which contribute to morbidity and mortality:

- **Factors produced by neoplastic plasma cells cause resorption of bone, the major pathologic feature of multiple myeloma.** Of particular importance, myeloma-derived factors upregulate the expression of the receptor activator of NF-κB ligand (RANKL) by bone marrow stromal cells, which in turn activate osteoclasts. Other factors released from tumor cells are potent inhibitors of osteoblast function. The net effect is increased bone resorption, leading to hypercalcemia and pathologic fractures.
- **Myeloma causes defects in humoral immunity.** Through uncertain mechanisms, myeloma cells compromise the function of normal B cells. Ironically, although the plasma has elevated levels of immunoglobulin owing to the presence of an M protein, the production of functional antibodies is often profoundly depressed. As a result, patients are at high risk for bacterial infections.
- **Renal dysfunction** stems from several pathologic effects of myeloma that may occur alone or in combination. Most important are *obstructive proteinaceous casts* that often form in the distal convoluted tubules and the collecting ducts. The casts consist mostly of Bence Jones proteins along with variable amounts of complete immunoglobulin, proteins secreted from tubular epithelium, and albumin. *Light chain deposition* in the glomeruli or the interstitium, either as amyloid or linear deposits, may also contribute to renal damage. Completing the assault is hypercalcemia, which may lead to dehydration and renal stones, and an increased incidence of bacterial pyelonephritis, which stems in part from the hypogammaglobulinemia.

MORPHOLOGY AND ANCILLARY FINDINGS

Morphology. Multiple myeloma usually manifests with **multifocal destructive skeletal lesions** that most commonly involve the vertebral column, ribs, skull, pelvis, femur, clavicle, and scapula. The lesions arise in the medullary cavity, erode cancellous bone, and progressively destroy the bone cortex. Bone destruction often leads to **pathologic fractures,** most frequently in the vertebral column or femur. The bone lesions usually appear as **punched-out defects** 1 to 4 cm in diameter (Fig. 10.28A). Microscopic examination of the marrow shows increased numbers of plasma cells, which usually constitute greater than 30% of the cellularity. Myeloma cells may resemble normal plasma cells but more often show abnormal features such as prominent nucleoli or cytoplasmic inclusions **(Russell bodies)** containing immunoglobulin (Fig. 10.28B). With disease progression, myeloma cells may spread to the viscera and other soft tissue sites, and in terminal stages a leukemic picture may emerge.

Renal involvement **(myeloma kidney)** is associated with proteinaceous casts consisting mostly of Bence Jones proteins that obstruct the distal convoluted tubules and the collecting ducts. Multinucleate giant cells derived from macrophages usually surround the casts. Very often the **epithelial cells adjacent to the casts become necrotic or atrophic** owing to the toxic effects of Bence Jones proteins. Other common pathologic processes involving the kidney include **metastatic calcification,** stemming from bone resorption and hypercalcemia; **light chain (AL) amyloidosis,** involving the renal glomeruli and vessel walls; and **bacterial pyelonephritis,** secondary to the increased susceptibility to bacterial infections. Rarely, infiltrates of neoplastic plasma cells are seen in the renal interstitium.

Laboratory Studies. Laboratory analyses typically show increased levels of immunoglobulins in the blood and/or Bence Jones proteins in the urine. Free light chains and an M protein component are observed together in 60% to 70% of cases, whereas in about 20% of patients only free light chains are present. Around 1% of myelomas are nonsecretory; hence, the absence of a detectable M component does not completely exclude the diagnosis.

Clinical Features. Clinical findings stem mainly from (1) the effects of plasma cells on the skeleton; (2) the production of excessive immunoglobulins, which often have abnormal physicochemical properties; (3) the suppression of humoral immunity; and (4) renal insufficiency.

Bone resorption often leads to pathologic fractures and chronic pain. The attendant hypercalcemia can give rise to neurologic manifestations, such as confusion, weakness, and lethargy, and contributes to renal dysfunction. Decreased production of normal immunoglobulins sets the stage for recurrent bacterial infections. Of great significance is renal insufficiency, which trails only infections as a cause of death. Renal failure occurs in up to 50% of patients and is positively correlated with the level of Bence Jones proteinuria, highlighting the importance of free light chains in renal disease. Certain light chains are also prone to cause amyloidosis of the AL type (Chapter 5), which can exacerbate renal dysfunction and deposit in other tissues as well.

The diagnosis rests on radiologic and laboratory findings, including assays that detect and quantify M proteins and Bence Jones proteins. It can be strongly suspected when imaging studies show typical bone lesions, but definitive diagnosis requires a bone marrow examination. Marrow involvement often gives rise to a normocytic normochromic anemia, sometimes accompanied by moderate leukopenia and thrombocytopenia.

The prognosis is variable. Patients with multiple bony lesions, if untreated, rarely survive for more than 6 to 12 months, whereas asymptomatic patients with a high plasma M component, so called "smoldering myeloma," may not require treatment for many years. The median survival is approximately 5 years. Although cures have yet to be achieved, advances in therapy offer hope. Myeloma cells are prone to accumulate misfolded, unpaired immunoglobulin chains and as a result are sensitive to inhibitors of the proteasome, a cellular organelle that degrades misfolded proteins. Misfolded proteins activate apoptotic pathways (Chapter 2) and proteasome inhibitors induce myeloma cell death by exacerbating this inherent tendency. Thalidomide-like drugs are also effective in treating myeloma by stimulating the degradation of specific prooncogenic myeloma cell proteins. Bisphosphonates, drugs that inhibit bone resorption, reduce pathologic fractures and limit the hypercalcemia. Hematopoietic stem cell transplantation prolongs life but is not curative. New CAR-T cell therapies using cytotoxic T cells engineered to recognize plasma cell

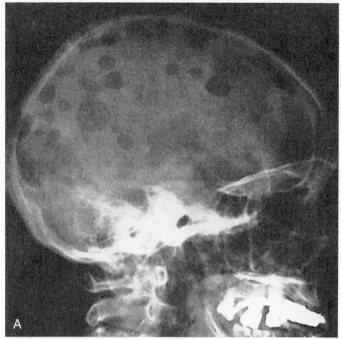

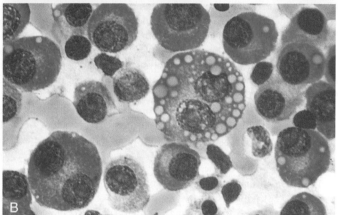

FIG. 10.28 Multiple myeloma. (A) Radiograph of the skull, lateral view. The sharply punched-out bone defects are most obvious in the calvaria. (B) Bone marrow aspirate. Normal marrow cells are largely replaced by plasma cells, including atypical forms with multiple nuclei, prominent nucleoli, and cytoplasmic droplets containing immunoglobulin (Russell bodies).

antigens have produced excellent results and are now available for use when other therapies fail.

Lymphoplasmacytic Lymphoma

Lymphoplasmacytic lymphoma is a B-cell neoplasm of older adults that usually presents in the sixth or seventh decade of life. Although bearing a superficial resemblance to CLL/SLL, it differs in that a substantial fraction of the tumor cells undergo terminal differentiation to plasma cells. Most commonly, the plasma cell component secretes monoclonal IgM, often in amounts sufficient to cause a hyperviscosity syndrome known as *Waldenström macroglobulinemia*. Unlike multiple myeloma, complications stemming from the secretion of free light chains (e.g., renal failure and amyloidosis) are relatively rare and bone destruction does not occur.

Pathogenesis. **Virtually all cases of lymphoplasmacytic lymphoma are associated with acquired activating mutations in *MYD88.*** The *MYD88* gene encodes an adaptor protein that participates in signaling events that activate NF-κB, which promotes the growth and survival of the tumor cells.

MORPHOLOGY AND ANCILLARY FINDINGS

Morphology. Typically, the marrow contains an infiltrate of lymphocytes, plasma cells, and plasmacytoid lymphocytes in varying proportions (eFig. 10.8), often accompanied by mast cell hyperplasia. Periodic acid-Schiff—positive inclusions containing immunoglobulin are frequently seen in the cytoplasm (**Russell bodies**) or the nucleus (**Dutcher bodies**) of some of the plasmacytoid cells. At diagnosis the tumor has usually disseminated to the lymph nodes, spleen, and liver. Infiltration of the nerve roots, meninges, and more rarely the brain may also occur with disease progression.

Immunophenotype. The lymphoid component expresses B-cell markers such as CD20 and surface immunoglobulin, whereas the plasma cell component secretes the same immunoglobulin that is expressed on the surface of the lymphoid cells. In almost all tumors, the secreted immunoglobulin is an IgM.

Clinical Features. The dominant presenting complaints are nonspecific and include weakness, fatigue, and weight loss. Approximately half the patients have lymphadenopathy, hepatomegaly, and splenomegaly. Anemia caused by marrow infiltration is common. About 10% of patients have autoimmune hemolysis caused by cold agglutinins, IgM antibodies that bind to red cells at temperatures of less than 37°C (discussed earlier).

Patients with IgM-secreting tumors have additional signs and symptoms stemming from the physicochemical properties of IgM. Because of its large size, at high concentrations IgM greatly increases the viscosity of the blood, giving rise to a *hyperviscosity syndrome* characterized by the following:

- *Visual impairment* associated with venous congestion, which is reflected by striking tortuosity and distention of retinal veins; retinal hemorrhages and exudates may also contribute to problems with vision
- *Neurologic problems* such as headaches, dizziness, deafness, and stupor, all stemming from sluggish venous blood flow
- *Bleeding* related to the formation of complexes between macroglobulins and clotting factors as well as interference with platelet function
- *Cryoglobulinemia* resulting from the precipitation of IgM at low temperatures, which produces symptoms such as Raynaud phenomenon and cold urticaria

Lymphoplasmacytic lymphoma is an indolent disease. Because most IgM is intravascular, symptoms caused by the high IgM levels (e.g., hyperviscosity and hemolysis) can be alleviated by plasmapheresis. Tumor growth can be controlled with low doses of chemotherapeutic drugs and immunotherapy with anti-CD20 antibody, and recent work has shown that BTK inhibitors are also effective. Transformation to large-cell lymphoma occurs but is uncommon. With new therapies such as BTK inhibitors, the median survival is approximately 10 years.

Before ending our review of lymphoid and plasma cell neoplasms, it is worthwhile pausing to summarize the manner in which common driver mutations in specific entities produce changes in cellular

behavior that exemplify particular hallmarks of cancer (Fig. 10.29). Such alterations not only highlight important pathogenic principles but are also increasingly the targets of effective therapies, such as antibodies that block PD-1 (Hodgkin lymphoma) and drugs that antagonize BCL2 (chronic lymphocytic leukemia and other B-cell tumors).

Histiocytic Neoplasms

Langerhans Cell Histiocytosis

The term *histiocytosis* is an "umbrella" designation for a variety of proliferative disorders of dendritic cells or macrophages. Some, such as very rare histiocytic sarcomas, are highly malignant neoplasms. Others, such as most histiocytic proliferations in lymph nodes, are completely benign and reactive. Between these two extremes lie a group of uncommon tumors composed of Langerhans cells, collectively called *Langerhans cell histiocytosis.* As described in Chapter 5, Langerhans cells are immature dendritic cells found in the epidermis; similar cells are found in many other organs, where they function to capture antigens and display them to T cells.

Langerhans cell proliferations take on different clinical forms, but all are believed to be variations of the same basic disorder. The proliferating Langerhans cells express MHC class II antigens, CD1a, and langerin. Langerin is a transmembrane protein found in *Birbeck granules,* cytoplasmic pentalaminar rodlike tubular structures that in electron micrographs have a characteristic periodicity and sometimes a dilated terminal end ("tennis racket" appearance). Under the light microscope, the proliferating Langerhans cells do not resemble their normal dendritic counterparts. Instead, they have abundant, often vacuolated cytoplasm and vesicular folded nuclei (eFig. 10.9), an appearance more akin to that of tissue macrophages (called histiocytes by morphologists)—hence the term *Langerhans cell histiocytosis.*

Langerhans cell histiocytosis can be grouped into two relatively distinctive clinicopathologic entities.

- *Multisystem Langerhans cell histiocytosis (Letterer-Siwe disease)* usually occurs in children younger than 2 years of age. It typically manifests with multifocal cutaneous lesions that grossly resemble seborrheic skin eruptions and are composed of Langerhans cells. Most affected patients have hepatosplenomegaly, lymphadenopathy, pulmonary lesions, and (later in the course) destructive osteolytic bone lesions. Extensive marrow infiltration often leads to pancytopenia and predisposes the patient to recurrent bacterial infections. The disease is rapidly fatal if untreated. With intensive chemotherapy, 50% of patients survive 5 years.
- *Unisystem Langerhans cell histiocytosis (eosinophilic granuloma)* may be unifocal or multifocal. It is characterized by expanding accumulations of Langerhans cells, usually within the medullary cavities of bones or less commonly in the skin, lungs, or stomach. The Langerhans cells are admixed with variable numbers of lymphocytes, plasma cells, neutrophils, and eosinophils, which are usually prominent. Virtually any bone may be involved; the calvaria, ribs, and femur are most commonly affected. *Unifocal disease* most often involves a single bone. It may be asymptomatic or cause pain, tenderness, and pathologic fracture. It is an indolent disorder that may heal spontaneously or be cured by local excision or irradiation. *Multifocal unisystem disease* usually affects children and typically manifests with multiple erosive bony masses that sometimes extend into soft tissues. In about 50% of cases, involvement of the posterior pituitary stalk of the hypothalamus leads to diabetes insipidus. The combination of calvarial bone defects, diabetes insipidus, and exophthalmos is referred to as the *Hand-Schüller-*

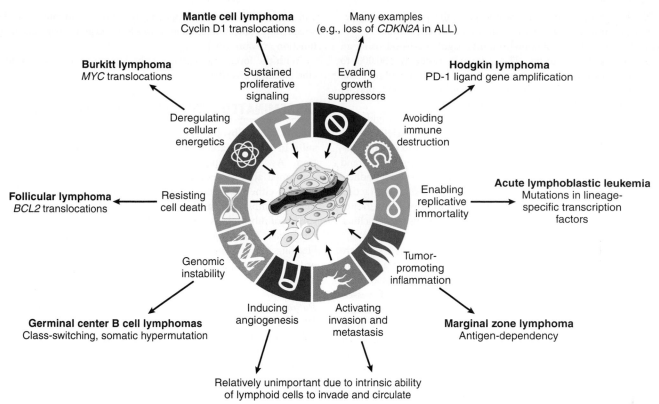

FIG. 10.29 Cancer hallmarks exemplified by particular lymphoid neoplasms. Some of the best characterized pathogenic mechanisms in lymphoid malignancies are summarized here, including dysregulation of MYC in Burkitt lymphoma (leading to Warburg metabolism and rapid cell growth); dysregulation of BCL2 in follicular lymphoma (leading to resistance to apoptosis); PD-1 ligand gene amplification in Hodgkin lymphoma (leading to evasion of host immunity); events leading to loss of cell cycle control (cyclin D1 rearrangements in mantle cell lymphoma and loss of the *CDKN2A* gene in acute lymphoblastic leukemia [ALL]); mutations in various transcription factors, particularly in ALL, that block differentiation and enhance "leukemia stem cell" self-renewal; and chronic immune stimulation, in marginal zone lymphoma. By contrast, because lymphoid cells normally circulate throughout the body, there is relatively little selective pressure in lymphoid malignancies for aberrations that increase angiogenesis or activate invasion and metastasis. *ALL,* Acute lymphoblastic leukemia; *PD-1,* programmed cell death protein 1.

Christian triad. Many patients experience spontaneous regressions; others are treated effectively with chemotherapy.

A clue to the pathogenesis of Langerhans cell tumors lies in the discovery that the different clinical forms are frequently associated with an acquired mutation in the serine/threonine kinase BRAF, which leads to hyperactivity of the kinase. This same mutation is found in a variety of other tumors, including hairy cell leukemia (described earlier), benign nevi, melanoma, papillary thyroid carcinoma, and some colon cancers (Chapter 6). BRAF is a component of the RAS signaling pathway that drives cellular proliferation and survival, effects that likely contribute to the growth of neoplastic Langerhans cells. Notably, BRAF inhibitor therapy is effective in tumors with BRAF mutations and has emerged as a targeted therapy for these disorders.

BLEEDING DISORDERS

These disorders are characterized clinically by abnormal bleeding, which may appear spontaneously or follow an inciting event (e.g., trauma or surgery). A review of the laboratory tests used to evaluate patients with a suspected bleeding disorder along with the underlying principles is presented next, followed by consideration of specific disorders of coagulation. We conclude with a discussion of a few clinically important complications of blood product transfusion.

The most important tests for investigation of suspected coagulopathies are the following:

- *Prothrombin time* (PT). This test assesses the extrinsic and common coagulation pathways (Chapter 3). It measures the time (in seconds) needed for plasma to clot after addition of tissue thromboplastin (e.g., brain extract) and Ca^{2+} ions. A prolonged PT can result from deficiencies of factor V, VII, X, prothrombin, or fibrinogen, or the presence of an acquired inhibitor (typically an antibody) that interferes with the extrinsic pathway.
- *Partial thromboplastin time* (PTT). This test assesses the intrinsic and common coagulation pathways. It measures the time (in seconds) needed for the plasma to clot after the addition of kaolin, cephalin, and Ca^{2+}. Kaolin activates the contact-dependent factor XII and cephalin substitutes for platelet phospholipids. Prolongation of PTT can be caused by deficiencies of factor V, VIII, IX,

X, XI, XII, prothrombin, or fibrinogen, or the presence of an acquired inhibitor that interferes with the intrinsic pathway.

- *Platelet count.* This is obtained on anticoagulated blood using an electronic particle counter. The reference range is 150,000 to 450,000/μL. Counts outside this range must be confirmed by visual inspection of a peripheral blood smear, as the electronic platelet count may be thrown off by a number of artifacts.
- *Tests of platelet function.* At present no single test provides an adequate assessment of the complex functions of platelets. Aggregation tests that measure the response of platelets to certain agonists and qualitative and quantitative tests of von Willebrand factor (vWF) (which you will recall is required for platelet adherence to collagen) are both commonly used in clinical practice. Instrument-based assays that provide quantitative measures of platelet function are not yet available for routine use in the clinic.

In addition to these standard tests, more specialized tests are available that measure the levels of specific clotting factors and fibrin split products or assess the presence of circulating anticoagulants.

Bleeding disorders may stem from abnormalities of vessels (including their supportive connective tissue), platelets, or coagulation factors, alone or in combination. Bleeding resulting from *vascular fragility* is seen with vitamin C deficiency (scurvy) (Chapter 7), amyloidosis affecting blood vessels (Chapter 5), chronic glucocorticoid use, rare inherited conditions affecting the connective tissues, and a large number of infectious and hypersensitivity vasculitides. Some of these conditions are discussed in other chapters; others are beyond the scope of this book. Bleeding that results purely from vascular fragility is characterized by the "spontaneous" appearance of petechiae and ecchymoses in the skin and mucous membranes (probably resulting from minor trauma). In most instances laboratory tests of coagulation are normal.

Bleeding may result from systemic conditions that inflame or damage endothelial cells. If severe enough, such insults convert the vascular lining to a prothrombotic surface that activates coagulation throughout the circulatory system, a condition known as *disseminated intravascular coagulation* (DIC) (discussed in the next section). Paradoxically, in DIC, platelets and coagulation factors are often used up faster than they can be replaced, resulting in deficiencies that may lead to severe bleeding (a condition referred to as *consumptive coagulopathy*).

Deficiencies of platelets (thrombocytopenia) are an important cause of bleeding. These occur in a variety of clinical settings that are discussed later. Other bleeding disorders stem from qualitative defects in platelet function. Such defects may be acquired, as in uremia and certain myeloproliferative neoplasms and after aspirin ingestion; or inherited, as in von Willebrand disease and other rare congenital disorders. The clinical signs of inadequate platelet function include easy bruising, nosebleeds (epistaxis), excessive bleeding from minor trauma, and menorrhagia.

In bleeding disorders stemming from defects in one or more coagulation factors, the PT, PTT, or both are prolonged. Unlike platelet defects, petechiae and mucosal bleeding are usually absent. Instead, hemorrhages tend to occur in parts of the body that are subject to trauma, such as the joints of the lower extremities. Massive hemorrhage may occur after surgery, dental procedures, or severe trauma. This category includes the hemophilias, an important group of inherited coagulation disorders.

It is not uncommon for bleeding to occur as a consequence of a mixture of defects. This is the case in DIC, in which both thrombocytopenia and coagulation factor deficiencies contribute to bleeding,

and in von Willebrand disease, a fairly common inherited disorder in which both platelet function and (to a lesser degree) coagulation factor function are abnormal.

With the foregoing overview as background, we now turn to specific bleeding disorders.

DISSEMINATED INTRAVASCULAR COAGULATION (DIC)

DIC is caused by the systemic activation of coagulation and results in the formation of thrombi throughout the microcirculation. As a consequence, platelets and coagulation factors are consumed and, secondarily, fibrinolysis is activated. Thus, DIC can give rise either to tissue hypoxia and microinfarcts caused by myriad microthrombi or to a bleeding disorder related to pathologic activation of fibrinolysis and depletion of the elements required for hemostasis (*consumptive coagulopathy*). This entity probably causes bleeding more commonly than all the congenital coagulation disorders combined, as it occurs as a complication of a wide variety of disorders.

Pathogenesis. Before discussing specific disorders associated with DIC, we must first consider in a general way the pathogenic mechanisms by which intravascular clotting occurs. Reference to earlier comments on normal hemostasis (Chapter 3) may be helpful at this point. Recall that clotting can be initiated by either the extrinsic pathway, which is triggered by the release of tissue factor (tissue thromboplastin), or the intrinsic pathway, which involves the activation of factor XII by surface contact, collagen, or negatively charged substances. Both pathways lead to the generation of thrombin. Clotting is normally limited by the rapid clearance of activated clotting factors by the liver, the action of endogenous anticoagulants (e.g., protein C), and the concomitant activation of fibrinolytic factors.

DIC is usually triggered by either (1) the release of tissue factor or procoagulants into the circulation or (2) widespread endothelial cell damage (Fig. 10.30). Thromboplastic substances can be released into the circulation from a variety of sources—for example, the placenta in obstetric complications or certain types of cancer cells, particularly those of acute promyelocytic leukemia and adenocarcinomas. Cancer cells may also provoke coagulation in other ways, such as by releasing proteolytic enzymes or expressing tissue factor. In bacterial sepsis (an important cause of DIC), microbial endotoxins or exotoxins stimulate the expression of tissue factor on monocytes. Activated monocytes also release IL-1 and tumor necrosis factor, both of which stimulate the expression of tissue factor on endothelial cells and simultaneously decrease the expression of thrombomodulin. The latter, as discussed, activates protein C, an anticoagulant (Chapter 3). The net result of these alterations is the enhanced generation of thrombin and the blunting of inhibitory pathways that limit coagulation.

Severe endothelial cell injury can initiate DIC by causing the release of tissue factor and by exposing subendothelial collagen and bound vWF. However, even subtle forms of endothelial damage can unleash procoagulant activity by stimulating tissue factor expression and downregulating the expression of anticoagulant factors such as thrombomodulin. Widespread endothelial injury can be produced by the deposition of antigen-antibody complexes (e.g., in systemic lupus erythematosus), by temperature extremes (e.g., after heat stroke or burn injury), or by infections (e.g., resulting from meningococci or rickettsiae). As discussed in Chapter 3, endothelial injury is an important consequence of the systemic inflammatory response

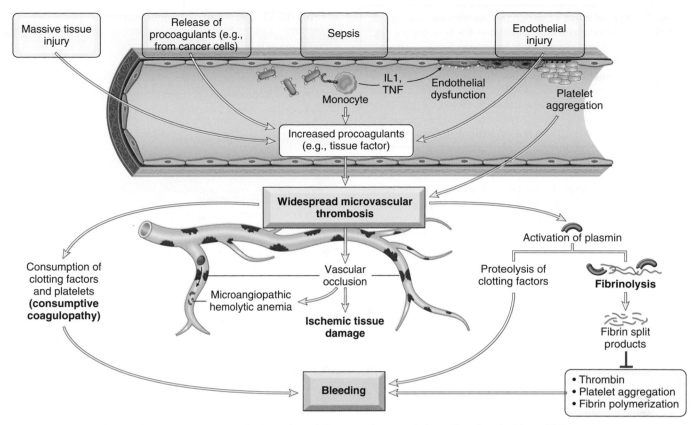

FIG. 10.30 Pathophysiology of disseminated intravascular coagulation. *IL-1*, Interleukin-1; *TNF*, tumor necrosis factor.

syndrome triggered by sepsis and other systemic insults, and, not surprisingly, DIC is a frequent complication of this syndrome.

Disorders associated with DIC are listed in Table 10.10. Of these, DIC is most often associated with sepsis, obstetric complications,

Table 10.10 Major Disorders Associated With Disseminated Intravascular Coagulation

Obstetric Complications
Abruptio placentae
Retained nonviable fetus
Septic abortion
Amniotic fluid embolism
Eclampsia
Infections
Sepsis (gram-negative and gram-positive)
Meningococcemia
Rocky Mountain spotted fever
Histoplasmosis
Aspergillosis
Malaria
Neoplasms
Carcinomas of pancreas, prostate, lung, and stomach
Acute promyelocytic leukemia
Massive Tissue Injury
Trauma
Burns
Extensive surgery
Miscellaneous
Acute intravascular hemolysis, snakebite, giant hemangioma, shock, heat stroke, vasculitis, aortic aneurysm, liver disease

malignancy, and major trauma (especially to the brain). Trauma to the brain releases negatively charged membrane components that activate the intrinsic arm of the coagulation cascade. The initiating events in these conditions are sometimes multiple and often interrelated. For example, in obstetric conditions, tissue factor derived from the placenta, a retained nonviable fetus, or amniotic fluid may enter the circulation, and coexistent shock, hypoxia, and acidosis may lead to endothelial injury.

Whatever its cause, DIC has two consequences. First, there is widespread fibrin deposition within the microcirculation. The associated obstruction leads to ischemia in the more severely affected or vulnerable organs and hemolysis as red cells undergo mechanical injury while passing through vessels narrowed by fibrin thrombi *(microangiopathic hemolytic anemia)*. Second, because of the depletion of platelets and clotting factors and the secondary release of plasminogen activators, there is a superimposed bleeding tendency. Plasmin cleaves not only fibrin (fibrinolysis) but also factors V and VIII, thereby reducing their activity. Fibrinolysis creates fibrin degradation products that inhibit platelet aggregation, have antithrombin activity, and impair fibrin polymerization, all of which contribute to the bleeding tendency (see Fig. 10.30).

MORPHOLOGY

In DIC, **microthrombi** are most often found in the arterioles and capillaries of the kidneys, adrenals, brain, and heart, but no organ is spared. The glomeruli contain small fibrin thrombi. These may be associated with only a subtle, reactive swelling of the endothelial cells or varying degrees of focal glomerulitis. The microvascular occlusions give rise to small infarcts in the renal cortex. In severe cases, the entire cortex may become ischemic, leading to bilateral renal cortical necrosis. Involvement of the adrenal glands can produce the **Waterhouse-Friderichsen syndrome** (Chapter 18). Microinfarcts are also commonly encountered in the brain and are often surrounded by microscopic or gross foci of hemorrhage. Similar changes may be seen in the heart and the anterior pituitary. DIC may contribute to the development of **Sheehan postpartum pituitary necrosis** (Chapter 20). The bleeding tendency associated with DIC is manifested not only by larger-than-expected hemorrhages near foci of infarction but also by diffuse petechiae and ecchymoses on the skin, serosal linings of the body cavities, epicardium, endocardium, lungs, and mucosal lining of the urinary tract.

Clinical Features. As might be imagined, depending on the balance between clotting and bleeding tendencies, the range of possible clinical manifestations is enormous. Clinically, DIC is divided into acute and chronic presentations. Acute DIC is more likely to be fulminant and to be associated with marked coagulation test abnormalities, whereas chronic DIC may be associated with mild laboratory abnormalities and little to no clinical symptoms. In general, acute DIC (e.g., that associated with obstetric complications) is dominated by bleeding, whereas chronic DIC (e.g., as occurs in patients with adenocarcinoma) tends to manifest with signs and symptoms related to thrombosis. The abnormal clotting is usually confined to the microcirculation, but large vessels are involved on occasion. The manifestations of DIC may be minimal, or there may be shock, acute renal failure, dyspnea, cyanosis, convulsions, and coma. Most often, the onset of DIC is heralded by the appearance of petechiae and ecchymoses on the skin. These may be the only manifestations, or there may be severe hemorrhage into the gut or urinary tract. Laboratory evaluation shows thrombocytopenia and prolongation of the PT and PTT (from depletion of platelets, clotting factors, and fibrinogen). Fibrin split products are increased in the plasma.

The prognosis varies widely depending on the nature of the underlying disorder and the severity of the intravascular clotting and fibrinolysis. Acute DIC may be life threatening and must be treated aggressively with anticoagulants such as heparin or the coagulants contained in fresh frozen plasma. Conversely, chronic DIC is sometimes identified unexpectedly by laboratory testing. In either circumstance, definitive treatment must be directed at the underlying cause.

THROMBOCYTOPENIA

Isolated thrombocytopenia is associated with a bleeding tendency and normal coagulation tests. A count less than 150,000 platelets/µL is generally considered thrombocytopenia. However, only when platelet counts fall to 20,000 to 50,000 platelets/µL is there an increased risk of posttraumatic bleeding; spontaneous bleeding is unlikely until counts fall below 5,000 platelets/µL. Most bleeding occurs from small, superficial blood vessels and produces *petechiae* or *ecchymoses* in the skin, the mucous membranes of the gastrointestinal and urinary tracts, and other sites. Larger hemorrhages into the central nervous system are a major hazard in those with markedly depressed platelet counts.

The major causes of thrombocytopenia are listed in Table 10.11. Clinically important thrombocytopenia is confined to disorders with reduced production or increased destruction of platelets. When the cause is the accelerated destruction of platelets, the bone marrow usually shows a compensatory increase in the number of megakaryocytes. Also of note, thrombocytopenia is one of the most common hematologic manifestations of AIDS. It can occur early in the course of HIV infection and has a multifactorial basis, including immune

Table 10.11 Causes of Thrombocytopenia

Decreased Production of Platelets
Generalized Bone Marrow Dysfunction
Aplastic anemia: congenital and acquired
Marrow infiltration: leukemia, disseminated cancer
Selective Impairment of Platelet Production
Drug-induced: alcohol, thiazides, cytotoxic drugs
Infections: measles, HIV infection
Ineffective Megakaryopoiesis
Megaloblastic anemia
Paroxysmal nocturnal hemoglobinuria
Decreased Platelet Survival
Immunologic Destruction
Autoimmune: Immune thrombocytopenic purpura, systemic lupus erythematosus
Alloimmune: posttransfusion and neonatal
Drug-associated: quinidine, heparin, sulfa compounds
Infections: infectious mononucleosis, HIV infection, cytomegalovirus infection
Nonimmunologic Destruction
Disseminated intravascular coagulation
Thrombotic thrombocytopenic purpura
Hemolytic uremic syndrome
Microangiopathic hemolytic anemias
Sequestration
Hypersplenism
Dilutional
Multiple transfusions (e.g., for massive blood loss)

DIC, Disseminated intravascular coagulation; *HIV,* human immunodeficiency virus.

complex—mediated platelet destruction, antiplatelet autoantibodies, and HIV-mediated suppression of megakaryocyte development and survival. Notably, the incidence of thrombocytopenia has fallen sharply in those receiving effective antiretroviral therapy.

Immune Thrombocytopenic Purpura

Immune thrombocytopenic purpura (ITP) includes two clinical subtypes. *Chronic ITP* is a relatively common disorder that most often affects women between the ages of 20 and 40 years. *Acute ITP* is seen mostly in children after viral infections. It is self-limited and will not be discussed further.

Antibodies directed against platelet membrane glycoproteins IIb/IIIa or Ib/IX complexes are detected in roughly 80% of cases of chronic ITP. The spleen is an important site of antiplatelet antibody production and the major site of destruction of the IgG-coated platelets. Although splenomegaly is not a feature of uncomplicated chronic ITP, the importance of the spleen in the premature destruction of platelets is proved by the benefits of splenectomy, which normalizes the platelet count and induces a complete remission in more than two-thirds of patients. The bone marrow usually contains increased numbers of megakaryocytes, a finding common to all forms of thrombocytopenia caused by accelerated platelet destruction.

The onset of chronic ITP is insidious. Common findings include petechiae, easy bruising, epistaxis, gum bleeding, and hemorrhage after minor trauma. Fortunately, more serious intracerebral or subarachnoid hemorrhages are uncommon. The diagnosis rests on the clinical features, the presence of thrombocytopenia, examination of the marrow, and the exclusion of secondary ITP. Reliable clinical tests for antiplatelet antibodies are not available. Treatment usually involves the use of immunosuppressive agents and, in some cases, splenectomy.

Heparin-Induced Thrombocytopenia

This special type of drug-induced thrombocytopenia (discussed in more detail in Chapter 3) merits brief mention because of its clinical importance. Moderate to severe thrombocytopenia develops in 3% to 5% of patients after 1 to 2 weeks of treatment with unfractionated heparin. The disorder is caused by IgG antibodies that bind platelet factor 4 in a heparin-dependent fashion. The resultant immune complexes bind to platelet Fc receptors and trigger platelet activation, thereby exacerbating the condition that heparin is used to treat—thrombosis. Both venous and arterial thromboses occur, even in the setting of marked thrombocytopenia, and may cause severe morbidity (e.g., loss of limbs) and death. Cessation of heparin therapy breaks the cycle of platelet activation and consumption. The risk of this complication is lowered (but not prevented entirely) by use of low-molecular-weight heparin preparations.

Thrombotic Microangiopathies: Thrombotic Thrombocytopenic Purpura and Hemolytic Uremic Syndrome

The term *thrombotic microangiopathies* encompasses a spectrum of clinical syndromes that include thrombotic thrombocytopenic purpura (TTP) and hemolytic uremic syndrome (HUS). As originally defined, TTP is associated with the pentad of fever, thrombocytopenia, microangiopathic hemolytic anemia, transient neurologic deficits, and renal failure. HUS is also associated with microangiopathic hemolytic anemia and thrombocytopenia but is distinguished from TTP by the absence of neurologic symptoms, the dominance of acute renal failure, and frequent occurrence in children (Chapter 12). These distinctions sometimes blur, as many adults with TTP lack one or more of the five criteria, and some patients with HUS have fever and neurologic dysfunction.

Fundamental to both HUS and TTP is the widespread formation of platelet-rich thrombi in the microcirculation. The mechanisms of platelet activation differ, however; in HUS, it may stem from abnormal activation of complement or from endothelial damage by certain toxins, whereas in TTP it is caused by congenital or acquired deficiency of a metalloprotease called ADAMTS13, which negatively regulates the activity of von Willebrand factor (described later). Regardless of cause, consumption of platelets leads to thrombocytopenia, and the narrowing of blood vessels by the thrombi results in a microangiopathic hemolytic anemia. All the thrombotic microangiopathies produce renal damage of variable severity, and their pathogenesis is discussed in greater detail in Chapter 12.

It is important to note that although DIC and the thrombotic microangiopathies share features such as microvascular occlusion and microangiopathic hemolytic anemia, they are pathogenically distinct. Furthermore, unlike in DIC, in TTP and HUS activation of the coagulation cascade is not of primary importance, and so the results of laboratory tests of coagulation (e.g., the PT and PTT tests) are usually normal.

COAGULATION DISORDERS

Coagulation disorders result from either congenital or acquired deficiencies of clotting factors. Acquired deficiencies are most common and often involve several factors simultaneously. As discussed in Chapter 7, vitamin K is required for the synthesis of prothrombin and clotting factors VII, IX, and X, and its deficiency causes a severe coagulation defect. The liver synthesizes several coagulation factors and also removes many activated coagulation factors from the circulation; thus, hepatic parenchymal diseases are common causes of complex hemorrhagic diatheses. As already discussed, DIC may also lead to multiple concomitant factor deficiencies. Rarely, autoantibodies may cause acquired deficiencies limited to a single factor.

Hereditary deficiencies of many coagulation factors occur. Hemophilia A (a deficiency of factor VIII) and hemophilia B (Christmas disease, a deficiency of factor IX) are X-linked traits, whereas other deficiencies are autosomal recessive disorders. Of the inherited deficiencies, only von Willebrand disease, hemophilia A, and hemophilia B are sufficiently common to warrant further consideration.

Deficiencies of Factor VIII–von Willebrand Factor Complex

Hemophilia A and von Willebrand disease are caused by qualitative or quantitative defects involving the factor VIII–vWF complex. As background for subsequent discussion of these disorders, it is useful to review the structure and function of these two proteins (Fig. 10.31).

As described earlier, factor VIII is an essential cofactor for activated factor IX, a component of the intrinsic coagulation pathway that in turn activates factor X. Circulating factor VIII binds noncovalently to vWF, which exists as large multimers of up to 20 megadaltons in weight. Endothelial cells are the major source of plasma vWF, whereas most factor VIII is synthesized in the liver. vWF is found in the plasma (in association with factor VIII), in platelet granules, in endothelial cells within cytoplasmic vesicles called Weibel-Palade bodies, and in the subendothelium, where it binds to collagen.

When endothelial cells are stripped away by trauma or injury, subendothelial vWF is exposed and binds platelets, mainly through glycoprotein Ib and to a lesser degree through glycoprotein IIb/IIIa (see Fig. 10.31). The most important function of vWF is to facilitate the adhesion of platelets to damaged blood vessel walls, a crucial early event in the formation of a hemostatic plug. Inadequate platelet adhesion is believed to underlie the bleeding tendency in von Willebrand disease. In addition to its role in platelet adhesion, vWF also stabilizes factor VIII; thus, vWF deficiency leads to a secondary deficiency of factor VIII.

The various forms of von Willebrand disease are diagnosed by measuring the quantity, size, and function of vWF. vWF function is assessed using the *ristocetin platelet agglutination test*. Ristocetin enhances the bivalent binding of vWF and platelet membrane glycoprotein Ib, creating interplatelet "bridges" that cause platelets to clump (agglutination), an event that can be measured easily. Thus, ristocetin-dependent platelet agglutination serves as a useful bioassay for vWF.

With this background we now turn to the discussion of diseases resulting from deficiencies of the factor VIII–vWF complex.

von Willebrand Disease

It is estimated that approximately 1% of people in the United States have von Willebrand disease, making it the most common inherited bleeding disorder. von Willebrand disease is transmitted as an autosomal dominant disorder. It usually presents as spontaneous bleeding from mucous membranes, excessive bleeding from wounds, and menorrhagia. It is underrecognized, as the diagnosis requires sophisticated tests and the clinical manifestations often are quite mild.

People with von Willebrand disease have compound defects in platelet function and coagulation, but in most cases only the platelet defect produces clinical findings. The exceptions are in rare patients with homozygous von Willebrand disease, in whom there is a

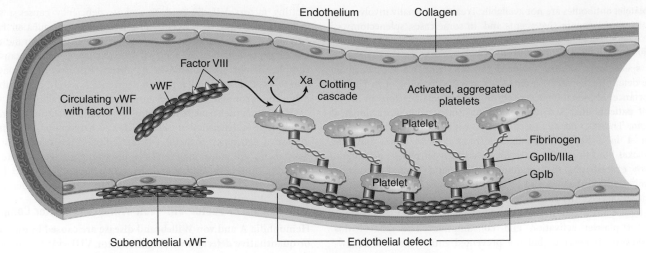

FIG. 10.31 Structure and function of factor VIII–von Willebrand factor (vWF) complex. Factor VIII and vWF circulate as a complex. vWF is also present in the subendothelial matrix of normal blood vessels. Following its activation by thrombin, factor VIII dissociates from vWF and takes part in the coagulation cascade by forming a complex with activated factor IX *(not shown)* that activates factor X. vWF causes adhesion of platelets to subendothelial collagen, primarily through the glycoprotein Ib (GpIb) platelet receptor. Aggregation of platelets occurs through bridging interactions involving platelet glycoprotein IIb/IIIa and fibrinogen.

concomitant deficiency of factor VIII severe enough to produce features resembling those of hemophilia (described later).

The effects of the causative mutations vary, allowing von Willebrand disease to be divided into several subtypes:

- *Type 1* is the classic and most common variant of von Willebrand disease. It is an autosomal dominant disorder in which the quantity of circulating vWF is reduced. There is also a measurable but clinically insignificant decrease in factor VIII levels.
- *Type II* is divided into several subtypes characterized by the selective loss of high–molecular-weight multimers of vWF. Because these large multimers are the most active form, there is a functional deficiency of vWF. In type IIA, the high–molecular-weight multimers are not synthesized, leading to a true deficiency. In type IIB, abnormal "hyperfunctional" high–molecular-weight multimers are synthesized that are rapidly removed from the circulation. These high–molecular-weight multimers cause spontaneous platelet aggregation (a situation reminiscent of the very-high–molecular-weight multimer aggregates seen in TTP; Chapter 12); indeed, some people with type IIB von Willebrand disease have mild chronic thrombocytopenia, presumably resulting from platelet consumption.

Hemophilia A: Factor VIII Deficiency

Hemophilia A is the most common hereditary cause of serious bleeding. It is an X-linked recessive disorder caused by reduced factor VIII activity. It primarily affects males. Much less commonly, excessive bleeding occurs in heterozygous females, presumably due to preferential inactivation of the X chromosome carrying the normal factor VIII gene (unfavorable lyonization). Approximately 30% of cases are caused by new mutations; in the remainder, there is a positive family history. Severe hemophilia A is observed in people with marked deficiencies of factor VIII (activity levels <1% of normal). Milder deficiencies may only become apparent in the face of trauma or other hemostatic stresses. The varying degrees of factor VIII deficiency are explained by the existence of many different causative mutations, including deletions, inversions, hand splice junction mutations. In

about 10% of patients, the factor VIII protein levels are normal, but the coagulant activity is low because of a mutation in factor VIII that causes a loss of function.

In symptomatic cases there is a tendency toward easy bruising and hemorrhage after trauma or operative procedures. In addition, "spontaneous" hemorrhages are frequently encountered in tissues that are subject to mechanical stress, particularly the joints, where recurrent bleeds *(hemarthroses)* lead to progressive deformities that can be crippling. Petechiae are characteristically absent.

Specific assays for factor VIII are used to confirm the diagnosis. Typically, patients with hemophilia A have a prolonged PTT that is corrected by mixing the patient's plasma with normal plasma. Specific factor assays are then used to confirm the deficiency of factor VIII.

In approximately 15% of those with severe hemophilia A, replacement therapy is complicated by the development of neutralizing antibodies against factor VIII, probably because factor VIII is seen by the immune system as a "foreign" antigen. In these persons, the PTT fails to correct in mixing studies. Recently, the problem of factor VIII inhibitors has been circumvented by a new treatment with a bispecific antibody that binds factor IX to factor X, thereby bypassing the need for factor VIII altogether. This antibody treatment appears to be more effective at reducing bleeding and is easier to administer than factor VIII but (like factor VIII infusion) is expensive.

Hemophilia B: Factor IX Deficiency

Severe factor IX deficiency is an X-linked disorder that is indistinguishable clinically from hemophilia A but much less common. As with hemophilia A, the PTT is prolonged. The diagnosis is made using specific assays of factor IX. It is treated by infusion of recombinant factor IX.

COMPLICATIONS OF TRANSFUSION

Blood products often are rightly called "the gift of life," permitting people to survive traumatic injuries and procedures such as hematopoietic stem cell transplantation and complex surgical procedures that would otherwise prove fatal. Over 5 million red cell transfusions are given in U.S. hospitals each year. Thanks to improved screening of donors, blood products (red cells, platelets, and fresh-frozen plasma) are safer than ever before.

Nevertheless, complications still occur. Most are minor and transient. The most common is referred to as a *febrile nonhemolytic reaction,* which takes the form of fever and chills, sometimes with mild dyspnea, within 6 hours of a transfusion of red cells or platelets. It is thought that these reactions are caused by inflammatory mediators derived from donor leukocytes. The frequency of these reactions increases with the storage age of the product and is decreased by measures that limit donor leukocyte contamination. Symptoms respond to antipyretics and are short lived.

Other transfusion reactions are uncommon or rare but can have severe and sometimes fatal consequences and therefore merit brief discussion.

Allergic Reactions

Severe, potentially fatal, allergic reactions may occur when blood products containing certain antigens are given to previously sensitized recipients. These are most likely to occur in patients with IgA deficiency, which has a frequency of 1:300 to 1:500 people. The reaction is triggered by IgG antibodies that recognize IgA in the infused blood product. Fortunately, most patients with IgA deficiency do not develop such antibodies, and severe reactions are rare, occurring in 1 in 20,000 to 1 in 50,000 transfusions. *Urticarial allergic reactions* may be triggered by the presence of an allergen in the donated blood product that is recognized by IgE antibodies in the recipient. These are more common, occurring in 1% to 3% of transfusions, but they are generally mild.

Hemolytic Reactions

Acute hemolytic reactions are usually caused by preformed IgM antibodies against donor red cells that fix complement. They most commonly stem from an error in patient identification or tube labeling that allows a patient to receive an ABO incompatible unit of blood. Preexisting "natural" IgM antibodies, usually against blood group antigens A or B, bind to red cells and rapidly induce complement-mediated lysis, intravascular hemolysis, and hemoglobinuria associated with fever, shaking chills, and flank pain. The direct Coombs test is positive unless all the donor red cells have lysed. The signs and symptoms are due to complement activation rather than hemolysis per se, as osmotic lysis of red cells (e.g., by mistakenly infusing red cells and 5% dextrose in water simultaneously) produces hemoglobinuria without any other symptoms. In severe cases the process may rapidly progress to DIC, shock, renal failure, and death.

Delayed hemolytic reactions are caused by antibodies that recognize red cell antigens that the recipient was sensitized to previously, for example, through a previous blood transfusion. These are typically caused by IgG antibodies and are associated with a positive direct Coombs test and laboratory features of hemolysis (e.g., low haptoglobin and elevated LDH). Antibodies to blood group antigens such as Rh, Kell, and Kidd sometimes fix complement, resulting in severe and potentially fatal reactions identical to those seen with ABO mismatches. Other antibodies that do not fix complement typically result in extravascular hemolysis and relatively mild signs and symptoms.

Transfusion-Associated Circulatory Overload

The leading cause of transfusion-related death, transfusion-associated circulatory overload (TACO), is caused by fluid/volume overload due to transfusion and is much more likely in patients with cardiovascular and pulmonary disease. It occurs in up to 1% of transfused patients overall but is more common in elderly patients who are seriously ill, such as ICU patients. Risk is greatest in those receiving multiple units of blood products over a short period of time. With reductions in other complications of transfusion, TACO is now believed to be the most common cause of transfusion-related mortality.

TACO presents with respiratory distress within 6 to 12 hours of transfusion. Treatment involves cessation of transfusions and initiation of supportive measures.

Transfusion-Related Acute Lung Injury

Transfusion-related acute lung injury (TRALI) is a severe, frequently fatal complication in which factors in a transfused blood product trigger the activation of neutrophils in the lung microvasculature. The incidence is low, probably less than 1 per 10,000 transfusions.

Current thinking about TRALI favors a "two-hit" hypothesis. This proposes that neutrophils of the recipient are primed for activation by the recipient's underlying clinical condition. This "priming" event has diverse causes, including smoking, sepsis, and shock, and leads to sequestration of neutrophils. The second hit involves activation of primed neutrophils by a factor present in the transfused blood product.

The leading "second hit" candidate is an antibody in the transfused blood product that recognizes antigens expressed on neutrophils. By far the most common antibodies associated with TRALI are those that bind MHC class I antigens. These antibodies are often found in multiparous women, in whom they are generated in response to paternal MHC antigens expressed by the fetus. Indeed, measures to exclude multiparous women from plasma donation have substantially lowered the incidence of TRALI.

The presentation is dramatic, with sudden onset of respiratory failure associated with diffuse bilateral pulmonary infiltrates during or soon after a transfusion. The treatment is largely supportive and the outcome is guarded; mortality is 5% in uncomplicated cases and up to 67% in those who are severely ill.

Infectious Complications

Virtually any infectious agent can be transmitted through blood products, but bacterial and viral infections are most likely to be so. Significant bacterial contamination (sufficient to produce symptoms) is much more common in platelet preparations than red cell preparations because platelets (unlike red cells) must be stored at room temperature, which favors growth of bacterial contaminants. Rates of bacterial infection secondary to platelet transfusion can be as high as 1 in 5000. Many of the symptoms (fever, chills, hypotension) resemble those of transfusion reactions, and it may be necessary to start broad-spectrum antibiotics prospectively in symptomatic patients while awaiting laboratory results. New guidelines in the United States that call for testing of all platelet products for the presence of bacteria will likely decrease this complication.

Advances in donor selection, donor screening, and infectious disease testing have dramatically decreased the incidence of viral transmission by blood products. However, on rare occasions when the donor is acutely infected, viruses can still be transmitted. Rates of transmission of HIV, hepatitis C, and hepatitis B are estimated to be 1 in 2 million, 1 in 1 million, and 1 in 500,000, respectively. There also remains a low risk of transmission of "exotic" infections such as West Nile virus, trypanosomiasis, and babesiosis.

DISORDERS OF THE SPLEEN AND THYMUS

SPLENOMEGALY

The spleen is frequently involved in a wide variety of systemic diseases. In virtually all instances the spleen responds by enlarging (splenomegaly), an alteration that produces a set of stereotypical signs and symptoms. Evaluation of splenic enlargement is aided by recognition of the usual limits of splenomegaly produced by specific disorders. It would be erroneous to attribute an enlarged spleen pushing into the pelvis to vitamin B_{12} deficiency, or to entertain a diagnosis of CML in the absence of splenomegaly. Disorders that may produce splenomegaly fall into several broad classes (Table 10.12).

The microscopic changes associated with these diseases are discussed in the relevant sections of this and other chapters.

A chronically enlarged spleen often removes excessive numbers of one or more of the formed elements of blood, resulting in anemia, leukopenia, or thrombocytopenia. This is referred to as *hypersplenism*, a state that can be associated with many of the diseases listed previously. In addition, platelets are particularly susceptible to *sequestration* in the interstices of the red pulp; as a result, thrombocytopenia is more prevalent and severe in persons with splenomegaly than is anemia or neutropenia.

DISORDERS OF THE THYMUS

As is well known, the thymus has a crucial role in T-cell maturation. It is not surprising, therefore, that the thymus can be involved by lymphomas, particularly those of T-cell lineage (discussed earlier in this chapter). The focus here is on the two most frequent (albeit still uncommon) disorders of the thymus: thymic hyperplasia and thymoma.

Thymic Hyperplasia

Thymic hyperplasia is often associated with the presence of lymphoid follicles, or germinal centers, within the medulla. These germinal centers contain reactive B cells, which are rare in normal thymuses. Thymic hyperplasia is found in most patients with *myasthenia gravis* and sometimes also in other autoimmune diseases, such as systemic lupus erythematosus and rheumatoid arthritis. The relationship between the thymus and myasthenia gravis is discussed in Chapter 20. Of significance, removal of the hyperplastic thymus is often beneficial early in the disease.

Thymoma

Thymomas are tumors of thymic epithelial cells. Several classification systems for thymoma based on cytologic and biologic criteria have been proposed. One simple and clinically useful classification is as follows:

- Benign or encapsulated thymoma: cytologically and biologically benign
- Malignant thymoma
  - *Type I:* cytologically benign but infiltrative and locally aggressive
  - *Type II* (thymic carcinoma): cytologically and biologically malignant

Table 10.12 Disorders Associated With Splenomegaly

I. Infections
Nonspecific splenitis of various blood-borne infections (particularly infectious endocarditis)
Infectious mononucleosis
Tuberculosis
Typhoid fever
Brucellosis
Cytomegalovirus
Syphilis
Malaria
Histoplasmosis
Toxoplasmosis
Trypanosomiasis
Schistosomiasis
Leishmaniasis
Echinococcosis
II. Congestive States Related to Portal Hypertension
Cirrhosis of the liver
Portal or splenic vein thrombosis
Cardiac failure
III. Lymphohematogenous Disorders
Hodgkin lymphoma
Non-Hodgkin lymphomas and lymphocytic leukemias
Myeloproliferative neoplasms
Hemolytic anemias
IV. Immunologic-Inflammatory Conditions
Rheumatoid arthritis
Systemic lupus erythematosus
V. Storage Diseases
Gaucher disease
Niemann-Pick disease
Mucopolysaccharidoses
VI. Miscellaneous Disorders
Amyloidosis
Primary neoplasms and cysts
Secondary neoplasms

Clinical Features. Thymomas are rare. They may arise at any age, but most occur in middle-aged adults. In a large series about 30% were asymptomatic; 30% to 40% produced local manifestations such as cough, dyspnea, and superior vena cava syndrome; and the remainder were associated with a systemic disease, most commonly myasthenia gravis, in which a concomitant thymoma is discovered in 15% to 20% of patients. Removal of the tumor often leads to improvement of myasthenia gravis. In addition, thymomas may be associated with several other paraneoplastic syndromes. These include (in rough order of frequency) pure red cell aplasia, hypogammaglobulinemia, and multiorgan autoimmunity. The latter resembles graft-versus-host disease.

■ RAPID REVIEW

Anemia

- Causes of anemia include blood loss (hemorrhage), increased red cell destruction (hemolysis), and decreased red cell production (marrow failure).

- *Microcytic anemias* are most often caused by iron deficiency or thalassemia.
- *Macrocytic anemias* may be caused by folate or vitamin B$_{12}$ deficiency. Anemia with macrocytosis may also be seen in the setting of an elevated reticulocyte count, such as in patients recovery from a bleeding episode.
- Certain *normocytic anemias* are associated with telltale changes in red cell shape (e.g., hereditary spherocytosis, sickle cell disease).
- Clinical manifestations of anemia depend on the tempo with which it develops and whether it is caused by a failure of red cell production or by increased red cell destruction.
- Acute onset anemia (e.g., from a large bleed) may present with shortness of breath, organ failure, and shock.
- Chronic onset anemia may appear insidiously, with slowly worsening pallor, fatigue, and lassitude.
- Extravascular hemolysis may be associated with jaundice and gallstones.
- With ineffective erythropoiesis, there may be iron overload leading to heart and endocrine failure.
- Severe congenital anemias are associated with growth retardation and if there is a hemolytic component bone deformities due to reactive marrow hyperplasia.

Hemolytic Anemia

- *Hereditary spherocytosis:* An autosomal dominant disorder caused by mutations that destabilize the red cell membrane skeleton, leading to loss of membrane and formation of spherocytes, which are removed in the spleen. It manifests with anemia, splenomegaly, and cholelithiasis.
- *Sickle cell anemia:* An autosomal recessive disorder resulting from a mutation in β-globin that causes deoxygenated hemoglobin to self-associate into long polymers that distort and damage the red cell. This leads to moderate to severe hemolytic anemia and periodic blockage of vessels by sickled cells that produce pain crises and tissue infarction. Patients are at high risk for bacterial infections and stroke.
- *Thalassemia:* An autosomal codominant disorder caused by mutations in α- or β-globin that reduce hemoglobin synthesis and results in a microcytic, hypochromic anemia. In β-thalassemia major, unpaired α-globin chains precipitate and lead to ineffective hematopoiesis.
- *Glucose-6-phosphate dehydrogenase (G6PD) deficiency:* An X-linked disorder caused by mutations that destabilize G6PD, making red cells susceptible to oxidant damage. Hemolytic triggers include drugs and infections.
- *Immunohemolytic anemia:* An acquired condition caused by antibodies against normal red cell constituents or antigens modified by haptens (such as drugs). Antibody binding results in red cell opsonization and extravascular hemolysis or (uncommonly) complement fixation and intravascular hemolysis.
- *Malaria:* An intracellular red cell parasite that causes chronic hemolysis of variable severity. Falciparum malaria may be fatal because of the propensity of infected red cells to adhere to small vessels in the brain (cerebral malaria).

Anemia of Diminished Erythropoiesis

- *Iron deficiency anemia:* Caused by chronic bleeding or inadequate iron intake, it leads to insufficient hemoglobin synthesis and hypochromic, microcytic red cells.
- *Anemia of chronic inflammation:* Caused by inflammatory cytokines, which increase hepcidin levels (sequestering iron in macrophages) and suppress erythropoietin production

- *Megaloblastic anemia:* Caused by deficiencies of folate or vitamin B$_{12}$, which lead to inadequate synthesis of thymidine and defective DNA replication. Findings include enlarged abnormal hematopoietic precursors (megaloblasts), ineffective hematopoiesis, macrocytic anemia, hypersegmented neutrophils, macroovalocytes, pancytopenia, and (with B$_{12}$ deficiency) spinal cord degeneration.
- *Aplastic anemia:* Caused by bone marrow failure due to diverse causes, including exposures to toxins and radiation, idiosyncratic reactions to drugs and viruses, immune-mediated marrow suppression, and inherited defects in telomerase and DNA repair factors
- *Myelophthisic anemia:* Caused by replacement of the bone marrow by infiltrative processes such as metastatic carcinoma and granulomatous disease. Findings include release of early marrow precursors into the blood (leukoerythroblastosis) and the appearance of teardrop-shaped red cells in peripheral smears.

Acute Leukemias

- Present acutely with symptoms related to cytopenias
- Three major subtypes, all associated with mutations that interfere with hematopoietic stem cell differentiation:
  - *AML:* A tumor of immature myeloid lineage cells, it is most common in adults over age 60. Acute promyelocytic leukemia (APL) is a notable subtype that is caused by a (15;17) translocation that produces a chimeric gene encoding a PML-RARA fusion protein. APL is marked by the presence of numerous cells with Auer rods and DIC and high curability with all-trans retinoic acid and arsenic salts. Other subtypes are difficult to treat, particularly in older individuals. Often arises from preexisting myeloid neoplasm, either MDS or a myeloproliferative neoplasm.
  - *B-ALL:* A neoplasm of precursor B cells, it is most common in children 2 to 11 years of age. A subset (mostly in adults) is associated with a (9;22) translocation that produces a chimeric gene encoding a constitutively active BCR-ABL tyrosine kinase; these tumors respond well to targeted therapy with tyrosine kinase inhibitors. Other tumors are highly responsive to chemotherapy, except infantile AMLs associated with *KMT2A* gene rearrangements and B-ALLs in older individuals that lack *BCR-ABL* fusion genes.
  - *T-ALL:* A neoplasm of precursor T cells, it is most common in adolescent males. It may present as a thymic mass without blood involvement and generally has an excellent prognosis except in older adults.

Myelodysplastic Syndromes

- Myeloid tumors characterized by disordered and ineffective hematopoiesis
- Caused by diverse driver mutations in genes encoding splicing factors, epigenetic regulators, and transcription factors involved in hematopoiesis
- Manifest with one or more cytopenias and dysplasia in one or more lineages in the marrow and peripheral blood
- Progresses in 10% to 40% of cases to AML

Myeloproliferative Neoplasms

- Myeloid tumors in which production of formed myeloid elements is increased, leading to high blood counts and extramedullary hematopoiesis
- Caused in many instances by acquired mutations that lead to constitutive activation of tyrosine kinases
- Several major subtypes are recognized:
  - *Chronic myeloid leukemia:* Caused by a t(9;22) that creates a fusion gene encoding a constitutively active BCR-ABL tyrosine

kinase, it presents with high granulocyte and platelet counts and splenomegaly. Without treatment, there is a high incidence of transformation to acute B lymphoblastic or myeloid leukemia, but the disease is very well controlled by BCR-ABL inhibitors.

- *Polycythemia vera:* Caused by activating mutations in the JAK2 tyrosine kinase, it presents with high red cell counts and often high platelet and granulocyte counts. Without treatment there is a high risk of thrombosis, but this can be prevented with periodic removal of red cells. Late in the course it may progress to a spent phase marked by marrow myelofibrosis.
- *Primary myelofibrosis:* Caused by activating mutations in the *JAK2, MPL* (which encodes the thrombopoietin receptor, a tyrosine kinase), or *CALR* genes (mutated CALR activates the thrombopoietin receptor). It may present with high granulocyte counts, thrombocytosis, and mild splenomegaly but then rapidly progresses to a phase of marrow fibrosis marked by cytopenias (particularly anemia), leukoerythroblastosis, and increasing splenomegaly.

Non-Hodgkin Lymphoma and Chronic Lymphoid Leukemias

- Classification is based on cell of origin and stage of differentiation.
- Most common types are B-cell tumors.
- Often associated with immune abnormalities
- Generally assumed to be disseminated at diagnosis
- Multiple subtypes are recognized:
  - *Small lymphocytic lymphoma/chronic lymphocytic leukemia:* Most common adult leukemia (CLL), this is an indolent CD5+ B-cell tumor. Characteristic findings include diffuse effacement of lymph nodes with proliferation centers and high-level expression of the antiapoptotic factor BCL2. It is associated with immune abnormalities and increased susceptibility to infection and autoimmune disorders. A small number of cases present without blood involvement (SLL). About 10% of cases transform to an aggressive B cell lymphoma.
  - *Follicular lymphoma:* The most common indolent lymphoma, it is caused in part by a (14;18) translocation that leads to overexpression of BCL2. In lymph nodes, it recapitulates the growth pattern of normal germinal center B cells. About 30% to 40% of cases transform to an aggressive B cell lymphoma.
  - *Mantle cell lymphoma:* This moderately aggressive CD5+ B-cell tumor is strongly associated with an (11;14) translocation that results in overexpression of cyclin D1.
  - *Extranodal marginal zone lymphoma:* This is a mature B-cell tumor arising at extranodal sites that are chronically inflamed due to autoimmune disease or infection (e.g., *H. pylori*). It remains localized for long periods and may regress if the inflammatory stimulus is removed.
  - *Diffuse large B-cell lymphoma:* This is a heterogeneous group of aggressive B-cell tumors that constitute the most common type of lymphoma in adults. Important driver mutations include rearrangements or mutations of the *BCL6* gene, a (14;18) translocation involving *BCL2*, and translocations involving *MYC*. Approximately 50% of patients are cured with aggressive chemotherapy.
  - *Burkitt lymphoma:* This is a very aggressive B-cell tumor that usually arises at extranodal sites and is nearly always associated with translocations involving the *MYC* proto-oncogene. A subset of cases is associated with EBV infection. It is curable with chemotherapy.
  - *Hairy cell leukemia:* This indolent B-cell tumor that takes its name from circulating cells with "hairy" cytoplasmic extensions

commonly presents with splenomegaly and cytopenias. It is strongly associated with *BRAF* mutations and shows excellent responses to chemotherapy and BRAF inhibitors.
- *Mycosis fungoides (MF)* and *Sézary syndrome (SS):* MF is an indolent tumor of CD4+ skin-homing T cells that responds well to topical therapy. SS is also a tumor of CD4+ T cells, but it presents with diffuse erythroderma and circulating tumor cells and pursues a more aggressive course.
- *Adult T-cell leukemia/lymphoma:* The only human cancer associated with a retrovirus (HTLV-1), this tumor of CD4+ T cells arises in chronically infected older adults. It is usually aggressive and responds poorly to therapy.
- *Peripheral T-cell lymphoma:* This term encompasses a heterogeneous group of mature T-cell neoplasms that often produce cytokines leading to systemic symptoms. They are generally aggressive and respond poorly to therapy.

Hodgkin Lymphomas

- B-cell tumors that are often associated with inflammatory symptoms
- Involved lymph nodes contain tumor giant cells called Reed-Sternberg (RS) cells and variants and abundant inflammatory cells, which are recruited by factors released from the RS cells and non-neoplastic cells
- A subset of cases are associated with EBV infection.
- Responds very well to chemotherapy and to immune checkpoint inhibitors

Plasma Cell Neoplasms and Related Entities

- *Multiple myeloma:* A relatively common plasma cell tumor associated with diverse translocations involving immunoglobulin genes. This tumor is associated with "CRAB" manifestations: hyper**c**alcemia; **r**enal disease; **a**nemia; and **b**one pain, due to pathologic fractures. The neoplastic plasma cells suppress normal humoral immunity, secrete partial immunoglobulins that may cause nephrotoxicity (Bence Jones proteins) and amyloid deposition, and cause lytic bone lesions.
- *Monoclonal gammopathy of uncertain significance (MGUS):* A common asymptomatic precursor of multiple myeloma defined by the presence of a clonal plasma cell population producing a serum M protein.
- *Lymphoplasmacytic lymphoma:* A B-cell tumor with plasma cell differentiation that secretes IgM, is strongly associated with *MYD88* mutations, and often causes a hyperviscosity syndrome (Waldenström macroglobulinemia)

Histiocytic Disorders

- May be reactive or neoplastic
- *Hemophagocytic lymphohistiocytosis (HLH)* is a reactive disorder also known as macrophage activation syndrome. It occurs in children with inherited defects in genes encoding components of the cytotoxic granules of T cells and NK cells that limit the killing of cells infected with viruses such as EBV. Failure to kill virally infected cells elicits a positive feedback loop that leads to overproduction of cytokines and excessive activation of macrophages, which often consume normal marrow elements. HLH may also occur in older adults with peripheral T-cell lymphoma, probably due to cytokine release from tumor cells.
- *Langerhans cell histiocytosis* is a neoplasm of dendritic cells that is often caused by activating mutations in the BRAF serine/threonine kinase. Most cases follow an indolent course.

Bleeding Disorders

- *Disseminated intravascular coagulation (DIC):* A syndrome caused by systemic activation of coagulation, DIC may be triggered by sepsis, major trauma, certain cancers, and obstetric complications. It leads to consumption of coagulation factors and platelets and may produce bleeding; vascular occlusion and tissue hypoxemia; or both.
- *Immune thrombocytopenic purpura (ITP):* Caused by destruction of platelets by autoantibodies, it may be triggered by drugs, infections, or lymphomas, or may be idiopathic.
- *Thrombotic thrombocytopenic purpura (TTP):* Manifests with thrombocytopenia, microangiopathic hemolytic anemia, renal failure, fever, and CNS involvement. TTP is caused by deficiencies of ADAMTS13, a metalloprotease that prevents the accumulation of hyperactive very-high–molecular-weight multimers of vWF in the blood. The deficiency of ADAMTS13 may be acquired (autoantibodies) or inherited.
- *Hemolytic uremic syndrome (HUS):* Manifesting with thrombocytopenia, microangiopathic hemolytic anemia, and renal failure, HUS is caused by deficiencies of complement regulatory proteins or exposure to agents that damage endothelial cells. The resulting injury initiates platelet activation, platelet aggregation, and microvascular thrombosis.
- *von Willebrand disease:* An autosomal dominant disorder caused by mutations in vWF, it typically manifests as mild to moderate bleeding disorder. The bleeding resembles that seen in ITP (mucosal bleeding, petechiae) because vWF is required for normal platelet function (primary hemostasis).
- *Hemophilia:* An X-linked disorder caused by mutations in either coagulation factor VIII (hemophilia A) or factor IX (hemophilia B), hemophilia presents with delayed bleeding after trauma, often into deep soft tissues or joints due to a defect in secondary hemostasis.

Complications of Transfusion

- *Febrile nonhemolytic reaction:* The most common complication transfusion, this reaction is usually mild and transient.
- *Allergic reactions:* These occur when blood products containing certain antigens are given to sensitized recipients and may be severe (IgG-meditated) or mild (IgE-mediated). The severe form occurs mainly in patients with IgA deficiency, while the mild form is much more common (1% to 3% of transfusions).
- *Hemolytic reactions:* These are caused by preformed IgM antibodies against donor red cells that fix complement and are most often due to ABO incompatibility. It presents with fever, shaking chills, flank pain, and hemoglobinuria and may rapidly progress to DIC, shock, renal failure, and death. The direct Coombs test is positive.
- *Delayed hemolytic reactions:* These occur in a previously sensitized transfusion recipient and are caused by antibodies that recognize donor red cell antigens. They are associated with a positive direct Coombs test and hemolysis and may be severe if antibody fixes complement.
- *Transfusion-associated circulatory overload:* The leading cause of transfusion-related death, it is caused by fluid/volume overload due to transfusion and is much more likely in patients with cardiovascular and pulmonary disease.
- *Transfusion-related acute lung injury (TRALI):* TRALI is a rare, severe, frequently fatal complication. The pathogenesis involves a "priming" event leading to pulmonary sequestration of the recipient's neutrophils and a "second hit" consisting of an antibody in the transfused blood product that recognizes antigens expressed on primed neutrophils. Antibodies associated with TRALI often bind MHC class I antigens.
- *Infectious complications of transfusion* are uncommon and include bacterial and viral infections.

Disorders of the Spleen and Thymus

- *Splenomegaly* has diverse causes, including neoplasms, infection, storage diseases, chronic hemolytic disorders, inflammation, and congestion. It commonly leads to thrombocytopenia due to platelet sequestration.
- *Thymic hyperplasia* is enlargement caused by lymphoid follicles, or germinal centers, within the medulla. It is associated with myasthenia gravis and sometimes other autoimmune diseases, which may remit if the thymus is removed.
- *Thymoma* is a neoplasm of thymic epithelial cells that may be benign or malignant and is sometimes associated with myasthenia gravis or paraneoplastic syndromes, which may remit if the thymus is removed.

■ **Laboratory Tests**

Test	Reference Values	Pathophysiology/Clinical Relevance
Activated partial thromboplastin time (aPTT), plasma	25—37 seconds	aPTT assesses the coagulation factors of the intrinsic (factors XII, XI, IX, and VIII) and the common (factors X, V, II, and fibrinogen) pathways. Deficiency of any of these factors can cause aPTT elevations. Heparin and antiphospholipid antibodies (lupus anticoagulant) cause isolated aPTT elevation. Since aPTT is a clot-based assay, anticoagulation therapy can result in elevated aPTT. In this test "a" refers to an activator (e.g., silica) that reduces clotting time and narrows the reference range.
ADAMTS13 activity, plasma	≥70%	ADAMTS13 is a circulating metalloproteinase synthesized primarily by the liver that cleaves ultra-large multimers of von Willebrand factor (vWF), thereby preventing excessive platelet aggregation. Inherited or acquired deficiencies of ADAMTS13 (the latter caused by autoantibodies) may lead to thrombotic thrombocytopenic purpura (TTP). This assay reports ADAMTS13 activity as a percentage of the activity seen in healthy individuals.
Antibody screen, serum	Negative	Antibodies against foreign red cell antigens (alloantibodies) may arise after exposure through blood transfusion, pregnancy, or transplantation. In an antibody screen, a patient serum sample is mixed with test red cells with known antigen profiles. If the antibody screen is positive, the blood bank identifies the specific antibodies and then selects banked cells that are safe for transfusion. A similar process may also be performed for platelets.
Basophil count, blood	$0.01—0.08 \times 10^9$/L	A basophil count is part of a complete blood count (CBC) with differential. Basophils are the least common WBC in the peripheral blood. Basophils are increased in myeloproliferative neoplasms (especially chronic myeloid leukemia), hypothyroidism, chronic inflammation, and autoimmune diseases.
Beta-2-microglobulin (B2M), serum	1.21—2.70 µg/mL	B2M is the constant light chain of HLA class I molecules, which are expressed on the surface of most nucleated cells. Serum B2M may be elevated in patients with plasma cell neoplasms, such as multiple myeloma, in which it is an indicator of a worse prognosis. Serum B2M may also be elevated in patients on long-term hemodialysis, in whom B2M may deposit as an amyloid. Risk of this complication has been decreased, but not eliminated, by improved hemodialysis protocols.
Cold agglutinin titer, serum	<1:64	Cold agglutinin syndrome is caused by IgM antibodies that bind red cells in peripheral parts of the body in which the temperature is <37°C. They may produce hemolysis or agglutination, leading to cyanosis of the ears, fingers, and toes. The blood specimen must be kept at 37—38°C before testing. When cold antibody hemolysis is suspected, a Coombs test for C3d on patient red cells is performed; if this is positive, cold agglutinin titer is done reflexively. Cold agglutinins may be associated with mycoplasma pneumonia, infectious mononucleosis, and hematologic malignancies.
Complete blood count (CBC), blood	See individual tests.	The CBC includes the red cell, white blood cell (WBC), and platelet counts and all the red cell indices (mean corpuscular volume, mean corpuscular hemoglobin, mean corpuscular hemoglobin concentration, red cell distribution width). A CBC with differential includes all the above tests plus a WBC differential count. The CBC is a general screening test to evaluate overall health, assess a wide range of hematologic disorders, and determine eligibility for medications and/or chemotherapy.
Cryoglobulins, serum	Negative	Cryoglobulins are immunoglobulins that precipitate at temperatures below 37°C. There are three subtypes: type I, monoclonal IgG or IgM; type II, a mixture of polyclonal and monoclonal immunoglobulins; and type III, polyclonal. Type I cryoglobulins are associated with lymphoplasmacytic lymphoma and multiple myeloma. Type II cryoglobulins are seen in the setting of chronic hepatitis C and autoimmune disorders such as SLE. Type III cryoglobulins are seen in some autoimmune diseases and infections. At low temperatures, cryoglobulins can precipitate in the skin of the extremities and occlude blood vessels, leading to purpura, skin necrosis, Raynaud phenomenon, arthralgias, and neuropathy.

Direct antiglobulin test (DAT, direct Coombs test), indirect antiglobulin test (indirect Coombs test), blood	Negative	The DAT assesses in vivo coating of red cells by IgG and complement C3d, opsonins that can cause extravascular hemolysis. In the DAT, the patient's red cells are incubated with antibodies specific for IgG or C3d, which causes the red cells to agglutinate if IgG and/or C3d are present on the surface of the red cells. In the indirect Coombs test, the patient's serum is first incubated with red cells with defined antigens, and anti-Ig is then added, which causes agglutination if antibodies against the test red cell antigens are present. The DAT is used to assess patients with suspected hemolysis, while the indirect Coombs test is used to guide the transfusion of red cells.
Eosinophil count, blood	$0.03-0.48 \times 10^9$/L	Eosinophils arise from precursor cells in the bone marrow and are relatively infrequent in the peripheral blood in healthy individuals. Eosinophils are increased in parasitic infections, allergic conditions, asthma, drug hypersensitivity, autoimmune and connective tissue disorders, eosinophilic granulomatosis with polyangiitis (formerly known as Churg-Strauss syndrome), myeloproliferative neoplasms, and some types of lymphoma.
Factor VIII (FVIII) activity assay, plasma	55%–200%	FVIII is a coagulation cofactor that is bound to and stabilized by von Willebrand factor (vWF) in the serum. It is an essential cofactor in factor X activation by factor IX. This test measures the activity of FVIII in patient plasma and is reported as a percentage relative to reference normal plasma. Hemophilia A is an X-linked recessive disorder caused by inherited FVIII deficiency; it presents with hemarthroses and prolonged bleeding. Rare patients with homozygous von Willebrand disease may present with low FVIII levels and hemophilia-like bleeding. Autoantibodies to FVIII can inhibit its function, resulting in acquired hemophilia.
Factor IX (FIX) activity assay, plasma	65%–140%	FIX is a protease that is part of the intrinsic coagulation pathway. It is activated by factor XIa or factor VIIa/tissue factor. In the presence of calcium, phospholipids, and factor VIIIa, FIXa activates factor X, which generates thrombin from prothrombin. Inherited FIX deficiency causes hemophilia B, also called Christmas disease, an X-linked recessive disorder that is clinically indistinguishable from hemophilia A.
Ferritin, serum	Male: 24–336 µg/L Female: 11–307 µg/L	Ferritin is found in serum and in the cytoplasm of tissue macrophages; it is the major storage protein for iron. Ferritin concentration varies with age and sex and correlates with total iron stores; therefore, ferritin levels are low in iron deficiency anemia and high in iron overload (e.g., hemochromatosis). Ferritin is often measured in combination with serum iron, transferrin saturation, and total iron binding capacity; these tests may be less precise and do not distinguish depleted iron stores from iron sequestration (e.g., anemia of chronic inflammation). Low serum ferritin is highly specific for iron deficiency anemia.
Folate, serum	≥4.0 µg/L	Folate is an essential water-soluble vitamin. It is a coenzyme for one carbon metabolism, which has an essential role in the synthesis of thymidine, one of the building blocks for DNA. Megaloblastic anemia (characterized by large, abnormally nucleated erythrocytes in the bone marrow) is the major clinical manifestation of folate deficiency. The peripheral blood picture is identical to that seen in vitamin B_{12} deficiency (see below). Low serum folate concentrations in pregnancy are associated with neural tube defects. Folate deficiency may be due to poor absorption (e.g., celiac disease), insufficient intake (e.g., chronic excess alcohol use), and medications (e.g., methotrexate).
Haptoglobin, serum	30–200 mg/dL	Haptoglobin is a serum protein produced by the liver that binds hemoglobin released from lysed red cells. Hemoglobin-haptoglobin complexes are rapidly removed from the circulation by macrophages. If the rate of hemolysis overwhelms the binding capacity of serum haptoglobin, free hemoglobin passes through the kidneys (hemoglobinuria). Serum haptoglobin levels are decreased in hemolytic anemias.
Hematocrit, blood	Males: 38%–49% Females: 35%–45%	Hematocrit (packed cell volume) is the percentage of blood volume that is taken up by packed red cells in a centrifuged sample. The hematocrit is decreased in anemia and increased in polycythemia. It may be falsely elevated in the setting of sickled red cells and severe hypertriglyceridemia. The hematocrit is approximately three times the hemoglobin (assuming the red blood cells are normal in size and shape).

Hemoglobin, blood	Males: 13.2—16.6 g/dL Females: 11.6—15.0 g/dL	Hemoglobin is the oxygen-carrying molecule in red cells. The hemoglobin molecule is a tetramer that after the first year of life consists of two α-globin chains and two β-globin chains. Each subunit contains a heme molecule composed of an iron ion in a porphyrin ring. Each heme molecule can bind one oxygen molecule. Hemoglobin is decreased in anemia and increased in polycythemia. Hemoglobin is approximately one-third the hematocrit (assuming the red cells are of normal size and shape).
Hemoglobin S (HbS), blood	Absent	HbS has a valine residue instead of a glutamate residue at position 6 of β-globin. HbS tends to aggregate and polymerize in the deoxygenated state resulting in sickling of red cells. Homozygosity for HbS results in sickle cell anemia (SCA), while heterozygosity for this allele results in sickle cell trait, which is usually asymptomatic. Hemoglobin proteins with a variety of mutations can be identified by electrophoresis or high performance liquid chromatography. Recent transfusion can lower HbS concentration and complicate diagnosis of sickle cell disease. Measurement of HbS pre- and posttransfusion is frequently used to monitor patients with SCA on regular transfusion protocols. In sickle cell trait, HbS typically makes up between 35% and 45% of total hemoglobin.
Heparin-PF4 IgG antibody, serum	Absent	Antibodies to heparin-platelet factor 4 (PF4) complexes form in some patients after heparin therapy, causing heparin-induced thrombocytopenia (HIT), generally beginning 5—10 days after therapy initiation. These patients are at risk for venous and arterial thromboembolism. While the test is sensitive (98%—100%), specificity is limited since not all anti-PF4 antibodies activate or deplete platelets.
Lactate dehydrogenase (LDH), serum	≥122—222 U/L	Lactate dehydrogenase is an enzyme that is present in almost all cells. High concentrations are present in the liver, muscle, and kidney; moderate concentrations are present in red cells. Serum LDH levels are increased in conditions associated with cell damage/death (e.g., myocardial infarction, liver disease, hemolytic anemia, pulmonary embolism) and with certain cancers (e.g., metastatic melanoma, lymphoma).
Lymphocyte count, blood	$0.95—3.07 \times 10^9$/L	Lymphocytes are a subset of white blood cells that includes T cells, B cells, and NK cells. Lymphocytes are the most plentiful circulating WBC type in young children, and the second most plentiful WBC type (after neutrophils) in healthy adults. The most important causes of significant lymphocytosis include viral infections, autoimmune diseases, and lymphocytic leukemias (e.g., chronic lymphocytic leukemia). Lymphocytopenia may be due to infections (especially HIV), immunosuppressive therapy, medications (e.g., corticosteroids), and inherited immunodeficiency syndromes. Lymphocyte subsets (e.g., CD4, CD8) can be determined by flow cytometry.
Mean corpuscular hemoglobin (MCH),[a] blood	26.5—34.0 pg	MCH is a measure of the average quantity of hemoglobin per red cell. It is calculated by dividing hemoglobin concentration by the red cell count (MCH = Hgb × 10/red cell count). MCH and mean corpuscular volume (MCV) are related such that when MCV is low, MCH is also low. When MCH is low, the oxygen-carrying capacity of the blood is reduced. The most common cause of low MCH is iron deficiency. Elevated MCH may be seen in megaloblastic anemia due to folate or vitamin B_{12} deficiency.
Mean corpuscular hemoglobin concentration (MCHC),[a] blood	Males: 31.5%—36.3% Females: 31.4%—36.0%	MCHC is the average concentration of hemoglobin per red cell. It is calculated by dividing hemoglobin by hematocrit (MCHC = Hb × 10/Hct). MCHC is increased in hereditary spherocytosis, homozygous hemoglobin C disease, and sickle cell anemia.
Mean corpuscular volume (MCV), blood	78.2—97.9 fL	MCV is directly measured by automated hematology analyzers or can be calculated from hematocrit and red cell count (MCV = Hct × 10/red cell count). Increased MCV (macrocytosis) can be seen in reticulocytosis (e.g., hemolytic anemia), megaloblastic anemia (e.g., vitamin B_{12} or folate deficiency), and many patients with myelodysplastic syndrome. MCV may be falsely elevated in the setting of red cell agglutination. Decreased MCV (microcytosis) is seen when there is inadequate hemoglobin synthesis (e.g., iron deficiency anemia, anemia of chronic disease, thalassemia).
Monocyte count, blood	$0.26—0.81 \times 10^9$/L	Monocytes are a component of the innate immune system. They circulate in the blood before differentiating into macrophages. Monocyte numbers increase in certain chronic infections (e.g., tuberculosis), forms of chronic inflammation (e.g., autoimmune disease), and certain myeloproliferative neoplasms (e.g., chronic myelomonocytic leukemia). Monocyte levels may be decreased in corticosteroid therapy, chemotherapy, some infections, and hairy cell leukemia.

Neutrophil count, blood	$1.56-6.45 \times 10^9/L$	Neutrophils are phagocytic white blood cells that are important in acute inflammation. They are the most plentiful WBC in the peripheral blood of adult patients. Absolute neutrophilia is seen in acute infections (especially bacterial and fungal), tissue necrosis, infusion of growth factor (granulocyte-colony stimulating factor; G-CSF), corticosteroid therapy, and chronic myeloid neoplasms. "Left shift" refers to the presence of an increased proportion of immature neutrophils ("band" forms) and is characteristic of acute infection. Neutropenia is primarily due to destruction or decreased production of neutrophils. Causes include medications (e.g., chemotherapy), radiation, certain infections, autoimmune disease, bone marrow failure, and hematologic malignancies (e.g., MDS, acute leukemia).
Platelet count, blood	Males: $135-317 \times 10^9/L$ Females: $157-371 \times 10^9/L$	Platelets are central to primary hemostasis. They interact with von Willebrand factor and exposed collagen to form a platelet plug at sites of endothelial injury. Causes of thrombocytopenia are sequestration (e.g., hypersplenism), increased consumption (e.g., heparin-induced thrombocytopenia, immune thrombocytopenic purpura, disseminated intravascular coagulation, thrombotic thrombocytopenic purpura), or decreased production (infiltration of bone marrow, leukemias, viral infections). Causes of thrombocytosis include inflammation, hyposplenism/splenectomy, iron deficiency, and myeloproliferative neoplasms. Even if counts are normal, platelets may be dysfunctional due to drugs (e.g., aspirin), uremia, and genetic diseases (e.g., Bernard-Soulier syndrome, Glanzmann thrombasthenia).
Prothrombin time (PT), plasma	PT: 9.4–12.5 seconds International normalized ratio (INR): 0.9–1.1	PT assesses the extrinsic pathway of the coagulation cascade and is therefore elevated when there is a quantitative or qualitative abnormality in factors VII, X, II (prothrombin), or I (fibrinogen). PT results may be standardized among laboratories by converting the value into an international normalized ratio (INR), where the normal value is 1. PT/INR is commonly used as a screening test or to monitor patients on warfarin therapy.
Red cell count, blood	Males: $4.35-5.65 \times 10^{12}/L$ Females: $3.92-5.13 \times 10^{12}/L$	Red cell count is the number of red cells per mL of blood. Red cell production is stimulated by erythropoietin (EPO), which is produced by the kidneys. Absolute polycythemia is due to increased production (e.g., polycythemia vera, EPO administration, EPO-producing tumors) whereas anemia may be due to decreased production (e.g., iron deficiency, infiltrative marrow processes) or increased destruction (e.g., sickle cell anemia, hereditary spherocytosis).
Red cell distribution width (RDW), blood	Males: 11.8%–14.5% Females: 12.2%–16.1%	RDW is a measure of the variability in red cell size. Increased RDW is seen when there is anisocytosis or when there is a dimorphic red population (i.e., two populations of differing size as is the case in recent transfusion in a patient with a microcytic anemia). The presence of reticulocytes also increases the RDW. In the setting of microcytic anemia, increased RDW suggests iron deficiency anemia. An increased RDW in the setting of macrocytosis is suggestive of vitamin B_{12} or folic acid deficiency, or myelodysplastic syndrome.
Reticulocyte count, blood	0.60%–2.71%	Reticulocytes are immature red cells that are anucleate but still contain ribosomes and RNA. They are slightly larger and more basophilic than mature red cells due to retained RNA. The reticulocyte count reports reticulocytes as a percentage of total number of red cells and reflects recent bone marrow erythropoietic function. Elevated reticulocyte count is a normal physiologic response to anemia of any cause. In patients with anemia, the reticulocyte count may be falsely elevated since it is reported as a percentage of red cells (which are low in anemia).
Total iron binding capacity (TIBC), serum	250–400 µg/dL	Serum iron is bound to transferrin, which is typically about one-third saturated with iron. When iron stores in the body are depleted (e.g., iron deficiency anemia), transferrin levels increase in the blood, increasing the total iron-binding capacity (TIBC). In iron overload, TIBC decreases since free transferrin diminishes. TIBC, serum iron, and percent saturation are often assessed in the setting of iron deficiency anemia; however, serum ferritin is more sensitive and more accurately reflects the body's iron stores.

Vitamin B$_{12}$, serum	180—914 ng/L	Vitamin B$_{12}$ (cobalamin) is a water-soluble vitamin. It is required for the conversion of homocysteine to methionine in a process that yields tetrahydrofolic acid (TH$_4$), which is required for the synthesis of deoxythymidine monophosphate (dTMP), a building block for DNA. The most common cause of vitamin B$_{12}$ deficiency is chronic atrophic gastritis (pernicious anemia), an autoimmune disease leading to the destruction of gastric parietal cells. Vitamin B$_{12}$ deficiency is also seen in strict vegetarians and individuals with disorders affecting the distal ileum (e.g., Crohn disease). Vitamin B$_{12}$ deficiency leads to megaloblastic anemia and neuropathy. The former is characterized by hypersegmented neutrophils, macrocytosis, anemia, leukopenia, and thrombocytopenia due to decreased DNA synthesis. Vitamin B$_{12}$ deficiency also causes a demyelinating disorder of the posterior spinal tracts that is characterized by burning pain or loss of sensation in the extremities, weakness, spasticity and paralysis, confusion, disorientation, and dementia. Neurologic symptoms may occur without any discernible hematologic changes in the blood.
von Willebrand factor (vWF) antigen, plasma	55%—200%	von Willebrand factor (vWF) is synthesized in endothelial cells and megakaryocytes. In primary hemostasis, vWF binds to platelet receptor GPIb-IX and subendothelial collagen, thereby promoting platelet adhesion to collagen. Testing for vWF quantity is generally combined with a functional assay of vWF (e.g., vWF:Ristocetin cofactor assay). Decreased levels or decreased function of vWF can be seen in inherited or acquired forms of von Willebrand disease.
White blood cell (WBC) count, blood	3.4—9.6 × 10^9/L	WBCs are counted using an automatic analyzer. Most labs perform an automated differential count as part of the WBC count. When abnormal cells are detected, a manual review of the blood smear is performed. Increased WBCs are most often due to infections or hematologic malignancies. A low WBC count is usually a reflection of impaired marrow production due to medications or an infiltrative marrow disorder (e.g., fibrosis, granulomas, neoplasms). In severe sepsis, there may be a paradoxical drop in the WBC count due to consumption.

Molecular Tests of Relevance in Hematologic Malignancies

Analyte	Method	Pathophysiology/Clinical Relevance
BCL2 gene rearrangement	The presence of a BCL2 rearrangement in follicular lymphoma is inferred by an immunohistochemical stain for BCL2 protein (which is not expressed in normal germinal center B cells) or is detected directly by performing FISH or by karyotyping.	BCL2 is an antiapoptotic protein. Its overexpression in follicular lymphoma is due to BCL2 gene rearrangement, most commonly a t(14;18) in which BCL2 is fused to part of the immunoglobulin heavy chain locus (IGH). BCL2 rearrangements are also seen in a subset of diffuse large B-cell lymphoma and in certain other aggressive B-cell lymphomas.
BCL6 gene rearrangement	The presence of a BCL6 rearrangement is detected directly by performing FISH or by karyotyping.	BCL6 is a transcription factor that is required for the differentiation of antigen-stimulated B cells into germinal center B cells. BCL6 rearrangements are seen in a subset of diffuse large B-cell lymphoma.
BCR-ABL fusion gene	The presence of a BCR-ABL fusion gene is detected directly by performing FISH or by karyotyping or is inferred by using RT-PCR to identify BCR-ABL fusion mRNAs.	BCR-ABL fusion genes encode a constitutively active ABL tyrosine kinase. These fusions are found in 100% of chronic myeloid leukemia and a significant subset of B-cell acute lymphoblastic leukemia/lymphoma. Tumors with BCR-ABL fusion genes respond well to ABL kinase inhibitors. Sensitive BCR-ABL RT-PCR tests can also be used to monitor treated patients for early disease recurrence.
BRAF mutation	DNA sequence analysis, either as a focused test or as part of a NextGen sequencing panel	These mutations lead to constitutive activation of BRAF, a serine/threonine kinase that participates in the MAPK/ERK signaling pathway. BRAF mutations are found in all cases of typical hairy cell leukemia, which is very responsive to BRAF inhibitors.
CALR mutation	DNA sequence analysis, usually as part of a NextGen sequencing panel	Mutated CALR encodes a secreted protein that stimulates the thrombopoietin receptor, a tyrosine kinase. CALR mutations are found in a subset of primary myelofibrosis and essential thrombocythemia.

CCND1 gene rearrangement	The presence of a *CCND1* rearrangement is inferred by an immunohistochemical stain for cyclin D1 protein, which is not expressed in normal B cells, or is detected directly by performing FISH or by karyotyping.	Cyclin D1 forms complexes with two cyclin-dependent kinases, CDK4 and CDK6, that phosphorylate and inactivate RB during the G1 phase of the cell cycle, thereby promoting progression to S phase. *CCND1* rearrangements are seen in >95% of mantle cell lymphomas and a subset of multiple myelomas.
IDH1/IDH2 gene mutation	DNA sequence analysis, usually as part of a NextGen sequencing panel	Mutated IDH1 and IDH2 acquire a new enzymatic activity that drives high level production of 2-hydroxyglutarate (2HG), a metabolite intermediate that inhibits enzymes such as TET2, a regulator of DNA methylation. Mutated *IDH1* or *IDH2* are found in a subset of AML, which respond to drugs that selectively inhibit mutated IDH1 or IDH2.
JAK2 gene mutation	DNA sequence analysis, either as a focused test or as part of a NextGen sequencing panel	JAK2 is a tyrosine kinase expressed by hematopoietic cells that participates in the JAK/STAT signaling pathway downstream of several cytokine receptors. Activating *JAK2* mutations are found in 100% of polycythemia vera cases and in about 50% of essential thrombocythemia and 50% of primary myelofibrosis cases.
MPL gene mutation	DNA sequence analysis, usually as part of a NextGen sequencing panel	*MPL* encodes the thrombopoietin receptor tyrosine kinase. *MPL* mutations that produce constitutive activation of thrombopoietin receptor are found in a subset of primary myelofibrosis and essential thrombocythemia.
MYC gene rearrangement	The presence of an *MYC* rearrangement is detected directly by performing FISH or by karyotyping.	*MYC* rearrangement occurs in essentially all Burkitt lymphoma and a subset of diffuse large B-cell lymphoma and other aggressive B-cell malignancies.
MYD88 gene mutation	DNA sequence analysis, usually as part of a NextGen sequencing panel	*MYD88* encodes a signaling molecule that participates in Toll-like receptor signaling. Activating mutations in MYD88 are observed in >95% of cases of lymphoplasmacytic lymphoma.
PML-RARA fusion gene	The presence of a *PML-RARA* fusion gene is usually detected directly by performing FISH.	*PML-RARA* fusion genes are found in acute promyelocytic leukemia (APL). They encode chimeric PML-RARA fusion proteins consisting of part of the retinoic acid receptor fused to part of the promyelocytic leukemia protein. The PML-RARA fusion protein blocks myeloid cell differentiation by interfering with the function of the normal retinoic acid receptor. High doses of all-trans retinoic acid (ATRA) or treatment with arsenic salts abrogate the function of the PML-RARA fusion protein, leading to differentiation of APL cells into neutrophils, which then die by apoptosis. ATRA and arsenic salts are now standard treatment for APL, which is curable in >90% of cases.

[a]Duke University Health Systems Clinical Laboratories reference values.

References values from https://www.mayocliniclabs.com/ by permission of Mayo Foundation for Medical Education and Research. All rights reserved.

Adapted from Deyrup AT, D'Ambrosio D, Muir J, et al. Essential Laboratory Tests for Medical Education. *Acad Pathol.* 2022;9. doi: 10.1016/j.acpath.2022.100046.

Lung

OUTLINE

The major function of the lung is to provide the body with oxygen and to remove carbon dioxide. Efficient gas exchange is enabled by the lung's

The contributions to this chapter by Dr. Aliya Husain, Department of Pathology, University of Chicago, Chicago, Illinois, in several previous editions of this book are gratefully acknowledged.

anatomy, which serves to maximize the surface area of air spaces through which oxygen is absorbed from the air and vessels through which it is transported throughout the body bound to hemoglobin, while minimizing the distance between these two compartments, and therefore merits brief review. The *trachea* branches to give rise to right and left mainstem *bronchi*, which in turn give rise to three main bronchi on the

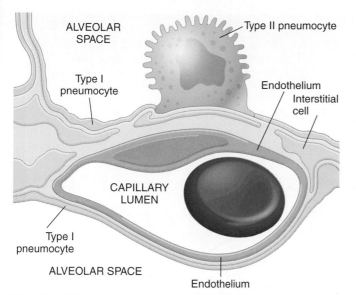

FIG. 11.1 Microscopic structure of the alveolar wall. Note that the basement membrane (yellow) is thin on one side and widened where it is continuous with the interstitial space.

right and two on the left. The main bronchi branch to give rise to progressively smaller airways, termed *bronchioles,* which are distinguished from bronchi by the lack of cartilage and submucosal glands within their walls. Further branching of bronchioles leads to *terminal bronchioles;* the part of the lung distal to the terminal bronchiole is called an *acinus.* Pulmonary acini are composed of *respiratory bronchioles* (emanating from the terminal bronchiole) that proceed into *alveolar ducts,* which immediately branch into *alveolar sacs,* the blind ends of the respiratory passages, whose walls are formed entirely of *alveoli,* the site of gas exchange. The alveolar walls (or alveolar septa) consist of the following components, proceeding from blood to air (Fig. 11.1):

- The *capillary endothelium* and *basement membrane*
- The *pulmonary interstitium,* composed of fine elastic fibers, small bundles of collagen, a few fibroblast-like cells, smooth muscle cells, mast cells, and rare mononuclear cells
- *Alveolar epithelium,* consisting of a continuous layer of two principal cell types: flattened, platelike type I pneumocytes covering 95% of the alveolar surface and rounded type II pneumocytes. The latter synthesize pulmonary surfactant and are the main cell type involved in repair of alveolar epithelium after damage to type I pneumocytes.

A few alveolar macrophages usually lie free within the alveolar space. In city dwellers, these macrophages often contain phagocytosed carbon particles.

Lung diseases can broadly be divided into those affecting the airways, the interstitium, or the pulmonary vascular system. This division into discrete compartments is deceptively simple, as disease in one compartment often causes secondary alterations of morphology and function in others.

ATELECTASIS (COLLAPSE)

Atelectasis is loss of lung volume caused by inadequate expansion of air spaces. Because atelectatic lung continues to be perfused, it produces a ventilation-perfusion imbalance and hypoxemia. On the basis of the underlying mechanism and its anatomic, atelectasis is classified into three forms:

- *Obstruction atelectasis* occurs when an obstruction prevents air from reaching distal airways. Air present distal to the obstruction

is gradually absorbed, leading to alveolar collapse. The most common cause of resorption atelectasis is postoperative intrabronchial mucous or mucopurulent plugs, but it may also result from foreign body aspiration (particularly in children), bronchial asthma, bronchiectasis, chronic bronchitis, or intrabronchial tumor, in which it may be the first sign of malignancy.
- *Compression atelectasis* is caused by the accumulation of fluid, blood, or air within the pleural cavity. A frequent cause is pleural effusions in the setting of congestive heart failure. Leakage of air into the pleural cavity (pneumothorax) also leads to compression atelectasis. Basal atelectasis, resulting from a failure to breathe deeply, commonly occurs in patients who are bedridden, in those with ascites, and during and after surgery.
- *Contraction atelectasis* (or cicatrization atelectasis) occurs when local or diffuse pulmonary or pleural fibrosis hampers lung expansion.

Atelectasis (except when caused by contraction) is potentially reversible and should be treated promptly to prevent hypoxemia and superimposed infection of the collapsed lung.

ACUTE LUNG INJURY AND ACUTE RESPIRATORY DISTRESS SYNDROME

Acute lung injury (ALI) is characterized by the abrupt onset of hypoxemia and bilateral pulmonary edema in the absence of cardiac failure (noncardiogenic pulmonary edema); if severe, ALI may lead to acute respiratory distress syndrome (ARDS). Both ARDS and ALI are associated with inflammation-induced increases in pulmonary vascular permeability, edema, and epithelial cell death. The histologic manifestation of these conditions is *diffuse alveolar damage.*

The definition of acute respiratory distress syndrome (ARDS) is evolving. Formerly considered to be the severe end of a spectrum of acute lung injury, it is now defined as respiratory failure occurring within 1 week of a known clinical insult with bilateral opacities on chest imaging that are not fully explained by effusions, atelectasis, cardiac failure, or fluid overload. It is graded based on the severity of blood hypoxemia. Causes are diverse; the shared feature is that all lead to extensive bilateral alveolar injury.

ARDS may occur in a multitude of clinical settings and is associated with primary pulmonary diseases and severe systemic inflammatory disorders such as sepsis. The most frequent triggers of ARDS are pneumonia (35%–45%) and sepsis (30%–35%) followed by aspiration, trauma (including brain injury, abdominal surgery, and multiple fractures), pancreatitis, and transfusion reactions. Notably, COVID-19 pneumonia (described later) progresses in a subset of patients to ARDS, which often requires intubation and mechanical ventilation. ARDS should not be confused with respiratory distress syndrome of the newborn; the latter is caused by a deficiency of surfactant in the setting of prematurity.

Pathogenesis. **The underlying basis of ARDS is injury to the epithelial and endothelial linings of the alveolar-capillary membrane.** Most research suggests that ARDS stems from an inflammatory reaction initiated by proinflammatory mediators (Fig. 11.2). Release of factors such as IL-1 and tumor necrosis factor (TNF) leads to endothelial activation and sequestration and activation of neutrophils in pulmonary capillaries. Neutrophils are thought to have an important role in the pathogenesis of ARDS. Histologic examination of lungs early in the disease process shows increased numbers of neutrophils within capillaries, the interstitium, and alveoli. Activated neutrophils release a variety of products (e.g., reactive oxygen

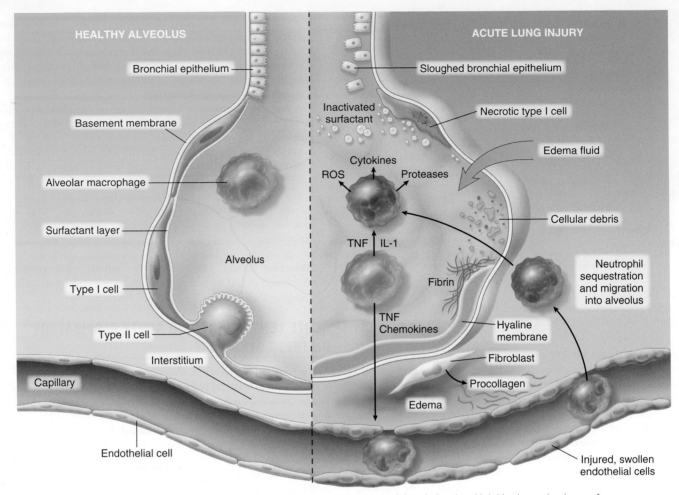

FIG. 11.2 Acute lung injury. The healthy alveolus *(left)* and the injured alveolus *(right)* in the early phase of acute lung injury and the acute respiratory distress syndrome. Under the influence of proinflammatory cytokines such as IL-1 and tumor necrosis factor *(TNF)* (released by macrophages), neutrophils are sequestered in the pulmonary microvasculature and then egress into the alveolar space, where they undergo activation. Activated neutrophils release mediators such as reactive oxygen species (ROS), cytokines, and proteases, which contribute to local tissue damage, accumulation of edema fluid, surfactant inactivation, and hyaline membrane formation. (Modified from Ware LB: Pathophysiology of acute lung injury and the acute respiratory distress syndrome. *Semin Respir Crit Care Med* 27:337, 2006.)

species, proteases) that damage the alveolar epithelium and endothelium. The assault on the endothelium and epithelium causes vascular leakiness and a loss of surfactant that stiffens the alveolar unit. Of note, the destructive forces unleashed by neutrophils can be counteracted by an array of endogenous antiproteases and antioxidants. In the end, it is the balance between these destructive and protective factors that determines the degree of tissue injury and clinical severity of ARDS.

MORPHOLOGY

In the **acute phase of ARDS,** the lungs are dark red, firm, airless, and heavy. Microscopic examination reveals capillary congestion, necrotic alveolar epithelial cells, interstitial and intraalveolar edema and hemorrhage, and (particularly with sepsis) collections of neutrophils in capillaries. The most characteristic finding is the presence of **hyaline membranes,** particularly lining the distended alveolar ducts (Fig. 11.3). Such membranes consist of fibrin-rich edema fluid admixed with remnants of necrotic epithelial cells. Overall, the picture is remarkably similar to that seen in

respiratory distress syndrome of the newborn (Chapter 4). In the **organizing stage,** type II pneumocytes proliferate vigorously in an attempt to regenerate the alveolar lining. Complete resolution is unusual; more commonly, the fibrin-rich exudates undergo organization, leading to fibrosis and alveolar septal thickening.

Clinical Features. It is estimated that acute lung injury or ARDS affects approximately 200,000 patients per year in the United States. In 85% of cases, it develops within 72 hours of the initial insult. ARDS is the underlying disorder in a sizable minority of patients who require mechanical ventilation. Imaging studies show bilateral ground glass opacities (eFig. 11.1). Predictors of poor prognosis include advanced age, bacteremia (sepsis), and the development of multiorgan failure. The overall mortality rate is about 40%, with death usually stemming from the underlying condition or superimposed infection. Death from respiratory failure is uncommon. Survivors frequently have decreased physical endurance due in part to lung function abnormalities.

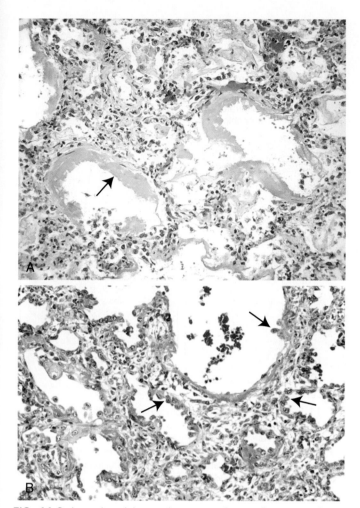

FIG. 11.3 Acute lung injury and acute respiratory distress syndrome. (A) Diffuse alveolar damage in the acute phase. Some alveoli are collapsed, while others are distended; many are lined by bright pink hyaline membranes *(arrow)*. (B) The healing stage is marked by resorption of hyaline membranes and thickening of alveolar septa by inflammatory cells, fibroblasts, and collagen. Numerous reactive type II pneumocytes *(arrows)* also are seen at this stage, associated with regeneration and repair.

OBSTRUCTIVE AND RESTRICTIVE PULMONARY DISEASES

Diffuse pulmonary diseases can be classified into two categories: (1) obstructive (airway) disease, characterized by an increase in resistance to air flow caused by partial or complete obstruction at any level; and (2) restrictive disease, marked by reduced expansion of lung parenchyma, and decreased total lung capacity.

The major diffuse obstructive disorders are *emphysema, chronic bronchitis, bronchiectasis,* and *asthma.* In patients with these diseases, the expiratory flow rate, measured as the forced expiratory volume at 1 second (FEV_1), is significantly decreased, whereas forced vital capacity (FVC) is either normal or slightly decreased. Thus, the ratio of FEV_1 to FVC is decreased. An FEV_1/FVC ratio of less than 0.7 generally indicates the presence of obstructive disease. Expiratory obstruction may result from airway narrowing, classically observed in asthma, or from loss of elastic recoil, seen in emphysema.

By contrast, in diffuse restrictive diseases, FVC is reduced and the expiratory flow rate is normal or reduced proportionately. Hence, the ratio of FEV_1 to FVC is near normal. Restrictive diseases fall into two broad categories: (1) disorders of chest wall expansion in the presence of normal lungs (e.g., severe obesity, diseases of the pleura, and neuromuscular disorders, such as the Guillain-Barré syndrome [Chapter 20]) and (2) acute or chronic interstitial lung diseases. The classic acute restrictive disease is ARDS, discussed earlier. Chronic restrictive diseases (discussed later) include the pneumoconioses, interstitial fibrosing disorders, and infiltrative conditions such as sarcoidosis.

OBSTRUCTIVE LUNG (AIRWAY) DISEASES

In their prototypical forms, the four major disorders in this group—emphysema, chronic bronchitis, asthma, and bronchiectasis—have distinct clinical and anatomic characteristics (Table 11.1). However, emphysema and chronic bronchitis cooccur so frequently that they are typically considered together under the rubric of *chronic obstructive pulmonary disease.* Their close association is not surprising, as cigarette smoking is the major underlying cause of both emphysema and chronic bronchitis.

Chronic Obstructive Pulmonary Disease

Chronic obstructive pulmonary disease (COPD), a major public health problem, is defined by the World Health Organization

Table 11.1 Disorders Associated With Airflow Obstruction

Clinical Entity	Anatomic Site	Major Pathologic Changes	Etiology	Signs/Symptoms
Emphysema	Acinus	Air space enlargement, wall destruction	Tobacco smoke	Dyspnea
Chronic bronchitis	Bronchus	Mucous gland hypertrophy and hyperplasia, hypersecretion	Tobacco smoke, air pollutants	Cough, sputum production
Bronchiectasis	Bronchus	Airway dilation and scarring	Persistent or severe infections	Cough, purulent sputum, fever
Asthma	Bronchus	Smooth muscle hypertrophy and hyperplasia, excessive mucus, inflammation	Immunologic or undefined causes	Episodic wheezing, cough, dyspnea
Small airway disease, bronchiolitis[a]	Bronchiole	Inflammatory scarring, partial obliteration of bronchioles	Tobacco smoke, air pollutants	Cough, dyspnea

[a]Can be present in all forms of obstructive lung disease or occur by itself.

(WHO) as "a common, preventable and treatable disease that is characterized by persistent respiratory symptoms and airflow limitation that is due to airway and/or alveolar abnormalities caused by exposure to noxious particles or gases." COPD affects more than 10% of the U.S. adult population over the age of 40 years. It is the fourth leading cause of death in this country, the third leading cause of death worldwide, and is rising in frequency due to increases in cigarette smoking in parts of Africa and Asia. Overall, 35% to 50% of heavy smokers develop COPD; conversely, about 80% of COPD is attributable to smoking. Women appear to be more susceptible than men to developing COPD. Additional risk factors include poor lung development early in life, exposure to environmental and occupational pollutants, airway hyperresponsiveness, and certain genetic polymorphisms.

Although emphysema and chronic bronchitis often occur together as part of COPD, it is useful to discuss these patterns of lung injury and associated functional abnormalities individually to highlight the pathophysiologic basis of different causes of airflow obstruction (Fig. 11.4). We will conclude our discussion by returning to the clinical features of COPD.

Emphysema

Emphysema is characterized by permanent enlargement of the air spaces distal to the terminal bronchioles, accompanied by destruction of their walls but without significant fibrosis. It is classified according to its anatomic distribution. As discussed earlier, the acinus is the structure distal to terminal bronchioles, and a cluster of three to five acini is called a *lobule* (Fig. 11.5A). There are four patterns of emphysema: (1) centriacinar, (2) panacinar, (3) distal acinar, and (4) irregular. Only the first two types are associated with COPD, with centriacinar emphysema being about 20 times more common than panacinar disease.

- *Centriacinar (centrilobular) emphysema.* The distinctive feature of centriacinar emphysema is involvement of the central or proximal parts of the acini with sparing of the distal alveoli. Thus, both emphysematous and normal air spaces exist within the same acinus and lobule (Fig. 11.5B). The lesions are more common and severe in the upper lobes, particularly in the apical segments. In advanced centriacinar emphysema the distal acinus is also

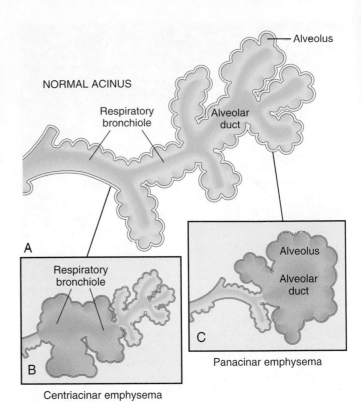

FIG. 11.5 Major patterns of emphysema. (A) Diagram of normal structure of the acinus, the fundamental unit of the lung. (B) Centriacinar emphysema with dilation that initially affects the respiratory bronchioles. (C) Panacinar emphysema with initial distention of all the peripheral structures (i.e., the alveolus and alveolar duct); the disease later extends to affect the respiratory bronchioles.

involved, making it difficult to differentiate from panacinar emphysema. Centroacinar emphysema is most common in individuals who smoke cigarettes, in whom it is often accompanied by chronic bronchitis.

- *Panacinar (panlobular) emphysema.* In panacinar emphysema, the acini are uniformly enlarged, from the level of the respiratory bronchiole to the terminal blind alveoli (Fig. 11.5C). In contrast to centriacinar emphysema, panacinar emphysema occurs more commonly in the lower lung zones and is associated with α1-antitrypsin deficiency.
- *Distal acinar (paraseptal) emphysema.* In this form of emphysema, the part of the acinus distal to the respiratory bronchiole is primarily affected. It tends to be found near the pleura, along the lobular connective tissue septa, and at the margins of the lobules adjacent to areas of fibrosis, scarring, or atelectasis, and is usually more severe in the upper half of the lungs. The characteristic finding is multiple enlarged air spaces ranging in diameter from less than 0.5 mm to more than 2.0 cm, sometimes forming cystic structures, that with further enlargement give rise to *bullae*. The cause is unknown; it comes to attention most often in young adults who present with spontaneous pneumothorax.
- *Irregular emphysema.* Irregular emphysema, so named because the acinus is irregularly involved, is almost invariably associated with scarring. In most cases it occurs in small foci and is clinically insignificant.

Pathogenesis. **Inhaled cigarette smoke and other noxious particles cause lung damage and inflammation, which, particularly in patients**

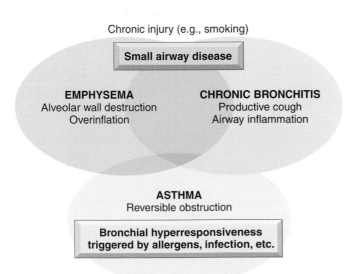

FIG. 11.4 Schematic representation of overlap between chronic obstructive lung diseases.

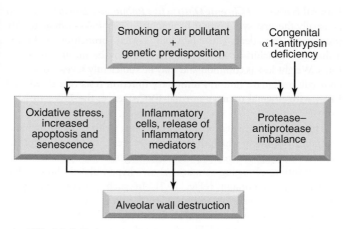

FIG. 11.6 Pathogenesis of emphysema. See text for details.

bronchioles to collapse during expiration. **This leads to functional airflow obstruction in the absence of mechanical obstruction.**

MORPHOLOGY

The diagnosis and classification of emphysema depend largely on the macroscopic appearance of the lung. Typical **panacinar emphysema** produces pale, voluminous lungs that often obscure the heart when the anterior chest wall is removed at autopsy. The macroscopic features of **centriacinar emphysema** are less impressive. Until late stages, the lungs are a deeper pink than in panacinar emphysema and less voluminous; the upper two-thirds of the lungs are more severely affected than the lower lungs. Histologic examination reveals **destruction of alveolar walls without fibrosis, leading to enlarged air spaces** (Fig. 11.7). Due to alveolar loss, the number of alveolar capillaries is diminished. Terminal and respiratory bronchioles may be deformed because of the loss of septa that tether these structures in the parenchyma. Bronchiolar inflammation and submucosal fibrosis are often present in advanced disease.

with a genetic predisposition, result in parenchymal destruction. Factors that influence the development of emphysema include the following (Fig. 11.6):

- *Inflammatory cells and mediators:* A wide variety of inflammatory mediators have been implicated (including leukotriene B_4, the chemokine IL-8, the cytokine tumor necrosis factor [TNF], and others). These serve to recruit additional inflammatory cells from the circulation (chemotactic factors), amplify the inflammatory process (proinflammatory cytokines), and induce structural changes (growth factors). The inflammatory cells present in lesions include neutrophils, macrophages, and CD4+ and CD8+ T cells. It is not known what antigens the T cells are specific for.
- *Protease–antiprotease imbalance:* Several proteases are released from the inflammatory cells and epithelial cells that break down connective tissues. In patients who develop emphysema, there is a relative deficiency of protective antiproteases (discussed below).
- *Oxidative stress:* Reactive oxygen species are present in cigarette smoke, which also contains particles and other substances that stimulate the release of additional reactive oxygen species from inflammatory cells such as macrophages and neutrophils. These cause tissue damage and inflammation (Chapter 2).
- *Airway infection:* Although infection is not thought to play a role in the initiation of tissue destruction, bacterial and/or viral infections cause acute exacerbations.

The idea that proteases are important is based in part on the observation that an inherited deficiency of the antiprotease α1-antitrypsin predisposes to emphysema, an effect that is compounded by smoking. About 1% of patients with emphysema have this defect. α1-antitrypsin, normally present in serum, tissue fluids, and macrophages, is a major inhibitor of proteases (particularly elastase) secreted by neutrophils during inflammation. It is encoded by the proteinase inhibitor *(Pi)* locus on chromosome 14. The *Pi* locus is polymorphic, and approximately 0.01% of the U.S. population is homozygous for the *Z* allele, a genotype that is associated with markedly decreased serum levels of α1-antitrypsin. More than 80% of these individuals develop symptomatic panacinar emphysema, which occurs at an earlier age and is of greater severity if the individual smokes.

Protease-mediated damage of extracellular matrix has a central role in the airway obstruction seen in emphysema. Small airways are normally held open by the elastic recoil of the lung parenchyma, and the loss of elastic tissue in the walls of alveoli that surround respiratory bronchioles reduces radial traction and thus causes the respiratory

Chronic Bronchitis

Chronic bronchitis is defined by the presence of a persistent productive cough for at least 3 consecutive months in at least 2 consecutive years. Thus its definition is based on clinical features, as opposed to emphysema which is defined anatomically. It is common among people who smoke cigarettes and urban dwellers in smog-ridden cities. In early stages of chronic bronchitis, the cough produces mucoid sputum, but airflow is not obstructed. Some patients with chronic bronchitis have evidence of hyperresponsive airways, with intermittent bronchospasm and wheezing (asthmatic bronchitis), while other patients with bronchitis, especially those who smoke heavily, develop chronic outflow obstruction, usually with associated emphysema.

Pathogenesis. **The distinctive feature of chronic bronchitis is hypersecretion of mucus, beginning in the large airways.** Although the most important cause is cigarette smoking, other air pollutants, such as sulfur dioxide and nitrogen dioxide, may contribute. These

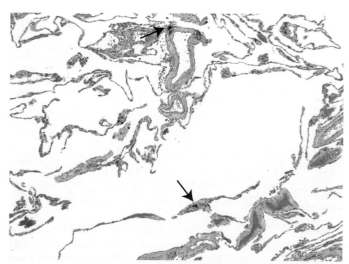

FIG. 11.7 Pulmonary emphysema. There is marked enlargement of the air spaces, with destruction of alveolar septa but without fibrosis. Note the presence of black anthracotic pigment *(arrows)*.

environmental irritants induce (1) hypertrophy of mucous glands in the trachea and bronchi; (2) an increase in mucin-secreting goblet cells in the epithelial surfaces of smaller bronchi and bronchioles; and (3) inflammation marked by the infiltration of macrophages, neutrophils, and lymphocytes. In contrast with asthma (described later), eosinophils are not seen in chronic bronchitis. Whereas the mucus hypersecretion primarily involves the large bronchi, the airflow obstruction in chronic bronchitis results from small airway disease (*chronic bronchiolitis*) induced by mucous plugging of the bronchiolar lumen, inflammation, and bronchiolar wall fibrosis.

It is postulated that many of the effects of environmental irritants on respiratory epithelium are mediated by local release of cytokines such as IL-13 from T cells. The expression of mucins in bronchial epithelium and the production of neutrophil elastase are also increased as a consequence of exposure to tobacco smoke. Microbial infection is often present but has a secondary role, chiefly by maintaining inflammation and exacerbating symptoms.

MORPHOLOGY

Grossly, the mucosal lining of the larger airways is usually **hyperemic and swollen** by edema fluid and is covered by a layer of mucinous or mucopurulent **secretions.** The smaller bronchi and bronchioles may also be filled with secretions. The diagnostic feature of chronic bronchitis in the trachea and larger bronchi is **enlargement of the mucus-secreting glands** (Fig. 11.8). The magnitude of the increase in size is assessed by the ratio of the thickness of the submucosal gland layer to that of the bronchial wall (the Reid index—normally 0.4). Variable numbers of inflammatory cells, largely lymphocytes and macrophages but sometimes also admixed neutrophils, are frequently seen in the bronchial mucosa. **Chronic bronchiolitis** (small airway disease), characterized by goblet cell metaplasia, mucus plugging, inflammation, and fibrosis, is also seen. In severe cases, there may be complete obliteration of the lumen as a consequence of fibrosis **(bronchiolitis obliterans).** It is the submucosal fibrosis that leads to luminal narrowing and airway obstruction. Emphysematous changes often coexist.

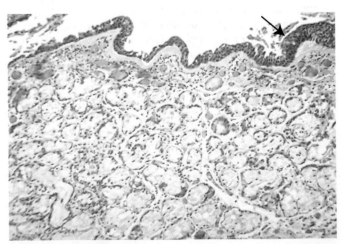

FIG. 11.8 Chronic bronchitis. The lumen of the bronchus is above. Note the marked thickening of the mucous gland layer (approximately twice normal) and squamous metaplasia *(arrow)* of lung epithelium. (From the Teaching Collection of the Department of Pathology, University of Texas, Southwestern Medical School, Dallas, Texas.)

Clinical Features of Chronic Obstructive Pulmonary Disease. *Dyspnea* is usually the first symptom; it begins insidiously but is often steadily progressive. In patients with underlying chronic bronchitis or chronic asthmatic bronchitis, cough and wheezing may be the initial symptoms. Weight loss is common and may be sufficiently severe to suggest an occult malignant tumor. **Pulmonary function tests reveal reduced FEV$_1$ with normal or near-normal FVC. Hence, the FEV$_1$ to FVC ratio is reduced.**

The classic presentation of emphysema with no "bronchitic" component is one in which the patient is barrel-chested and dyspneic, with obviously prolonged expiration, sitting forward in a hunched-over position. Imaging studies show hyperinflated lungs that "flatten" the diaphragm (eFig. 11.2). In such patients, air space enlargement is severe and diffusion capacity is low. Dyspnea and hyperventilation are prominent, so until very late in the disease, gas exchange is adequate and blood gas values are relatively normal. Hypoxia-induced vascular spasm and loss of capillary surface area from alveolar destruction cause the gradual development of *secondary pulmonary hypertension,* which in 20% to 30% of patients leads to right-sided congestive heart failure (cor pulmonale, Chapter 9).

At the other end of the clinical spectrum is a patient with pronounced chronic bronchitis and a history of recurrent infections. The course is quite variable. In some patients, cough and sputum production persist indefinitely without ventilatory dysfunction, while others develop significant outflow obstruction. Dyspnea is usually less prominent than in those with "pure" emphysema, and in the absence of increased respiratory drive the patient may retain carbon dioxide, becoming hypoxic and often cyanotic. The majority of patients with this type of COPD are overweight or obese, which may further decrease ventilation, particularly during sleep. Patients with severe chronic bronchitis have more frequent exacerbations, more rapid disease progression, and poorer outcomes than those with emphysema alone. Progressive COPD is marked by the development of pulmonary hypertension, sometimes leading to cardiac failure (Chapter 9); recurrent infections; and ultimately respiratory failure. Approximately 10% to 30% of patients have obstructive sleep apnea; the pathogenic relationship between these two disorders is incompletely understood.

Emphysematous Conditions Other Than COPD

Several other conditions marked by abnormal air spaces or accumulations of air within the lungs or other tissues merit brief mention:

- *Compensatory emphysema* is the dilation of residual alveoli in response to loss of lung substance elsewhere, such as through surgical removal of a diseased lung or lobe.
- *Obstructive overinflation* is expansion of the lung due to air trapping. A common cause is subtotal obstruction of an airway by a tumor or foreign object. Obstructive overinflation may be life threatening if expansion of the affected portion produces compression of the remaining normal lung.
- *Bullous emphysema* refers to large subpleural blebs or bullae (spaces >1 cm in diameter in the distended state) (Fig. 11.9). Such blebs stem from a localized accentuation of one of the four forms of pulmonary emphysema (discussed previously); most often the blebs are subpleural and prone to rupture, leading to pneumothorax.
- *Mediastinal (interstitial) emphysema* is caused by entry of air into the interstitium of the lung, from where it may then track to the mediastinum and sometimes the subcutaneous tissue. It may occur when a sudden increase in intraalveolar pressure (as with vomiting or violent coughing) causes alveolar rupture, allowing air to dissect into the interstitium. It may also occur in patients on respirators

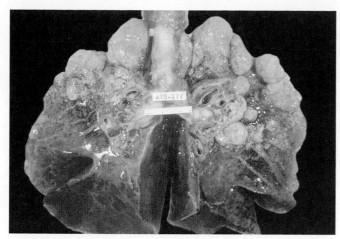

FIG. 11.9 Bullous emphysema with large apical and subpleural bullae. (From the Teaching Collection of the Department of Pathology, University of Texas Southwestern Medical School, Dallas, Texas.)

who have partial bronchiolar obstruction or in individuals with a perforating injury (e.g., a fractured rib). If the interstitial air reaches the subcutaneous tissue, there can be marked swelling of the head and neck and crackling crepitation *(subcutaneous emphysema)* over the chest. In most instances the air is resorbed spontaneously after the site of entry seals.

Asthma

Asthma is a chronic inflammatory disorder of the airways that causes recurrent episodes of bronchospasm characterized by wheezing, breathlessness, chest tightness, and cough, particularly at night and/or early in the morning. The hallmarks of asthma are the following:
- Intermittent, reversible airway obstruction
- Chronic bronchial inflammation with eosinophils
- Bronchial smooth muscle cell hypertrophy and hyperreactivity
- Increased mucus secretion

In patients with severe airway hyperreactivity, trivial stimuli may be sufficient to trigger attacks. Many cells play a role in the inflammatory response, in particular eosinophils, mast cells, macrophages, lymphocytes, neutrophils, and epithelial cells. Of note, asthma has increased in incidence significantly in more affluent countries over the past four decades. One proposed explanation for this trend is the *hygiene hypothesis,* according to which a lack of exposure to microbes and potential allergens in early childhood results in hyperreactivity to immune stimuli later in life. Attractive as it seems, there is no mechanistic basis for this hypothesis.

Pathogenesis. **Major factors contributing to the development of asthma include genetic predisposition to type I hypersensitivity (atopy), acute and chronic airway inflammation, and bronchial hyperresponsiveness to a variety of stimuli.** Asthma may be subclassified as *atopic* (marked by evidence of allergen sensitization) or *nonatopic.* In both types, episodes of bronchospasm are triggered by diverse exposures, such as respiratory infections (especially viral), airborne irritants (e.g., smoke, fumes), and environmental stresses. There are varying patterns of inflammation—eosinophilic (most common), neutrophilic, mixed inflammatory, and pauci-granulocytic—that are associated with differing etiologies, immunopathologies, and responses to treatment.

Both atopic and nonatopic forms of asthma are caused by activation of mast cells and eosinophils, which release mediators that induce bronchoconstriction, inflammation, and mucus production. The difference lies in how these are triggered—by immune mechanisms involving Th2 cells and IgE in the atopic form (discussed below) and by infection or nonimmunologic stimuli in the nonatopic form.

Asthma shows familial clustering, but the role of genetics in asthma is complex. Genome-wide association studies have identified a large number of genetic variants associated with asthma risk, some in genes encoding factors like the IL-4 receptor that are clearly involved in asthma pathogenesis. However, the precise contribution of asthma-associated genetic variants to the development of disease remains to be determined.

Atopic Asthma

This is the most common type of asthma and is a classic example of type I IgE-mediated hypersensitivity reaction (Chapter 5). It usually begins in childhood. A positive family history of atopy and/or asthma is common, and the onset of asthmatic attacks is often preceded by allergic rhinitis, urticaria, or eczema. Attacks may be triggered by allergens in dust, pollen, animal dander, or food, or by infections. The diagnosis depends on the presence of typical episodic symptoms and documentation of airflow limitation that is corrected by treatment with bronchodilators. Skin testing with the offending antigen results in an immediate wheal-and-flare reaction. In addition, immunoassays can be used to identify the presence of IgE antibodies that recognize specific allergens.

The classic atopic form is associated with activation of type 2 helper T (Th2) cells, which release cytokines that account for most of the observed features—specifically, increased production of IgE from B cells (stimulated by IL-4 and IL-13); increased recruitment and activation of eosinophils (stimulated by IL-5); and increased mucus production (stimulated by IL-13). IgE binds to Fc receptors on submucosal mast cells, sensitizing these cells to allergens that cross-link IgE molecules and stimulate the release of mast cell granule contents and the secretion of cytokines and other mediators. These mediators set in motion events that lead to two waves of reaction, an early (immediate) phase and a late phase (Fig. 11.10):
- The *early phase reaction* is dominated by bronchoconstriction, increased mucus production, and vasodilation. Bronchoconstriction is triggered by mediators released from mast cells, including histamine, prostaglandin D_2, and leukotrienes C_4, D_4, and E_4, and also by reflex neural pathways.
- The *late-phase reaction* is inflammatory in nature. Inflammatory mediators stimulate epithelial cells to produce chemokines (including eotaxin, a potent chemoattractant of eosinophils) that promote the recruitment of Th2 cells, eosinophils, and other leukocytes, thus amplifying an inflammatory reaction that is initiated by resident immune cells.
- Repeated bouts of inflammation lead to structural changes in the bronchial wall that are collectively referred to as *airway remodeling.* These changes include hypertrophy of bronchial smooth muscle and mucus glands and increased vascularity and deposition of subepithelial collagen, which may occur several years before symptoms begin.
- In addition, recent experimental work has shown that *Charcot-Leyden crystals* (eFig. 11.3), derived from a protein produced by eosinophils called galectin-10 and frequently seen in the airway mucous of patients with asthma, may be an important proinflammatory factor.

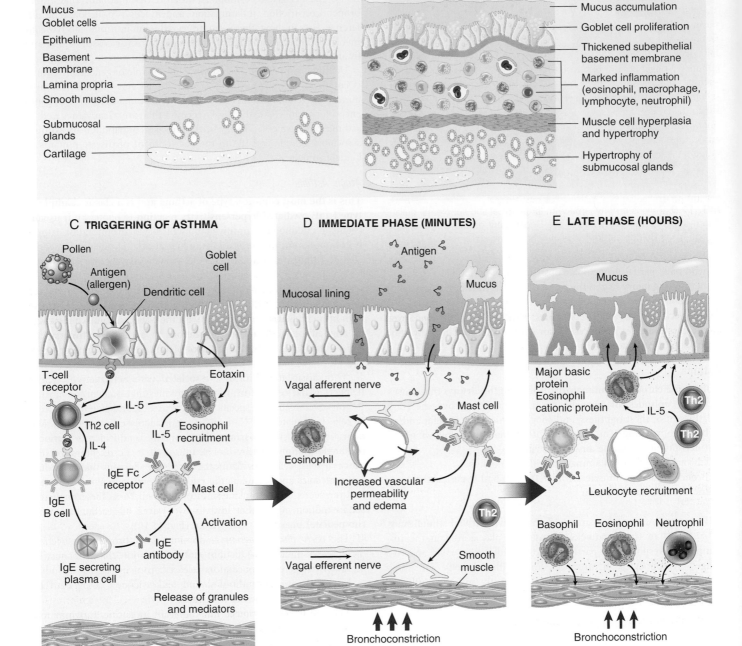

FIG. 11.10 (A and B) Comparison of a healthy airway and an airway involved by asthma. The asthmatic airway is marked by accumulation of mucus in the bronchial lumen secondary to an increase in the number of mucus-secreting goblet cells in the mucosa and hypertrophy of submucosal glands; intense chronic inflammation due to recruitment of eosinophils, macrophages, and other inflammatory cells; thickened basement membrane; and hypertrophy and hyperplasia of smooth muscle cells. (C) Inhaled allergens (antigen) elicit a Th2-dominated response favoring IgE production and eosinophil recruitment. (D) On reexposure to antigen (Ag), the immediate reaction is triggered by antigen-induced crosslinking of IgE bound to Fc receptors on mast cells. These cells release mediators that directly and via neuronal reflexes induce bronchospasm, increased vascular permeability, mucus production, and recruitment of leukocytes. The latter (i.e., leukocyte recruitment) is the dominant finding in late phase reaction. (E) Leukocytes recruited to the site of reaction (neutrophils, eosinophils, and basophils; lymphocytes and monocytes) release additional mediators that initiate the late phase of asthma. Several factors released from eosinophils (e.g., major basic protein, eosinophil cationic protein) also cause damage to the epithelium.

Nonatopic Asthma

Patients with nonatopic forms of asthma do not have evidence of allergen sensitization, and skin test results are usually negative. A positive family history of asthma is less common. Respiratory infections due to viruses (e.g., rhinovirus, parainfluenza virus) and inhaled air pollutants (e.g., sulfur dioxide, ozone, nitrogen dioxide) are common triggers. Also important are other environmental triggers, such as cold air, stress, and exercise. It is thought that virus-induced inflammation of the respiratory mucosa lowers the threshold of the subepithelial vagal receptors to irritants. Although the connections are not well understood, the ultimate humoral and cellular mediators of airway obstruction (e.g., eosinophils) are common to both atopic and nonatopic variants of asthma, so treatment is similar.

Drug-Induced Asthma

Several pharmacologic agents provoke asthma, aspirin being the most striking example. Patients with aspirin sensitivity present with recurrent rhinitis, nasal polyps, urticaria, and bronchospasm. The precise pathogenesis is unknown but is likely to involve some abnormality in prostaglandin metabolism stemming from inhibition of cyclooxygenase by aspirin.

Occupational Asthma

Occupational asthma may be triggered by fumes (e.g., epoxy resins, plastics), organic and chemical dusts (e.g., wood, cotton, platinum), gases (e.g., toluene), and other chemicals. Asthma attacks usually develop after repeated exposure to the inciting antigen(s).

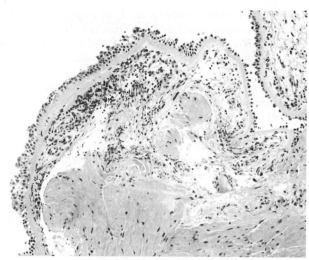

FIG. 11.11 Bronchial biopsy specimen from an asthmatic patient showing subbasement membrane fibrosis, eosinophilic inflammation, and smooth muscle hyperplasia.

> ## MORPHOLOGY
>
> The morphologic changes in asthma have been described in individuals who die due to severe attacks and in mucosal biopsy specimens of individuals challenged with allergens. In fatal cases, the lungs are distended due to air trapping (overinflation), and there may be small areas of atelectasis. The most striking finding is occlusion of bronchi and bronchioles by thick, tenacious **mucous plugs** containing whorls of shed epithelium (**Curschmann spirals**). Numerous eosinophils and **Charcot-Leyden crystals** (see eFig. 11.3) are also present. Other characteristic morphologic changes in asthma (Fig. 11.10B), collectively called airway remodeling, include
> * Thickening of airway wall
> * Subbasement membrane fibrosis (Fig. 11.11)
> * Increased submucosal vascularity
> * An increase in size of the submucosal glands and goblet cell metaplasia of the airway epithelium
> * Hypertrophy and/or hyperplasia of bronchial muscle

Clinical Features. An attack of asthma is characterized by severe dyspnea and wheezing due to bronchoconstriction and mucus plugging, which leads to trapping of air in distal air spaces and progressive hyperinflation of the lungs. In the usual case, attacks last from 1 to several hours and subside either spontaneously or with therapy. Intervals between attacks are characteristically free from overt respiratory difficulties, but persistent subtle deficits can be detected by pulmonary function tests. Occasionally a severe paroxysm occurs that does not respond to therapy and persists for days and even weeks (*status asthmaticus*). The associated hypercapnia, acidosis, and severe hypoxia may be fatal, although in most cases the condition is more disabling than lethal.

Patients with relatively mild episodic disease are usually treated symptomatically with bronchodilators (such as beta-agonist drugs) and glucocorticoids, sometimes in combination with leukotriene inhibitors (recall that leukotrienes are potent bronchoconstrictors). In patients with more severe disease who have elevated eosinophil counts, high IgE levels, and other evidence of a heightened Th2 response, antibodies that block the action of specific immune mediators (such as IL-4, IL-5, and IgE) are beneficial.

Bronchiectasis

Bronchiectasis is the permanent dilation of bronchi and bronchioles caused by destruction of smooth muscle and supporting elastic tissue; it typically results from or is associated with chronic necrotizing infections. It is not a primary disorder, as it always occurs secondary to persistent infection or obstruction caused by a variety of conditions. Bronchiectasis gives rise to a characteristic symptom complex dominated by cough and expectoration of copious amounts of purulent sputum. Diagnosis depends on an appropriate history and radiographic demonstration of bronchial dilation. The conditions that most commonly predispose to bronchiectasis include:
* *Bronchial obstruction.* Common causes are tumors, foreign bodies, and impaction of mucus. In these conditions, bronchiectasis is localized to the obstructed lung segment. Bronchiectasis may also complicate atopic asthma and chronic bronchitis.
* *Congenital or hereditary conditions,* for example:
  * *Cystic fibrosis,* in which widespread severe bronchiectasis results from obstruction caused by abnormally viscid mucus and secondary infections (Chapter 4)
  * *Immunodeficiency states,* particularly immunoglobulin deficiencies, in which localized or diffuse bronchiectasis develops because of recurrent bacterial infections
  * *Primary ciliary dyskinesia* (also called *immotile cilia syndrome*), a rare autosomal recessive disorder that is frequently associated with bronchiectasis and sterility in males. It is caused by inherited abnormalities of cilia, thereby impairing mucociliary clearance of the airways, leading to persistent infections
* *Necrotizing, or suppurative, pneumonia,* particularly with virulent organisms such as *Staphylococcus aureus* or *Klebsiella* spp.,

predisposes affected patients to development of bronchiectasis. Post-tuberculosis bronchiectasis continues to be a significant cause of morbidity in endemic areas. Advanced bronchiectasis has also been reported after SARS-CoV-2 pneumonia.

Pathogenesis. **Two intertwined processes contribute to bronchiectasis: obstruction and chronic infection.** Either may be the initiator. For example, obstruction caused by a foreign body may impair clearance of secretions, providing a favorable substrate for superimposed infection. The resultant inflammatory damage to the bronchial wall and the accumulating exudate further distend the airways, leading to irreversible dilation. Conversely, a persistent necrotizing infection in the bronchi or bronchioles may lead to poor clearance of secretions, obstruction, and inflammation with peribronchial fibrosis and traction on the bronchi, culminating again in full-blown bronchiectasis.

MORPHOLOGY

Bronchiectasis usually affects the lower lobes bilaterally, particularly the most vertical air passages. When caused by tumors or aspiration of foreign bodies, it may be sharply localized to a single segment of the lungs. Usually, the most severe involvement is found in the more distal bronchi and bronchioles. The airways may be **dilated** to as much as four times their usual diameter and can be seen on gross examination almost to the pleural surface (Fig. 11.12). By contrast, in healthy lungs, the bronchioles cannot be followed by eye beyond a point 2 to 3 cm from the pleura.

The histologic findings vary with the activity and chronicity of the disease. In severe active cases, an intense acute and chronic inflammatory exudate within the walls of the bronchi and bronchioles leads to desquamation of lining epithelium and extensive areas of ulceration. Typically, sputum

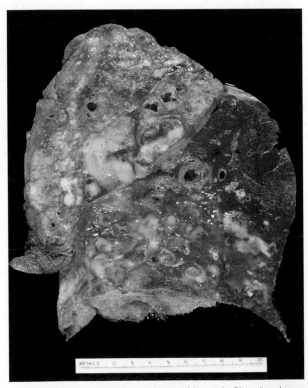

FIG. 11.12 Bronchiectasis in a patient with cystic fibrosis who underwent lung resection for transplantation. Cut surface of lung shows markedly dilated bronchi filled with purulent mucus that extend to subpleural regions.

cultures reveal mixed flora; the usual organisms include staphylococci, streptococci, pneumococci, enteric organisms, anaerobic and microaerophilic bacteria, and (particularly in children) *Haemophilus influenzae* and *Pseudomonas aeruginosa.*

When healing occurs, the lining epithelium may regenerate completely; however, the injury usually cannot be repaired, and abnormal dilation and scarring persist. Fibrosis of the bronchial and bronchiolar walls and peribronchiolar fibrosis develop in more chronic cases. In some instances, the necrosis destroys the bronchial or bronchiolar walls, producing an abscess cavity.

Clinical Features. **Bronchiectasis is characterized by severe, persistent cough associated with expectoration of mucopurulent, sometimes foul-smelling, sputum.** Other common symptoms include dyspnea, rhinosinusitis, and hemoptysis. Symptoms are often episodic and are precipitated by upper respiratory tract infections or the introduction of new pathogenic agents. Severe widespread bronchiectasis may lead to significant obstructive ventilatory defects, with hypoxemia, hypercapnia, pulmonary hypertension, and cor pulmonale. However, with current treatment, outcomes have improved and severe complications of bronchiectasis, such as brain abscess, amyloidosis (Chapter 5), and cor pulmonale, occur less frequently now than in the past. Resection of the affected part of lung is needed in some cases.

CHRONIC INTERSTITIAL (RESTRICTIVE, INFILTRATIVE) LUNG DISEASES

Chronic interstitial lung diseases are a heterogeneous group of disorders characterized by bilateral, often patchy, pulmonary fibrosis mainly affecting the walls of alveoli. Many of the entities in this group are of unknown cause and pathogenesis; some have both an intraalveolar and an interstitial component. Chronic interstitial lung diseases are categorized based on clinicopathologic and histologic features (Table 11.2), but the histologic features among the various entities often overlap. The similarity in clinical signs, symptoms, radiographic findings, and pathophysiologic and histologic

Table 11.2 Major Categories of Chronic Interstitial Lung Disease

Fibrosing
Idiopathic pulmonary fibrosis/usual interstitial pneumonia
Nonspecific interstitial pneumonia
Cryptogenic organizing pneumonia
Collagen vascular disease-associated
Pneumoconiosis
Therapy-associated (drugs, radiation)
Granulomatous
Sarcoidosis
Hypersensitivity pneumonia
Eosinophilic
Loeffler syndrome
Drug allergy—associated
Idiopathic chronic eosinophilic pneumonia
Smoking-Related
Desquamative interstitial pneumonia
Respiratory bronchiolitis

changes justify their consideration as a group. The shared hallmark of these disorders is reduced lung compliance (stiff lungs), which in turn necessitates increased effort to breathe (dyspnea). Furthermore, damage to the alveolar epithelium and interstitial vasculature produces abnormalities in the ventilation-perfusion ratio, leading to hypoxia. Chest radiographs show small nodules, irregular lines, or "ground-glass shadows." With progression, patients may develop respiratory failure, pulmonary hypertension, and cor pulmonale (Chapter 9). When advanced, the etiology of the underlying diseases may be difficult to determine because all these disorders result in diffuse scarring and gross destruction of the lung, referred to as *end-stage* or *"honeycomb" lung.*

Fibrosing Diseases

Idiopathic Pulmonary Fibrosis (Usual Interstitial Pneumonia)

Idiopathic pulmonary fibrosis (IPF) refers to a pulmonary disorder of unknown etiology that is characterized by patchy, progressive bilateral interstitial fibrosis. The radiologic and histologic pattern of fibrosis is referred to as usual interstitial pneumonia (UIP), which is required for the diagnosis of IPF. Because its etiology is unknown, it is also known as *cryptogenic organizing alveolitis.* Males are affected more often than females, and it is a disease of older adults, virtually never occurring before 50 years of age. Of note, similar pathologic changes in the lung may be present in entities such as asbestosis, collagen vascular diseases, and other conditions, and IPF is therefore a diagnosis of exclusion.

Pathogenesis. **The interstitial fibrosis that characterizes IPF is believed to result from repeated injury and defective repair of alveolar epithelium, often in a genetically predisposed individual** (Fig. 11.13). The cause of the injury is obscure; a variety of sources have been proposed, including chronic gastroesophageal reflux. However, only a small fraction of individuals with reflux or who have been exposed to other proposed environmental triggers develop IPF; thus, other unknown factors must have an important role. The clearest etiologic clues come from genetic studies. Germline mutations leading to loss of telomerase function are associated with increased risk, suggesting that cellular senescence contributes to a profibrotic phenotype. Approximately 35% of affected individuals have a genetic variant in the *MUC5B* gene that alters the production of mucin, while a smaller number of affected patients have germline mutations in surfactant genes. These genes are only expressed in lung epithelial cells, suggesting that epithelial cell abnormalities are key initiators of IPF. It is hypothesized that abnormal epithelial repair at the sites of chronic injury and inflammation gives rise to exuberant fibroblastic or myofibroblastic proliferation and collagen deposition. Although the mechanisms of fibrosis are incompletely understood, excessive activation of profibrotic factors such as TGF-β is likely to be involved. One school of thought holds that alveolar macrophages with an M2 phenotype (Chapter 2) have a central role in driving fibrosis due to their ability to secrete cytokines that promote fibroblast activation.

the interlobular septa. The earliest lesions demonstrate exuberant fibroblastic proliferation **(fibroblastic foci)** (Fig. 11.15). Over time these areas become more collagenous and less cellular. A typical finding is the coexistence of both early and late lesions. The dense fibrosis causes collapse of alveolar walls and formation of cystic spaces **(honeycomb fibrosis)** lined by hyperplastic type II pneumocytes or bronchiolar epithelium. The interstitial inflammation consists of alveolar septal infiltrates of lymphocytes and occasional plasma cells, mast cells, and eosinophils. Secondary pulmonary hypertensive changes (intimal fibrosis and medial thickening of pulmonary arteries) are often present.

Clinical Features. IPF usually presents with the gradual onset of a nonproductive cough and progressive dyspnea. On physical examination, most patients have characteristic "dry" or "velcro-like" crackles during inspiration. Cyanosis, cor pulmonale, and peripheral edema may develop in later stages of the disease. The characteristic clinical and radiologic findings (i.e., subpleural and basilar fibrosis, reticular abnormalities, and "honeycombing") are often diagnostic

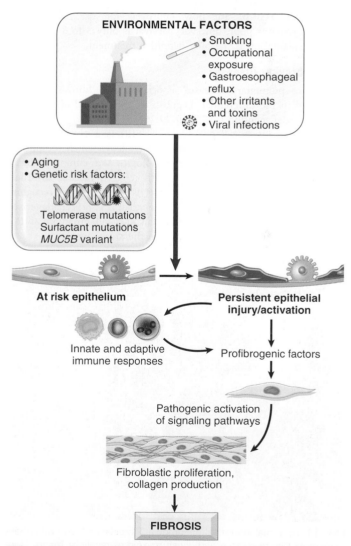

FIG. 11.13 Proposed pathogenic mechanisms in idiopathic pulmonary fibrosis. *MUC5B*, Mucin 5B. See text for details.

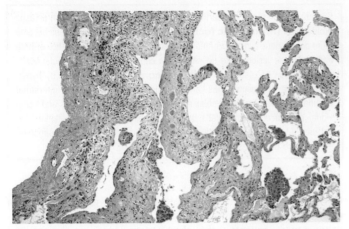

FIG. 11.14 Usual interstitial pneumonia. The fibrosis, which varies in intensity, is more pronounced in the subpleural region.

(eFig. 11.4). Antiinflammatory therapies have proven to be of little use, in line with the idea that inflammation is of secondary pathogenic importance. By contrast, antifibrotic therapies such as nintedanib, a tyrosine kinase inhibitor, and pirfenidone, an inhibitor of TGF-β, are now approved for use. The overall prognosis remains poor, however; survival is only 3 to 5 years, and lung transplantation is the only definitive treatment.

Other Fibrosing Diseases

Other rare pulmonary diseases associated with fibrosis must be considered in the differential diagnosis of IPF, several of which are worthy of brief mention (see Table 11.2).

• *Nonspecific interstitial pneumonia* (NSIP) is a chronic bilateral interstitial lung disease of unknown etiology, which (despite its name) has distinct radiologic, histologic, and clinical features, including a frequent association with collagen vascular disorders such as rheumatoid arthritis. NSIP is important to recognize because it has a much better prognosis than IPF. It is characterized by mild to moderate interstitial chronic inflammation and/or fibrosis that is patchy but uniform in the areas involved.

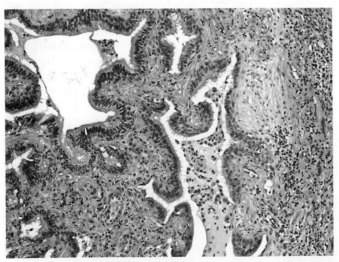

FIG. 11.15 Usual interstitial pneumonia. Fibroblastic focus with fibers running parallel to surface and bluish myxoid extracellular matrix. Honeycombing is present to the left.

• *Cryptogenic organizing pneumonia* is a second uncommon entity associated with fibrosis. It presents with cough and dyspnea, and chest radiographs show subpleural or peribronchial patchy areas of airspace consolidation consisting of intraalveolar plugs of loose organizing connective tissue. Some patients recover spontaneously, while most require treatment, usually with oral steroids.

• The differential diagnosis of fibrosing pulmonary disorders also includes *autoimmune disorders* such as systemic sclerosis, rheumatoid arthritis, and systemic lupus erythematosus, all of which may be complicated by diffuse pulmonary fibrosis.

Pneumoconioses

Pneumoconiosis is a term originally coined to describe lung disorders caused by inhalation of mineral dusts. The term has since been broadened to include diseases induced by organic and inorganic particulates, and some experts also regard chemical fume- and vapor-induced lung diseases as pneumoconioses. The mineral dust pneumoconioses—most commonly caused by inhalation of coal dust, silica, and asbestos—usually stem from exposure in the workplace. In the case of asbestos, an increased risk for cancer extends to the family members of asbestos workers and to individuals exposed outside of the workplace.

Pathogenesis. The reaction of the lung to mineral dusts depends on the size, shape, and solubility of the particles and their inherent proinflammatory properties. For example, particles greater than 5 to 10 μm are unlikely to reach distal airways, and particles smaller than 0.5 μm move into and out of alveoli, often without significant deposition and injury. Particles that are 1 to 5 μm in diameter are of greatest concern as they tend to lodge at the bifurcation of the distal airways. Coal dust is relatively inert, and large amounts must be deposited in the lungs before lung disease is clinically detectable. Silica, asbestos, and beryllium stimulate greater immune response than coal dust, resulting in fibrotic reactions at lower concentrations.

The pulmonary alveolar macrophage is a key cellular element in the initiation and perpetuation of inflammation, lung injury, and fibrosis. Following phagocytosis by macrophages, many particles activate the inflammasome and induce production of the proinflammatory cytokine IL-1 as well as the release of other factors. These factors initiate an inflammatory response that leads to fibroblast proliferation and collagen deposition. Some of the inhaled particles may reach the lymphatics either by direct drainage or within migrating macrophages and thereby initiate an immune response to components of the particulates and/or to self proteins that are modified by the particles. This leads to an amplification and extension of the local reaction. Tobacco smoking worsens the effects of all inhaled mineral dusts, more so with asbestos than other particles.

Coal Workers' Pneumoconiosis

Dust reduction in coal mines has greatly reduced the incidence of coal dust–induced disease; however, there is an increasing prevalence of coal workers' pneumoconiosis (CWP) in older miners in the United States, particularly in the region known as Appalachia. The spectrum of lung findings in coal workers is wide, ranging from *asymptomatic anthracosis*, in which carbon pigment deposits without a perceptible cellular reaction; to *simple CWP*, in which macrophages accumulate with little to no pulmonary dysfunction; to *complicated CWP* or *progressive massive fibrosis (PMF)*, in which fibrosis is extensive and lung function is compromised (see Table 11.3). Although statistics vary, it seems that less than 10% of cases of simple CWP progress to

PMF. Of note, PMF is a generic term that is applied to confluent pulmonary fibrosis; it may arise in any of the pneumoconioses discussed here.

Although coal is mainly carbon, coal mine dust contains a variety of trace metals, inorganic minerals, and crystalline silica. In general, the risk of CWP is higher in miners working in areas in which coal has higher levels of contaminating chemicals and minerals.

MORPHOLOGY

Pulmonary anthracosis is the most innocuous coal-induced pulmonary lesion in coal miners and is also commonly seen in urban dwellers and individuals who smoke tobacco. Inhaled carbon pigment is engulfed by alveolar or interstitial macrophages, which then accumulate in the connective tissue along the pulmonary and pleural lymphatics and in draining lymph nodes.

Simple CWP is characterized by the presence of **coal macules** and larger **coal nodules**. The coal macule consists of dust-laden macrophages and small amounts of collagen fibers arrayed in a delicate network. Although these lesions are scattered throughout the lung, the upper lobes and upper zones of the lower lobes are more heavily involved. In due course, **centrilobular emphysema** may occur.

Complicated CWP (PMF) occurs on a background of simple CWP by coalescence of coal nodules and generally develops over many years. It is characterized by multiple, dark black scars larger than 2 cm and sometimes up to 10 cm in diameter that consist of dense collagen and pigment (Fig. 11.16).

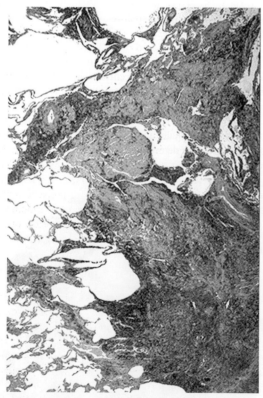

FIG. 11.16 Progressive massive fibrosis in a coal worker. A large amount of black pigment is associated with fibrosis. (From Klatt EC: *Robbins and Cotran Atlas of Pathology*, ed 2, Philadelphia, 2009, Elsevier, p 121.)

Clinical Features. CWP is usually a benign disease that produces little decline in lung function. In those in whom PMF develops, there is increasing pulmonary dysfunction, pulmonary hypertension, and cor pulmonale. Progression from CWP to PMF has been linked to exposure to higher coal dust levels and to total dust burden. Once established, PMF tends to progress even in the absence of further exposure. After taking smoking-related risk into account, there is no increased frequency of lung carcinoma in coal miners, a feature that distinguishes CWP from both silica and asbestos exposures (discussed next).

Silicosis

Silicosis is currently the most prevalent chronic occupational disease in the world. It is caused by inhalation of crystalline silica, mostly in occupational settings. Workers involved in sandblasting and hard-rock mining are at particularly high risk. Silica occurs in both crystalline and amorphous forms, but crystalline forms (including quartz, cristobalite, and tridymite) are by far the most toxic and fibrogenic. Of these, quartz is most commonly implicated in silicosis. After inhalation, silica particles are ingested by alveolar macrophages, leading to lysosomal damage, activation of the inflammasome, and release of inflammatory mediators, including IL-1, TNF, lipid mediators, oxygen-derived free radicals, and fibrogenic cytokines.

MORPHOLOGY

Silicotic nodules in their early stages are tiny, barely palpable, discrete, pale-to-black (if coal dust is present) nodules in the upper zones of the lungs (Fig. 11.17). Microscopically, silicotic nodules have **concentrically arranged hyalinized collagen fibers** surrounding an amorphous center. The "whorled" appearance of the collagen fibers is quite characteristic (Fig. 11.18). Examination of the nodules by **polarized microscopy reveals weakly birefringent silica** particles, primarily in the center of the nodules. As the disease progresses, individual nodules may coalesce into hard, collagenous scars, with eventual progression to PMF. The intervening lung parenchyma may be compressed or overexpanded, and a honeycomb pattern may develop. Fibrotic lesions may also occur in hilar lymph nodes and the pleura.

Clinical Features. Silicosis is usually detected in asymptomatic workers on routine chest radiographs, which typically show a fine nodularity in the upper zones of the lung. Shortness of breath does not develop until late in the course, after PMF is present. Many patients with PMF develop pulmonary hypertension and cor pulmonale. The disease is slowly progressive, often impairing pulmonary function to a degree that severely limits physical activity. Silicosis is associated with an increased susceptibility to tuberculosis, perhaps because crystalline silica may inhibit the ability of pulmonary macrophages to kill phagocytosed mycobacteria. Nodules of silicotuberculosis often contain a central zone of caseation. Most evidence suggests that silicosis is also associated with modestly increased risk of lung cancer.

Asbestos-Related Diseases

Asbestos is a family of crystalline hydrated silicates with a fibrous geometry. Occupational exposure to asbestos is linked to multiple pulmonary pathologies, including (1) parenchymal interstitial fibrosis (*asbestosis*); (2) localized fibrous plaques, or, rarely, diffuse fibrosis in the pleura; (3) pleural effusions; (4) lung carcinoma; (5) malignant pleural and peritoneal mesothelioma; and (6) laryngeal carcinoma. An increased incidence of asbestos-related cancers in family members of

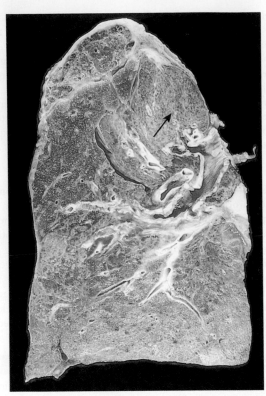

FIG. 11.17 Advanced silicosis, seen in a transected lung. Scarring has contracted the upper lobe into a small dark mass that is discolored due to the presence of carbon dust *(arrow)*. Note the dense pleural thickening. (Courtesy of Dr. John Godleski, Brigham and Women's Hospital, Boston, Massachusetts.)

effects of asbestos on the mesothelium are mediated by free radicals induced by asbestos fibers, which preferentially localize in the distal lung close to the mesothelial layer. It is also likely that toxic chemicals adsorbed onto the asbestos fibers contribute to their pathogenicity. For example, the adsorption of carcinogens in tobacco smoke onto asbestos fibers may be the basis for the strong synergy between tobacco smoking and the development of lung carcinoma in asbestos workers.

MORPHOLOGY

Asbestosis is marked by **diffuse pulmonary interstitial fibrosis** and the presence of **asbestos bodies,** golden brown, fusiform or beaded rods with a translucent center. They consist of asbestos fibers coated with an iron-containing proteinaceous material (Fig. 11.19). Apparently, asbestos bodies are formed when macrophages attempt to phagocytose asbestos fibers; the iron "crust" is derived from ferritin.

   In contrast with CWP and silicosis, asbestosis begins in the lower lobes and subpleurally, spreading to the middle and upper lobes of the lungs as the fibrosis progresses. Contraction of the fibrous tissue distorts the normal architecture, creating enlarged air spaces enclosed within thick fibrous walls; eventually, the affected regions become honeycombed. Simultaneously, fibrosis develops in the visceral pleura, causing adhesions between the lungs and the chest wall. The scarring may trap and narrow pulmonary arteries and arterioles; this, along with worsening lung function, may lead to pulmonary hypertension and cor pulmonale.

   Pleural plaques are the most common manifestation of asbestos exposure. They consist of well-circumscribed plaques of dense collagen (Fig. 11.20), often containing calcium. They develop most frequently on the anterior and posterolateral aspects of the **parietal pleura** and over the domes of the diaphragm. Uncommonly, asbestos exposure induces pleural effusion or diffuse pleural fibrosis.

asbestos workers is due to residual asbestos particles on the workers' clothing.

Pathogenesis. **As with silica crystals, once phagocytosed by macrophages, asbestos fibers activate the inflammasome and damage phagolysosomal membranes, stimulating the release of proinflammatory factors and fibrogenic mediators.** In addition to cellular and fibrotic lung reactions, asbestos probably also functions as both a tumor initiator and a promoter. Some of the oncogenic

Clinical Features. The clinical findings in asbestosis are indistinguishable from those of any other chronic interstitial lung disease. Progressively worsening dyspnea appears 10 to 20 years after exposure. It is usually accompanied by cough and production of sputum. The disease may remain static or progress to congestive heart failure, cor pulmonale, and death. Pleural plaques are usually asymptomatic and are detected on radiographs as circumscribed calcific densities.

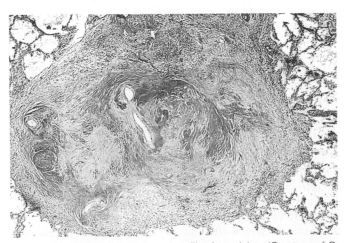

FIG. 11.18 Coalescent collagenous silicotic nodules. (Courtesy of Dr. John Godleski, Brigham and Women's Hospital, Boston, Massachusetts.)

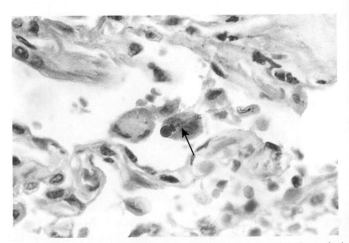

FIG. 11.19 High-power detail of an asbestos body, revealing the typical beading and knobbed ends *(arrow)*.

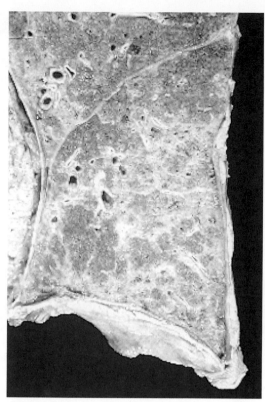

FIG. 11.20 Asbestosis. Markedly thickened visceral pleura covers the lateral and diaphragmatic surface of the lung. Note also severe interstitial fibrosis diffusely affecting the lower lobe of the lung.

People exposed to asbestos have a markedly increased risk of developing lung carcinoma and malignant mesothelioma. The risk for developing lung carcinoma is increased about 5-fold for asbestos workers, while the relative risk for mesothelioma, normally a very rare tumor (2—17 cases per 1 million individuals), is more than 1000 times greater. Concomitant cigarette smoking greatly increases the risk for lung carcinoma but not for mesothelioma. Lung or pleural cancer associated with asbestos exposure carries a particularly poor prognosis.

Drug- and Radiation-Induced Pulmonary Disease

Drugs can cause a variety of acute and chronic alterations of lung structure and function. For example, *bleomycin,* an anticancer agent, causes pneumonitis and interstitial fibrosis through direct toxic effects and by stimulating the influx of inflammatory cells into the alveoli. *Amiodarone,* an antiarrhythmic agent, is also associated with pneumonitis and fibrosis. *Radiation pneumonitis* is a well-known complication of irradiation of pulmonary and other thoracic tumors. *Acute radiation pneumonitis,* which typically occurs 1 to 6 months after therapy in as many as 20% of patients, is manifested by fever, dyspnea out of proportion to the volume of irradiated lung, pleural effusion, and pulmonary infiltrates in the irradiated lung bed. These signs and symptoms may resolve with corticosteroid therapy or progress to *chronic radiation pneumonitis,* associated with pulmonary fibrosis.

Granulomatous Diseases

Sarcoidosis

Sarcoidosis is a multisystem disease of unknown etiology characterized by noncaseating granulomatous inflammation in many tissues and organs. We discuss it here because one presentation of sarcoidosis is as a restrictive lung disease. Other diseases, including mycobacterial and fungal infections and berylliosis, may also produce noncaseating granulomas; therefore, the histologic diagnosis of sarcoidosis is one of exclusion. Although sarcoidosis can manifest in many ways, bilateral hilar lymphadenopathy or lung involvement (or both), visible on chest radiographs, is the major finding at presentation in most cases. Eye and skin involvement each occurs in about 25% of cases and are occasionally the presenting feature of the disease.

Sarcoidosis occurs throughout the world, affecting both genders and all age groups. There are, however, certain interesting epidemiologic trends:

- A consistent predilection for adults younger than 40 years of age
- A high incidence in Danish and Swedish populations and in the United States among people of African descent (in whom the frequency is 2 to 3 times higher than in those of European descent)
- A higher prevalence among nonsmokers, an association that is virtually unique to sarcoidosis among pulmonary diseases

Pathogenesis. **Although the etiology of sarcoidosis remains unknown, several lines of evidence suggest that it is a disease of disordered immune regulation in genetically predisposed individuals exposed to undefined environmental agents.** The role of each of these contributory influences is summarized in the following discussion.

Several immunologic abnormalities in sarcoidosis suggest the development of a cell-mediated response to an unidentified antigen. The process is driven by CD4+ helper T cells. These immunologic "clues" include the following:

- Intraalveolar and interstitial accumulation of CD4+ Th1 cells
- Oligoclonal expansion of CD4+ Th1 T cells within the lung as determined by analysis of T-cell receptor rearrangements
- Increases in Th1 cytokines such as IL-2 and IFN-γ, resulting in T-cell proliferation and macrophage activation, respectively
- Increases in several cytokines in the local environment (IL-8, TNF, macrophage inflammatory protein-1α) that favor recruitment of additional T cells and monocytes and contribute to the formation of granulomas
- Interestingly, levels of CD4+ helper T cells in the blood are often low, a finding associated with anergy to common skin test antigens such as *Candida* or purified protein derivative (PPD), an *M. tuberculosis* antigen

After lung transplantation, sarcoidosis recurs in the new lungs in at least one-third of patients. Several putative "antigens" have been proposed as the inciting agent for sarcoidosis, but there is no concrete evidence linking sarcoidosis to any specific antigen or infectious agent.

MORPHOLOGY

The cardinal histopathologic feature of sarcoidosis is the **nonnecrotizing epithelioid granuloma** (Fig. 11.21). This is a discrete, compact collection of epithelioid macrophages rimmed by an outer zone rich in CD4+ T cells. It is not uncommon to see intermixed multinucleate giant cells formed by fusion of macrophages. Early on, a thin layer of laminated fibroblasts is found peripheral to the granuloma; over time, these proliferate and lay down collagen that replaces the entire granuloma with a hyalinized scar. Two other microscopic features are sometimes seen in the granulomas: (1) **Schaumann bodies,** laminated concretions composed of calcium and proteins, and (2) **asteroid bodies,** stellate inclusions enclosed within giant cells. Their presence is not required for diagnosis of sarcoidosis, and they may be found in granulomas seen in other disorders. Rarely, foci of central necrosis may be present in sarcoid granulomas, especially in the nodular form.

The **lungs** are involved at some stage of the disease in 90% of patients. The granulomas predominantly involve the interstitium rather than air spaces and have a tendency to localize in the connective tissue around bronchioles and pulmonary venules and in the pleura ("lymphangitic" distribution). Bronchoalveolar lavage fluid contains abundant CD4+ T cells. In 5% to 15% of patients, the granulomas are eventually replaced by **diffuse interstitial fibrosis,** resulting in a so-called "honeycomb lung."

Intrathoracic **hilar and paratracheal lymph nodes** are enlarged in 75% to 90% of patients, while one-third present with peripheral lymphadenopathy. The nodes are characteristically painless and have a firm, rubbery texture. Unlike in tuberculosis, lymph nodes in sarcoidosis are "nonmatted" (nonadherent) and do not undergo necrosis.

Skin lesions are encountered in approximately 25% of patients. **Erythema nodosum,** a hallmark of acute sarcoidosis, presents as bilateral raised, red, tender nodules on the anterior aspects of the legs. It is a form of panniculitis marked by infiltrates of chronic inflammatory cells and fibrosis; classic sarcoidal granulomas are uncommon in these lesions. Alternatively, sarcoid may involve the skin as discrete painless subcutaneous nodules; these lesions usually contain typical noncaseating granulomas.

Involvement of the eye and lacrimal glands occurs in about one-fifth to one-half of patients. The ocular involvement takes the form of **iritis** or **iridocyclitis** and may be unilateral or bilateral. As a consequence, corneal opacities, glaucoma, and (less commonly) total loss of vision may develop. The posterior uveal tract is also affected, with resultant **choroiditis, retinitis,** and **optic nerve involvement.** These ocular lesions are frequently accompanied by inflammation in the lacrimal glands, with suppression of lacrimation **(sicca syndrome). Unilateral or bilateral parotitis with painful enlargement of the parotid glands** occurs in fewer than 10% of patients with sarcoidosis; some develop xerostomia (dry mouth). Combined uveoparotid involvement is designated **Mikulicz syndrome.**

The spleen may appear unaffected grossly, but in about three-fourths of cases, it contains granulomas. In approximately 10%, it becomes clinically enlarged. **The liver** demonstrates microscopic granulomas, usually in the portal triads, about as often as the spleen, but only about one-third of patients demonstrate hepatomegaly or abnormal liver function. Involvement of **bone marrow** is reported in as many as 40% of patients, although it rarely causes severe manifestations.

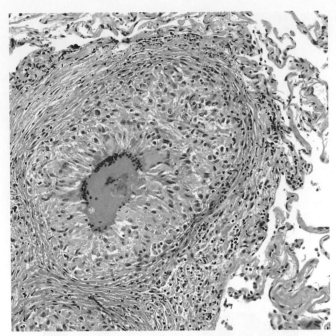

FIG. 11.21 Sarcoidosis. A characteristic noncaseating granuloma with a large central multinucleated giant cell is present. (From Diagnostic Pathology: Thoracic and ExpertPath. Copyright Elsevier 2022.)

that are consistent with the disease, the exclusion of other disorders with similar presentations, and the identification of noncaseating granulomas in involved tissues. In particular, tuberculosis must be excluded.

Sarcoidosis follows an unpredictable course characterized by either chronic progressive disease or periods of activity interspersed with remissions. Remissions may be spontaneous or initiated by steroid therapy and are often permanent. Overall, 65% to 70% of affected individuals recover with minimal or no residual manifestations. Another 20% develop permanent lung dysfunction or visual impairment. Of the remaining 10% to 15%, most succumb to progressive pulmonary fibrosis and cor pulmonale.

Clinical Features. In many affected individuals, the disease is entirely asymptomatic, discovered on routine chest films as bilateral hilar adenopathy or as an incidental finding at autopsy. In others, peripheral lymphadenopathy, cutaneous lesions, eye involvement, splenomegaly, or hepatomegaly may be presenting manifestations. In about two-thirds of symptomatic cases, there is gradual appearance of respiratory symptoms (e.g., shortness of breath, dry cough, or vague substernal discomfort) or constitutional signs and symptoms (e.g., fever, fatigue, weight loss, anorexia, night sweats). Laboratory findings may include hypercalcemia and hypercalciuria, both related to production of biologically active vitamin D by the macrophages that form the granulomas.

A definitive test for sarcoidosis does not exist. Establishing the diagnosis requires the presence of clinical and radiologic findings

Hypersensitivity Pneumonitis

Hypersensitivity pneumonitis is an immunologically mediated lung disease that primarily affects the alveoli and is therefore often called *allergic alveolitis.* It is associated with diverse occupational and household exposures. Most often it results from heightened sensitivity to inhaled antigens such as those found in moldy hay (Table 11.3). Because the damage occurs at the level of alveoli, it manifests predominantly as a restrictive lung disease associated with variable decreases in diffusion capacity, lung compliance, and total lung volume.

Several lines of evidence suggest that hypersensitivity pneumonitis is an immunologically mediated disease:

- Bronchoalveolar lavage specimens show increased numbers of CD4+ and CD8+ T lymphocytes.
- Most affected patients have specific antibodies against the offending antigen in their serum.
- Deposits of complement and immunoglobulins have been demonstrated within pulmonary vessel walls.
- Noncaseating granulomas are found in the lungs of two-thirds of affected patients.

Table 11.3 Sources of Antigens Causing Hypersensitivity Pneumonitis

Source of Antigen	Types of Exposures
Mushrooms, fungi, yeasts	Contaminated wood, humidifiers, central hot air heating ducts, peat moss plants
Bacteria (Thermophilic actinomycetes)	Dairy barns (farmer's lung)
M. avium complex (MAC)	Metalworking fluids, sauna, hot tub
Birds	Pigeons, dove feathers, ducks, parakeets
Chemicals	Isocyanates (auto painters), zinc, dyes

From Lacasse Y, Girard M, Cormier Y: Recent advances in hypersensitivity pneumonitis, *Chest* 142:208, 2012.

MORPHOLOGY

The histopathologic picture in both acute and chronic forms of hypersensitivity pneumonitis includes patchy mononuclear cell infiltrates in the pulmonary interstitium, particularly around bronchioles. Lymphocytes predominate, but plasma cells and epithelioid macrophages are also present. In acute forms of the disease, variable numbers of neutrophils may also be seen. **Poorly formed (noncohesive) granulomas,** without necrosis, are present in more than two-thirds of cases, usually in a peribronchiolar location (Fig. 11.22). In advanced chronic cases, bilateral, upper-lobe-dominant interstitial fibrosis (UIP pattern) occurs.

Clinical Features. Hypersensitivity pneumonitis may manifest either as an acute reaction, with fever, cough, dyspnea, and constitutional signs and symptoms arising 4 to 8 hours after exposure, or as a chronic disease characterized by insidious onset of cough, dyspnea, malaise, and weight loss. With the acute form, the diagnosis is usually obvious because of the temporal relationship of symptom onset and exposure to the inciting antigen. When antigenic exposure is eliminated after acute attacks of the disease, complete resolution of pulmonary symptoms occurs within days. Failure to remove the inciting agent from the environment eventually results in irreversible chronic interstitial pulmonary disease.

Pulmonary Eosinophilia

A number of disorders are characterized by pulmonary infiltrates rich in eosinophils, which are recruited to the lung by local release of chemotactic factors. These diverse diseases generally are of immunologic origin, but their etiology is not understood. They sometimes have known associations such as with helminth infections, drugs such as Allopurinol, and vasculits, but most often are idiopathic. Their clinical course is varied, but when chronic they may culminate in interstitial fibrosis.

Smoking-Related Interstitial Diseases

In addition to obstructive lung disease (COPD), smoking is also associated with restrictive or interstitial lung diseases. *Desquamative interstitial pneumonia (DIP)* and *respiratory bronchiolitis* are two related examples of smoking-associated interstitial lung disease. The most striking histologic feature of DIP is the accumulation of large numbers of macrophages containing dusty-brown pigment (*smokers' macrophages*) in the air spaces (Fig. 11.23). The alveolar septa are thickened by a sparse inflammatory infiltrate (usually lymphocytes);

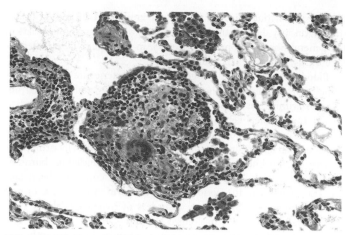

FIG. 11.22 Hypersensitivity pneumonitis, histologic appearance. Loosely formed interstitial granulomas and chronic inflammation are characteristic.

interstitial fibrosis, when present, is mild. Pulmonary function tests usually show a mild restrictive abnormality. Overall, patients with DIP have a good prognosis and an excellent response to steroids and smoking cessation; however, some patients progress despite therapy. Respiratory bronchiolitis is a common disorder of people who smoke that is characterized by the presence of pigmented intraluminal macrophages similar to those in DIP, but in a "bronchiolocentric" distribution (first- and second-order respiratory bronchioles). Mild peribronchiolar fibrosis is also seen. As with DIP, affected patients present with gradual onset of dyspnea and dry cough, symptoms that recede with smoking cessation.

DISEASES OF PULMONARY VESSELS

Pulmonary Embolism, Hemorrhage, and Infarction

Thromboemboli to the pulmonary arteries cause approximately 100,000 deaths per year in the United States and often complicate the course of other diseases. The true incidence of nonfatal pulmonary embolism is not known. Some cases undoubtedly occur outside the hospital in ambulatory patients, in whom the emboli are small, clinically silent, and not detected. Even among hospitalized patients,

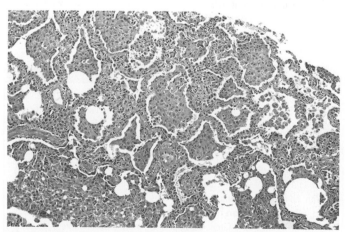

FIG. 11.23 Desquamative interstitial pneumonia. There is accumulation of large numbers of macrophages within the alveolar spaces with only slight fibrous thickening of the alveolar walls.

no more than one-third of pulmonary emboli are diagnosed before death. Autopsy data on the incidence vary widely, ranging from 1% in the general hospital population to 30% in individuals dying after severe burns, trauma, or fractures.

Blood clots that occlude large pulmonary arteries are almost always embolic in origin. More than 95% of pulmonary emboli arise from thrombi within the deep veins of the legs that have propagated to involve the popliteal vein and the larger veins above it. The influences that predispose to venous thrombosis are discussed in Chapter 3; the following risk factors are paramount: (1) surgery, especially orthopedic surgery on the knee or hip; (2) severe trauma (including burns or multiple fractures); (3) disseminated cancer; (4) congestive heart failure; (5) for women, the period around parturition or the use of oral contraception pills; (6) primary disorders of hypercoagulability (e.g., factor V Leiden); and (7) prolonged bed rest.

The pathophysiologic consequences of pulmonary thromboembolism depend largely on the size of the embolus, which in turn dictates the size of the occluded pulmonary artery, and the cardiopulmonary status of the patient. There are two important consequences of pulmonary arterial occlusion: (1) an acute increase in pulmonary artery pressure resulting from blockage of flow and vasospasm caused by neurogenic mechanisms and/or release of mediators (e.g., thromboxane A_2, serotonin) and (2) ischemia of the downstream pulmonary parenchyma. Thus, occlusion of a major vessel results in an abrupt increase in pulmonary artery pressure, diminished cardiac output, right-sided heart failure *(acute cor pulmonale)*, and sometimes sudden death. If smaller vessels are occluded, the result is less severe and may be clinically silent. In those who are symptomatic, hypoxemia develops through several mechanisms:

- *Perfusion of atelectatic lung zones.* Alveolar collapse occurs in ischemic areas because of a reduction in surfactant production and because pain associated with embolism leads to reduced movement of the chest wall, leading to mismatch of blood flow and ventilation (V/Q mismatch).
- *Decreased cardiac output causes a widening of the difference between arterial and venous oxygen saturation.*
- *Right-to-left shunting* of blood may occur through a patent foramen ovale, present in 30% of individuals.

Recall that the lungs are oxygenated not only by the pulmonary arteries but also by bronchial arteries and directly from air in the alveoli. Thus, ischemic necrosis (infarction) is the exception rather than the rule, occurring in as few as 10% of patients with thromboemboli. It occurs only if there is compromise in cardiac function or bronchial circulation, or if the region of the lung at risk is underventilated as a result of underlying pulmonary disease.

MORPHOLOGY

The consequences of pulmonary embolism depend on the size of the embolic mass and the general state of the circulation. A large embolus may embed in the main pulmonary artery or its major branches or lodge astride the bifurcation as a **saddle embolus** (Fig. 11.24). Smaller emboli become lodged in medium-sized and small pulmonary arteries. With adequate circulation and bronchial arterial flow, the vitality of the parenchyma is maintained, but alveolar hemorrhage may occur as a result of ischemic damage to the endothelial cells.

With compromised cardiovascular status, as may occur with congestive heart failure, **infarction** results. The more peripheral the embolic occlusion, the higher the risk for infarction. About three-fourths of all infarcts affect the lower lobes and more than one-half are multiple. Characteristically, infarcts are wedge-shaped, with their base at the pleural surface and the apex pointing toward the hilus of the lung. Pulmonary infarcts are hemorrhagic and

appear as raised red-blue areas of coagulative necrosis when acute (red infarcts) (Fig. 11.25). The adjacent pleural surface is often covered by a fibrinous exudate. The occluded vessel is usually located near the apex of the infarcted area. Extravasated red cells begin to lyse within 48 hours, and the infarct gradually becomes brownish as hemosiderin is produced. In time, fibrosis begins at the margins and eventually converts the infarct into a scar.

Clinical Features. The clinical consequences of pulmonary thromboembolism can be summarized as follows:

- Most (60% to 80%) are clinically silent because they are small; the bronchial circulation sustains the viability of the affected lung parenchyma, and the embolic mass is rapidly removed by fibrinolytic activity.
- In 5% of cases, acute right-sided heart failure, cardiovascular collapse (shock), or death occurs suddenly. Massive pulmonary embolism is one of the few causes of virtually instantaneous death. These severe consequences typically happen when more than 60% of the pulmonary vasculature is obstructed by a large embolus or multiple simultaneous smaller emboli.
- Obstruction of small to medium pulmonary branches (10% to 15% of cases) causes pulmonary infarction if some element of circulatory insufficiency is present. Typically, individuals who sustain infarctions present with dyspnea.
- In a small subset of patients (accounting for <3% of cases), recurrent "showers" of emboli lead to pulmonary hypertension, chronic right-sided heart failure, and, with time, pulmonary vascular sclerosis and progressively worsening dyspnea.

Emboli usually resolve, thanks to endogenous fibrinolytic activity that leads to their complete dissolution. However, a small, relatively

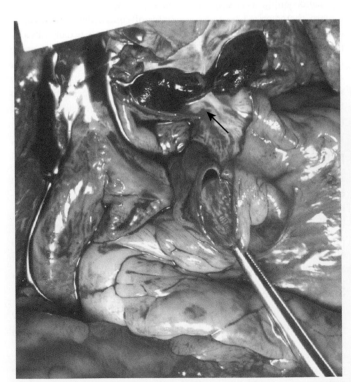

FIG. 11.24 Large saddle embolus from the femoral vein lying astride the main left and right pulmonary arteries. (Courtesy of Dr. Linda Margraf, Department of Pathology, University of Texas Southwestern Medical School, Dallas, Texas.)

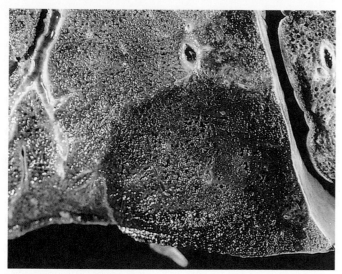

FIG. 11.25 A small, roughly wedge-shaped hemorrhagic pulmonary infarct of recent occurrence.

innocuous embolus may presage a larger one, and patients who have experienced one pulmonary embolism have a 30% chance of having a second. Prophylactic therapy includes anticoagulation, early ambulation of postoperative and postparturient patients, application of elastic stockings, intermittent pneumatic calf compression, and isometric leg exercises for bedridden patients. Those who develop pulmonary embolism are given anticoagulation therapy. Patients with massive pulmonary embolism who are hemodynamically unstable (e.g., shock, acute right heart failure) are candidates for thrombolytic therapy.

Nonthrombotic pulmonary emboli come in several uncommon but potentially lethal forms, such as air, fat, and amniotic fluid embolism (Chapter 3). Intravenous substance use is often associated with foreign body embolism in the pulmonary microvasculature; the presence of magnesium trisilicate (talc) in the intravenous mixture elicits a granulomatous response within the interstitium or pulmonary arteries. Involvement of the interstitium may lead to fibrosis, while vascular involvement leads to pulmonary hypertension. Residual talc crystals can be demonstrated within the granulomas using polarized light. Bone marrow embolism (denoted by the presence of hematopoietic and fat elements within a pulmonary artery) may occur after trauma and in patients with bone infarction secondary to sickle cell anemia.

Pulmonary Hypertension

The pulmonary circulation is normally one of low resistance, and pulmonary blood pressures are only about one-eighth of systemic pressures. **Pulmonary hypertension (defined as pressures of 25 mm Hg or more at rest) may be caused by a decrease in the cross-sectional area of the pulmonary vascular bed or, less commonly, by increased pulmonary vascular blood flow.**

Pathogenesis. On the basis of pathogenesis, the World Health Organization has divided pulmonary hypertension into 5 groups, each associated with different disorders. The most important of these associations are the following:

- *Chronic obstructive or interstitial lung diseases* (group 3). These diseases obliterate alveolar capillaries, increasing pulmonary resistance to blood flow and thereby pulmonary blood pressure.

- *Congenital or acquired heart disease* (group 2). Mitral stenosis, for example, causes an increase in left atrial pressure and pulmonary venous pressure that is eventually transmitted to the arterial side of the pulmonary vasculature, leading to hypertension.
- *Recurrent thromboemboli* (group 4). Recurrent pulmonary emboli may reduce the functional cross-sectional area of the pulmonary vascular bed, which in turn leads to an increase in pulmonary vascular resistance and hypertension.
- *Autoimmune diseases* (group 1). Several diseases (most notably systemic sclerosis) involve the pulmonary vasculature and/or the interstitium, leading to increased vascular resistance and pulmonary hypertension.
- *Obstructive sleep apnea* (also group 3) is a common disorder associated with obesity and hypoxemia. As the incidence of obesity increases, it is an increasingly significant contributor to the development of pulmonary hypertension and cor pulmonale.
- *Schistosomiasis* (group 5) in its chronic hepatosplenic form may be the most common cause of pulmonary hypertension worldwide. The mechanism is unclear; embolization of eggs and portopulmonary hypertension due to liver cirrhosis are suspected causes.

Rarely, *idiopathic pulmonary arterial hypertension* is diagnosed when known causes are excluded. This name is a misnomer, however, as up to 80% of "idiopathic" pulmonary hypertension (also referred to as *primary pulmonary hypertension*) has a genetic basis, sometimes being inherited in families as an autosomal dominant trait with incomplete penetrance. As is often the case, investigating the molecular basis of this uncommon familial form of the disease has provided new pathogenic insights, in this instance by illuminating the role of bone morphogenetic protein (BMP), a member of the TGF-β superfamily. Inactivating germline mutations in the gene encoding bone morphogenetic protein receptor 2 (BMPR2) are found in 75% of familial cases of pulmonary hypertension and 25% of sporadic cases. More recently, mutations in other components of the BMPR2 pathway have been identified in affected patients. Details remain to be clarified, but it appears that defects in BMPR2 signaling lead to dysfunction of endothelium and proliferation of vascular smooth muscle cells in the pulmonary vasculature. Because only 10% to 20% of individuals with *BMPR2* mutations develop disease, it is likely that modifier genes and/or environmental triggers also contribute to the pathogenesis of the disorder.

MORPHOLOGY

Regardless of their etiology, all forms of pulmonary hypertension are associated with **medial hypertrophy of the pulmonary muscular and elastic arteries, pulmonary arterial sclerosis, and right ventricular hypertrophy.** The vessel changes may involve the entire arterial tree, from the main pulmonary arteries down to the arterioles (Fig. 11.26). In severe cases, sclerotic thickening is seen in the pulmonary artery and its major branches. The arterioles and small arteries are most prominently affected by medial hypertrophy and intimal fibrosis, sometimes narrowing the lumens to pinpoint channels. An uncommon but characteristic pathologic change is the **plexiform lesion,** so called because a tuft of capillary formations is present, producing a network, or web, that spans the lumens of dilated thin-walled small arteries and may extend outside the vessel.

Other findings in the lung may point to the underlying etiology. For example, the presence of organizing recanalized thrombi favors recurrent pulmonary emboli as the cause, whereas parenchymal lung disease (pulmonary fibrosis, emphysema, chronic bronchitis) suggests chronic hypoxia as the triggering event.

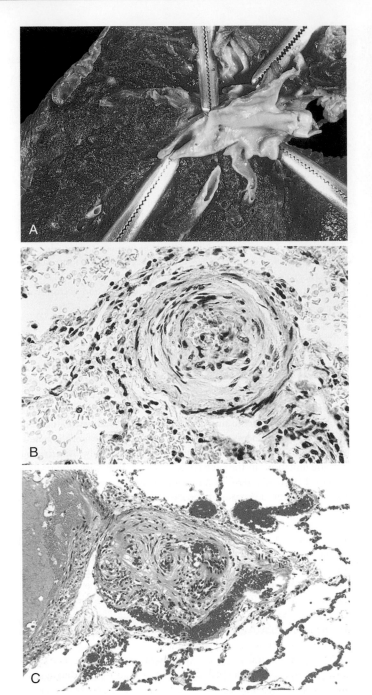

FIG. 11.26 Vascular changes in pulmonary hypertension. (A) Patchy sclerotic thickening, a change usually limited to large pulmonary arteries. (B) Marked medial hypertrophy. (C) Plexiform lesion characteristic of advanced pulmonary hypertension seen in small arteries.

Clinical Features. Pulmonary hypertension produces symptoms when the disease is advanced. Idiopathic pulmonary hypertension is most common in women 20 to 40 years of age. The presenting features are usually dyspnea and fatigue, but some patients have anginal chest pain. Over time, respiratory distress, cyanosis, and right ventricular hypertrophy appear, and death from decompensated cor pulmonale, often with superimposed thromboembolism and pneumonia, ensues within 2 to 5 years in 80% of patients.

Treatment choices depend on the underlying etiology. For those with secondary disease, therapy is directed at the primary cause

(e.g., thromboembolic disease or hypoxemia). A variety of vasodilators have been used with varying success in those with group 1 disease or refractory disease belonging to other groups. Lung transplantation is a definitive treatment for selected patients.

Diffuse Pulmonary Hemorrhage Syndromes

Pulmonary hemorrhage is a dramatic complication of some interstitial lung disorders. Among these so-called "pulmonary hemorrhage syndromes" are (1) Goodpasture syndrome, (2) granulomatosis with polyangiitis, and (3) idiopathic pulmonary hemosiderosis, a rare disorder of unknown etiology seen mostly in children. Only the first two entities will be discussed briefly.

Goodpasture Syndrome

Goodpasture syndrome is an uncommon autoimmune disease in which lung and kidney injury is caused by circulating autoantibodies against type IV collagen, a component of the basement membranes of renal glomeruli and pulmonary alveoli. The antibodies trigger destruction and inflammation of the basement membranes in pulmonary alveoli and renal glomeruli, giving rise to *necrotizing hemorrhagic interstitial pneumonitis* and *rapidly progressive glomerulonephritis*.

> ### MORPHOLOGY
>
> The lungs are heavy and have areas of red-brown consolidation due to **alveolar hemorrhage.** Microscopic examination shows focal necrosis of alveolar walls associated with intraalveolar hemorrhage, fibrous thickening of septa, and hypertrophic type II pneumocytes. There is abundant **hemosiderin,** a residuum of earlier episodes of hemorrhage (Fig. 11.27). A characteristic **linear pattern of immunoglobulin deposition** (usually IgG), a hallmark diagnostic finding in renal biopsy specimens (Chapter 12), may also be seen along alveolar septa in the lung.

Clinical Features. Most cases of Goodpasture syndrome occur in patients in their teens or twenties. In contrast to many other autoimmune diseases, there is a male preponderance. The majority of patients are active smokers. Plasmapheresis and immunosuppressive therapy have markedly improved a once-dismal prognosis. Plasma exchange removes offending antibodies, and immunosuppressive drugs inhibit antibody production. With severe renal disease, renal transplantation is eventually required.

Granulomatosis and Polyangiitis

More than 80% of patients with granulomatosis and polyangiitis (formerly *Wegener granulomatosis*) develop upper respiratory or pulmonary manifestations at some time in their course (Chapter 8). The lung lesions are characterized by a combination of necrotizing vasculitis ("angiitis") and parenchymal necrotizing granulomatous inflammation. The signs and symptoms stem from involvement of the upper respiratory tract (chronic sinusitis, epistaxis, nasal perforation) and the lungs (cough, hemoptysis, chest pain). Antineutrophil cytoplasmic antibodies (PR3-ANCAs) are present in approximately 90% of cases (Chapter 8).

PULMONARY INFECTIONS

In the United States, pulmonary infections in the form of pneumonia are responsible for approximately one-sixth of all deaths, a

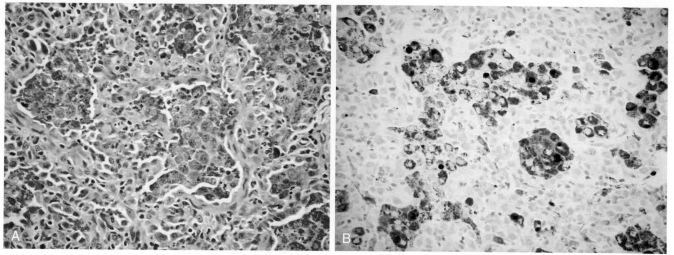

FIG. 11.27 Diffuse alveolar hemorrhage. (A) Lung biopsy specimen demonstrates large numbers of intra-alveolar hemosiderin-laden macrophages on a background of thickened fibrous septa. (B) The tissue has been stained with Prussian blue, an iron stain that highlights the abundant intracellular hemosiderin. (From the Teaching Collection of the Department of Pathology, Children's Medical Center, Dallas, Texas.)

toll that has risen during the COVID-19 pandemic. Pneumonia can be broadly defined as any infection in the lung. Normally, the lung parenchyma remains sterile because of a number of immune and nonimmune defense mechanisms that extend throughout the respiratory system from the nasopharynx to the alveolar air spaces (Fig. 11.28). The vulnerability of the lung to infection despite these defenses is not surprising because (1) many microbes are airborne and readily inhaled into the lungs; (2) nasopharyngeal flora is regularly aspirated during sleep, even by healthy individuals; and (3) lung diseases often lower local immune defenses.

The importance of immune defenses in preventing pulmonary infections is emphasized by the impact of inherited or acquired defects in innate immunity (including neutrophil and complement defects) or adaptive immunity (e.g., humoral immunodeficiency), all of which increase the incidence of bacterial pneumonia. For example, patients with mutations in MYD88, an adaptor protein required for signaling by Toll-like receptors, are extremely susceptible to severe necrotizing pneumococcal infections, while patients with congenital defects in IgA production (the major immunoglobulin in airway secretions) are at increased risk for pneumonias caused by encapsulated organisms such as pneumococcus and *H. influenzae*. On the other hand, defects in Th1 cell–mediated immunity lead mainly to increased infections with intracellular microbes such as atypical mycobacteria. Much more commonly, environmental stresses interfere with pulmonary immune defense mechanisms. For example, cigarette smoke compromises mucociliary clearance and pulmonary macrophage function, alcohol impairs neutrophil function as well as cough and epiglottic reflexes (thereby increasing the risk for aspiration), and exposure to air pollution may impair the function of macrophages and epithelial cells.

Bacterial pneumonias are classified according to the specific etiologic agent or, if no pathogen can be isolated, by the clinical setting in which the infection occurs. Specific clinical settings are associated with a fairly distinct group of pathogens (summarized in Table 11.4). Thus, consideration of the clinical setting can be a helpful guide when antimicrobial therapy must be given empirically.

Community-Acquired Bacterial Pneumonias

Bacterial pneumonias often follow a viral upper-respiratory tract infection. *S. pneumoniae* (pneumococcus) is the most common cause of community-acquired acute pneumonia and is discussed first, followed by other relatively common pathogens.

Streptococcus pneumoniae. Pneumococcal infections occur with increased frequency in two clinical settings: (1) chronic diseases such as chronic heart failure, COPD, or diabetes, and (2) congenital or acquired defects in immune responses. In addition, decreased or absent splenic function greatly increases the risk for overwhelming pneumococcal sepsis. The spleen contains the largest collection of phagocytes in the body and is the major organ responsible for removal of pneumococci from the blood. The spleen is also a major site of production of antipolysaccharide antibodies, the dominant protective antibodies against encapsulated bacteria. Notably, the overall incidence of pneumococcal pneumonia is decreasing, in part due to widespread use of pneumococcal vaccination, which results in both a decline in the individual rates of pneumococcal pneumonia and produces herd immunity in the population.

The presence of numerous neutrophils in sputum containing gram-positive, lancet-shaped diplococci supports the diagnosis of pneumococcal pneumonia, but *S. pneumoniae* is part of the endogenous flora in 20% of adults, and therefore false-positive results may be obtained. Isolation of pneumococci from blood cultures is more specific but less sensitive (in the early phase of illness, only 20% to 30% of patients have positive blood cultures). Pneumococcal vaccines containing capsular polysaccharides from the common serotypes are useful in preventing pneumococcal sepsis in individuals at high risk.

Haemophilus influenzae. Encapsulated *H. influenzae* type B is an important cause of community-acquired pneumonia and invasive infection in children worldwide, but its impact has been dramatically diminished in higher-resource parts of the world by vaccination in infancy against this organism. "Nontypeable" (unencapsulated) forms of *H. influenzae* remain important causes of community-acquired pneumonias in children and adults. Adults at high risk for developing infections include those with chronic pulmonary diseases such as cystic

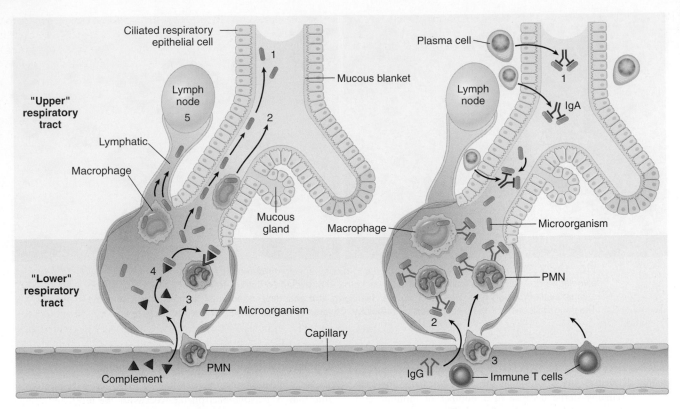

A INNATE IMMUNE DEFENSES   B ADAPTIVE IMMUNE DEFENSES

FIG. 11.28 Lung defense mechanisms. (A) Innate defenses against infection: *1,* In the healthy lung, removal of microbial organisms depends on entrapment in the mucous blanket and removal by means of the muco-ciliary elevator; *2,* phagocytosis by alveolar macrophages can kill and degrade organisms and remove them from the air spaces by migrating onto the mucociliary elevator; or *3,* phagocytosis and killing by neutrophils recruited by macrophage factors; *4,* complement may enter the alveoli and be activated by the alternative pathway to produce the opsonin C3b, which enhances phagocytosis; *5,* organisms, including those ingested by phagocytes, may reach the draining lymph nodes to initiate immune responses. (B) Additional mechanisms operate after development of adaptive immunity: *1,* Secreted IgA can block attachment of the microorganism to epithelium in the upper respiratory tract; *2,* in the lower respiratory tract, serum antibodies (IgM, IgG) are present in the alveolar lining fluid and activate complement more efficiently by the classic pathway, yielding C3b *(not shown)*; in addition, IgG is an opsonin; *3,* the accumulation of immune T cells is important for con-trolling infections by viruses and other intracellular microorganisms. *PMN,* Neutrophil.

fibrosis, bronchiectasis, and particularly COPD; *H. influenzae* is one of the most common bacterial causes of acute exacerbations of COPD.

Moraxella catarrhalis. *M. catarrhalis* is a cause of bacterial pneu-monia in older adults, particularly in those with cardiopulmonary dis-ease, diabetes, or immunodeficiency. It is the second most common bacterial cause of acute exacerbation of COPD. Along with *S. pneumoniae* and *H. influenzae,* *M. catarrhalis* is one of the three most frequent causes of otitis media (infection of the middle ear) in children.

Staphylococcus aureus. *S. aureus* is an important cause of sec-ondary bacterial pneumonia in children and healthy adults after viral respiratory illnesses (e.g., measles in children and influenza in both children and adults). Staphylococcal pneumonia is associated with a high incidence of complications such as lung abscess and empyema. Staphylococcal pneumonia occurring in association with right-sided staphylococcal endocarditis is a serious complication of intravenous substance use. It is also an important cause of hospital-acquired pneumonia (discussed later).

Klebsiella pneumoniae. *K. pneumoniae* is the most frequent cause of gram-negative bacterial pneumonia. *Klebsiella*-related pneumonia frequently afflicts individuals with chronic diseases that impair host defenses. Thick and gelatinous sputum is characteristic, as the organism produces an abundant viscid capsular polysaccharide that the patient may have difficulty expectorating.

Pseudomonas aeruginosa. Although discussed here with community-acquired pathogens because of its association with infections in cystic fibrosis, *P. aeruginosa* infection is most often acquired in hospital settings (discussed later). *Pseudomonas* pneumonia is also common in individuals who are neutropenic, usually secondary to chemotherapy or leukemic involvement of the bone marrow; in patients with extensive burns; and in patients requiring mechanical ventilation. Other risk factors include lung parenchymal abnormalities, repeated courses of antibiotics, and glucocorticoid use. *P. aeruginosa* has a propensity to invade blood vessels at the site of infection, with consequent extrapulmonary spread. *Pseudomonas* bacteremia is a fulminant disease, with death often occurring within a matter of days. Histologic examination reveals organisms invading the walls of necrotic blood vessels *(Pseudomonas vasculitis),* leading to secondary coagulative necrosis of the pulmonary parenchyma.

Table 11.4 The Pneumonia Syndromes and Implicated Pathogens

Community-Acquired Bacterial Pneumonia

Streptococcus pneumoniae
Haemophilus influenzae
Moraxella catarrhalis
Staphylococcus aureus
Legionella pneumophila
Enterobacteriaceae (*Klebsiella pneumoniae*) and *Pseudomonas* spp.
Mycoplasma pneumoniae
Chlamydia pneumoniae
Coxiella burnetii (Q fever)

Community-Acquired Viral Pneumonia

COVID-19 (SARS-CoV-2), respiratory syncytial virus, human metapneumovirus, parainfluenza virus (children); influenza A and B (adults); adenovirus (military recruits)

Health Care–Associated Pneumonia

Staphylococcus aureus, methicillin-sensitive or methicillin-resistant
Pseudomonas aeruginosa
Streptococcus pneumoniae

Hospital-Acquired Pneumonia

Gram-negative rods belonging to Enterobacteriaceae (*Klebsiella* spp., *Serratia marcescens*, *Escherichia coli*) and *Pseudomonas* spp.
S.aureus (usually methicillin-resistant)

Aspiration Pneumonia

Anaerobic oral flora (Bacteroides, Prevotella, Fusobacterium, Peptostreptococcus), admixed with aerobic bacteria (*S. pneumoniae*, *S. aureus*, *H. influenzae*, and *Pseudomonas aeruginosa*)

Chronic Pneumonia

Nocardia
Actinomyces
Granulomatous: *Mycobacterium tuberculosis* and atypical mycobacteria, *Histoplasma capsulatum*, *Coccidioides immitis*, *Blastomyces dermatitidis*

Necrotizing Pneumonia and Lung Abscess

Anaerobic bacteria (extremely common) with or without admixed aerobic infection
S. aureus, *K. pneumoniae*, *Streptococcus pyogenes*, and type 3 pneumococcus (uncommon)

Pneumonia in the Immunocompromised Host

Cytomegalovirus
Pneumocystis jiroveci
Mycobacterium avium complex (MAC)
Invasive aspergillosis
Invasive candidiasis
"Usual" bacterial, viral, and fungal organisms (listed above)

Legionella pneumophila. *L. pneumophila* is the agent of Legionnaire disease, an eponym for the epidemic and sporadic forms of pneumonia caused by this organism. *Pontiac fever* is a related self-limited upper respiratory tract infection caused by *L. pneumophila*, without pneumonia. *L. pneumophila* flourishes in artificial aquatic environments, such as industrial cooling systems and in shower heads, sink faucets, and hot tubs, among others. The usual mode of transmission is inhalation of aerosolized organisms or aspiration of contaminated drinking water. *Legionella* pneumonia is common in individuals with cardiac, renal, immunologic, or hematologic disease. Patients with organ transplants are particularly susceptible. *Legionella* pneumonia may be quite severe, frequently requiring hospitalization, and has a fatality rate of 30% to 50% in individuals who are immunocompromised. Rapid diagnosis is facilitated by demonstration of *Legionella* antigens in the urine or by a positive fluorescent antibody test on sputum samples; culture remains the standard diagnostic assay. PCR-based tests can be used on bronchial secretions in atypical cases.

Mycoplasma pneumoniae. Mycoplasma infections are particularly common among children and young adults. They occur sporadically or as local epidemics in closed communities (e.g., schools, military camps, prisons). Assays for *Mycoplasma* antigens and polymerase chain reaction (PCR) testing for *Mycoplasma* DNA are available.

MORPHOLOGY

Bacterial pneumonia has two patterns of anatomic distribution: lobular bronchopneumonia and lobar pneumonia (Fig. 11.29). In the context of pneumonias, the term "consolidation," used frequently, refers to "solidification" of the lung due to replacement of the air by exudate in the alveoli. Patchy consolidation of the lung is the dominant characteristic of **bronchopneumonia,** while consolidation of a large portion of a lobe or of an entire lobe defines **lobar pneumonia** (Fig. 11.30). These anatomic categorizations may be difficult to apply in individual cases because patterns overlap, and patchy involvement may evolve to become confluent over time, producing complete lobar consolidation. Moreover, the same organisms may produce either pattern depending on patient susceptibility. Most important from the clinical standpoint are identification of the causative agent and determination of the extent of disease.

In **lobar pneumonia,** four stages of the inflammatory response have classically been described. In the first stage of **congestion,** the lung is heavy, wet, and red. It is characterized by vascular engorgement, intraalveolar fluid with few neutrophils, and often numerous bacteria. The stage of **red hepatization** that follows is characterized by massive confluent exudation, as neutrophils, red cells, and fibrin fill the alveolar spaces (Fig. 11.31A). On gross examination, the lobe is red, firm, and airless, with a liverlike consistency, hence the term *hepatization*. The stage of **gray hepatization** that follows is marked by progressive disintegration of red cells and the persistence of a fibrinosuppurative exudate (Fig. 11.31B), resulting in a color change to grayish brown. In the final stage of **resolution,** the exudate within the alveolar spaces is broken down by enzymatic digestion to produce granular, semifluid debris that is resorbed, ingested by macrophages, expectorated, or organized by fibroblasts (Fig. 11.31C). Extension of the pneumonia to the lung periphery often produces a pleural fibrinous reaction **(pleuritis)**. This may resolve or undergo organization, leaving fibrous thickening or permanent adhesions.

In **bronchopneumonia** there are focal areas of consolidation resulting from acute suppurative inflammation. The consolidation may be confined to one lobe but is more often multilobar and frequently bilateral and basal because of the tendency of secretions to gravitate to the lower lobes. Well-developed lesions are slightly elevated, dry, granular, gray-red to yellow, and poorly delimited at their margins. Histologically, a neutrophil-rich exudate fills the bronchi, bronchioles, and adjacent alveolar spaces (see Fig. 11.31A).

Complications of pneumonia include (1) tissue destruction and necrosis, causing **abscess formation;** (2) spread of infection to the pleural cavity, causing pleuritis and the intrapleural fibrinosuppurative reaction known as **empyema;** and (3) **bacteremic dissemination** to the heart valves, pericardium, brain, kidneys, spleen, or joints, variously causing abscesses, endocarditis, meningitis, or suppurative arthritis.

Clinical Features. The major symptoms of typical community-acquired acute bacterial pneumonia are abrupt onset of high fever, shaking chills, and cough producing mucopurulent sputum; occasionally, patients have hemoptysis. When pleuritis is present, it

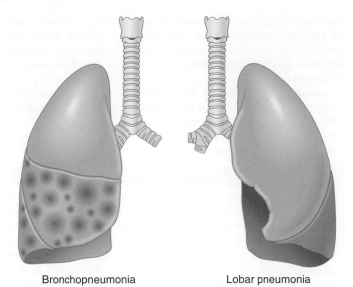

FIG. 11.29 The anatomic distribution of bronchopneumonia and lobar pneumonia affecting the lower lobes of the lung.

is accompanied by pleuritic pain and pleural friction rub. The whole lobe is radiopaque in lobar pneumonia, whereas there are focal opacities in bronchopneumonia.

The clinical course is markedly modified by the administration of effective antibiotics. Treated patients may be afebrile with few clinical signs 48 to 72 hours after the initiation of antibiotics. The identification of the organism and the determination of its antibiotic sensitivity are the keystones of therapy. Fewer than 10% of patients with pneumonia severe enough to merit hospitalization succumb, and in most such instances death results from a complication, such as empyema,

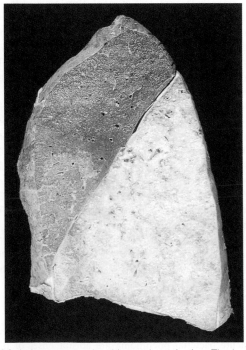

FIG. 11.30 Lobar pneumonia with gray hepatization. The lower lobe is uniformly consolidated.

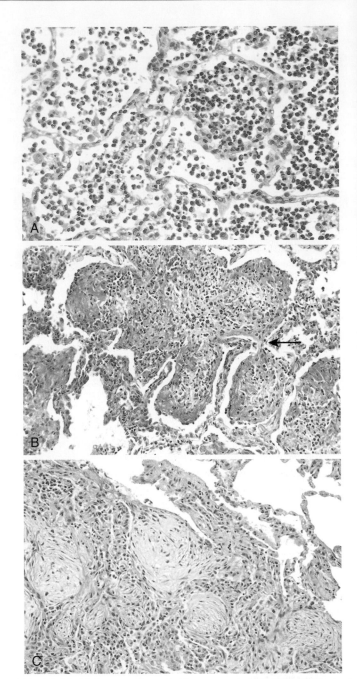

FIG. 11.31 (A) Acute pneumonia. The congested septal capillaries and extensive neutrophil exudation into alveoli correspond to early red hepatization. Fibrin nets have not yet formed. (B) Early organization of intraalveolar exudates, seen in areas to be streaming through the pores of Kohn *(arrow)*. (C) Advanced organizing pneumonia, featuring transformation of exudates to fibromyxoid masses richly infiltrated by macrophages and fibroblasts.

meningitis, endocarditis, or pericarditis, or to some predisposing influence, such as debility or chronic excess alcohol use.

Community-Acquired Viral Pneumonias

Prior to the COVID-19 pandemic, the most common causes of community-acquired viral pneumonias were influenza types A and B, the respiratory syncytial viruses, human metapneumovirus, adenovirus, rhinoviruses, rubeola virus, and varicella virus (see

Table 11.5). During the year 2020, SARS-CoV-2, the agent of COVID-19, rapidly became the leading cause of community-acquired viral pneumonia in most parts of the world.

All these viruses share a propensity to infect and damage respiratory epithelium, producing an inflammatory response. When the process extends to alveoli, there is usually interstitial inflammation, but some outpouring of fluid into alveolar spaces may also occur, so on chest films the changes may mimic those of bacterial pneumonia. As a result, it is not possible to distinguish bacterial and viral pneumonia based on radiologic appearance alone. Moreover, damage leading to necrosis of the respiratory epithelium inhibits mucociliary clearance and predisposes to secondary bacterial infections. Such serious complications of viral infection are more likely in infants, older adults, malnourished patients, individuals who are immunocompromised, and those who drink alcohol excessively.

We will first review the common morphologic and clinical features of viral pneumonias and then cover two of the most important causes of severe viral pneumonia, influenza viruses and coronaviruses.

MORPHOLOGY

The morphologic patterns in viral pneumonias are similar. The process may be patchy or it may involve whole lobes bilaterally or unilaterally. Macroscopically, the affected areas are red-blue and congested. On histologic examination, the **inflammatory reaction is largely confined to the walls of the alveoli** (Fig. 11.32). The septa are widened and edematous; they usually contain a mononuclear inflammatory infiltrate of lymphocytes, macrophages, and, occasionally, plasma cells. In the classic case, alveolar spaces in viral pneumonias are free of cellular exudate. In severe cases, however, diffuse alveolar damage with hyaline membranes may develop. In less severe, uncomplicated cases, resolution of the disease is followed by reconstitution of the normal architecture. Superimposed bacterial infection results in a mixed histologic picture.

Clinical Features. The course of viral pneumonia is extremely varied. It may masquerade as an upper respiratory tract infection or "chest cold" that goes undiagnosed or manifest as a fulminant, life-threatening

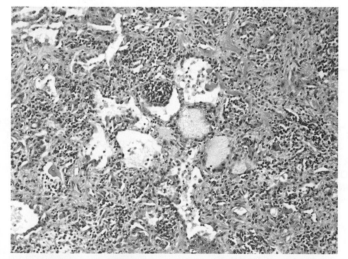

FIG. 11.32 Viral pneumonia. The thickened alveolar walls are infiltrated with lymphocytes and some plasma cells, which are spilling over into alveolar spaces. Note the focal alveolar edema *(center)* and early fibrosis *(upper right).*

infection. The initial presentation is usually that of an acute, nonspecific febrile illness characterized by fever, headache, malaise, and, later, cough with minimal sputum. In those who develop symptomatic pneumonia, the presence of the inflammatory exudate in alveolar walls prevents oxygenation of blood flowing through the affected air spaces, which in turn causes mismatch of ventilation and perfusion. As a result, the degree of respiratory distress is often out of proportion to the physical and radiographic findings.

Influenza Viruses

Influenza causes frequent epidemics and periodic pandemics. The influenza virus has a single-stranded RNA genome divided into eight separate segments that are held together by a nucleoprotein that determines the virus type—A, B, or C. The surface of the virus consists of a lipid bilayer containing viral hemagglutinin (H) and neuraminidase (N) proteins, which determine the subtype (e.g., H1N1, H3N2). Host antibodies to hemagglutinin and neuraminidase prevent and ameliorate, respectively, infection with the influenza virus. The type A viruses infect humans, pigs, horses, and birds and are the major cause of pandemic and epidemic influenza outbreaks. Epidemics of influenza emerge when new subtypes acquire mutations of the hemagglutinin and neuraminidase antigens that allow the virus to escape most host antibodies *(antigenic drift)*. Pandemics, which last longer and are more widespread than epidemics, occur when both the hemagglutinin and neuraminidase coding sequences are altered by recombination with animal viruses *(antigenic shift)*, creating a new virus against which the population has little to no preexisting immunity. Commercially available influenza vaccines are imperfect but provide reasonable protection against the infection, especially in vulnerable infants and in older adults.

Insight into future pandemics has come from studying the past. DNA analysis of viral genomes retrieved from the lungs of a soldier who died in the great 1918 influenza pandemic that killed 20 million to 40 million individuals worldwide identified swine influenza sequences, consistent with this virus having its origin in an antigenic shift. The first flu pandemic of this century, in 2009, also resulted from an antigenic shift involving a virus of swine origin. It caused particularly severe infections in young adults, apparently because older adults had antibodies against past influenza strains that conveyed partial protection. Comorbidities such as diabetes, heart disease, lung disease, and immunocompromise were also associated with a higher risk for severe infection.

What then might be the source of the next great flu pandemic? One concern is centered on avian influenza, which normally infects birds. One avian strain, type H5N1, has spread throughout the world in wild and domestic birds. As of December 2019 approximately 860 H5N1 influenza virus infections (from 15 countries) were reported to the World Health Organization (WHO). These infections resulted in high mortality, mainly due to pneumonia, even in adolescents and young adults. Nearly all cases have been acquired by close contact with domestic birds. Fortunately, the transmission of the current H5N1 avian virus is inefficient. However, if H5N1 influenza recombines with an influenza that is highly infectious for humans, a strain might emerge that is capable of sustained human-to-human transmission (and, thus, of causing the next great influenza pandemic).

Coronaviruses

Coronaviruses are enveloped, positive-sense RNA viruses that infect humans and several other vertebrate species. Weakly pathogenic coronaviruses cause mild coldlike upper respiratory tract infections, while highly pathogenic ones may cause severe, often fatal, pneumonia. An example of a highly pathogenic type is SARS-CoV-2 (severe acute respiratory syndrome coronavirus 2), a strain that is responsible for the first great pandemic of the 21st century, a viral disease called COVID-19.

Pathogenesis. Highly pathogenic coronaviruses like SARS-CoV-2 have viral spike proteins that bind the protein angiotensin-converting enzyme 2 (ACE2), which is found on the surface of nasopharyngeal epithelium and type 2 alveolar epithelial cells. Following exposure, the virus is taken up into ACE2-expressing cells and replicates rapidly, such that presymptomatic or newly symptomatic individuals are most likely to spread the infection to others. Transmission is mainly through respiratory droplets that are produced by coughing, sneezing, talking, or singing and is most likely to occur indoors in poorly ventilated spaces.

The outcome of SARS-CoV-2 infection is highly variable, ranging from asymptomatic infection, particularly in children and younger adults, to severe disease that leads to rapid progressive pneumonia and pulmonary failure. The major risk factors for severe disease include the following:

- *Age.* Although COVID-19 can be lethal at any age, it is particularly deadly in the elderly, especially those older than 75 years.
- *Comorbidities.* These include obesity, smoking, diabetes, and chronic cardiac, pulmonary, and renal disease.
- *Socioeconomic background, socially defined race, and gender.* Males are at higher risk for severe disease, as well as African Americans, Hispanics, and South Asian Americans. Some studies that have controlled for comorbidities suggest that the association with African and Hispanic descent is largely due to underlying health and economic disparities, not genetic factors.
- *Laboratory abnormalities.* These include lymphopenia, thrombocytopenia, and evidence of coagulopathy or hepatic, cardiac, or renal damage.
- *Genetic factors.* Several studies have detected an association between the type A blood group and severe disease, while others have identified germline mutations in genes encoding components of the type I interferon pathway in a subset of patients with severe disease.

The pathogenesis of COVID-19 remains to be completely elucidated, but a working model is shown in Fig. 11.33. Viral infection of type 2 alveolar epithelium may cause damage through direct cytopathic effects of the virus as well as through the ensuing immune response. Individuals who develop severe disease generally have higher viral loads early in the course, indicating an inability to control the virus early on. In some individuals, this failure may be due to autoantibodies or genetic variants that interfere with type I interferon signaling, or to less well-defined alterations in the immune system that occur with aging or in the presence of comorbid conditions such as obesity and diabetes. It is hypothesized that large numbers of SARS-CoV-2–infected cells elicit an excessive immune response marked by high levels of cytokines such as interferon-γ, IL-6, and TNF, setting off an inflammatory cascade sometimes referred to as cytokine storm. This in turn produces dysfunction not only in the lung but in multiple other organ systems, including the heart and kidneys, features that are reminiscent of the systemic inflammatory response syndrome (SIRS, Chapter 2). In those who are severely affected, this pro-inflammatory state persists even after viral loads fall, perhaps because ongoing tissue damage causes more inflammation. A relatively unusual feature of severe COVID-19 is a high propensity for venous and arterial thrombosis. The cause is incompletely understood, but it has been noted that thrombosis often occurs in the setting of very high levels of plasma fibrinogen and markedly elevated blood viscosity, a well-known risk factor for thrombosis.

MORPHOLOGY

In addition to features seen in other viral pneumonias (described previously), severe cases of COVID-19 may show additional findings. The coagulopathy that accompanies the disease may cause venous thromboembolism and arterial thrombosis, leading to limb ischemia and stroke, as well as the formation of microthrombi in the inflamed lung that may exacerbate pulmonary dysfunction. Myocarditis and inflammatory infiltrates in the CNS have also been reported, but whether these are direct or indirect effects of COVID-19 is unclear.

Clinical Features. The onset of COVID-19 resembles that of other causes of viral pneumonia, with the exception that it is likely to be associated with loss of smell and taste, apparently because of infection of olfactory epithelial cells. The diagnosis is readily made by PCR-based assays for the viral genome or by more rapid (but less

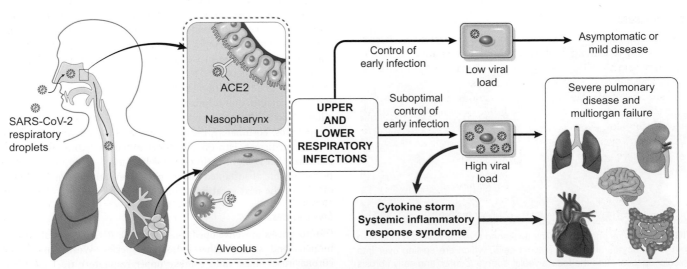

FIG. 11.33 Pathogenesis of COVID-19. *SARS-CoV-2,* Severe acute respiratory syndrome coronavirus 2. See text for details.

sensitive) assays for viral proteins. Those with symptomatic pneumonia benefit from treatment with immunosuppressive steroids, in line with the idea that severe disease involves an overexuberant immune response. Low-dose anticoagulants also improve outcomes, presumably by countering the procoagulant state that is induced by COVID-19. The availability of highly effective vaccines to SARS-CoV-2 is reducing the spread of this virus, but not before COVID-19 took a terrible toll of millions of lives worldwide. The pandemic has also seen the emergence of new strains of SARS-CoV-2; some, such as the Omicron variant, are more easily spread, making it probable that (like influenza) SARS-CoV-2 will persist and become an endemic seasonal respiratory infection.

Hospital-Acquired Pneumonias

Hospital-acquired, or nosocomial, pneumonias are defined as pulmonary infections acquired during a hospital stay. These infections not only have an adverse impact on the clinical course of ill patients but also add considerably to the burgeoning cost of health care. Hospital-acquired infections are common in patients with severe underlying disease and those who are immunosuppressed or are on prolonged antibiotic regimens. Patients on mechanical ventilation are a particularly high-risk group, and infections acquired in this setting are given the designation *ventilator-associated pneumonia*. Gram-negative rods (members of *Enterobacteriaceae* and *Pseudomonas* spp.) and *S. aureus* are the most common isolates; unlike community-acquired pneumonias, *S. pneumoniae* is not a common pathogen in the hospital setting.

Aspiration Pneumonia

Aspiration pneumonia occurs in patients who are debilitated or those who aspirate gastric contents while unconscious (e.g., after a stroke) or during repeated vomiting. Those affected typically have abnormal gag and swallowing reflexes. The resultant pneumonia is partly chemical, due to the irritating effects of the gastric acid, and partly bacterial. Typically, more than one organism is recovered on culture, aerobes being more common than anaerobes (Table 11.5). Aspiration pneumonia is often necrotizing, pursues a fulminant clinical course, and is a frequent cause of death in individuals predisposed to aspiration. In those who survive, abscess formation is a common complication. By contrast, microaspiration occurs in many individuals, especially those with gastroesophageal reflux, and may exacerbate other lung diseases but does not lead to pneumonia.

Lung Abscess

Lung abscess refers to a localized area of suppuration within the pulmonary parenchyma that results in the formation of one or more large cavities. The causative organism may be introduced into the lung by any of the following mechanisms:

- *Aspiration of infective material* from carious teeth or infected sinuses or tonsils. This may occur during oral surgery, anesthesia, coma, or alcoholic intoxication, or in debilitated patients with depressed cough reflexes.
- *Aspiration of gastric contents*, usually together with infectious organisms originating in the oropharynx
- *As a complication of necrotizing bacterial pneumonias*, particularly those caused by *S. aureus, Streptococcus pyogenes, K. pneumoniae, Pseudomonas* spp., and, rarely, type 3 pneumococci. Mycotic infections and bronchiectasis also may lead to lung abscesses.
- *Bronchial obstruction*, particularly due to neoplasms, especially lung cancer. Impaired drainage, distal atelectasis, and aspiration of blood and tumor fragments all contribute to the development

of abscesses. An abscess also may form within an excavated necrotic portion of a tumor. It may be preceded by bronchiectasis.
- *Septic embolism*, from infective endocarditis of the right side of the heart
- In addition, lung abscesses may result from *hematogenous spread of bacteria* in disseminated pyogenic infection. This occurs most characteristically in staphylococcal bacteremia and often results in multiple lung abscesses.
- Finally, selected pathogens can generate or colonize cavitary lesions and radiographically mimic lung abscess. Culprit pathogens include fungi (e.g., *Aspergillus* spp., *Cryptococcus* spp., *Histoplasma capsulatum, Blastomyces dermatitidis, Coccidioides* spp., the agents of mucormycosis), *Mycobacterium tuberculosis*, nontuberculous mycobacteria (e.g., *M. avium, M. kansasii, M. abscessus*), and parasites (e.g., *Entamoeba histolytica, Paragonimus westermani, Echinococcus* [hydatid cyst]). Pyogenic bacteria can also superinfect cavities caused by mycobacterial, fungal, and parasitic infections, leading to accumulation of liquid in an otherwise empty cavity.

Anaerobic bacteria are present in almost all lung abscesses, and they are the exclusive isolates in one-third to two-thirds of cases. The most frequently encountered anaerobes are commensals normally found in the oral cavity, principally species of *Prevotella, Fusobacterium, Bacteroides, Peptostreptococcus,* and microaerophilic streptococci.

MORPHOLOGY

Abscesses range in diameter from a few millimeters to large cavities 5 to 6 cm across. The location and number of abscesses in any particular case depend on their mode of development. Pulmonary abscesses resulting from aspiration of infective material are **more common on the right side** (with its more vertical airways) than on the left and are usually single. They tend to occur in the posterior segment of the right upper lobe and in the apical segments of the right lower lobe, locations that reflect the probable path of aspirated material in a recumbent individual. Abscesses that develop in the course of pneumonia or bronchiectasis are often multiple, basal, and scattered. Septic emboli and abscesses arising from hematogenous seeding are commonly multiple and may affect any region of the lungs.

As the focus of suppuration enlarges it almost inevitably ruptures into airways. The resulting partial drainage of the abscess cavity may produce an air-fluid level on radiographic examination. Occasionally, abscesses rupture into the pleural cavity, producing bronchopleural fistulas that may result in **pneumothorax** or **empyema**. Other complications arise from embolization of septic material to the brain, giving rise to meningitis or brain abscess. On histologic examination, depending on the chronicity of the lesion, the suppurative focus is surrounded by mononuclear infiltrates (lymphocytes, plasma cells, macrophages) and variable degrees of fibrous scarring.

Clinical Features. The manifestations of a lung abscess are much like those of bronchiectasis and include a prominent cough that usually yields copious amounts of foul-smelling, purulent, or sanguineous sputum; occasionally, hemoptysis occurs. Spiking fever and malaise are common. Clubbing of the fingers, weight loss, and anemia may appear. Abscesses occur in 10% to 15% of patients with lung cancer; thus, when a lung abscess is found in an older adult, underlying carcinoma must be considered. Secondary amyloidosis (Chapter 5) may develop in chronic cases. Treatment includes antibiotic therapy and, if needed, surgical drainage or resection. Overall, the mortality rate is in the range of 10%.

Tuberculosis

Tuberculosis is a communicable chronic granulomatous disease caused by *Mycobacterium tuberculosis*. It usually involves the lungs but may affect any organ or tissue in the body.

Epidemiology. **The World Health Organization (WHO) considers tuberculosis (TB) to be the most common cause of death resulting from an endemic infectious agent.** It is estimated in 2021 that 1.3 million people died of TB worldwide and that there were 5.8 million new cases. In the Western world, deaths from TB peaked in 1800 and steadily declined throughout the 1800s and 1900s. However, in 1984 this decline reversed abruptly due to the increased incidence of TB in people infected with HIV. As a consequence of intensive public health surveillance and TB prophylaxis among individuals who are immunocompromised, the incidence of TB in U.S.-born individuals again started to decline in 1992. Nevertheless, as of 2019 there were an estimated 13 million cases of latent tuberculosis in the United States.

TB flourishes in the settings of poverty, crowding, and chronic debilitating illness. In the United States, TB is a disease of older adults, the urban poor, the foreign-born, and patients with AIDS. African Americans, American Indians, the Inuit (from the Arctic), and Hispanics have a higher incidence of tuberculosis than European Americans, most likely due to lack of access to care and socioeconomic factors such as multifamily housing. Certain diseases also increase the risk, such as diabetes, Hodgkin lymphoma, chronic lung disease (particularly silicosis), chronic renal failure, malnutrition, alcohol use disorder, and immunosuppression. In areas of the world where HIV infection is prevalent, HIV infection is a dominant risk factor for the development of TB.

It is important that *infection* be differentiated from *disease*. Infection implies seeding of a focus with organisms, which may or may not cause clinically significant tissue damage (i.e., disease). Infection is usually acquired by direct person-to-person transmission of organisms in airborne droplets from an individual with active disease to a susceptible host. In most newly infected individuals, an asymptomatic focus of pulmonary infection appears that is self-limited and, upon resolution, leaves (if anything) a tiny, fibrocalcific nodule at the site. As discussed later, bacteria spread from the primary focus to various other sites in the body but the infection remains latent. Viable organisms may remain dormant in such foci for decades and possibly for the life of the host. Such individuals are infected but do not have active disease and therefore cannot transmit organisms to others. But if immune defenses are lowered, the infection may reactivate to produce communicable and potentially life-threatening disease.

Infection with *M. tuberculosis* typically leads to the development of delayed hypersensitivity. This can be detected by either IFN-γ release assays (IGRAs) or the tuberculin (purified protein derivative [PPD], or Mantoux) skin test. IGRAs are in vitro tests in which T cells from the patient are stimulated with protein antigens from *M. tuberculosis* and production of IFN-γ is measured to assess the level of T-cell immunity. The tuberculin skin test is performed by intracutaneous injection of a purified protein derivative of *M. tuberculosis,* which induces a visible and palpable induration in infected individuals that peaks in 48 to 72 hours. A positive IGRA or tuberculin test signifies T cell—mediated immunity to mycobacterial antigens but does not differentiate between infection and active disease. Recognized limitations of both tests are false-negative reactions (anergy) that may be produced by certain viral infections, sarcoidosis, malnutrition, Hodgkin lymphoma, immunosuppression, and (notably) overwhelming active tuberculous disease. False-positive reactions may result from infection by atypical mycobacteria.

About 80% of the population in certain Asian and African countries is tuberculin positive; by contrast, in 2019 approximately 5% of the U.S. population was positive. In general, 3% to 4% of individuals acquire active TB during the first year after "tuberculin conversion" and no more than 15% do so thereafter. Thus, only a small fraction of those who contract an infection develop active disease.

Etiology. Mycobacteria are slender rods that are acid fast (i.e., they have a high content of complex lipids that bind tightly to the Ziehl-Neelsen [carbol fuchsin] stain). *M. tuberculosis hominis* is responsible for most cases of TB, which is spread by individuals with active disease. Transmission is primarily through inhalation of airborne organisms in aerosols generated by expectoration or by exposure to contaminated secretions. Oropharyngeal and intestinal TB contracted by drinking milk contaminated with *Mycobacterium bovis* is now rare except in countries with tuberculous dairy cows where unpasteurized milk is consumed. Other mycobacteria, particularly *Mycobacterium avium complex,* are much less virulent than *M. tuberculosis* and rarely cause disease in immunocompetent individuals but may cause disseminated disease in patients with AIDS and rare inherited deficiencies of cell-mediated immunity.

Pathogenesis. The course of TB in a newly exposed immunocompetent individual is dictated by the development of cell-mediated immunity, which confers resistance to the organism and results in development of tissue hypersensitivity to tubercular antigens. The typical pathologic features such as caseating granulomas and cavitation are the result of the destructive tissue hypersensitivity of the host immune response. Because the effector cells for both protective immunity and damaging hypersensitivity are the same, the appearance of tissue hypersensitivity also signals the acquisition of immunity. The sequence of events from inhalation of the infectious inoculum to containment of the primary focus is illustrated in Fig. 11.34 and can be outlined as follows:

- *Entry into macrophages.* A virulent strain of mycobacteria gains entry to macrophage endosomes, a process mediated by several macrophage receptors, including the mannose receptor and complement receptors that recognize components of mycobacterial cell walls.
- *Replication in macrophages.* Once internalized, the organisms inhibit normal microbicidal responses by preventing the fusion of the lysosomes with the phagocytic vacuole, allowing the mycobacterium to persist in the vacuoles and proliferate. Thus, during the earliest phase of primary TB (the first 3 weeks) in a nonsensitized patient, the bacilli proliferate unchecked within pulmonary alveolar macrophages and air spaces, eventually resulting in bacteremia and seeding of the organisms to multiple sites. Despite the bacteremia, most individuals at this stage are asymptomatic or have a mild flu-like illness.
- *Development of cell-mediated immunity.* This occurs approximately 3 weeks after exposure. Mycobacterial antigens reach the draining lymph nodes and are processed and presented to CD4+ T cells by dendritic cells and macrophages. Under the influence of macrophage-secreted IL-12, CD4+ T cells of the Th1 subset are generated that secrete IFN-γ.
- *T cell—mediated macrophage activation and killing of bacteria.* IFN-γ released by the Th1 cells is crucial for activating macrophages. Activated macrophages, in turn, release a variety of mediators and upregulate expression of genes with important anti-mycobacterial effects, including (1) TNF, which is responsible for recruitment of

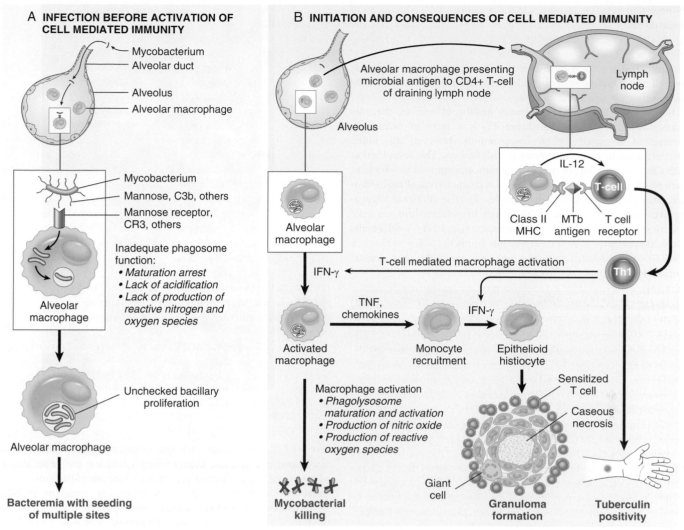

A INFECTION BEFORE ACTIVATION OF CELL MEDIATED IMMUNITY

- Mycobacterium
- Alveolar duct
- Alveolus
- Alveolar macrophage

- Mycobacterium
- Mannose, C3b, others
- Mannose receptor, CR3, others

Inadequate phagosome function:
- *Maturation arrest*
- *Lack of acidification*
- *Lack of production of reactive nitrogen and oxygen species*

Alveolar macrophage

Alveolar macrophage

Unchecked bacillary proliferation

Bacteremia with seeding of multiple sites

B INITIATION AND CONSEQUENCES OF CELL MEDIATED IMMUNITY

Alveolar macrophage presenting microbial antigen to CD4+ T-cell of draining lymph node

Alveolus

Lymph node

IL-12

Class II MHC — MTb antigen — T cell receptor

T-cell

Alveolar macrophage

IFN-γ

T-cell mediated macrophage activation

Th1

TNF, chemokines

IFN-γ

Activated macrophage

Monocyte recruitment

Epithelioid histiocyte

Macrophage activation
- *Phagolysosome maturation and activation*
- *Production of nitric oxide*
- *Production of reactive oxygen species*

Sensitized T cell

Caseous necrosis

Giant cell

Mycobacterial killing

Granuloma formation

Tuberculin positivity

FIG. 11.34 Sequence of events in the natural history of primary pulmonary tuberculosis. This sequence commences with inhalation of virulent strains of *Mycobacterium* and culminates in the development of immunity and delayed hypersensitivity to the organism. (A) Events occurring in the first 3 weeks after exposure. (B) Events thereafter. The development of resistance to the organism is accompanied by conversion to a positive result on tuberculin skin testing. Cells and bacteria are not drawn to scale. *CR3*, Complement receptor 3; *IFN-γ*, interferon γ; *MHC*, major histocompatibility complex; *MTb*, *Mycobacterium* tuberculosis; *TNF*, tumor necrosis factor.

monocytes, which are activated to develop into the macrophages that characterize the granulomatous response; (2) inducible nitric oxide synthase (iNOS), which raises nitric oxide (NO) levels, helping to create reactive nitrogen intermediates that appear to be particularly important in killing of mycobacteria; and (3) antimicrobial peptides (defensins) that are also toxic to mycobacteria.

- *Granulomatous inflammation and tissue damage.* **In addition to stimulating macrophages to kill mycobacteria, the Th1 response orchestrates the formation of granulomas.** Macrophages activated by IFN-γ differentiate into the "epithelioid histiocytes" that aggregate to form granulomas; some epithelioid cells may fuse to form giant cells. Activated macrophages also secrete TNF and chemokines, which promote recruitment of more monocytes. The importance of TNF is underscored by the fact that patients with rheumatoid arthritis and inflammatory bowel disease being treated with TNF antagonists are at increased risk for TB reactivation. In many individuals, the T-cell response halts the infection before

significant tissue destruction or illness occurs. In other individuals with immune deficits due to age or immunosuppression, however, the immune response is insufficient to hold the infection at bay.

In summary, immunity to a tubercular infection is primarily mediated by Th1 cells, which stimulate macrophages to kill mycobacteria. This immune response, while largely effective, comes at the cost of hypersensitivity and accompanying tissue destruction. Defects in any of the steps of a Th1 T-cell response (including IL-12, IFN-γ, TNF, or nitric oxide production) result in poorly formed granulomas, absence of resistance, and disease progression. Individuals with inherited mutations in any component of the T-cell response are extremely susceptible to infections with mycobacteria. Reactivation of the infection or reexposure to the bacilli in a previously sensitized host results in rapid mobilization of a defensive reaction but also increased tissue necrosis. By contrast, the loss of hypersensitivity (indicated by tuberculin negativity in an *M. tuberculosis*–infected patient) is an ominous sign of fading resistance to the organism and is a harbinger of severe disease.

Primary Tuberculosis

Primary TB is the form of disease that develops in a previously unexposed and therefore unsensitized patient. About 5% of those newly infected develop significant disease.

In the large majority of otherwise healthy individuals, the only short-term consequence of primary TB is a focus of pulmonary scarring, as discussed earlier. Uncommonly, however, this initial infection leads to *progressive primary tuberculosis*. This complication occurs in patients who are overtly immunocompromised or who have more subtle defects in host defenses, as is characteristic of individuals with severe acute malnutrition (Chapter 7). The incidence of progressive primary TB is particularly high in patients who are HIV positive with significant immunosuppression (i.e., CD4+ T cell counts below 200 cells/μL). Immunosuppression blunts the ability to mount a CD4+ T cell—mediated response and as a result the characteristic granulomatous reaction to TB is absent.

MORPHOLOGY

In countries in which bovine TB and infected milk have largely disappeared, primary TB almost always begins in the lungs. The inhaled bacilli usually implant in the distal air spaces of the lower part of the upper lobe or in the upper part of the lower lobe, typically close to the pleura. During the development of sensitization, a 1-cm to 1.5-cm area of gray-white consolidation appears that is called the **Ghon focus.** In the majority of cases, the center of this focus undergoes caseous necrosis. Tubercle bacilli, either free or within phagocytes, travel via the lymphatic vessels to the regional lymph nodes, which also often caseate. This combination of parenchymal and nodal lesions is called the **Ghon complex** (Fig. 11.35). Lymphatic and hematogenous dissemination to other parts of the body also occurs during the first few weeks. Development of cell-mediated immunity controls the infection in approximately 95% of cases. Therefore, the Ghon complex undergoes progressive fibrosis, and calcification often follows (detectable as a **Ranke complex** on radiograph). Despite seeding of other organs, no lesions develop. Histologically, sites of overt infection are involved by a characteristic inflammatory reaction marked by the presence of caseating and noncaseating granulomas, which consist of epithelioid macrophages and multinucleate giant cells (Fig. 11.36A to C). In those who do not mount an effective immune response due to immunocompromise, progressive primary tuberculosis may develop. Lesions in such individuals often lack granulomas and instead consist of sheets of macrophages containing numerous bacilli (Fig. 11.36D).

Secondary Tuberculosis (Reactivation Tuberculosis)

Secondary TB is the pattern of disease that arises in a previously sensitized host. It may appear shortly after primary TB but more commonly arises from reactivation of dormant primary lesions many decades after initial infection, particularly when host resistance is weakened. It may also result from reinfection, which may occur either because the protection afforded by the primary disease has waned or because of exposure to a large inoculum of virulent bacilli. Whatever the source of the organisms, only a few patients (<5%) with primary disease develop secondary TB.

Secondary pulmonary TB is classically localized to the apex of one or both upper lobes. The reason is obscure but may relate to high oxygen tension in the apices. Because of the preexistence of hypersensitivity, the bacilli elicit a prompt tissue response that tends to wall off the focus. As a result, regional lymph nodes are less prominently

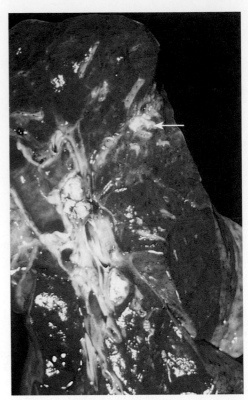

FIG. 11.35 Primary pulmonary tuberculosis, Ghon complex. The gray-white parenchymal focus *(arrow)* is under the pleura in the lower part of the upper lobe. Hilar lymph nodes with caseation are seen *(left).*

involved than in primary TB. On the other hand, the infection and associated inflammation often undergo cavitation and erode into and disseminate along airways. Such changes are an important source of infectivity, as affected patients produce sputum containing the bacilli.

Secondary TB should always be an important diagnostic consideration in HIV-positive patients who present with pulmonary disease. Although an increased risk for TB exists at all stages of HIV disease, the manifestations differ depending on the degree to which the patient is immunocompromised. For example, patients who are less severely immunocompromised (CD4+ T cell counts >300 cells/μL) present with "usual" secondary TB (apical disease with cavitation), while those who are more significantly immunocompromised (CD4+ T cell counts below 200 cells/μL) more often present with a clinical picture that resembles progressive primary TB (lower and middle lobe consolidation, hilar lymphadenopathy, and noncavitary disease). The extent to which the patient is immunocompromised also determines the frequency of extrapulmonary involvement, rising from 10% to 15% in patients who are mildly immunocompromised to greater than 50% in those with severe immune deficiency.

MORPHOLOGY

The initial lesion of secondary TB is usually a small focus of consolidation, less than 2 cm in diameter, within 1 to 2 cm of the **apical pleura.** Such foci are sharply circumscribed, firm, gray to yellow areas with a variable amount of central caseation and peripheral fibrosis. In cases that resolve, the initial parenchymal focus undergoes progressive fibrous encapsulation, leaving only fibrocalcific scars. Histologically, active lesions show characteristic coalescent nodules with central caseation. Although tubercle bacilli can be demonstrated by appropriate methods in early exudative and caseous phases of granuloma formation, it is usually impossible to find them in the late, fibrocalcific stages.

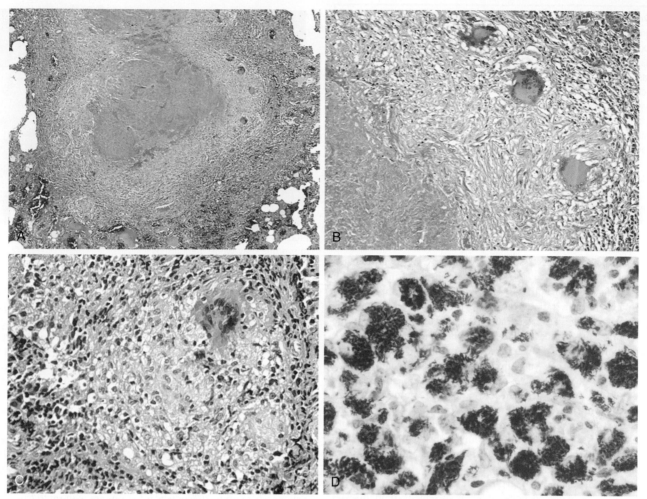

FIG. 11.36 The morphologic spectrum of tuberculosis. A characteristic tubercle at low magnification (A) and at higher power (B) shows central granular caseation surrounded by epithelioid and multinucleate giant cells. This is the usual response in individuals who develop cell-mediated immunity to the organism. (C) Occasionally, even in immunocompetent patients, tubercular granulomas may not show central caseation; hence, irrespective of the presence or absence of caseous necrosis, use of special stains for acid-fast organisms is indicated when granulomas are present. (D) In this specimen from a patient who is immunocompromised, sheets of macrophages packed with mycobacteria are seen (acid-fast stain).

Localized, apical, secondary pulmonary TB may heal with fibrosis either spontaneously or after therapy, or the disease may progress and extend along several different pathways. In **progressive pulmonary TB,** the apical lesion and the area of caseation expands. Erosion into a bronchus evacuates the caseous center, creating a ragged, **irregular cavity lined by caseous material** that is poorly walled off by fibrous tissue (Fig. 11.37). Erosion of blood vessels results in hemoptysis. With adequate treatment, the process may be arrested, although healing by fibrosis often distorts the pulmonary architecture. Irregular cavities, now free of caseous necrosis, may remain intact or collapse and become fibrotic. If the treatment is inadequate or host defenses are impaired, the infection may spread by direct extension and by dissemination through airways, lymphatic channels, and the vascular system. **Miliary pulmonary disease** occurs when organisms reach the bloodstream through lymphatic vessels and then recirculate to the lung via the pulmonary arteries. The lesions appear as small (2-mm) foci of yellow-white consolidation scattered through the lung parenchyma (the word *miliary* is derived from the resemblance of these foci to millet seeds). With progressive pulmonary TB, the pleural cavity is invariably involved and serous **pleural effusions, tuberculous empyema,** or **obliterative fibrous pleuritis** may develop.

Endobronchial, endotracheal, and **laryngeal TB** may develop when infective material is spread either through lymphatic channels or from expectorated infectious material. The mucosal lining may be studded with minute granulomatous lesions, sometimes apparent only on microscopic examination.

Systemic miliary TB ensues when the organisms disseminate hematogenously throughout the body. Systemic miliary TB is most prominent in the liver, bone marrow, spleen, adrenal glands, meninges, kidneys, fallopian tubes, and epididymis (Fig. 11.38).

Isolated-organ TB may appear after hematogenous seeding to any organ or tissue and may be the presenting manifestation of TB. Relatively common sites of isolated involvement include the meninges, kidneys, adrenal glands, bones, and fallopian tubes. When the vertebrae are affected, the condition is referred to as **Pott disease.** Paraspinal "cold" abscesses may extend along the tissue planes to present as an abdominal or pelvic mass.

Lymphadenitis is the most frequent form of extrapulmonary TB, usually occurring in the cervical region ("scrofula"). Lymphadenopathy tends to be unifocal, and most patients do not have concurrent extranodal disease. Patients who are HIV positive, on the other hand, almost always have multifocal disease, systemic symptoms, and either pulmonary or other organ involvement by active TB.

In years past, **intestinal TB** contracted by drinking contaminated milk was fairly common as a primary focus of TB. In higher-income countries today, intestinal TB is more often a complication of protracted advanced secondary TB, occurring due to the swallowing of coughed-up infective material. Typically, the organisms are trapped in mucosal lymphoid aggregates of the small and large bowel, which then undergo inflammatory enlargement with ulceration of the overlying mucosa, particularly in the ileum.

The many patterns of TB are depicted in Fig. 11.39.

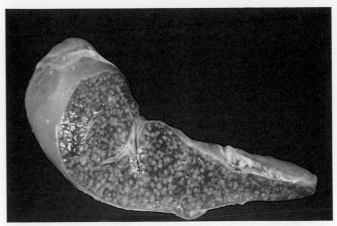

FIG. 11.38 Miliary tuberculosis of the spleen. The cut surface shows numerous gray-white granulomas.

Clinical Features. Localized secondary TB may be asymptomatic. When manifestations appear, they are usually insidious in onset, with gradual development of both systemic and localizing symptoms and signs. Systemic manifestations related to the release of cytokines by activated macrophages (e.g., TNF and IL-1) often appear early in the disease course and include malaise, anorexia, weight loss, and fever. Commonly, the fever is low grade and remittent (appearing late each afternoon and then subsiding) and is often accompanied by night sweats. With progressive pulmonary involvement, increasing amounts of sputum, at first mucoid and later purulent, appear. When cavitation is present, the sputum contains tubercle bacilli. Some degree of hemoptysis is present in about half of pulmonary TB cases. Pleuritic pain may result from extension of the infection to the pleural surfaces. Extrapulmonary manifestations of TB are legion and depend on the organ system involved (e.g., tuberculous salpingitis may present as infertility, tuberculous meningitis with headache and neurologic deficits, spine involvement [Pott disease] with back pain and paraplegia).

The diagnosis of pulmonary disease is based in part on the history and on physical and radiographic findings of consolidation or cavitation in the apices of the lungs. Ultimately, however, tubercle bacilli must be identified. The most common method for diagnosis of active mycobacterial infection remains detection of organisms in sputum by acid-fast staining or by staining with fluorescent auramine

rhodamine. Conventional cultures for mycobacteria require up to 10 weeks, but liquid media—based radiometric assays that detect mycobacterial metabolism are able to provide an answer within 2 weeks. PCR amplification can be performed on liquid growth media, as well as on tissue sections, to identify the mycobacterium. However, culture remains the standard diagnostic modality because it can identify the occasional PCR-negative case and also allows testing of drug susceptibility. Of concern, multidrug resistance (MDR), defined as resistance of mycobacteria to two or more of the primary drugs used for treatment of TB, is becoming more common, and the WHO estimated that 465,000 individuals had multidrug-resistant TB in 2019, representing approximately 3% of new cases and 20% of previously treated cases. The epicenter of this troubling development lies in Eastern Europe, Russia, several areas of Africa, and parts of Asia, regions where up to 20% of new infections are with multidrug-resistant strains. Of even greater concern, approximately 5% to 10% of such cases exhibit extensive multidrug resistance, defined by resistance to many of the antibiotics in current use against TB.

The prognosis is determined by the extent of the infection (localized versus widespread), the immune status of the host, and the antibiotic sensitivity of the organism. The prognosis is guarded in those with multidrug-resistant TB. Amyloidosis may develop in persistent cases.

Nontuberculous Mycobacterial Disease

Nontuberculous mycobacteria most commonly cause localized pulmonary disease in immunocompetent elderly individuals. In the United States, strains implicated most frequently include *Mycobacterium avium-intracellulare* (also called *M. avium* complex), *Mycobacterium kansasii*, and *Mycobacterium abscessus*. Nontuberculous mycobacterial infection often manifests as upper lobe cavitary disease, mimicking tuberculosis, especially in patients with a history of smoking, COPD, or chronic excess alcohol use.

In individuals who are immunocompromised (primarily patients who are HIV-seropositive), *M. avium* complex infection manifests as a disseminated disease associated with systemic signs and symptoms (e.g., fever, night sweats, weight loss). Enlargement of the liver and spleen due to the presence of numerous macrophages bearing intracellular bacilli is common, as are gastrointestinal symptoms such as diarrhea and malabsorption. The pattern of pulmonary involvement is often indistinguishable from that seen with TB in patients with AIDS. Disseminated *M. avium* complex infection in patients with AIDS tends to occur late in the clinical course, when CD4+ T cell counts have fallen below

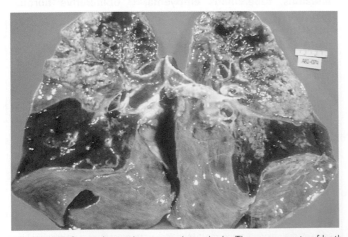

FIG. 11.37 Secondary pulmonary tuberculosis. The upper parts of both lungs are riddled with gray-white areas of caseation and multiple areas of softening and cavitation.

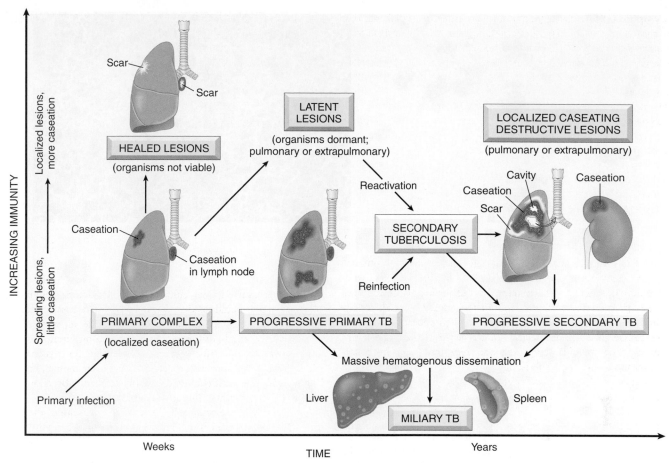

FIG. 11.39 The natural history and spectrum of tuberculosis. *TB*, Tuberculosis. (Adapted from a sketch provided by Dr. R.K. Kumar, The University of New South Wales, School of Pathology, Sydney, Australia.)

100 cells/μL. Hence, in such patients, tissue examination does not reveal granulomas; instead, sheets of macrophages filled with mycobacteria are seen. *M. avium* complex infections are also encountered in elderly patients, presumably because of waning immunity, but in this context the infections typically remain localized to the lung and follow a relatively benign course.

Fungal Pneumonias

Infections caused by dimorphic fungi, which include *Histoplasma capsulatum, Coccidioides immitis,* and *Blastomyces dermatitidis,* may manifest as isolated pulmonary disease in immunocompetent individuals or disseminated disease in individuals who are immunocompromised. Because of overlap in their clinical presentations, infections caused by these fungi are considered together in this section.

Epidemiology. Each of the dimorphic fungi has a typical geographic distribution, as follows:

- *Histoplasma capsulatum* is endemic in the Ohio and central Mississippi River valleys and along the Appalachian Mountains in the southeastern United States. Warm, moist soil containing droppings from bats and birds provides an ideal medium for the growth of the mycelial form, which produces infectious spores.
- *Coccidioides immitis* is endemic in the southwestern and far western regions of the United States, particularly in California's San Joaquin Valley, where coccidial infection is known as "valley fever."
- *Blastomyces dermatitidis* has a distribution in the United States that overlaps with those in which histoplasmosis is found.

MORPHOLOGY

The yeast forms are fairly distinctive, allowing each of these fungi to be identified in tissue sections:

- *H. capsulatum:* Round to oval, small yeast forms measuring 2 to 5 μm in diameter (Fig. 11.40A)
- *C. immitis:* Thick-walled, nonbudding spherules, 20 to 60 μm in diameter, often filled with small endospores (Fig. 11.40B)
- *B. dermatitidis:* Round to oval yeast forms (5 to 25 μm in diameter) that reproduce by characteristic broad-based budding (Fig. 11.40C and D)

Manifestations may take the form of (1) acute (primary) pulmonary infection, (2) chronic (granulomatous) pulmonary disease, or (3) disseminated miliary disease. The primary pulmonary nodules, composed of aggregates of macrophages filled with organisms, are associated with similar lesions in the regional lymph nodes. These lesions evolve into small granulomas with multinucleate giant cells and may develop central necrosis and, later, fibrosis and calcification. The similarity to primary tuberculosis is striking, and differentiation requires identification of the yeast forms (best seen with silver stains).

In infants or adults who are immunocompromised, particularly those with HIV infection, disseminated disease (analogous to miliary tuberculosis) may develop. Under these circumstances, well-formed granulomas are absent and instead focal collections of phagocytes containing yeast forms are seen within the liver, spleen, lymph nodes, gastrointestinal tract, and bone marrow. The adrenal glands and meninges may also be involved, and in a minority of cases ulcers form in the nose and mouth, on the tongue, or in the larynx.

Cutaneous infections with disseminated *Blastomyces* organisms frequently induce striking epithelial hyperplasia, which may be mistaken for squamous cell carcinoma. Blastomycosis also has a characteristic proclivity for infecting bone.

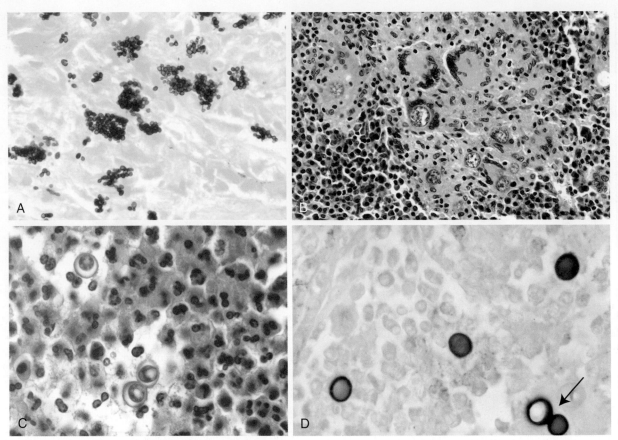

FIG. 11.40 (A) *Histoplasma capsulatum* yeast forms fill phagocytes in a lymph node of a patient with disseminated histoplasmosis (silver stain). (B) Coccidioidomycosis with intact spherules within multinucleated giant cells. (C) Blastomycosis, with rounded budding yeasts, larger than neutrophils. Note the characteristic thick wall and nuclei (not seen in other fungi). (D) Silver stain highlights the broad-based budding seen in *Blastomyces dermatitidis* organisms *(arrow)*.

Clinical Features. The clinical symptoms and signs resemble those of a "flulike" syndrome and are most often self-limited. In the vulnerable host, chronic cavitary pulmonary disease develops, with a predilection for the upper lobe, resembling the secondary form of tuberculosis. Spread to lymph nodes may produce perihilar masslike lesions that resemble bronchogenic carcinoma radiologically. At this stage, manifestations may include cough, hemoptysis, dyspnea, and chest pain.

Disseminated disease produces a febrile illness marked by hepatosplenomegaly, anemia, leukopenia, and thrombocytopenia.

Pneumonia in the Immunocompromised Host

Pneumonia is one of most common and serious complications in individuals with compromised immune systems. Some of the responsible pathogens also cause disease in immunocompetent individuals, but with manifestations that are typically much less severe than in those with defective immunity. Other pathogens are almost purely "opportunistic," virtually never causing significant disease in immunocompetent individuals. The opportunistic pulmonary pathogens include (1) bacteria (e.g., *Mycobacterium avian intracellulare*); (2) viruses (e.g., cytomegalovirus and herpesvirus); and (3) fungi (e.g., *P. jiroveci, Candida* spp., *Aspergillus* spp., and *Cryptococcus neoformans*). Here we discuss some of the pathogens that are most problematic in those with compromised immune systems.

Cytomegalovirus

Depending on the age and the immune status of the host, infection by cytomegalovirus (CMV), a member of the herpesvirus family, may manifest in various forms. Cells infected by the virus exhibit gigantism of both the cytoplasm and the nucleus. The nucleus typically contains a large inclusion surrounded by a clear halo ("owl's eye"), an appearance that inspired the name of the classic form of symptomatic disease in neonates—*cytomegalic inclusion disease.* Although cytomegalic inclusion disease involves many organs, CMV infections are discussed here because CMV pneumonitis is a serious problem in adults who are immunocompromised, particularly those with AIDS and recipients of allogeneic hematopoietic stem cell transplants.

Transmission of CMV may occur by several age-dependent mechanisms:

- A fetus may be infected transplacentally from a newly acquired or reactivated infection in the mother (congenital CMV infection).
- The virus may be transmitted to the infant through cervical or vaginal secretions at birth, or later through the breast milk of a mother with an active infection (perinatal CMV infection).
- Preschool children, especially in day care centers, may acquire it through saliva. Toddlers can readily transmit the virus to their parents.
- In patients older than 15 years of age, the venereal route is the dominant mode of transmission, but spread may also occur

through contact with respiratory secretions and by the fecal-oral route.

- Iatrogenic transmission may occur at any age through organ transplantation or blood transfusion.

CMV infects a wide range of cells in various tissues, including epithelium, endothelium, neurons, and macrophages. **Infected cells are strikingly enlarged, often to a diameter of 40 μm, and exhibit cellular and nuclear pleomorphism.** Prominent intranuclear basophilic inclusions spanning half the nuclear diameter are usually set off from the nuclear membrane by a clear halo (Fig. 11.41). Smaller basophilic inclusions are also frequently seen in the cytoplasm.

Clinical Features. The clinical outcome of CMV infection depends on the age and immune status of the host. As discussed in Chapter 4, perinatal CMV infection may lead to serious disseminated disease involving the brain, retina, heart, and other tissues. By contrast, infections are nearly always asymptomatic in healthy young children and adults. In surveys around the world, 50% to 100% of adults demonstrate anti-CMV antibodies in the serum, indicating previous exposure. The most common clinical manifestation of CMV infection in immunocompetent hosts beyond the neonatal period is an infectious mononucleosis—like illness marked by fever, atypical lymphocytosis, lymphadenopathy, and hepatomegaly accompanied by abnormal liver function test results, suggesting mild hepatitis. Most patients recover from CMV mononucleosis without sequelae, although excretion of the virus may occur in body fluids for months to years. Irrespective of the presence or absence of symptoms during acute infection, once infected, an individual is seropositive for life. The virus remains latent within leukocytes, which is the major reservoir of reactivation infection.

Immunosuppression-related CMV infection occurs most commonly in transplant recipients and in patients with AIDS and may represent a new infection or reactivation of a latent infection. CMV is the most common opportunistic viral pathogen in patients with AIDS. Disseminated CMV infections in individuals who are immunocompromised

primarily affect the lungs, gastrointestinal tract, and retina; the central nervous system is usually spared. In the lung, infection is associated with typical cytomegalic changes, mononuclear cell infiltrates, and foci of necrosis and may be of sufficient severity to cause acute respiratory distress syndrome. Intestinal necrosis and ulceration may develop and may be extensive, leading to the formation of "pseudomembranes" (Chapter 13) and debilitating diarrhea. CMV retinitis, the most common form of opportunistic CMV disease, may occur alone or in combination with involvement of the lungs and intestinal tract. Diagnosis of CMV infection may be made by demonstration of characteristic viral inclusions in tissue sections, viral culture, rising antiviral antibody titers, or PCR—based detection of CMV DNA. The latter has revolutionized the approach to monitoring patients for early evidence of infection after transplantation.

Pneumocystis

P. jiroveci (previously *P. carinii*) is an opportunistic infectious fungus. Serologic evidence indicates that virtually all individuals are exposed to *Pneumocystis* during the first few years of life, but in most the infection remains latent. Reactivation with development of clinical disease occurs almost exclusively in individuals who are immunocompromised. Indeed, patients with untreated AIDS are extremely susceptible to *P. jiroveci*, as are severely malnourished infants and patients receiving high doses of immunosuppressive drugs. In patients with AIDS, the risk for *P. jiroveci* infection increases in inverse proportion to the CD4+ T cell count and is particularly high in those with counts of less than 200 cells/μL. *Pneumocystis* infection is largely confined to the lung, where it produces an interstitial pneumonitis. It often is found together with CMV infection, possibly because CMV interferes with the function of alveolar macrophages and T cells.

Involved areas of the lung contain a characteristic **intraalveolar, foamy, pink-staining exudate** ("cotton candy" exudate) in H&E-stained sections (Fig. 11.42A). The septa are thickened by edema and a sparse mononuclear infiltrate. Special stains (e.g., silver stains) are required to visualize the organism, seen as **round- to cup-shaped cysts** (4 to 10 μm in diameter) within the alveolar exudates (see Fig. 11.42B).

Clinical Features. The diagnosis of *Pneumocystis* pneumonia should be considered in any immunocompromised patient with respiratory symptoms and abnormal findings on chest radiograph. Fever, dry cough, and dyspnea occur in 90% to 95% of patients. Radiographic evidence of bilateral perihilar and basilar infiltrates is typical. Hypoxia is frequent; pulmonary function studies show a restrictive lung defect. The most sensitive and effective method of diagnosis is to identify the organism in sputum or bronchoalveolar lavage fluid using immunostains. If treatment is initiated before involvement is widespread, the outlook is good; however, because residual organisms are likely to persist, particularly in patients with AIDS, relapses are common unless the underlying immunodeficiency is corrected or prophylactic therapy is given.

Candidiasis

Candida species encompass the group of fungi that are most commonly associated with human disease. Most disease is caused by *C. albicans*, a normal inhabitant of the oral cavity, gastrointestinal tract, and vagina in many individuals. Systemic candidiasis (with associated pneumonia) is restricted to patients who are immunocompromised; it has protean manifestations.

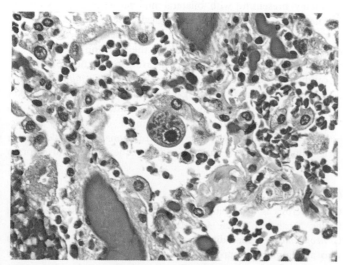

FIG. 11.41 Cytomegalovirus infection of the lung. A distinct nuclear inclusion and multiple cytoplasmic inclusions are seen in an enlarged cell.

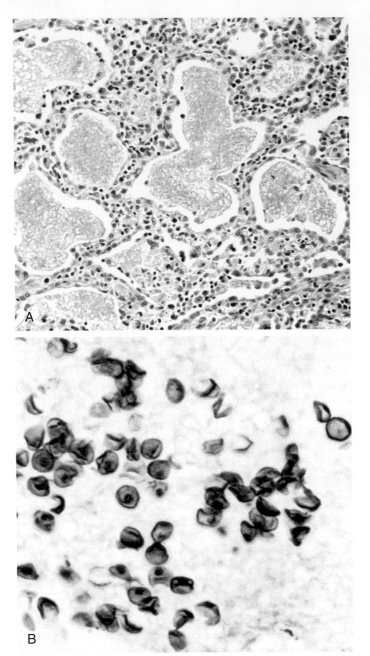

FIG. 11.42 *Pneumocystis* pneumonia. (A) The alveoli are filled with a characteristic foamy acellular exudate. (B) Silver stain demonstrates cup-shaped and round cysts within the exudate.

MORPHOLOGY

In tissue sections, *C. albicans* demonstrates yeastlike forms (blastoconidia), pseudohyphae, and true hyphae (Fig. 11.43A). Pseudohyphae are an important diagnostic clue; these are budding yeast cells joined end to end at constrictions that simulate the appearance of true fungal hyphae. The organisms may be visible with routine H&E stains, but a variety of special "fungal" stains (Gomori methenamine-silver, periodic acid—Schiff) are used to better highlight the pathogens. *Candida* pneumonia is marked by the presence of invasion of tissues by yeast and pseudohyphae and the presence of a predominant neutrophilic inflammatory response.

Clinical Features. Candidiasis may involve the mucous membranes, skin, and deep organs (invasive candidiasis). Among these varied presentations, the following merit brief mention:

- *Superficial infection of the oral cavity (thrush).* This is the most common presentation. Proliferation of the fungi on the mucosal surface creates gray-white, dirty-looking pseudomembranes composed of matted organisms, inflammatory cells, and tissue debris. Deep to the surface, there are mucosal hyperemia and inflammation. Thrush is seen in newborns, debilitated patients, children receiving oral corticosteroids for asthma, and patients receiving courses of broad-spectrum antibiotics that destroy normal bacterial flora. The other major risk group includes patients who are HIV positive; thus, patients with oral thrush not associated with an obvious underlying condition should be evaluated for HIV infection.
- *Vaginitis* is extremely common in women, especially those who are diabetic, pregnant, or on oral contraceptive pills.
- *Esophagitis* is common in patients with AIDS and in those with hematolymphoid malignancies. These patients present with dysphagia (painful swallowing) and retrosternal pain; endoscopy demonstrates white plaques and pseudomembranes resembling those found on other mucosal surfaces.
- *Skin infection* may manifest in many different forms, including infection of the nail (*onychomycosis*); nail folds (*paronychia*); hair follicles (*folliculitis*); moist, intertriginous skin such as armpits or webs of the fingers and toes (*intertrigo*); and penile skin (*balanitis*). *Diaper rash* is a cutaneous candidal infection seen in the perineum in the region of contact with wet diapers.
- *Chronic mucocutaneous candidiasis* is characterized by persistent infection of the mucous membranes, skin, hair, and nails. It is associated with a variety of underlying T-cell defects. These include *Job syndrome*, an inherited condition associated with a defect in Th17 T-cell responses, which are important in controlling fungal infections in particular by recruiting neutrophils (Chapter 5).
- *Invasive candidiasis* is defined by bloodborne dissemination of organisms to various tissues or organs. Common patterns include (1) renal abscess; (2) myocardial abscess and endocarditis; (3) brain involvement (e.g., meningitis, parenchymal microabscesses); (4) endophthalmitis (virtually any eye structure can be involved); (5) hepatic abscesses; and (6) *Candida* pneumonia, usually presenting with bilateral nodular infiltrates resembling *Pneumocystis* pneumonia radiologically (see earlier). The major risk factors for invasive disease are neutropenia, recent treatment with chemotherapy (which damages the gut), and the presence of central venous catheters. An increasing proportion of invasive candidiasis is caused by species other than *C. albicans*, which are often resistant to antifungal agents. Patients with acute leukemias who are profoundly neutropenic after chemotherapy are particularly prone to the development of systemic disease. *Candida* endocarditis is the most common fungal endocarditis, usually occurring in patients with prosthetic heart valves or in intravenous drug users.

Cryptococcosis

Cryptococcosis is caused by *C. neoformans* or, in Australia and the Pacific Northwest of the United States and Canada, by *C. gattii*. *C. neoformans*—related disease almost exclusively manifests in hosts who are immunocompromised, particularly patients with AIDS or hematolymphoid malignancies. By contrast, *C. gattii* is able to cause disease in individuals who are not significantly immuncompromised.

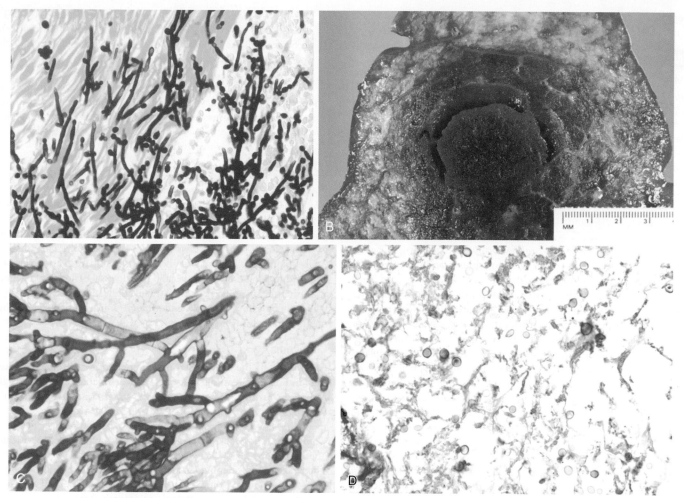

FIG. 11.43 The morphology of fungal infections. (A) *Candida* organism has pseudohyphae and budding yeasts (silver stain). (B) Invasive aspergillosis (gross appearance) of the lung in a patient who received a hematopoietic stem cell transplant. (C) Gomori methenamine-silver (GMS) stain shows septate hyphae with acute-angle branching, consistent with *Aspergillus*. (D) Cryptococcosis of the lung in a patient with AIDS. The organisms are somewhat variable in size. (B, Courtesy of Dr. Dominick Cavuoti, Department of Pathology, University of Texas Southwestern Medical School, Dallas, Texas.)

MORPHOLOGY

The fungus, a 5- to 10-μm yeast, has a thick, gelatinous capsule and reproduces by budding (see Fig. 11.43D). Sites of involvement are marked by a variable tissue response, which ranges from large collections of gelatinous organisms with a minimal or absent inflammatory cell infiltrate (so-called **cryptococcomas**) to a granulomatous reaction (in less immunocompromised hosts). In the central nervous system these fungi grow in gelatinous masses within the meninges or expand the perivascular Virchow-Robin spaces, producing so-called "**soap-bubble lesions**" (Chapter 21). Identification of the capsule is a key diagnostic clue. In routine H&E stains, the capsule is not directly visible but often a clear "halo" representing the area occupied by the capsule can be seen surrounding the individual fungi. Periodic acid–Schiff staining effectively highlights the fungal capsule.

Clinical Features. Cryptococcus is most likely to be acquired by inhalation of aerosolized contaminated soil or bird droppings. The fungus initially localizes in the lungs and then disseminates to other sites, particularly the meninges. Cryptococcosis usually manifests as pulmonary, central nervous system, or disseminated disease. Cough and dyspnea are the most common pulmonary symptoms. Common CNS symptoms include headache and neck stiffness that may evolve to a variety of focal or global neurologic deficits. *C. gattii* appears to be more likely than *C. neoformans* to cause large cryptococcal masses, even in immunocompetent individuals, that may mimic the appearance of a neoplasm. The diagnosis is made by visualization of the organism in tissue or CSF samples or through the cryptococcal antigen latex agglutination assay, which is positive in serum or CSF in more than 95% of patients infected with the organism. This test detects cryptococcal polysaccharide antigen by agglutination of latex beads coated with antibodies to the antigen. The prognosis is excellent in those with disease confined to the lung but more guarded in those with CNS disease.

Opportunistic Molds

Mucormycosis and aspergillosis are uncommon infections that are almost always limited to patients who are immunocompromised. They are particularly common in the setting of hematolymphoid malignancy and profound neutropenia, high-dose immunosuppressive therapy, recent hematopoietic stem cell transplantation, or, in the case of mucormycosis, poorly controlled diabetes.

Clinical Features. In *rhinocerebral mucormycosis,* zygomycetes have a propensity to colonize the nasal cavity or sinuses and then spread by direct extension into the brain, orbit, and other head and neck structures. Patients with diabetic ketoacidosis are most likely to develop a fulminant invasive form of rhinocerebral mucormycosis. Pulmonary mucormycosis may be localized (e.g., cavitary lesions) or may manifest radiologically with diffuse "miliary" involvement.

Aspergillus infection may take several forms. *Invasive aspergillosis* preferentially localizes to the lungs, and infection most often manifests as a necrotizing pneumonia (Fig. 11.43B). Systemic dissemination, especially to the brain, is a complication that is often fatal. *Allergic bronchopulmonary aspergillosis* occurs in patients with asthma who develop an exacerbation of symptoms caused by a type I hypersensitivity reaction against the fungus growing in the bronchi. Such patients often have circulating IgE antibodies against *Aspergillus* and peripheral eosinophilia. *Aspergilloma* ("fungus ball") formation occurs by fungal colonization of preexisting pulmonary cavities (e.g., dilated bronchi or lung cysts, posttuberculosis cavitary lesions). These masses may act as ball valves to occlude the cavity, thereby predisposing the patient to infection and hemoptysis.

Pulmonary Disease in Human Immunodeficiency Virus Infection

Pulmonary disease is a leading contributor to morbidity and mortality in individuals who are HIV positive. Although the use of antiretroviral agents and chemoprophylaxis has markedly decreased the incidence of opportunistic infections, the plethora of entities that may present with pulmonary findings in patients who are HIV positive makes diagnosis and treatment a challenge. The following considerations may be helpful when considering such patients.

- In addition to opportunistic infections, patients who are HIV positive are at increased risk for bacterial pneumonias and TB. The implicated bacteria include *S. pneumoniae, S. aureus, H. influenzae,* and gram-negative rods. Bacterial pneumonias in individuals who are infected with HIV are more common, more severe, and more often associated with bacteremia than in those without HIV infection.
- Not all pulmonary infiltrates in individuals who are HIV positive are infectious. A host of noninfectious diseases, including Kaposi sarcoma (Chapters 5 and 8), non-Hodgkin lymphoma (Chapter 10), and lung cancer occur with increased frequency and must be excluded.
- The CD4+ T cell count is useful in narrowing the differential diagnosis. As a rule of thumb, bacterial and tubercular infections occur with normal or mildly suppressed CD4+ counts (more than 200

cells/μL); *Pneumocystis* pneumonia usually occurs at CD4+ T cell counts below 200 cells/μL, while CMV and *M. avium* complex infections are uncommon until the very late stages of the disease (CD4+ T cell counts below 50 cells/μL).

Finally, one must remember that pulmonary disease in individuals who are HIV positive may result from more than one cause and that even common pathogens may be responsible for disease with atypical manifestations.

LUNG TUMORS

Roughly 95% of primary lung tumors are carcinomas; the remaining 5% span a miscellaneous group that includes carcinoid, mesenchymal malignancies (e.g., fibrosarcoma, leiomyosarcoma), lymphomas, and a few benign lesions. The most common benign tumor is "hamartoma," which shows up as a small (1 to 4 cm), discrete "coin lesion" on chest imaging. It consists mainly of mature cartilage admixed with fat, fibrous tissue, and blood vessels. Clonal cytogenetic abnormalities have been demonstrated, indicating this is actually a benign neoplasm; the name *hamartoma* (which implies a developmental anomaly) is a misnomer.

Carcinoma

Carcinoma of the lung is strongly associated with tobacco smoking and is the leading cause of cancer-related death in high-resource countries. It has long held this position among males in the United States, accounting for about one-third of cancer deaths in men, and since 1987 has been the leading cause of cancer deaths in women as well. American Cancer Society estimates for 2022 include approximately 237,000 new cases of lung cancer and 130,000 deaths. The peak incidence of lung cancer is in individuals in their fifties and sixties. At diagnosis, more than 50% of patients already have distant metastases, while an additional one-fourth have disease in the regional lymph nodes. The overall prognosis remains very poor: the 5-year survival rate for all stages of lung cancer combined is about 20%, and even when disease is localized to the lung at diagnosis, the 5-year survival rate is only 50%. On a hopeful note, targeted therapeutics and immune checkpoint inhibitors have improved survival in a subset of tumors.

The four major histologic types of lung carcinoma are adenocarcinoma, squamous cell carcinoma, small cell carcinoma (a subtype of neuroendocrine carcinoma), and large cell carcinoma (Table 11.5). In some cases, there is a combination of histologic patterns (e.g., small cell carcinoma and adenocarcinoma). Squamous cell and small cell carcinoma have the strongest association with smoking, but there is also an association with adenocarcinoma. As tobacco smoking has decreased in the United States, adenocarcinoma has replaced squamous cell carcinoma as the most common primary lung tumor in recent years. Adenocarcinoma is also by far the most common primary lung tumor arising in women, in never-smokers, and in individuals younger than 45 years of age.

Until recently, lung carcinoma was classified into two broad groups: small cell lung cancer (SCLC) and nonsmall cell lung cancer (NSCLC), the latter including adenocarcinoma, squamous cell carcinoma, and large cell carcinoma. The reason for this historic division is that relative to SCLC, NSCLCs are more likely to be resectable and as a group respond poorly to conventional chemotherapy. In recent years, however, effective therapies that target specific oncoproteins that are found in a subset of NSCLC have emerged and immunotherapy approaches (checkpoint blockade, discussed in Chapter 6) are now

Table 11.5 Histologic Classification of Malignant Epithelial Lung Tumors (2021 WHO Classification, Simplified Version)

Adenocarcinoma
　Acinar, papillary, micropapillary, solid, lepidic predominant, mucinous subtypes
Squamous cell carcinoma
Large cell carcinoma
Neuroendocrine carcinoma
　Small cell carcinoma
　Carcinoid tumor
Mixed carcinomas
　Adenosquamous carcinoma
　Small cell carcinoma and other types
Other unusual morphologic variants
　Sarcomatoid carcinoma
　　Spindle cell carcinoma
　　Giant cell carcinoma

approved for a subset of NSCLC, providing another treatment option. In part because of these clinical advances, the older classification of lung carcinoma was replaced in 2015 by a World Health Organization classification, a simplified version of which is shown in Table 11.5.

Pathogenesis. **Like other cancers, smoking-related carcinomas of the lung arise by a stepwise accumulation of driver mutations that produce neoplastic cells possessing the hallmarks of cancer.** The occurrence of molecular changes is not random but tends to follow an order that parallels the histologic progression toward cancer. Thus, inactivation of one or more putative tumor suppressor genes located on the short arm of chromosome 3 (3p) is a very common early event, whereas mutations in the *TP53* tumor suppressor gene and the *KRAS* oncogene occur relatively late. Certain genetic changes, such as loss of chromosomal material on 3p, are found even in benign bronchial epithelium of people who smoke but do not have lung cancer, suggesting that large areas of the respiratory mucosa are mutagenized by exposure to carcinogens ("field effect"). On this fertile soil, cells that accumulate additional mutations ultimately develop into cancer.

A subset of adenocarcinomas, particularly those arising in nonsmoking women, harbor mutations that activate the epidermal growth factor receptor (EGFR), a receptor tyrosine kinase that stimulates downstream progrowth pathways involving RAS, PI3K, and other signaling molecules. The frequency of this mutation varies in different populations. Of note, these tumors are sensitive to drugs that inhibit EGFR signaling, although the response is often short lived. *EGFR* and *KRAS* mutations (in 30% of adenocarcinomas) are mutually exclusive, as might be expected since KRAS lies downstream of EGFR. Other "targetable" mutations have been described at a low frequency in adenocarcinomas (4% to 6% overall), including mutations that activate other tyrosine kinases, such as ALK, ROS1, HER2, and MET. Recently, drugs have been developed that target a subset of mutated forms of KRAS. Each of these mutated proteins is optimally targeted by a different drug, which has spurred a new era of "personalized" lung cancer treatment, in which the genetics of the tumor guide therapy.

With regard to carcinogenic influences, **there is strong evidence that cigarette smoking and, to a much lesser extent, other environmental carcinogens are the main culprits responsible for the mutations that give rise to lung cancers.** About 90% of lung cancers

occur in individuals who are currently smoking or who have stopped recently. Moreover, there is a nearly linear correlation between the frequency of lung cancer and pack-years of cigarette smoking. The increased risk is 60 times greater among individuals who smoke heavily (two packs a day for 20 years) than among nonsmokers. For unclear reasons, women are more susceptible to carcinogens in tobacco smoke than men. Although cessation of smoking decreases the risk for developing lung cancer over time, it never returns to baseline levels, and genetic changes that predate the full development of lung cancer can persist for many years in the bronchial epithelium of people who formerly smoked. Passive smoking (proximity to people who are smoking cigarettes) also increases the risk for developing lung cancer, as does smoking of pipes and cigars, albeit only modestly.

Other carcinogenic influences associated with occupational exposures act in concert with smoking and may sometimes be solely responsible for lung cancer; examples include work in uranium mines, work with asbestos, and inhalation of dusts containing arsenic, chromium, nickel, or vinyl chloride. A cardinal example of a synergistic interaction between two carcinogens is found in asbestos and tobacco smoking: exposure to asbestos in nonsmokers increases the risk for developing lung cancer 5-fold, whereas in individuals who smoke heavily who are exposed to asbestos the risk is elevated approximately 55-fold.

Even though smoking and other environmental influences are paramount in the causation of lung cancer, not all individuals exposed to tobacco smoke develop cancer (about 11% of individuals who smoke heavily do). It is very likely that the mutagenic effect of carcinogens is modified by genetic factors. Recall that many chemicals require metabolic activation via the P-450 monooxygenase enzyme system for conversion into ultimate carcinogens (Chapter 6). Individuals with certain polymorphisms involving the P-450 genes have an increased capacity to activate procarcinogens found in cigarette smoke and are thus exposed to larger doses of carcinogens and incur a greater risk of developing lung cancer. Similarly, individuals whose peripheral blood lymphocytes undergo chromosomal breakages after exposure to tobacco-related carcinogens (mutagen sensitive genotype) have a greater than 10-fold increased risk for developing lung cancer over control subjects.

By analogy to the adenoma—carcinoma sequence in the colon (Chapter 13), it is proposed that some invasive adenocarcinomas of the lung arise through an atypical adenomatous hyperplasia—adenocarcinoma in situ—invasive adenocarcinoma sequence. Studies of lung injury models in mice have identified a population of multipotent cells in the lung periphery at the bronchioloalveolar duct junction, termed *bronchioalveolar stem cells (BASCs)*. After lung injury, multipotent BASCs proliferate and replenish the normal cell types (bronchiolar Clara cells and alveolar cells) found in this location, thereby facilitating epithelial regeneration. It is postulated that BASCs incur the first mutation that initiates the changes that eventuate in full-blown malignancy.

The sequential morphologic changes leading to development of squamous cell carcinomas are well documented; there is a linear correlation between the intensity of exposure to cigarette smoke and the appearance of ever more worrisome epithelial changes that begin with rather innocuous basal cell hyperplasia and squamous metaplasia and progress to squamous dysplasia and carcinoma in situ, before culminating in invasive cancer. Squamous cell carcinomas tend to occur in the central parts of the lung and likely originate from basal squamous cells with stem cell-like properties.

By contrast, precursor lesions for small cell carcinoma have not been clearly described. These tumors are also distinct from other forms of lung carcinoma in virtually always having loss of function mutations in both *TP53* and *RB,* the two most important tumor suppressor genes (Chapter 6). Small cell carcinoma is marked by high growth rates and early development of widespread metastases. Some of the salient pathologic and clinical differences between small cell carcinoma and common forms of nonsmall cell carcinoma are summarized in Table 11.6.

MORPHOLOGY

Carcinomas of the lung begin as small lesions that are typically firm and gray-white. They may arise as intraluminal masses, invade the bronchial mucosa, or form large bulky masses pushing into adjacent lung parenchyma. **Adenocarcinoma** is usually **peripherally located** (Fig. 11.44A) but may also occur closer to the hilum. In general, adenocarcinoma grows more slowly and forms smaller masses than do the other subtypes but also tends to metastasize widely at an early stage. It may assume a variety of growth patterns, including **acinar (gland-forming)** (Fig. 11.44B); **papillary; mucinous** (which is often multifocal and may manifest as pneumonia-like consolidation); and **solid** types. Immunohistochemical stains for markers such as TTF-1, a transcription factor that is relatively specific for lung adenocarcinoma, may be helpful in establishing the diagnosis (Fig. 11.44B).

The putative precursor of adenocarcinoma is **atypical adenomatous hyperplasia** (eFig. 11.5A), which is thought to progress in a stepwise fashion to adenocarcinoma in situ, minimally invasive adenocarcinoma, and invasive adenocarcinoma. Atypical adenomatous hyperplasia appears as a well-demarcated focus of epithelial proliferation (with a diameter of 5 mm or less) composed of cuboidal to low-columnar cells that demonstrate nuclear hyperchromasia, pleomorphism, and prominent nucleoli. Genetic analyses have shown that atypical adenomatous hyperplasia is monoclonal and shares many molecular aberrations with adenocarcinomas (e.g., *KRAS* mutations).

Adenocarcinoma in situ (AIS) (previously called bronchioloalveolar carcinoma) often presents as a single nodule in peripheral parts of the lung. The key features of adenocarcinoma in situ are diameter of 3 cm or less, growth along preexisting structures, and preservation of alveolar architecture (eFig. 11.5B). The tumor cells, which may be nonmucinous, mucinous, or mixed, grow in a monolayer along the alveolar septa (referred to as lepidic spread) which serve as a scaffold. By definition, adenocarcinoma in situ does not demonstrate destruction of alveolar architecture or stromal invasion with desmoplasia, features that would merit the diagnosis of invasive adenocarcinoma.

Squamous cell carcinoma is more common in men than in women and is closely correlated with a smoking history; it tends to **arise centrally in major bronchi** (Fig. 11.44D) and to spread first to local hilar nodes. On average, dissemination outside the thorax occurs later than with other histologic types. Large lesions may undergo central necrosis, giving rise to **cavitation.** Squamous cell carcinoma is often preceded by the development of **bronchial squamous metaplasia or dysplasia,** which then transforms to **carcinoma in situ,** over a period of several years (eFig. 11.6). At this time, atypical cells may be identified in cytologic smears of sputum or in bronchial lavage fluids or brushings, although the lesion is asymptomatic and undetectable on radiographs. Eventually, the small neoplasm reaches a symptomatic stage, when a well-defined tumor mass begins to obstruct the lumen of a major bronchus, often producing distal atelectasis and infection. Simultaneously, the lesion invades the surrounding lung. On histologic examination, these tumors range from well-differentiated neoplasms with keratin pearls (Fig. 11.44C) and intercellular bridges to poorly differentiated neoplasms exhibiting only minimal squamous cell features.

Large cell carcinoma is an undifferentiated epithelial tumor that lacks the cytologic features of neuroendocrine carcinoma and shows no evidence of glandular or squamous differentiation (Fig. 11.44E). It is a diagnosis of exclusion and accounts for only about 10% of cases. The tumor cells typically have large nuclei, prominent nucleoli, and moderate amounts of cytoplasm.

Small cell carcinoma generally appears as a pale gray, **centrally located mass** that extends into the lung parenchyma. The tumor cells are relatively small and round to fusiform in shape and have scant cytoplasm and finely granular chromatin with a salt-and-pepper appearance (Fig. 11.44F). Numerous mitotic figures are present, as is necrosis, which may be extensive. The tumor cells are fragile and often show fragmentation and "crush artifact" in small biopsy specimens, releasing DNA that stains blue (Azzapardi effect, see Fig. 11.44F). These tumors express a variety of neuroendocrine markers and may secrete polypeptide hormones that may result in paraneoplastic syndromes (see later). By the time of diagnosis, most have metastasized to hilar and mediastinal lymph nodes. In the 2021 WHO Classification, small cell lung carcinoma is grouped together with large cell neuroendocrine carcinoma, another very aggressive tumor that exhibits neuroendocrine morphology and expresses neuroendocrine markers (synaptophysin, chromogranin, and CD56).

Mixed patterns (e.g., adenosquamous carcinoma, mixed adenocarcinoma and small cell carcinoma) are seen in 10% or less of lung carcinomas.

All lung cancer subtypes tend to spread to lymph nodes in the carina, the mediastinum, and the neck (scalene nodes) and clavicular regions, and, sooner or later, to distant sites. Involvement of the left supraclavicular node (Virchow node) is particularly characteristic and sometimes calls attention to an occult primary tumor. These cancers, when advanced, often extend into the pleural or pericardial space, leading to inflammation and effusions. They may compress or infiltrate the superior vena cava to cause superior vena cava syndrome. Apical neoplasms may invade the brachial or cervical sympathetic plexus, causing severe pain in the distribution of the ulnar nerve or Horner syndrome (ipsilateral enophthalmos, ptosis, miosis, and anhidrosis). Such neoplasms are sometimes called **Pancoast tumors,** and the combination of clinical findings is known as **Pancoast syndrome.** Pancoast tumor is often accompanied by destruction of the first and second ribs and sometimes the thoracic vertebrae. As with other carcinomas, tumor-node-metastasis (TNM) staging is used to indicate the size and spread of the primary neoplasm.

Clinical Features. Carcinomas of the lung are insidious lesions that in many cases are unresectable at the time of diagnosis. In some patients, chronic cough and expectoration call attention to localized disease that may be cured surgically. By the time other symptoms, such as hoarseness, chest pain, superior vena cava syndrome, pericardial or pleural effusion, or persistent atelectasis or pneumonitis, appear, the prognosis is poor. Too often, the tumor presents with symptoms caused by metastatic spread to distant sites such as the brain (neurologic changes), liver (hepatomegaly), or bones (pain). Although the adrenal glands may be nearly obliterated by metastatic disease, adrenal insufficiency (Addison disease) is uncommon, because islands of cortical cells sufficient to maintain adrenal function usually persist.

Overall, squamous cell carcinoma and adenocarcinoma carry a more favorable prognosis than small cell carcinoma. When squamous cell carcinoma or adenocarcinoma is detected before metastasis or local spread (as in high-risk patients undergoing surveillance imaging), cure is possible by lobectomy or pneumonectomy. Unresectable adenocarcinomas with targetable mutations in tyrosine kinases such as EGFR may show remarkable responses to specific inhibitors. A few of these patients have long-term remissions lasting for years, but relapse within months to a year is typical. Resistant tumors are found to have new mutations that either alter the drug target themselves (e.g., an additional mutation in *EGFR* that prevents drug binding) or circumvent tumor dependence on the drug target. Immune checkpoint inhibitors improve outcomes in nonsmall cell carcinomas, and are

Table 11.6 Comparison of Small Cell Lung Carcinoma and Nonsmall Cell Lung Carcinoma (Adenocarcinoma and Squamous Cell Carcinoma)

Feature	Small Cell Lung Carcinoma	Nonsmall Cell Lung Carcinoma
Morphology		
Microscopic appearance	Scant cytoplasm; small, hyperchromatic nuclei with fine chromatin pattern; indistinct nucleoli; diffuse sheets of cells	Abundant cytoplasm; pleomorphic nuclei with coarse chromatin pattern; prominent nucleoli; glandular or squamous architecture
Neuroendocrine Markers		
Dense core granules on electron microscopy; expression of chromogranin, synaptophysin, and CD56	Present	Absent
Epithelial Markers		
Epithelial membrane antigen, carcinoembryonic antigen, and cytokeratin intermediate filaments	Present	Present
Mucin	Absent	Present in adenocarcinomas
Peptide hormone production	Adrenocorticotropic hormone, anti-diuretic hormone, gastrin-releasing peptide, calcitonin	Parathyroid hormone—related peptide (PTH-rp) in squamous cell carcinoma
Tumor Suppressor Gene Abnormalities		
3p deletions	>90%	>80%
RB mutations	~90%	~20%
p16/CDKN2A mutations	~10%	>50%
TP53 mutations	>90%	>50%
Dominant Oncogene Abnormalities		
KRAS mutations	Rare	~30% (adenocarcinomas)
EGFR mutations	Absent	~20% (adenocarcinomas, nonsmokers, women)
ALK rearrangements	Absent	4%—6% adenocarcinomas, nonsmokers, often have signet ring morphology
Response to Therapy		
Response to chemotherapy and radiotherapy	Often complete response but invariably recur	Incomplete
Response to checkpoint inhibitor therapy	Unresponsive	Responsive

particularly effective when combined with chemotherapy, a new therapeutic approach.

By contrast, the prognosis and treatment of small cell carcinoma have changed little. Small cell carcinoma has invariably spread by the time it is detected, even when the primary tumor is small and appears to be localized. Thus, surgical resection is not curative. Small cell carcinoma is very sensitive to radiotherapy and chemotherapy but invariably recurs, and as of yet targeted therapies are unavailable. The median survival with treatment is only 1 year and only 5% of patients are alive at 10 years. Despite a very high mutation burden, these tumors are less responsive to immune checkpoint inhibitors than nonsmall cell lung cancers. Work is ongoing to understand and overcome resistance to immunotherapy.

In addition to the direct effects of the tumor cells, it is estimated that 3% to 10% of patients with lung cancer develop a *paraneoplastic syndrome* (Chapter 6). The manifestations include (1) hypercalcemia caused by secretion of a parathyroid hormone—related peptide; (2) Cushing syndrome (from increased production of adrenocorticotropic hormone); (3) syndrome of inappropriate secretion of antidiuretic hormone; (4) neuromuscular syndromes, including a myasthenic syndrome, peripheral neuropathy, and polymyositis; (5) clubbing of the fingers and hypertrophic pulmonary osteoarthropathy; and (6) coagulation abnormalities, including migratory thrombophlebitis,

nonbacterial endocarditis, and disseminated intravascular coagulation. Hypercalcemia is most often encountered with squamous cell carcinoma, the hematologic syndromes with adenocarcinoma, and the neurologic syndromes with small cell carcinoma, but exceptions abound.

Carcinoid Tumors

Carcinoid tumors are malignant tumors composed of cells that contain dense-core neurosecretory granules in their cytoplasm and occasionally secrete hormonally active polypeptides. They are best thought of a low-grade neuroendocrine carcinoma and are subclassified as typical or atypical; both are often resectable and curable. They may occur as part of the multiple endocrine neoplasia syndrome (Chapter 18). Bronchial carcinoids tend to occur in younger adults (mean 40 years) and represent about 5% of all pulmonary neoplasms.

> ## MORPHOLOGY
>
> Most carcinoids originate in main bronchi and grow in one of two patterns: (1) as a polypoid, spherical intraluminal mass (Fig. 11.45A); or (2) as a mucosal plaque penetrating the bronchial wall to fan out in the peribronchial tissue—the so-called **collar-button lesion.** Even penetrating lesions push into the lung substance along a broad front and are well demarcated.

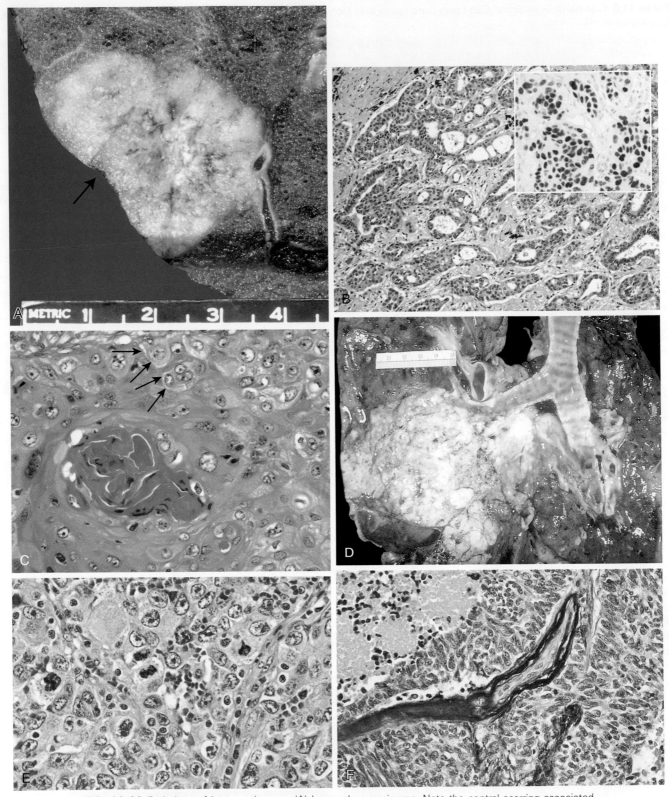

FIG. 11.44 Pathology of lung carcinomas. (A) Lung adenocarcinoma. Note the central scarring associated with anthracotic pigments and pleural puckering *(arrow)*. (B) Gland-forming adenocarcinoma; inset shows staining for thyroid transcription factor 1 (TTF-1), which is characteristic. (C) Well-differentiated squamous cell carcinoma, showing keratinization, pearls, and intercellular bridges *(arrows)*. (D) Squamous cell carcinoma appearing as a central (hilar) mass that is invading contiguous parenchyma. (E) Large cell carcinoma, consisting of sheets of large cells without gland formation or squamous differentiation. (F) Small cell carcinoma with small deeply basophilic cells and areas of necrosis *(top left)*. Note basophilic staining of vascular walls due to encrustation by DNA from necrotic tumor cells (Azzopardi effect). (A, From Diagnostic Pathology: Familial Cancer Syndromes and ExpertPath. Copyright Elsevier 2022.)

Peripheral carcinoids are less common. Although 5% to 15% of carcinoids have metastasized to the hilar nodes at presentation, distant metastases are rare. Histologically, **typical carcinoids,** like their counterparts in the intestinal tract, are composed of nests of uniform cells with regular round nuclei and "salt-and-pepper" chromatin, absent or rare mitoses, and little pleomorphism (Fig. 11.45B). **Atypical carcinoid** tumors display a higher mitotic rate and small foci of necrosis. These tumors have a higher incidence of lymph node and distant metastasis than typical carcinoids. Unlike typical carcinoids, the atypical tumors have *TP53* mutations in 20% to 40% of cases. Typical carcinoid, atypical carcinoid, and large cell neuroendocrine and small cell carcinoma can be viewed as a continuum of increasing histologic aggressiveness and malignant potential within the spectrum of pulmonary neuroendocrine neoplasms.

Clinical Features. Most carcinoid tumors manifest with signs and symptoms related to their intraluminal growth, including cough, hemoptysis, and recurrent bronchial and pulmonary infections. Peripheral tumors are often asymptomatic and are discovered incidentally on chest radiographs. Only rarely do pulmonary carcinoids induce the *carcinoid syndrome,* characterized by intermittent attacks of diarrhea, flushing, and cyanosis. The reported 5- and 10-year survival rates for typical carcinoids are above 85%, while these rates drop to 56% and 35%, respectively, for atypical carcinoids.

PLEURAL LESIONS

Disease of the pleura is usually a complication of underlying pulmonary disease. Secondary infections and pleural adhesions are common findings at autopsy. Important primary disorders are (1) intrapleural bacterial infections and (2) *malignant mesothelioma,* a neoplasm of the pleura.

Pleural Effusion and Pleuritis

Pleural effusions (fluids in the pleural space) may be either transudates or exudates. When the effusion is a transudate, the condition is termed *hydrothorax.* Congestive heart failure (either right-sided or left-sided) is the most common cause of bilateral hydrothorax. An exudate, characterized by protein content greater than 30 g/L and, often, inflammatory cells, suggests pleuritis. The four principal causes of

pleural exudate formation are (1) bacterial infection (*suppurative pleuritis* or *empyema*), either through direct extension of a pulmonary infection or bloodborne seeding; (2) cancer (lung carcinoma, metastatic neoplasms to the lung or pleural surface, mesothelioma); (3) pulmonary infarction; and (4) viral pleuritis. Other less common causes of pleural exudative effusions are systemic lupus erythematosus, rheumatoid arthritis, and uremia, as well as previous thoracic surgery. Malignant effusions are characteristically large and frequently bloody (*hemorrhagic pleuritis).* Cytologic examination may reveal the malignant cells.

Whatever the cause, transudates and serous exudates are usually resorbed without residual effects if the inciting cause is controlled or remits. By contrast, fibrinous, hemorrhagic and suppurative exudates may lead to fibrous organization, yielding adhesions or fibrous pleural thickenings that sometimes undergo calcification.

Pneumothorax, Hemothorax, and Chylothorax

Pneumothorax refers to the presence of air or other gas in the pleural sac. It may occur in young, apparently healthy adults, usually men without any known pulmonary disease (primary or spontaneous pneumothorax), or as a result of some thoracic or lung disorder (secondary pneumothorax). Secondary pneumothorax occurs when a pulmonary lesion situated close to the pleural surface ruptures, allowing inspired air to gain access to the pleural cavity. Responsible pulmonary lesions include emphysema, lung abscess, tuberculosis, carcinoma, and many other, less common processes. Mechanical ventilatory support with high pressure may also trigger secondary pneumothorax.

There are several possible complications of pneumothorax. Some air leaks only permit air to move into the pleural cavity, leading to an increase in intrapleural pressure (*tension pneumothorax*) that shifts the mediastinum (eFig. 11.7). Compromise of the pulmonary circulation may follow and may even be fatal. If the leak seals and the lung is not reexpanded within a few weeks (either spontaneously or through medical or surgical intervention), scarring may occur that prevents the lung from ever fully reexpanding. In these cases, serous fluid collects in the pleural cavity, creating *hydropneumothorax.* With prolonged collapse, the lung becomes vulnerable to infection, as does the pleural cavity when communication between it and the lung persists. Empyema is thus an important complication of pneumothorax (*pyopneumothorax).*

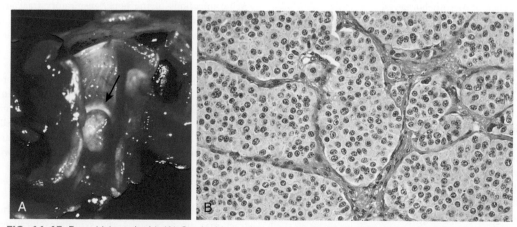

FIG. 11.45 Bronchial carcinoid. (A) Carcinoid growing as a spherical, pale mass *(arrow)* protruding into the lumen of the bronchus. (B) Histologic appearance demonstrating small, rounded, uniform nuclei and moderate cytoplasm. (Courtesy of Dr. Thomas Krausz, Department of Pathology, University of Chicago Pritzker School of Medicine, Chicago, Illinois.)

Hemothorax, the collection of whole blood (in contrast with bloody effusion) in the pleural cavity, may be a complication of a ruptured intrathoracic aortic aneurysm, an event that is almost always fatal. In contrast to bloody pleural effusions, with hemothorax, the blood clots within the pleural cavity.

Chylothorax is a pleural collection of milky lymphatic fluid containing microglobules of lipid. The total volume of fluid may not be large, but chylothorax is always significant because it implies obstruction of the major lymph ducts, usually by an intrathoracic cancer (e.g., a primary or secondary mediastinal neoplasm, such as a lymphoma).

Malignant Mesothelioma

Despite its rarity, malignant mesothelioma has assumed great importance because it is highly related to exposure to airborne asbestos. It is a cancer of mesothelial cells, usually arising in the parietal or visceral pleura; it also occurs much less commonly in the peritoneum and pericardium. Approximately 80% to 90% of individuals with this cancer have a history of exposure to asbestos. Those who work directly with asbestos (e.g., shipyard workers, miners, insulators) are at greatest risk, but individuals whose only exposure is living in proximity to an asbestos factory or living with an asbestos worker are also at increased risk (due to particle contamination of the worker's clothing). The latency period for development of malignant mesothelioma after exposure to asbestos is long, often 25 to 40 years, suggesting that causative driver mutations are acquired slowly over an extended period of time. As stated earlier, the combination of cigarette smoking and asbestos exposure greatly increases the risk for developing lung carcinoma, but it does not increase the risk for developing malignant mesothelioma, one of the many puzzles in cancer biology.

Once inhaled, asbestos fibers remain in the body for life. Thus, the lifetime risk after exposure does not diminish over time (unlike with smoking, in which the risk decreases after cessation). It has been hypothesized that asbestos fibers preferentially gather near the mesothelial cell layer, where they generate reactive oxygen species that cause DNA damage and mutations. Sequencing of mesothelioma genomes has revealed multiple driver mutations, many of which cluster in pathways involved in DNA repair, cell cycle control, and growth factor signaling. Of interest, one of the most commonly mutated genes in sporadic mesothelioma, *BAP1*, encodes a tumor suppressor involved in DNA repair that is also the target of germline mutations in families showing a high incidence of mesothelioma.

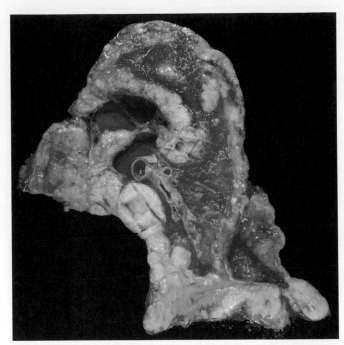

FIG. 11.46 Malignant mesothelioma. Note the thick, firm, white pleural tumor encasing the bisected lung.

Clinical Features. Malignant mesothelioma remains a nearly uniformly fatal disease. Most patients present with gradually worsening nonspecific pulmonary symptoms such as cough and dyspnea. As the disease advances, the tumor may impinge on local structures, leading to superior vena cava syndrome or heart failure. Imaging reveals thickening of the pleura and often pleural effusion, sometimes accompanied by a shift of the mediastinum toward the affected lung due to its underinflation. Even with extrapleural pneumonectomy and chemotherapy, most patients succumb due to respiratory failure or invasion of heart and pericardium in 12 to 18 months.

LESIONS OF THE UPPER RESPIRATORY TRACT

Acute Infections

Acute infections of the upper respiratory tract are among the most common afflictions of humans, most frequently manifesting as the "common cold." The clinical features are well known: nasal congestion accompanied by watery discharge; sneezing; scratchy, dry, sore throat; and a slight increase in temperature that is more pronounced in young children. The most common pathogens are rhinoviruses, but coronaviruses, respiratory syncytial viruses, parainfluenza and influenza viruses, adenoviruses, enteroviruses, and sometimes even group A β-hemolytic streptococci have been implicated. In a significant number of cases (around 40%), the organism cannot be identified. Most of these infections occur in the fall and winter and are self-limited (usually lasting for 1 week or less). In a minority of cases, colds are complicated by the development of bacterial otitis media or sinusitis.

In addition to the common cold, infections of the upper respiratory tract may produce signs and symptoms localized to the pharynx, epiglottis, or larynx. *Acute pharyngitis,* manifesting as a sore throat, may be caused by a host of agents. Mild pharyngitis with minimal physical findings frequently accompanies a cold and is the most common form of pharyngitis. More severe forms with tonsillitis, associated with marked hyperemia and exudates, occur with β-hemolytic streptococcal and adenovirus infections. Streptococcal tonsillitis is important to recognize and treat early because of the associated potential for development of peritonsillar abscesses or for progression to poststreptococcal glomerulonephritis (Chapter 12) and acute rheumatic fever (Chapter 9). Coxsackievirus A infection may produce pharyngeal vesicles and ulcers *(herpangina)*. Infectious mononucleosis, caused by Epstein-Barr virus (EBV), is an important cause of pharyngitis.

Acute bacterial epiglottitis is a syndrome predominantly affecting young children who have an infection of the epiglottis caused by *H. influenzae*, in which pain and airway obstruction are the major findings. The onset is abrupt. Failure to appreciate the need to maintain an open airway for a child with this condition can have fatal consequences. The advent of vaccination against *H. influenzae* has greatly decreased the incidence of this disease in resource-rich parts of the world.

Acute laryngitis may result from inhalation of irritants, allergic reactions, and agents that produce the common cold. Brief mention should be made of two uncommon but important forms of laryngitis: *tuberculous* and *diphtheritic*. The former is almost always a consequence of protracted active tuberculosis, during which infected sputum is coughed up. Diphtheritic laryngitis is rare in resource-rich countries because of the widespread immunization of young children against diphtheria toxin but remains a serious health problem in resource-limited parts of the world. After it is inhaled, *Corynebacterium diphtheriae* implants on the mucosa of the upper airways, where it elaborates a powerful exotoxin that causes necrosis of the mucosal epithelium, accompanied by a dense fibrinopurulent exudate, to create the classic superficial, dirty-gray pseudomembrane of diphtheria. The major hazards of this infection are sloughing and aspiration of the pseudomembrane (causing obstruction of major airways) and absorption of bacterial exotoxins (producing myocarditis, peripheral neuropathy, or other tissue injury).

In children, parainfluenza virus is the most common cause of laryngotracheobronchitis, more commonly known as *croup*, but other agents such as respiratory syncytial virus may also precipitate this condition. Although self-limited, croup may cause frightening inspiratory stridor and harsh persistent cough. In occasional cases, the laryngeal inflammatory reaction may narrow the airway sufficiently to result in respiratory failure. Another bacterial pathogen that can cause laryngotracheobronchitis is *Bordtella pertussis*, the cause of whooping cough. This agent secretes a number of toxins that induce epithelial cell death and induce a characteristic cough that can persist for weeks. Viral infections in the upper respiratory tract predispose the patient to secondary bacterial infection, particularly by staphylococci and streptococci.

Nasopharyngeal Carcinoma

Nasopharyngeal carcinoma is a rare neoplasm that merits comment because of (1) its strong epidemiologic links to EBV and (2) its high frequency in certain populations, particularly Southern China, suggesting that germline genetics have an important role in its pathogenesis. It is thought that EBV has the capacity to infect nasopharyngeal epithelium and that, in some susceptible individuals, this leads to transformation of the epithelial cells.

Nasopharyngeal carcinoma has three histologic variants: keratinizing squamous cell carcinoma, nonkeratinizing squamous cell carcinoma, and undifferentiated carcinoma; the last-mentioned is the most common and the one most closely linked with EBV (eFig. 11.8). The tumor cells contain EBV genomes and express several EBV proteins, including latent membrane protein-1 (LMP1), which generates

oncogenic signals that active the NF-κB pathway. The undifferentiated tumors are composed of large epithelial cells with indistinct cell borders ("syncytial" growth) and prominent eosinophilic nucleoli and are often heavily infiltrated by T cells, which are believed to be responding to viral antigens. Nasopharyngeal carcinomas invade locally, spread to cervical lymph nodes, and then metastasize to distant sites. They tend to be radiosensitive, and 5-year survival rates of 50% are reported, even for patients with advanced disease. Responses to immune checkpoint inhibitors also have been reported, providing a new therapeutic strategy for tumors that do not respond to conventional therapy.

Laryngeal Tumors

A variety of nonneoplastic, benign and malignant neoplasms of epithelial and mesenchymal origin may arise in the larynx, but only vocal cord nodules, papillomas, and squamous cell carcinomas are sufficiently common to merit comment. In all these conditions, the most common presenting feature is hoarseness.

Nonmalignant Lesions

Vocal cord nodules ("polyps") are smooth, hemispherical protrusions (usually <0.5 cm in diameter) that are most often located on the true vocal cords. The nodules are composed of fibrous tissue and covered by stratified squamous mucosa that is usually intact but may be ulcerated from trauma caused by contact with the other vocal cord. These lesions occur chiefly in individuals who smoke heavily or singers (singer's nodes), suggesting that they are the result of chronic irritation or overuse.

Laryngeal papilloma or *squamous papilloma* of the larynx is a benign neoplasm, usually located on the true vocal cords, that forms a soft, raspberry-like excrescence rarely more than 1 cm in diameter. Histologically, it consists of multiple slender, fingerlike projections supported by central fibrovascular cores and covered by an orderly stratified squamous epithelium. When the papilloma is on the free edge of the vocal cord, trauma may lead to ulceration that can be accompanied by hemoptysis.

Papillomas are usually single in adults but are often multiple in children, in whom the condition is referred to as *recurrent respiratory papillomatosis* due to the tendency to recur after excision. These lesions are caused by human papillomavirus (HPV) types 6 and 11 and often spontaneously regress at puberty. Cancerous transformation is rare. The most likely cause for their occurrence in children is vertical transmission from an infected mother during delivery. Therefore, the recent availability of an HPV vaccine that can protect women of reproductive age against infection with types 6 and 11 provides an opportunity for prevention of laryngeal papillomatosis in children.

Carcinoma of the Larynx

Carcinoma of the larynx represents only 2% of all cancers. It most commonly occurs after 40 years of age and is more common in men than in women (M : F ratio of 7 : 1). Environmental factors are very important in its causation: nearly all cases occur in people who smoke, and alcohol and asbestos exposure may also have roles. Human papillomavirus sequences have been detected in about 15% of tumors, which tend to have a better prognosis than other carcinomas.

About 95% of laryngeal cancers are squamous cell carcinomas. Rarely, adenocarcinomas are seen. The tumor develops directly on the vocal cords (glottic tumors) in 60% to 75% of cases or may arise above the cords (supraglottic; 25% to 40%) or below the cords (subglottic; <5%). Laryngeal squamous cell carcinoma appears as a pearly gray, wrinkled plaque that undergoes ulceration and can fungate with tumor progression (Fig. 11.47). The glottic tumors are usually

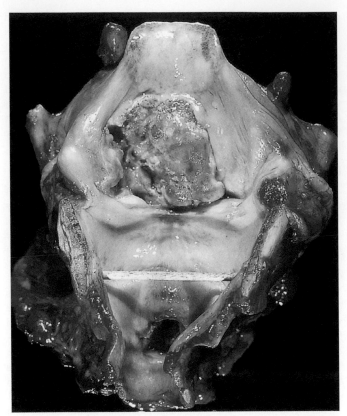

FIG. 11.47 Laryngeal squamous cell carcinoma arising in a supraglottic location (above the true vocal cord). (From Fletcher, C.D., Diagnostic Histopathology of Tumors, 5th edition, Elsevier, Philadelphia, 2021, Fig. 4B.9B.)

keratinizing, well to moderately differentiated squamous cell carcinomas. As expected with lesions arising from recurrent exposure to environmental carcinogens, adjacent mucosa may demonstrate squamous cell hyperplasia and foci of dysplasia or even carcinoma in situ.

Carcinoma of the larynx usually presents with persistent hoarseness. The location of the tumor within the larynx has a significant bearing on prognosis. About 90% of glottic tumors are confined to the larynx at diagnosis because these tumors interfere with vocal cord mobility and cause symptoms early in their course and also because the glottic region has a sparse lymphatic supply, making spread less likely. By contrast, the supraglottic larynx is rich in lymphatics and nearly one-third of supraglottic tumors metastasize to regional (cervical) lymph nodes. Subglottic tumors have the worst prognosis because they tend to produce few symptoms until they are advanced. With surgery, radiation therapy, or combination treatment, many patients can be cured, but about one-third die of the disease. The usual cause of death is widespread metastases and cachexia, sometimes complicated by pulmonary infection.

■ RAPID REVIEW

Acute Lung Injury and Acute Respiratory Distress Syndrome

- *Acute lung injury* (ALI): New onset pulmonary inflammation with alveolar/endothelial damage
- *Acute respiratory distress syndromes* (ARDS): Clinical syndrome of respiratory insufficiency caused by diffuse alveolar damage

- ARDS triggers include sepsis, severe trauma, or diffuse pulmonary infection.
- Neutrophils and their products have a central role in endothelial and epithelial injury.
- Histologic findings include alveolar edema, epithelial necrosis, neutrophil accumulation, and presence of hyaline membranes.

Chronic Obstructive Pulmonary Disease (COPD)

- Most commonly manifests as emphysema and/or chronic bronchitis, which often coexist
- Smoking is the major risk factor for COPD.
- COPD is typically progressive and may lead to worsening pulmonary function and cor pulmonale (right-sided heart failure).
- COPD is characterized by functional outflow obstruction due to loss of elastic tissue in alveolar walls; it is associated with reduced FEV_1 and normal or near normal FVC.
- *Emphysematous COPD* is characterized by enlargement of air spaces distal to terminal bronchioles that is caused by destruction of elastic support structures by proteases released from inflammatory cells, particularly neutrophils.
- Emphysema subtypes include *centriacinar* (most common: smoking-related) and *panacinar* (seen in α_1-antitrypsin deficiency).
- Emphysema is marked by increased chest volume, dyspnea, and relatively normal blood oxygenation at rest.
- *Chronic bronchitis* is defined by persistent productive cough for at least 3 consecutive months in at least 2 consecutive years.
- Mucus production in bronchitis stems from hyperplasia of tracheal and large airway mucous glands, whereas airway obstruction stems from small airway inflammation (chronic bronchiolitis).
- Histologic findings include enlargement of mucus-secreting glands, goblet cell metaplasia, inflammation, and bronchiolar wall fibrosis.
- Bronchitic patients tend to develop hypoxemia and hypercapnia.

Asthma

- Characterized by reversible bronchoconstriction caused by airway hyperresponsiveness to a variety of stimuli
- *Atopic asthma:* A Th2 and IgE-mediated immunologic reaction to environmental allergens that has an early-phase (immediate) reaction triggered by release of mast cell contents and a late-phase reaction triggered by inflammatory cells and cytokines
- Th2 cytokines (IL-4, IL-5, and IL-13) are important mediators of atopic asthma.
- *Nonatopic asthma:* Triggers include viral infections, inhaled air pollutants, exposure to cold, and even exercise.
- Eosinophils are key inflammatory cells in almost all subtypes of asthma, and eosinophil products (such as major basic protein) contribute to airway damage.
- Airway remodeling (subbasement membrane thickening and hypertrophy of bronchial glands and smooth muscle) may add an irreversible component to the airway obstruction.

Chronic Interstitial Lung Diseases

- Diffuse interstitial fibrosis gives rise to restrictive lung diseases characterized by reduced forced expiratory volume (FEV), reduced forced vital capacity (FVC), and normal FEV to FVC ratio.
- Diseases that cause diffuse interstitial fibrosis are marked by chronic alveolar injury and increased local release of fibrogenic cytokines such as TGF-β.

- *Idiopathic pulmonary fibrosis* (IPF), also called usual interstitial pneumonia, is prototypic and is characterized by patchy interstitial fibrosis, fibroblastic foci, and formation of cystic spaces (honeycomb lung).
- IPF is associated with germline mutations in telomerase and particular genetic variants in mucin and surfactant, both of which are expressed by alveolar epithelium.

Pneumoconioses

- Chronic fibrosing diseases resulting from exposure to organic and inorganic particulates
- Pathogenesis: the phagocytosis of dust particulates by pulmonary alveolar macrophages leads to inflammasome activation and release of inflammatory mediators and fibrogenic cytokines.
- *Coal dust—induced disease* varies from asymptomatic to simple coal workers' pneumoconiosis to progressive massive fibrosis (PMF).
- *Silicosis* is the most common pneumoconiosis in the world and is most commonly caused by inhalation of crystalline silica (e.g., quartz).
  - Manifestations of silicosis range from asymptomatic silicotic nodules to PMF.
  - Silicosis is associated with an increased susceptibility to tuberculosis and possibly lung cancer.
- *Asbestos* exposure is linked to interstitial fibrosis (asbestosis), localized fibrous plaques, pleural effusions, lung cancer, and malignant mesothelioma.
- Cigarette smoking and asbestos exposure combine to synergistically increase the risk of lung cancer.
- Family members of workers exposed to asbestos are also at increased risk for cancer.

Sarcoidosis

- Sarcoidosis is a multisystem granulomatous disease of unknown etiology.
- The classic (but not specific) histologic feature is well-formed non-necrotizing granulomas.
- Sarcoid is caused by an unknown immune stimulus that drives sustained activation of CD4+ Th1 cells in the lung and other tissues.
- Clinical manifestations include:
  - Lung involvement (90%), which starts as granulomatous disease and may progress to diffuse interstitial fibrosis.
  - Other clinical features include lymphadenopathy, eye involvement (sicca syndrome [dry eyes], iritis, or iridocyclitis), skin lesions (erythema nodosum, painless subcutaneous nodules), and visceral involvement (liver, skin, bone marrow).

Pulmonary Embolism (PE)

- Most pulmonary artery thrombi are embolic and usually arise from the deep lower leg veins.
- Risk factors for PE are those associated with deep venous thrombosis and include prolonged bed rest, knee or hip surgery, severe trauma, congestive heart failure, oral contraceptives, disseminated cancer, and genetic variants leading to hypercoagulability (e.g., Factor V Leiden).
- PE has a wide range of consequences, ranging from clinically silent (60% to 80%) to hypoxemia, shortness of breath, pleuritic pain, and possible infarction (15% to 35%) to acute right-sided heart failure, shock, and sudden death (5%).
- Risk for recurrence of PE is generally high.

Community-Acquired Pneumonia (CAP)

- May be bacterial or viral

- Two overlapping patterns of bacterial pneumonia, lobar and bronchopneumonia (patchy)
- Lobar pneumonias evolve through four morphologic stages: congestion, red hepatization, gray hepatization, and resolution.
- *S. pneumoniae* (pneumococcus) is the most common bacterial cause of CAP and usually has a lobar pattern of involvement.
- Other common causes of bacterial CAP in various settings include *H. influenzae* and *M. catarrhalis* (acute exacerbations of COPD), *S. aureus* (secondary to viral respiratory infections), *K. pneumoniae* (patients who are debilitated/malnourished), *P. aeruginosa* (cystic fibrosis, burn victims, patients with neutropenia), and *L. pneumophila* (particularly in organ transplant recipients).
- *Viral pneumonias* are characterized by respiratory distress out of proportion to the clinical and radiologic signs and inflammation that is predominantly confined to alveolar septa.
- Common causes of viral pneumonia include SARS-CoV-2 (COVID-19), influenza A and B, respiratory syncytial virus, human metapneumovirus, parainfluenza virus, and adenovirus.

Tuberculosis (TB)

- Chronic granulomatous disease caused by *M. tuberculosis* that usually affects the lungs
- Initial exposure results in a cellular immune response that confers resistance and leads to hypersensitivity.
- Th1 CD4+ T cells have a crucial role in cell-mediated immunity against mycobacteria.
- The hallmark of the tissue reaction to TB is granulomas, usually with caseous necrosis.
- *Primary pulmonary TB* in immunocompetent individuals is usually asymptomatic and leads to lesions in a subpleural focus and in draining lymph nodes that undergo healing. In states of immunodeficiency, primary progressive tuberculosis that involves large parts of lung can occur.
- *Secondary (reactivation) TB* arises in previously exposed individuals when host immune defenses are compromised and usually manifests as cavitary lesions in the lung apices. In states of immune deficiency secondary TB can also be progressive.
- In the setting of immunodeficiency (e.g., in individuals infected with HIV) progressive primary and secondary TB can result in life-threatening forms of disease (e.g., miliary TB and tuberculous meningitis).

Carcinoma of the Lung

- Smoking is the most important risk factor in all types.
- Three major genetically distinct histologic subtypes:
  - *Adenocarcinoma:* Most common, more prevalent in women and nonsmokers, it arises from precursor lesions such as atypical adenomatous hyperplasia and adenocarcinoma in situ and is associated with tyrosine kinase mutations (e.g., *EGFR*).
  - *Squamous cell carcinoma:* Arises from precursor lesions such as squamous dysplasia and squamous cell carcinoma in situ, often within areas of squamous metaplasia
  - *Small cell carcinoma:* Usually metastatic at presentation, it is best treated with chemotherapy and is strongly associated with *TP53* and *RB* mutations.
- Lung cancers commonly cause a variety of paraneoplastic syndromes.
- Because of a high burden of mutations caused by carcinogens in tobacco smoke, lung cancers express tumor neoantigens and are responsive to immune checkpoint inhibitor therapy.

■ Laboratory Tests

Test	Reference Value	Pathophysiology/Clinical Relevance
Acid-fast bacillus testing, variable specimens (e.g., sputum, tissue)	Negative	Unlike most bacteria, acid-fast organisms (e.g., *Mycobacterium tuberculosis* and *M. avium-intracellulare* complex) retain certain stains when exposed to acid alcohol due to their cell wall characteristics (e.g., the Ziehl-Neelsen stain). For sputum samples, the most sensitive tests use the fluorochrome auramine-O or auramine-rhodamine dyes; organisms are identified by fluorescence microscopy. In tissue samples, staining is performed with carbol fuchsin dyes (e.g., the Ziehl-Neelsen stain), and organisms are identified by light microscopy.
α1-antitrypsin (AAT), serum	100–190 mg/dL	The α1-antitrypsin (AAT) protein is produced by hepatocytes and inhibits neutrophil serine proteases, most notably neutrophil elastase. AAT deficiency is caused by mutations that result in misfolding of the protein and its accumulation in the liver. Consequent low serum levels of AAT in lung alveolar cells render them vulnerable to destructive proteases (e.g., neutrophil elastase), thereby increasing risk for panacinar emphysema. AAT serum measurements and protease inhibitor (Pi) phenotyping are important parts of the diagnostic workup for symptomatic patients. PiZZ type is the most common clinically relevant form with loss of up to 90% serum AAT.
PD-L1 expression, tumor tissue	Varies depending on tumor type, PD-L1 clone, scoring methods	Expression of PD-L1 on tumor cells allows tumors to evade killing by PD-1-expressing tumor-specific CD8+ T cells. Immunohistochemistry for PD-L1 is performed in multiple tumor types (e.g., melanoma, nonsmall cell lung cancer) to predict treatment response to PD-L1 inhibitors ("checkpoint inhibitors"). However, even lung cancers that do not express PD-L1 may respond to checkpoint inhibitors, possibly because of targeting of PD-L1 expressed on infiltrating immune cells such as macrophages.

Molecular Tests of Relevance in Lung Cancer		
Analyte	Method	Pathophysiology/Clinical Relevance
ALK gene rearrangement	In lung cancer, may be detected directly by FISH or DNA sequencing, or inferred from immunohistochemistry	ALK is a receptor tyrosine kinase that is not normally expressed in lung epithelium. Rearrangements that result in expression of constitutively active forms of ALK are seen in approximately 4% of nonsmall cell lung cancers and are enriched in cancers arising in nonsmokers and younger patients. These cancers are responsive to treatment with ALK inhibitors.
BRAF gene mutation	Targeted DNA sequencing or Next-Gen sequencing panels	*BRAF* encodes a serine/threonine kinase in the ERK/MAPK signaling pathway. Mutations that lead to constitutive BRAF activation are found in 1% to 3% of nonsmall cell lung cancers. Tumors with the most common *BRAF* mutation, which results in an amino acid substitution at valine 600, respond to regimens that include BRAF inhibitors.
EGFR gene mutation	Targeted DNA sequencing or Next-Gen sequencing panels	EGFR (epidermal growth factor receptor) is a receptor tyrosine kinase (RTK). Point mutations that cause constitutive activation of EGFR are found in approximately 15% of lung adenocarcinomas and are enriched in tumors arising in nonsmokers. Monoclonal antibody and small molecule inhibitors of EGFR are effective treatments for *EGFR*-mutated lung cancer.
MET gene abnormalities	Amplifications are detected by FISH, mutations by Next-Gen sequencing	*MET* encodes a receptor tyrosine kinase. The *MET* gene is amplified or contains mutations that stabilize the MET protein in 5% to 7% of nonsmall cell lung cancers and is altered in up to 20% of *EGFR*-mutated tumors that become resistant to EGFR inhibitors. Tumors with *MET* alterations are sensitive to MET inhibitors.
RAS gene mutation	Next-Gen sequencing	Activating *RAS* mutations are seen in 20% to 25% of lung adenocarcinomas and are enriched in tumors arising in people who smoke. These mutations are mutually exclusive with mutations in tyrosine receptor genes, which participate in the same signaling pathway. Approximately 50% of *RAS* mutations in lung cancers produce a glycine to cysteine substitution in residue 12 of RAS, a form of mutated RAS that can be effectively targeted by inhibitors that covalently bind the altered cysteine residue.
RET gene rearrangement	FISH or Next-Gen sequencing	*RET1* encodes a receptor tyrosine kinase that is constitutively activated as a consequence of *RET1* rearrangement in 1% to 2% of lung adenocarcinomas and is enriched in tumors arising in younger patients and nonsmokers. Tumors with *RET1* rearrangements are sensitive to particular tyrosine kinase inhibitors.
ROS1 gene rearrangement	Most commonly detected by FISH	*ROS1* encodes a receptor tyrosine kinase that is constitutively activated as a consequence of *ROS1* rearrangement in 1% to 2% of lung adenocarcinomas and is enriched in tumors arising in younger patients and nonsmokers. Tumors with *ROS1* rearrangements are sensitive to particular tyrosine kinase inhibitors.

References values from https://www.mayocliniclabs.com/ by permission of Mayo Foundation for Medical Education and Research. All rights reserved.

Adapted from Deyrup AT, D'Ambrosio D, Muir J, et al. Essential Laboratory Tests for Medical Education. *Acad Pathol.* 2022;9. doi: 10.1016/j.acpath.2022.100046.

Kidney

The well-known quotation "What is man…but an ingenious machine for turning, with infinite artfulness, the wine of Shiraz into urine" gives rather dramatic importance to the renal apparatus. In reality, the kidney is responsible for the following:

- *Excretion of soluble wastes*, which are filtered out of the plasma; this is the primary function of glomeruli.
- *Maintenance of ion balance.* Renal tubules absorb water and salts and thus regulate their concentration in the plasma.
- *Regulation of blood pressure.* The juxtaglomerular apparatus produces the hormone renin in response to reduced arterial flow or pressure. Renin in turn activates angiotensin, which constricts peripheral blood vessels and indirectly increases renal tubular reabsorption of sodium and water, which increases fluid volume; both these alterations serve to maintain normal blood pressure.
- *Hormone secretion.* The kidney produces erythropoietin, which regulates the hematocrit. The enzyme α_1 hydroxylase, also produced in the kidney, is responsible for producing the active form of vitamin D.

These functions depend on the coordinated actions of the four main structural components of the kidney:

- *Glomeruli* are the filtration units of the kidney. Their structure is described later, when we consider glomerular diseases.
- *Tubules* reabsorb water, small molecules, and ions that have been filtered through the glomeruli.
- The *interstitium* provides the scaffold that supports glomeruli and tubules.
- *Blood vessels* deliver arterial blood to glomeruli and return venous blood to the circulation.

These components function in a coordinated manner, so pathologic alterations in one usually affect the other structures. Nevertheless, we discuss them separately, mainly because diseases initially affecting different components usually differ in their pathogenesis. For example, most glomerular diseases are immunologically mediated, whereas

The contributions of Dr. Anthony Chang, Department of Pathology, University of Chicago, and Dr. Zoltan Laszik, Department of Pathology, University of California San Francisco, to previous editions of this chapter are gratefully acknowledged.

tubular and interstitial disorders are more often caused by toxic or infectious agents. Because these disorders are typically associated with inflammation, they are called glomerulonephritis (GN) and tubulointerstitial nephritis (TIN), respectively. When chronic kidney disease progresses to its most advanced stage, so-called end-stage renal disease, all four compartments of the kidney are usually damaged.

CLINICAL MANIFESTATIONS OF RENAL DISEASES

The clinical manifestations of renal disease reflect the underlying pathophysiology (Table 12.1). Before discussing individual diseases, we summarize the principal clinical features of renal disorders.

- *Nephrotic syndrome* is caused by glomerular alterations that result in increased glomerular permeability. It is characterized by the following:
  - *Proteinuria*, with daily protein loss in the urine of 3.5 g or more in adults (said to be in the "nephrotic range"), due to leakage of plasma proteins through an abnormally permeable glomerular basement membrane
  - *Hypoalbuminemia*, with plasma albumin levels dropping below 3 g/dL because of urinary loss of proteins, particularly albumin because it has a lower molecular weight than globulins
  - *Generalized edema*, because of decreased plasma colloid osmotic pressure due to the hypoalbuminemia, leading to leakage of fluid from the blood into extravascular spaces
  - *Hyperlipidemia and lipiduria*. The cause of the hyperlipidemia is unclear but is thought to be due to a combination of increased hepatic lipoprotein synthesis, abnormal transport of circulating lipid particles, and decreased lipid catabolism. The associated lipiduria reflects the increased permeability of the glomerular basement membrane (GBM) to lipoproteins.
- *Nephritic syndrome* is caused by glomerular inflammation and is characterized by the following:
  - *Hematuria* (red cells and red cell casts in urine) and white blood cells in the urine due to leakage through injured glomerular capillary walls
  - *Proteinuria* (usually in the subnephrotic range) with or without edema
  - *Azotemia* (defined below) resulting from reduced glomerular filtration rate (GFR)
  - *Hypertension* caused by activation of the renin-angiotensin system
  - *Rapidly progressive glomerulonephritis (RPGN)* is an acute and rapidly worsening subtype of nephritic syndrome resulting from diverse causes. Morphologically, it is usually accompanied by the formation of crescents in glomeruli and is hence also called *crescentic GN.*
- *Acute kidney injury* is manifested by a rapid decline (hours to days) in GFR secondary to intrinsic diseases of the kidney or extrarenal causes. The latter may be prerenal (reduced fluid volume and therefore reduced glomerular perfusion) or postrenal (obstruction to the outflow tract). Acute kidney injury (AKI) was previously called acute renal failure, but AKI is now preferred because the damage is of varying severity and is not always associated with renal failure. AKI may present with reduced or no urine output (*oliguria* or *anuria*, respectively), hypertension, and other signs of renal dysfunction. Laboratory tests reveal an increase in blood urea nitrogen (BUN) and serum creatinine and are collectively termed *azotemia*. When the azotemia is severe enough to cause clinical signs and symptoms, the term *uremia* is used.
- *Chronic kidney disease* (previously called chronic renal failure) results from any underlying disorder that causes progressive renal injury and scarring in the kidney. It is characterized by various metabolic and electrolyte abnormalities such as hyperphosphatemia, dyslipidemia, and metabolic acidosis. Because of the kidney's functional reserve, the ongoing renal scarring is often asymptomatic until it is advanced, when symptoms of uremia develop. Chronic kidney disease may progress to *end-stage renal disease* when renal function is irreversibly lost due to severe progressive scarring in the kidney from any cause, and the only available treatment options are dialysis and transplantation.
- *Asymptomatic hematuria* may occur in nephritis, vascular diseases, and renal cancer. It is usually microscopic; its main significance is that it provides a warning sign for an underlying disease.

DISEASES OF GLOMERULI

The glomerulus consists of an anastomosing network of capillaries invested by two layers of epithelium. The visceral epithelium (composed of podocytes) is part of the capillary wall, whereas the parietal epithelium encircles Bowman space (urinary space), the cavity in which the plasma filtrate collects. The parietal epithelium is continuous with tubular epithelium. The glomerular capillary wall consists of the following components (Fig. 12.1):

- Fenestrated *endothelial cells,* with openings between cells that are 70 to 100 nm in diameter. These openings (fenestrae) make the endothelium permeable to antibodies, other proteins, and small molecules, but they are too small to allow passage of blood cells.
- The *glomerular basement membrane* (GBM) consists of collagen (mostly type IV), laminin, polyanionic proteoglycans, fibronectin,

Table 12.1 Clinical Manifestations of Renal Diseases

Clinical Syndrome	Major Manifestations	Examples of Diseases
Glomerular syndromes		
Nephrotic syndrome	Proteinuria, hypoalbuminemia, hyperlipidemia, edema	Primary renal diseases: minimal change disease, membranous nephropathy Systemic diseases: diabetes
Nephritic syndrome	Hematuria, mild proteinuria, renal failure, hypertension	Primary renal diseases: postinfectious GN, MPGN type 1, RPGN Systemic diseases: SLE
Acute kidney injury	Abrupt onset of renal failure, oliguria/anuria	Acute tubular injury, thrombotic microangiopathy
Chronic kidney disease	Progressive renal failure (uremia)	Chronic glomerular or tubulointerstitial disease, nephrosclerosis

Other clinical manifestations that are discussed elsewhere include hypertension (Chapter 8) and secondary hyperparathyroidism (Chapter 18).

GN, Glomerulonephritis; *MPGN,* membranoproliferative glomerulonephritis; *RPGN,* rapidly progressive glomerulonephritis; *SLE,* systemic lupus erythematosus; *TMA,* thrombotic microangiopathy.

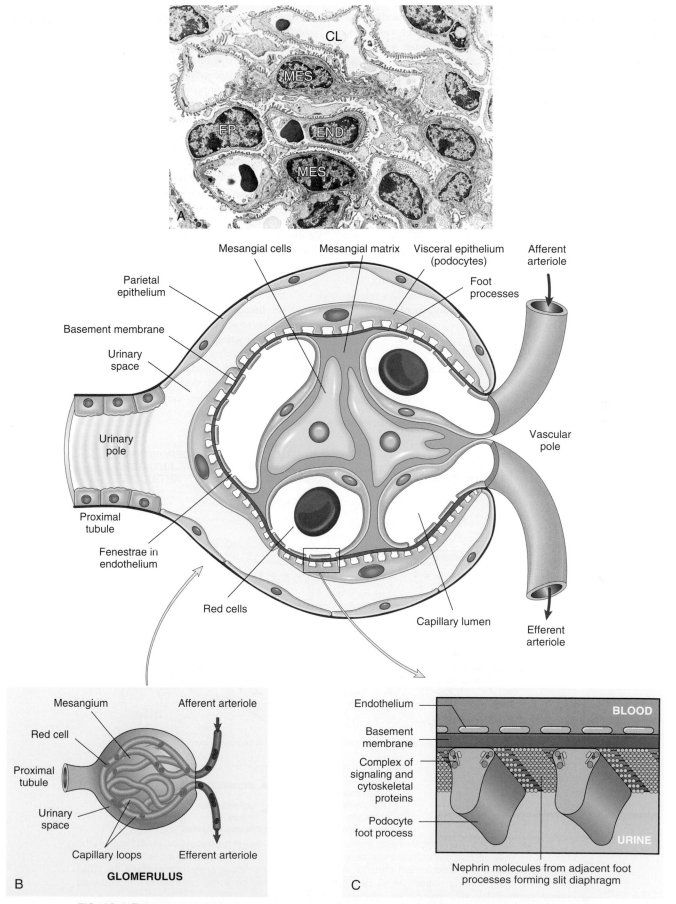

FIG. 12.1 The normal glomerulus. (A) Low-power electron micrograph of rat glomerulus. *CL,* Capillary lumen; *END,* endothelium; *EP,* epithelial cell; *MES,* mesangium. (B) Schematic diagram of a normal glomerulus showing the components. (C) A detailed view of the glomerular capillary wall.

and several other glycoproteins. It is located between endothelial cells and podocytes and prevents the passage of large molecules, especially anionic proteins, and cells into the Bowman space.

- *Podocytes* (visceral epithelial cells) are specialized cells that possess interdigitating foot processes embedded in and adherent to the outer layer of the GBM. Adjacent foot processes are separated by 20- to 30-nm-wide gaps, which are bridged by a thin *slit diaphragm,* a structure composed mainly of the proteins nephrin and podocin that maintains the selective permeability of the glomerular filtration barrier.
- *Mesangial cells* are contractile mesenchymal cells that lie in the extracellular matrix between the capillaries that supports the glomerular tuft. These cells can proliferate and produce extracellular matrix components, such as collagen, as well as cytokines that promote leukocyte recruitment and growth factors.

Normally, the glomerular filtration system is permeable to water and small solutes and almost completely impermeable to molecules of the size and molecular charge of albumin (a 70-kDa protein). This selective permeability discriminates among protein molecules mainly according to size (the larger, the less permeable) and charge (the more cationic, the more permeable).

Mechanisms of Glomerular Injury and Disease

Immune mechanisms underlie most types of glomerular diseases. Antibodies may bind to the GBM by several mechanisms (Fig. 12.2): (1) subendothelial or subepithelial deposition of circulating antigen-antibody complexes; (2) antibodies binding to extrinsic molecules planted within the glomerulus or scattered intrinsic glomerular antigens, producing an appearance of in situ immune complex formation; and (3) anti-GBM antibodies binding to continuously distributed intrinsic GBM antigens. The deposition of immune complexes or antibodies initiates complement and/or Fc receptor mediated inflammation and leukocyte activation (Chapter 5), resulting in glomerular injury that is characteristic of nephritis (nephritic syndrome). In some cases, the antibodies or immune complexes disrupt the glomerular permeability barrier enough to cause the nephrotic syndrome, even without overt inflammation. Subendothelial deposits tend to be associated with greater inflammation, presumably because of easier access of complement proteins and leukocytes from the blood, whereas subepithelial complexes often produce proteinuria with little or no inflammation, possibly because they interfere with the function of the slit diaphragm or epithelial cells. A consistent morphologic finding in all cases of nephrotic syndrome is fusion of epithelial foot processes. It is unclear if this is a cause or an effect of proteinuria.

Deposition of Circulating Immune Complexes. It has long been known that GN may be caused by deposition of preformed immune complexes. Because fluid from the blood passes through the GBM at high pressure (to produce urine) and the GBM is a continuous barrier, it is a common site of deposition of circulating immune complexes. Hence, the kidneys are often involved in systemic immune complex diseases (type III hypersensitivity). Examples include systemic lupus erythematosus, in which the antigens are endogenous nucleoproteins, or the GN that follows certain bacterial (streptococcal), viral

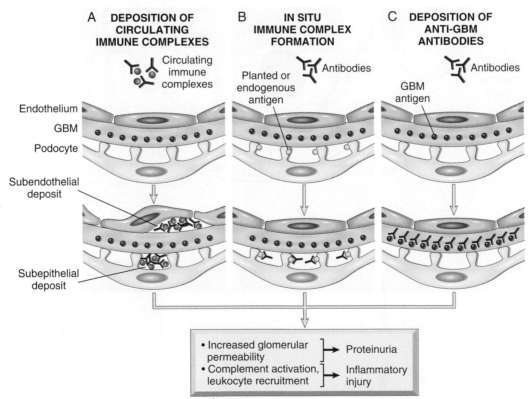

FIG. 12.2 Mechanisms of glomerular injury. Immune complexes formed in the circulation (A) or locally in the glomerulus (B) may deposit in the glomerular basement membrane (GBM), producing a granular pattern of staining for antibodies and complement proteins. Antibodies against antigens present throughout the GBM (C) produce a linear staining pattern. In all cases, the outcome may be some combination of increased glomerular permeability, inflammation, and glomerular injury.

(hepatitis B), parasitic (*Plasmodium falciparum* malaria), and other infections, in which the antigens are exogenous. Often the inciting antigen is unknown.

The hallmark of immune complex-mediated GN is the appearance of deposits of immunoglobulins and complement, which can be demonstrated by immunofluorescence and electron microscopy. By immunofluorescence microscopy, these deposits appear *granular*, to which some pathologists give the rather picturesque description of "lumpy-bumpy" (Fig. 12.3A). Electron microscopy reveals electron-dense immune deposits in the GBM; these may be subendothelial, subepithelial, or in the mesangium.

Formation of Immune Complexes In Situ. Binding of antibodies to extrinsic molecules planted in the GBM or intrinsic glomerular antigens in a patchy distribution produces the appearance of in situ immune complex formation. In both cases the bound antibodies appear granular by immunofluorescence microscopy. Membranous nephropathy is the classic example of glomerular disease resulting from local formation of immune complexes containing antibodies reactive with endogenous antigens. In this disorder, complexes formed in the subepithelial portion of the GBM cause profound loss of glomerular permeability, resulting in the nephrotic syndrome, with little or no inflammation.

Deposition of Antiglomerular Basement Membrane Antibody. Antibody-mediated GN results from the glomerular deposition of autoantibodies directed against protein components of the GBM. The best-characterized disease in this group is anti-GBM antibody—mediated GN, also known as *Goodpasture disease*. In this type of injury, antibodies are directed against intrinsic GBM antigens. The distribution of these antigens is continuous, creating a *linear* pattern of staining when visualized with immunofluorescence microscopy (Fig. 12.3B). This form of GN is an example of type II hypersensitivity (Chapter 5).

Other Mechanisms of Glomerular Injury. Several other mechanisms may cause glomerular injury.

- *Unregulated activation of complement* may be triggered by autoantibodies against complement components or inherited abnormalities of complement regulatory proteins. The ensuing complement-mediated injury may affect several tissues, including the kidney. Two forms of GN (dense deposit disease and C3 GN) and one form of a systemic disease with significant renal manifestations (complement-mediated thrombotic microangiopathy, also known as atypical hemolytic uremic syndrome) belong to this category.

- *Other recruited or intrinsic cells* may contribute to glomerular injury. Resident glomerular cells, especially *mesangial cells*, may be stimulated by antibodies and immune complexes to secrete cytokines and other mediators that can contribute to glomerular inflammation. Activated *T lymphocytes* have also been implicated in experimental models of glomerular injury, but there is little evidence for this in human diseases. *Platelets* may aggregate and release mediators, including prostaglandins, growth factors, and TGF-β, which may stimulate collagen deposition (glomerulosclerosis).

- *Podocyte injury.* Because of the role of podocytes in maintaining the permeability barrier of the GBM, injury to these cells is an important cause of glomerular disease. Podocyte injury can be induced by antibodies to podocyte antigens; by toxins; possibly by certain cytokines; or by still poorly characterized circulating factors, as in some cases of focal segmental glomerulosclerosis (discussed later). Podocyte injury produces morphologic changes including effacement of foot processes, vacuolization, and retraction and detachment of cells from the GBM, and the resulting disruption of normal slit diaphragms often results in proteinuria. Inherited mutations in the structural components of slit diaphragms, such as nephrin and podocin, are also associated with functional alterations that lead to rare hereditary forms of nephritis.

- *Loss of nephrons* itself exacerbates glomerular injury. Once renal disease, glomerular or otherwise, destroys sufficient nephrons to reduce the GFR to 30% to 50% of normal, the remaining glomeruli undergo progressive scarring, called *glomerulosclerosis*, leading eventually to end-stage renal disease. The loss of nephrons triggers adaptive changes to maintain renal function, including glomerular enlargement, and increased blood flow and transcapillary pressure (capillary hypertension). These alterations are ultimately maladaptive, resulting in endothelial and

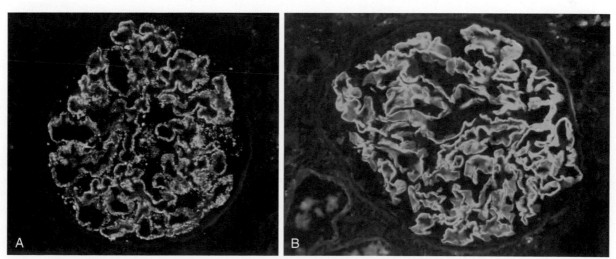

FIG. 12.3 Patterns of deposition of immune complexes as seen by immunofluorescence microscopy. (A) Granular, characteristic of immune complex deposition. (B) Linear, characteristic of antiglomerular basement membrane (anti-GBM) antibody deposition. (A, Courtesy of Dr. J. Kowalewska, Department of Pathology, University of Washington, Seattle, Washington.)

podocyte injury, increased glomerular permeability to proteins (even in the absence of primary glomerular disease), and accumulation of proteins and lipids in the mesangial matrix. Subsequently, there may be capillary obliteration and finally segmental (affecting a portion of a glomerulus) or global (affecting the entire glomerulus) sclerosis of glomeruli. The latter results in further reduction of nephron mass, initiating a cycle of progressive scarring and loss of function.

We now turn to a consideration of specific types of GN and the syndromes they produce (Table 12.2). We divide these diseases into those that primarily cause the nephrotic syndrome and those associated with manifestations of the nephritic syndrome; some diseases do not fit into either category. The diagnosis and classification of glomerular diseases are based largely on morphology, so renal biopsy is a mainstay of the diagnosis and management of these disorders.

Table 12.2 Summary of Major Primary Glomerular Diseases

Disease	Most Frequent Clinical Presentation	Pathogenesis	Glomerular Pathology		
			Light Microscopy	Fluorescence Microscopy	Electron Microscopy
Minimal change disease	Nephrotic syndrome	Unknown; podocyte injury	Normal	Negative	Effacement of foot processes; no deposits
Focal segmental glomerulosclerosis	Nephrotic syndrome; nonnephrotic range proteinuria	Unknown; reaction to loss of renal mass; plasma factor?	Focal and segmental sclerosis and hyalinosis	Usually negative; IgM and C3 may be present in areas of scarring	Effacement of foot processes; epithelial denudation
Membranous nephropathy	Nephrotic syndrome	In situ immune complex formation; PLA2R antigen in most cases of primary disease	Diffuse capillary wall thickening and subepithelial "spike" formation	Granular IgG and C3 along GBM	Subepithelial deposits
Membranoproliferative glomerulonephritis (MPGN) type I	Nephrotic/nephritic syndrome	Immune complex	Membranoproliferative pattern; GBM splitting	Granular IgG, C3, C1q, and C4 along GBM and mesangium	Subendothelial deposits
C3 glomerulopathy (dense deposit disease and C3 glomerulonephritis)	Nephrotic/nephritic syndrome; nonnephrotic proteinuria	Activation of alternative complement pathway; antibody-mediated or hereditary defect in regulation	Mesangial proliferative or membranoproliferative patterns	C3	Mesangial, intramembranous and subendothelial electron-dense or "waxy" deposits
Acute postinfectious glomerulonephritis	Nephritic syndrome	Immune complex mediated; circulating or planted antigen	Diffuse endocapillary proliferation; leukocytic infiltration	Granular IgG and C3 along GBM and mesangium	Primarily subepithelial humps
IgA nephropathy	Recurrent hematuria or proteinuria	Immune complexes containing IgA	Mesangial or focal endocapillary proliferative glomerulonephritis	IgA ± IgG, IgM, and C3 in mesangium	Mesangial and paramesangial dense deposits
Rapidly progressive glomerulonephritis	Rapid onset of nephritic syndrome, usually with proteinuria; progression to renal failure	Varies: autoantibodies against collagen type IV α3 chain (anti-GBM antibodies); immune complexes; no immune deposits	Extracapillary proliferation with crescents; necrosis	Linear or granular IgG and C3; fibrin in crescents	Immune complexes or no deposits; GBM disruptions; fibrin

GBM, Glomerular basement membrane; *IgA*, immunoglobulin A; *IgG*, immunoglobulin G; *IgM*, immunoglobulin M; *PLA2R*, phospholipase A2 receptor.

Table 12.3 Causes of Nephrotic Syndrome

Cause	Prevalence (%)[a]	
	Children	Adults
Primary Glomerular Disease		
Minimal change disease	65	10
Focal segmental glomerulosclerosis	10	35
Membranous nephropathy	5	30
Membranoproliferative glomerulonephritis	10	10
IgA nephropathy and others	10	15
Systemic Diseases With Renal Manifestations		
Diabetes		
Amyloidosis		
Systemic lupus erythematosus		
Drug ingestion (e.g., gold, penicillamine, heroin)		
Infections (e.g., malaria, syphilis, hepatitis B, HIV)		
Malignancy (e.g., carcinoma, melanoma)		
Miscellaneous (e.g., bee sting allergy, hereditary nephritis)		

HIV, Human immunodeficiency virus.

[a]Approximate prevalence of primary disease is 95% of the cases in children and 60% in adults. Approximate prevalence of systemic disease is 5% of the cases in children and 40% in adults.

Disorders Presenting With the Nephrotic Syndrome

Many primary glomerular diseases cause the nephrotic syndrome, but in adults this syndrome is most often secondary to diabetes, amyloidosis, and systemic lupus erythematosus (Table 12.3). The renal lesions produced by amyloidosis are discussed in Chapter 5 and those caused by diabetes in Chapter 18. Because of the great increase of type 2 diabetes associated with obesity, diabetic nephropathy is now the most common cause of chronic kidney disease in the United States. Here we discuss primary glomerular diseases.

Minimal Change Disease

Minimal change disease, a relatively benign disorder, is the most frequent cause of the nephrotic syndrome in children and is characterized by glomeruli that have a normal appearance by light microscopy. It may develop at any age but is most common between 1 and 7 years of age. In most cases it is idiopathic, but it is also seen in association with certain infections, therapeutic drugs, and neoplasms.

Pathogenesis. The leading hypothesis for the pathogenesis of minimal change disease is that circulating molecules injure podocytes and cause proteinuria secondary to foot process effacement. Since foot process effacement is common to many causes of nephrotic syndrome, it is not entirely clear whether it is the primary lesion or is secondary to proteinuria. An immune mechanism is suspected mainly because of the clinical response to steroids. Although there are reports of "permeability factors" secreted by patients' lymphocytes and other cells, none has been characterized biochemically or established as being causative. Recent work points to a potential pathogenic role for antibodies against slit diaphragm proteins, but this also remains to be proven. Thus, the pathogenesis of the disease remains unknown.

MORPHOLOGY

The glomeruli are histologically normal (accounting for the name of the disease), and no deposits of antibody or complement are seen by immunofluorescence (Fig. 12.4A). The cells of the proximal convoluted tubules often are heavily laden with protein droplets and lipids due to tubular reabsorption of the molecules that have leaked through the diseased glomeruli. The only morphologic glomerular abnormality is the **diffuse effacement of podocyte foot processes,** visible by electron microscopy (Fig. 12.4B). Other ultrastructural changes in podocytes include vacuolization, microvillus formation, and occasional focal detachments, suggesting some form of podocyte injury. Steroid therapy reverses these podocyte alterations, and proteinuria remits concomitantly.

Clinical Features. The disease typically manifests with abrupt development of the nephrotic syndrome in an otherwise healthy child. Renal function is usually preserved. The protein loss affects mainly smaller plasma proteins, chiefly albumin (selective proteinuria). The prognosis for children with this disorder is favorable. More than 90% of children respond to a short course of corticosteroid therapy; however, proteinuria recurs in more than two-thirds of the initial responders, and some of these individuals become steroid

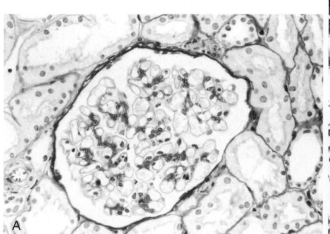
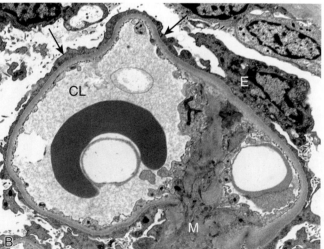

FIG. 12.4 Minimal change disease. (A) Glomerulus showing normal basement membranes and absence of proliferation (PAS stain, which highlights polysaccharides and glycoproteins). (B) Ultrastructural characteristics of minimal change disease include effacement of foot processes *(arrows)* and absence of deposits. *CL,* Capillary lumen; *E,* epithelial cell; *M,* mesangium.

dependent. Less than 5% develop chronic kidney disease over time, most often focal segmental glomerulosclerosis (FSGS), suggesting that minimal change disease and FSGS are stages in a continuum of progressive glomerular disease. Because of its responsiveness to therapy in children, minimal change disease must be differentiated from other causes of the nephrotic syndrome. Adults with this disease also respond to steroid therapy, but the response is slower than in children and relapses are more common.

Focal Segmental Glomerulosclerosis

Focal segmental glomerulosclerosis (FSGS) is characterized by sclerosis of some (but not all) glomeruli (focal) that involves only a part of each affected glomerulus (segmental). It is not a specific disease entity but a pattern of injury that is often found in adults and children with the nephrotic syndrome. Several forms of FSGS are recognized.

- *Primary,* with no identifiable predisposing cause. Primary FSGS accounts for about 30% of all cases of the nephrotic syndrome in the United States. It is a frequent cause of nephrotic syndrome in children and an increasingly common cause in adults. It is also the primary glomerular disorder that most commonly progresses to end-stage renal disease in the United States.
- *Secondary* to diverse insults, including the following:
  - A *maladaptive response to nephron loss.* Loss of functional renal mass may result from any form of chronic kidney disease. It is also seen in severely obese patients who develop proteinuria. In all these conditions, there is increased filtration pressure in residual glomeruli, and this is believed to result in FSGS.
  - *Infections.* FSGS is seen in 5% to 10% of patients infected with HIV; however, the incidence is decreasing with improved antiviral therapy.
  - *Drug use,* specifically heroin use, and, less commonly, various therapeutic agents.
- *Genetic.* The inherited forms vary in incidence in different populations and usually have an autosomal recessive pattern of inheritance. Over 60 genes have been implicated, some of which encode proteins involved in podocyte function, such as nephrin, podocin, and cytoskeletal proteins.

Pathogenesis. Injury to podocytes is the likely initiating event of primary FSGS. Injury may manifest initially as foot process fusion, associated with increased glomerular permeability, and may progress to loss of podocytes and slit diaphragms. The source of the injury remains unknown. As with minimal change disease, permeability-inducing factors produced by lymphocytes have been proposed, but they remain undefined. The recurrence of proteinuria in some patients following renal transplantation for FSGS, sometimes within a day or less, supports the idea that a circulating mediator leads to podocyte damage. Entrapment of plasma proteins and lipids and ECM deposition in glomeruli lead to obliteration of the capillaries and consequent glomerulosclerosis.

MORPHOLOGY

Primary FSGS initially affects the juxtamedullary glomeruli, but with progression, most glomeruli may be affected. The lesions involve some tufts within a glomerulus while sparing others (Fig. 12.5). The affected glomerular segments exhibit **obliterated capillary lumina, increased mesangial matrix, deposition of hyaline material,** and foamy (lipid-laden) macrophages. Immunofluorescence microscopy often reveals nonspecific trapping of immunoglobulins, usually IgM, and complement in the areas of sclerosis. On electron microscopy, the podocytes exhibit **effacement of foot processes.** With time, progression leads to global sclerosis of the glomeruli, pronounced tubular atrophy, and interstitial fibrosis, which, in advanced disease, is difficult to differentiate from other forms of chronic glomerular disease.

A morphologic variant called **collapsing glomerulopathy** is characterized by collapse of the glomerular tuft and epithelial cell hyperplasia. This is a more severe manifestation of FSGS that carries a particularly poor prognosis.

Clinical Features. FSGS must be distinguished from minimal change disease because the clinical course and response to therapy are markedly different. Both are associated with the nephrotic syndrome, but the incidence of hematuria and hypertension is higher in individuals with FSGS. Also, unlike minimal change disease, FSGS-associated proteinuria is nonselective, and in general the response to corticosteroid therapy is poor. At least 50% of patients with FSGS develop end-stage renal disease within 10 years of diagnosis.

Membranous Nephropathy

Membranous nephropathy is characterized by subepithelial deposits of antigen-antibody complexes along the GBM. It usually presents in adults between the ages of 30 and 60 years and follows an indolent and slowly progressive course.

Up to 80% of cases of membranous nephropathy are primary, caused by autoantibodies against podocyte antigens. In the

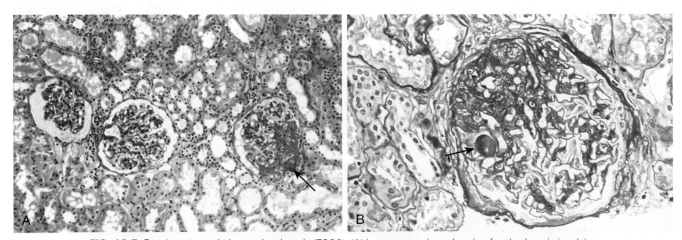

FIG. 12.5 Focal segmental glomerulosclerosis (FSGS). (A) Low-power view showing focal sclerosis involving one of three glomeruli *(arrow).* (B) Involvement of a segment of a glomerulus, with sclerosis and hyaline deposit *(arrow).*

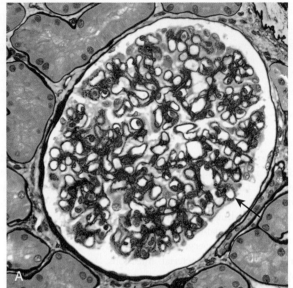

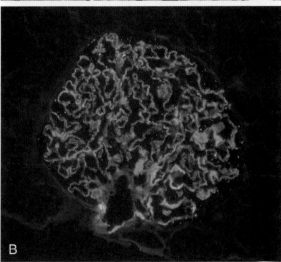

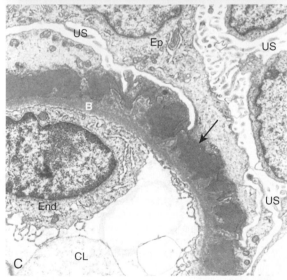

FIG. 12.6 Membranous nephropathy. (A) Diffuse thickening of the glomerular basement membrane without proliferation of cells or inflammation (silver stain, which highlights proteins in the GBM). (B) Granular deposits of IgG by immunofluorescence along the GBM. (C) Subepithelial deposits *(arrow)*, effacement of foot processes, and the presence of spikes of basement membrane material between the immune deposits. *B,* Basement membrane; *CL,* capillary lumen; *End,* endothelium; *Ep,* epithelial cell; *US,* urinary space. (B, Courtesy of Dr. Vighnesh Walavalkar, Department of Pathology, University of California San Francisco.)

remainder, the disease is secondary to other conditions, including the following:

- *Infections* (e.g., chronic hepatitis B, syphilis, schistosomiasis, malaria)
- *Malignant neoplasms,* particularly carcinomas of various sites and B cell tumors such as chronic lymphocytic leukemia
- *Autoimmune diseases, particularly systemic lupus erythematosus*
- *Exposure to inorganic salts* (gold, mercury)
- *Drugs* (e.g., penicillamine, captopril, nonsteroidal antiinflammatory agents)

Pathogenesis. **Primary membranous nephropathy is an autoimmune disease in which autoantibodies form in situ immune complexes usually with endogenous glomerular antigens.** Circulating autoantibodies against the podocyte antigen phospholipase A$_2$ receptor (PLA2R) are present in 70% to 80% of patients, and in the rest, antibodies against several other glomerular antigens have been detected, but it is not established if any of these are causative. Complement proteins are also detected; however, the mechanism for complement activation is unclear since the most common autoantibody is of the IgG4 isotype, which is a poor activator of the classical complement pathway.

MORPHOLOGY

The main histologic feature of membranous nephropathy is **diffuse thickening of the capillary wall** (Fig. 12.6A). Immunofluorescence microscopy shows **granular deposits** of immunoglobulins and complement along the GBM (Fig. 12.6B). By electron microscopy, the thickening is seen to be caused by **subepithelial deposits** between the GBM and epithelial cells; the intervening small protrusions of GBM matrix produce a **spike and dome pattern** (see Fig. 12.6B). As the disease progresses, the spikes enclose the deposits, which become incorporated into the GBM. In addition, as in other causes of nephrotic syndrome, the podocytes show **effacement of foot processes.** With further progression, glomeruli may become sclerosed.

Clinical Features. Most cases of membranous nephropathy present as nephrotic syndrome, usually without antecedent illness. In contrast to minimal change disease, the proteinuria is nonselective and usually fails to respond to corticosteroid therapy. Serologic detection of anti-PLA2R is helpful in making a diagnosis and the titer is useful in monitoring response to therapy. Membranous nephropathy follows a notoriously variable and often indolent course. Overall, although proteinuria persists in greater than 60% of patients, only about 40% progress to renal failure over a period of 2 to 20 years. An additional 10% to 30% of cases have a more benign course with partial or complete remission of proteinuria.

Membranoproliferative Glomerulonephritis

Membranoproliferative GN (MPGN) is a pattern of glomerular injury characterized by thickening of the GBM and mesangial hypercellularity. It accounts for 5% to 10% of cases of idiopathic nephrotic syndrome in children and adults. In the past, MPGN was subclassified into two types (I and II) on the basis of distinct pathologic findings. These are now recognized to be distinct entities, termed *MPGN type I*, which is defined by the presence of immune complexes, and *dense deposit disease* (formerly *MPGN type II*), in which there is complement activation without immune complexes. MPGN type I is far more common (about 80% of cases) and is the focus here. Dense deposit disease will be discussed later along with the related condition of C3 glomerulonephritis.

Pathogenesis. **Type I MPGN may be caused by deposition of circulating immune complexes or by in situ immune complex formation with a planted antigen** with activation of both classical and alternative complement pathways. In many cases, an underlying disorder can be identified, such as infection (e.g., hepatitis B and C), autoimmune disease (e.g., SLE), or monoclonal gammopathy. The disease is idiopathic in a minority of patients.

MORPHOLOGY

By light microscopy the glomeruli are large and show **hypercellularity caused by proliferation of mesangial cells and capillary endothelial cells and by infiltrating leukocytes;** these changes often accentuate the glomerular lobules (Fig. 12.7A). The GBM is thickened,

and the glomerular capillary wall often shows a double contour, or "tram track," appearance. This "splitting" of the GBM is due to its disruption by interposed mesangial and inflammatory cells and the deposition of mesangial matrix and immune complexes. By immunofluorescence microscopy, granular deposits of IgG and complement proteins are often present (Fig. 12.7B). By electron microscopy, **discrete deposits** are seen in the GBM and occasionally in the mesangium (Fig. 12.7C).

Clinical Features. Most patients with primary MPGN present as adolescents or young adults with hematuria and varying degrees of proteinuria. The disease usually follows a slowly progressive, unremitting course. Treatment with steroids, immunosuppressive agents, and antiplatelet drugs has not proven to be of any benefit. MPGN may also occur in association with other disorders (secondary MPGN), such as systemic lupus erythematosus, hepatitis B and C, chronic liver disease, and chronic bacterial infections. Indeed, many so-called "idiopathic" cases are believed to be associated with hepatitis C and related cryoglobulinemia. These secondary cases of MPGN are more common in adults; treatment of the underlying disease may resolve the kidney lesions.

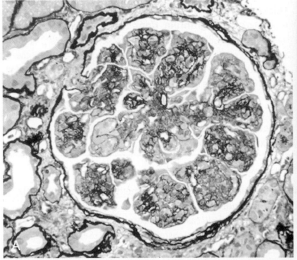
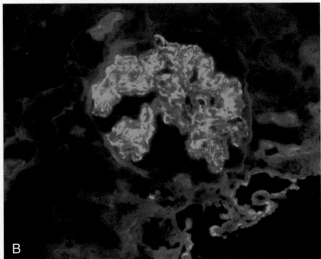
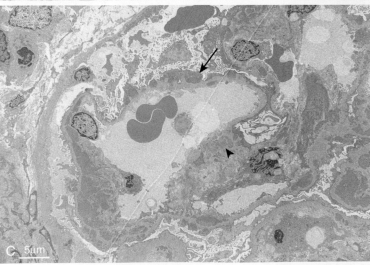

FIG. 12.7 Membranoproliferative glomerulonephritis (MPGN). (A) Mesangial cell proliferation, increased mesangial matrix (staining black with silver stain), basement membrane thickening with segmental splitting, accentuation of lobular architecture, swelling of cells lining peripheral capillaries, and influx of leukocytes (endocapillary proliferation) (silver stain). (B) Granular deposits of IgG in the GBM and mesangium. (C) Electron-dense deposits in the glomerular capillary wall between duplicated (split) basement membranes *(arrow)* and in mesangial regions *(arrowhead)*. (B, C, Courtesy of Dr. Vighnesh Walavalkar, Department of Pathology, University of California San Francisco.)

C3 Glomerulopathy

The term *C3 glomerulopathy* encompasses two conditions characterized by excessive activation of the complement system, *dense deposit disease* (formerly called *MPGN type II*), in which deposits are seen in the GBM by electron microscopy, and *C3 glomerulonephritis*, in which deposits are less prominent. These are rare diseases with shared clinical, morphologic, and pathogenic features that may represent a spectrum of injury.

Pathogenesis. **Complement dysregulation due to acquired or hereditary abnormalities of the alternative pathway of complement activation is the underlying cause of dense deposit disease and C3 GN.** Some patients have an activating autoantibody against C3 convertase, called *C3 nephritic factor (C3NeF)*, that causes uncontrolled cleavage of C3 by the alternative complement pathway. In other patients, autoantibodies to or mutations in various complement regulatory proteins, such as Factor H, Factor I, and membrane cofactor protein (MCP) are the cause of unregulated activation of the alternative pathway of complement.

MORPHOLOGY

Although glomerular changes in dense deposit disease and C3 GN vary from relatively subtle to severe, the classic light microscopic presentation is similar to that seen in MPGN type I. The glomeruli are hypercellular, the capillary walls show duplicated basement membranes, and the mesangial matrix is increased (Fig. 12.8A). By immunofluorescence microscopy, in both dense deposit disease and C3 GN there is **mesangial and glomerular capillary wall staining for C3** (Fig. 12.8B). IgG and the early components of the classical complement pathway (C1q and C4) are usually absent in both conditions. By electron microscopy, in C3 GN there are mesangial and subendothelial electron-dense "waxy" deposits (Fig. 12.8C). By contrast, in the aptly named dense deposit disease, the GBM is transformed into an irregular, ribbonlike, electron-dense structure, resulting from the deposition of C3-containing material (Fig. 12.8D).

Clinical Features. Dense deposit disease is usually seen in children and young adults, whereas C3 GN is more common in adults. In both

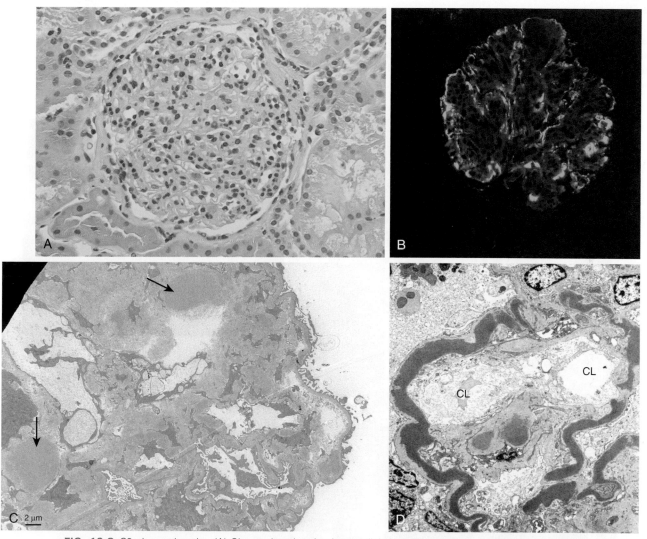

FIG. 12.8 C3 glomerulopathy. (A) Glomerulus showing hypercellularity and increased mesangial matrix. (B) Granular deposits of C3b in the GBM and mesangium. (C) "Waxy" electron-dense deposits in the mesangium *(arrows)*. (D) In dense deposit disease, there are dense homogeneous deposits within the basement membrane. (A, Courtesy of Dr. Zoltan Laszik, Department of Pathology, University of California San Francisco; C, Courtesy of Dr. Vighnesh Walavalkar, Department of Pathology, University of California San Francisco.)

diseases, patients present with variable proteinuria or hematuria and usually mild azotemia. Serum C3 levels are typically reduced. Both diseases carry a poor prognosis and almost one-third of patients progress to end-stage renal failure. The diseases tend to recur in up to 85% of patients after renal transplantation.

Disorders Presenting With the Nephritic Syndrome

Glomerular diseases that present with the nephritic syndrome are usually associated with significant inflammation in the glomeruli, which damages capillary walls, leading to leakage of red cells (hematuria), and decreased GFR, which results in oliguria and azotemia.

Acute Postinfectious Glomerulonephritis

Acute postinfectious GN is characterized by glomerular deposition of immune complexes resulting in inflammation and damage to glomeruli. The classic pattern is seen in poststreptococcal GN, but other bacterial infections, such as pneumococcus and staphylococcus, as well as viral infections, such as mumps, measles, chickenpox, and hepatitis B and C, may be the inciting event. The incidence of the disease has decreased in higher-income countries because of antibiotic treatment of the initial infection, and more than 90% of cases are now seen in lower-income countries.

Pathogenesis. **Postinfectious GN is caused by glomerular deposition of immune complexes consisting of microbial antigens and specific antibodies, resulting in complement activation by the classical pathway and subsequent inflammation.** In children, it most often follows infection by certain "nephritogenic" strains of β-hemolytic streptococci. Streptococcal antigens implicated in the formation of the complexes include streptococcal exotoxin B, a highly immunogenic protein that has been detected in the GBM deposits. In older adults, GN may develop following and even concurrent with active staphylococcal infection. Typical features of immune complex disease, such as hypocomplementemia and granular deposits of IgG and complement on the GBM, are seen. The immune complexes may be preformed circulating complexes of streptococcal antigens and antibodies that deposit in the GBM or may be formed in situ by antibody binding to streptococcal antigens deposited in the GBM.

MORPHOLOGY

By light microscopy, the most characteristic change in postinfectious GN is **increased cellularity** of the glomerular tufts that affects nearly all glomeruli—hence the term *diffuse GN* (Fig. 12.9A). The increased cellularity is caused by proliferation of endothelial and mesangial cells and by infiltrating neutrophils and monocytes. Sometimes there is necrosis of the capillary walls. In a few cases, crescents (discussed later) may be observed within the urinary space, formed in response to the severe injury. Immunofluorescence studies reveal **granular deposits of IgG and complement** within the capillary walls and some mesangial areas (Fig. 12.9B). Electron microscopy shows subendothelial, intramembranous, or, most often, **subepithelial deposits** nestled against the GBM forming "humps" (Fig. 12.9C). These deposits are usually cleared over a period of about 2 months after resolution of the infection.

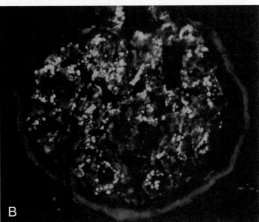

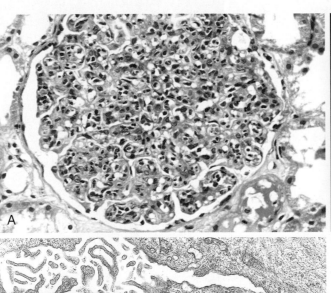

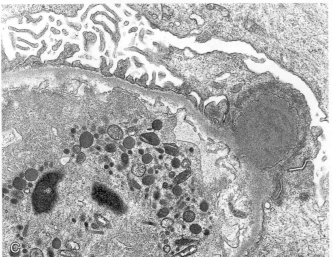

FIG. 12.9 Acute poststreptococcal glomerulonephritis. (A) Glomerular hypercellularity due to intracapillary leukocytes and possibly proliferation of intrinsic glomerular cells. (B) Immunofluorescent stain demonstrates discrete, coarsely granular deposits of IgG (and C3), corresponding to deposit seen in (C). (C) Typical electron-dense subepithelial deposit and a neutrophil in the lumen. (A, C, Courtesy of Dr. H. Rennke, Brigham and Women's Hospital, Boston. B, Courtesy of Dr. J. Kowaleska, Cedars-Sinai Medical Center, Los Angeles.)

Clinical Features. Poststreptococcal GN is a representative example of postinfectious GN. The typical case develops in a child 1 to 4 weeks after recovery from a group A streptococcal infection, but in rare instances the disease develops during the infection. In most cases, the initiating infection is localized to the pharynx or skin. The clinical presentation varies from asymptomatic to mild hematuria to acute nephritic syndrome with edema, hypertension, and mild to moderate azotemia. Some degree of proteinuria is often present, and it is occasionally severe enough to produce the nephrotic syndrome. Serum complement levels are low during the active phase of the disease, and serum anti–streptolysin O antibody titers are elevated in post-streptococcal cases.

More than 95% of affected children eventually recover renal function, but some develop rapidly progressive GN owing to severe injury with crescent formation (see later), or chronic renal disease from secondary scarring. In adults, the prognosis is more guarded, with 15% to 50% of affected individuals developing chronic renal disease over a few years or 1 to 2 decades, depending on the clinical and histologic severity.

Rapidly Progressive (Crescentic) Glomerulonephritis

Rapidly progressive GN (RPGN) is a clinical syndrome with diverse etiologies characterized by acute renal failure, features of the nephritic syndrome, and often severe oliguria. In many cases, renal biopsy reveals the presence of glomerular crescents; hence, the disease is also called *crescentic GN.*

Pathogenesis. In most cases, the glomerular injury of RPGN is immunologically mediated. Three forms are recognized:

- *Anti-GBM antibody–mediated crescentic GN* (Goodpasture disease) is characterized by linear deposits of IgG and, in many cases, C3, in the GBM (type II hypersensitivity, Chapter 5). In some patients, the anti-GBM antibodies also bind to pulmonary alveolar capillary basement membranes and lead to pulmonary hemorrhages, which, when associated with renal failure, is known as *Goodpasture syndrome* (Chapter 11).
- *Immune complex–mediated crescentic GN* may complicate any of the immune complex nephritides, including postinfectious GN, systemic lupus erythematosus, IgA nephropathy, and Henoch-Schönlein purpura. In other cases, immune complexes are demonstrated but the underlying cause is undetermined. This type of RPGN frequently shows cellular proliferation and influx of leukocytes within the glomerular tuft (proliferative GN), in addition to crescent formation. A consistent finding is the characteristic granular pattern of staining of the GBM and/or mesangium for immunoglobulin and/or complement on immunofluorescence studies.
- *Pauci-immune crescentic GN* is defined by the lack of detectable anti-GBM antibody or immune complex deposition. The presence of circulating antineutrophil cytoplasmic antibodies (PR3-ANCA) in some cases of crescentic GN suggests that these are a component of a systemic vasculitis (Chapter 8). In many cases, however, pauci-immune crescentic GN is idiopathic.

addition to crescents, cellular proliferation is seen within the capillary loops and/or in the mesangial areas in cases with immune complex-mediated pathogenesis. Immunofluorescence studies reveal the characteristic strong **linear staining** with IgG and C3 along the GBM in anti-GBM antibody-mediated disease (see Fig. 12.3B), a **granular pattern** of glomerular staining in immune complex-mediated GN, and no staining in pauci-immune GN. Electron microscopy shows electron-dense immune complex deposits within the glomeruli in immune complex—mediated GN. Electron microscopy may show **ruptures in the GBM,** signifying severe glomerular injury (Fig. 12.10B). The crescents eventually obliterate Bowman's space and over time may undergo scarring, resulting in progressive glomerulosclerosis.

Clinical Features. The onset of RPGN resembles other causes of the nephritic syndrome, but oliguria and azotemia are more pronounced. Proteinuria sometimes approaching the nephrotic range may occur.

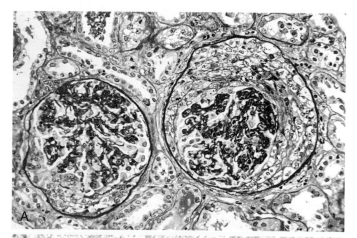

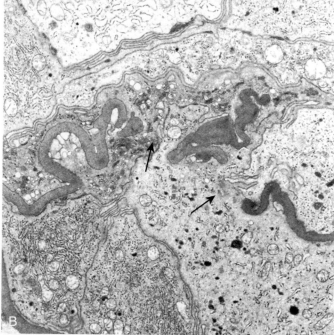

FIG. 12.10 Crescentic glomerulonephritis (A) Compressed glomerular tufts and crescent-shaped mass of proliferating epithelial cells and leukocytes within the Bowman capsule (PAS stain). (B) Electron micrograph showing characteristic wrinkling of glomerular basement membrane with focal disruptions *(arrows)*. (A, Courtesy of Dr. M. A. Venkatachalam, University of Texas Health Sciences Center, San Antonio, Texas.)

Some affected individuals become anuric and require long-term dialysis or transplantation. If untreated, RPGN can lead to renal failure within a period of weeks to months. The prognosis is roughly correlated to the fraction of involved glomeruli (patients in whom crescents are present in less than 80% of the glomeruli have a more favorable prognosis), and the severity of renal failure at diagnosis. All forms are treated with immunosuppressive agents; plasmapheresis may also benefit those with anti-GBM antibody GN and ANCA-related pauci-immune crescentic GN.

Lupus Nephritis

Systemic lupus erythematosus (SLE) is an autoimmune disease in which patients make autoantibodies against their own nuclear proteins and many other self antigens. The pathogenesis, lesions, and clinical features of the disease are discussed in Chapter 5. Much of the pathology is caused by immune complexes composed of nuclear antigens and specific antibodies; in fact, SLE is the prototype of a human systemic immune complex disease (type III hypersensitivity, Chapter 5). Glomeruli are the major site of deposition of immune complexes and bear the brunt of the lesions; the renal involvement in SLE is discussed here.

MORPHOLOGY

According to the currently accepted classification, six patterns of glomerular disease are recognized in lupus nephritis. There is overlap within these classes and lesions may evolve from one class to another over time. Thus, the exact percentage of patients with each of the six classes of lesions is difficult to determine; suffice it to say that class I is least common and class IV is most common.

- **Minimal mesangial lupus nephritis** (class I) is very uncommon and is characterized by immune complex deposition in the mesangium, identified by immunofluorescence and by electron microscopy, but without structural changes by light microscopy. This pattern is not diagnosed often because patients are usually asymptomatic and have normal urinalysis results and serum creatinine levels, so biopsy is rarely done.
- **Mesangial proliferative lupus nephritis** (class II) is characterized by mesangial cell proliferation, often accompanied by accumulation of mesangial matrix, and granular mesangial deposits of immunoglobulin and complement without involvement of glomerular capillaries. These patients may have proteinuria or microscopic hematuria but almost never develop nephrotic syndrome or renal failure.
- **Focal lupus nephritis** (class III) is defined by involvement of fewer than 50% of all glomeruli. The lesions may be segmental or global. Affected glomeruli may exhibit swelling and proliferation of endothelial and mesangial cells associated with leukocyte accumulation, capillary necrosis, and hyaline thrombi. Often, there is extracapillary proliferation associated with focal necrosis and crescent formation (Fig. 12.11A). The clinical presentation ranges from mild hematuria and proteinuria to acute renal insufficiency. Red cell casts in the urine are common when the disease is active. Some patients progress to diffuse glomerulonephritis. The active inflammatory lesions can heal completely or lead to chronic global or segmental glomerular scarring.
- **Diffuse lupus nephritis** (class IV) is the most common and most severe form of lupus nephritis. The lesions are identical to those in class III but differ in extent; in diffuse lupus nephritis, half or more of the glomeruli are affected. Involved glomeruli show proliferation of endothelial, mesangial, and epithelial cells (Fig. 12.11B), with the latter sometimes producing crescents that fill Bowman's space. Subendothelial immune complex deposits may create a circumferential thickening of the capillary wall, forming "wire-loop" structures on light microscopy (Fig. 12.11C). Immune complexes can be detected by electron microscopy (Fig. 12.11D)

and immunofluorescence (Fig. 12.11E). Lesions may progress to scarring of glomeruli. Patients with diffuse glomerulonephritis are usually symptomatic, showing hematuria as well as proteinuria. Hypertension and mild to severe renal insufficiency are also common.
- **Membranous lupus nephritis** (class V) is characterized by diffuse thickening of the capillary walls due to deposition of subepithelial immune complexes, similar to idiopathic membranous nephropathy. The immune complexes are usually accompanied by increased production of basement membrane-like material, resulting in "spikes" between the deposited immune complexes, visible by silver stain. This lesion is usually accompanied by severe proteinuria and nephrotic syndrome and may occur concurrently with focal or diffuse lupus nephritis.
- **Advanced sclerosing lupus nephritis** (class VI) is characterized by sclerosis of more than 90% of the glomeruli and represents end-stage renal disease.

Changes in the **interstitium and tubules** are frequently present. Rarely, tubulointerstitial lesions may be the dominant abnormality. Discrete immune complexes similar to those in glomeruli are present in the tubular or peritubular capillary basement membranes in many lupus nephritis patients. Sometimes, there are well-organized B-cell follicles in the interstitium, associated with plasma cells that may be sources of autoantibodies.

Clinical Features. SLE has protean clinical manifestations (Chapter 5). The renal manifestations usually present as a mixed nephrotic/nephritic picture. Patients may develop hematuria with red cell casts and proteinuria that is severe enough to produce full-blown nephrotic syndrome. Kidney involvement portends a poor prognosis, and renal failure is a frequent cause of death.

Other Glomerular Diseases

Some diseases present most often with gross or microscopic hematuria that may progress to renal failure, but without the severe proteinuria characteristic of the nephrotic syndrome or the inflammatory lesions of nephritis. Two of these entities are described next.

IgA Nephropathy

The hallmark of IgA nephropathy is the mesangial deposition of IgA-anti-IgA immune complexes. It is one of the most common causes of recurrent hematuria and is the most common primary glomerular disease revealed by renal biopsy worldwide.

Pathogenesis. **IgA nephropathy is caused by immune complexes consisting of poorly glycosylated (galactose-deficient) IgA and autoantibodies against this IgA.** A genetic component is probably involved, since more than 25% of blood relatives of patients have increased serum levels of this form of IgA. There is an increased incidence in HLA-identical siblings as well as an increased frequency of certain HLA and complement genotypes in these populations. The abnormal IgA tends to aggregate and deposit in the mesangium. Instead of galatose, this IgA contains N-acetylgalactosamine, which may be recognized as foreign and elicit an autoimmune response. IgG and IgA autoantibodies may form immune complexes with circulating IgA, which also deposit in the mesangium, where they activate the complement system and initiate glomerular injury. By itself, the deposited IgA cannot activate the classical complement pathway, and activation by the alternative and lectin pathways has been suggested. Infections increase mucosal production of IgA, accounting for the association of the disease with antecedent infection. Patients with celiac disease, in which intestinal mucosal

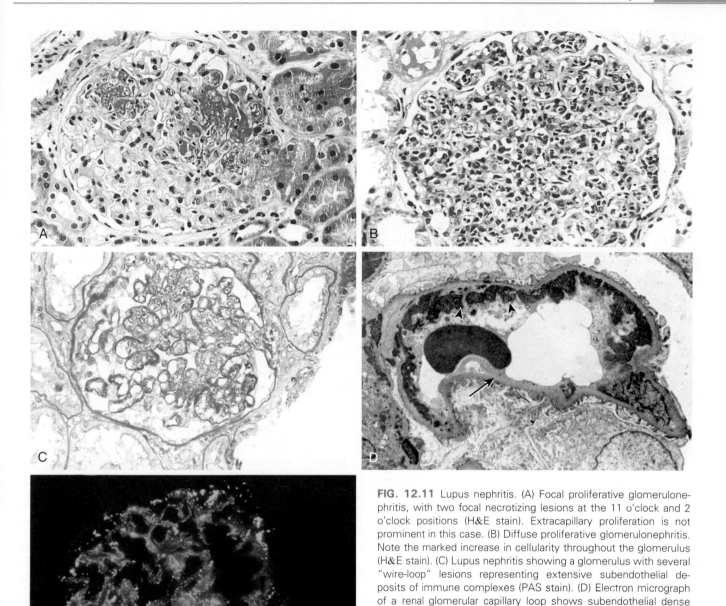

FIG. 12.11 Lupus nephritis. (A) Focal proliferative glomerulonephritis, with two focal necrotizing lesions at the 11 o'clock and 2 o'clock positions (H&E stain). Extracapillary proliferation is not prominent in this case. (B) Diffuse proliferative glomerulonephritis. Note the marked increase in cellularity throughout the glomerulus (H&E stain). (C) Lupus nephritis showing a glomerulus with several "wire-loop" lesions representing extensive subendothelial deposits of immune complexes (PAS stain). (D) Electron micrograph of a renal glomerular capillary loop shows subendothelial dense deposits *(arrowhead)* on basement membrane *(arrow)* that correspond to "wire loops" seen by light microscopy. (E) Deposition of IgG antibody in a granular pattern, detected by immunofluorescence. (A to C, Courtesy of Dr. Helmut Rennke, Department of Pathology, Brigham and Women's Hospital, Boston, Massachusetts. D, Courtesy of Dr. Edwin Eigenbrodt, Department of Pathology, University of Texas, Southwestern Medical School, Dallas, Texas. E, Courtesy of Dr. Jean Olson, Department of Pathology, University of California, San Francisco, California.)

immune responses against food antigens are common, are prone to IgA nephropathy, as are patients with liver disease in which there is defective hepatobiliary clearance of IgA complexes.

MORPHOLOGY

Histologically, the lesions in IgA nephropathy vary considerably. The glomeruli may appear normal or may show any of the following: mesangial widening and hypercellularity (Fig. 12.12A); segmental inflammation confined to some glomeruli (focal proliferative GN); diffuse mesangial proliferation (mesangioproliferative GN); or (rarely) overt crescentic GN. The characteristic immunofluorescence picture is of **mesangial deposition of IgA** (Fig. 12.12B), often with C3 and the alternative pathway protein properdin and smaller amounts of IgG or IgM. Early components of the classical complement pathway are usually absent. Electron microscopy confirms the presence of dense mesangial deposits.

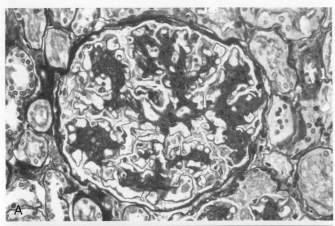

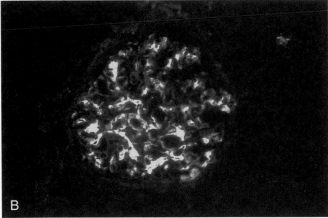

FIG. 12.12 IgA nephropathy. (A) Light microscopy showing mesangial proliferation and matrix increase. (B) Characteristic deposition of IgA, principally in mesangial regions, detected by immunofluorescence.

Clinical Features. IgA nephropathy most often affects children and young adults. The classic presentation of IgA nephropathy is macroscopic hematuria after an infection of the respiratory or, less commonly, gastrointestinal or urinary tract, seen in 40% to 50% of patients, especially those under the age of 40; 30% to 40% of patients have asymptomatic microscopic hematuria. The course is highly variable. The hematuria typically lasts for several days and initially subsides but then recurs periodically, usually in the setting of a viral infection. Less than 10% of patients present with nephrotic syndrome or rapidly progressive GN. Many patients maintain normal renal function for decades but slow progression to end-stage renal disease occurs in 25% to 50% of cases over a period of 20 years. Recurrence of IgA deposits in transplanted kidneys is frequent.

Hereditary Nephritis

Hereditary nephritis refers to a group of glomerular diseases caused by mutations in genes encoding type IV collagen, the major GBM protein. The most common of these rare diseases are *Alport syndrome* and *thin basement membrane disease.* In Alport syndrome, nephritis is accompanied by sensorineural deafness and various eye disorders, including lens dislocation, posterior cataracts, and corneal dystrophy. Thin basement membrane disease is the most common cause of benign familial hematuria.

Pathogenesis. Alport syndrome is most often an X-linked disease caused by mutations in the *COL4A5* gene on the X chromosome,

which encodes the α5 chain of type IV collagen, a major component of the GBM. Rare autosomal recessive or dominant forms are linked to defects in the genes that encode the α3 or α4 chains of type IV collagen. Type IV collagen is also crucial for maintaining the structure of the cochlea and lens, explaining the association of Alport syndrome with deafness and eye disorders. In 40% of patients, thin basement membrane disease is associated with heterozygous mutations in the genes encoding the α3 and α4 chains; the cause is unknown in the remainder.

MORPHOLOGY

In Alport disease, there are no specific lesions on histologic examination but electron microscopy reveals a **thin, attenuated GBM** early in the course that, over time, develops irregular foci of thickening and thinning with pronounced splitting and lamination of the lamina densa, giving rise to a "basketweave" appearance (eFig. 12.1). Immunohistochemical staining demonstrates the absence of type IV collagen in the GBM. In contrast to Alport syndrome, uniform thinning of the GBM is the only morphologic finding in thin basement membrane disease.

Clinical Features. Individuals with hereditary nephritis present at 5 to 20 years of age with gross or microscopic hematuria and proteinuria and progress to overt renal failure by the age of 20 to 50 years. Due to the prevalence of X-linked disease, Alport syndrome is most common in males, who are also at higher risk for end-stage renal disease and deafness than affected females. Individuals with thin basement membrane disease usually present with persistent asymptomatic hematuria and follow a benign, nonprogressive course.

DISEASES AFFECTING TUBULES AND INTERSTITIUM

Most forms of tubular injury also involve the interstitium, so the two are considered together. There are three major categories of these diseases: (1) infection of the kidney and urinary tract (*pyelonephritis*), (2) other (noninfectious) inflammation involving the tubules and interstitium (*tubulointerstitial nephritis*), and (3) ischemic or toxic tubular injury, leading to *acute tubular injury* and the clinical syndrome of *acute kidney injury.*

Acute Pyelonephritis

Acute pyelonephritis is suppurative inflammation of the kidney and the renal pelvis caused by bacterial infection. It is an important manifestation of urinary tract infection (UTI), which can involve the lower urinary tract (cystitis, prostatitis, urethritis) or upper urinary tract (pyelonephritis), or both. The majority of cases of pyelonephritis are associated with infections of the lower urinary tract, most of which remain localized and do not spread to the kidney.

Pathogenesis. **The principal causative organisms in acute pyelonephritis are enteric gram-negative bacilli that are normal inhabitants of the intestinal tract.** *Escherichia coli* is by far the most common; others include *Proteus, Klebsiella, Enterobacter,* and *Pseudomonas.* Recurrent infections may occur, especially in individuals who undergo urinary tract manipulations or have congenital or acquired anomalies of the lower urinary tract (see later).

Ascending infection from the lower urinary tract is the most important and frequent route by which bacteria reach the kidney (Fig. 12.13). Less commonly, infection is hematogenous (e.g., secondary to sepsis or bacterial endocarditis). Pyelonephritis is

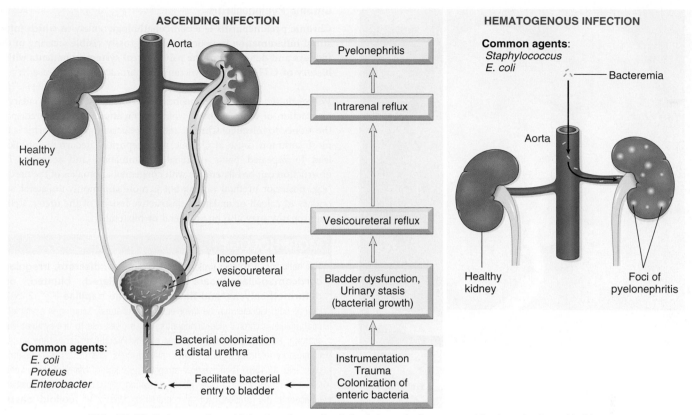

ASCENDING INFECTION

Aorta

Pyelonephritis

Intrarenal reflux

Healthy kidney

Incompetent vesicoureteral valve

Vesicoureteral reflux

Bladder dysfunction, Urinary stasis (bacterial growth)

Common agents:
E. coli
Proteus
Enterobacter

Bacterial colonization at distal urethra

Facilitate bacterial entry to bladder

Instrumentation Trauma Colonization of enteric bacteria

HEMATOGENOUS INFECTION

Common agents:
Staphylococcus
E. coli

Bacteremia

Aorta

Healthy kidney

Foci of pyelonephritis

FIG. 12.13 Pathways of renal infection. Ascending infection results from a combination of urinary bladder infection, vesicoureteral reflux, and intrarenal reflux and spreads from calyces into the renal cortex. Hematogenous infection, which is less common, results from bacteremic spread, leading to foci of pyelonephritis that may develop into abscesses.

more common in women because the proximity of the female urethra to the rectum predisposes to colonization by enteric bacteria. Adhesion of bacteria to mucosal surfaces is followed by colonization of the distal urethra (and the introitus in females). Further growth may allow the organisms to reach the bladder, a pathway of spread that may be enhanced by procedures such as urethral instrumentation, including catheterization and cystoscopy. The bacteria then ascend along the ureters to infect the renal pelvis and parenchyma.

Normally, bladder urine is sterile because of the antimicrobial properties of the bladder mucosa and the flushing mechanism associated with periodic voiding of urine. Outflow obstruction and bladder dysfunction produce stasis, allowing bacteria to multiply undisturbed, without being flushed out. Hence, UTI is particularly frequent among patients with urinary tract obstruction, as may occur with benign prostatic hyperplasia and uterine prolapse. The frequency of UTI is also increased in diabetes because of the increased susceptibility to infection and neurogenic bladder dysfunction, which can lead to urine stasis, and during pregnancy, due to urine stasis caused by pressure exerted on the bladder and ureters by the enlarging uterus.

Incompetence of the vesicoureteral valve, resulting in vesicoureteral reflux (VUR), is an important cause of ascending infection. The reflux allows bacteria to ascend the ureter into the renal pelvis. VUR is present in 20% to 40% of young children with UTI, usually due to a congenital defect that results in incompetence of the ureterovesical valve. VUR can also be acquired in individuals with a flaccid bladder resulting from spinal cord injury or with

bladder dysfunction secondary to diabetes. VUR results in residual urine in the bladder after voiding, which favors bacterial growth. Furthermore, VUR affords a ready mechanism by which infected bladder urine can be propelled into the renal pelvis and renal parenchyma. Additional risk factors for acute pyelonephritis include preexisting renal conditions with renal scarring and intraparenchymal obstruction and also immunosuppressive therapy and immunodeficiency.

MORPHOLOGY

One or both kidneys may be involved. The affected kidney may be normal in size or enlarged. Typically, **discrete, yellowish, raised abscesses** are grossly apparent on the renal surface (Fig. 12.14A). The characteristic histologic feature is **neutrophil-rich inflammation** initially limited to tubules (Fig. 12.14B) and later spreading to the interstitium. Neutrophils may extend from the tubules into the collecting ducts, giving rise to white blood cell casts in the urine. Typically, the glomeruli are not affected.

When obstruction is prominent, pus does not drain and may fill the renal pelvis, calyces, and ureter, producing **pyonephrosis.**

Papillary necrosis is a rare form of pyelonephritis seen in patients with three predisposing conditions: diabetes, urinary tract obstruction, and sickle cell anemia. This lesion is marked by ischemic and suppurative necrosis of the tips of the renal papillae (eFig. 12.2).

Clinical Features. Acute pyelonephritis is often associated with predisposing conditions, as described earlier under Pathogenesis. After

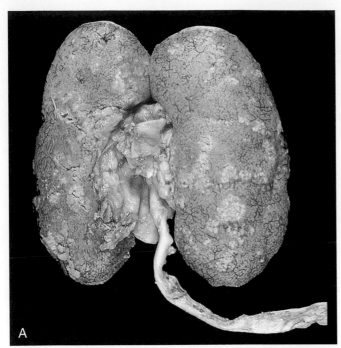

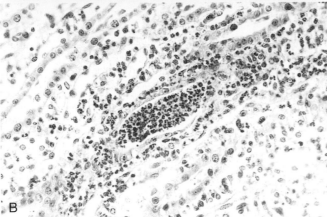

FIG. 12.14 Acute pyelonephritis. (A) The cortical surface shows grayish white areas of inflammation and abscess formation. (B) Neutrophilic exudates within tubules and interstitium.

the first year of life (by which time congenital anomalies in males are usually diagnosed) and up to approximately 40 years of age, infections are much more frequent in females. Up to 6% of pregnant women develop bacteriuria sometime during pregnancy, and 20% to 40% of these women eventually develop UTI if not treated. With increasing age, the incidence in males rises as a result of the development of prostatic hyperplasia and attendant bladder obstruction.

The onset of uncomplicated acute pyelonephritis is usually sudden, with pain at the costovertebral angle and systemic evidence of infection (chills, fever, nausea, and malaise), and localizing urinary tract signs (dysuria, frequency, and urgency). The urine may appear turbid due to abundant neutrophils (*pyuria*). The disease is usually unilateral and hence does not give rise to renal failure. When predisposing factors are present, the disease may become recurrent or chronic and is more likely to be bilateral. The development of papillary necrosis is associated with a worse prognosis.

Chronic Pyelonephritis

Chronic pyelonephritis is a clinicopathologic entity in which interstitial inflammation is associated with grossly visible scarring of the kidneys and deformity of the pelvicalyceal system in patients with a history of UTI. It is a known cause of chronic kidney disease.

Pathogenesis. Chronic pyelonephritis develops most often secondary to obstruction or reflux, both of which, as mentioned earlier, predispose the kidney to infection. Chronic reflux—associated pyelonephritis is the most common cause of chronic pyelonephritis. Recurrent infections lead to repeated bouts of renal inflammation and scarring. The obstruction can be bilateral, as with congenital anomalies of the urethra (e.g., posterior urethral valves), but is more commonly unilateral, secondary to calculi or unilateral obstructive lesions of the ureter. Reflux nephropathy may also be unilateral or bilateral.

MORPHOLOGY

The hallmark of chronic pyelonephritis is **coarse, discrete, irregular corticomedullary scars overlying dilated, blunted, or deformed calyces, and flattening of the papillae** (Fig. 12.15A). One or both kidneys may be involved. When bilateral, scarring is asymmetrical, unlike in chronic glomulonephritis, which gives rise to fine symmetrical scarring. Microscopic changes include patchy interstitial fibrosis and an inflammatory infiltrate of lymphocytes, plasma cells, and occasionally neutrophils (Fig. 12.15B). Tubules show atrophy and dilation. Many of the dilated tubules contain pink to blue, glassy-appearing casts that are PAS-positive (indicating the presence of glycoproteins), known as **colloid casts** because they resemble the colloid inside thyroid follicles (Chapter 18). Glomeruli are normal or show variable sclerosis.

Clinical Features. Many patients with chronic pyelonephritis present with gradual onset of renal insufficiency while others have signs of kidney disease detected on routine laboratory tests. In some cases, hypertension may be the presenting symptom. Radiologic studies show that affected kidneys are asymmetrically contracted, with variable blunting and deformity of the calyces. Bacteria may or may not be detected in the urine. If the disease is bilateral and progressive, tubular dysfunction leads to an inability to concentrate the urine (*hyposthenuria*), manifested by polyuria and nocturia.

As noted earlier, some individuals with chronic pyelonephritis or reflux nephropathy ultimately develop secondary glomerulosclerosis, associated with proteinuria; eventually, these injuries all contribute to progression of chronic kidney disease.

Tubulointerstitial Nephritis

Tubulointerstitial nephritis (TIN) is a generic term for noninfectious inflammatory kidney diseases that primarily involve the interstitium and tubules. Although pyelonephritis also involves these structures, it is considered a separate entity because of its association with ascending bacterial infections. TIN may be caused by immune reactions to drugs, irradiation, some infections, and systemic autoimmune disorders.

Drug-Induced Tubulointerstitial Nephritis

Acute drug-induced TIN occurs as an adverse reaction to a variety of drugs. It is associated most frequently with penicillins (ampicillin), other antibiotics (rifampin), diuretics (furosemide), proton pump inhibitors (omeprazole), nonsteroidal antiinflammatory agents, cimetidine and immune checkpoint inhibitors.

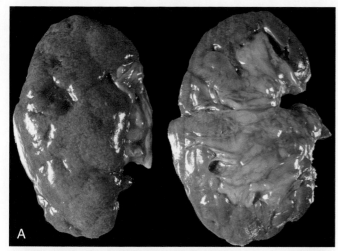

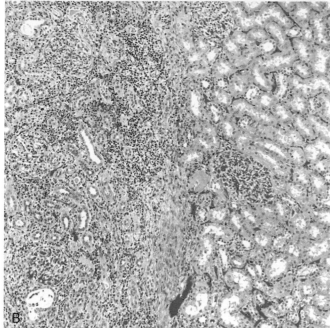

FIG. 12.15 Chronic pyelonephritis. (A) Shrunken kidney with irregular, coarse scars. (B) Focus of chronic inflammation with tubular atrophy and interstitial fibrosis (*left* part of micrograph).

Pathogenesis. Many features of the disease suggest a hypersensitivity reaction, including a latent period between drug exposure and lesion development, eosinophilia and rash; the idiosyncratic nature of the drug reaction (i.e., the lack of dose dependence); and the recurrence of the reaction upon reexposure to the same or other similar drugs. Serum IgE levels are sometimes increased, suggesting immediate (type I) hypersensitivity. In other cases, the nature of the inflammatory infiltrate and the presence of positive skin tests to drugs suggest a T cell–mediated (type IV) hypersensitivity reaction.

The most likely sequence of pathogenic events is that the drugs are secreted by tubules and covalently bind to some cytoplasmic or extracellular component of tubular cells, creating immunogenic neoantigens. The resultant tubulointerstitial injury is then caused by immune reactions to these neoantigens that injure tubular cells or their basement membranes.

The interstitium shows pronounced edema and infiltration by mononuclear cells, principally lymphocytes and macrophages (Fig. 12.16). Eosinophils and neutrophils may be present, often in large numbers. With some drugs (e.g., thiazides, rifampin), a T cell–mediated reaction may give rise to interstitial nonnecrotizing granulomas with giant cells. The glomeruli appear normal except in some cases caused by nonsteroidal antiinflammatory agents, in which the hypersensitivity reaction also leads to podocyte foot process effacement and the nephrotic syndrome.

Clinical Features. The disease begins 1 to 2 weeks after exposure to the drug and is characterized by fever, eosinophilia (which may be transient), rash (in 15% to 25% of individuals), and renal dysfunction. Urinary findings include hematuria, minimal or no proteinuria, and presence of white cells (sometimes including eosinophils). A rising serum creatinine or acute kidney injury with oliguria develops in about 50% of cases, particularly in older patients. Clinical recognition of drug-induced kidney injury is imperative, because withdrawal of the offending drug is followed by recovery, although it may take several months for renal function to return to normal.

Acute Tubular Injury

Acute tubular injury (ATI) is characterized by damage to tubular epithelial cells and an acute decline in renal function, often associated with shedding of granular casts and tubular cells into the urine. The older term *acute tubular necrosis* is not used because frank necrosis is rarely seen in the kidney. The constellation of changes, broadly termed *acute kidney injury,* manifests clinically as decreased GFR and concurrent elevation of serum creatinine. ATI is the most common cause of acute kidney injury and may produce oliguria (defined as urine output of <400 mL/day).

Pathogenesis. There are two forms of ATI that differ in their underlying causes but result in similar outcomes (Fig. 12.17).

- *Ischemic ATI* is most often the result of inadequate blood flow to the kidney, often in the setting of marked hypotension and shock. Initiating events include severe trauma, blood loss, acute pancreatitis, and septicemia. Ischemia to tubules may also result from reduced intrarenal blood flow, as in small vessel vasculitis, malignant hypertension, and thrombotic microangiopathies. Mismatched blood transfusions and other hemolytic crises, as well as myoglobinuria, also produce a clinical picture resembling that of ischemic ATI.
- *Nephrotoxic ATI* is caused by a variety of poisons, including heavy metals (e.g., mercury) and organic chemicals (e.g., ethylene glycol), a multitude of drugs such as gentamicin and other antibiotics, and radiographic contrast agents.

Proximal tubular epithelial cells are particularly sensitive to ischemia and toxins because of several factors, including elevated intracellular concentrations of various molecules that are resorbed in the proximal tubule, exposure to high concentrations of luminal solutes that are concentrated by the resorption of water from the glomerular filtrate, and a high rate of oxygen consumption, which is required to generate the ATP that is needed for transport and reabsorption functions.

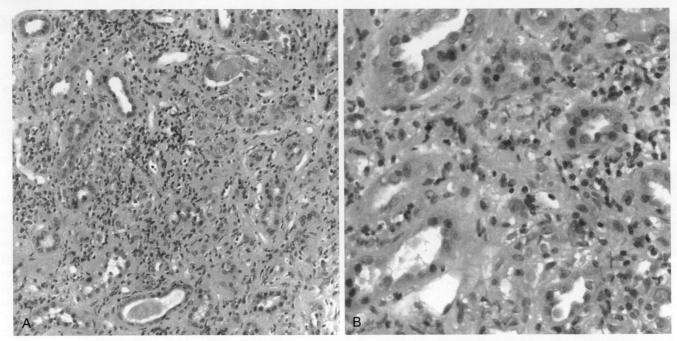

FIG. 12.16 Drug-induced tubulointerstitial nephritis. (A) Chronic inflammatory infiltrate in the interstitium with tubular injury. (B) Prominent eosinophilic infiltrate.

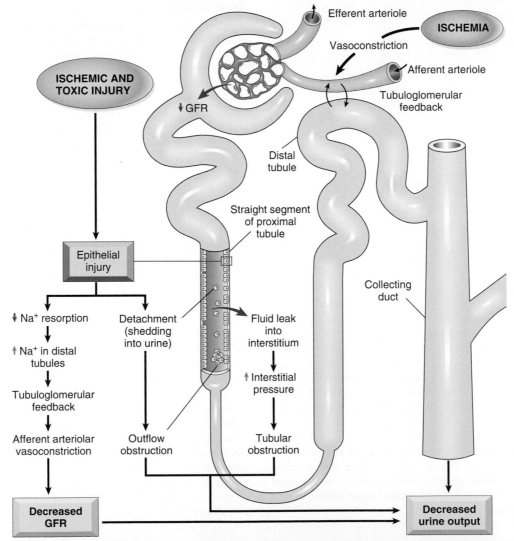

FIG. 12.17 Postulated sequence in ischemic and toxic acute tubular injury. Injury to tubular epithelium leads to decreased glomerular filtration rate (GFR) and obstruction to tubules, resulting in decreased urine output (oliguria and ultimately anuria).

Ischemia and toxins damage the plasma membrane of tubular epithelial cells, resulting in decreased sodium reabsorption by proximal tubules and hence increased sodium delivery to distal tubules. This triggers a tubuloglomerular feedback mechanism involving the renin-angiotensin pathway that causes *intrarenal vasoconstriction,* which decreases glomerular blood flow and oxygen delivery to the tubules in the outer medulla (thick ascending limb and straight segment of the proximal tubule). The reduced GFR further decreases blood flow and causes more ischemic tubular injury. Necrosis and detachment of epithelial cells from the basement membranes and their shedding into the urine can block the outflow of urine, increasing intratubular pressure and thereby exacerbating the decline in GFR. Additionally, fluid from the damaged tubules may leak back into the interstitium, resulting in decreased urine output, increased interstitial pressure, and collapse of the tubules.

If the precipitating cause is corrected, the patchiness of tubular necrosis and the maintained integrity of the basement membrane allow regeneration of preserved epithelial cells and recovery of function. If the injury is prolonged and severe, the acute lesions may progress to chronic kidney disease.

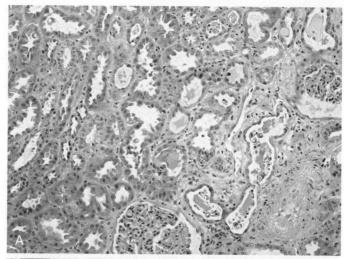

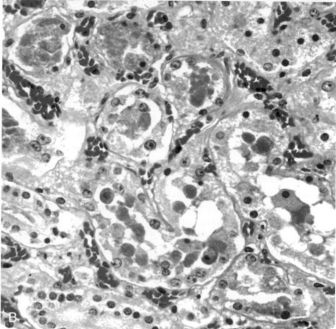

FIG. 12.18 Acute tubular injury. (A) Detachment of tubular epithelial cells from their underlying basement membranes, and granular casts. (B) Necrotic tubular epithelial cells and cellular debris in tubular lumens. Congestion of peritubular capillaries is prominent.

MORPHOLOGY

Ischemic ATI is characterized by lesions in the straight portions of the proximal tubule and the ascending thick limbs, but no segment of the proximal or distal tubules is spared. There is often a variety of **tubular alterations,** including attenuation of proximal tubular brush borders, blebbing and sloughing of brush borders, vacuolization of cells, and detachment and sloughing of epithelial cells from their underlying basement membranes into the lumen (Fig. 12.18). A common finding is the presence of **proteinaceous casts** in the distal tubules and collecting ducts, which consist of Tamm-Horsfall protein (normally secreted by tubular epithelium) and plasma proteins. The interstitium usually shows generalized edema along with a mild inflammatory infiltrate consisting of neutrophils, lymphocytes, and plasma cells. The histologic picture of **nephrotoxic ATI** is similar, but overt necrosis is usually more prominent in the proximal tubule than in ischemic ATI. Regenerating tubular epithelial cells may contain mitotic figures.

Clinical Features. The course of ischemic ATI is initially dominated by the inciting event. Affected patients often present with manifestations of acute kidney injury, including oliguria, decreased GFR, and increased serum creatinine. Electrolyte abnormalities, acidosis, and the signs and symptoms of uremia and fluid overload are common complications. The prognosis depends on the severity and nature of the underlying injury and the presence or absence of comorbid conditions. In the absence of supportive treatment or dialysis, patients may die. With supportive care, patients usually survive and have a good chance of recovering renal function. During the early phase of recovery there is diuresis with loss of electrolytes because the tubular epithelium has not fully recovered. In those with pre-existing chronic kidney disease, complete recovery is less frequent, and progression to end-stage renal disease is unfortunately common.

DISEASES INVOLVING BLOOD VESSELS

Systemic vascular diseases, such as atherosclerosis, hypertension, and various forms of vasculitis, also affect renal blood vessels and often have deleterious effects on renal function (Chapter 8). Conversely, the kidney is involved in the pathogenesis of both primary and secondary hypertension. This section covers the renal lesions associated with hypertension.

Hypertensive Renal Disease

Systemic hypertension has significant pathologic and functional effects on the kidneys. As discussed in Chapter 8, long-standing hypertension has been called essential or benign, but the term *primary hypertension* is now preferred. A small fraction of these patients develops rapid increases in blood pressure that cause organ damage, so-called *malignant hypertension,* a medical emergency. The renal manifestations of chronic and malignant hypertension are similar but with some significant differences.

Pathogenesis. The arterial lesions associated with primary hypertension are the result mainly of endothelial dysfunction and platelet activation (Chapter 8).

- Long-standing hypertension causes *endothelial injury*, leading to increased permeability of the vessels to plasma proteins and platelet deposition. Growth factors produced by platelets and other cells stimulate proliferation of vascular smooth muscle cells and synthesis of extracellular matrix proteins, resulting in medial and intimal thickening. Hemodynamic effects of high blood pressure and aging may exacerbate these changes.
- Platelets deposited on the injured endothelium are activated to produce growth factors and may trigger repeated bouts of thrombus formation.

The extravasation of plasma proteins through injured endothelium and increased deposition of basement membrane matrix in the vessel wall lead to the morphologic alteration known as *hyaline arteriosclerosis*. The narrowing of blood vessels causes ischemia with subsequent tubular atrophy and interstitial fibrosis (scarring), producing changes in the gross appearance of the kidney called *nephrosclerosis*. Nephrosclerosis may develop in any disease in which chronic ischemia leads to atrophy and fibrosis. Some degree of nephrosclerosis, albeit mild, is present in many individuals older than 60 years of age. The frequency and severity of these lesions increase with age, especially when hypertension or diabetes is present. Many primary renal diseases cause hypertension; hence, nephrosclerosis is often superimposed on other primary kidney diseases.

In patients with severe "malignant" hypertension, the proliferation of vascular smooth muscle cells produces a morphologic appearance known as *hyperplastic arteriosclerosis*. In addition, the vascular injury may be sufficient to produce *fibrinoid necrosis* of arterioles and small arteries associated with intravascular thrombosis.

The ischemia caused by these vascular alterations activates the renin-angiotensin system, which functions to increase vascular tone and systemic blood pressure. Thus, hypertension acts on the kidneys to cause more hypertension, setting up a vicious cycle.

There is considerable clinical and morphologic overlap between severe hypertension and thrombotic microangiopathy (TMA, discussed later). However, the best-defined forms of primary TMA result from inherited or acquired abnormalities in coagulation or platelets that are not associated with hypertension, so these entities are pathogenically distinct.

MORPHOLOGY

In nephrosclerosis caused by long-standing hypertension, the kidneys are **symmetrically atrophic**. Typically, the renal surface shows diffuse, fine granularity (Fig. 12.19A). Microscopically, a prominent change is homogeneous, pink hyaline thickening of the arteriole walls, known as **hyaline arteriosclerosis**, with loss of underlying cellular detail and narrowing of vessel lumina (Fig. 12.19B). Diffuse tubular atrophy and interstitial fibrosis are present, but inflammatory infiltrates are absent or scant (Fig. 12.19C). In advanced cases, the glomeruli also become sclerosed. Larger blood vessels (interlobar and arcuate arteries) show intimal thickening with replication of internal elastic lamina along with fibrous thickening of the media.

In patients with malignant hypertension, the kidneys may be normal in size or shrunken, depending on the duration and severity of the hypertension. Small, **pinpoint petechial hemorrhages** may appear on the cortical surface from rupture of arterioles or glomerular capillaries, giving the kidney a **flea-bitten appearance**. Damage to the small vessels is manifested as **fibrinoid necrosis** of the arterioles (Fig. 12.20A). The vessel walls show a homogeneous, granular eosinophilic appearance masking underlying detail. In the interlobular arteries and larger arterioles, marked proliferation of intimal

cells produces an "onion-skin" appearance (Fig. 12.20B). This lesion, called **hyperplastic arteriosclerosis**, causes narrowing and even obliteration of arterioles and small arteries. Necrosis may also involve glomeruli, sometimes with microthrombi within the glomeruli.

Clinical Features. Most patients with long-standing hypertension show some functional renal impairment, such as loss of urine concentrating ability or a diminished GFR. Mild proteinuria is a frequent finding, but renal failure or uremia is rare. However, people with severe blood pressure elevations or a second underlying disease, especially diabetes, are at increased risk of renal failure. There are reports of a higher prevalence of this condition in persons of African descent in the United States and South Africa.

The full-blown syndrome of malignant hypertension is characterized by papilledema, encephalopathy, cardiovascular abnormalities, and renal failure. Most often, the early symptoms are related to increased intracranial pressure and include headache, nausea, vomiting, and visual impairment, particularly the development of scotomas or "spots". At the onset of rapidly mounting blood pressure, there is marked proteinuria and microscopic, or sometimes macroscopic, hematuria, but no significant alteration in renal function. Soon, however, acute kidney injury develops. The syndrome is a medical emergency that requires prompt and aggressive antihypertensive therapy before irreversible renal lesions develop. About 50% of patients survive at least 5 years; 90% of deaths are caused by uremia, and the other 10% are caused by cerebral hemorrhage or cardiac failure.

Thrombotic Microangiopathies

The term thrombotic microangiopathy (TMA) refers to lesions seen in various clinical syndromes characterized by microvascular thrombosis accompanied by microangiopathic hemolytic anemia, thrombocytopenia, and, in some cases, renal failure. The disorder may be primary (with no other underlying disease) or secondary to other known diseases. Primary forms of TMA include *Shiga toxin–mediated hemolytic uremic syndrome (HUS); complement-mediated TMA*, previously known as *atypical HUS*; *thrombotic thrombocytopenic purpura (TTP)*; and some of the *drug-mediated TMAs*.

Pathogenesis. **The major pathogenic factors in the thrombotic microangiopathies are endothelial cell injury and platelet activation and aggregation.** They can be caused by diverse insults, including external toxins, drugs, autoantibodies, and inherited mutations, all of which lead to small vessel thrombosis in the capillaries and arterioles of various organs. Vascular insufficiency results in ischemic injury and organ dysfunction. The classic manifestations of thrombotic microangiopathy are platelet-rich thrombi in small vessels, thrombocytopenia caused by platelet consumption, and microangiopathic hemolytic anemia due to mechanical injury (shearing) of red cells as they pass through vascular channels narrowed by thrombi. The secondary forms are associated with various underlying disorders, such as severe hypertension, systemic sclerosis, pregnancy, chemotherapy, antiphospholipid antibodies, and transplant rejection, with less well-defined etiology and pathogenesis. Only the three major forms of primary thrombotic microangiopathies (Table 12.4) are discussed here.

- *Shiga toxin—mediated HUS.* As many as 75% of cases follow intestinal infection with Shiga toxin—producing *E. coli*, such as occurs following ingestion of contaminated food (e.g., beef). Many of the remaining cases are linked to infection with *Shigella dysenteriae*,

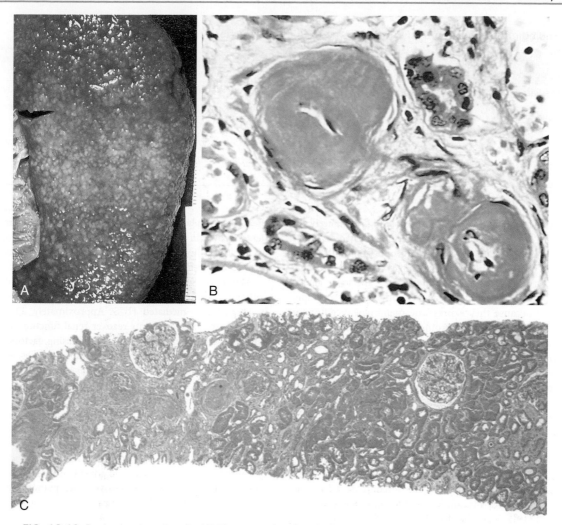

FIG. 12.19 Benign nephrosclerosis. (A) The external surface is finely granular because of scarring. (B) Two arterioles with hyaline deposition, marked thickening of the walls, and a narrowed lumen. (C) Tubular atrophy resulting from vascular narrowing, and interstitial fibrosis (stained blue). (B, Courtesy of Dr. M. A. Venkatachalam, Department of Pathology, University of Texas Health Sciences Center, San Antonio, Texas; C, Courtesy of Dr. Vighnesh Walavalkar, Department of Pathology, University of California San Francisco.)

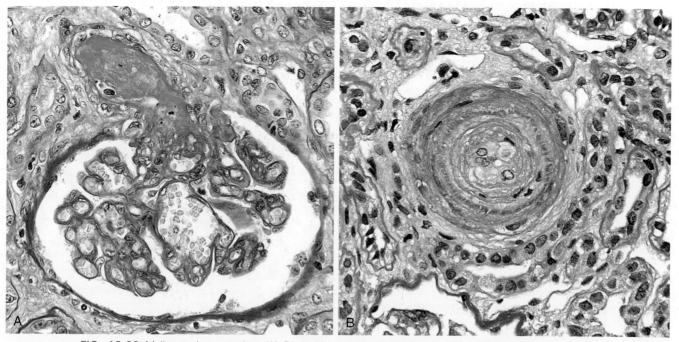

FIG. 12.20 Malignant hypertension. (A) Fibrinoid necrosis of afferent arteriole. (B) Hyperplastic arteriolosclerosis (onion-skin lesion), typically seen in cases with long-standing hypertension.

Table 12.4 Etiologic Classification of the Major Forms of Primary Thrombotic Microangiopathy

	Forms	Etiology
Shiga toxin–mediated HUS	Acquired	Shiga toxin–producing *E. coli*, *Shigella dysenteriae* serotype 1
Complement-mediated TMA	Inherited	Complement dysregulation due to genetic abnormalities (relatively common)
	Acquired	Acquired complement dysregulation due to autoantibodies (rare)
TTP	Inherited	Genetic ADAMTS13 deficiency (rare)
	Acquired	ADAMTS13 deficiency due to autoantibodies (relatively common)

ADAMTS13, A disintegrin and metalloproteinase with a thrombospondin type 1 motif, member 13; *HUS,* hemolytic uremic syndrome; *TMA,* thrombotic microangiopathy; *TTP,* thrombotic thrombocytopenic purpura.

which also produces Shiga toxin. At low doses, Shiga toxin activates endothelial cells, leading to leukocyte adhesion, increased endothelin production, and decreased nitric oxide production (both favoring vasoconstriction), as well as other changes that may promote platelet adhesion and activation. At high doses, the toxin causes endothelial cell death. Renal glomerular endothelial cells are especially vulnerable because they express the membrane receptor for Shiga toxin. Endothelial injury promotes microvascular thrombosis, which tends to be most prominent in glomerular capillaries, afferent arterioles, and interlobular arteries.

- *Complement-mediated TMA* is caused by acquired or hereditary abnormalities of factors that negatively regulate the alternative pathway of complement. Their absence leads to excessive activation of complement, with ensuing microvascular injury and microvascular thrombosis. Some of these cases were earlier grouped under "atypical HUS."
- *TTP* is caused by acquired or inherited deficiencies in ADAMTS13 a plasma protease that cleaves von Willebrand factor (vWF) multimers into smaller sizes (Chapter 10). Acquired defects in ADAMTS13 are caused by inhibitory autoantibodies directed against ADAMTS13, while inherited deficiencies stem from mutations in the gene encoding ADAMTS13. Deficiencies of ADAMTS13 result in the formation of abnormally large vWF multimers that activate platelets spontaneously, leading to platelet aggregation and thrombosis in multiple organs, including the kidney.

MORPHOLOGY

The morphologic lesions are similar in all forms of TMA. **Thrombi** are seen in glomerular capillaries (Fig. 12.21), arterioles, and sometimes the larger arteries in severe cases. Additional glomerular changes in HUS resulting from endothelial injury include widening of the subendothelial space, duplication or splitting of the GBM, and lysis of mesangial cells. Cortical necrosis may occur in severe cases. If TMA persists, scarring of glomeruli may develop. Except for varying amounts of fibrinogen in the glomeruli and arterioles, immunofluorescence studies are typically negative for immunoglobulins and complement.

Clinical Features. The principal clinical manifestations of TMA are fever, thrombocytopenia, hemolytic anemia, transient neurologic deficits, and renal failure. Shiga toxin–associated HUS is one of the main causes of acute kidney injury in children. It is characterized by the sudden onset, usually after a gastrointestinal or flulike prodromal episode, of bleeding manifestations (especially hematemesis and melena), severe oliguria, hematuria, microangiopathic hemolytic anemia, and (in some individuals) prominent neurologic changes. If

the acute kidney injury is managed properly with dialysis, most patients recover in a matter of weeks. The long-term prognosis (over 15 to 25 years), however, is not uniformly favorable, as about 25% of affected children eventually develop renal insufficiency.

The onset of complement-mediated TMA is usually sudden, without prodromal diarrhea. The outcome is significantly poorer than in Shiga toxin–mediated HUS. Approximately 20% succumb, and only 60% to 70% of patients recover renal function. Plasma exchange can be used to temporarily restore missing factors (in those with inherited disease) or remove pathogenic antibodies. An antibody that blocks complement activation is effective in reducing thrombosis and improving renal function and is now the first-line therapy in complement-mediated HUS.

The typical onset of TTP is also sudden, with a dominant involvement of the central nervous system; the kidneys are less commonly involved than in Shiga toxin– and complement-mediated HUS. Without therapy, TTP is usually rapidly fatal, with survival rates of approximately 10%. With the advent of plasma exchange therapy, which replaces ADAMTS13 and removes pathogenic antibodies, the prognosis has improved dramatically. In those who survive, residual renal abnormalities are rare.

CHRONIC KIDNEY DISEASE

Chronic kidney disease is a term that describes a final common pathway of progressive nephron loss that can be seen in any type of severe renal disease. Alterations in the function of remaining intact nephrons eventually become maladaptive and cause further scarring.

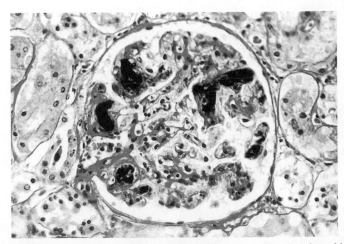

FIG. 12.21 Thrombotic microangiopathy. Fibrin stain showing thrombi *(red)* in the glomerular capillaries.

This ultimately results in an end-stage kidney with sclerosed glomeruli, tubules, interstitium, and vessels, regardless of the site of the original injury. Unless the disorder is treated with dialysis or transplantation, death from uremia, electrolyte disturbances, or other complications results.

Pathogenesis. As progressive renal damage destroys more and more nephrons, adaptive mechanisms are initiated that try to maintain renal function. One adaptation to the decrease in glomerular filtration rate is hyperfiltration by the remaining functional glomeruli, which, as discussed earlier, involves hemodynamic changes that ultimately lead to more glomerular damage. Until a critical loss of nephrons occurs, an increase in the rate of excretion of solutes per nephron due to increased plasma concentrations (for creatinine), decreased tubular reabsorption (for sodium, phosphate, and calcium), or increased tubular secretion (for potassium and hydrogen ions) helps to maintain homeostasis until the late stages of chronic kidney disease. The rate of functional decline varies based on the original disease; however, renal function often deteriorates progressively even when the original insult is controlled. Hypertension, regardless of the etiology, results in more rapid decline of renal function.

Chronic kidney disease is about five times more common in African-Americans than in European-Americans. Recently, polymorphisms in the *APOL1* gene have been identified that increase the risk of kidney disease and also confer resistance to trypanosomiasis, suggesting that these alleles arose because of selection pressure in sub-Saharan regions where trypanosome infection is endemic. Although how APOL1 contributes to resistance to the parasite infection or to kidney disease is unknown, these findings have led to clinical trials of APOL1 inhibitors in patients with renal disease.

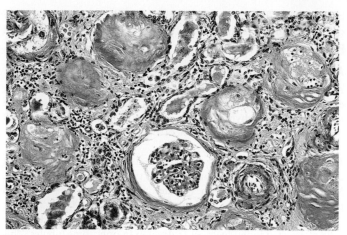

FIG. 12.22 Chronic kidney disease. Replacement of virtually all glomeruli by collagen (stained blue in this trichrome stain), with tubular atrophy and interstitial fibrosis. (Courtesy of Dr. M.A. Venkatachalam, Department of Pathology, University of Texas Health Sciences Center, San Antonio, Texas.)

prognosis is poor; progression to uremia and death is the rule unless the patient is treated with dialysis or transplantation.

CYSTIC DISEASES

Cystic diseases of the kidney are a heterogeneous group that includes hereditary, developmental, and acquired disorders. They often present diagnostic problems for clinicians, radiologists, and pathologists and occasionally can be confused with malignant tumors. Some forms, such as adult polycystic disease, are major causes of chronic kidney disease.

The underlying defect in hereditary cystic diseases is in the cilia-centrosome complex of tubular epithelial cells. Thus, these are examples of *ciliopathy*. Such defects may interfere with fluid absorption or cellular maturation, resulting in cyst formation. A brief overview of simple cysts, the most common form, is presented next, followed by a more detailed discussion of polycystic kidney disease. Renal dysplasia, the most common form of cystic renal disease in childhood, is discussed later.

Simple Cysts

Simple cysts are generally innocuous lesions that occur as multiple or single cystic spaces of variable size. Commonly, they are 1 to 5 cm in diameter; translucent; lined by a gray, glistening, smooth membrane; and filled with clear fluid. On microscopic examination, these membranes are lined by a single layer of cuboidal epithelium, which in many instances becomes flattened or atrophic. The cysts are usually confined to the cortex. Rarely, massive cysts may be as large as 10 cm in diameter.

Simple cysts are a common postmortem finding of no clinical significance. The main importance of cysts lies in their differentiation from tumors, when they are discovered either incidentally or during evaluation of hematuria or flank pain. Radiographic studies show that in contrast with renal tumors, renal cysts have smooth contours and are almost always avascular, and by ultrasonography cysts produce fluid signals rather than solid tissue signals.

Acquired cystic kidney disease occurs in patients with end-stage renal disease who have undergone dialysis for many years. Multiple cysts may be present in both the cortex and the medulla and some may

Clinical Features. Chronic kidney disease may develop insidiously and only be discovered late in its course, as it is often asymptomatic. Frequently, renal disease is first diagnosed by the detection of proteinuria, hypertension, or azotemia on routine medical examination. Findings related to the underlying disorder may precede development of chronic kidney disease. Some degree of proteinuria is present in almost all cases. When the initial glomerular disease caused the nephrotic syndrome, progressive glomerulosclerosis may lessen the protein loss as the disease advances. Hypertension is very common and must be controlled medically to prevent more rapid deterioration of renal function. Although microscopic hematuria is usually present, grossly bloody urine is infrequent at this late stage. The long-term bleed, causing hematuria. The risk for renal neoplasms, particularly cystic ones, in this setting is over 100 times greater than in the general population.

Autosomal Dominant (Adult) Polycystic Kidney Disease

Adult polycystic kidney disease is characterized by multiple expanding cysts affecting both kidneys that ultimately destroy the intervening parenchyma. It is seen in approximately 1 in 500 to 1000 individuals and accounts for 10% of cases of chronic kidney disease.

Pathogenesis. Adult polycystic disease is an autosomal dominant disorder caused by mutations in one of two genes, *PKD1* and *PKD2*. Mutations in *PKD1*, which encodes a cell membrane—associated protein called *polycystin-1*, are the cause in 85% to 90% of families. Although mutations of the *PKD1* gene are present in all renal tubular cells of affected individuals, cysts develop in only some tubules. This is most likely due to a requirement for loss of the second allele, an apparently sporadic somatic event, for cyst development to occur. Polycystin-1 localizes to the primary cilium of tubular cells (as do nephrocystins linked to medullary cystic disease, discussed later). Cilia are hairlike organelles that project into the lumina from the apical surface of tubular cells, where they serve as sensors of fluid flow. Current evidence suggests that reduction of polycystin-1 function below a critical threshold produces defects in mechanosensing by tubular epithelial cells that perturb downstream signaling events involving calcium influx. This in turn leads to altered cell polarity, increased proliferation, and increased fluid secretion, promoting the formation of cysts that progressively enlarge over time.

The *PKD2* gene, implicated in 10% to 15% of cases, encodes *polycystin-2*. Although structurally distinct, polycystins-1 and -2 are believed to act together by forming heterodimers. Thus, mutation in either gene gives rise to essentially the same phenotype, although patients with *PKD2* mutations have a slower rate of disease

progression compared to patients with *PKD1* mutations. Loss of the wild-type copy of *PKD2* also appears to be necessary for cyst formation in this subtype of the disease.

Clinical Features. Polycystic kidney disease in adults usually does not produce symptoms until the fourth decade of life, by which time the kidneys are quite large and the condition may be identified by abdominal palpation. The most common presenting symptom is flank pain or a heavy, dragging sensation. Acute distention of a cyst, either by intracystic hemorrhage or by obstruction, may cause excruciating pain. Intermittent gross hematuria is common. The most important complications, because of their deleterious effect on already marginal renal function, are hypertension and urinary infection. Hypertension of variable severity develops in about 75% of individuals with this disorder.

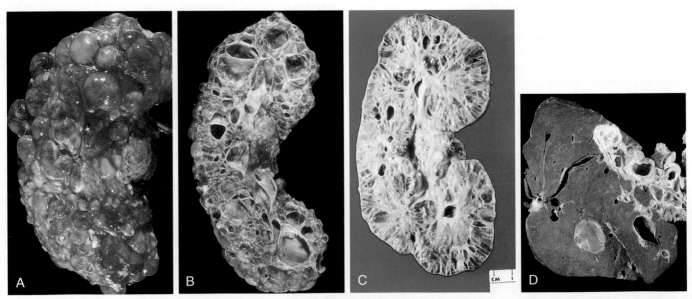

FIG. 12.23 Polycystic kidney disease. (A and B) Autosomal dominant adult polycystic kidney disease (ADPKD) viewed from the external surface and bisected. The kidney is markedly enlarged and contains numerous dilated cysts. (C) Autosomal recessive childhood PKD, showing smaller cysts and dilated channels at right angles to the cortical surface. (D) Liver cysts associated with PKD.

The condition is slowly progressive and, over time, most patients require dialysis or kidney transplantation. Ultimately, about 40% of adult patients die of coronary or hypertensive heart disease, 25% of infection, 15% of a ruptured saccular aneurysm or hypertensive intracerebral hemorrhage, and the rest of other causes.

Autosomal Recessive (Childhood) Polycystic Kidney Disease

The childhood form of polycystic kidney disease is a rare autosomal recessive disorder that is genetically distinct from adult polycystic kidney disease. It occurs in approximately 1 in 20,000 live births. Perinatal, neonatal, infantile, and juvenile subcategories have been defined, depending on age at presentation and the presence of associated hepatic lesions. Perinatal and neonatal forms are most common. All types result from mutations in the *PKHD1* gene, which encodes a putative membrane receptor protein called *fibrocystin*. Fibrocystin is found in cilia in tubular epithelial cells, but its function remains unknown. Serious manifestations are usually present at birth, and young infants may die quickly from hepatic or renal failure. Patients who survive infancy develop liver cirrhosis (congenital hepatic fibrosis).

MORPHOLOGY

In autosomal recessive polycystic kidney disease, **numerous small cysts** in the cortex and medulla give the kidney a spongelike appearance (Fig. 12.23C). Dilated, elongated channels at right angles to the cortical surface completely replace the medulla and cortex. The cysts have a uniform lining of cuboidal cells, reflecting their origin from the collecting tubules. The disease is invariably bilateral. In almost all cases, findings include multiple epithelium-lined **liver cysts** and proliferation of portal bile ducts (Fig. 12.23D).

Medullary Diseases With Cysts

Two major types of cystic disease affect the medulla: nephronophthisis-medullary cystic disease complex, which is almost always associated with renal dysfunction, and medullary sponge kidney, a relatively common and usually innocuous condition.

Nephronophthisis—medullary cystic disease complex is an underappreciated cause of chronic kidney disease; in aggregate, its various forms are now thought to be the most common genetic cause of end-stage renal disease in children and young adults. Four variants are recognized on the basis of the timing of onset: infantile, juvenile, adolescent, and adult, of which the juvenile form is the most common. At least 13 gene loci (*NHP1* to *NHP13*) have been identified for autosomal recessive forms of the nephronophthisis complex. The majority of these genes encode proteins that are components of the epithelial ciliary apparatus, suggesting that the pathogenesis involves ciliary dysfunction. Approximately 15% to 20% of children with juvenile nephronophthisis have extrarenal manifestations, which most often appear as retinal abnormalities, including retinitis pigmentosa, and even early-onset blindness in the most severe form. Other abnormalities found in some individuals include oculomotor apraxia, intellectual disability, cerebellar malformations, and liver fibrosis.

Medullary sponge kidney is a usually asymptomatic congenital disorder likely resulting from a developmental abnormality. It is characterized by dilation of terminal collecting ducts associated with medullary cysts of variable size. Symptomatic cases are often associated with renal stones, discussed later.

MORPHOLOGY

Grossly, kidneys with nephronophthisis-medullary cystic disease complex are **small and contracted.** Numerous small cysts lined by flattened or cuboidal epithelium are present, typically at the corticomedullary junction (eFig. 12.3). Other pathologic changes are nonspecific but often include a chronic tubulointerstitial nephritis with tubular atrophy and thickened tubular basement membranes and progressive interstitial fibrosis.

Clinical Features. The initial manifestations of nephronophthisis-medullary cystic disease are usually polyuria and polydipsia, a consequence of diminished tubular function. Progression to end-stage renal disease ensues over a variable period of 2 to 10 years. The disease is difficult to diagnose because there are no serologic markers, and the cysts may be too small to be seen with radiologic imaging. Adding to this difficulty, cysts may not be apparent on renal biopsy if the corticomedullary junction is not well sampled. A positive family history and unexplained chronic renal failure in young patients should lead to suspicion of the diagnosis.

Multicystic Renal Dysplasia

Multicystic dysplasia is the most common form of renal cystic disease in childhood. The term *dysplasia* in this context refers to a developmental rather than a preneoplastic lesion. Because renal dysplasia is often associated with obstruction in the lower urinary tract, increased hydrostatic pressure in the developing kidney is thought to play a role in its development. Most cases are unilateral, but both kidneys may be involved. The kidney is usually grossly distorted; the cysts range from microscopic to several centimeters in diameter (eFig. 12.4). The histologic hallmarks are ducts and tubules lined by epithelial cells and surrounded by cuffs of cellular mesenchyme. The affected kidney is generally nonfunctional.

URINARY TRACT OBSTRUCTION

Obstructive lesions of the urinary tract increase susceptibility to infection and to stone formation, and unrelieved obstruction almost always leads to permanent renal atrophy, termed hydronephrosis or obstructive uropathy. There are many causes of obstruction (Fig. 12.24), most of which can be cured surgically. Here we discuss renal stones (urolithiasis) and hydronephrosis; other disorders that may cause urinary obstruction are discussed in Chapters 16 and 17.

Renal Stones (Urolithiasis)

Urolithiasis refers to calculus formation at any level in the urinary collecting system; most often, calculi arise in the kidney. Symptomatic urolithiasis is more common in men than in women. Kidney stones occur frequently; it is estimated that by 70 years of age, 11% of men and 5.6% of women in the United States will have developed a symptomatic kidney stone. A familial tendency toward stone formation has long been recognized.

Pathogenesis. **Renal stones form when the urinary concentration of the stone's constituents exceeds their solubility in urine (supersaturation).** The cause of stone formation is often obscure, particularly in the case of calcium-containing stones; predisposing conditions include the concentration of the solute, changes in urine pH, and bacterial

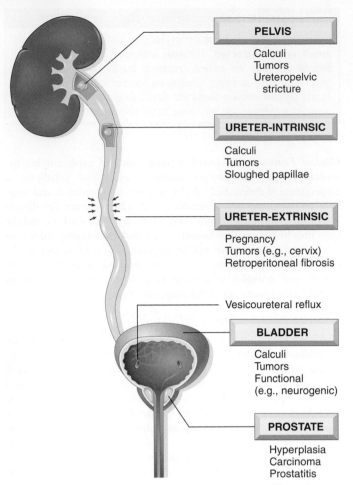

PELVIS
Calculi
Tumors
Ureteropelvic
stricture

URETER-INTRINSIC
Calculi
Tumors
Sloughed papillae

URETER-EXTRINSIC
Pregnancy
Tumors (e.g., cervix)
Retroperitoneal fibrosis

Vesicoureteral reflux

BLADDER
Calculi
Tumors
Functional
(e.g., neurogenic)

PROSTATE
Hyperplasia
Carcinoma
Prostatitis

FIG. 12.24 Causes of urinary tract obstruction.

Table 12.5 Prevalence of Various Types of Renal Stones

Stone	Distribution (%)
Calcium oxalate and/or calcium phosphate	80
Idiopathic hypercalciuria (50%)	
Hypercalcemia and hypercalciuria (10%)	
Hyperoxaluria (5%)	
Enteric (4.5%)	
Primary (0.5%)	
Hyperuricosuria (20%)	
No known metabolic abnormality (15% to 20%)	
Struvite (Mg, NH_3, PO_4)	10
Renal infection	
Uric acid	6–7
Associated with hyperuricemia	
Associated with hyperuricosuria	
Idiopathic (50% of uric acid stones)	
Cystine	1–2
Others or unknown	±1–2

acid stones, however, have neither hyperuricemia nor increased urine urate but demonstrate an unexplained tendency to excrete a persistently acidic urine with a pH <5.5. This low pH favors uric acid stone formation. Cystine stones are almost invariably associated with a genetically determined defect in the renal transport of certain amino acids, including cystine. Like uric acid stones, cystine stones are more likely to form when the urine is relatively acidic.

MORPHOLOGY

Stones are unilateral in about 80% of patients. Common sites of formation are the renal pelvis and calyces and the bladder. Multiple stones are often found in one kidney. Calculi tend to be small (average diameter, 2–3 mm) and may be smooth or jagged (eFig. 12.5). Occasionally, progressive accretion of salts leads to the development of branching structures known as **staghorn calculi,** which create a cast of the renal pelvis and calyceal system. These massive stones are usually composed of magnesium ammonium phosphate.

Clinical Features. Stones may be present without producing symptoms or significant renal damage. This is particularly true with large stones lodged in the renal pelvis. Smaller stones may pass into the ureter, where they can lodge and produce excruciating pain, known as renal or ureteral colic, characterized by paroxysms of flank pain radiating toward the groin. Often there is associated gross hematuria. Stones may obstruct urine flow or produce sufficient trauma to cause ulceration and bleeding. In either case, they predispose the patient to bacterial infection. In most cases, the diagnosis is readily made radiologically.

Hydronephrosis

Hydronephrosis is dilation of the renal pelvis and calyces, with accompanying atrophy of the parenchyma, caused by obstruction to the outflow of urine. The obstruction may be sudden or insidious, and it may occur at any level of the urinary tract, from the urethra to the renal pelvis. The most common causes are categorized as follows:

infections. Risk factors include diet, dehydration, infections, and genetic predisposition. There are three major types of renal stones based on the predominant mineral constituent (Table 12.5). In all cases, an organic matrix of mucoprotein is present that makes up about 2.5% of the stone by weight.

- *Calcium stones.* About 80% of renal stones are composed of calcium oxalate alone or mixed with calcium phosphate. Half of the patients who develop calcium stones have hypercalciuria that is not associated with hypercalcemia. Most patients in this group absorb calcium from the gut in excessive amounts (absorptive hypercalciuria) and excrete it in the urine, and some have a primary renal defect in calcium reabsorption (renal hypercalciuria). Alkaline urine predisposes to formation of calcium phosphate stones.
- *Magnesium stones.* About 10% are composed of magnesium ammonium phosphate (struvite). They almost always occur in individuals with a persistently alkaline urine secondary to UTIs. In particular, infections with urea-splitting bacteria, such as *Proteus vulgaris* and staphylococci, predispose individuals to urolithiasis. Moreover, bacteria may serve as particulate nidi for the formation of any kind of stone. In vitamin A deficiency, desquamated cells from the metaplastic epithelium of the collecting system act as nidi.
- *Uric acid and cystine stones.* Approximately 6% to 9% are either uric acid or cystine stones. Gout and treatment of certain cancers, such as acute leukemias, lead to high urine uric acid levels and the possibility of uric acid stones. About half of individuals with uric

- *Congenital,* such as atresia of the urethra, valve formations in either the ureter or urethra, an aberrant renal artery compressing the ureter, abnormal position of the kidney with torsion, or kinking of the ureter
- *Acquired*
  - *Foreign bodies* (e.g., calculi or sloughed necrotic papillae)
  - *Proliferative lesions* (e.g., benign prostatic hyperplasia, carcinoma of the prostate, bladder tumors [papilloma and carcinoma], contiguous malignant disease [retroperitoneal lymphoma, and carcinoma of the cervix or uterus])
  - *Inflammatory lesions* (e.g., prostatitis, ureteritis, urethritis, and retroperitoneal fibrosis)
  - *Neurogenic,* such as paralysis of the bladder following spinal cord damage
  - *Pregnancy,* in which hydronephrosis is mild

Bilateral hydronephrosis occurs only when the obstruction is below the level of the ureters. If blockage is at the ureters or above, the lesion is unilateral. Sometimes obstruction is complete, allowing no urine to pass; usually it is only partial.

Pathogenesis. Even with complete obstruction, glomerular filtration persists for some time, and the filtrate subsequently diffuses back into the renal interstitium and perirenal spaces and ultimately returns to the lymphatic and venous systems. Because of the continued filtration, the affected calyces and pelvis become dilated, often markedly so. The unusually high pressure thus generated in the renal pelvis and transmitted back through the collecting ducts compresses the renal vasculature and produces arterial insufficiency and venous stasis. The most severe effects are seen in the papillae, which are subjected to the greatest increases in pressure. Hence, the initial functional disturbances are largely tubular, manifested primarily by impaired concentrating ability. Only later does glomerular filtration begin to diminish. In addition to functional changes, the obstruction may also trigger an interstitial inflammatory reaction, leading eventually to interstitial fibrosis.

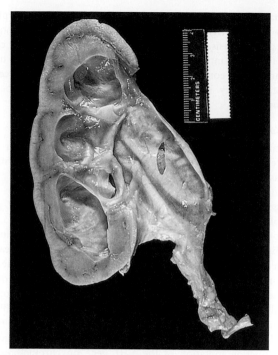

FIG. 12.25 Hydronephrosis of the kidney, with marked dilation of the pelvis and calyces and thinning of renal parenchyma.

silent for long periods unless the other kidney is also dysfunctional or has been removed. Often the enlarged kidney is discovered on routine physical examination. Sometimes the underlying cause of the hydronephrosis, such as renal calculi or an obstructing tumor, produces symptoms that uncover the hydronephrosis. Removal of obstruction usually permits full return of function within a few weeks; however, with longstanding obstruction the changes become irreversible.

NEOPLASMS

Many types of benign and malignant neoplasms occur in the urinary tract. In general, benign neoplasms such as small cortical papillary adenomas (<0.5 cm in diameter), which are found in up to 40% of adults in autopsies, have no clinical significance. The most common malignant neoplasm of the kidney is renal cell carcinoma, followed in frequency by nephroblastoma (Wilms tumor) and by primary neoplasms of the calyces and pelvis. Neoplasms of the lower urinary tract are about twice as common as renal cell carcinomas. They are discussed in Chapter 16.

Renal Cell Carcinoma

Renal cell carcinomas are derived from the renal tubular epithelium and therefore are located predominantly in the cortex. These neoplasms represent 80% to 85% of all primary malignant neoplasms of the kidney and 2% to 3% of all cancers in adults, or about 65,000 cases per year in the United States; 40% of patients die of the disease. Carcinomas of the kidney are most common from the sixth to seventh decades, and men are affected about twice as often as women. The risk for developing these neoplasms is higher in patients who smoke, have hypertension, are obese, or have had occupational exposure to cadmium. The risk is increased 30-fold in individuals with acquired polycystic disease as a complication of chronic dialysis.

> **MORPHOLOGY**
>
> With subtotal or intermittent obstruction, the kidney may be massively enlarged (lengths in the range of 20 cm), and the organ may consist almost entirely of the greatly distended pelvicalyceal system (Fig. 12.25). The renal parenchyma itself is compressed and atrophied, with obliteration of the papillae and flattening of the pyramids. By contrast, when obstruction is sudden and complete, glomerular filtration is compromised relatively early, and renal function may cease while dilation is comparatively mild. Depending on the level of the obstruction, one or both ureters also may be dilated **(hydroureter).**
>
> On microscopic examination, the early lesions show tubular dilation and atrophy followed by loss of the glomeruli and replacement of the renal parenchyma by fibrous tissue. In uncomplicated cases, the accompanying inflammatory reaction is minimal. Superimposed pyelonephritis, however, is common.

Clinical Features. Bilateral hydronephrosis leads to anuria and renal failure. When the obstruction is distal to the bladder, the dominant symptoms are those of bladder distention. Paradoxically, incomplete bilateral obstruction causes polyuria rather than oliguria as a result of defects in tubular concentrating mechanisms, and this may obscure the true nature of the lesion. Unilateral hydronephrosis may remain

Renal cell carcinomas are classified on the basis of morphology and growth patterns. However, recent advances in the understanding of the genetic basis of renal carcinomas have led to a new classification that takes into account the molecular origins of these tumors. The three most common forms, discussed next, are clear cell carcinoma, papillary renal cell carcinoma, and chromophobe renal carcinoma.

Clear Cell Carcinoma

Clear cell carcinoma is the most common type, accounting for 65% of renal cell carcinomas. Histologically, it is composed of cells with clear cytoplasm.

Pathogenesis. **Loss or inactivation of both copies of the *VHL* gene is the molecular hallmark of clear cell carcinoma.** Although most cases are sporadic, they also occur in familial forms or in association with von Hippel-Lindau (VHL) disease. The study of VHL disease has provided important insights into the pathogenesis of clear cell carcinoma. VHL disease is an autosomal dominant disorder characterized by a predisposition to a variety of neoplasms, especially hemangioblastomas of the cerebellum and retina. Bilateral, often multiple, clear cell carcinomas develop in 40% to 60% of affected individuals. The disease is caused by an inherited germline loss-of-function mutation of the *VHL* gene on chromosome 3p25. Tumors are initiated by loss or silencing of the second allele by somatic mutation or hypermethylation. *VHL* gene function is also lost in the majority of sporadic clear cell carcinomas, which often have monoallelic deletions of a segment on chromosome 3p that harbors the *VHL* gene and mutation or inactivation of the second, nondeleted allele. The VHL protein causes the oxygen-dependent degradation of hypoxia-inducible factors (HIFs); in the absence of VHL, HIFs are stabilized and levels remain high even under normoxic conditions. HIFs are transcription factors that stimulate the expression of vascular endothelial growth factor (VEGF), an important angiogenic protein that supports the vascularization of tumors (Chapter 6). HIF also collaborates with MYC to alter cellular metabolism in a way that promotes cell growth. In addition, recent deep sequencing of clear cell carcinoma genomes has revealed frequent loss-of-function mutations in genes that encode proteins that regulate histone methylation. These findings suggest that changes in the epigenome play an important role in the genesis of this subtype of renal carcinoma.

Papillary Renal Cell Carcinoma

Papillary renal cell carcinoma accounts for 10% to 15% of all renal cancers and displays a characteristic papillary growth pattern. These neoplasms are frequently multifocal and bilateral and appear as early-stage tumors.

Pathogenesis. Like clear cell carcinomas, papillary renal cell carcinoma occurs in familial and sporadic forms. The unifying feature in both forms are genetic abnormalities that increase that function of MET, a tyrosine kinase receptor encoded by the *MET* gene on chromosome 7q. In sporadic tumors, increased MET function often stems from increased *MET* copy number or from somatic activating mutations in *MET*, whereas familial cases are typically caused by germline activating *MET* mutations. The net effect in all instances is an increase in MET signaling, which spurs abnormal growth of proximal tubular epithelial cells.

Chromophobe Renal Cell Carcinoma

Chromophobe renal cell carcinoma is the least common form, representing 5% of renal cell carcinomas. It arises from intercalated cells of collecting ducts. The lightly eosinophilic tumor cells are pale (chromophobe) but do not appear clear as in clear cell carcinomas. These neoplasms frequently display multiple losses of entire chromosomes leading to extreme hypoploidy. The critical changes in gene function that lead to oncogenesis have yet to be determined. In general, chromophobe renal cell cancers have a favorable prognosis.

MORPHOLOGY

Clear cell carcinomas are usually large, solitary, spherical masses 3 to 15 cm in diameter when symptomatic; high-resolution radiographic techniques may detect smaller lesions incidentally. They can arise anywhere in the cortex. The cut surface is **yellow to orange** (due to abundant lipid), **with areas of necrosis and prominent cystic softening or hemorrhage** (Fig. 12.26). The margins of the tumor are well defined, but in some cases local spread creates satellite lesions. As the tumor enlarges, it may fungate through the walls of the collecting system, extending through the calyces and pelvis as far as the ureter. Even more frequently, the **tumor invades the renal vein** and grows as a solid column within this vessel, sometimes extending in serpentine fashion as far as the inferior vena cava and even into the right side of the heart. Occasionally, direct invasion into the perinephric fat and adrenal gland may be seen. In most cases, because of the presence of large amounts of lipid and glycogen, **the neoplastic cells appear clear, with a vacuolated appearance and distinct cell membranes.** The cells are arranged in nests separated by a delicate, fibrovascular stroma. The nuclei are usually small and round (Fig. 12.27A). In another morphologic variant, the tumor cells have granular cytoplasm and resemble tubular epithelium. Other cases are anaplastic, with numerous

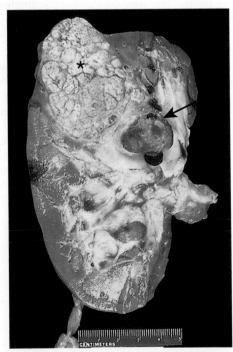

FIG. 12.26 Renal cell carcinoma. Representative cross-section showing yellowish, spherical neoplasm *(asterisk)* in one pole of the kidney. Note the tumor in the dilated, thrombosed renal vein *(arrow).*

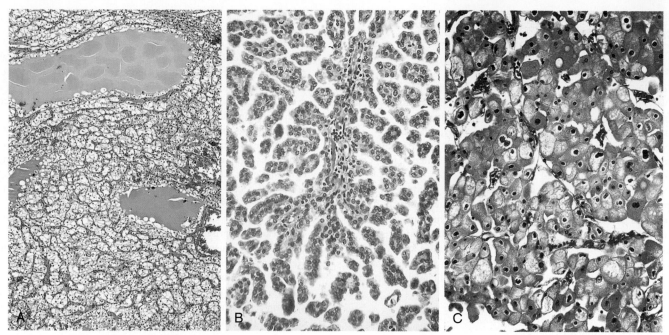

FIG. 12.27 Renal cell carcinoma. (A) Clear cell type. (B) Papillary type. (C) Chromophobe type. (From Fletcher, C.D., Diagnostic Histopathology of Tumors, 5th edition, Elsevier, Philadelphia, 2021, Figs. 12A.14, 12A.16, 12A.24.)

mitotic figures and markedly enlarged, hyperchromatic, pleomorphic nuclei. The cellular arrangement varies widely, with cells forming abortive tubules or clustering in cords or disorganized masses. The stroma is usually scant but highly vascularized.

Papillary renal cell carcinomas tend to be bilateral and multiple. They may also show necrosis, hemorrhage, and cystic degeneration but are less vibrantly orange-yellow than clear cell carcinomas due to their lower lipid content. Cuboidal to low columnar cells with eosinophilic to clear cytoplasm line papillae with fibrovascular cores (Fig. 12.27B).

Chromophobe renal cell carcinoma appears tan-brown on gross examination. The cells usually have eosinophilic cytoplasm mixed with pale granular cells with very prominent, distinct cell membranes and often perinuclear haloes (Fig. 12.27C).

Clinical Features. Renal cell carcinomas have several peculiar clinical characteristics that create challenging diagnostic problems. The signs and symptoms vary, but the triad of painless hematuria, a palpable abdominal mass, and dull flank pain is characteristic (though all three are seen in only 10% of cases). Hematuria is the most frequent presenting manifestation, occurring in more than 50% of cases. Macroscopic hematuria tends to be intermittent and fleeting, superimposed on a persistent microscopic hematuria. Less commonly, the tumor may declare itself by virtue of its size, manifesting as flank pain and a palpable mass. Small tumors may be detected incidentally radiographically. Extrarenal manifestations are fever and polycythemia, which, because they are nonspecific, may be misinterpreted for some time before the underlying renal tumor is appreciated. Polycythemia affects 5% to 10% of affected individuals and is due to production of erythropoietin by the neoplastic cells. Uncommonly, other paraneoplastic syndromes, including hypercalcemia, hypertension, Cushing syndrome, or feminization or masculinization (Chapter 6), are present. Symptoms referable to metastatic disease may also bring the patient to clinical attention; common locations for metastases are the lungs and the bones.

Other Renal Tumors

Oncocytoma

Oncocytoma, a benign tumor that arises from the intercalated cells of collecting ducts, represents 3% to 7% of renal neoplasms. Oncocytomas are characterized by abundant mitochondria, providing the basis for their tan color and their finely granular eosinophilic cytoplasm, seen histologically (eFig. 12.6). A central stellate scar is another feature. The tumor cells may contain multiple chromosomal abnormalities, including loss of chromosomes 1 and Y, and rearrangements involving the cyclin D1 locus. These tumors also harbor disruptive mutations that lead to loss of complex I, a key component of the electron transport chain that is required for oxidative phosphorylation. This, in turn, appears to activate feedback loops that increase mitochondrial proliferation, which is responsible for the characteristic morphology. Multiple oncocytomas may be seen in patients with tuberous sclerosis (Chapter 21). It is important, and often difficult, to distinguish these tumors from renal cell carcinoma. In 10% to 30% of patients with multiple oncocytic nodules, there may be a coexisting renal cell carcinoma, so careful monitoring is needed.

Angiomyolipoma

This benign tumor arising from perivascular cells (pericytes) constitutes 1% to 2% of renal tumors. It is seen most often as part of the tuberous sclerosis complex (Chapter 21). The tumors are often discovered as incidental lesions.

Wilms Tumor

Although Wilms tumor is rare in adults, it is the third most common solid (nonhematologic) cancer in children younger than 10 years of age. Wilms tumor, like retinoblastoma, may arise sporadically or be familial, with the susceptibility to tumorigenesis inherited as an autosomal dominant trait. This neoplasm is discussed in Chapter 4 along with other tumors of childhood.

■ RAPID REVIEW

Clinical Manifestations of Renal Diseases

Major clinical correlates of kidney diseases include the following:

- *Nephrotic syndrome* is caused by glomerular alterations that result in increased permeability, leading to proteinuria (>3.5 g/24 hours), hypoalbuminemia, generalized edema, and hyperlipidemia.
- *Nephritic syndrome* is caused by glomerular injury associated with inflammation, leading to hematuria (usually microscopic), mild proteinuria, azotemia, and hypertension.
- *Acute kidney injury* is caused by renal diseases or extrarenal abnormalities (e.g., reduced fluid volume, urinary tract obstruction), and is characterized by reduced urine output, hypertension, and laboratory signs of renal compromise (azotemia or uremia).
- *Chronic kidney disease* results from scarring of the kidney secondary to glomerular, tubulointerstitial, or vascular disease and is characterized by electrolyte abnormalities (metabolic acidosis), uremia, and progressive renal failure.

Diseases of Glomeruli

Mechanisms of Glomerular Injury

Most often mediated by antibodies and immune complexes, which activate complement and recruit leukocytes, that cause inflammation, or disrupt the glomerular permeability barrier. They are deposited in glomeruli by three mechanisms:

- *Deposition of circulating immune complexes:* Glomeruli are a common site of immune complex deposition; this creates a granular pattern of staining for antibodies and complement.
- *In situ immune complex formation:* Antibodies bind to patchily distributed intrinsic or planted antigens in the GBM, also producing a granular staining pattern.
- *Binding of anti-GBM antibodies:* Antibodies against uniformly distributed glomerular antigens bind to the GBM, creating a linear staining pattern.

Disorders Presenting With the Nephrotic Syndrome

Primary glomerular diseases producing the nephrotic syndrome include the following:

- *Minimal change disease:* Selective proteinuria (loss of mostly albumin); unknown pathogenesis; histologically normal glomeruli, fusion of foot processes by electron microscopy; good response to steroids
- *Focal segmental glomerulosclerosis (FSGS):* Scarring of segments of some glomeruli; primary form likely results from injury to podocytes possibly due to circulating factors, other cases may be secondary to loss of renal mass, infections, drug reactions, or genetic causes; nonselective proteinuria, poor response to steroids
- *Membranous nephropathy:* In situ immune complex formation by antibodies binding to various podocyte or GBM antigens; most often primary; nephrotic syndrome may progress to renal failure
- *Membranoproliferative glomerulonephritis:* Immune complex–mediated injury with GBM thickening and mesangial hypercellularity; progressive course
- *C3 glomerulopathy:* Consists of dense deposit disease, in which deposits are seen in the GBM, and C3 GN, in which deposits are scant; caused by excessive, dysregulated complement activation

Disorders Presenting With the Nephritic Syndrome

- *Acute postinfectious glomerulonephritis:* Typically occurs after streptococcal infection in children and young adults but may occur following other infections; caused by glomerular deposition of immune complexes, leading to complement activation and neutrophilic inflammation
- *Rapidly progressive glomerulonephritis:* Clinical manifestation of severe glomerular injury caused by anti-GBM antibodies or immune complexes; glomeruli show severe damage with formation of epithelial crescents

Other Glomerular Diseases

- *IgA nephropathy:* Characterized by mesangial deposits of immune complexes comprised of poorly glycosylated IgA and IgG anti-IgA antibody; causes recurrent, usually asymptomatic, hematuria
- *Hereditary nephritis:* Caused by mutations in genes encoding GBM type IV collagen; manifests as hematuria and slowly progressing proteinuria and declining renal function. Two forms are Alport syndrome (hearing and visual disorders in addition to renal disease) and thin basement membrane disease.

Diseases Affecting Tubules and Interstitium

- *Acute pyelonephritis:* Bacterial infection caused most often by ascending infection as a result of reflux, obstruction, or other abnormality of the urinary tract and less commonly by hematogenous spread of bacteria; characterized by purulent inflammation with abscess formation in the kidneys, sometimes with papillary necrosis
- *Chronic pyelonephritis:* Usually associated with urinary obstruction or reflux; results in scarring of the pelvicalyceal system and the interstitium of the involved kidney and gradual development of chronic kidney disease
- *Tubulointerstitial nephritis:* Inflammatory lesions of the tubules and interstitium not associated with ascending bacterial infection but most often caused by hypersensitivity reactions to therapeutic drugs
- *Acute tubular injury* (ATI): Ischemic or toxic damage to tubules, leading to oliguria and azotemia. Characterized morphologically by injury or necrosis of segments of the tubules (typically the proximal tubules), proteinaceous casts in distal tubules, and interstitial edema.

Diseases Involving Blood Vessels

- *Nephrosclerosis:* Chronic renal damage associated with hypertension, characterized by hyaline arteriosclerosis and narrowing of vascular lumina with resultant ischemic tubular atrophy and interstitial fibrosis
- *Severe (malignant) hypertension:* Acute kidney injury associated with severely elevated blood pressure. Characteristic vascular lesions are fibrinoid necrosis and hyperplasia of arterial smooth muscle cells; petechial hemorrhages appear on the cortical surface.
- *Thrombotic microangiopathies:* Disorders characterized by platelet-rich thrombi in glomeruli and small vessels resulting in acute kidney injury; three major types:
  - *Shiga toxin–associated hemolytic uremic syndrome (HUS),* usually caused by gastrointestinal toxin–producing *E. coli* infections. The toxin is believed to damage endothelial cells, leading to thrombus formation.
  - *Complement-mediated HUS,* caused by defects in complement regulatory proteins that may be inherited (genetic) or acquired (due to autoantibodies); excessive complement activation causes endothelial injury.

- *Thrombotic thrombocytopenia purpura (TTP),* caused by inherited or acquired defects in ADAMTS13, a plasma protease that cleaves von Willebrand factor (vWF), leading to accumulation of abnormally large vWF multimers that activate platelets, leading to thrombi formation.

Chronic Kidney Disease

End result of progressive nephron loss from any cause, leading to glomerular obliteration, tubular atrophy, and interstitial fibrosis.

Cystic Diseases

- *Simple cysts:* Usually incidental findings of no clinical consequence
- *Autosomal dominant (adult) polycystic kidney disease:* Caused by mutations in the genes encoding polycystin-1 or polycystin-2 (*PKD1* and *PKD2*, respectively), which are involved in functions of cilia; kidneys may be extremely large and contain many variably sized cysts
- *Autosomal recessive (childhood) polycystic kidney disease:* Caused by mutations in the gene encoding fibrocystin *(PKHD1),* also found in cilia; kidneys contain numerous small cysts; strongly associated with liver cysts
- *Nephronophthisis—medullary cystic disease complex:* Autosomal recessive disease, a cause of chronic kidney disease in children

and young adults; associated with mutations in genes that encode epithelial cell proteins called *nephrocystins* that may be involved in ciliary function; kidneys are contracted and contain multiple small cysts

Urinary Tract Obstruction

- *Renal stones:* May be composed of calcium or magnesium salts or urate; form when concentration of constituents exceed solubility in urine
- *Hydronephrosis:* Dilation of renal pelvis and calyces caused by outflow obstruction; may lead to parenchymal atrophy

Renal Cell Carcinoma

Renal cell carcinomas account for 2% to 3% of all cancers in adults and are classified into three main types:

- *Clear cell carcinoma* is the most common type; associated with loss or inactivation of the VHL tumor suppressor protein; tumors frequently invade the renal vein
- *Papillary renal cell carcinoma* is frequently associated with increased expression and activating mutations of the *MET* oncogene; tend to be bilateral and multiple; show variable papilla formation
- *Chromophobe renal cell carcinoma* is less common; neoplastic cells have eosinophilic cytoplasm.

■ Laboratory Tests[b]

Test	Reference Values	Pathophysiology/Clinical Relevance
Bicarbonate,[a] serum	Males ≥18 years, females ≥10 years: 22–29 mEq/L	Bicarbonate is an important buffer that maintains acid-base balance and the proper pH of epithelial secretions. Serum bicarbonate concentration is used to calculate pH in the Henderson-Hasselbalch equation to evaluate an acid-base disorder. Bicarbonate levels are low in metabolic acidosis and respiratory alkalosis and elevated in metabolic alkalosis and respiratory acidosis. If serum levels are sufficiently high, metabolic alkalosis will result. Causes of increased serum bicarbonate include gastric HCl loss (e.g., due to vomiting) and K+ loss. Dysfunctional CFTR (mutated in cystic fibrosis) results in decreased bicarbonate levels in luminal secretions.
Blood urea nitrogen (BUN), serum	Males ≥18 years: 8–24 mg/dL Females ≥18 years: 6–21 mg/dL	Ammonia is generated when proteins are catabolized. The liver metabolizes this ammonia to urea, which is released into the blood and then eliminated by the kidneys, thereby removing nitrogen from the body. BUN may be elevated in conditions affecting the urinary tract (e.g., acute glomerulonephritis, polycystic kidney disease, urinary obstruction due to benign prostatic hyperplasia), dehydration, and congestive heart failure, the latter due to decreased renal perfusion. BUN is also elevated in liver diseases. BUN alone is not very informative by itself; a BUN/creatinine ratio (normal 10–15 : 1) is more useful in monitoring renal health (see below).
Chloride,[a] serum	≥18 years: 98–107 mmol/L	Chloride is part of the basic metabolic panel (BMP: Cl, Na, glucose, BUN, K, CO_2, creatinine). It reflects the body's ability to maintain fluid homeostasis and acid-base balance. It is the primary anion in the extracellular fluid and is necessary for transmitting action potentials in neurons. Alkalosis is seen with low chloride levels, while acidosis is associated with high chloride levels. Causes of decreased chloride include vomiting, diarrhea, diabetic ketoacidosis, syndrome of inappropriate ADH secretion (SIADH), metabolic alkalosis, and heart failure. Causes of increased chloride include renal failure, dehydration, diabetes insipidus, and respiratory alkalosis.
Creatinine, serum	Males ≥15 years: 0.7–1.3 mg/dL Females ≥18 years: 0.6–1.0 mg/dL	Creatinine is derived from creatine (primarily synthesized in kidney and liver) and phosphocreatine. A fairly constant proportion of creatinine (related to skeletal muscle mass and metabolism) is released into blood, and creatinine is freely filtered by the glomerulus and serum levels can be used to calculate glomerular filtration rate (GFR). Both serum BUN and creatinine levels vary in inverse proportion to GFR, with the normal ratio being 10–15 : 1. When there is a disproportionate rise in BUN (higher ratio), it suggests prerenal failure. When the relative ratio is tilted toward creatinine, it is indicative of renal failure caused by intrinsic diseases of the kidney that affect GFR.

Phospholipase A2 receptor (PLA2R) antibody	Negative	Membranous nephropathy (MN) is a renal disease in which immune complexes deposit along the subepithelial surface of the glomerular basement membrane. In about 70% of cases of MN, the antibodies in the complexes are directed against the podocyte PLA2R protein. The PLA2R antibody levels correlate with risk of disease progression. PLA2R antibody levels can also be used to monitor response to treatment.
Potassium, serum[a]	3.6—5.2 mmol/L	Potassium is the main intracellular cation, while sodium is the main extracellular cation. The Na+/K+ ATPase membrane pump maintains the concentrations of these 2 cations in their respective compartments. Plasma level is regulated by the kidney. Both hypo- and hyperkalemia can lead to cardiac arrhythmias. Important causes of hypokalemia include medications (e.g., diuretics), vomiting, diarrhea, and diabetic ketoacidosis. Hyperkalemia may be due to medications (e.g., ACE inhibitors), Addison disease, renal failure (decreased excretion), and extracellular potassium shift (e.g., secondary to diabetic ketoacidosis). Extensive cellular destruction (e.g., trauma, burns, hemolysis) can also lead to hyperkalemia. Potassium may appear falsely elevated in hemolyzed blood samples.
Renin activity, plasma	Adults, normal sodium diet 0.6—4.3 ng/mL/hr	The renal juxtaglomerular apparatus produces renin, an enzyme that converts angiotensinogen to angiotensin I, which is then further converted to angiotensin II. Angiotensin II stimulates the zona glomerulosa of the adrenal cortex to release aldosterone, which increases Na+ reabsorption. Consequent water reabsorption causes a rise in systemic (and therefore renal) blood pressure. Renin secretion by the kidney is stimulated by a fall in glomerular blood pressure, by decreased sodium concentration at the macula, and by stimulation of sympathetic outflow to the kidney. Plasma renin activity (PRA) is measured as part of the diagnosis and treatment of hypertension. Interpretation is dependent on salt intake, posture, time of day, and certain medications. Renal disease, especially unilateral renal artery stenosis, results in elevated aldosterone and renin.
Sodium, serum[a]	135—145 mmol/L	Na+ is the main extracellular cation while K+ is the main intracellular cation. The Na+/K+ ATPase membrane pump maintains the concentrations of these 2 cations in their respective locations. When extracellular Na+ levels decrease, water shifts into cells and vice versa. With chronically low levels of Na+, cells adapt and patients may be asymptomatic, but acute hyponatremia can result in seizures or brain herniation due to cerebral edema. Hyponatremia is usually due to excess hydration, not insufficient intake, and can be seen in renal failure, primary polydipsia, thiazide diuretics, SIADH, and adrenal insufficiency. Rapid correction of hyponatremia can lead to osmotic demyelination syndrome. Hypernatremia is often due to fluid depletion (e.g., vomiting, diarrhea, dehydration, osmotic diuresis in uncontrolled diabetes). Symptoms include signs of dehydration such as thirst, headache, lethargy, and weakness. When untreated, severe hypernatremia can cause spasms, seizure, and coma.

[a]These electrolytes are part of basic metabolic panels used to monitor and diagnose a variety of disorders, not only kidney diseases.

[b]The assistance of Dr. Samantha Gunning, Department of Medicine, University of Chicago for review of this table is gratefully acknowledged.

References values from https://www.mayocliniclabs.com/ by permission of Mayo Foundation for Medical Education and Research. All rights reserved.

Adapted from Deyrup AT, D'Ambrosio D, Muir J, et al. Essential Laboratory Tests for Medical Education. *Acad Pathol.* 2022;9. doi: 10.1016/j.acpath.2022.100046.

Oral Cavity and Gastrointestinal Tract

OUTLINE

The contributions to this chapter by Dr. Jerrold R. Turner, Department of Pathology, Brigham and Women's Hospital, Boston, Massachusetts, in several previous editions of this book are gratefully acknowledged.

The gastrointestinal tract is a hollow tube consisting of the esophagus, stomach, small intestine, colon, rectum, and anus. Each region has complementary, highly integrated functions that regulate the intake, processing, and absorption of ingested nutrients and the disposal of waste products. The intestines are also where the immune system encounters a diverse array of antigens derived from food and endogenous gut microbes that must be tolerated as well as pathogens that may contaminate food and drink that must be eliminated. It should then come as no surprise that the gastrointestinal tract is commonly involved in a wide spectrum of infectious and inflammatory processes. In this chapter, we discuss diseases that affect each part of the gastrointestinal tract. Disorders that typically involve more than one region, such as Crohn disease, are considered according to the region they involve most frequently. We begin our discussion with diseases of the oral cavity, since that is where the journey of food begins.

ORAL CAVITY

Pathologic conditions of the oral cavity can be broadly divided into diseases affecting teeth and their support structures, oral mucosa, salivary glands, and the jaw. Discussed next are the more common conditions affecting these sites. Odontogenic cysts and tumors (benign and malignant), which are derived from the epithelial and/or mesenchymal tissues associated with tooth development, are also described briefly.

DISEASES OF TEETH AND SUPPORTING STRUCTURES

Bacteria in the oral cavity are directly or indirectly responsible for the most common disorders of the teeth and gums, caries, gingivitis, and periodontitis.

Caries

Dental caries result from focal demineralization of tooth structure (enamel and dentin) caused by acids generated during the fermentation of sugars by bacteria. Worldwide, caries is the main cause of tooth loss before 35 years of age. In the past, caries was pervasive in high-resource countries where there is ready access to foods containing large amounts of refined carbohydrates. However, the rate of caries has dropped markedly in countries such as the United States due to improved oral hygiene and fluoridation of drinking water. Fluoride is incorporated into the crystalline structure of enamel, forming fluoroapatite, which is resistant to degradation by bacterial acids. With the globalization of the world's economy, processed foods are being increasingly consumed in lower-resource countries, and as a result the rate of caries is increasing in these regions of the world.

Gingivitis

Inflammation involving the squamous mucosa, or gingiva, and associated soft tissues that surround teeth is called gingivitis. The most frequent cause is poor oral hygiene, which facilitates buildup of dental plaque and calculus between and on the surfaces of teeth. Dental plaque is a sticky biofilm composed of bacteria, salivary proteins, and desquamated epithelial cells. As it accumulates, plaque becomes mineralized to form calculus, or tartar. Subgingival plaque and associated bacteria lead to chronic gingivitis, marked by erythema, edema, and bleeding. Gingivitis may occur at any age but is most prevalent and severe in adolescence, where it is present in 40% to 60% of individuals, after which the incidence tapers off. Fortunately, gingivitis can be reversed, primarily by regular brushing and flossing of teeth and periodic cleaning, which reduces accumulation of plaque and calculus.

Periodontitis

Periodontitis is an inflammatory process that affects the supporting structures of the teeth (periodontal ligaments), alveolar bone, and cementum. With progression, periodontitis may result in destruction of periodontal ligaments and alveolar bone and, eventually, tooth loss. Periodontitis is associated with poor oral hygiene that affects the composition of gingival bacteria. Facultative gram-positive organisms are associated with healthy teeth, whereas anaerobic and microaerophilic gram-negative bacteria colonize plaque within areas of active periodontitis. Bacterial species that are closely associated with periodontitis include *Aggregatibacter (Actinobacillus) actinomycetemcomitans*, *Porphyromonas gingivalis*, and *Prevotella intermedia*.

ORAL INFLAMMATORY LESIONS

Aphthous Ulcers (Canker Sores)

These common superficial mucosal ulcerations affect up to 40% of the population. They are more frequent in the first two decades of life, are extremely painful, and often recur. The cause is unknown; they tend to be familial and may be associated with celiac disease, inflammatory bowel disease, and Behçet disease, a rare vasculitic disorder. These ulcers can be solitary or multiple; typically, they are shallow and have a hyperemic base covered by a thin exudate that is rimmed by a narrow zone of erythema (Fig. 13.1). In most cases they resolve spontaneously in 7 to 10 days.

Herpes Simplex Virus Infections

Herpes simplex virus causes a self-limited primary infection that may reactivate if host resistance is compromised. Most orofacial herpetic infections are caused by herpes simplex virus type 1 (HSV-1), with the remainder being caused by HSV-2, a type that is more highly

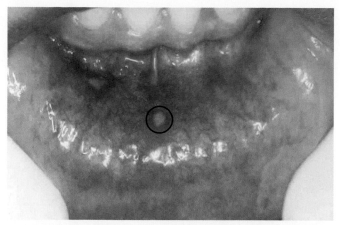

FIG. 13.1 Aphthous ulcer. Single ulceration with an erythematous halo surrounding a grayish fibrinopurulent membrane *(circle)*.

associated with genital herpes. Primary infections typically occur in children between 2 and 4 years of age and are often asymptomatic. However, in 10% to 20% of cases primary infection manifests as acute herpetic gingivostomatitis, with abrupt onset of vesicles and ulcerations throughout the oral cavity.

Most adults harbor latent HSV-1, which may reactivate, resulting in a so-called "cold sore" or recurrent herpetic stomatitis. Factors associated with HSV reactivation include trauma, allergies, exposure to ultraviolet light and extremes of temperature, upper respiratory tract infections, pregnancy, menstruation, and immunosuppression. Recurrent lesions usually occur at the site of primary inoculation or in adjacent mucosa innervated by the same axon and typically appear as groups of small (1- to 3-mm) vesicles. The lips *(herpes labialis)*, nasal orifices, buccal mucosa, gingiva, and hard palate are the most common locations. Less often, the reactivated infection involves the cornea, producing pain, blurred vision, and photophobia. Lesions typically resolve spontaneously within 7 to 10 days, but patients who are immunocompromised and those with corneal involvement often require antiviral therapy. Morphologically, the lesions resemble those seen in esophageal herpes (see Fig. 13.8) and genital herpes (Chapter 16). The infected cells become ballooned and have large eosinophilic intranuclear inclusions. Adjacent cells commonly fuse to form large multinucleated polykaryons.

Oral Candidiasis (Thrush)

Candidiasis is the most common fungal infection of the oral cavity. *Candida albicans* is a normal component of the oral flora and only produces disease under unusual circumstances. Predisposing factors include:

- Immunosuppression
- The presence of certain strains of *C. albicans*
- A permissive oral microbial flora (microbiota)

Broad-spectrum antibiotics that alter the normal microbiota may promote oral candidiasis, which most commonly appears as a pseudomembranous form known as *thrush*. Thrush is characterized by a superficial, curdlike, gray to white inflammatory membrane composed of matted organisms enmeshed in a fibrinosuppurative exudate that can be readily scraped off to reveal an underlying erythematous base. In individuals who are mildly immunosuppressed or debilitated (e.g., patients with diabetes), the infection usually remains superficial, but spread to deep sites may be seen with more severe immunosuppression, such as in organ or hematopoietic stem cell transplant

recipients and patients with neutropenia, chemotherapy-induced immunosuppression, or AIDS.

PROLIFERATIVE AND NEOPLASTIC LESIONS OF THE ORAL CAVITY

Stromal Proliferative Lesions

Fibromas are submucosal nodular fibrous tissue masses that form when chronic irritation (trauma from teeth or dentures) results in reactive connective tissue hyperplasia (Fig. 13.2A). They occur most often on the buccal mucosa along the bite line. Treatment consists of surgical excision and removal of the source of irritation.

Pyogenic granuloma (Fig. 13.2B) is an inflammatory lesion typically found on the gingiva of children, young adults, and pregnant women (Chapter 8). The lesions are highly vascular, giving them a red to purple color, and often ulcerated. In some cases, their growth may be so rapid as to suggest a malignant neoplasm. However, histologic examination demonstrates a proliferation of capillaries similar to those seen in granulation tissue. Pyogenic granulomas may regress or undergo fibrosis, sometimes associated with calcification. Complete surgical excision is the definitive treatment.

Leukoplakia and Erythroplakia

Leukoplakia and erythroplakia are squamous lesions of the oropharynx that may be precursors of squamous cell carcinoma. The

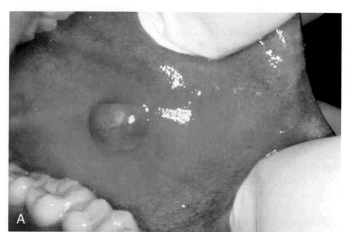

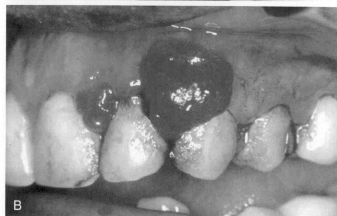

FIG. 13.2 Stromal proliferations. (A) Fibroma, appearing as a pink exophytic nodule on the buccal mucosa. (B) Pyogenic granuloma, seen as an erythematous hemorrhagic exophytic mass arising from the gingival mucosa.

terms are reserved for lesions that arise in the absence of any known cause; accordingly, lesions caused by chronic irritation or entities such as lichen planus and candidiasis are not leukoplakia. Approximately 3% of the world's population has leukoplakic lesions, of which 5% to 25% are dysplastic and at risk for progression to squamous cell carcinoma. Thus, until proven otherwise by histologic evaluation, leukoplakia is considered precancerous. A related, less common entity, *erythroplakia*, is associated with a much greater risk for malignant transformation than leukoplakia. Leukoplakia and erythroplakia are most common in adults between 40 and 70 years of age and have a 2 : 1 male predominance. Although the etiology is multifactorial, the most important risk factor is tobacco use, including smokeless tobacco.

MORPHOLOGY

Leukoplakia typically appears as a well-demarcated gray-white plaque (Fig. 13.3A). On histologic examination leukoplakia and erythroplakia show a spectrum of epithelial changes ranging from a hyperplastic, hyperkeratotic but orderly squamous epithelium to lesions with marked dysplasia, sometimes associated with carcinoma in situ (Fig. 13.3B). Dysplastic lesions are often associated with an underlying inflammatory cell infiltrate consisting of lymphocytes and macrophages. The most severe dysplastic changes are associated with erythroplakia, which undergoes malignant transformation in more than 50% of cases. Grossly, erythroplakia appears as a red, velvety, sometimes eroded, flat or slightly depressed lesion.

Squamous Cell Carcinoma

Approximately 95% of cancers of the oral cavity are squamous cell carcinomas, with the remainder largely consisting of adenocarcinomas of salivary glands. Oral squamous cell carcinoma is an aggressive epithelial malignancy. The overall incidence of oral squamous cell carcinoma has risen since the 1980s, despite a decline in tobacco use, due to an increase in human papillomavirus–associated cancers, which are now believed to outnumber those related to alcohol and tobacco in the United States and Europe.

Pathogenesis. **Squamous cancers of the oropharynx arise through two distinct pathogenic pathways, one involving exposure to carcinogens and the other to infection with high-risk variants of human papilloma virus (HPV).** Carcinogen exposure in the United States and Europe mainly stems from chronic use of alcohol and/or tobacco (both smoked and chewed), while in India and Southeast Asia, chewing of betel nuts and leaves (paan) are predisposing factors. DNA sequencing of tobacco-associated cancers has revealed a mutational signature consistent with exposure to carcinogens. The most commonly mutated genes include *TP53*, genes that regulate proliferation (e.g., *RAS*), and genes that regulate squamous differentiation (e.g., *NOTCH*). The elevated risk for development of additional primary tumors in these patients has led to the concept of "field cancerization"; this hypothesis suggests that multiple neoplastic clones develop independently as a result of years of chronic mucosal exposure to carcinogens.

By contrast, HPV-related tumors tend to occur in the tonsillar crypts and harbor oncogenic "high-risk" HPV subtypes, particularly HPV-16. Exposure to HPV occurs through orogenital sex. As was discussed in Chapter 6, high-risk subtypes of HPV express the viral oncoproteins E6 and E7, which inhibit the critical tumor suppressors p53 and RB, respectively. HPV-associated tumors carry far fewer mutations than those associated with tobacco exposure and often overexpress p16, a cyclin-dependent kinase inhibitor.

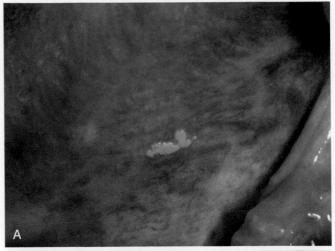

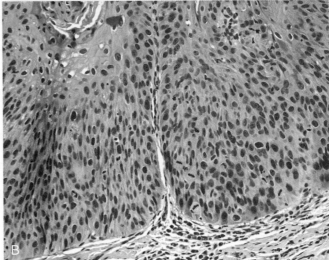

FIG. 13.3 Leukoplakia. (A) Gross appearance of leukoplakia is highly variable. In this example, the lesion is smooth with well-demarcated borders and minimal elevation. (B) Histologic appearance of leukoplakia showing dysplasia, characterized by nuclear and cellular pleomorphism and loss of normal maturation.

MORPHOLOGY

Squamous cell carcinoma may arise anywhere in the oral cavity. **The most common locations for carcinogen-associated cancers are the ventral surface of the tongue, floor of the mouth, lower lip, soft palate, and gingiva** (Fig. 13.4A). In early stages, these cancers may appear as raised, firm pearly plaques or irregular, roughened, or verrucous mucosal thickenings. The surrounding mucosa may show leukoplakia or erythroplakia. By contrast, **HPV-associated cancers arise in the tonsil or the back of the tongue.** As these lesions enlarge, they typically form ulcerated and protruding masses that have irregular and indurated or rolled borders. Histologic patterns range from well-differentiated keratinizing neoplasms (Fig. 13.4B) to anaplastic, sometimes sarcomatoid, tumors. However, the degree of histologic differentiation, as determined by the relative degree of keratinization, does not correlate with biologic behavior. Typically, oral squamous cell carcinoma infiltrates locally before it metastasizes. The cervical lymph nodes are the most common sites of regional metastasis; frequent sites of distant metastases include the mediastinal lymph nodes, lungs, and liver.

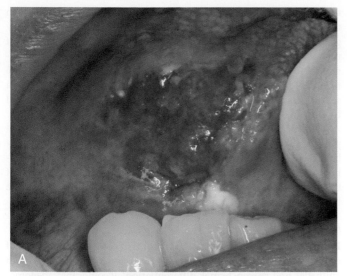

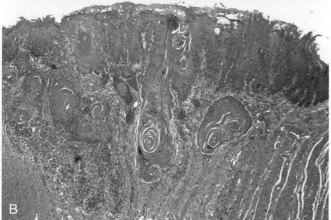

FIG. 13.4 Oral squamous cell carcinoma. (A) Gross appearance demonstrating ulceration and induration of the oral mucosa. (B) Histologic appearance showing numerous nests and islands of malignant keratinocytes invading the underlying connective tissue stroma.

Clinical Features. Despite advances in treatment of oral squamous cell carcinoma, the overall survival at 5 years is only 50%, in large part because it is often diagnosed at an advanced stage. Multiple primary tumors may be present at initial diagnosis but more often are detected later, in an estimated 3% to 7% of patients per year. Therefore, surveillance and early detection of new premalignant lesions are critical for the long-term survival of patients diagnosed with oral squamous cell carcinoma.

Advanced stages of disease are treated with a combination of surgery, radiation, and chemotherapy. Tumors that arise in the setting of carcinogen exposure are responsive to immune checkpoint inhibitors, presumably because they harbor a high burden of tumor neoantigens. The prognosis for patients with HPV-positive tumors is better than for those with HPV-negative tumors, possibly because HPV-positive tumors are less genetically heterogeneous. The HPV vaccine is protective against cervical cancer and if widely adopted should also sharply reduce the frequency of HPV-associated oral squamous cell carcinoma.

DISEASES OF SALIVARY GLANDS

There are three major salivary glands—parotid, submandibular, and sublingual—and numerous minor salivary glands distributed throughout the oral mucosa. Inflammatory or neoplastic disease may develop within any of these.

Xerostomia

Xerostomia **is defined as a dry mouth resulting from a decrease in the production of saliva.** Its incidence varies among populations but has been reported in more than 20% of individuals older than 70 years of age. It is a major feature of the autoimmune disorder Sjögren syndrome, in which it is usually accompanied by dry eyes (Chapter 5). A lack of salivary secretions is also a major complication of radiation therapy. However, xerostomia is most frequently observed as a side effect of many commonly used medications, including anticholinergic, antidepressant/antipsychotic, diuretic, antihypertensive, sedative, muscle relaxant, analgesic, and antihistaminic agents. Nontherapeutic drugs such as methamphetamine, cocaine, and cannabis can also cause xerostomia. On examination, the oral cavity may reveal only dry mucosa and/or atrophy of the papillae of the tongue, with fissuring and ulcerations, or, in Sjögren syndrome, concomitant inflammatory enlargement of the salivary glands. Complications of xerostomia include increased rates of dental caries and candidiasis, as well as difficulty in swallowing and speaking.

Sialadenitis

Inflammation of the salivary gland, referred to as *sialadenitis,* **may be induced by trauma, viral or bacterial infection, or autoimmune disease.** The most common viral sialadenitis is *mumps,* a paramyxovirus infection that predominantly involves the parotid glands. Mumps produces interstitial inflammation marked by a mononuclear inflammatory infiltrate. While mumps is usually a self-limited benign condition in children, in adults the virus may cause pancreatitis or orchitis; the latter sometimes results in sterility.

Mucocele is the most common inflammatory lesion of salivary glands. It results from blockage or rupture of a salivary gland duct, with consequent leakage of saliva into the surrounding connective tissue stroma. Mucocele occurs most often in toddlers and young and old adults and typically manifests as a fluctuant swelling of the lower lip that may change in size, particularly in association with meals (Fig. 13.5A). Histologic examination demonstrates a cyst-like space lined by granulation tissue or fibrous connective tissue and filled with mucin and inflammatory cells, particularly macrophages (Fig. 13.5B). Complete excision of the lesion and the minor salivary gland is the definitive treatment.

Bacterial sialadenitis is a common infection that most often involves the major salivary glands, particularly the submandibular glands. Duct obstruction by stones *(sialolithiasis)* is a common antecedent to infection; it may also be induced by impacted food debris or by edema secondary to injury. Dehydration and decreased secretory function may also predispose to formation of stones and consequent bacterial invasion. The most frequent pathogens are *Staphylococcus aureus* and *Streptococcus viridans.* Bacterial sialoadenitis may produce nonspecific interstitial inflammation of the affected glands or, when caused by staphylococci or other pyogens, may lead to suppuration and abscess formation.

Autoimmune sialadenitis, better known as Sjögren syndrome, is discussed in Chapter 5.

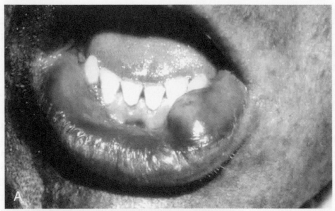

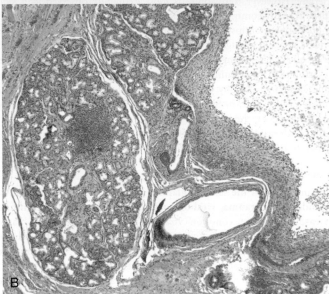

FIG. 13.5 Mucocele. (A) Fluctuant fluid-filled lesion on the lower lip after trauma. (B) Cystlike cavity *(right)* filled with mucinous material and lined by organizing granulation tissue. The normal gland acini are seen on the *left*.

Neoplasms

Despite their relatively simple morphology, the salivary glands give rise to at least 30 histologically distinct tumors (Table 13.1), a small number of which account for more than 90% of cases. Salivary gland tumors are relatively uncommon, representing less than 2% of human

Table 13.1 Histopathologic Classification and Prevalence of the Most Common Benign and Malignant Salivary Gland Tumors

Benign	Malignant
Pleomorphic adenoma (50%)	Mucoepidermoid carcinoma (15%)
Warthin tumor (5%)	Acinic cell carcinoma (6%)
Oncocytoma (2%)	Adenocarcinoma NOS (6%)
Cystadenoma (2%)	Adenoid cystic carcinoma (4%)
Basal cell adenoma (2%)	Malignant mixed tumor (3%)

NOS, Not otherwise specified.

Data from Ellis GL, Auclair PL, Gnepp DR: *Surgical Pathology of Salivary Glands,* vol 25, *Major Problems in Pathology,* Philadelphia, 1991, Saunders.

tumors. Approximately 65% to 80% arise within the parotid, 10% in the submandibular gland, and the remainder in the minor salivary glands, including the sublingual glands. Approximately 15% to 30% of tumors in the parotid glands are malignant. By contrast, approximately 40% of submandibular, 50% of minor salivary gland, and 70% to 90% of sublingual tumors are cancerous. Thus, the likelihood that a salivary gland tumor is malignant seems to be inversely proportional to the size of the gland.

Salivary gland tumors usually occur in adults. Parotid gland neoplasms cause swelling in front of and below the ear. Benign tumors may be present for months to several years before coming to clinical attention, while cancers more often come to attention promptly because of their more rapid growth. However, the only reliable way to differentiate benign from malignant lesions is through histopathologic evaluation.

Pleomorphic Adenoma

Pleomorphic adenoma is a benign tumor that consists of a mixture of ductal (epithelial) and myoepithelial cells and often exhibits both epithelial and mesenchymal differentiation. Pleomorphic adenomas represent about 60% of parotid gland tumors, are less common in the submandibular glands, and are relatively rare in the minor salivary glands.

MORPHOLOGY

Pleomorphic adenomas typically manifest as rounded, well-demarcated masses of several centimeters in greatest dimension. Although they are encapsulated, in some locations (particularly the palate), the capsule is not fully developed, and expansile growth produces protrusions into the surrounding tissues. The cut surface is gray-white and typically contains myxoid and blue translucent chondroid areas. Their most striking histologic feature is their characteristic heterogeneity. Epithelial elements are dispersed throughout the tumor stroma, which may contain variable mixtures of myxoid, hyaline, chondroid (cartilaginous), and even osseous tissue. In some pleomorphic adenomas, the epithelial elements predominate; in others, they are present only in widely dispersed foci. This histologic diversity has given rise to the alternative, albeit less preferred, name *mixed tumor.* **Epithelial elements resembling ductal or myoepithelial cells are arranged in ducts, acini, irregular tubules, strands, or sheets. These are typically dispersed within a mesenchyme-like background of loose myxoid tissue containing islands of cartilage and, rarely, foci of bone** (Fig. 13.6). Sometimes the epithelial cells form well-developed ducts lined by cuboidal to columnar cells with an underlying layer of deeply chromatic, small myoepithelial cells. In other instances, there may be strands or sheets of myoepithelial cells. Islands of well-differentiated squamous epithelium may also be present. In most cases, no epithelial dysplasia or mitotic activity is evident. No difference in biologic behavior has been observed between the tumors composed largely of epithelial elements and those composed largely of mesenchymal elements.

Clinical Features. Pleomorphic adenoma presents as a slow-growing, painless, mobile, discrete mass. Recurrence occurs in 25% of cases after simple enucleation of the tumor and in 4% of cases after wider resection and stems from a failure to remove minute extensions of tumor into surrounding soft tissues.

Carcinoma arising in a pleomorphic adenoma is referred to variously as a *carcinoma ex pleomorphic adenoma* or *malignant mixed tumor.* The incidence of malignant transformation increases from 2% in tumors present for less than 5 years to almost 10% in those present for more than 15 years. These cancers usually take the form of an

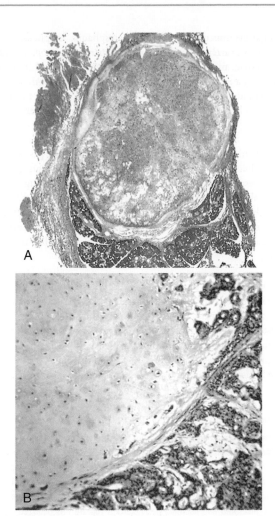

FIG. 13.6 Pleomorphic adenoma. (A) Low-power view showing a well-demarcated tumor with adjacent, deeply staining, normal salivary gland parenchyma. (B) High-power view showing epithelial cells as well as myoepithelial cells within chondroid matrix material.

adenocarcinoma or undifferentiated carcinoma. Unfortunately, they are among the most aggressive malignant neoplasms of salivary glands, with mortality rates of 30% to 50% at 5 years.

Mucoepidermoid Carcinoma

Mucoepidermoid carcinoma is composed of variable mixtures of squamous cells, mucus-secreting cells, and intermediate cells. This neoplasm represents about 15% of all salivary gland tumors. While it mainly occurs in the parotids (60%–70%), it also accounts for a large fraction of salivary gland neoplasms in the other glands, particularly the minor salivary glands. Overall, mucoepidermoid carcinoma is the most common primary malignant tumor of the salivary glands.

MORPHOLOGY

Mucoepidermoid carcinomas may be up to 8 cm in diameter and, although apparently circumscribed, lack well-defined capsules and are often infiltrative. The cut surface is pale gray to white and frequently demonstrates small, mucinous cysts. On histologic examination, these tumors contain cords, sheets, or cysts lined by squamous, mucous, or intermediate cells (eFig. 13.1). The latter is a hybrid cell type with squamous features and mucin-filled vacuoles, which are most easily detected with mucin stains. Cytologically, the tumor cells may be benign appearing or highly anaplastic and unmistakably malignant.

Clinical Features. Clinical course and prognosis depend on histologic grade. Low-grade tumors may invade locally and recur in about 15% of cases but metastasize only rarely and afford a 5-year survival rate of over 90%. By contrast, high-grade neoplasms and, to a lesser extent, intermediate-grade tumors are invasive and difficult to excise. As a result, they recur in 25% to 30% of cases, and about 30% metastasize to distant sites. The 5-year survival rate is only 50%.

ODONTOGENIC CYSTS AND TUMORS

Odontogenic cysts are derived from remnants of odontogenic epithelium present within the jaws. In contrast to the rest of the skeleton, epithelium-lined cysts are quite common in the jaws and may be either inflammatory, developmental, or neoplastic in origin. Only the most common lesions are considered here.

Dentigerous cysts originate around the crown of an unerupted tooth and are thought to result from a developmental defect involving of the dental follicle (primordial tissue that makes the enamel surface of teeth). They are lined by a thin, stratified squamous epithelium and are typically associated with a dense chronic inflammatory infiltrate in the surrounding connective tissue. Complete removal is curative.

Keratocystic odontogenic tumor is a neoplasm that occurs most frequently in individuals between 10 and 40 years of age, predominantly in males and typically in the posterior mandible. Previously considered to be a developmental aberration, it is now known to have clonal chromosomal aberrations and often harbors loss-of-function mutations in tumor suppressor genes, including *PTCH1*. As would be expected, individuals with *nevoid basal cell carcinoma syndrome,* which is caused by germline mutations in *PTCH1*, are at increased risk for keratocystic odontogenic tumor. On histologic examination, the cyst lining consists of a thin layer of keratinized squamous epithelium with a prominent basal cell layer. It is locally aggressive and has a high recurrence rate. Effective treatment requires complete surgical removal.

The *periapical cyst* has an inflammatory etiology. This common lesion occurs at the tooth apex as a result of long-standing pulpitis, which may be caused by advanced caries or trauma. Necrosis of the pulpal tissue may traverse the length of the root and exit the apex of the tooth into the surrounding alveolar bone, leading to a periapical abscess. Over time, granulation tissue (with or without an epithelial lining) may develop. Periapical inflammatory lesions persist due to bacterial infection or necrotic tissue in the area. Successful treatment consists of complete removal of the offending material followed by restoration or extraction of the tooth.

Odontogenic tumors are a complex group of lesions with diverse histologic appearances and clinical behaviors. Most are true neoplasms, either benign or malignant. They are derived from odontogenic epithelium, ectomesenchyme, or both. The two most common and clinically significant tumors are ameloblastoma and odontoma.

Ameloblastoma arises from odontogenic epithelium. It is typically cystic and slow growing and, despite being locally invasive, has an indolent course. The cysts are lined by palisading columnar epithelium that sometimes undergoes squamous differentiation and that overlies a loose stroma with stellate cells (eFig. 13.2). *Odontoma*, the most common type of odontogenic tumor, arises from epithelium but shows extensive deposition of enamel and dentin. It is cured by local excision.

ESOPHAGUS

The esophagus develops from the cranial portion of the foregut. It is a hollow, highly distensible muscular tube that extends from the epiglottis to the gastroesophageal junction, located just above the diaphragm. Acquired diseases of the esophagus range from lethal cancers to the persistent "heartburn" of gastroesophageal reflux, which may be chronic and incapacitating or merely an occasional annoyance.

OBSTRUCTIVE AND VASCULAR DISEASES

Mechanical Obstruction

Atresia, fistulas, and duplications may occur in any part of the gastrointestinal tract, including the esophagus (eFig. 13.3). When they involve the esophagus, they are discovered shortly after birth, usually because of regurgitation during feeding, warranting prompt surgical repair. Absence, or agenesis, of the esophagus is extremely rare; atresia, in which a thin, noncanalized cord replaces a segment of esophagus, is more common. It occurs most frequently at or near the tracheal bifurcation and is usually associated with a fistula connecting the upper or lower esophageal pouches to a bronchus or the trachea. This abnormal connection may result in aspiration, suffocation, pneumonia, or severe fluid and electrolyte imbalances.

Esophageal stenosis may be congenital or (more commonly) acquired. When acquired, the narrowing is generally caused by fibrous thickening of the submucosa and atrophy of the muscularis propria due to inflammation and scarring secondary to chronic gastroesophageal reflux, systemic sclerosis, irradiation, ingestion of caustic agents, or other forms of severe injury. Stenosis-associated dysphagia is usually progressive: difficulty eating solids typically occurs long before problems with swallowing liquids appear.

Functional Obstruction

Efficient delivery of food and fluids to the stomach requires coordinated waves of peristaltic contractions. *Esophageal dysmotility* interferes with this process and can take several forms, all characterized by dyscoordinated contraction or spasm of the muscularis. Because it increases esophageal wall stress, spasm also can cause small diverticula to form. Esophageal dysmotility can be separated into several forms depending on the nature of the contractile abnormalities.

Achalasia is characterized by the triad of incomplete lower esophageal sphincter (LES) relaxation, increased LES tone, and esophageal aperistalsis. Primary achalasia is caused by degeneration of distal esophageal inhibitory neurons and is, by definition, idiopathic. Loss of neural innervation due to damage within the esophagus, the extraesophageal vagus nerve, or the dorsal motor nucleus of the vagus may lead to secondary achalasia. This occurs in Chagas disease, in which *Trypanosoma cruzi* infection causes destruction of the myenteric plexus, failure of LES relaxation, and esophageal dilatation. As mentioned in Chapter 9, *T.cruzi* is an important cause of myocarditis in South and Central America. Achalasia-like disease may also be caused by diabetic autonomic neuropathy, infiltrative disorders such as malignancy, amyloidosis and sarcoidosis, and lesions of dorsal motor nuclei, which may be due to polio or surgical ablation.

Ectopia

Ectopic tissues (developmental rests) are common in the gastrointestinal tract. The most frequent site of ectopic gastric mucosa is the upper third of the esophagus, where it is referred to as an *inlet patch*. Although such tissue is generally asymptomatic, acid released by ectopic gastric mucosa may lead to dysphagia, esophagitis, Barrett esophagus, or, rarely, adenocarcinoma. *Gastric heterotopia,* patches of ectopic gastric mucosa in the small bowel (e.g., within a *Meckel diverticulum,* a remnant of the omphalomesenteric duct that is present in approximately 2% of individuals) or the colon, may present with occult blood loss due to local injury caused by acid secretion.

Esophageal Varices

Before returning to the heart, venous blood from the gastrointestinal tract is delivered to the liver via the portal vein. This circulatory pattern is responsible for the first-pass effect, in which drugs and other materials absorbed in the intestines are processed by the liver before entering the systemic circulation. **Diseases that impede portal blood flow cause portal hypertension and may lead to the development of esophageal varices, an important cause of massive, life-threatening bleeding.**

Pathogenesis. One of the few sites where the splanchnic and systemic venous circulations communicate is the esophagus. Portal hypertension induces development of collateral channels that allow portal blood to shunt into the caval system. However, the increased blood flow enlarges and dilates subepithelial and submucosal venous plexi within the distal esophagus. These vessels, termed *varices,* develop in 50% of patients with cirrhosis, most commonly in association with alcohol-related liver disease. Worldwide, hepatic schistosomiasis is the second most common cause of varices. A more detailed consideration of portal hypertension is provided in Chapter 14.

MORPHOLOGY

Varices are most commonly detected during endoscopy (Fig. 13.7A and B) and appear as tortuous dilated veins within the submucosa of the distal esophagus and proximal stomach (Fig. 13.7C and D). The overlying mucosa can be intact or ulcerated and necrotic, particularly if rupture has occurred.

Clinical Features. Varices are often asymptomatic, but their rupture can lead to massive hematemesis and death and constitutes a medical emergency. Despite intervention, as many as 20% of patients die from the first bleeding episode, either as a direct consequence of hemorrhage or due to hepatic coma triggered by hypovolemic shock and metabolic disturbances. Among those who survive, additional episodes of hemorrhage, each potentially fatal, occur in as many as 60% of cases.

ESOPHAGITIS

Esophageal Lacerations

The most common esophageal lacerations are *Mallory-Weiss tears,* which are often induced by severe retching or vomiting. Normally, a reflex relaxation of the gastroesophageal musculature precedes the antiperistaltic contractile wave associated with vomiting. This relaxation may fail during prolonged vomiting and, as a result, the refluxing gastric contents may cause the esophageal wall to stretch and tear. Patients usually present with hematemesis.

The roughly linear lacerations of Mallory-Weiss syndrome are longitudinally oriented and usually cross the gastroesophageal junction (Fig. 13.8A). These superficial tears generally heal quickly without intervention. By contrast, transmural esophageal tears (*Boerhaave syndrome*) result in severe mediastinitis and usually require prompt surgical intervention.

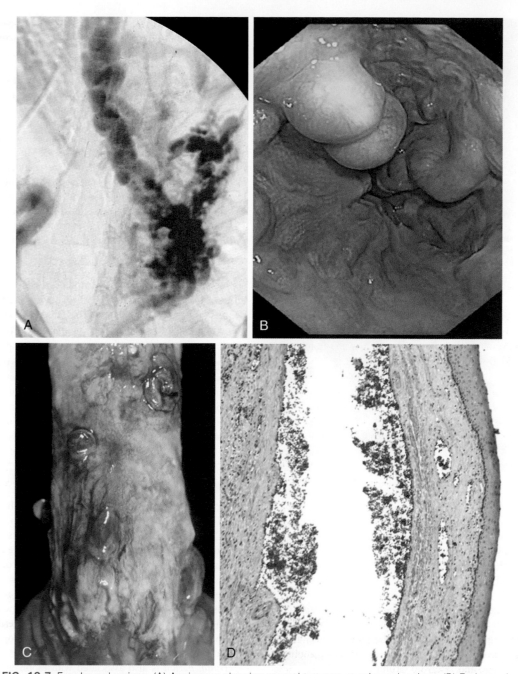

FIG. 13.7 Esophageal varices. (A) Angiogram showing several tortuous esophageal varices. (B) Endoscopic view of esophageal varices, readily visible as bulging submucosal vessels. (C) Collapsed varices are present in this postmortem specimen corresponding to the angiogram in (A). The polypoid areas are sites of variceal hemorrhage that were ligated with bands. (D) Dilated varices beneath intact squamous mucosa.

Chemical Esophagitis and Iatrogenic Esophageal Injury

The stratified squamous mucosa of the esophagus may be damaged by a variety of irritants including alcohol, corrosive acids or alkalis, excessively hot fluids, and heavy smoking. Medicinal pills, most commonly doxycycline and bisphosphonates, may adhere to the esophageal lining and dissolve in the esophagus rather than passing immediately into the stomach, resulting in *pill-induced esophagitis*. Esophagitis due to chemical injury generally causes only self-limited pain, particularly odynophagia (pain with swallowing).

Hemorrhage, stricture, or perforation may occur in severe cases. Iatrogenic esophageal injury may be caused by cytotoxic chemotherapy, radiation therapy, or graft-versus-host disease. The morphologic changes are nonspecific, consisting of ulceration and acute inflammation. Irradiation also causes blood vessel damage, adding an element of ischemic injury.

Infectious Esophagitis

Infectious esophagitis may occur in otherwise healthy individuals but is most frequent in those who are debilitated or immunocompromised. In

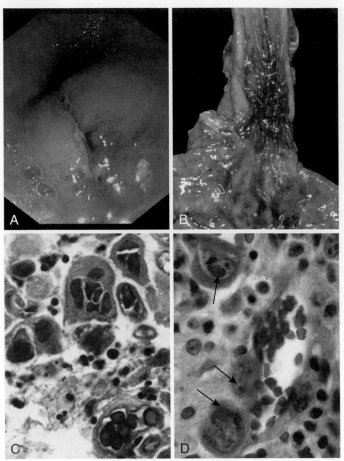

FIG. 13.8 Traumatic and viral esophagitis. (A) Endoscopic view of a longitudinally oriented Mallory-Weiss tear. These superficial lacerations can range from millimeters to several centimeters in length. (B) Postmortem specimen with multiple herpetic ulcers in the distal esophagus. (C) Multinucleate squamous cells containing herpesvirus nuclear inclusions. (D) Cytomegalovirus-infected endothelial cells with nuclear and cytoplasmic inclusions *(arrows)*. (Endoscopic image courtesy of Dr. Ira Hanan, The University of Chicago, Chicago, Illinois.)

these patients, esophageal infection by herpes simplex viruses, cytomegalovirus (CMV), or fungal organisms is common. Among fungi, *Candida* is the most common pathogen. The esophagus may also be involved in desquamative skin diseases, such as bullous pemphigoid and epidermolysis bullosa, and rarely by Crohn disease.

Infection by fungi or bacteria may be primary or complicate a preexisting ulcer. Nonpathogenic oral bacteria are frequently found in ulcer beds, while pathogenic organisms, which account for about 10% of infectious esophagitis cases, may invade the lamina propria and cause necrosis of the overlying mucosa. Candidiasis is characterized by adherent, grayish white pseudomembranes composed of densely matted fungal hyphae and inflammatory cells covering the esophageal mucosa, similar to that seen in the oral cavity.

The endoscopic appearance often provides a clue to the identity of the infectious agent in viral esophagitis. Herpes simplex virus (HSV) typically produces punched-out ulcers (Fig. 13.8B), and histopathologic analysis demonstrates nuclear viral inclusions within a rim of degenerating epithelial cells at the ulcer edge (Fig. 13.8C). By contrast, CMV causes shallower ulcerations. Biopsy of CMV lesions shows the characteristic nuclear and cytoplasmic inclusions within endothelial

cells and stromal cells (Fig. 13.8D). Immunohistochemical staining for HSV and CMV antigens may be a useful diagnostic tool.

Reflux Esophagitis

Reflux of gastric contents is the most frequent cause of esophagitis and the most common gastrointestinal ailment with which patients present in the outpatient setting in the United States. The associated clinical condition is termed *gastroesophageal reflux disease (GERD).* The stratified squamous epithelium of the esophagus is resistant to abrasion from foods but is sensitive to acid. Mucosal protection to acid is afforded by mucin and bicarbonate secreted from submucosal glands in the proximal and distal esophagus. More importantly, high lower-esophageal sphincter tone protects against reflux of acidic gastric contents, which are under positive pressure.

Pathogenesis. **Reflux of gastric fluids is central to the development of mucosal injury in GERD.** In some cases, duodenal bile reflux may exacerbate the damage. Conditions that decrease lower esophageal sphincter tone or increase abdominal pressure contribute to GERD and include alcohol and tobacco use, obesity, central nervous system depressants, pregnancy, hiatal hernia (discussed later), delayed gastric emptying, and increased gastric volume. In many cases, no definitive cause of reflux is identified.

MORPHOLOGY

By endoscopy erythema may be the only alteration. In mild GERD the mucosal histology is often unremarkable. With more significant disease, eosinophils are recruited to the squamous mucosa, followed by neutrophils, which are usually associated with more severe injury (Fig. 13.9A). Basal zone hyperplasia and elongation of lamina propria papillae may also be seen.

Clinical Features. GERD is most common in those over 40 years of age. The most frequent symptoms are heartburn, dysphagia, and, less often, noticeable regurgitation of sour-tasting gastric contents. Rarely, chronic GERD is punctuated by attacks of severe chest pain that may be mistaken for heart disease. Treatment with proton pump inhibitors reduces gastric acidity and typically provides symptomatic relief. While the severity of symptoms is not closely related to the degree of histologic change, the latter tends to increase with disease duration. Complications include esophageal ulceration, hematemesis, melena, stricture development, and Barrett esophagus, a precursor lesion to esophageal carcinoma (see below).

Hiatal hernia is also associated with esophageal reflux. It is characterized by separation of the diaphragmatic crura and protrusion of the stomach into the thorax through the resulting gap. Congenital hiatal hernias are recognized in infants and children, but many are acquired in later life. They are symptomatic in fewer than 10% of adults. Because hiatal hernia may lead to LES incompetence, when present symptoms often resemble GERD.

Eosinophilic Esophagitis

Eosinophilic esophagitis is a chronic immunologic disorder characterized clinically by symptoms related to esophageal dysfunction and histologically by the presence of eosinophilic inflammation. Symptoms include food impaction and dysphagia in adults and feeding intolerance or GERD-like symptoms in children. The cardinal histologic feature is epithelial infiltration by large numbers of eosinophils, particularly superficially (Fig. 13.9B) and at sites far from the

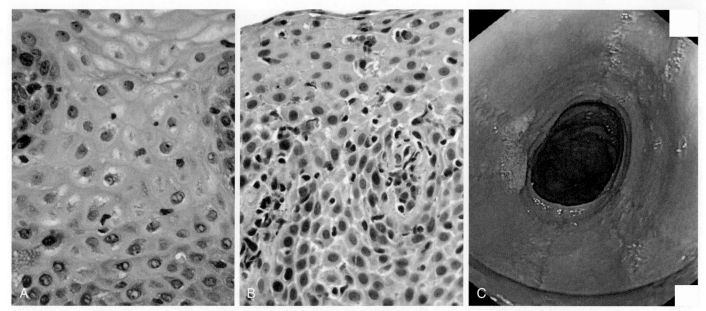

FIG. 13.9 Esophagitis. (A) Reflux esophagitis with scattered intraepithelial eosinophils. (B) Eosinophilic esophagitis with numerous intraepithelial eosinophils and scattered eosinophilic microabscesses. (C) Endoscopy reveals circumferential rings in the proximal esophagus of this patient with eosinophilic esophagitis. (Endoscopic image courtesy of Dr. Ira Hanan, The University of Chicago, Chicago, Illinois.)

gastroesophageal junction. Their abundance can help to differentiate eosinophilic esophagitis from GERD, Crohn disease, and other causes of esophagitis. Endoscopically evident rings in the upper and mid portions of the esophagus (Fig. 13.9C) may also help to distinguish eosinophilic esophagitis from GERD. Patients with eosinophilic esophagitis are typically refractory to proton pump inhibitor treatment. Most patients are atopic, and many have atopic dermatitis, allergic rhinitis, asthma, or modest peripheral eosinophilia. Treatments include dietary restrictions to prevent exposure to food allergens (e.g., cow's milk, soy products) and corticosteroids.

Barrett Esophagus

Barrett esophagus is a complication of chronic GERD that is characterized by intestinal metaplasia of the esophageal mucosa and an increased risk for development of adenocarcinoma. The incidence of Barrett esophagus is rising: it is estimated to occur in as many as 10% of individuals with symptomatic GERD. Patients typically present between 40 and 60 years of age and males are affected more than females. Molecular studies indicate that Barrett epithelium shares many acquired driver mutations with adenocarcinoma, consistent with the view that Barrett esophagus is a precursor of cancer. In keeping with this, epithelial dysplasia, considered to be a precursor lesion, develops in 0.2% to 1% of individuals with Barrett esophagus each year; its incidence increases with duration of symptoms and increasing patient age. Although the vast majority of esophageal adenocarcinoma is associated with Barrett esophagus, most individuals with Barrett esophagus do not develop esophageal cancer.

MORPHOLOGY

Barrett esophagus is recognized endoscopically as tongues or patches of reddish, velvety mucosa extending upward from the gastroesophageal junction (Fig. 13.10A). This metaplastic mucosa alternates with residual smooth, pale pink or gray squamous (esophageal) mucosa proximally and interfaces with light-brown columnar (gastric) mucosa distally (Fig. 13.10B and C). High-resolution endoscopes have increased the sensitivity of Barrett esophagus detection.

The defining feature of intestinal metaplasia is the presence of goblet cells, which have distinct mucin vacuoles that stain pale blue by H&E and impart the shape of a wine goblet to the remaining cytoplasm (Fig. 13.10C). Dysplasia is classified as low grade or high grade based on morphologic criteria.

Clinical Features. Diagnosis of Barrett esophagus is usually prompted by GERD symptoms and requires endoscopy and biopsy. Most experts require both endoscopic evidence of abnormal mucosa more than 1 cm above the gastroesophageal junction and histologically documented intestinal metaplasia for diagnosis of Barrett esophagus. The optimal management is a matter of debate, but most clinicians recommend periodic surveillance endoscopy with biopsy to screen for dysplasia. Dysplasia is often treated and more advanced lesions, including high-grade dysplasia and intramucosal carcinoma, always require therapeutic intervention. Available modalities include surgical resection *(esophagectomy)*, radiofrequency ablation, and endoscopic mucosectomy.

ESOPHAGEAL TUMORS

Adenocarcinoma and squamous cell carcinoma account for the majority of esophageal tumors. Worldwide, squamous cell carcinoma is more common, but adenocarcinoma is on the rise. Other rare tumors are not discussed here.

Adenocarcinoma

Esophageal adenocarcinoma typically arises in a background of Barrett esophagus and long-standing GERD. Risk for development of adenocarcinoma is greater in patients with documented dysplasia and in those who use tobacco, are obese, or who have had previous radiation therapy. In the United States, esophageal adenocarcinoma is seven times

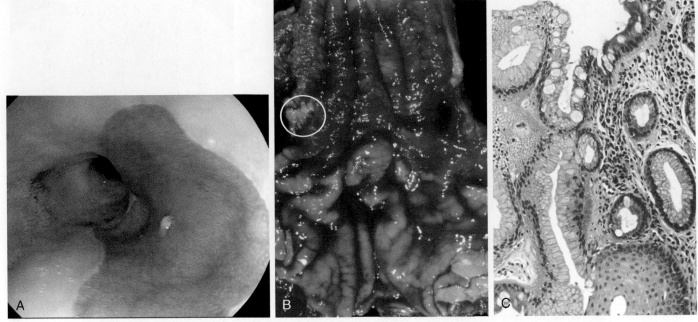

FIG. 13.10 Barrett esophagus. (A) Barrett esophagus at endoscopy, seen as a patch of reddish mucosa. (B) Gross image of Barrett esophagus (compare to Fig. 13.7C). Only a focal area of paler squamous mucosa *(circle)* remains within the predominantly metaplastic, reddish mucosa of the distal esophagus. (C) Histologic appearance of the gastroesophageal junction in Barrett esophagus. Note the transition between esophageal squamous mucosa *(lower right)* and metaplastic mucosa containing goblet cells *(upper)*. (Endoscopic image courtesy of Dr. Priya Kathpalia, University of California at San Francisco, San Francisco, California.)

more common in men than in women and is more common in individuals of European descent. Incidence varies worldwide, with rates being highest in Western countries, including the United States, the United Kingdom, Canada, Australia, and the Netherlands, and lowest in Korea, Thailand, Japan, and Ecuador. In countries where esophageal adenocarcinoma is more common, the incidence has increased more rapidly than for almost any other cancer. As a result, esophageal adenocarcinoma, which represented less than 5% of esophageal cancers before 1970, now accounts for half of all esophageal cancers in some Western countries, including the United States. This increase is largely attributed to the increased incidence of GERD and associated Barrett esophagus.

Pathogenesis. **Molecular studies suggest that the progression of Barrett esophagus to adenocarcinoma occurs over an extended period through the stepwise acquisition of genetic and epigenetic changes.** This model is supported by the observation that epithelial clones identified in nondysplastic Barrett metaplasia persist and accumulate mutations during progression to dysplasia and invasive carcinoma. Chromosomal abnormalities and *TP53* mutation are often present in the early stages of esophageal adenocarcinoma. Additional genetic changes and inflammation are thought to contribute to tumor progression.

MORPHOLOGY

Esophageal adenocarcinoma usually occurs in the distal third of the esophagus and may invade the adjacent gastric cardia (Fig. 13.11A). Early lesions often appear as flat or raised patches in otherwise intact mucosa, while advanced tumors tend to form large exophytic masses, infiltrate diffusely, or ulcerate and invade deeply. On microscopic examination, Barrett esophagus is frequently present adjacent to the tumor. Tumors typically produce mucin and form glands (Fig. 13.11B).

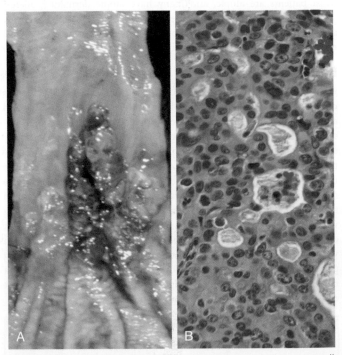

FIG. 13.11 Esophageal adenocarcinoma. (A) Adenocarcinoma usually occurs distally and, as in this case, often involves the gastric cardia. (B) Esophageal adenocarcinoma growing as back-to-back glands containing blue-gray mucin.

Clinical Features. Patients most commonly present with pain or difficulty in swallowing, progressive weight loss, chest pain, or vomiting. By the time signs and symptoms appear, the tumor has usually invaded submucosal lymphatic vessels. As a result of the advanced stage at diagnosis, the overall 5-year survival rate is less than 25%. By contrast, 5-year survival is close to 80% in the few patients with adenocarcinoma limited to the mucosa or submucosa.

Squamous Cell Carcinoma

In the United States, esophageal squamous cell carcinoma typically occurs in adults older than 45 years of age and affects males four times more frequently than females. Risk factors include alcohol and tobacco use, caustic esophageal injury, achalasia, Plummer-Vinson syndrome (iron deficiency anemia, dysphagia, and esophageal webs), frequent consumption of very hot beverages, and previous radiation therapy to the mediastinum. The incidence of esophageal squamous cell carcinoma can vary by more than 100-fold between and within countries, being more common in rural and lower resource areas. The countries with highest incidences are Iran, central China, Hong Kong, Argentina, Brazil, and South Africa.

Pathogenesis. **A majority of esophageal squamous cell carcinomas in Europe and the United States is associated with the use of alcohol and tobacco, the effects of which synergize to increase risk.** However, esophageal squamous cell carcinoma is also common in some regions where alcohol and tobacco use are uncommon due to religious or societal norms. In these areas, nutritional deficiencies and exposure to polycyclic hydrocarbons, nitrosamines, and other mutagenic compounds, such as those found in fungus-contaminated foods, are suspected to be the risk factors. HPV infection has also been implicated in esophageal squamous cell carcinoma in high-risk regions. DNA sequencing of esophageal squamous cell carcinoma has identified frequent mutations in genes that regulate squamous differentiation (e.g., *TP63* and *NOTCH*) as well as genes encoding regulators of proliferation (e.g., cyclins, cyclin-dependent kinases, RB).

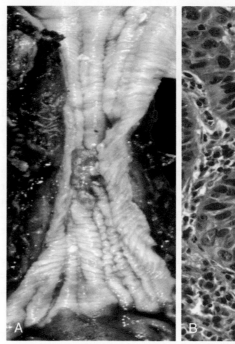

FIG. 13.12 Esophageal squamous cell carcinoma. (A) Squamous cell carcinoma most frequently is found in the mid esophagus, where it commonly causes strictures. (B) Squamous cell carcinoma composed of nests of malignant cells that partially recapitulate the stratified organization of squamous epithelium.

Clinical Features. Manifestations of squamous cell carcinoma of the esophagus appear insidiously and include dysphagia, odynophagia (pain on swallowing), and obstruction. As with other forms of esophageal obstruction, patients may unconsciously adjust to the progressively increasing obstruction by altering their diet from solid to liquid foods. Extreme weight loss and debilitation may occur as consequences of impaired nutrition and tumor-associated cachexia. As with adenocarcinoma, hemorrhage and sepsis may accompany tumor ulceration. Occasionally, squamous cell carcinoma of the upper and mid esophagus presents with symptoms caused by aspiration of food via a tracheoesophageal fistula.

Although 5-year survival rates are 75% for patients with superficial esophageal carcinoma, they are much lower for patients with advanced tumors. Since most tumors are detected at an advanced stage, the overall 5-year survival rate is only approximately 10%.

STOMACH

Disorders of the stomach are a frequent source of disease, with inflammatory and neoplastic lesions being the most common. In the United States, symptoms related to gastric acidity account for nearly one-third of health care spending on gastrointestinal disease. In addition, despite a decreasing incidence in certain locales, including the United States, gastric cancer remains a leading cause of death worldwide.

The stomach is divided into four major anatomic regions: the cardia, fundus, body, and antrum. The cardia is lined mainly by mucin-secreting *foveolar cells* that form shallow glands. The antral glands are similar but also contain endocrine cells, such as *G cells* that release gastrin to stimulate luminal acid secretion by *parietal cells* within the gastric fundus and body. The well-developed glands of the body and fundus also contain *chief cells*, which produce and secrete digestive enzymes such as pepsin.

GASTROPATHY AND ACUTE GASTRITIS

Gastritis results from mucosal injury. When neutrophils are present, the lesion is referred to as *acute gastritis*. When cell injury and regeneration are present but inflammatory cells are rare or absent, the term *gastropathy* is applied. Agents that cause gastropathy include nonsteroidal antiinflammatory drugs, alcohol, bile, and stress-induced injury. Acute mucosal erosion or ulceration, such as Curling ulcers or lesions following disruption of gastric blood flow, for example, in portal hypertension, can also cause gastropathy that typically progresses to gastritis. The term *hypertrophic gastropathy* is applied to a specific group of diseases exemplified by Ménétrier disease and Zollinger-Ellison syndrome (discussed later).

Both gastropathy and acute gastritis may be asymptomatic or cause variable degrees of epigastric pain, nausea, and vomiting. In more severe cases, there may be mucosal erosion, ulceration, hemorrhage, hematemesis, melena or, rarely, massive blood loss.

Pathogenesis. The gastric lumen normally has a pH close to 1—more than 1 million times more acidic than the blood. This harsh environment aids digestion but also has the potential to damage the mucosa. Several mechanisms have evolved to protect the gastric mucosa from "self-digestion" (Fig. 13.13). Surface foveolar cells produce a thin layer of mucus that is resistant to acid and has a neutral pH due to secretion of bicarbonate ions by surface epithelial cells. This mucus layer also protects the mucosa from potential physical damage caused by food particles. In addition, any protons that diffuse back into the lamina

propria are buffered by the rich blood supply of the gastric mucosa. Gastropathy, acute gastritis, and chronic gastritis may occur after disruption of these protective mechanisms. The main causes include:

- *Nonsteroidal antiinflammatory drugs* (NSAIDs) inhibit cyclooxygenase (COX)-dependent synthesis of prostaglandins E_2 and I_2, which protect the gastric lining by stimulating mucus and bicarbonate secretion, mucosal blood flow, and epithelial restitution.
- The gastric injury that occurs in uremic patients and those infected with urease-secreting *H. pylori* may be due to inhibition of gastric bicarbonate transporters by ammonium ions.
- *Aging*, which is associated with reduced mucin and bicarbonate secretion, has been suggested to explain the increased susceptibility of older adults to gastritis.
- *Hypoxemia and decreased oxygen delivery* may account for an increased incidence of gastropathy and acute gastritis at high altitudes.
- *Ingestion of harsh chemicals*, particularly acids or bases, either accidentally or in suicide attempts, leads to severe gastric mucosal damage as a result of direct injury to epithelial and stromal cells. Direct cellular damage also contributes to gastritis induced by excessive alcohol consumption, NSAID use, and radiation therapy. Agents that inhibit cell division, such as those used in cancer chemotherapy, may cause generalized mucosal damage due to insufficient epithelial renewal.

MORPHOLOGY

Histologically, gastropathy and mild acute gastritis may be difficult to recognize since the lamina propria shows only moderate edema and slight vascular congestion. The surface epithelium is intact, but hyperplasia of

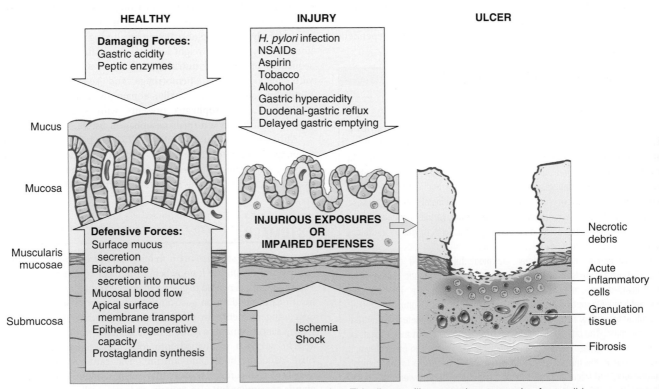

FIG. 13.13 Mechanisms of gastric injury and protection. This diagram illustrates the progression from mild forms of injury to ulceration that may occur with acute or chronic gastritis. Ulcers include layers of necrotic debris, inflammation, and granulation tissue; scarring, which develops over time, is present only in chronic lesions. *NSAIDs,* Nonsteroidal antiinflammatory drugs.

foveolar mucus cells is typically present. Neutrophils, lymphocytes, and plasma cells are not prominent.

The presence of neutrophils above the basement membrane in contact with epithelial cells is abnormal in all parts of the gastrointestinal tract and signifies active inflammation or, at this site, gastritis (rather than gastropathy). The term **active inflammation** is preferred over acute inflammation throughout the luminal gastrointestinal tract since neutrophils may be present in both acute and chronic disease states. With more severe mucosal damage, erosions and hemorrhage develop. Hemorrhage may manifest as dark punctae in an otherwise hyperemic mucosa. Concurrent presence of erosion and hemorrhage is termed **acute erosive hemorrhagic gastritis.**

Stress-Related Mucosal Disease

Stress-related gastric injury occurs in patients with severe trauma, extensive burns, intracranial disease, major surgery, serious medical diseases, and other forms of severe physiologic stress. More than 75% of critically ill patients develop endoscopically visible gastric lesions during the first 3 days of their illness. In some cases, the ulcers are given specific names based on location and clinical associations. Examples are as follows:

- *Stress ulcers*, which may occur in critically ill patients with shock, sepsis, or severe trauma
- *Curling ulcers*, which may occur in the proximal duodenum of individuals who have suffered severe burns or trauma
- *Cushing ulcers*, which may occur in the stomach, duodenum, or esophagus of patients with CNS injury, such as stroke; these have a high incidence of perforation

Pathogenesis. Stress-related gastric mucosal injury is most often due to ischemia caused by systemic hypotension or reduced gastric blood flow resulting from splanchnic vasoconstriction. The decrease in blood flow appears to reduce the secretion of bicarbonate while also diminishing buffering by blood, setting the stage for mucosal injury. In patients who are severely ill, systemic acidosis may also contribute to mucosal injury by lowering the intracellular pH of mucosal cells. CNS injury may lead to the formation of Cushing ulcers by stimulation of vagal nuclei, which transmit parasympathetic impulses that promote acid hypersecretion.

MORPHOLOGY

Stress-related gastric mucosal injury ranges from shallow erosions caused by superficial epithelial damage to deep lesions that penetrate the mucosa. Acute ulcers are round and typically less than 1 cm in diameter. The ulcer base is frequently stained brown to black by acid-digested extravasated red cells. Unlike peptic ulcers, which arise in the setting of chronic injury and are typically solitary lesions at the interface of the body and antrum, acute stress ulcers can be found anywhere in the stomach and are often multiple. They are sharply demarcated, with essentially normal adjacent mucosa, although there may be suffusion of blood into the mucosa and submucosa and some inflammatory reaction. The scarring and thickening of blood vessels that characterize chronic peptic ulcers are absent. Healing with complete reepithelialization occurs days or weeks after the injurious factors are removed.

Clinical Features. Ulcers are associated with nausea, vomiting, melena, and coffee-ground hematemesis. Bleeding from superficial gastric erosions or ulcers sufficient to require transfusion develops in 1% to 4% of these patients. Other complications, including perforation, also may occur. Prophylaxis with proton pump inhibitors may blunt the impact of stress ulceration, but the most important determinant of outcome is the severity of the underlying condition.

CHRONIC GASTRITIS

The most common cause of chronic gastritis is infection with the bacillus *Helicobacter pylori*. Autoimmune gastritis, typically associated with gastric atrophy, is the most common cause in patients without *H. pylori* infection. Chronic NSAID use is a third important cause of gastritis in some populations, as discussed later. Less common causes include radiation injury and chronic bile reflux.

The signs and symptoms associated with chronic gastritis are typically less severe but more persistent than those of acute gastritis. Nausea and upper abdominal discomfort may occur, sometimes with vomiting, but hematemesis is uncommon.

Helicobacter pylori Gastritis

The discovery of the association of *H. pylori* with peptic ulcer disease revolutionized the understanding of chronic gastritis. These spiral-shaped bacilli are present in gastric biopsy specimens from almost all patients with duodenal ulcers and a majority of those with gastric ulcers or chronic gastritis. Acute *H. pylori* infection is subclinical in most cases, and it is the subsequent chronic gastritis that ultimately brings the affected person to medical attention.

Epidemiology. In the United States, *H. pylori* infection is associated with lower economic status, residence in areas with poor sanitation, and birth outside of the United States. Infection is typically acquired in childhood and may persist for life. Improved sanitation in many areas likely explains why *H. pylori* infection rates among younger individuals today are markedly lower than they were in similarly aged individuals 30 years ago. Worldwide, colonization rates vary from less than 10% to more than 80% as a function of age, geography, and social factors.

Pathogenesis. *H. pylori* organisms have adapted to the ecologic niche provided by gastric mucus. Although *H. pylori* may invade the gastric mucosa, colonization appears to be sufficient to produce disease. Four features are linked to *H. pylori* virulence:
- *Flagella,* which allow the bacteria to move in viscous mucus
- *Urease,* which generates ammonia from endogenous urea, thereby elevating local gastric pH around the organisms and protecting the bacteria from the acidic pH of the stomach
- *Adhesins,* which enhance bacterial adherence to surface foveolar cells
- *Toxins,* such as those encoded by cytotoxin-associated gene A (*CagA*) and *CagE*. These factors appear to stimulate the release of cytokines such as IL-8, a potent chemotactic factor for neutrophils, and thereby initiate and sustain innate and adaptive immune responses that lead to mucosal damage.

H. pylori infection first establishes itself in the antrum, where the organisms and associated inflammation stimulate G cells to release gastrin, resulting in hyperacidity and an increased risk of peptic ulcer disease (discussed later). With time, however, in some patients the infection spreads to involve the body of the stomach, an event that may lead to loss of parietal cell function, gastric atrophy, and intestinal metaplasia, a precursor of gastric adenocarcinoma.

Gastric biopsy specimens stained with H&E or Giemsa generally demonstrate *H. pylori* in individuals who are infected (Fig. 13.14A); immunohistochemical stains that are specific for the organism are also useful. The organism is concentrated within mucus overlying foveolar cells in the surface and neck regions of glands. The inflammatory reaction includes a variable number of neutrophils within the lamina propria, including some that cross the basement membrane to involve the epithelium (Fig. 13.14B) and accumulate in the lumen of gastric pits to create pit abscesses. The regenerative changes associated with repair of mucosal damage may give rise to **hyperplastic polyps,** which are composed of elongated foveolar glands with active or chronically inflamed stroma. The superficial lamina propria includes large numbers of plasma cells, often in clusters or sheets, as well as increased numbers of lymphocytes and macrophages. When intense, inflammatory infiltrates may create thickened rugal folds, mimicking infiltrative malignant lesions. Chronic inflammation may lead to the appearance of **inflammatory polyps**. Submucosal lymphoid aggregates, some with germinal centers, are frequently present (Fig. 13.14C) and represent an induced form of **mucosa-associated lymphoid tissue** (MALT) that has the potential to transform into lymphoma. **Intestinal metaplasia,** characterized by the presence of goblet cells and columnar absorptive cells (Fig. 13.14D), may also occur and is associated with increased risk of gastric adenocarcinoma. *H. pylori* shows tropism for gastric foveolar epithelium and is generally not found in areas of intestinal metaplasia, acid-producing mucosa of the gastric body, or duodenal epithelium. Antral biopsies are therefore preferred for evaluation of *H. pylori* gastritis.

Clinical Features. In addition to histologic and immunohistochemical identification of the organism, several diagnostic tests have been developed, including a noninvasive serologic test for *H. pylori* antibodies, a stool test for the organism, and the urea breath test, based on the generation of ammonia by bacterial urease. Gastric biopsy specimens can also be analyzed by the rapid urease test, bacterial culture, or polymerase chain reaction (PCR) assay for *H. pylori* DNA. Effective treatments include combinations of antibiotics and proton pump inhibitors. Patients with *H. pylori* gastritis usually improve after treatment, but relapses may occur due to incomplete eradication or reinfection.

Autoimmune Gastritis

Autoimmune gastritis accounts for less than 10% of cases of chronic gastritis. In contrast to *H. pylori*–associated gastritis, autoimmune gastritis typically spares the antrum and induces gastric atrophy (Table 13.2). Autoimmune gastritis is characterized by the following:

- *Antibodies to parietal cells and intrinsic factor* that can be detected in serum and gastric secretions
- *Reduced serum pepsinogen I levels*
- *Antral endocrine cell hyperplasia*
- *Vitamin B₁₂ deficiency* leading to pernicious anemia and neurologic changes
- *Impaired gastric acid secretion (achlorhydria)*

Pathogenesis. **Autoimmune gastritis causes immune-mediated loss of parietal cells and subsequent reductions in acid and intrinsic factor secretion.** There is an association with other autoimmune diseases, suggesting some common genetic or environmental risk factor. The loss of parietal cells has been attributed to autoreactive T-cells, and the serum of affected patients contains autoantibodies

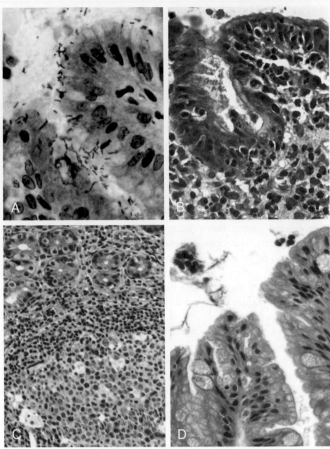

FIG. 13.14 *H. pylori* gastritis. (A) Spiral-shaped *H. pylori* bacilli are highlighted in this Warthin-Starry silver stain. Organisms are abundant within surface mucus. (B) Intraepithelial and lamina propria neutrophils are prominent. (C) Lymphoid aggregates with germinal centers and abundant subepithelial plasma cells within the superficial lamina propria are characteristic of *H. pylori* gastritis. (D) Intestinal metaplasia, recognizable as the presence of goblet cells admixed with gastric foveolar epithelium, can develop and is a risk factor for gastric adenocarcinoma.

that block intrinsic factor function (Chapter 10). Deficient acid secretion stimulates gastrin release, resulting in hypergastrinemia and hyperplasia of antral gastrin-producing G cells. Lack of intrinsic factor disables ileal vitamin B₁₂ absorption, leading to B₁₂ deficiency and megaloblastic anemia, a disease called *pernicious anemia* (Chapter 10).

Autoimmune gastritis is characterized by **damage of oxyntic (acid-producing) mucosa** within the body and fundus. Damage to the antrum and cardia is typically absent or mild. Due to diffuse atrophy, the oxyntic mucosa of the body and fundus appears markedly thinned and rugal folds are lost. Neutrophils may be present, but the inflammatory infiltrate is more commonly composed of lymphocytes, macrophages, and plasma cells and is centered on the gastric glands. Parietal and chief cell loss can be extensive, and **intestinal metaplasia** may develop. Hyperplasia of gastrin-secreting G cells is associated with an increased risk of gastric carcinoid tumors, histologic features of which are described later.

Table 13.2 Characteristics of *Helicobacter pylori*–Associated and Autoimmune Gastritis

Feature	*H. pylori*–Associated	Autoimmune
Location	Antrum	Body
Inflammatory infiltrate	Neutrophils, subepithelial plasma cells, germinal centers	Lymphocytes, macrophages
Acid production	Increased to slightly decreased	Decreased
Gastrin	Normal to markedly increased	Markedly increased
Other lesions	Hyperplastic/inflammatory polyps	Neuroendocrine hyperplasia
Serology	Antibodies to *H. pylori*	Antibodies to parietal cells (H^+,K^+-ATPase, intrinsic factor)
Sequelae	Peptic ulcer, adenocarcinoma, lymphoma	Atrophy, pernicious anemia, adenocarcinoma, carcinoid tumor
Associations	Lower economic status, residence in rural areas	Autoimmune disease; thyroiditis, diabetes, Graves disease

Clinical Features. The median age at diagnosis is 60 years and there is a slight female predominance. Patients may present with dyspepsia or symptoms related to vitamin B_{12} deficiency or iron deficiency, the latter because gastric acid and digestive enzymes are required for optimal iron uptake. Antibodies to parietal cells and intrinsic factor are uniformly present, whereas vitamin B_{12} deficiency and pernicious anemia develop in only a minority of patients.

COMPLICATIONS OF CHRONIC GASTRITIS

There are several important complications of chronic gastritis: peptic ulcer disease, mucosal atrophy, and intestinal metaplasia and dysplasia.

Peptic Ulcer Disease

Peptic ulcer disease (PUD) is most often associated with *H. pylori* infection or NSAID use. The imbalances of mucosal defenses and damaging forces that cause chronic gastritis (see Fig. 13.13) are also responsible for PUD. In the United States, NSAID use is becoming the most common cause of gastric ulcers as *H. pylori* infection rates fall and low-dose aspirin use in the aging population increases. PUD may occur in any portion of the gastrointestinal tract exposed to acidic gastric juices but is most common in the gastric antrum and first portion of the duodenum. Peptic (acid-induced) injury may occur in the esophagus as a result of acid reflux (GERD) or acid secretion by ectopic gastric mucosa. Peptic injury in the small intestine may also be associated with gastric heterotopia, such as may be seen within a Meckel diverticulum.

Epidemiology. PUD is common and is a frequent cause of physician visits worldwide. More than 4 million individuals in the United States are treated for this condition each year. The lifetime risk for developing an ulcer is approximately 10% for males and 4% for females.

Pathogenesis. **More than 70% of PUD cases are associated with *H. pylori* infection;** in these individuals, PUD generally develops on a background of chronic gastritis. Because only 5% to 10% of individuals infected with *H. pylori* develop ulcers, it is probable that host factors as well as variation among *H. pylori* strains contribute to PUD development.

Hyperacidity, which may be caused by *H. pylori* infection, parietal cell hyperplasia, excessive secretory responses, or loss of signals that inhibit acid secretion, is central to the pathogenesis of PUD. For example, *Zollinger-Ellison syndrome,* characterized by multiple peptic ulcerations in the stomach, duodenum, and even jejunum, is caused by tumors that produce gastrin constitutively, leading to massive acid production. Cofactors in peptic ulcerogenesis include chronic NSAID use; cigarette smoking, which reduces mucosal blood flow and healing; and high-dose corticosteroids, which suppress prostaglandin synthesis and impair healing. Peptic ulcers are more frequent in individuals with alcohol-related cirrhosis, chronic obstructive pulmonary disease, chronic renal failure, and hyperparathyroidism. In the latter two conditions, hypercalcemia stimulates gastrin production and thereby increases acid secretion.

> ## MORPHOLOGY
>
> Peptic ulcers are four times more common in the proximal duodenum than in the stomach. Duodenal ulcers usually occur within a few centimeters of the pyloric valve and involve the anterior duodenal wall. Gastric peptic ulcers are predominantly located near the interface of the body and antrum. The classic peptic ulcer is a round to oval, **sharply punched-out defect** (Fig. 13.15A and B). The ulcer base is smooth and clean as a result of peptic digestion of exudate and on histologic examination is composed of highly vascular granulation tissue (Fig. 13.15C).

Clinical Features. Peptic ulcers occur most often in middle-aged to older adults without obvious precipitating conditions other than chronic gastritis. They are solitary in more than 80% of patients. A majority of peptic ulcers come to clinical attention after incidents of epigastric burning or aching pain, although a significant fraction manifest with complications such as iron deficiency anemia, hemorrhage, or perforation. Pain tends to occur 1 to 3 hours after meals during the day, is worse at night, and is relieved by alkali or food. Nausea, vomiting, bloating, and belching may be present. Healing may occur with or without therapy, but the tendency to develop additional ulcers remains.

PUD causes much more morbidity than mortality. A variety of surgical approaches were formerly used to treat PUD, but current therapies are aimed at *H. pylori* eradication with antibiotics and neutralization of gastric acid, usually through use of proton pump inhibitors. These efforts have markedly reduced the need for surgical management, which is reserved primarily for treatment of ulcers with uncontrollable bleeding or perforation.

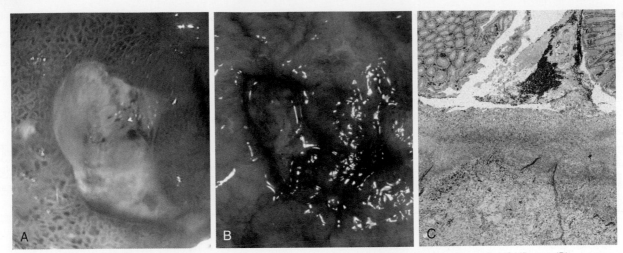

FIG. 13.15 Peptic ulcer disease. (A) Endoscopic view of typical antral ulcer associated with NSAID use. (B) Gross view of a similar ulcer that was resected due to gastric perforation, presenting as free air under the diaphragm. Note the clean edges. (C) The necrotic ulcer base is composed of granulation tissue overlaid by degraded blood. (Endoscopic image courtesy of Dr. Ira Hanan, The University of Chicago, Chicago, Illinois.)

Mucosal Atrophy and Intestinal Metaplasia

Long-standing chronic gastritis may be associated with mucosal atrophy and intestinal metaplasia, recognized by the presence of goblet cells. Intestinal metaplasia is strongly associated with development of gastric adenocarcinoma, a risk that may be exacerbated by the achlorhydria of gastric mucosal atrophy, as this appears to permit overgrowth of bacteria that produce carcinogenic nitrosamines. Intestinal metaplasia caused by chronic *H. pylori* gastritis may regress after eradication of the organism, but it is unclear if this lowers the risk of adenocarcinoma.

Dysplasia

Chronic gastritis exposes the epithelium to inflammation-related free radical damage and results in sustained attempts at repair, leading to increased epithelial proliferation. Over time, this can lead to the accumulation of genetic alterations that result in carcinoma. Preinvasive in situ lesions can be recognized histologically as dysplasia, which is marked by variations in epithelial cell size, shape, and orientation along with coarse chromatin texture, hyperchromasia, and nuclear enlargement. These overlap with and are sometimes difficult to distinguish from injury-associated regenerative changes.

GASTRIC POLYPS AND TUMORS

Gastric Polyps

Polyps are identified in up to 5% of upper gastrointestinal tract endoscopies. Although many different types of polyps occur in the stomach, only the more common types are described here.

Inflammatory and Hyperplastic Polyps

Up to 75% of gastric polyps are considered to be inflammatory or hyperplastic in origin. This distinction is artificial, however, as inflammatory and hyperplastic polyps lie at opposite ends of the morphologic spectrum of a single entity with varying degrees of inflammation. These polyps most commonly affect individuals between 50 and 60 years of age and usually arise in a background of chronic gastritis, which initiates the injury that leads to reactive

hyperplasia and polyp formation. If associated with *H. pylori* gastritis, polyps may regress after bacterial eradication. The frequency with which dysplasia, a precancerous in situ lesion, develops in these polyps correlates with size: there is a significant increase in risk with polyps larger than 1.5 cm.

Fundic Gland Polyps

Fundic gland polyps occur sporadically and in individuals with familial adenomatous polyposis (FAP). Polyps associated with FAP may show dysplasia, but almost never progress to become malignant. The incidence of sporadic lesions has increased markedly as a result of the widespread use of proton pump inhibitors. This likely results from increased gastrin secretion in response to reduced acidity, leading to gastrin-driven glandular hyperplasia. Fundic gland polyps are nearly always asymptomatic and are usually an incidental finding. These well-circumscribed polyps occur in the gastric body and fundus, are often multiple, and are composed of cystically dilated, irregular glands lined by flattened parietal and chief cells.

Gastric Adenoma

Gastric adenoma represents up to 10% of gastric polyps and is an important precursor to gastric adenocarcinoma. Its incidence increases with age and varies among different populations in parallel with that of gastric adenocarcinoma. Patients are usually between 50 and 60 years of age and males are affected three times more often than females. Gastric adenomas almost always occur on a background of chronic gastritis with atrophy and intestinal metaplasia and exhibit epithelial dysplasia, which can be classified as low or high grade (eFig. 13.4). The risk for development of adenocarcinoma is related to the size of the adenoma and is particularly elevated with lesions greater than 2 cm in diameter. Overall, the risk of malignant transformation is far greater than with colonic polyps, and areas of carcinoma may be present in up to 30% of gastric adenomas at the time of excision.

Gastric Adenocarcinoma

Adenocarcinoma is the most common malignancy of the stomach, accounting for more than 90% of all gastric cancers. Worldwide, it is estimated to account for 8% of all deaths from cancer. Early symptoms resemble those of chronic gastritis, including dyspepsia, dysphagia, and nausea. As a result, the cancer is often diagnosed at advanced stages when clinical manifestations such as weight loss, anorexia, altered bowel habits, anemia, and hemorrhage trigger diagnostic evaluation. There are two types of gastric adenocarcinoma: (1) diffuse, which is characterized by signet ring cells and infiltrative growth, and (2) intestinal, which typically forms a mass or ulcer and is composed of malignant glands. These two types have different etiologies and presentations.

Epidemiology. Gastric cancer rates vary markedly with geography, likely due predominantly to environmental factors. The incidence is up to 20 times higher in Japan, Chile, Costa Rica, and Eastern Europe than in North America, Northern Europe, Africa, and Southeast Asia. This has led to the implementation of endoscopic screening programs in older adults in regions of high incidence, such as Japan and Korea, which are designed to detect early, resectable gastric cancers limited to the mucosa and submucosa. Notably, the incidence of gastric cancer is lower in Japanese migrants to the United States than in Japanese natives, highlighting the importance of environmental exposures. Screening programs are not cost effective in regions in which the incidence is low, and less than 20% of cases are detected at an early stage in North America and Northern Europe.

Gastric cancer is more common in lower socioeconomic groups and in individuals with multifocal mucosal atrophy and intestinal metaplasia. Peptic ulcer disease does not impart an increased risk for development of gastric cancer, but patients who have had partial gastrectomies for peptic ulcer disease have a slightly higher risk for developing cancer in the residual gastric stump as a result of hypochlorhydria, bile reflux, and chronic gastritis.

In the United States and other Western countries, gastric cancer rates have dropped by more than 85% since the early 20th century, likely reflecting decreased exposure to environmental factors (e.g., *H. pylori* infection and carcinogens in food) implicated in the development of gastric cancer. However, one form of gastric adenocarcinoma, cancer of the gastric cardia, is rising in incidence. This trend is probably related to increased rates of Barrett esophagus and may reflect the growing prevalence of obesity and chronic gastroesophageal reflux disease in the United States.

Pathogenesis. Gastric cancers are genetically heterogeneous, but certain molecular alterations are frequently found. We will consider these first and then discuss the role of two infectious agents, *H. pylori* and Epstein-Barr virus.

- *Mutations.* While the majority of gastric cancers are not hereditary, mutations identified in familial gastric cancer have provided important insights into the pathogenesis of sporadic cases. Germline mutations in *CDH1*, which encodes E-cadherin, a protein that contributes to epithelial intercellular adhesion, are associated with familial gastric cancers, usually of the diffuse type. Notably, somatic mutations in *CDH1* are present in about 50% of sporadic diffuse gastric tumors, and E-cadherin expression is drastically decreased in the rest, often by methylation of the *CDH1* promoter. Thus, the loss of E-cadherin function is a key step in the development of diffuse gastric cancer. By contrast, patients with familial adenomatous polyposis caused by germline loss of function mutations in the adenomatous polyposis coli gene (*APC*), a negative regulator of the WNT pathway, are at increased risk for development of intestinal-type gastric cancer. Sporadic intestinal-type gastric cancer is associated with several genetic abnormalities, including acquired gain-of-function mutations of β-catenin, a protein that is negatively regulated by the APC protein, further implicating hyperactive WNT signaling in this subtype of gastric carcinoma. In addition, *TP53* mutations are present in a majority of sporadic gastric cancers of both histologic types, which also exhibit amplification of the gene encoding the HER2 tyrosine kinase in approximately 10% to 20% of cases.

- *H. pylori.* Chronic gastritis, most commonly due to *H. pylori* infection, promotes the development and progression of cancers, another example of the prooncogenic effect of certain types of chronic inflammation (Chapter 6). These oncogenic effects may be related to increased epithelial proliferation in response to chronic damage, epigenetic changes associated with intestinal metaplasia, and suppression of local adaptive immunity, an alteration that may be seen in chronically inflamed tissues.

- *Epstein-Barr virus (EBV).* Up to 10% of gastric adenocarcinomas are associated with Epstein-Barr virus (EBV) infection. Although the precise role of EBV in the development of gastric adenocarcinomas remains to be defined, it is notable that EBV episomes in these tumors are clonal, supporting the hypothesis that infection precedes neoplastic transformation. Further, *TP53* mutations are uncommon in EBV-positive gastric tumors, suggesting that the molecular pathogenesis of these cancers is distinct from that of other gastric adenocarcinomas. Morphologically, EBV-positive tumors tend to occur in the proximal stomach, usually have diffuse growth pattern, and are often associated with a marked lymphocytic infiltrate.

MORPHOLOGY

Gastric adenocarcinomas are classified according to their gross and histologic appearance into intestinal and diffuse types. **Intestinal-type cancers** tend to be bulky (Fig. 13.16A) and are composed of glandular structures, features resembling those of esophageal and colonic adenocarcinomas. Intestinal-type adenocarcinomas typically grow along broad cohesive fronts to form either an exophytic mass or an ulcerated tumor. The neoplastic cells often contain apical mucin vacuoles, and abundant mucin may be present in gland lumina.

Diffuse gastric cancers display an infiltrative growth pattern (Fig. 13.16B) and are composed of dyscohesive cells with large mucin vacuoles that expand the cytoplasm and push the nucleus to the periphery, creating a **signet ring cell** appearance (Fig. 13.16C). These cells permeate the mucosa and stomach wall individually or in small clusters. A mass may be difficult to appreciate in diffuse gastric cancer, but these infiltrative tumors often evoke a **desmoplastic** reaction that stiffens the gastric wall and causes diffuse rugal flattening, imparting a "leather bottle" appearance termed **linitis plastica**.

Clinical Features. The increased prevalence of gastric cancer in geographic areas where risk is elevated stems from an increased incidence in the intestinal type and associated precursor lesions. In these geographic areas, the mean age at presentation is 55 years and the male-to-female ratio is 2 : 1. By contrast, the incidence of diffuse gastric cancer is relatively uniform across countries, there are no identified precursor lesions, and the disease occurs at similar frequencies in males and females. Of note, the decrease in gastric cancer incidence over the past 100 years applies only to the intestinal type, which is most closely associated with atrophic gastritis and intestinal metaplasia. As a result, the incidence of intestinal and diffuse types of gastric cancers is now similar in some regions.

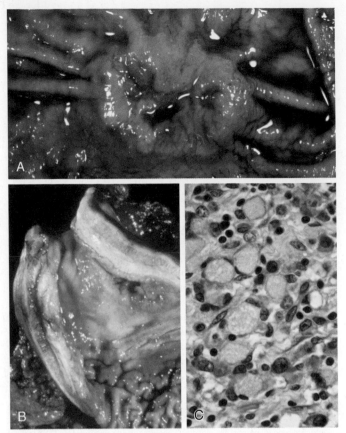

FIG. 13.16 Gastric adenocarcinoma. (A) Intestinal-type adenocarcinoma consisting of an elevated mass with heaped-up borders and central ulceration. Compare with the peptic ulcer in Fig. 13.15A. (B) Linitis plastica due to diffuse adenocarcinoma. The gastric wall is markedly thickened, and rugal folds are partially lost. (C) Signet ring cells in diffuse adenocarcinoma with large cytoplasmic mucin vacuoles and peripherally displaced, crescent-shaped nuclei.

The depth of invasion and the extent of nodal and distant metastasis at the time of diagnosis (tumor stage) are the most powerful prognostic indicators. Local invasion into the duodenum, pancreas, and retroperitoneum is often seen. When possible, surgical resection remains the preferred treatment. With surgical resection, the 5-year survival rate for early gastric cancer may exceed 90%, even if lymph node metastases are present. However, most gastric cancers are discovered at advanced stage in the United States, and the overall 5-year survival rate is less than 30%, in large part because current chemotherapy regimens have limited impact. This may change at least somewhat for the better with the advent of individualized therapies. For example, patients whose tumors overexpress HER2 tyrosine kinase benefit from treatment with agents that inhibit HER2 signaling.

Gastric Lymphoma

Although extranodal lymphomas may arise in virtually any tissue, they do so most commonly in the gastrointestinal tract, including the stomach. In allogeneic hematopoietic stem cell and organ transplant recipients, the bowel is also the most frequent site for Epstein-Barr virus–positive B-cell lymphoproliferations. Nearly 5% of all gastric malignancies are primary lymphomas, the most common of which are indolent extranodal marginal zone B-cell lymphomas. In the gut, these tumors are often referred to as lymphomas of mucosa-associated lymphoid tissue (MALT) or MALTomas. This entity and the second most common primary lymphoma of the gut, diffuse large B-cell lymphoma, are discussed in Chapter 10.

Neuroendocrine (Carcinoid) Tumor

Neuroendocrine tumors, also referred to as carcinoid tumors, are neoplasms that arise from the neuroendocrine cells that are located in many organs, including the endocrine pancreas and the gut. In some instances, these tumors arise in settings in which hormones drive hyperplasia of neuroendocrine cells, such as gastric carcinoids that occur in autoimmune gastritis and associated hypergastrinemia. A majority of these tumors are found in the gastrointestinal tract, with more than 40% occurring in the small intestine. The tracheobronchial tree and lungs are the next most commonly involved sites (Chapter 11). These tumors were historically called "carcinoid" because they are slower growing than carcinomas. The current WHO classification refers to these tumors as low- or intermediate-grade neuroendocrine tumors. These tumors are identical to tumors at other sites such as the lung, where they retain the same carcinoid (Chapter 11). High-grade neuroendocrine tumors, termed *neuroendocrine carcinoma*, resemble small cell carcinoma of the lung (Chapter 11) and, in the gastrointestinal tract, are most common in the jejunum.

MORPHOLOGY

Neuroendocrine tumors are intramural or submucosal masses that create small polypoid lesions (Fig. 13.17A). The tumors are grossly yellow or tan in appearance and elicit an intense desmoplastic reaction that may cause kinking of the bowel and obstruction. On histologic examination, they are composed of islands, trabeculae, strands, glands, or sheets of uniform cells with scant, pink granular cytoplasm and a round-to-oval stippled nucleus (Fig. 13.17B).

Clinical Features. The peak incidence of neuroendocrine tumors is in the sixth decade, but they may appear at any age. Symptoms are determined by the hormones they produce. For example, the *carcinoid*

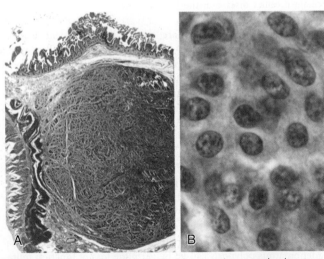

FIG. 13.17 Gastrointestinal carcinoid tumor (neuroendocrine tumor). (A) Carcinoid tumors often form a submucosal nodule composed of tumor cells embedded in dense fibrous tissue. (B) High magnification shows the bland cytology that typifies neuroendocrine tumors. The chromatin texture, with fine and coarse clumps, frequently assumes a "salt-and-pepper" pattern.

syndrome is caused by vasoactive substances secreted by the tumor that lead to cutaneous flushing, sweating, bronchospasm, colicky abdominal pain, diarrhea, and right-sided cardiac valvular fibrosis. When tumors are confined to the intestine, the vasoactive substances released are metabolized to inactive forms by the liver—a "first-pass" effect similar to that seen with oral drugs. Thus, carcinoid syndrome occurs in less than 10% of patients and is strongly associated with hepatic metastatic disease.

The most important prognostic factor for gastrointestinal neuroendocrine tumors is location:

- *Foregut neuroendocrine (carcinoid) tumors* found within the stomach, duodenum proximal to the ligament of Treitz, and esophagus rarely metastasize and are generally cured by resection. Rare gastrin-producing neuroendocrine tumors, also termed *gastrinomas*, may present with symptoms related to increased acid production, including pain and/or bleeding from gastroduodenal ulcers, refractory gastroesophageal reflux, and diarrhea due to inactivation of pancreatic enzymes by excessive gastric acid. This constellation of findings is referred to as *Zollinger-Ellison syndrome.*
- *Midgut neuroendocrine (carcinoid) tumors* arise in the jejunum and ileum, are often multiple, and tend to be aggressive. In these tumors, depth of local invasion, size, and the presence of necrosis and mitoses are associated with poor outcome.
- *Hindgut neuroendocrine (carcinoid)* tumors arising in the appendix and colorectum are typically discovered incidentally. Those in the appendix occur at any age and almost uniformly pursue a benign course. Rectal tumors tend to produce polypeptide hormones and may manifest with abdominal pain and weight loss. Because they are usually discovered when small, metastasis of rectal neuroendocrine tumors is uncommon.

Gastrointestinal Stromal Tumor

Gastrointestinal stromal tumor (GIST) is the most common mesenchymal tumor of the abdomen and most frequently arises in the stomach. The term stromal is a historical mistake, as GIST is now recognized to arise from the interstitial cells of Cajal, the pacemaker cells of the gastrointestinal muscularis propria. A wide variety of other mesenchymal neoplasms also occur in the stomach. Many are named for the cell type they most closely resemble; for example, smooth muscle tumors are called *leiomyomas* or *leiomyosarcomas*, nerve sheath tumors are termed *schwannomas*, and those resembling glomus bodies in the nail beds and at other sites are termed *glomus tumors*. Only GIST is sufficiently frequent to merit further discussion.

Pathogenesis. **The most common driver mutation in GIST is a gain-of-function mutation in the gene encoding the receptor tyrosine kinase KIT.** These are present in 75% to 85% of all GISTs. An additional 8% of GISTs have mutations that activate a related receptor tyrosine kinase, platelet-derived growth factor receptor A (PDGFRA). For unknown reasons, GISTs bearing *PDGFRA* mutations are overrepresented in the stomach. *KIT* and *PDGFRA* gene mutations are mutually exclusive, reflecting their ability to activate the same downstream signaling pathways, which drive cell growth (Chapter 6). Germline mutations in these genes are present in rare individuals, who have a propensity to develop multiple GISTs as well as diffuse hyperplasia of Cajal cells.

In rare GISTs without *KIT* or *PDGFRA* mutations, genes encoding components of the mitochondrial succinate dehydrogenase (SDH) complex are most commonly affected. These mutations result in loss of SDH function and confer increased risk for both GIST and

paraganglioma. One mutant allele is often inherited, with the second copy of the gene being either mutated or otherwise silenced in the tumor. The loss of SDH causes a number of metabolic changes, including increased production of reactive oxygen species, activation of hypoxia inducible factor (HIF), and increased dependency on glycolysis for ATP production; how these alterations lead to transformation is uncertain.

> ### MORPHOLOGY
>
> Primary gastric GISTs usually form a solitary, well-circumscribed, fleshy, submucosal mass. Metastases may form multiple small serosal nodules or fewer large nodules in the liver; spread outside of the abdomen is uncommon. GISTs may be composed of thin, elongated **spindle cells** or plumper **epithelioid cells** (eFig. 13.5). The most useful diagnostic marker is KIT, which is immunohistochemically detectable in 95% of these tumors.

Clinical Features. The peak incidence of gastric GIST is around 60 years of age, with less than 10% occurring in individuals younger than 40 years of age. GIST is slightly more common in males. It may present with symptoms related to mass effects or mucosal ulceration, intestinal obstruction, or gastrointestinal bleeding. Complete surgical resection is the primary treatment for localized gastric GIST.

Prognosis correlates with tumor size, mitotic index, and location, with gastric GISTs being somewhat less aggressive than those arising in the small intestine. Recurrence or metastasis is rare for gastric GISTs less than 5 cm in diameter but common for mitotically active tumors larger than 10 cm. Tumors that are unresectable or metastatic often respond, sometimes for years, to tyrosine kinase inhibitors that are active against KIT and PDGFRA, such as imatinib. Unfortunately, as in chronic myeloid leukemia (Chapter 10), resistance to imatinib eventually arises due to outgrowth of subclones with additional mutations in KIT or PDGFRA. In some instances, these tumors respond to different tyrosine kinase inhibitors that bypass resistance to imatinib.

SMALL AND LARGE INTESTINES

The small intestine and colon are the principal sites of nutrient absorption and are exposed to the diverse array of antigens that are present in food and in gut microbes, which create a unique ecosystem referred to as the *microbiome*. The intestines may become involved by a wide variety of vascular, mechanical, infectious, inflammatory, and neoplastic disorders. Many of these diseases affect nutrient and water transport, perturbations that may cause malabsorption and diarrhea. The colon is also the most common site of gastrointestinal neoplasia in Western populations. We will begin our discussion with disorders that lead to mechanical obstruction of the bowel.

INTESTINAL OBSTRUCTION

Obstruction of the gastrointestinal tract may occur at any level, but the small intestine is most often involved because of its relatively narrow lumen. Collectively, *hernias, intestinal adhesions, intussusception,* and *volvulus* account for 80% of mechanical obstructions (Fig. 13.18), while tumors and infarction account for most of the remainder. The clinical manifestations of intestinal obstruction include abdominal pain and distention, vomiting, and constipation. Surgical intervention is usually required in cases involving mechanical obstruction or severe

Herniation **Adhesions**

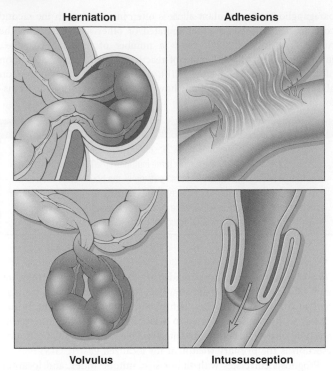

Volvulus **Intussusception**

FIG. 13.18 Intestinal obstruction. The four major mechanical causes of intestinal obstruction are (1) herniation of a segment in the umbilical or inguinal regions, (2) adhesion between loops of intestine, (3) volvulus, and (4) intussusception.

infarction. Volvulus and adhesions between bowel loops are illustrated in Fig. 13.18. Brief comments are made next about other causes of obstruction.

Intussusception

Intussusception occurs when a segment of the intestine, constricted by a wave of peristalsis, telescopes into the immediately distal segment. Once trapped, the invaginated segment is propelled by peristalsis and pulls the mesentery along. Intussusception is the most common cause of intestinal obstruction in children younger than 2 years of age. There is usually no underlying anatomic defect and the child is otherwise healthy. Other cases are associated with viral infection and rotavirus vaccines and may be related to reactive hyperplasia of Peyer patches, which can act as the leading edge of the intussusception. If left untreated, intussusception may progress to intestinal obstruction, compression of mesenteric vessels, and infarction. Contrast enemas are diagnostically useful and are also effective in correcting intussusception in infants and young children. However, surgical intervention is necessary when an intraluminal mass or tumor serves as the initiating point of traction, as is typical in older children and in adults.

Hirschsprung Disease

Hirschsprung, **also known as congenital aganglionic megacolon,** *disease* **occurs in approximately 1 of 5000 live births and stems from a congenital defect in colonic innervation.** It may be isolated or occur in combination with other developmental abnormalities. It is more common in males but tends to be more severe in females. Siblings of those affected are at increased risk for development of Hirschsprung disease.

Patients typically present as neonates with failure to pass meconium in the immediate postnatal period followed by obstructive constipation. The major threats to life are enterocolitis, fluid and electrolyte disturbances, perforation, and peritonitis. Surgical resection of the aganglionic segment with anastomosis of the normal colon to the rectum is effective, although it may take years for patients to attain normal bowel function and continence.

Pathogenesis. The enteric neuronal plexus develops from neural crest cells that migrate into the bowel wall during embryogenesis. **Hirschsprung disease results when the migration of neural crest cells from cecum to rectum is disrupted.** This produces a distal intestinal segment that lacks both the *Meissner submucosal plexus* and the *Auerbach myenteric plexus* ("aganglionosis") and thus fails to develop coordinated peristaltic contractions. Loss-of-function mutations in the RET receptor tyrosine kinase account for the majority of familial cases and approximately 15% of sporadic cases. Mutations in other genes involved in the development of neural crest cells have been identified in cases without *RET* mutations, and individuals with trisomy 21 are also at increased risk for uncertain reasons.

MORPHOLOGY

Hirschsprung disease always affects the rectum, but the length of the additional involved segments varies. Most cases are limited to the rectum and sigmoid colon, but severe disease can involve the entire colon. The aganglionic region may have a grossly normal or contracted appearance, while the normally innervated proximal colon may undergo progressive dilation as a result of functional distal obstruction (Fig. 13.19). Diagnosis is made by histologically confirming the absence of ganglion cells in the affected segment.

Abdominal Hernia

Any weakness or defect in the wall of the peritoneal cavity may permit protrusion of a serosa-lined pouch of peritoneum called a

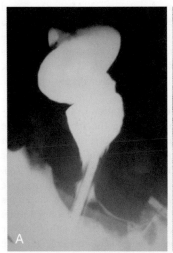
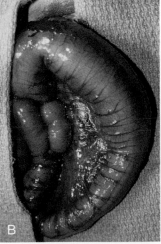

FIG. 13.19 Hirschsprung disease. (A) Preoperative barium enema study showing constricted rectum *(bottom)* and dilated sigmoid colon. Ganglion cells were absent in the rectum, but present in the sigmoid colon. (B) Corresponding intraoperative appearance of the dilated sigmoid colon. (Courtesy of Dr. Aliya Husain, The University of Chicago, Chicago, Illinois.)

hernia sac. Acquired hernias most commonly occur anteriorly, through the inguinal and femoral canals or umbilicus, or at sites of surgical scars. These are of concern because of the risk of visceral protrusion *(external herniation)*. This is most likely to occur with inguinal hernias, which tend to have narrow orifices and large sacs. Small bowel loops herniate most often, but portions of omentum or large bowel may also herniate and become entrapped. Pressure at the neck of the outpouching bowel may impair venous drainage, leading to stasis and edema. These changes increase the bulk of the herniated loop, leading to permanent entrapment *(incarceration)* and, over time, arterial and venous compromise *(strangulation)*, which may result in infarction.

VASCULAR DISORDERS OF BOWEL

Ischemic Bowel Disease

The majority of the GI tract is supplied by the celiac, superior mesenteric, and inferior mesenteric arteries. As they approach the intestinal wall, the superior and inferior mesenteric arteries ramify into the mesenteric arcades. Interconnections between arcades and collateral vessels make it possible for the small intestine and colon to tolerate slowly progressive loss of blood supply from one artery. By contrast, acute compromise of any major vessel may lead to infarction of segments of intestine. In a large majority of cases, acute obstruction is caused by thrombosis or embolism. The most important risk factor for thrombosis is severe atherosclerosis. Obstructive emboli most commonly originate from aortic atheromas or cardiac mural thrombi. Mesenteric venous thrombosis, which can also lead to ischemic disease, is uncommon but can result from inherited or acquired hypercoagulable states, invasive neoplasms, cirrhosis, trauma, or abdominal masses that compress the portal drainage. Intestinal hypoperfusion may also occur in the absence of vascular obstruction in the setting of cardiac failure, shock, dehydration, or use of vasoconstrictive drugs.

Pathogenesis. **The severity of vascular compromise, the time frame of its development, and the vessels that are affected are the major factors that determine the severity of ischemic bowel disease.** At the onset of vascular compromise, some hypoxic injury occurs, but intestinal epithelial cells are relatively resistant to short-term hypoxia. Ironically, the greatest damage appears to be initiated by restoration of the blood supply *(reperfusion injury)*. While the mechanisms of reperfusion injury are incompletely understood, they may involve free radical production, neutrophil infiltration, and locally produced inflammatory mediators (Chapter 1).

Two aspects of intestinal vascular anatomy also contribute to the distribution of ischemic damage:

- *Watershed zone* refers to intestinal segments at the end of their respective arterial supplies that are particularly susceptible to ischemia. These zones include the splenic flexure, where the superior and inferior mesenteric arterial circulations terminate, and to a lesser extent the sigmoid colon and rectum, where the inferior mesenteric, pudendal, and iliac arterial circulations end. Generalized hypotension or hypoxemia may cause localized injury at these vulnerable sites, and ischemic disease should be considered in the differential diagnosis for focal colitis of the splenic flexure or rectosigmoid colon.
- *Patterns of intestinal microvessels.* Intestinal capillaries run alongside the glands from the crypts to the surface before making a hairpin turn and returning to empty into the postcapillary venules.

This configuration leaves the surface epithelium particularly vulnerable to ischemic injury.

MORPHOLOGY

While there is increased susceptibility of watershed zones, **mucosal and mural infarction** may involve any level of the gut from stomach to anus. Involvement is frequently segmental and patchy, and the affected mucosa is hemorrhagic and often ulcerated. The bowel wall is thickened by edema. With severe disease, pathologic changes include extensive mucosal and submucosal hemorrhage and necrosis. Damage is more pronounced with acute arterial thrombosis, which often leads to **transmural infarction.** Blood-tinged mucus or blood accumulates within the lumen. Coagulative necrosis of the muscularis propria occurs within 1 to 4 days and may be associated with purulent serositis and perforation.

Microscopic examination of ischemic intestine demonstrates **atrophy** or **sloughing of surface epithelium** (Fig. 13.20A). By contrast, crypts may be hyperproliferative. Inflammatory infiltrates are initially absent in acute ischemia, but neutrophils are recruited within hours of reperfusion. Chronic ischemia is accompanied by fibrous scarring of the lamina propria (Fig. 13.20B) and, uncommonly, stricture formation. In acute phases of ischemic damage, bacterial superinfection and enterotoxin release may induce pseudomembrane formation that can resemble *Clostridium difficile*—associated pseudomembranous colitis (discussed later).

Clinical Features. Ischemic bowel disease most commonly occurs in older adults with coexisting cardiac or vascular disease. Acute transmural infarction typically manifests with sudden, severe abdominal pain and tenderness, sometimes accompanied by nausea, vomiting, and bloody diarrhea or grossly melanotic stool. This presentation may progress to shock and vascular collapse within hours due to blood loss from the ischemic bowel. Peristaltic sounds diminish or disappear, and muscular spasm affecting abdominal muscles creates boardlike rigidity of the abdominal wall. Because these physical signs overlap with those of other abdominal emergencies, including acute pancreatitis, acute appendicitis, perforated ulcer, and acute cholecystitis, the diagnosis of intestinal infarction may be delayed or missed, with disastrous consequences. As the mucosal barrier breaks down, bacteria enter the circulation and sepsis may develop; the mortality rate in cases complicated by sepsis exceeds 50%.

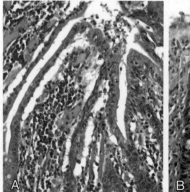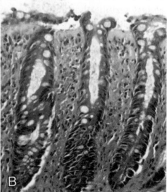

FIG. 13.20 Ischemia. (A) Characteristic attenuated and partially detached villous epithelium in acute jejunal ischemia. Note the hyperchromatic nuclei of proliferating crypt cells. (B) Chronic colonic ischemia with atrophic surface epithelium and fibrotic lamina propria.

The overall progression of ischemic enteritis depends on the underlying cause and severity of injury:

- *Mucosal and mural infarctions* alone may not be fatal. However, these may progress to more extensive, transmural infarction if the vascular supply is not restored by correcting the underlying cause or (in chronic disease) the development of an adequate collateral blood supply.
- *Chronic ischemia* may masquerade as inflammatory bowel disease, with episodes of bloody diarrhea interspersed with periods of healing.
- *Cytomegalovirus (CMV) infection* causes ischemic gastrointestinal disease as a consequence of viral infection of endothelial cells. CMV infection may be a complication of immunosuppressive therapy.
- *Radiation enterocolitis* occurs when the gastrointestinal tract is irradiated. In addition to epithelial damage, radiation-induced vascular injury may produce ischemic disease.
- *Necrotizing enterocolitis* is an idiopathic disorder of the small and large intestines that may result in transmural necrosis (Chapter 4). It is the most common acquired gastrointestinal emergency of neonates, particularly those who are premature or of low birth weight. Its occurrence is often associated with initiation of oral feeding. Although the pathogenesis of necrotizing enterocolitis is not defined, ischemic injury is thought to contribute.

Angiodysplasia

Angiodysplasia is characterized by malformed submucosal and mucosal blood vessels. It occurs most often in the cecum or right colon and usually presents after the sixth decade of life. Although it affects less than 1% of the adult population, angiodysplasia accounts for 20% of major episodes of lower intestinal bleeding.

As with all lower gastrointestinal bleeding, in most instances the blood is maroon or bright red in color. This is in distinction to upper gastrointestinal bleeding, which tends to produce black, tarry stools *(melena)* and so-called coffee ground emesis. These distinctions are not absolute, as a very brisk upper gastrointestinal bleed may produce red blood per rectum and bleeds from the right colon sometimes produce dark stools.

Hemorrhoids

Hemorrhoids are dilated anal and perianal collateral vessels that connect the portal and caval venous systems to relieve elevated venous pressure within the hemorrhoidal plexus. Thus, although hemorrhoids are less serious than esophageal varices, the pathogenesis of these lesions is similar. They are common, affecting about 5% of the population. Frequent predisposing factors include constipation and associated straining (which increase intraabdominal and venous pressures), venous stasis of pregnancy, and portal hypertension.

Collateral vessels within the inferior hemorrhoidal plexus are located below the anorectal line and are termed *external hemorrhoids,* while those that result from dilation of the superior hemorrhoidal plexus within the distal rectum are referred to as *internal hemorrhoids.* On histologic examination, hemorrhoids consist of thin-walled, dilated submucosal vessels beneath the anal or rectal mucosa. These vessels are subject to trauma, which leads to rectal bleeding. In addition, they can become thrombosed and inflamed.

Hemorrhoids often manifest with pain and self-limited rectal bleeding, particularly bright red blood seen on toilet paper. When they develop as a result of portal hypertension, the implications are more ominous. Hemorrhoidal bleeding is generally not a medical emergency; treatment options include sclerotherapy, rubber band ligation, and infrared coagulation. In severe cases, hemorrhoids may be removed surgically.

DIARRHEAL DISEASE

Diarrhea is defined as the passage of loose or watery stools, typically of amounts greater than 200 grams per day. In severe cases, stool volume can exceed 14 L per day and, without fluid resuscitation, result in death. Worldwide, diarrheal diseases are estimated to cause the deaths of 1.5 to 2 million children under 5 years of age annually. Diarrhea is a common symptom of many intestinal diseases, including those due to infection, inflammation, ischemia, malabsorption, and nutritional deficiency. It is subclassified into four major categories:

- *Secretory diarrhea* is characterized by isotonic stool and persists during fasting.
- *Osmotic diarrhea,* such as that occurring with lactase deficiency, is due to osmotic force exerted by unabsorbed luminal solutes. The diarrheal fluid is at least 50 mOsm more concentrated than plasma and the condition abates with fasting.
- *Malabsorptive diarrhea* caused by inadequate nutrient absorption is associated with steatorrhea and is relieved by fasting.
- *Exudative diarrhea* is due to inflammatory disease and characterized by purulent, bloody stools that continue during fasting.

We begin our discussion with malabsorptive diarrhea. Other disorders associated with secretory and exudative types of diarrhea (e.g., cholera and inflammatory bowel disease, respectively) are addressed in separate sections.

Malabsorptive Diarrhea

Malabsorption manifests most commonly as chronic diarrhea and is characterized by defective absorption of fats, fat- and water-soluble vitamins, proteins, carbohydrates, electrolytes, minerals, and water. Chronic malabsorption causes weight loss, anorexia, abdominal distention, borborygmi (a rumbling or gurgling noise of the intestines), and muscle wasting. A hallmark of malabsorption is *steatorrhea,* characterized by excessive fecal fat and bulky, frothy, greasy, yellow or clay-colored stools. The most common chronic malabsorptive disorders in Western countries are pancreatic insufficiency, celiac disease, and Crohn disease. Environmental enteric dysfunction, or environmental enteropathy, which has a malabsorptive component, is another cause that is pervasive in some lower-resource countries.

Malabsorption results from a disturbance in at least one of the four phases of nutrient absorption:

- *Intraluminal digestion,* in which proteins, carbohydrates, and fats are broken down into absorbable forms
- *Terminal digestion,* which involves the hydrolysis of carbohydrates and peptides by disaccharidases and peptidases, respectively, in the brush border of the small-intestinal mucosa
- *Transepithelial transport,* in which nutrients, fluid, and electrolytes are transported across and processed within the small-intestinal epithelium
- *Lymphatic transport* of absorbed lipids

In many malabsorptive disorders, a defect in one of these processes predominates, but more than one usually contributes (Table 13.3). As a result, malabsorption syndromes resemble each other more than they differ. Signs and symptoms include diarrhea (from nutrient

Table 13.3 Defects in Malabsorptive and Diarrheal Disease

Disease	Intraluminal Digestion	Terminal Digestion	Transepithelial Transport	Lymphatic Transport
Celiac disease		+	+	
Tropical sprue		+	+	
Chronic pancreatitis	+			
Cystic fibrosis	+			
Primary bile acid malabsorption	+		+	
Carcinoid syndrome			+	
Autoimmune enteropathy		+	+	
Disaccharidase deficiency		+		
Mycobacterial infection, Whipple disease				+
Abetalipoproteinemia			+	
Viral gastroenteritis		+	+	
Bacterial gastroenteritis		+	+	
Parasitic gastroenteritis		+	+	
Inflammatory bowel disease	+	+	+	

+, Indicates that the process can be abnormal in the disease indicated. Other processes are not typically affected.

malabsorption and excessive intestinal secretion), flatus, abdominal pain, and weight loss. Inadequate absorption of vitamins and minerals may result in anemia and mucositis due to pyridoxine, folate, or vitamin B_{12} deficiency; bleeding due to vitamin K deficiency; osteopenia and tetany due to calcium, magnesium, or vitamin D deficiency; and neuropathy due to vitamin A or B_{12} deficiency. A variety of endocrine and skin disturbances may also occur. Mycobacterial infection, which may lead to lymphatic transport defects, is discussed with infectious causes of diarrhea in the next section.

Cystic Fibrosis

Cystic fibrosis is discussed in greater detail in Chapter 4; only the associated malabsorption is considered here. Due to mutations of the epithelial cystic fibrosis transmembrane conductance regulator (CFTR), individuals with cystic fibrosis have defects in intestinal and pancreatic ductal ion transport. This abnormality interferes with bicarbonate, sodium, and water secretion, ultimately resulting in inadequate luminal hydration. In the pancreas, luminal dehydration results in the production of abnormally viscous mucus, which obstructs the ducts and leads to autodigestion of the pancreas and eventually exocrine pancreatic insufficiency in more than 80% of patients. The failure of nutrient digestion in the small bowel in turn results in osmotic diarrhea, which can be effectively treated in most patients with oral digestive enzyme supplements. Lipase deficiency can lead to steatorrhea.

Celiac Disease

Celiac disease, also known as *celiac sprue* or *gluten-sensitive enteropathy*, is an immune-mediated enteropathy triggered by the ingestion of gluten-containing cereals, such as wheat, rye, or barley, in genetically predisposed individuals. Oats do not contain gluten but are sometimes added to this list as oats processed in factories that also process wheat, rye, or barley may be cross-contaminated. Celiac disease is found globally and has a worldwide estimated prevalence of about 1%. The primary treatment for celiac disease is a *gluten-free diet*, which results in symptomatic improvement for most patients.

Pathogenesis. **Celiac disease is an intestinal immune reaction to gluten, the major storage protein of wheat and similar grains.** Digestion of gluten by luminal and brush border enzymes produces a 33–amino acid peptide known as gliadin that is resistant to further proteolysis (Fig. 13.21). Deamidation of gliadin by tissue transglutaminase in the lamina propria increases its binding to HLA-DQ2 and HLA-DQ8 class II MHC molecules expressed on antigen-presenting cells, allowing gliadin to be presented to CD4+ T cells. These activated CD4+ T cells produce cytokines such as interferon-γ that likely contribute to the tissue damage and characteristic mucosal histopathology. An antibody response follows, leading to the production of antibodies against tissue transglutaminase, deamidated gliadin, and, perhaps due to cross-reactive epitopes, cardiac endomysium. Whether these antibodies contribute to celiac disease pathogenesis or are merely markers of immune activation remains controversial, but their levels are well correlated with the presence of celiac disease and response to a gluten-free diet.

In addition to CD4+ cells, there is an accumulation of CD8+ cells that are not specific for gliadin but that may play an ancillary role in causing tissue damage. It is thought that some gliadin peptides induce epithelial cells to produce cytokines such as IL-15, which in turn trigger activation and proliferation of CD8+ intraepithelial lymphocytes. These T cells are proposed to kill enterocytes that have been induced by various stressors to express molecules such as MIC-A, a surface glycoprotein, that may be recognized by activated CD8+ T cells and NK cells expressing the NKG2D receptor. The resulting epithelial damage is then predicted to increase the movement of gliadin peptides across the epithelium and their deamidation by tissue transglutaminase, perpetuating the cycle of disease. Whatever the precise mechanism, the epithelial injury leads to blunting of villi and altered epithelial cell differentiation, both of which may contribute to malabsorption.

While nearly all individuals eat grain and are exposed to gluten and gliadin, most do not develop celiac disease. Thus, host factors determine whether celiac disease develops. Among these, HLA proteins seem to be critical, since almost all individuals with celiac disease express HLA-DQ2 or HLA-DQ8. There is also an association with

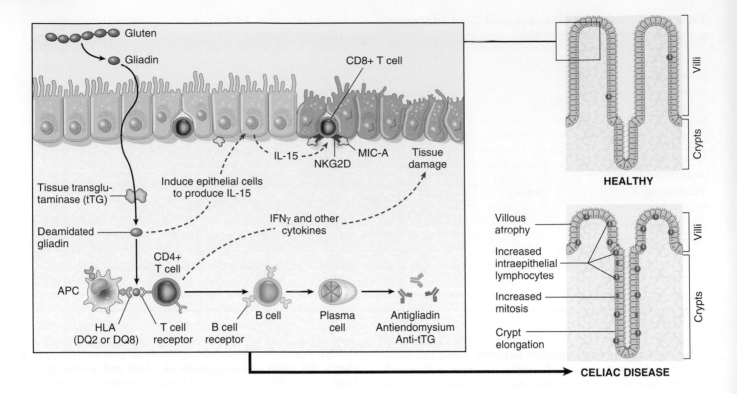

FIG. 13.21 A model for the pathogenesis of celiac disease *(left)*. CD4+ T cells are stimulated by antigen-presenting cells displaying deamidated gliadin peptides to produce a variety of cytokines that stimulate antibody production from B cells. The source of the epithelial damage (denoted by *dotted lines*) is less certain. Cytokines such as interferon-γ produced by the CD4+ T cells may directly damage epithelial cells. Alternatively, deamidated gliadin may induce epithelial cells to produce IL-15, stimulating intraepithelial CD8+ T cells expressing the NKG2D receptor to recognize and kill epithelial cells expressing the molecule MIC-A (MHC class I polypeptide-related sequence A). The resulting morphologic alterations *(right)* include varying degrees of villous atrophy, increased numbers of intraepithelial lymphocytes, and epithelial proliferation with crypt elongation.

other immune diseases including type 1 diabetes, thyroiditis, and Sjögren syndrome.

MORPHOLOGY

Biopsy specimens from the second portion of the duodenum or proximal jejunum, which are exposed to the highest concentrations of dietary gluten, are generally diagnostic. The histopathology is characterized by **crypt hyperplasia, villous atrophy** (Fig. 13.22), and increased intraepithelial lymphocytes (eFig. 13.6). The loss of mucosal and brush-border surface area due to villous atrophy probably accounts for the malabsorption. In addition, increased rates of epithelial turnover, reflected in increased crypt mitotic activity, may limit the ability of absorptive enterocytes to fully differentiate and express proteins necessary for terminal digestion and transepithelial transport. Other histologic findings may include increased numbers of plasma cells, mast cells, and eosinophils, especially within the upper part of the lamina propria. It should be noted that intraepithelial lymphocytosis and villous atrophy can be present in other disorders, including viral enteritis. Therefore, serologic findings, combined with histologic examination, are most specific for diagnosis of celiac disease.

Clinical Features. Pediatric celiac disease, which affects male and female children equally, usually manifests between 6 and 24 months of

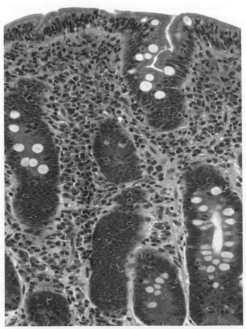

FIG. 13.22 Celiac disease. Advanced cases of celiac disease show complete loss of villi, or total villous atrophy. Note the dense plasma cell infiltrates in the lamina propria and intraepithelial lymphocytes.

age (after introduction of gluten to the diet) with irritability, abdominal distention, anorexia, diarrhea, failure to thrive, weight loss, or muscle wasting. Older children, by contrast, are more likely to present with abdominal pain, nausea, vomiting, bloating, or constipation. A characteristic pruritic, blistering skin lesion, *dermatitis herpetiformis,* is present in as many as 10% of patients (Chapter 22).

In adults, celiac disease manifests most commonly between 30 and 60 years of age with anemia (due to iron deficiency and, less commonly, B$_{12}$ and folate deficiency), diarrhea, bloating, and fatigue. Many cases, however, escape clinical attention for extended periods because of atypical presentations, and some patients have silent celiac disease, defined as positive serology and villous atrophy without symptoms.

Noninvasive serologic tests are generally performed before biopsy. The most sensitive tests identify the presence of IgA antibodies to tissue transglutaminase or IgA or IgG antibodies to deamidated gliadin. Antiendomysial antibodies are highly specific but less sensitive than other antibodies.

Patients with celiac disease have an elevated risk of small bowel malignancy. The most common celiac disease–associated cancer is *enteropathy-associated T-cell lymphoma,* an aggressive tumor of intraepithelial T lymphocytes. *Small-intestinal adenocarcinoma* is also more frequent in individuals with celiac disease. Thus, when symptoms such as abdominal pain, diarrhea, and weight loss recur despite a strict gluten-free diet, the differential diagnosis includes cancer or *refractory sprue,* in which the response to a gluten-free diet is lost. Gluten exposure is the most common cause of recurrent symptoms; most individuals with celiac disease do well with dietary restrictions and die of unrelated causes.

Environmental Enteric Dysfunction

The term environmental enteric dysfunction, or environmental enteropathy, refers to a syndrome of impaired intestinal function that is prevalent in areas with poor sanitation infrastructure and suboptimal hygiene. It is most common in parts of sub-Saharan Africa, such as Zambia; aboriginal populations within northern Australia; southern India; and some groups living in poverty in South America and Asia. Because of its tendency to occur in a belt close to the equator, it has also been referred to as *tropical enteropathy* or *tropical sprue.* Its etiology is uncertain. Some work has implicated small intestinal colonization by toxigenic coliform bacteria, but oral antibiotic treatment and nutritional supplementation do not usually fully reverse the syndrome. Small intestinal biopsy specimens show blunted villi and chronic inflammation, including intraepithelial lymphocytes, findings similar to those seen in celiac disease, which must be excluded by serologic studies. Although relatively well tolerated in adults, environmental enteropathy may cause sufficient malabsorption to stunt the growth and impair the cognitive development of affected children.

Lactase (Disaccharidase) Deficiency

The term "lactase deficiency" sounds like a descriptor of an abnormality, but in fact expression of lactase wanes following weaning in virtually all mammals. An exception is found in people who descended from certain populations in Africa, Europe, and the Middle East who have acquired mutations that lead to persistent, lifelong lactase expression.

Lactase deficiency gives rise to osmotic diarrhea following the consumption of lactose-rich foods, such as dairy products. The disaccharidases, including lactase, are located in the apical brush border membrane of villous absorptive epithelial cells. Lactase deficiency is of several types:

- *Congenital lactase deficiency* is a rare autosomal recessive disorder caused by mutations in the gene encoding lactase. It manifests as explosive diarrhea with watery, frothy stools and abdominal distention after milk ingestion. Symptoms abate when exposure to milk and milk products is terminated.
- *Acquired lactase deficiency,* as mentioned, is caused by the loss of lactase gene expression early in childhood and is very common, being estimated to affect roughly two-thirds of the world's population and about one-half of adults in the United States. The acquired deficiency typically manifests after the age of weaning from breast milk.
- *Transient lactase deficiency* is caused by small bowel injury, as may occur due to infectious or inflammatory insults, and is reversible if the cause of the injury remits.

Abetalipoproteinemia

Abetalipoproteinemia is a rare autosomal recessive disease marked by an inability of enterocytes to secrete triglyceride-rich chylomicrons. This transepithelial transport defect is caused by mutation of the gene encoding *microsomal triglyceride transfer protein* and renders enterocytes incapable of exporting lipoproteins, free fatty acids, and fat-soluble vitamins. Abetalipoproteinemia manifests in infancy. The clinical picture is dominated by failure to thrive, diarrhea, and steatorrhea. Deficiencies of essential fatty acids and fat-soluble vitamins lead to defects in coagulation (due to vitamin K deficiency) and skeletal, CNS, and retinal abnormalities. A characteristic finding in peripheral blood smears is the presence of acanthocytic red cells (*spur cells*), owing to an alteration in the lipid content of red cell membranes.

Microscopic Colitis

Microscopic colitis encompasses two idiopathic entities, *collagenous colitis* and *lymphocytic colitis.* Both manifest with chronic, nonbloody, watery diarrhea without weight loss. Findings on radiologic and endoscopic studies are typically normal. Collagenous colitis, which occurs primarily in middle-aged and older women, is characterized by the presence of a dense subepithelial collagen layer, increased numbers of intraepithelial lymphocytes, and a mixed inflammatory infiltrate within the lamina propria. Lymphocytic colitis is histologically similar, but the subepithelial collagen layer is of normal thickness and the increase in intraepithelial lymphocytes tends to be greater. Lymphocytic colitis is associated with celiac disease and, like celiac disease, is more frequent in those with the HLA-DQ2 haplotype. It is also associated with several other autoimmune diseases, including Hashimoto thyroiditis, type I diabetes, and certain forms of arthritis.

Graft-Versus-Host Disease

Graft-versus-host disease occurs after allogeneic hematopoietic stem cell transplantation (Chapter 5). The small bowel and colon are involved in most cases. Graft-versus-host disease is caused by donor T cell–mediated damage to the recipient's epithelial cells. The lymphocytic infiltrate in the lamina propria is typically sparse, suggesting that cytokines secreted by T cells may be the major mediators of tissue injury. Epithelial apoptosis, particularly of crypt cells, is the most common histologic finding. Intestinal graft-versus-host disease often manifests as watery diarrhea.

Infectious Enterocolitis

Globally, infectious enterocolitis is responsible for more than 1 million deaths annually and greater than 10% of deaths in children younger than 5 years of age. Enterocolitis presents with a broad range of signs and symptoms, including diarrhea, abdominal pain, urgency, perianal discomfort, incontinence, and hemorrhage. Bacterial

Table 13.4 Features of Bacterial Enterocolitides

Infection Type	Distribution	Reservoir	Transmission	Epidemiology	Affected GI Sites	Symptoms	Complications
Cholera	India, Africa	Shellfish	Fecal-oral, water	Sporadic, endemic, epidemic	Small intestine	Severe watery diarrhea	Dehydration, electrolyte imbalances
Campylobacter spp.	Higher-resource countries	Chickens, sheep, pigs, cattle	Poultry, milk, other foods	Sporadic; children, travelers	Colon	Watery or bloody diarrhea	Reactive arthritis, Guillain-Barré syndrome
Shigellosis	Worldwide, endemic in lower-resource countries	Humans	Fecal-oral, food, water	Children, migrant workers, travelers, nursing homes	Left colon, ileum	Bloody diarrhea	Reactive arthritis, urethritis, conjunctivitis, hemolytic-uremic syndrome
Salmonellosis	Worldwide	Poultry, farm animals, reptiles	Meat, poultry, eggs, milk	Children, older adults	Colon, small intestine	Watery or bloody diarrhea	Sepsis, abscess
Enteric (typhoid) fever	India, Mexico, Philippines	Humans	Fecal-oral, water	Children, adolescents, travelers	Small intestine	Bloody diarrhea, fever	Chronic infection, carrier state, encephalopathy, myocarditis, intestinal perforation
Yersinia spp.	Northern and central Europe	Pigs, cows, puppies, cats	Pork, milk, water	Clustered cases	Ileum, appendix, right colon	Abdominal pain, fever, diarrhea	Reactive arthritis, erythema nodosum
Enterotoxigenic *E. coli*	Lower-resource countries	Unknown	Food or fecal-oral	Infants, adolescents, travelers	Small intestine	Severe watery diarrhea	Dehydration, electrolyte imbalances
Enteropathogenic *E. coli*	Worldwide	Humans	Fecal-oral	Infants	Small intestine	Watery diarrhea	Dehydration, electrolyte imbalances
Enterohemorrhagic *E. coli*	Worldwide	Widespread, includes cattle	Beef, milk, produce	Sporadic and epidemic	Colon	Bloody diarrhea	Hemolytic-uremic syndrome
Enteroinvasive *E. coli*	Lower-resource countries	Unknown	Cheese, other foods, water	Young children	Colon	Bloody diarrhea	Unknown
Enteroaggregative *E. coli*	Worldwide	Unknown	Unknown	Children, adults, travelers	Colon	Nonbloody diarrhea, afebrile	Poorly defined
Pseudomembranous colitis (*C. difficile*)	Worldwide	Humans, hospitals	Antibiotics allow emergence	Immunocompromised antibiotic-treated	Colon	Watery diarrhea, fever	Relapse, toxic megacolon
Whipple disease	Rural > urban	Unknown	Unknown	Rare	Small intestine	Malabsorption	Arthritis, CNS disease
Mycobacterial infection	Worldwide	Unknown	Unknown	Immunocompromised endemic	Small intestine	Malabsorption	Pneumonia, infection at other sites

CNS, Central nervous system; *GI*, gastrointestinal.

infections, such as enterotoxigenic *Escherichia coli,* are frequently responsible, but the most common pathogens vary with age, nutrition, host immune status, and environment (Table 13.4). For example, epidemics of cholera are common in areas with poor sanitation as a result of inadequate public health measures, natural disasters (e.g., the Haitian earthquake of 2010), or war. Pediatric infectious diarrhea, which may result in severe dehydration and metabolic acidosis, is commonly caused by enteric viruses. A summary of the epidemiology and clinical features of selected causes of bacterial enterocolitis is presented in Table 13.4. Representative bacterial, viral, and parasitic enterocolitides are discussed next.

Cholera

Vibrio cholerae organisms are comma-shaped, gram-negative bacteria that cause cholera, a disease that has been endemic in the Ganges Valley of India and Bangladesh for all recorded history. *V. cholerae* is transmitted primarily by contaminated drinking water. However, person-to-person transmission also occurs and in rare instances it can be transmitted in seafood. There is a marked seasonal variation in most locales due to rapid growth of *Vibrio* bacteria at warm temperatures. The only animal reservoirs are shellfish and plankton.

Pathogenesis. **Vibrio organisms cause disease by producing a potent toxin that interferes with the absorptive function of enterocytes.** Flagellar proteins are necessary for efficient colonization of the gut by *Vibrio* organisms, and a secreted metalloproteinase with hemagglutinin activity is important for shedding in the stool. Disease is caused by a preformed enterotoxin known as *cholera toxin* composed of five B subunits that direct endocytosis and an enzymatically active A subunit. After uptake into the endoplasmic reticulum, a fragment of the A subunit is transported into the cytosol, where it interacts with host factors to ribosylate and activate the G protein $G_{s\alpha}$. This stimulates adenylate cyclase, leading to increases in intracellular cyclic adenosine monophosphate (cAMP), which binds and activates the cystic fibrosis transmembrane conductance regulator (CFTR). In enterocytes, activation of CFTR leads to the outflow of chloride ions into the lumen of the gut, creating an osmotic gradient that produces massive *secretory diarrhea.* Mucosal biopsy specimens show only minimal morphologic alterations.

Clinical Features. Most exposed individuals are asymptomatic or suffer only mild diarrhea; unlike many other forms of infectious enterocolitis, fever is uncommon. In those with severe disease, there is abrupt onset of watery diarrhea and vomiting after an incubation period of 1 to 5 days. The volume of diarrhea may reach 1 L per hour, leading to dehydration, hypotension, electrolyte imbalances, muscle cramping, anuria, shock, loss of consciousness, and death. Most deaths occur within the first 24 hours of presentation. The mortality rate for untreated severe cholera is 50% to 70%, but with simple fluid replacement more than 99% of patients survive.

Campylobacter Enterocolitis

Campylobacter jejuni is a common cause of acute diarrhea worldwide and is a major foodborne pathogen in the United States. In resource-limited countries, it is often endemic and frequently afflicts visitors from resource-rich areas (so-called *"traveler's diarrhea"*). Most infections are associated with ingestion of raw or undercooked meat; unpasteurized milk or contaminated water are also culpable in some cases.

Pathogenesis. The number of organisms ingested, the virulence of the infecting strain, and host immunity determine whether *Campylobacter*

ingestion results in disease. Virulence factors appear to influence disease development by contributing to four properties: motility, adherence, toxin production, and invasion. Flagella allow *Campylobacter* to be motile and facilitate adherence, colonization, and mucosal invasion. Cytotoxins that cause epithelial damage and a cholera toxin—like enterotoxin are also elaborated by some *C. jejuni* isolates. Dysentery (bloody diarrhea) is generally associated with invasion and only occurs with a small minority of *Campylobacter* strains. *Enteric fever* occurs when bacteria proliferate within the lamina propria and mesenteric lymph nodes.

Campylobacter infection may result in reactive arthritis, primarily in patients with the HLA-B27 allele. Other extraintestinal complications include erythema nodosum and Guillain-Barré syndrome (Chapter 20), a flaccid paralysis caused by autoimmunity-driven inflammation of peripheral nerves that develops in 0.1% or less of individuals infected with *Campylobacter.*

> ### MORPHOLOGY
>
> *Campylobacter, Shigella, Salmonella,* and many other bacterial infections, including *Yersinia* and *E. coli,* all induce a similar microscopic picture, termed **acute self-limited colitis.** The histology of acute self-limited colitis includes prominent lamina propria and intraepithelial neutrophil infiltrates (Fig. 13.23A); **cryptitis** (neutrophil infiltration of the crypts) and **crypt abscesses** (crypts with accumulations of luminal neutrophils) may also be present. The preservation of crypt architecture in most cases is helpful in distinguishing these infections from inflammatory bowel disease (Fig. 13.23B). Specific diagnosis is primarily by stool culture, but molecular tests are becoming more widely available.

Clinical Features. Ingestion of as few as 500 *C. jejuni* organisms may cause disease after an incubation period of up to 8 days. Watery diarrhea, either acute or with onset after an influenza-like prodrome, is

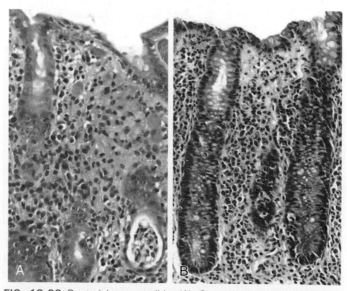

FIG. 13.23 Bacterial enterocolitis. (A) *Campylobacter jejuni* infection produces acute, self-limited colitis. Neutrophils can be seen within surface and crypt epithelium, and a crypt abscess is present *(lower right).* (B) Enteroinvasive *Escherichia coli* infection is similar to other acute, self-limited colitides. Note the maintenance of normal crypt architecture and spacing, despite abundant intraepithelial neutrophils.

the primary manifestation, and dysentery develops in 15% to 50% of patients. Patients may shed bacteria for 1 month or more after clinical resolution. The disease is usually self-limited and antibiotic therapy is generally not required. The fatality rate is low and mainly confined to older adults and those with HIV, in whom *C. jejuni* infection may lead to severe, debilitating illness.

Shigellosis

Shigella is one of the most common causes of bloody diarrhea (dysentery). Shigellae are gram-negative, unencapsulated, nonmotile, facultative anaerobes that are highly transmissible by the fecal-oral route or through ingestion of contaminated water and food. The infective dose is fewer than 100 organisms, and each gram of stool contains as many as 10^9 organisms during acute phases of the disease.

In the United States, the incidence of *Shigella* infection has declined over the past several decades, but it remains an important cause of disease, particularly in underserved populations and among individuals living in poverty. The burden of disease is greater in lower-resource countries in which *Shigella* is endemic, particularly in children under 5 years of age, in whom it is an important cause of morbidity and mortality. Globally, it is estimated that there are approximately 170 million cases of *Shigella* annually, resulting in approximately 160,000 deaths.

Pathogenesis. *Shigella* organisms are resistant to the harsh acidic environment of the stomach, which partially explains the very low infective dose. Once in the intestine, organisms are taken up by M (microfold) epithelial cells, which are specialized for sampling and uptake of luminal antigens. After intracellular proliferation, the bacteria escape into the lamina propria. These bacteria then infect epithelial cells through the basolateral membranes, which express bacterial receptors. Alternatively, luminal organisms may elaborate factors that directly modulate epithelial tight junctions to expose basolateral bacterial receptors and enable binding. This may be mediated by virulence proteins, some of which are directly injected into the host cytoplasm. Certain *Shigella dysenteriae* serotypes also produce the Shiga toxin Stx, which inhibits eukaryotic protein synthesis and causes host cell death.

> ### MORPHOLOGY
>
> *Shigella* infections are most prominent in the rectosigmoid colon, but the ileum may also be involved, perhaps reflecting the abundance of M cells in the epithelium overlying Peyer patches. The histologic appearance in early cases is similar to other acute self-limited colitides. In more severe cases, the mucosa is hemorrhagic and ulcerated, and pseudomembranes may be present. Perhaps because of the tropism for M cells, which acts to localize the damage, aphthous-appearing ulcers similar to those in Crohn disease may also occur. Distinguishing *Shigella* infection from chronic inflammatory bowel disease is challenging, particularly if there is distortion of crypt architecture.

Clinical Features. **Shigella causes self-limited disease characterized by about 6 days of diarrhea, fever, and abdominal pain.** After an incubation period of 1 to 7 days, the initial watery diarrhea progresses to a dysenteric phase in approximately 50% of patients. Nausea and vomiting are notably absent and the diarrhea is commonly described as frequent, small volume, and bloody. Constitutional symptoms can persist for as long as 1 month. A subacute presentation may also occur in a subset of adults. Antibiotic treatment shortens the clinical course and reduces the duration over which organisms are shed in the stool,

but antidiarrheal medications are contraindicated because they can prolong symptoms by delaying bacterial clearance.

Complications of *Shigella* infection are uncommon and include *reactive arthritis*, a triad of sterile arthritis, urethritis, and conjunctivitis that preferentially affects HLA-B27–positive men between 20 and 40 years of age. Hemolytic uremic syndrome, which is typically associated with *enterohemorrhagic Escherichia coli (EHEC)*, may also occur after infection with shigellae that secrete Shiga toxin.

Escherichia coli

Escherichia coli are gram-negative bacilli that colonize the healthy gastrointestinal tract; most are nonpathogenic, but a subset cause human disease. The latter are classified according to morphology, pathogenesis, and in vitro behavior (see Table 13.4). Here we summarize their pathogenic mechanisms:

- *Enterotoxigenic E. coli (ETEC)*, the principal cause of traveler's diarrhea, are spread by the fecal-oral route. They express a heat-labile toxin that is similar to cholera toxin and a heat-stable toxin that increases intracellular cyclic GMP, an alteration that also promotes the development of secretory diarrhea.
- *Enteropathogenic E. coli (EPEC)* are characterized by their ability to attach tightly to the enterocyte apical membranes and cause local loss (effacement) of microvilli. The bacterial proteins necessary for attachment and effacement are encoded by a large genomic pathogenicity island, the locus of enterocyte effacement. This locus also encodes proteins that inject bacterial effector proteins into the epithelial cell cytoplasm. EPEC can cause endemic diarrhea as well as diarrheal outbreaks, particularly in children younger than 2 years of age.
- *Enterohemorrhagic E. coli (EHEC)* are subclassified as O157:H7 and non-O157:H7 serotypes. Outbreaks of *E. coli* O157:H7 in high-resource countries have been associated with the consumption of milk, vegetables, and inadequately cooked ground beef. Both O157:H7 and non-O157:H7 serotypes produce Shiga-like toxins and can cause dysentery. They can also trigger hemolytic-uremic syndrome (Chapter 12).
- *Enteroinvasive E. coli (EIEC)* resemble *Shigella* bacteriologically but do not produce toxins. They invade the gut epithelial cells and cause a bloody diarrhea.
- *Enteroaggregative E. coli (EAEC)* attach to enterocytes by adherence fimbriae but do not invade. Although they cause symptoms by producing heat-labile toxin and Shiga-like toxins, histologic damage is minimal.

Salmonellosis

Salmonella species are divided into *Salmonella typhi*, the causative agent of typhoid fever, and nontyphoid *Salmonella* strains that cause gastroenteritis. Nontyphoid *Salmonella* infection, usually due to *Salmonella enteritidis*, is quite common: more than 1 million cases occur each year in the United States and result in approximately 2000 deaths. It is even more prevalent in lower resource parts of the world; worldwide, *Salmonella* is estimated to cause 550 million episodes of diarrheal illness each year, including 220 million cases in children. Infection is most common in young children and older adults, with a peak incidence in summer and fall. Transmission is usually through contaminated food, particularly raw or undercooked meat, poultry, eggs, and milk. Symptoms usually appear rapidly, within 8 to 72 hours of exposure, and typically consist of diarrhea, nausea, vomiting, fever, and abdominal cramping.

Pathogenesis. **Salmonellae possess virulence genes that, like Shigella and enteropathogenic E. coli, encode proteins capable of transferring bacterial proteins into M cells and enterocytes.** The transferred proteins activate host cell Rho GTPases (regulators of cytoskeletal organization), thereby triggering actin rearrangement and bacterial uptake into phagosomes, where the bacteria proliferate. Salmonellae also secrete a molecule that induces epithelial release of a chemoattractant eicosanoid that draws neutrophils into the lumen and potentiates mucosal damage. Very few viable *Salmonella* organisms are necessary to cause infection in healthy individuals; reduced gastric acid, as in individuals with atrophic gastritis or those on acid-suppressive therapy, further reduces the size of the inoculum that is required to produce disease.

Typhoid Fever

Typhoid fever, also referred to as *enteric fever*, affects up to 30 million individuals worldwide each year. It is caused by *Salmonella typhi* and *Salmonella paratyphi*. Infection by *S. typhi* is more common in endemic areas, where children and adolescents are most often affected. By contrast, *S. paratyphi* predominates in lower-resource countries and travelers to those areas. Humans are the sole reservoir for *S. typhi* and *S. paratyphi,* and transmission occurs from person to person or via contaminated food or water. Gallbladder colonization may be associated with gallstones and a chronic carrier state. Acute infection is associated with anorexia, abdominal pain, bloating, nausea, vomiting, and bloody diarrhea followed by a short asymptomatic phase that gives way to bacteremia and fever with flulike symptoms. It is during this phase that detection of organisms by blood culture may prompt antibiotic treatment and prevent further disease progression. Cultures are positive in 90% of cases during the febrile phase. Without such treatment, the febrile phase is followed by up to 2 weeks of sustained high fevers with abdominal tenderness that may mimic appendicitis. *Rose spots,* small erythematous maculopapular lesions, are seen on the chest and abdomen. Systemic dissemination may cause *extraintestinal complications* including encephalopathy, meningitis, seizures, endocarditis, myocarditis, pneumonia, and cholecystitis.

Like *S. enteritidis, S. typhi* and *S. paratyphi* are taken up by M cells and then engulfed by mononuclear cells in the underlying lymphoid tissue. This causes Peyer patches in the terminal ileum to enlarge into plateaulike elevations up to 8 cm in diameter. Mucosal shedding creates oval ulcers oriented along the long axis of the ileum. However, unlike *S. enteritidis, S. typhi* and *S. paratyphi* can disseminate via lymphatic and blood vessels. This causes reactive hyperplasia of draining lymph nodes, in which bacteria-containing phagocytes accumulate. In addition, the red pulp of the spleen expands due to prominent phagocyte hyperplasia. Randomly scattered small foci of parenchymal necrosis with macrophage aggregates, termed *typhoid nodules,* may be found in the liver, bone marrow, and lymph nodes.

Pseudomembranous Colitis

Pseudomembranous colitis caused by *Clostridioides difficile* is an important cause of morbidity and mortality in the hospital setting. It can be placed in the categories of *antibiotic-associated colitis* or *antibiotic-associated diarrhea*. While antibiotic-associated diarrhea may also be caused by other organisms such as *Salmonella, C. perfringens* type A, or *S. aureus,* of these only *C. difficile* causes pseudomembrane formation. *C. difficile* is an anaerobic, gram-positive, spore-forming bacillus. It is likely that disruption of the normal colonic microbiota by antibiotics allows *C. difficile* overgrowth. Almost any antibiotic may be responsible; the most important factors for disease development are the frequency of antibiotic use and its effect on colonic microbiota. Toxins released by *C. difficile* cause the ribosylation of small GTPases and lead to

disruption of the epithelial cytoskeleton, tight junction barrier loss, cytokine release, and apoptosis.

MORPHOLOGY

Fully developed *C. difficile*—associated colitis is accompanied by formation of **pseudomembranes** (Fig. 13.24A), made up of an adherent layer of inflammatory cells and debris at sites of colonic mucosal injury. The surface epithelium is denuded, and the superficial lamina propria contains a dense infiltrate of neutrophils and occasional fibrin thrombi within capillaries. Damaged crypts are distended by a mucopurulent exudate that "erupts" to the surface in a fashion reminiscent of a volcano (Fig. 13.24B).

Clinical Features. In addition to antibiotic exposure, risk factors for *C. difficile*—associated colitis include age greater than 65 years, use of proton pump inhibitors, hospitalization, and immunosuppression. The organism is particularly prevalent in hospitals; as many as 20% of hospitalized adults are colonized with *C. difficile* (a rate 10 times higher than in the general population), but most colonized patients are free of disease. Individuals with *C. difficile*—associated colitis usually present with watery diarrhea and abdominal cramping; dehydration, fever, and leukocytosis are seen in more severe cases. Fecal leukocytes and occult blood may be present, but grossly bloody diarrhea is rare. Diagnosis of *C. difficile*—associated colitis in symptomatic patients is made with a positive nucleic acid amplification test and a positive stool test for *C. difficile* toxin; patients with only a positive nucleic amplification test are considered to be colonized. Regimens of selected antibiotics are generally effective treatments, but antibiotic-resistant and hypervirulent *C. difficile* strains are increasingly common. In patients with severe or recurrent disease, fecal microbial transplantation may clear the infection, speaking to the role of a disturbed microbiome in the pathogenesis of *C. difficile* colitis.

Mycobacterial Infection

Mycobacterial species, including *M. tuberculosis, M. bovis,* and *M. avium* species, may infect the gastrointestinal tract primarily or

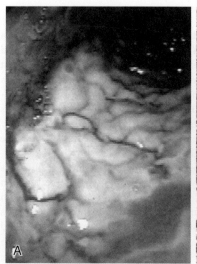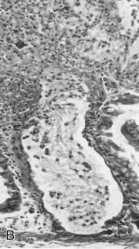

FIG. 13.24 *Clostridioides difficile* colitis. (A) The colon is coated by tan pseudomembranes composed of neutrophils, dead epithelial cells, and inflammatory debris (endoscopic view). (B) Typical pattern of neutrophils emanating from a crypt is reminiscent of a volcanic eruption.

as part of a disseminated infection. Gastrointestinal tuberculosis is rare in Western countries, except in individuals who are immuno-compromised, in whom *M. avium* infection is most common. In areas in which intestinal disease is endemic, including India and Pakistan, *M. bovis* is the usual cause. Risk factors for *M. bovis* infection include consumption of unpasteurized dairy products. Clinical features of *M. bovis* infection are similar to those caused by *M. tuberculosis*. Any part of the gut may be affected, but infection is most common in the ileocecal region, which is involved in 75% of cases.

Intestinal mycobacterial infection usually induces a granulomatous host response with caseous necrosis, often associated with systemic symptoms such as fever and night sweats. With chronicity, fibrosis, mucosal ulceration, and bleeding may develop. The granulomas may extend through the full thickness of the bowel, potentially leading to perforation, stenoses, or strictures. Patients may also develop perito-neal dissemination with ascites. By contrast, because *M. avium* infection typically affects individuals who are immunocompromised, granulomas may be absent. Instead, *M. avium* tends to accumulate in macrophages within the lamina propria. In some cases, the sheetlike expansion of macrophages may compress lymphatic vessels in the small bowel, leading to malabsorption. Such cases may mimic Whipple disease, a rare infection caused by *Tropheryma whipplei*, clinically and morphologically but can be easily distinguished by acid-fast stains, as *M. avium* is acid-fast and *T. whipplei* is not.

Norovirus

Norovirus (also known as Norwalk virus) causes approximately half of all gastroenteritis outbreaks worldwide and is a common cause of sporadic gastroenteritis in high-resource countries. It is very infec-tious; ingestion or inhalation of as few as 10 viral particles can transmit the disease. Local outbreaks are usually related to contaminated food or water, whereas person-to-person transmission underlies most sporadic cases. Infections spread easily within schools, hospitals, and nursing homes as well as other settings where people are packed closely together, such as cruise ships. After a short incubation period, affected individuals develop nausea, vomiting (often severe), explosive watery diarrhea, and abdominal pain. Biopsy morphology is nonspe-cific. The disease is self-limited.

Rotavirus

Rotavirus is most common cause of severe childhood diarrhea and diarrhea-related deaths worldwide. Children between 6 and 24 months of age are most vulnerable. Protection in the first 6 months of life is due to the presence of antibodies to rotavirus in breast milk, while protection beyond 2 years of age is due to im-munity that develops after the first infection. Like norovirus, it is highly infectious; the estimated minimal infective inoculum is only 10 viral particles. Rotavirus selectively infects and destroys mature (absorptive) enterocytes in the small intestine, and the villus sur-face is then first repopulated by immature secretory cells. This change in functional capacity results in loss of absorptive function and net secretion of water and electrolytes, compounded by an osmotic diarrhea from incompletely absorbed nutrients. Rotavirus infection becomes symptomatic after a short incubation period and manifests as several days of vomiting and watery diarrhea. Fortu-nately, the introduction of effective vaccines in 2006 has substan-tially reduced the burden of rotavirus disease in higher-resource countries and is beginning to have a positive impact in lower-resource countries as well.

Parasitic Disease

Parasitic disease and protozoal infections affect over half of the world's population on a chronic or recurrent basis. Intestinal parasites infesting humans include nematodes, such as the round-worms *Ascaris* and *Strongyloides*, hookworms, pinworms, cestodes (e.g., flatworms and tapeworms), trematodes (flukes), and protozoa. Some of the more common parasites are discussed briefly.

- *Ascaris lumbricoides.* This nematode is spread by human fecal-oral contamination and infects more than 1 billion individuals world-wide. Ingested eggs hatch in the intestine and the larvae penetrate the intestinal mucosa. From there, the larvae migrate via the splanchnic circulation to the liver, creating hepatic abscesses, and then through the systemic circulation to the lung, where they may cause pneumonitis. From the lung, larvae migrate up the tra-chea to the oropharynx and are swallowed, allowing them to again reach the intestine and mature into adult worms. Diagnosis is made by detection of eggs in the stool.
- *Strongyloides. Strongyloides* is widely found in tropical and subtrop-ical regions worldwide. The larvae of *Strongyloides* live in ground soil contaminated by feces. The larvae can penetrate unbroken skin of a person walking barefoot. From here the blood stream carries them to the lungs, from which they travel to the trachea and the oropharynx, allowing them to be swallowed and to reach the intestines, where they mature into adult worms. Unlike other intestinal worms, whose life cycle requires an ovum or larval stage outside the human, the eggs of *Strongyloides* can hatch within the intestine and release larvae that penetrate the mucosa, creating a cycle of *autoinfection*. Hence, *Strongyloides* infection may persist for life and immunocompromised individuals may develop overwhelming infections. The disease is asymptomatic in immunocompetent individuals.
- *Necator americanus* and *Ancylostoma duodenale.* These hook-worms infect more than 500 million individuals worldwide and cause significant morbidity. Infection is initiated by larval penetra-tion of the skin. After further development in the lungs, the larvae migrate up the trachea and are swallowed. Once in the duodenum, the larvae mature and the adult worms attach to the mucosa, suck blood, and reproduce. Hookworms are a leading cause of iron defi-ciency anemia in low-resource parts of the world. The diagnosis is made by detecting the eggs in stool.
- *Giardia lamblia.* This flagellated protozoan, also referred to as *Giardia duodenalis* or *Giardia intestinalis*, is the most common pathogenic parasite in humans. It is spread by fecally contaminated water or food. Infection may occur after ingestion of as few as 10 cysts and is characterized by acute or chronic malabsorptive diar-rhea. Because cysts are resistant to chlorine, *Giardia* organisms are endemic in unfiltered public and rural water supplies. In the acidic environment of the stomach, excystation occurs and tropho-zoites are released. Secretory IgA and mucosal IL-6 responses are important for clearance of *Giardia* infections. Individuals who are immunocompromised, particular those who fail to mount anti-body responses, are often severely affected. *Giardia* evades immune clearance through continuous modification of its major surface an-tigen, variant surface protein, and can persist for months or years while causing intermittent symptoms. *Giardia* infection reduces expression of brush border enzymes, including lactase, and causes microvillous damage and apoptosis of small-intestinal epithelial cells. *Giardia* trophozoites are noninvasive and can be identified in duodenal biopsy specimens or stool preps by their characteristic pear shape (eFig. 13.7A). The diagnosis is made with tests on stool for *Giardia*-specific antigens or nucleic acids.

- *Cryptosporidium.* Along with *Giardia*, *Cryptosporidium* is one of the most common enteric parasites of humans. Infections in higher-resource countries have been linked to contaminated public water supplies, whereas in lower-resource countries infection is associated with poor sanitary conditions and overcrowding; in these areas, *Cryptosporidium* is an important cause of childhood diarrhea and is responsible for as many as 200,000 deaths per year, a toll that may be second only to rotavirus. The organisms are typically found on the surface of small bowel epithelial cells (see eFig. 13.7B) and characteristically lead to secretory diarrhea and malabsorption. The diagnosis is made by identifying the organisms in stool preps by morphology or with tests for *Cryptosporidium*-specific nucleic acids.
- *Entamoeba histolytica.* This protozoan causes amebiasis and is spread by fecal-oral transmission, primarily in low-resource parts of the world with poor sanitation. Areas with high rates of infection include Mexico, parts of Central and South America, Africa, and India. In some areas the prevalence of infection may be as high as 50%.

  Amebiasis most often affects the cecum and ascending colon (see eFig. 13.7C, D). Dysentery develops when the amebae attach to the colonic epithelium, induce apoptosis, invade crypts, and burrow laterally into the lamina propria. The resulting damage leads to recruitment of neutrophils and creates a flask-shaped ulcer with a narrow neck and broad base. Parasites penetrate splanchnic vessels and embolize to the liver to produce abscesses in about 40% of patients with amebic dysentery. *Amebic liver abscesses*, which may exceed 10 cm in diameter, have a scant inflammatory reaction at their margins and a shaggy fibrinous lining. The abscesses persist after the acute intestinal illness has passed, and on rare occasions the parasites may subsequently spread to the lung, heart, kidneys, or brain. Individuals with amebiasis may present with abdominal pain, bloody diarrhea, or weight loss. Occasionally, acute necrotizing colitis and megacolon occur, both of which are associated with significant mortality.

INFLAMMATORY INTESTINAL DISEASE

Sigmoid Diverticulitis

In general, the term diverticular disease is a misnomer, as it usually refers to acquired pseudodiverticula rather than true diverticula. Colonic diverticula are rare in individuals younger than 30 years of age but rise in incidence sharply thereafter; their prevalence approaches 50% in Western adult populations older than 60 years of age. Diverticula are generally multiple, a condition referred to as *diverticulosis*. This disease is much less common in lower-resource countries, probably because of dietary differences.

Pathogenesis. **Colonic diverticula develop due to elevated intraluminal pressure.** The location of diverticula is explained by the unique structure of the colonic muscularis propria, where nerves, arterial vasa recta, and their connective tissue sheaths penetrate the inner circular muscle coat to create discontinuities in the muscle wall. In other parts of the intestine, these gaps are reinforced by the external longitudinal layer of the muscularis propria, but in the colon, this muscle layer is discontinuous, being gathered into three bands termed *taeniae coli*. This creates a point of structural weakness through which the mucosa and submucosa may herniate outward in response to high intracolonic luminal pressures. Most diverticula occur in the narrowest part of the colon, the sigmoid, which experiences the highest pressures during peristaltic contractions. The pathogenesis also appears to involve exaggerated peristaltic contractions and spasmodic sequestration of bowel segments. The etiology of these abnormal contractions is unknown, but they are hypothesized to be associated with consumption of Western diets high in red meat and low in fiber. Other risk factors include a sedentary lifestyle, obesity, smoking, and use of certain medications, including steroids and opiates.

MORPHOLOGY

Colonic diverticula are small, flasklike outpouchings, usually 0.5 to 1 cm in diameter, that occur in a regular distribution between the taeniae coli (Fig. 13.25A and B). They are most common in the sigmoid colon, but other regions of the colon may also be affected. The diverticula have a thin wall composed of a flattened or atrophic mucosa, compressed submucosa, and attenuated muscularis propria—often, this last component is totally absent (Fig. 13.25C and D). Obstruction of diverticula and stasis of contents leads to inflammation, producing **diverticulitis** and peridiverticulitis. Because the wall of the diverticulum is supported only by the muscularis mucosa and a thin layer of subserosal adipose tissue, inflammation, increased pressure, and mucosal ulceration within an obstructed diverticulum may result in **perforation**. With or without perforation, recurrent diverticulitis may cause segmental colitis, fibrotic thickening in and around the colonic wall, or stricture formation.

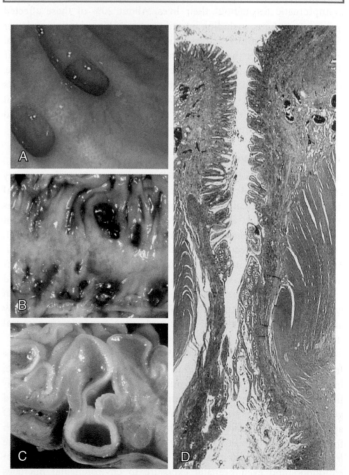

FIG. 13.25 Sigmoid diverticular disease. (A) Endoscopic view of two sigmoid diverticula. Compare to (B). (B) Gross examination of a resected sigmoid colon shows regularly spaced stool-filled diverticula. (C) Cross-section showing the outpouching of mucosa beneath the muscularis propria. (D) Low-power photomicrograph of a sigmoid diverticulum showing protrusion of the mucosa and submucosa through the muscularis propria. (Endoscopic image courtesy of Dr. Ira Hanan, The University of Chicago, Chicago, Illinois.)

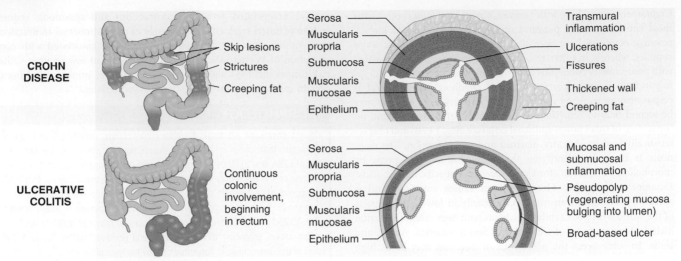

FIG. 13.26 Distribution and types of lesions in inflammatory bowel disease. The distinction between Crohn disease and ulcerative colitis is based primarily on morphology.

Clinical Features. Most individuals with diverticular disease remain asymptomatic throughout their lives. About 20% of those affected develop symptoms, including intermittent cramping, continuous lower abdominal discomfort, constipation, and diarrhea. Longitudinal studies have shown that while diverticula may regress early in their development, they often become larger and more numerous over time. Whether a high-fiber diet prevents such progression or protects against diverticulitis is unclear. Even when diverticulitis occurs, it most often resolves spontaneously or after antibiotic treatment, and relatively few patients require surgical intervention for perforation.

Inflammatory Bowel Disease

Inflammatory bowel disease (IBD) is a chronic inflammatory condition triggered by the host immune response to intestinal microbes in genetically predisposed individuals. IBD encompasses two entities, *Crohn disease* and *ulcerative colitis.* The distinction between Crohn disease and ulcerative colitis is based, in large part, on the distribution of affected sites and the morphologic expression of disease at those sites (Fig. 13.26; Table 13.5). Ulcerative colitis is limited to the colon and rectum and involves only the mucosa and submucosa. By contrast, Crohn disease, also referred to as *regional enteritis* (because of frequent ileal involvement), may involve any area of the gastrointestinal tract and often produces transmural inflammation.

Epidemiology. Both ulcerative colitis and Crohn disease frequently present in adolescents or in young adults. Worldwide, incidence varies according to a number of factors including population density (rural versus city), the extent of industrialization, and geography, as IBD is more prevalent in higher latitude locations. IBD appears to be increasing in incidence, including in regions in which the prevalence was historically low. One proposed explanation is the *hygiene hypothesis,* first applied to asthma, which suggests that childhood and even prenatal exposure to environmental microbes stimulates the immune system in a way that prevents excessive reactions. Applied to IBD, it suggests that a reduced frequency of enteric infections early in life due to improved hygiene results in inadequate development of regulatory processes that limit mucosal immune responses. While attractive and commonly stated, firm evidence is lacking and hence the increasing incidence of IBD remains mysterious.

Pathogenesis. **IBD appears to result from the combined effects of alterations in host interactions with intestinal microbiota, intestinal epithelial dysfunction, and aberrant mucosal immune responses.**

Table 13.5 Features of Crohn Disease and Ulcerative Colitis

Feature	Crohn Disease	Ulcerative Colitis
Morphology		
Bowel region affected	Ileum ± colon	Colon only
Rectal involvement	Sometimes	Always
Distribution	Skip lesions	Diffuse
Stricture	Yes	Rare
Bowel wall appearance	Thick	Thin
Inflammation	Transmural	Limited to mucosa and submucosa
Pseudopolyps	Moderate	Marked
Ulcers	Deep, knifelike	Superficial, broad-based
Lymphoid reaction	Marked	Moderate
Fibrosis	Marked	Mild to none
Serositis	Yes	No
Granulomas	Yes (~35%)	No
Fistulas/sinuses	Yes	No
Clinical		
Perianal fistula	Yes (in colonic disease)	No
Fat/vitamin malabsorption	Yes	No
Malignant potential	Yes	Yes
Recurrence after surgery	Common	No
Toxic megacolon	No	Yes

NOTE: Not all features may be present in a single case.

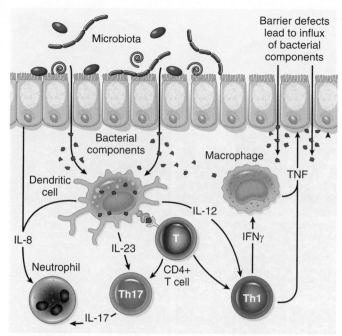

FIG. 13.27 A model of pathogenesis of inflammatory bowel disease (IBD). *IFN-γ*, Interferon gamma; *TNF*, tumor necrosis factor. See text for details.

This view is supported by epidemiologic, genetic, and clinical studies as well as data from laboratory models of IBD (Fig. 13.27). The associated factors can be broken down into four categories, as follows:

- *Genetic factors.* Risk for disease is increased when there is an affected family member. In Crohn disease, the concordance rate for monozygotic twins is approximately 50%. By contrast, concordance of monozygotic twins for ulcerative colitis is approximately 20%, suggesting that genetic factors are less dominant in this form of IBD.
  - Molecular linkage analyses of affected families have identified *NOD2* (nucleotide oligomerization binding domain 2) as a susceptibility gene in Crohn disease. *NOD2* encodes a protein that binds to intracellular bacterial peptidoglycans and subsequently activates NF-κB. Some studies suggest that the disease-associated form of NOD-2 is ineffective at defending against intestinal bacteria. This defect allows increased numbers of bacteria to penetrate past the epithelium into the intestinal wall, where they trigger inflammatory reactions. However, disease develops in less than 10% of individuals carrying specific *NOD2* polymorphisms, and these polymorphisms are uncommon in patients of African and Asian descent with Crohn disease; therefore, other factors are also important.
  - The search for IBD-associated genes using genome-wide association studies (GWAS) and other approaches have identified over 200 genes with nucleotide variants that are associated with IBD. In addition to *NOD2* (discussed previously), multiple variants associated with risk lie in autophagy-related genes. The latter encode components of the autophagosome pathway and, like NOD-2, are involved in host cell responses to intracellular bacteria, supporting the hypothesis that inadequate defense against luminal bacteria is important in the pathogenesis of IBD. However, none of these genes is associated with ulcerative colitis, and the associations hold mainly for people of European descent.

- *Abnormal mucosal immune responses.* How altered mucosal immunity contributes to the pathogenesis of ulcerative colitis and Crohn disease is still being deciphered, but it is notable that immunosuppressive and immunomodulatory agents are mainstays of IBD therapy, supporting a role for inappropriately sustained immune responses in these diseases. It is proposed that the initial trigger is the presentation of microbial antigens to CD4+ helper T cells, which are induced to differentiate into Th1 and Th17 cells by cytokines such as IL-12 and IL-23 (see Fig. 13.27). These then activate macrophages, recruit neutrophils, and release proinflammatory cytokines such as TNF. The presence of microbial antigens in the lamina propria may stem from defects in epithelial barrier function that are exacerbated by inflammation (see below). Whether the disease takes the form of ulcerative colitis or Crohn disease likely depends upon differences in the cytokine milieu that is induced in response to microbial products. Defects in regulatory T cells, especially the IL-10-producing subset that dampens the immune response, may also contribute to the inflammation; consistent with this idea, rare individuals with mutations in the IL-10 or IL-10 receptor genes are susceptible to severe, early-onset colitis. Other data suggest that mucosal production of the Th2-derived cytokine IL-13 is increased in ulcerative colitis, and, to a lesser degree, in Crohn disease. Thus, defective immune regulation likely contributes to the chronic inflammation in IBD. Notably, patients with IBD benefit from treatment with antibodies that inhibit TNF or IL-12/IL-23, supporting a role for these cytokines in its pathogenesis. The contribution of true autoimmunity is unclear, and no initiating or target self antigens have been definitively identified.

- *Epithelial defects.* A variety of epithelial defects have been described in Crohn disease, ulcerative colitis, or both. For example, defects in intestinal epithelial tight junction barrier function occur in patients with Crohn disease and a subset of their healthy first-degree relatives. This barrier dysfunction cosegregates with disease-associated *NOD2* polymorphisms, and experimental models demonstrate that barrier dysfunction can activate innate and adaptive mucosal immunity and sensitize subjects to disease. Interestingly, Paneth cell granules, which contain antimicrobial peptides that affect the composition of luminal microbiota, are abnormal in some patients with Crohn disease, suggesting a mechanism in which a defective "crosstalk" between the epithelium and the microbiota contributes to disease pathogenesis.

- *Changes in the microbiota.* The quantity of microbial organisms in the gastrointestinal lumen is enormous, amounting to as many as 10^{12} organisms/mL of fecal material in the colon (50% of fecal mass). There is significant interindividual variation in the composition of the microbiota, which is modified by diet and disease. Microbial transfer may either promote or reduce disease in animal models of IBD, and clinical trials suggest that probiotic (beneficial) bacteria or even fecal microbial transplants from healthy individuals may benefit patients with IBD.

We will discuss next the morphologic and clinical features of each of the two forms of IBD.

Crohn Disease

MORPHOLOGY

The most common sites of Crohn disease at presentation are the **terminal ileum, ileocecal valve,** and **cecum.** Disease is limited to the small intestine in about 40% of cases; the small intestine and the colon are both involved in 30% of patients; and the remainder of cases are characterized by colonic involvement only. Infrequently, Crohn disease may involve the esophagus or stomach. The presence of **skip lesions** (multiple, separate, sharply delineated areas of disease interspersed with areas of normal mucosa) is characteristic of Crohn disease and distinguishes Crohn disease from ulcerative colitis. Strictures are common (Fig. 13.28A).

The earliest lesion is the **aphthous ulcer;** these may progress, become multiple, and coalesce into elongated, serpentine ulcers oriented along the long axis of the bowel. Edema and loss of normal mucosal folds are common. Sparing of interspersed mucosa results in a coarsely textured, **cobblestone** appearance, in which diseased tissue is depressed below the level of normal mucosa (Fig. 13.28B). Those with colon involvement are susceptible to developing **toxic megacolon** before fibrosis develops, which prevents dilatation of the colon. **Fissures** frequently develop between mucosal folds and may extend deeply to become sites of perforation or fistula tracts. The intestinal wall is thickened as a consequence of transmural edema, inflammation, submucosal fibrosis, and hypertrophy of the muscularis propria, all of which contribute to formation of **strictures.** In cases with extensive transmural disease, mesenteric fat frequently becomes adherent to the serosal surface **(creeping fat)** (Fig. 13.28C).

The microscopic features of active Crohn disease include abundant neutrophils that infiltrate and damage crypt epithelium. Clusters of neutrophils within a crypt are referred to as a **crypt abscess** and are often associated with crypt destruction. Ulceration is common in Crohn disease, and there may be an abrupt transition between ulcerated and normal mucosa. Repeated cycles of crypt destruction and regeneration lead to **distortion of mucosal architecture;** the normally straight and parallel crypts take on branching shapes and unusual orientations to one another (Fig. 13.29A). Epithelial metaplasia, another consequence of chronic injury, often takes the form of gastric antral-appearing glands (pseudopyloric metaplasia). **Paneth cell metaplasia** may occur in the left colon, where Paneth cells are normally absent. These architectural and metaplastic changes may persist, even when active inflammation has resolved. Mucosal atrophy, with loss of crypts, may follow years of disease. **Noncaseating granulomas** (Fig. 13.29B), a hallmark of Crohn disease, are found in approximately 35% of cases and may arise in areas of active disease or uninvolved regions in any layer of the intestinal wall (Fig. 13.29C). Granulomas also may be found in mesenteric lymph nodes and sometimes even the skin, representing extraintestinal manifestations of Crohn disease. Importantly, the absence of granulomas does not preclude the diagnosis.

Clinical Features. The clinical manifestations of Crohn disease are extremely variable. In most patients, disease begins with intermittent attacks of relatively mild diarrhea, fever, and abdominal pain.

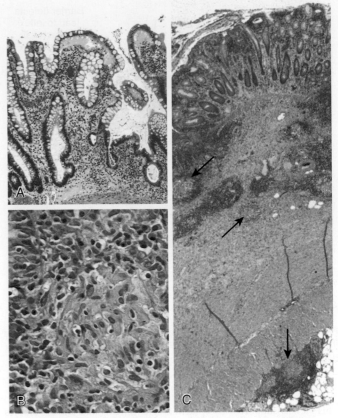

FIG. 13.29 Microscopic pathology of Crohn disease. (A) Haphazard crypt organization results from repeated injury and regeneration. (B) Noncaseating granuloma. (C) Transmural Crohn disease with markedly thickened wall and submucosal and serosal granulomas *(arrows)*.

Approximately 20% of patients present acutely with right lower quadrant pain and fever, features that mimic acute appendicitis or bowel perforation. Patients with colonic involvement may present with bloody diarrhea and abdominal pain, suggesting a colonic infection. Periods of disease activity are typically interrupted by asymptomatic intervals that last for weeks to many months. Disease reactivation may be associated with a variety of external triggers, including physical or emotional stress, specific dietary items, NSAID use, and cigarette smoking.

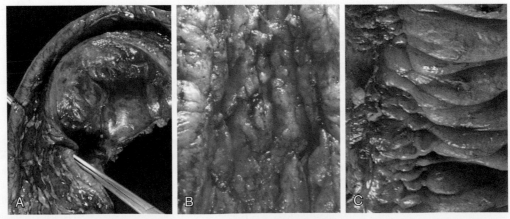

FIG. 13.28 Gross pathology of Crohn disease. (A) Small-intestinal stricture. (B) Linear mucosal ulcers and thickened intestinal wall. (C) Creeping fat.

Iron deficiency anemia due to blood loss may develop in individuals with colonic disease, while extensive small bowel disease and associated malabsorption may result in hypoalbuminemia, generalized nutrient malabsorption, or vitamin B_{12} deficiency. Fibrosing strictures, particularly of the terminal ileum, are common and require surgical resection. Disease often recurs at the site of anastomosis, and as many as 40% of patients require additional resections within 10 years. Fistulas can develop between loops of bowel and may also involve the urinary bladder, vagina, and abdominal or perianal skin. Perforations and peritoneal abscesses may also occur.

Extraintestinal manifestations of Crohn disease include uveitis, migratory polyarthritis, sacroiliitis, ankylosing spondylitis, erythema nodosum, and clubbing of the fingertips, any of which may develop before intestinal disease is recognized. Pericholangitis and primary sclerosing cholangitis may occur in those with Crohn disease but are more common in patients with ulcerative colitis. As discussed later, the risk for development of colonic and small intestinal adenocarcinoma is increased in patients with long-standing colonic Crohn disease.

Ulcerative Colitis

> ## MORPHOLOGY
>
> Ulcerative colitis always involves the rectum and extends proximally in a continuous fashion to involve part or all of the colon (Fig. 13.30A). Skip lesions are not seen. Disease of the entire colon is termed **pancolitis** (Fig. 13.30B). Disease limited to the rectum or rectosigmoid may be referred to descriptively as **ulcerative proctitis** or **ulcerative proctosigmoiditis.** The small intestine is normal, although mild mucosal inflammation of the distal ileum **(backwash ileitis)** may be present in severe cases.
>
> On gross evaluation, involved colonic mucosa may be slightly red and granular appearing or exhibit extensive **broad-based ulcers.** The transition between diseased and uninvolved colon is abrupt (Fig. 13.30C). Ulcers are aligned along the long axis of the colon but typically do not replicate the serpentine ulcers of Crohn disease. Isolated islands of regenerating mucosa

> often bulge into the lumen to create small elevations, termed **pseudopolyps.** Chronic disease may lead to **mucosal atrophy** and a flat, smooth mucosal surface lacking normal folds. Unlike in Crohn disease, mural thickening is absent, the serosal surface is normal, and strictures do not occur. However, inflammation and inflammatory mediators may damage the muscularis propria and disturb neuromuscular function, leading to colonic dilation and **toxic megacolon,** which carries a significant risk for perforation. Patients with toxic megacolon are quite sick with fever, tachycardia, hypotension.
>
> Histologic features of mucosal disease in ulcerative colitis are similar to colonic Crohn disease and include inflammatory infiltrates, crypt abscesses, crypt distortion, and epithelial metaplasia. However, skip lesions are absent, and inflammation is generally limited to the mucosa and superficial submucosa (Fig. 13.30D). In severe cases, mucosal damage may be accompanied by ulcers that extend more deeply into the submucosa, but the muscularis propria is rarely involved. Submucosal fibrosis, mucosal atrophy, and distorted mucosal architecture remain as residua of healed disease, but the histologic pattern may also revert to near normal after prolonged remission. Granulomas are not present.
>
> Some extraintestinal manifestations of ulcerative colitis overlap with those of Crohn disease, including migratory polyarthritis, sacroiliitis, ankylosing spondylitis, uveitis, skin lesions, pericholangitis, and primary sclerosing cholangitis.

Clinical Features. Ulcerative colitis is a relapsing disorder characterized by attacks of bloody, stringy, often mucoid diarrhea associated with lower abdominal pain and cramps that are temporarily relieved by defecation. These symptoms may persist for days, weeks, or months before they subside, and occasionally the initial attack may be sufficiently severe to constitute a medical or surgical emergency. More than half of patients have mild disease, but almost all experience at least one relapse during a 10-year period. Colectomy cures intestinal disease, but extraintestinal manifestations may persist.

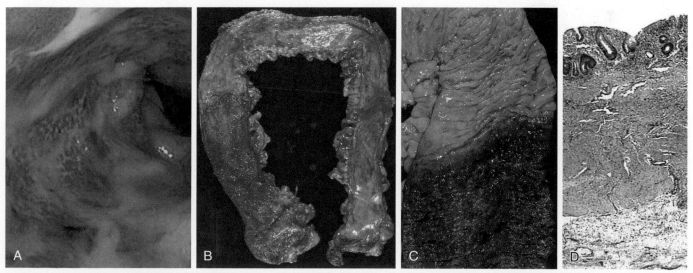

FIG. 13.30 Pathology of ulcerative colitis. (A) Endoscopic view of severe ulcerative colitis with ulceration and adherent mucopurulent material. (B) Total colectomy with pancolitis showing active disease, with red, granular mucosa in the cecum *(left)* and smooth, atrophic mucosa distally *(right)*. (C) Sharp demarcation between active ulcerative colitis *(bottom)* and normal *(top)*. (D) This full-thickness histologic section shows that disease is limited to the mucosa. Compare with Fig. 13.29C. (Endoscopic image courtesy of Dr. Ira Hanan, The University of Chicago, Chicago, Illinois.)

The factors that trigger ulcerative colitis are not known; infectious enteritis precedes disease onset in some cases. The onset of symptoms may occur shortly after smoking cessation in some patients, and smoking may partially relieve symptoms. However, studies of nicotine as a therapeutic agent have been disappointing.

Therapy is focused on antiinflammatory agents. Individuals with mild disease are often treated with glucocorticoids or aminosalicylates. Patients with more severe disease often benefit from treatment with biologic agents, such as antibodies that bind and neutralize TNF or IL-12/IL-23.

Colitis-Associated Neoplasia

One of the most serious long-term complications of ulcerative colitis and colonic Crohn disease is the development of adenocarcinoma. This risk is confined to the colon in patients with ulcerative colitis, but those with Crohn disease are also at increased risk of small intestinal adenocarcinoma. This process begins as dysplasia, which, just as in Barrett esophagus and chronic gastritis, is part of the progression to carcinoma. The risk for development of dysplasia is related to several factors:

- *Duration of disease.* Risk increases beginning 8 to 10 years after disease initiation.
- *Extent of involvement.* Patients with involvement of the entire colon are at greater risk than those with only partial involvement.
- *Inflammation.* Greater frequency and severity of active inflammation (characterized by the presence of neutrophils) may increase risk. This is another example of the enabling effect of inflammation on carcinogenesis (Chapter 6).

To facilitate early detection of neoplasia, patients are typically enrolled in colonoscopic surveillance programs approximately 8 years after diagnosis of IBD. An important exception to this approach is in patients with primary sclerosing cholangitis, who are at markedly greater risk for development of dysplasia; in this instance, surveillance is generally initiated at the time of diagnosis. Surveillance requires regular and extensive mucosal biopsy, which is costly and invasive. In many cases, dysplasia occurs in flat areas of mucosa that do not appear abnormal by eye. Thus, advanced endoscopic imaging techniques are being developed to try to improve the detection of early dysplastic changes.

COLONIC POLYPS AND NEOPLASTIC DISEASE

Polyps are most common in the colon and may also occur in the esophagus, stomach, or small intestine. Those without stalks are referred to as *sessile*. As sessile polyps enlarge, traction on the luminal protrusion may create a stalk. Polyps with stalks are termed *pedunculated*. In general, intestinal polyps can be classified as *nonneoplastic* or *neoplastic*. The most common neoplastic polyp is the adenoma, which has the potential to progress to cancer. Nonneoplastic colonic polyps can be further classified as inflammatory, hamartomatous, or hyperplastic.

Inflammatory Polyps

Inflammatory polyps are associated with the *solitary rectal ulcer syndrome*. Patients present with the triad of rectal bleeding, mucus discharge, and an inflammatory polyp on the anterior rectal wall. The underlying cause is impaired relaxation of the anorectal sphincter, creating a sharp angle at the anterior rectal shelf. This leads to recurrent abrasion and ulceration of the overlying rectal mucosa. With repeated cycles of injury and healing, a polypoid mass forms that is composed of inflamed and reactive mucosal tissue.

Hamartomatous Polyps

Hamartomatous polyps occur sporadically and as components of various genetically determined or acquired syndromes (Table 13.6). As described in Chapter 6, hamartomatous polyps are disorganized, tumorlike growths composed of mature cell types normally present at

Table 13.6 Gastrointestinal (GI) Polyposis Syndromes

Syndrome	Mean Age at Presentation (Years)	Mutated Gene(s)	GI Lesions	Selected Extragastrointestinal Manifestations
Peutz-Jeghers syndrome	10–15	LKB1/STK11	Arborizing polyps—small intestine > colon > stomach; colonic adenocarcinoma	Mucocutaneous pigmentation; increased risk for thyroid, breast, lung, pancreas, gonadal, and bladder cancers
Juvenile polyposis	<5	SMAD4, BMPR1A	Juvenile polyps; increased risk for gastric, small-intestinal, colonic, and pancreatic adenocarcinoma	Pulmonary arteriovenous malformations, digital clubbing
Cowden syndrome	<15	PTEN	Hamartomatous polyps, lipomas, ganglioneuromas, inflammatory polyps; increased risk for colon cancer	Benign skin tumors, benign and malignant thyroid and breast lesions
Tuberous sclerosis	Infancy to adulthood	TSC1, TSC2	Hamartomatous polyps (rectal)	Facial angiofibroma, cortical tubers, renal angiomyolipoma
Familial adenomatous polyposis (FAP)				
Classic FAP	10–15	APC	Multiple adenomas	Congenital RPE hypertrophy
Attenuated FAP	40–50	APC	Multiple adenomas	
Gardner syndrome	10–15	APC	Multiple adenomas	Osteomas, desmoids, skin cysts
Turcot syndrome	10–15	APC	Multiple adenomas	CNS tumors, medulloblastoma

CNS, Central nervous system; *RPE*, retinal pigment epithelium.

the site at which the polyp develops. Hamartomatous polyposis syndromes are rare but must be recognized because of associated intestinal and extraintestinal manifestations, the need to screen family members, and, in some instances, an increased risk of cancer.

Juvenile Polyps

Juvenile polyps are the most common type of hamartomatous polyp. They may be sporadic or syndromic. Sporadic juvenile polyps are usually solitary, whereas *juvenile polyposis*, an autosomal dominant syndrome, may be associated with dozens of polyps. Most juvenile polyps occur in children younger than 5 years. They are characteristically located in the rectum and usually manifest with rectal bleeding. In some cases, prolapse occurs and the polyp protrudes through the anal sphincter. Dysplasia occurs in a small proportion of juvenile polyps, and juvenile polyposis is associated with an increased risk for adenocarcinoma of the colon and other sites (see Table 13.6). This is not surprising, as juvenile polyposis is associated with germline mutations in genes that encode components of the TGFβ/BMP signaling pathway (e.g., *SMAD4*), which is frequently mutated in certain cancers. Colectomy may be required to limit the hemorrhage associated with polyp ulceration in juvenile polyposis.

> ### MORPHOLOGY
>
> Sporadic and syndromic juvenile polyps are similar in appearance. They are typically pedunculated, smooth-surfaced, reddish lesions less than 3 cm in diameter that display characteristic cystic spaces on cut sections. These spaces are dilated glands filled with mucin and inflammatory debris (Fig. 13.31A).

Peutz-Jeghers Syndrome

Peutz-Jeghers syndrome is a rare autosomal dominant disorder defined by the presence of multiple gastrointestinal hamartomatous polyps, mucocutaneous hyperpigmentation, and an increased risk for development of numerous malignancies. Included among the malignancies are cancers of the colon, pancreas, breast, lung, ovaries, uterus, and testes, as well as other unusual neoplasms. Germline loss-of-function mutations in the *LKB1/STK11* gene are present in approximately half of the patients with the familial form of Peutz-Jeghers syndrome. *LKB1/STK11* encodes a tumor suppressive protein kinase that regulates cellular metabolism, another example of the link between altered metabolism, abnormal cell growth, and cancer risk.

> ### MORPHOLOGY
>
> Hamartomatous polyps are most common in the small intestine, although they may also occur in the stomach, colon, and, rarely, in the bladder and lungs. On gross evaluation, the polyps are large and pedunculated with a lobulated contour. Histologic examination demonstrates a characteristic arborizing network of connective tissue, smooth muscle, lamina propria, and glands lined by normal-appearing intestinal epithelium (Fig. 13.31B).

Hyperplastic Polyps

Colonic hyperplastic polyps are common epithelial proliferations that typically occur in the sixth and seventh decades of life. Their pathogenesis is incompletely understood, but their formation is thought to result from decreased epithelial cell turnover and delayed shedding of surface epithelial cells, leading to a "pileup" of goblet cells. Although

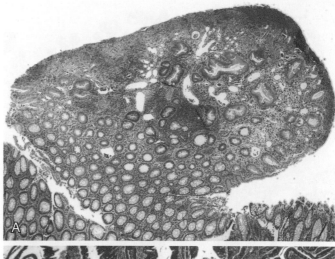

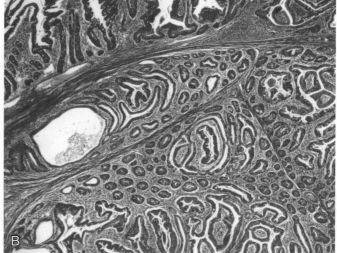

FIG. 13.31 Hamartomatous polyps. (A) Juvenile polyp. Note the surface erosion and cystically dilated crypts filled with mucus, neutrophils, and debris. (B) Peutz-Jeghers polyp. Complex glandular architecture and bundles of smooth muscle help to distinguish Peutz-Jeghers polyps from juvenile polyps.

these lesions have no malignant potential, they are difficult to distinguish endoscopically from sessile serrated adenomas, histologically similar lesions that do have malignant potential, and so are frequently biopsied.

> ### MORPHOLOGY
>
> Hyperplastic polyps are most commonly found in the left colon and are typically less than 5 mm in diameter. They are smooth, nodular protrusions of the mucosa, often on the crests of mucosal folds. They may occur singly but more frequently are multiple, particularly in the sigmoid colon and rectum. Histologically, they are composed of an expanded population of mature goblet and absorptive cells, crowding of which creates a serrated surface, which is the morphologic hallmark of these lesions (Fig. 13.32).

Adenomas

The most common and clinically important neoplastic polyps are colonic adenomas, which are precursor lesions of colorectal

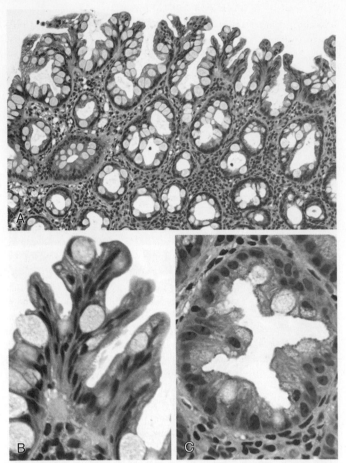

FIG. 13.32 Hyperplastic polyp. (A) Polyp surface with irregular tufting of epithelial cells. (B) Tufting results from epithelial overcrowding. (C) Epithelial crowding produces a serrated architecture when glands are cut in cross-section.

adenocarcinomas. There is no sex predilection, and they are present in nearly 50% of adults living in the Western world over 50 years of age. Because these polyps are precursors of colorectal cancer, current recommendations are that all adults in the United States undergo screening colonoscopy starting at 45 years of age. Since individuals with a family history are at risk for developing colon cancer earlier in life, they are typically screened at least 10 years before the youngest age at which a relative was diagnosed. While adenomas are less common in Asia, their frequency has risen (in parallel with an increasing incidence of colorectal adenocarcinoma) as Western diets and lifestyles become more common.

MORPHOLOGY

Typical adenomas range from 0.3 to 10 cm in diameter and can be **pedunculated** (Fig. 13.33A) or **sessile,** with both types having a velvety texture (Fig. 13.33B) and bumpy surface due to the abnormal epithelial growth pattern. Histologically, the cytologic hallmark is **epithelial dysplasia** (Fig. 13.34C), marked by nuclear hyperchromasia, elongation, and stratification. These changes are most easily appreciated at the surface of the adenoma because the epithelium fails to mature as cells migrate from the crypt. Pedunculated adenomas have slender fibromuscular stalks (Fig. 13.33C) containing prominent blood vessels derived from the submucosa. The stalk is usually covered by nonneoplastic epithelium, but dysplastic epithelium is sometimes present.

Adenomas may be classified as **tubular, tubulovillous,** or **villous** based on their architecture. Tubular adenomas tend to be small, pedunculated polyps composed of small, rounded, or tubular glands (Fig. 13.34A). By contrast, villous adenomas, which are often larger and sessile, are covered by slender villi (Fig. 13.34B). Tubulovillous adenomas have a mixture of tubular and villous elements. Although foci of invasion are more frequent in villous adenomas than in tubular adenomas, villous architecture alone does not increase cancer risk which is related to size, as discussed below.

The histologic features of **sessile serrated adenomas** overlap with those of hyperplastic polyps and these lesions typically lack dysplasia (Fig. 13.34D). Nevertheless, sessile serrated adenomas have a malignant potential similar to conventional adenomas. The most useful feature distinguishing sessile serrated adenoma from hyperplastic polyp is the presence of serrated architecture throughout the full length of the glands, including the crypt base, in association with crypt dilation and lateral growth (Fig. 13.34D). By contrast, serrated architecture is typically confined to the surface of hyperplastic polyps.

Although most colorectal adenomas behave in a benign fashion, a small proportion harbor invasive cancer at the time of detection. **Size is the most important characteristic that correlates with risk for**

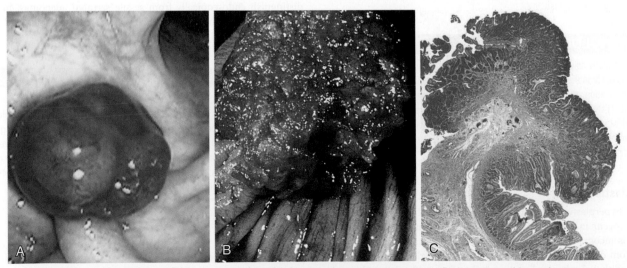

FIG. 13.33 Colonic adenomas. (A) Pedunculated adenoma (endoscopic view). (B) Adenoma with a velvety surface. (C) Low-magnification photomicrograph of a pedunculated tubular adenoma.

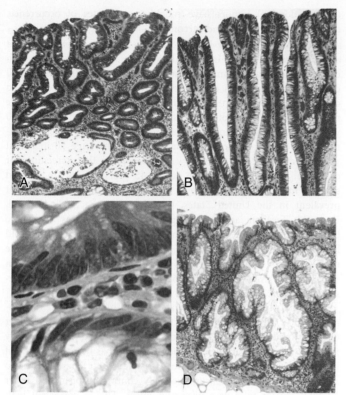

FIG. 13.34 Histologic appearance of colonic adenomas. (A) Tubular adenoma with a smooth surface and rounded glands. In this case, crypt dilation and rupture, with associated reactive inflammation, can be seen at the bottom of the field. (B) Villous adenoma with long, slender projections that are reminiscent of small-intestinal villi. (C) Dysplastic epithelial cells *(top)* with an increased nuclear-to-cytoplasmic ratio, hyperchromatic and elongated nuclei, and nuclear pseudostratification. Compare with the nondysplastic epithelium *(bottom)*. (D) Sessile serrated adenoma lined by goblet cells without typical cytologic features of dysplasia. This lesion is distinguished from a hyperplastic polyp by involvement of the crypts. Compare with the hyperplastic polyp in Fig. 13.32.

---

malignancy. For example, while cancer is extremely rare in adenomas less than 1 cm in diameter, some studies suggest that nearly 40% of lesions larger than 4 cm in diameter contain foci of invasive cancer. High-grade dysplasia is a second, less important risk factor for the presence of cancer in a polyp.

Familial Colonic Neoplasia Syndromes

Several syndromes associated with colonic polyps and increased rates of colon cancer have been described. The genetic bases of these disorders have been established and have provided insights that have greatly enhanced the understanding of sporadic colon cancer (Table 13.7).

Familial Adenomatous Polyposis

Familial adenomatous polyposis (FAP) is an autosomal dominant disorder marked by the appearance of numerous colorectal adenomas by the teenage years that is caused by mutation of the adenomatous polyposis coli *(APC)* gene. A count of at least 100 polyps is necessary for a diagnosis of classic FAP, and as many as several thousand may be present (Fig. 13.35). Except for their remarkable numbers, these growths are morphologically indistinguishable from sporadic adenomas. Colorectal adenocarcinoma develops in 100% of patients with untreated FAP, often before 30 years of age. As a result, prophylactic colectomy is standard therapy for individuals carrying *APC* mutations. However, patients remain at risk for extraintestinal manifestations, including neoplasia at other sites. Specific *APC* mutations are also associated with the development of other manifestations of FAP such as *Gardner syndrome* and *Turcot syndrome* (see Table 13.6). In addition to intestinal polyps, clinical features of Gardner syndrome include osteomas of the mandible, skull, and long bones; epidermal cysts; desmoid and thyroid tumors; and dental abnormalities, including unerupted and supernumerary teeth. Turcot syndrome is rarer and is characterized by intestinal adenomas and tumors of the central nervous system. Two-thirds of patients with Turcot syndrome have *APC* gene mutations and develop medulloblastomas. The remaining one-third have mutations in one of several genes involved in DNA repair and develop glioblastomas. The role of these base excision repair genes in carcinogenesis is discussed next.

Hereditary Nonpolyposis Colorectal Cancer

Hereditary nonpolyposis colorectal cancer (HNPCC), also known as *Lynch syndrome,* is an autosomal dominant condition marked by an increased risk for cancers of the colorectum, endometrium, stomach, ovary, ureters, brain, small bowel, hepatobiliary tract, and skin. Colon cancers in patients with HNPCC tend to occur at younger ages than do sporadic colon cancers and are often located in the right colon (see Table 13.7). In contrast to familial adenomatous polyposis, only a few adenomatous precursors are found in the colon of affected individuals. These precursors tend to be sessile serrated adenomas, which often give rise to adenocarcinomas with abundant mucin production.

Table 13.7 Common Patterns of Sporadic and Familial Colorectal Neoplasia

Etiology	Molecular Defect	Target Gene(s)	Transmission	Predominant Site(s)	Histology
Familial adenomatous polyposis	APC/WNT pathway	*APC*	Autosomal dominant	None	Tubular, villous; typical adenocarcinoma
Hereditary nonpolyposis colorectal cancer	DNA mismatch repair	*MSH2, MLH1*	Autosomal dominant	Right side	Sessile serrated adenoma; mucinous adenocarcinoma
Sporadic colon cancer (80%)	APC/WNT pathway	*APC*	None	Left side	Tubular, villous; typical adenocarcinoma
Sporadic colon cancer (10%–15%)	DNA mismatch repair	*MSH2, MLH1*	None	Right side	Sessile serrated adenoma; mucinous adenocarcinoma

FAP, Familial adenomatous polyposis.

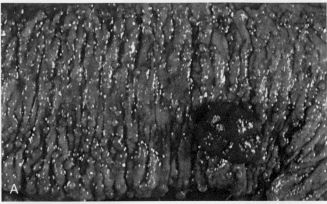

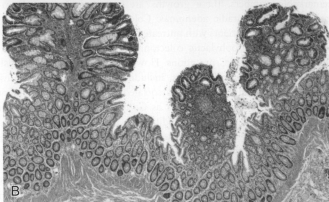

FIG. 13.35 Familial adenomatous polyposis. (A) Hundreds of small colonic polyps are present along with a dominant polyp *(right)*. (B) Three tubular adenomas are present in this single microscopic field.

HNPCC is caused by inherited germline mutations in genes that encode proteins responsible for the detection, excision, and repair of errors that occur during DNA replication. Five mismatch repair genes have been identified, but a majority of HNPCC cases are caused by mutations in *MSH2* or *MLH1*. Patients with HNPCC inherit one mutated DNA repair gene and one normal allele. When the second copy is lost through mutation or epigenetic silencing, the resulting defect in mismatch repair leads to the accumulation of mutations at rates up to 1000 times higher than normal, mostly in regions containing short repeating DNA sequences referred to as *microsatellite DNA*. The human genome contains approximately 50,000 to 100,000 microsatellites, which are prone to undergo expansion during DNA replication and are the most frequent sites of acquired mutations in HNPCC. Understanding of the genetic underpinnings of HNPCC has shed light on the mechanisms responsible for a subset of sporadic colon cancers, which also carry mutations in mismatch repair genes. The consequences of mismatch repair defects and the resulting *microsatellite instability* are discussed next in the context of colonic adenocarcinoma.

Adenocarcinoma

Adenocarcinoma of the colon is the most common malignancy of the gastrointestinal tract and is a major contributor to morbidity and mortality worldwide. By contrast, the small intestine, which accounts for 75% of the overall length of the gastrointestinal tract, is an uncommon site for benign and malignant tumors. Among malignant small-intestinal tumors, adenocarcinoma and carcinoid

(neuroendocrine) tumors have roughly equal rates of occurrence, followed by lymphoma and sarcoma.

Epidemiology. In the United States in 2022, it is estimated that approximately 151,000 individuals will be newly diagnosed with colorectal adenocarcinoma and that approximately 53,000 people will die of the disease. This represents nearly 15% of all cancer-related deaths, second only to lung cancer. Colorectal cancer incidence peaks at 60 to 70 years of age. Less than 20% of cases occur before 50 years of age, but for unclear reasons deaths from colorectal carcinoma have increased in individuals younger than age 50 in recent years, and as a result it is now recommended that screening for colorectal cancer begins at the age of 45 years. Males are affected slightly more often than females. Colorectal carcinoma is most prevalent in the United States, Canada, Australia, New Zealand, Denmark, Sweden, and other higher income countries that share lifestyles and diet. The incidence of this cancer is as much as 30-fold lower in India, South America, and Africa. In Japan, where the incidence was previously very low, the incidence has risen to an intermediate level (similar to those in the United Kingdom), presumably as a result of changes in lifestyle and diet.

The factors most closely associated with a high incidence of colorectal cancer are diets with a low intake of unabsorbable vegetable fiber and high intake of refined carbohydrates and fat. In addition to dietary modification, pharmacologic chemoprevention has become an area of interest. Colorectal cancer is also associated with obesity, tobacco smoking, and alcohol consumption. By contrast, aspirin and other NSAIDs appear to have a protective effect. This is consistent with studies showing that some NSAIDs cause polyp regression in patients with familial adenomatous polyposis in whom the rectum was left in place after colectomy. It is suspected that this effect is mediated by inhibition of the enzyme cyclooxygenase-2 (COX-2), which is highly expressed in 90% of colorectal carcinomas and 40% to 90% of adenomas and is known to promote epithelial proliferation, particularly in response to injury.

Pathogenesis. **Studies of colorectal carcinogenesis have provided fundamental insights into the general mechanisms of cancer evolution.** The combination of molecular events that lead to colonic adenocarcinoma is heterogeneous and includes genetic and epigenetic abnormalities. At least two distinct genetic pathways, the APC/β-catenin pathway and the microsatellite instability pathway, have been described. In simplest terms, mutations involving the APC/β-catenin pathway lead to increased WNT signaling, whereas those involving the microsatellite instability pathway are associated with defects in DNA mismatch repair (see Table 13.7). Both pathways involve the stepwise accumulation of multiple mutations, but the genes involved and the mechanisms by which the mutations accumulate differ. Epigenetic events, the most common of which is methylation-induced gene silencing, may enhance progression along both pathways.

- *APC/β-catenin pathway.* The classic *adenoma-carcinoma sequence,* which accounts for as many as 80% of sporadic colon tumors, typically involves mutation of the *APC* tumor suppressor early in the neoplastic process (Fig. 13.36). For adenomas to develop, both copies of the *APC* gene must be functionally inactivated, either by mutation or epigenetic silencing. APC is a key negative regulator of β-catenin, a component of the WNT signaling pathway (Chapter 6). The APC protein normally binds to and promotes the degradation of β-catenin. With loss of APC function, β-catenin accumulates and translocates to the nucleus, where it activates the

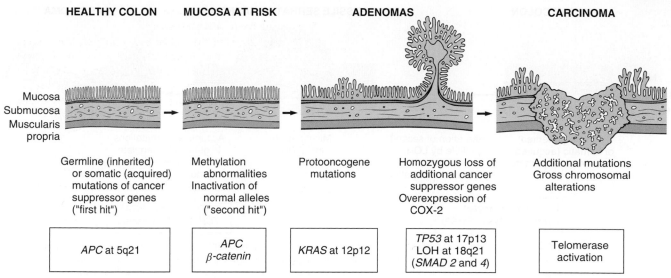

HEALTHY COLON	MUCOSA AT RISK	ADENOMAS	CARCINOMA

Mucosa
Submucosa
Muscularis
propria

Germline (inherited) or somatic (acquired) mutations of cancer suppressor genes ("first hit")	Methylation abnormalities Inactivation of normal alleles ("second hit")	Protooncogene mutations	Homozygous loss of additional cancer suppressor genes Overexpression of COX-2	Additional mutations Gross chromosomal alterations
APC at 5q21	*APC* β-catenin	*KRAS* at 12p12	*TP53* at 17p13 LOH at 18q21 (*SMAD 2* and *4*)	Telomerase activation

FIG. 13.36 Morphologic and molecular changes in the adenoma-carcinoma sequence. It is postulated that loss of one normal copy of the tumor suppressor gene *APC* occurs early. Individuals with familial adenomatous polyposis are born with one mutant allele, making them extremely prone to the development of colon cancer. Other mutations involving *KRAS*, *SMAD2*, and *SMAD4*, and the tumor suppressor gene *TP53*, as well as activation of telomerase, lead to the emergence of a full-blown cancer. Although there may be a preferred temporal sequence for these changes, it is the aggregate effect of the mutations, rather than their order of occurrence, that appears most critical. *APC*, Adenomatous polyposis coli; *COX-2*, cyclooxygenase-2; *LOH*, loss of heterozygosity.

transcription of genes, such as those encoding MYC and cyclin D1, that promote proliferation. This is followed by additional mutations, including activating mutations in *KRAS*, which also promote growth and prevent apoptosis. The conclusion that mutation of *KRAS* is a late event is supported by the observations that *KRAS* mutations are present in fewer than 10% of adenomas less than 1 cm in diameter, 50% of adenomas greater than 1 cm in diameter, and 50% of invasive adenocarcinomas. Neoplastic progression is also associated with mutations in other tumor suppressor genes such as *SMAD2* and *SMAD4*, which encode effectors of TGF-β signaling. Because TGF-β signaling normally inhibits the cell cycle, loss of these genes may allow unrestrained cell growth. The tumor suppressor gene *TP53* is mutated in 70% to 80% of colon cancers but is uncommonly affected in adenomas, suggesting that *TP53* mutations also occur at late stages of tumor progression. Loss of function of *TP53* and other tumor suppressor genes is often caused by chromosomal deletions, highlighting chromosomal instability as a hallmark of the APC/β-catenin pathway. Telomerase activation also likely plays a role in tumor progression.

- *Microsatellite instability pathway.* In patients with DNA mismatch repair deficiency (due to loss of mismatch repair genes, as discussed earlier), mutations accumulate in microsatellite repeats, a condition referred to as *microsatellite instability*. These mutations are generally silent because microsatellites are typically located in noncoding regions, but some microsatellite sequences are located in the coding or promoter regions of genes involved in regulation of cell growth, such as those encoding the type II TGF-β receptor and the proapoptotic protein BAX (Fig. 13.37). Because TGF-β inhibits colonic epithelial cell proliferation, type II TGF-β receptor mutations can contribute to uncontrolled cell growth, while loss of BAX may enhance the survival of genetically abnormal clones. In a subset of colon cancers with microsatellite instability, mutations in DNA mismatch repair genes are absent.

Instead, in these tumors the *MLH1* promoter region is hypermethylated, thereby reducing MLH1 expression and repair function. These features define the *CpG island hypermethylation phenotype* (CIMP). Activating mutations in the *BRAF* oncogene are common in these cancers, whereas *KRAS* and *TP53* are not typically mutated.

MORPHOLOGY

Overall, adenocarcinomas are distributed approximately equally over the entire length of the colon. **Tumors in the proximal colon often grow as polypoid, exophytic masses** that extend along one wall of the large-caliber cecum and ascending colon; these tumors rarely cause obstruction (Fig. 13.38A). By contrast, **carcinomas in the distal colon tend to be annular lesions that produce "napkin ring"** constrictions and luminal narrowing (Fig. 13.38B), sometimes to the point of obstruction. Both forms grow into the bowel wall over time and may be palpable as firm masses (Fig. 13.38C). The general microscopic characteristics of right- and left-sided colonic adenocarcinomas are similar. Most tumors are composed of tall columnar cells that resemble dysplastic epithelium found in adenomas (Fig. 13.39A). The invasive component of these tumors elicits a strong stromal desmoplastic response, which is responsible for their characteristic firm consistency. Some poorly differentiated tumors form few glands (Fig. 13.39B). Others produce abundant mucin that accumulates within the intestinal wall; these so-called mucinous carcinomas are associated with a poor prognosis. Tumors may also be composed of signet ring cells similar to those in gastric cancer (Fig. 13.39C).

Clinical Features. The availability of endoscopic screening combined with the recognition that most carcinomas arise within adenomas presents a unique opportunity for cancer prevention. Unfortunately, colorectal cancers develop insidiously and may therefore go

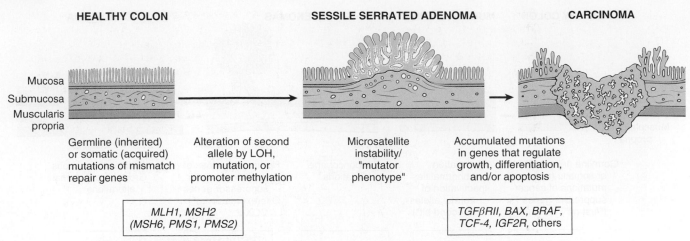

FIG. 13.37 Morphologic and molecular changes in the mismatch repair pathway of colon carcinogenesis. Defects in mismatch repair genes (most commonly *MLH1* or *MSH2*) result in microsatellite instability and permit accumulation of mutations in numerous genes. If these mutations affect genes involved in cell survival and proliferation, cancer may develop. *IGF2R,* Insulin-like growth factor 2 receptor; *LOH,* loss of heterozygosity; *TCF-4,* transcription factor-4; *TGFβRII,* transforming growth factor beta receptor II.

undetected for long periods. Cecal and other right-sided colon cancers are most often called to clinical attention by fatigue and weakness due to iron deficiency anemia. Thus, it is a clinical maxim that the underlying cause of iron deficiency anemia in an older male or postmenopausal female is gastrointestinal cancer until proven otherwise. Left-sided colorectal adenocarcinomas may produce occult bleeding, changes in bowel habits, or cramping, left lower-quadrant discomfort.

Although poorly differentiated and mucinous histologic patterns are associated with poor prognosis, the two most important prognostic factors are depth of invasion and the presence or absence of lymph node metastases. These factors form the core of the TNM (tumor-node-metastasis) classification and staging system from the American Joint Committee on Cancer (Chapter 6). Staging systems have become more complex with time, reflecting more nuanced treatment approaches and personalized therapeutic strategies. The most important considerations are:

- *Depth of invasion.* Tumors limited to the mucosa (i.e., those that do not cross the muscularis mucosae) have 5-year survival rates approaching 100%, while invasion into the submucosa or muscularis propria reduces 5-year survival to 95% and 70% to 90%, respectively (for tumors limited to the primary site). Invasion through the visceral serosal surface or into adjacent organs and tissues further reduces survival.

- *The presence of lymph node metastases* (Fig. 13.40A) also reduces survival. As a result, most cases with lymph node metastases receive radiation or chemotherapy. In some cases, these treatments may be administered prior to primary tumor resection, a process termed neoadjuvant therapy. Molecular characterization of the tumor can help guide the specific therapeutic approach.

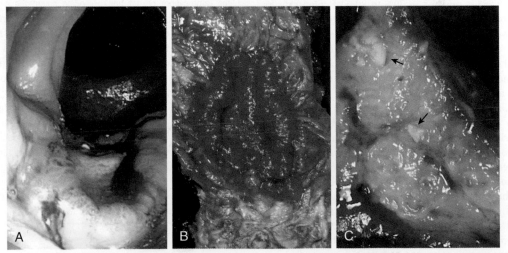

FIG. 13.38 Colorectal carcinoma. (A) Endoscopic view of ulcerated ascending colon adenocarcinoma. (B) Resected rectum showing a circumferential adenocarcinoma. Note the anal mucosa at the bottom of the image. (C) Cancer of the sigmoid colon that has invaded through the muscularis propria and is present within subserosal adipose tissue *(left).* Areas of chalky necrosis are present within the colon wall *(arrows).* (Endoscopic image courtesy of Dr. Ira Hanan, The University of Chicago, Chicago, Illinois.)

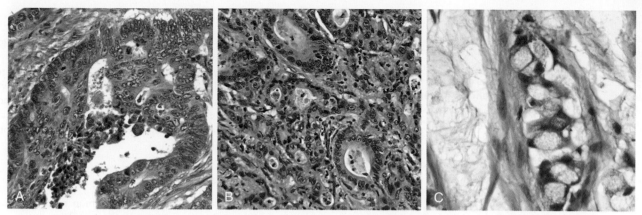

FIG. 13.39 Histologic appearance of colorectal carcinoma. (A) Well-differentiated adenocarcinoma. Note the elongated, hyperchromatic nuclei. Necrotic debris, present in the gland lumen, is typical. (B) Poorly differentiated adenocarcinoma forms a few glands but is largely composed of infiltrating nests of tumor cells. (C) Mucinous adenocarcinoma with signet ring cells and extracellular mucin pools.

- *Distant metastasis* to the lung (Fig. 13.40B), liver (Fig. 13.40C), or other sites also limits survival, and only 15% or fewer of patients with tumors at this stage are alive 5 years after diagnosis. Because of portal drainage of the colon, the liver is the most common site of metastatic lesions. However, the rectum does not drain by way of the portal circulation, and metastases from carcinomas of the anorectum region may circumvent the liver and lodge in the lung or other sites.

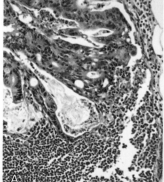
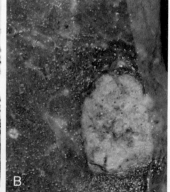
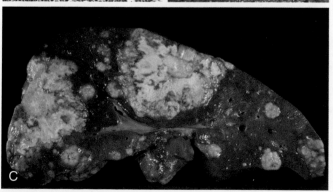

FIG. 13.40 Metastatic colorectal carcinoma. (A) Lymph node metastasis. Note the glandular structures within the subcapsular sinus. (B) Solitary subpleural nodule of colorectal carcinoma metastatic to the lung. (C) Liver containing two large and many smaller metastases. Note the central necrosis within metastases.

Regardless of stage, some patients with small numbers of metastases do well for years after resection of distant tumor nodules. This is particularly true of solitary metastases to the liver or lung and emphasizes the clinical and molecular heterogeneity of colorectal carcinomas. Tumors that exhibit microsatellite instability are often responsive to immune checkpoint inhibitor therapies, presumably because these tumors express particularly large numbers of tumor-specific neoantigens.

APPENDIX

The appendix is a true diverticulum of the cecum. Like any diverticulum, it is prone to acute and chronic inflammation, and acute appendicitis is a relatively common entity. Other lesions, including tumors, can also occur in the appendix but are far less common.

ACUTE APPENDICITIS

Acute appendicitis is most common in adolescents and young adults but may occur in any age group. The lifetime risk for appendicitis is 7%; males are affected slightly more often than females. Despite the prevalence of acute appendicitis, the diagnosis can be difficult to confirm preoperatively, and the condition may be confused with mesenteric lymphadenitis, acute salpingitis, ectopic pregnancy, mittelschmerz (pain associated with ovulation), and Meckel diverticulitis.

Pathogenesis. Acute appendicitis is thought to be initiated by a progressive increase in intraluminal pressure that compromises venous outflow. In 50% to 80% of cases, acute appendicitis is associated with luminal obstruction, usually by a small, stonelike mass of stool, or *fecalith,* or, less commonly, a gallstone, tumor, or mass of worms. Ischemic injury and stasis of luminal contents, which favor bacterial proliferation, trigger inflammatory responses including tissue edema and neutrophilic infiltration of the lumen, muscular wall, and periappendiceal soft tissues.

MORPHOLOGY

In early acute appendicitis, subserosal vessels are congested and a modest perivascular neutrophilic infiltrate is present within all layers of the wall. The inflammatory reaction transforms the normal glistening serosa into a dull, granular, erythematous surface. Although mucosal neutrophils and focal superficial ulceration are often present, these findings are not specific, and diagnosis of acute appendicitis requires neutrophilic infiltration of the muscularis propria. In more severe cases, focal abscesses may form within the wall **(acute suppurative appendicitis),** and these may even progress to large areas of hemorrhagic ulceration and gangrenous necrosis that extend to the serosa, creating **acute gangrenous appendicitis,** which is often followed by rupture and suppurative peritonitis.

Clinical Features. Typically, early acute appendicitis produces periumbilical pain that then moves to the right lower quadrant, followed by nausea, vomiting, low-grade fever, and a mildly elevated peripheral white blood cell count. A classic physical finding is *McBurney sign,* deep tenderness noted at a location two-thirds of the distance from the umbilicus to the right anterior superior iliac spine *(McBurney point).* These signs and symptoms, however, are often absent, creating difficulty in clinical diagnosis. Imaging studies such as CT scanning are helpful in narrowing the differential diagnosis.

TUMORS OF THE APPENDIX

Several tumors occur in the appendix, the most important of which are the following:

- *The most common tumor of the appendix is carcinoid,* a well-differentiated neuroendocrine tumor (discussed earlier). It is usually discovered incidentally at the time of surgery or on examination of a resected appendix. This neoplasm most frequently involves the distal tip of the appendix, where it produces a solid bulbous swelling up to 2 to 3 cm in diameter. Although intramural and transmural extension may be evident, nodal metastases are very infrequent and distant spread is exceptionally rare.
- *Adenomas and non–mucin-producing adenocarcinomas* occur in the appendix and may cause obstruction and enlargement that mimics the changes of acute appendicitis.
- *Mucinous cystadenoma* and *mucinous cystadenocarcinoma* also occur in the appendix. When they cause obstruction of the lumen, the appendix may be dilated by inspissated mucin, an appearance referred to as a *mucocele.* Rupture of the swollen appendix may lead to intraperitoneal seeding and spread. In women, the resulting peritoneal implants may be mistaken for mucinous ovarian tumors. In the most advanced cases, the abdomen fills with tenacious, semisolid mucin, a condition called *pseudomyxoma peritonei* (eFig. 13.8). This disseminated intraperitoneal disease may be held in check for years by repeated debulking but is ultimately fatal in most instances.

■ RAPID REVIEW

Diseases of Teeth and Supporting Structures

- *Caries:* Most common cause of tooth loss in individuals younger than 35 years of age, results from loss of tooth structure due to acids produced by fermentation of sugar by bacteria
- *Gingivitis:* Common and reversible inflammation of the mucosa surrounding the teeth associated with buildup of dental plaque and calculus
- *Periodontitis:* Chronic inflammatory condition associated with poor oral hygiene and altered oral microbiota that can lead to the destruction of tooth support structures and tooth loss

Oral Inflammatory Lesions

- *Aphthous ulcers:* Painful superficial ulcers of unknown etiology that are sometimes associated with systemic diseases
- *Herpes simplex virus:* Primary infection is self-limited and presents with vesicles (cold sores, fever blisters) that rupture and heal without scarring; persists in latent form in nerve ganglia and may reactivate
- *Oral candidiasis:* Occurs when the oral microbiota is altered (e.g., after antibiotic use); may become invasive in immunocompromised individuals

Lesions of the Oral Cavity

- *Fibroma* and *pyogenic granuloma:* Common reactive stromal lesions of the oral mucosa that present as small masses
- *Leukoplakia* and *erythroplakia:* Mucosal squamous plaques that may undergo malignant transformation (erythroplakia more commonly than leukoplakia)
- A majority of oral cavity cancers are squamous cell carcinomas, which fall into two classes: (1) those caused by carcinogen exposure (tobacco and alcohol use) and (2) those caused by high-risk HPV infection.

Diseases of Salivary Glands

- *Sialadenitis* (inflammation of the salivary glands): Can be caused by trauma, infection (such as mumps), or an autoimmune reaction
- *Pleomorphic adenoma:* A slow-growing neoplasm composed of a heterogeneous mixture of epithelial and mesenchymal cells that is benign but may recur; sometimes undergoes malignant transformation. Most common in parotid gland.
- *Mucoepidermoid carcinoma:* A malignant neoplasm of variable biologic aggressiveness that is composed of a mixture of squamous and mucous cells. Occurs both in parotid and minor salivary glands.

Odontogenic Cysts and Tumors

- The jaws are a common site of epithelium-lined cysts derived from odontogenic remnants.
- *Keratocystic odontogenic tumor:* A locally aggressive neoplasm with a high recurrence rate
- *Periapical cyst:* A reactive, inflammatory lesion associated with caries or dental trauma
- The most common odontogenic tumors are *ameloblastoma* and *odontoma.*

Diseases of the Esophagus

- *Esophageal obstruction* may occur due to mechanical or functional anomalies; mechanical causes include developmental defects, fibrotic strictures, and tumors.
- *Esophageal varices* are caused by dilation of collateral vessels in the context of portal hypertension and are prone to massive bleeding, which may be fatal.
- Vomiting if severe and prolonged may give rise to esophageal tears, which may be superficial and cross the GE junction *(Mallory-Weiss tear)* or transmural and prone to cause mediastinitis *(Boerhave syndrome).*
- *Achalasia,* characterized by incomplete lower esophageal sphincter relaxation, increased sphincter tone, and esophageal aperistalsis; is a common form of functional esophageal obstruction.

- *Esophagitis* can result from chemical or infectious mucosal injury; infections are most frequent in immunocompromised individuals.
- The most common cause of esophagitis is *gastroesophageal reflux disease (GERD)*, which must be differentiated from *eosinophilic esophagitis,* an immunologic disorder occurring mainly in atopic individuals.
- *Barrett esophagus,* which may develop in patients with chronic GERD, is defined by the presence of intestinal metaplasia and carries an increased risk for esophageal adenocarcinoma.
- *Esophageal squamous cell carcinoma* is associated with alcohol and tobacco use, caustic esophageal injury, achalasia, and Plummer-Vinson syndrome.

Acute and Chronic Gastritis

- *Gastritis* is mucosal inflammation; when the architecture of gastric glands is perturbed but inflammatory cells are absent or rare, the term *gastropathy* is applied.
- Causative factors in acute gastritis include any agent or disease that interferes with gastric mucosal protection.
- The most common cause of chronic gastritis is *H. pylori* infection; most remaining cases are caused by NSAIDs, alcohol use, or autoimmune gastritis.
- *H. pylori* gastritis typically affects the antrum and is associated with increased gastric acid production and chronic inflammation.
- *Autoimmune gastritis* causes atrophy of the gastric body oxyntic glands, which results in decreased gastric acid production, antral G-cell hyperplasia, achlorhydria, and vitamin B_{12} deficiency. Parietal cell and intrinsic factor antibodies are typically present.
- *Intestinal metaplasia* may develop in chronic gastritis and is a risk factor for gastric dysplasia and adenocarcinoma.
- *Peptic ulcer disease* may be caused by *H. pylori*—associated chronic gastritis and the resultant hyperchlorhydria, or NSAID use. Ulcers in the stomach or duodenum usually heal after suppression of gastric acid production, discontinuation of NSAID use or *H. pylori* eradication.

Gastric Polyps and Tumors

- *Inflammatory* and *hyperplastic gastric polyps* are reactive lesions associated with chronic gastritis. Risk for development of neoplasia increases with polyp size. Fundic gland polyps occur in association of proton pump inhibitor use.
- *Gastric adenomas* develop in a background of chronic gastritis with intestinal metaplasia and mucosal (glandular) atrophy and are precursor lesions of adenocarcinoma.
- *Gastric adenocarcinomas* are classified according to location and gross and microscopic appearance, which may be either intestinal type or diffuse (signet ring) type. Acquired or inherited E-cadherin loss is important in the pathogenesis of the diffuse type.
- The most important risk factor for gastric adenocarcinoma is chronic gastritis with intestinal metaplasia, which is often associated with *H. pylori* infection.
- *Primary gastric lymphomas* are most often derived from mucosa-associated lymphoid tissue, the development of which is induced by *H. pylori*—associated chronic gastritis.
- *Neuroendocrine tumors (carcinoids)* arise from the diffuse components of the endocrine system and are most common in the gastrointestinal tract, particularly the small intestine. Tumors of the small intestine tend to be most aggressive, while those of the appendix are almost always benign.

- *Gastrointestinal stromal tumor (GIST),* the most common mesenchymal tumor of the abdomen, occurs most often in the stomach. GISTs arise from the interstitial cells of Cajal and usually have activating mutations in either the KIT or PDGFRA receptor tyrosine kinases.

Intestinal Obstruction

- *Intussusception* is the most common cause of intestinal obstruction in children younger than 2 years of age and can usually be treated by barium enema or air enema.
- *Hirschsprung disease* is the result of defective neural crest cell migration during development from the cecum to the rectum. It gives rise to functional obstruction due to an absence of ganglion cells.
- *Abdominal herniation* may occur through any weakness or defect in the wall of the peritoneal cavity, including inguinal and femoral canals, umbilicus, and sites of surgical scarring.

Vascular Disorders of Bowel

- *Intestinal ischemia* may occur due to arterial or venous obstruction.
- Ischemic bowel disease resulting from hypoperfusion is most common at the splenic flexure, sigmoid colon, and rectum; these are watershed zones where two arterial circulations terminate.
- Systemic vasculitides and infectious diseases (e.g., CMV infection) may cause vascular disease that can result in chronic ischemia of the gastrointestinal tract.
- *Angiodysplasia* is a common cause of lower gastrointestinal bleeding in older adults.
- *Hemorrhoids* are collateral vessels that form in response to venous hypertension.

Malabsorptive Diarrhea

- *Diarrhea* can be characterized as secretory, osmotic, malabsorptive, or exudative.
- *Cystic fibrosis* leads to malabsorption by causing pancreatic insufficiency and deficient luminal breakdown of nutrients.
- *Celiac disease* is an immune-mediated enteropathy triggered by the ingestion of gluten-containing grains. The malabsorptive diarrhea in celiac disease is due to loss of brush border surface area and, possibly, abnormal enterocyte maturation.
- *Lactase deficiency* causes an osmotic diarrhea owing to the inability to break down or absorb lactose.
- *Abetalipoproteinemia* is characterized by an inability to secrete triglyceride-rich lipoproteins due to an inherited transepithelial transport defect.
- *Microscopic colitis* takes two forms, *collagenous colitis* and *lymphocytic colitis,* that both cause chronic watery diarrhea. The intestines are grossly normal, and the diseases are identified by their histologic features.

Infectious Enterocolitis

- *Vibrio cholera* releases a preformed toxin that causes massive chloride secretion, leading to secretory diarrhea.
- *Campylobacter jejuni* is the most common bacterial enteric pathogen in higher-resource countries and is also a frequent cause of traveler's diarrhea. Most isolates are noninvasive.

- *Salmonella* and *Shigella* spp. are invasive and associated with exudative bloody diarrhea (dysentery). *Salmonella* infection is a common cause of food poisoning. *S. typhi* can cause systemic disease (typhoid fever).
- *Pseudomembranous colitis* is often triggered by antibiotic therapy that disrupts the normal microbiota and allows *C. difficile* to colonize and grow. The organism produces toxins that disrupt epithelial function and cause necrosis.
- *Rotavirus* is a common cause of severe childhood diarrhea worldwide. The diarrhea is secondary to loss of mature enterocytes, resulting in malabsorption and increased fluid secretion. Rotavirus vaccine is protective.
- *Parasitic* and *protozoal* infections affect over half of the world's population on a chronic or recurrent basis. Among the important agents causing human disease are roundworms (*Ascaris* and *Strongyloides*), hookworms (*Necator* and *Ancylostoma*), and protozoa (*Giardia* and *Entamoeba*).

Inflammatory Bowel Disease (IBD)

- IBD is an umbrella term for Crohn disease and ulcerative colitis.
- IBD is thought to arise from a combination of host interactions with intestinal microbiota, intestinal epithelial dysfunction, and aberrant mucosal immune responses.
- *Crohn disease* most commonly affects the terminal ileum and cecum, but any site within the gastrointestinal tract can be involved; inflammation is transmural; skip lesions and noncaseating granulomas are common.
- *Ulcerative colitis* is limited to the colon, always involves the rectum, and ranges in extent from rectum-only disease to pancolitis; inflammation is confined to the mucosa; neither skip lesions nor granulomas are present.
- Both Crohn disease and ulcerative colitis may have extraintestinal manifestations.
- The risk for development of colonic epithelial dysplasia and adenocarcinoma is increased in patients who have had colonic IBD for more than 8 to 10 years.

Colonic Polyps, Adenomas, and Adenocarcinomas

- *Intestinal polyps* can be classified as nonneoplastic or neoplastic; nonneoplastic polyps can be further categorized as inflammatory, hamartomatous, or hyperplastic.

- *Inflammatory polyps* form as a result of chronic cycles of injury and healing.
- *Hamartomatous polyps* occur sporadically or as a part of genetic diseases (e.g., Peutz-Jeghers syndrome); in the latter case, they are often associated with increased risk for malignancy.
- *Hyperplastic polyps* are benign epithelial proliferations that are most common in the left colon and rectum and have no malignant potential; they must be distinguished from sessile serrated adenomas, which are precursors of colon cancer.
- *Neoplastic epithelial polyps* of the colon are termed adenomas. The hallmark feature of most of these lesions, which are the precursors of colonic adenocarcinomas, is dysplasia.
- *Sessile serrated adenomas* differ in lacking dysplasia and share some morphologic features with hyperplastic polyps.
- Familial adenomatous polyposis (FAP) and hereditary nonpolyposis colorectal cancer (HNPCC) are the most common forms of familial colon cancer.
  - FAP is caused by *APC* mutations; patients typically have hundreds of adenomas and develop colon cancer before 30 years of age.
  - HNPCC is caused by mutations in DNA mismatch repair genes that result in microsatellite instability. Patients with HNPCC have far fewer polyps and develop cancer at an older age than that typical for patients with FAP, but at a younger age than in patients with sporadic colon cancer.
- Most colonic cancers are adenocarcinomas that arise due to dysregulation of the APC-β-catenin pathway or due to mutations caused by microsatellite instability. The two most important prognostic factors are depth of invasion and the presence or absence of metastases to lymph nodes or distant organs.

Appendix

- Acute appendicitis is most common in children and adolescents. It is thought to be initiated by increased intraluminal pressure consequent to obstruction of the appendiceal lumen, which compromises venous outflow.
- The most common tumor of the appendix, the *carcinoid,* or *well-differentiated neuroendocrine tumor,* is most often discovered incidentally and is almost always benign.
- Mucinous tumors of the appendix may spread to the peritoneal cavity to produce widespread disease, often referred to as *pseudomyxoma peritonei.*

■ Laboratory Tests[a]

Test	Reference Values	Pathophysiology/Clinical Relevance
Deamidated gliadin IgG and IgA antibody, serum	Negative: <20.0 U Weak positive: 20.0–30.0 U Positive: >30.0 U	Deamidated gliadin antibody is a serum test for celiac disease in patients with IgA deficiency (approximately 2% of patients with celiac disease), who therefore lack IgA antibodies against tissue transglutaminase (tTG), which is the first-line serologic test for celiac disease. The sensitivity of this test is reduced if patients are on a gluten-free diet prior to testing.
Endomysial antibody, IgA, serum	Negative	IgA autoantibodies to the endomysium (connective tissue surrounding muscle cells) are elevated in 70% to 80% of patients with celiac disease or dermatitis herpetiformis. By comparison, anti-tTG autoantibodies have a sensitivity and specificity of 90% to 98% and 95% to 97%, respectively; therefore, this is often the first-line test in celiac disease assessment. This test is not useful in patients with IgA deficiency. Titer generally correlates with disease severity and declines with strict adherence to a gluten-free diet.
Helicobacter pylori breath test	Negative	*H. pylori* causes chronic gastritis and predisposes to peptic ulcer disease, gastric adenocarcinoma, and lymphoma. The organism produces urease, which neutralizes gastric acid and provides ammonia for bacterial protein synthesis. Patients with suspected *H. pylori* infection ingest a small amount of urea labeled with an isotope (e.g., nonradioactive carbon-13); if *H. pylori*–derived urease is present, urea is metabolized to isotope-labeled carbon dioxide, which is detected in the patient's breath. This high-sensitivity, high-specificity test may be used for diagnosis of *H. pylori* infection and for confirming *H. pylori* eradication. Antibiotics and drugs that suppress gastric acid production may cause false-negative results, while false-positive results may be seen in the setting of achlorhydria and infection with other urease-positive organisms.
Helicobacter pylori stool test	Negative	Two types of tests evaluate the presence of *H. pylori* shedding in the stool: (1) enzyme immunoassay or immunochromatography for bacterial antigens and (2) PCR for *H. pylori* bacterial sequences. These high-sensitivity, high-specificity tests may be used for diagnosis of *H. pylori* infection and for confirming *H. pylori* eradication. Antibiotics and drugs that suppress gastric acid production may cause false-negative results by suppressing *H. pylori* growth.
Intrinsic factor (IF) antibodies, serum	Negative	Intrinsic factor is secreted by gastric parietal cells and binds to vitamin B_{12}, facilitating its absorption in the terminal ileum. In pernicious anemia, autoantibodies to IF prevent vitamin B_{12} binding, leading to vitamin B_{12} deficiency. Vitamin B_{12} deficiency can manifest with megaloblastic anemia and neurologic symptoms. Although anti-IF antibodies are very specific, they are positive in only about 50% of patients with pernicious anemia.
Parietal cell antibodies, serum	Negative: <20.0 U Equivocal: 20.1–24.9 U Positive: >25.0 U	These are IgG antibodies that bind to the H^+/K^+ ATPase pump on gastric parietal cells. They are seen in autoimmune gastritis, an inflammatory condition that leads to loss of parietal cells, atrophy and metaplasia of the oxyntic mucosa, and, if chronic, pernicious anemia, caused by loss of intrinsic factor and decreased vitamin B_{12} absorption. Parietal cell antibodies are found in more than 90% of patients with pernicious anemia but are less specific than intrinsic factor antibodies.
Tissue transglutaminase (TTG) IgA antibody, serum	<4.0 U/mL (negative) 4.0–10.0 U/mL (weak positive) >10.0 U/mL (positive)	TTG deamidates gliadin, which binds with increased affinity to HLA-DQ2 and DQ8 molecules on antigen-presenting cells, leading to a CD4+ T-cell response. TTG autoantibodies are elevated in patients in celiac disease; this test is a first-line screening test in conjunction with biopsy to confirm diagnosis. Since it assesses the presence of IgA antibodies, it is negative in patients with IgA deficiency (about 2% of patients with celiac disease). The test may be negative if patients are on a gluten-free diet and is useful in monitoring adherence to a gluten-free diet.

Molecular Tests of Relevance in Gastrointestinal Cancer

Analyte	Method	Pathophysiology/Clinical Relevance
KIT mutation	Most commonly recognized in solid tumors by immunohistochemical staining for KIT; assessed in hematologic malignancies by DNA sequencing	Approximately 80% of gastrointestinal stromal tumors (GIST) have activating mutations in *KIT*, which encodes a receptor tyrosine kinase. *KIT* mutation correlates with strong immunohistochemical staining for KIT in GIST and is predictive of response to KIT inhibitors.

Microsatellite instability (MSI)/mismatch repair defect (MMS)	Usually assessed indirectly by immunohistochemical staining for MMR proteins (MLH1, MSH2, MSH6, PMS2); may be assessed directly by PCR amplification of microsatellites or DNA sequencing	About 2% to 3% of colorectal carcinomas arise in patients with germline defects in one of the DNA MMR genes (Lynch syndrome). Approximately 15% of sporadic colorectal carcinomas have MMR defects due to somatic hypermethylation of the *MLH1* promoter or acquired mutations in the same genes. MSI-high (MSI-H) colorectal carcinomas are often heavily infiltrated by T cells and are likely to respond to immune checkpoint inhibitors.

[a]The review of this table by Dr. Sonia S. Kupfer, Department of Medicine, University of Chicago, is greatly appreciated.

References values from https://www.mayocliniclabs.com/ by permission of Mayo Foundation for Medical Education and Research. All rights reserved.

Adapted from Deyrup AT, D'Ambrosio D, Muir J, et al. Essential Laboratory Tests for Medical Education. *Acad Pathol.* 2022;9. doi: 10.1016/j.acpath.2022.100046.

Liver and Gallbladder

LIVER

The healthy adult liver weighs 1400 to 1600 gm. It has a dual blood supply, with the portal vein providing 60% to 70% of hepatic blood flow and the hepatic artery supplying the remainder. The portal vein and the hepatic artery enter the inferior aspect of the liver through the hilum, or *porta hepatis*. Within the liver, the branches of the portal

veins, hepatic arteries, and bile ducts travel in parallel within *portal tracts,* ramifying through 10 to 12 orders of branches.

The most common terminology used to describe the hepatic microarchitecture is based on the lobular model (Fig. 14.1). This model divides the liver into lobules 1 to 2 mm in diameter that are centered on a terminal tributary of the hepatic vein and demarcated by portal tracts at their periphery. These lobules are often drawn as hexagonal structures, though the shapes are variable; nonetheless, it is a useful simplification. A second model divides the liver into triangular acini (see Fig. 14.1) based on the position of hepatocytes relative to their blood supply. The hepatocytes in the vicinity of the terminal hepatic vein are

The contributions to this chapter by Dr. Neil D. Theise, Department of Pathology at NYU Grossman School of Medicine, New York, New York, and the late Dr. Nelson Fausto, Department of Pathology, University of Washington, Seattle, Washington, in previous editions of this book are gratefully acknowledged.

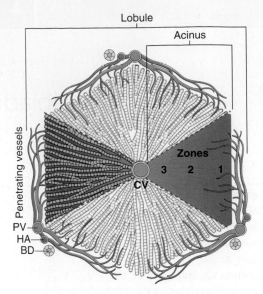

Lobule

Acinus

Zones
3 2 1

CV

Penetrating vessels

PV
HA
BD

FIG. 14.1 Models of liver anatomy. In the lobular model, the terminal hepatic vein (i.e., central hepatic vein) is at the center of a "lobule," while the portal tracts are at the periphery. Pathologists often refer to the regions of the parenchyma surrounding portal tract and central vein as "periportal" and "centrilobular," respectively. In the acinar model, on the basis of blood flow, three zones are defined, zone 1 being the closest to the blood supply and zone 3 being the farthest. *BD,* Bile duct; *CV,* central hepatic vein; *HA,* hepatic artery; *PV,* portal vein.

called *centrilobular*; those near the portal tract are *periportal*. **Division of the lobular parenchyma into zones is an important concept because each zone differs with respect to its metabolic activities and susceptibility to various forms of hepatic injury.**

Within the lobule, hepatocytes are organized into anastomosing sheets or "plates" extending from the portal tracts to the terminal hepatic veins. Between the trabecular plates of hepatocytes are vascular *sinusoids*. Blood flows through the sinusoids and exits into the terminal hepatic veins through numerous orifices in the vein wall. Hepatocytes are thus bathed by well-mixed portal venous blood on one side and hepatic arterial blood on the other. The sinusoids are lined by a fenestrated endothelium that overlies a perisinusoidal space (the *space of Disse*) into which abundant hepatocyte microvilli protrude. Attached to the luminal face of the sinusoids are scattered *Kupffer cells*, specialized long-lived tissue macrophages that arise early in embryogenesis. Another specialized cell type, the *hepatic stellate cell*, is found in the space of Disse and has a role in the storage of vitamin A. Between abutting hepatocytes are *bile canaliculi*, channels 1 to 2 μm in diameter that are formed by grooves in the plasma membranes of adjacent hepatocytes and are separated from the vascular space by tight junctions. These channels drain successively into the intralobular *canals of Hering*, periportal *bile ductules*, and finally into the *terminal bile ducts* within the portal tracts.

GENERAL FEATURES OF LIVER DISEASE

The most important primary diseases of the liver are viral hepatitis, alcohol-related liver disease, nonalcoholic fatty liver disease, and hepatocellular carcinoma. The liver is also frequently damaged secondarily in a variety of common disorders, such as heart failure, disseminated cancer, and extrahepatic infections. The large functional reserve of the liver reduces the clinical impact of mild liver damage, but severe diffuse liver disease can be life-threatening.

With the rare exception of fulminant hepatic failure, liver disease is an insidious process in which the signs and symptoms of hepatic decompensation appear weeks, months, or even years after the onset of injury. The hepatic injury may be imperceptible to the patient and manifest only as laboratory test abnormalities (Table 14.1); liver injury and healing may also be subclinical. Hence, individuals with hepatic abnormalities who are referred to hepatologists most frequently have chronic liver disease.

Mechanisms of Injury and Repair

Injured hepatocytes may show several potentially reversible changes, such as accumulation of fat (steatosis) and bilirubin (cholestasis); when injury is not reversible, hepatocytes die by necrosis or apoptosis. Necrosis (Fig. 14.2) is commonly seen following hepatic injury caused by hypoxia and ischemia. Apoptotic cell death (Fig. 14.3) predominates in viral, autoimmune, and drug- and toxin-induced hepatitides.

Widespread death of hepatocytes may produce confluent necrosis. This may be seen in acute toxic or ischemic injuries or in severe chronic viral or autoimmune hepatitis. Confluent necrosis begins as a zone of hepatocyte dropout around the central vein. With increasing severity, necrosis "bridges" central veins and portal tracts or adjacent portal tracts.

Regeneration to replace lost hepatocytes takes place primarily by mitotic replication of hepatocytes adjacent to those that have died. In more severe forms of acute liver injury, hepatic stem cells located in a niche near the canal of Hering may also begin to divide. The differentiating progeny of these tissue stem cells produce ductlike structures, called *ductular reactions*, a morphologic marker of stem cell–mediated liver regeneration.

Table 14.1 Laboratory Evaluation of Liver Disease

Test Category	Blood Measurement[a]
Hepatocyte integrity	Cytosolic hepatocellular enzymes[b] *Serum aspartate aminotransferase* (AST) *Serum alanine aminotransferase* (ALT) *Serum lactate dehydrogenase* (LDH)

Biliary excretory function	Substances normally secreted in bile[b]
	 Serum bilirubin
	   Total: unconjugated plus conjugated
	   Direct: conjugated only
	 Urine bilirubin
	 Serum bile acids
	 Plasma membrane enzymes (from damage to bile canaliculus)[b]
	   Serum alkaline phosphatase
	   Serum γ-glutamyl transpeptidase (GGT)

Hepatocyte synthetic function	Proteins secreted into the blood
	   Serum albumin[c]
	 Coagulation factors
	   Prothrombin time (PT)[b]
	   Partial thromboplastin time (PTT)[b]
	 Hepatocyte metabolism
	   Serum ammonia[b]
	   Aminopyrine breath test (hepatic demethylation)[c]

[a]Most commonly used tests are in italics.

[b]An elevation suggests liver disease.

[c]A decrease suggests liver disease.

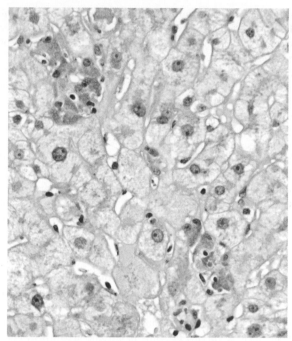

FIG. 14.2 Hepatocyte necrosis. This PAS-D—stained biopsy shows clusters of pigmented hepatocytes with eosinophilic cytoplasm indicative of hepatocytes undergoing necrosis. *PAS-D,* Periodic acid—Schiff stain after diastase digestion.

Scar formation may follow severe acute injury but occurs more often as a reaction to chronic injury. When there is severe injury that causes death of large numbers of hepatocytes and the dropout of liver cells, the underlying reticulin may collapse, precluding orderly regeneration of hepatocytes and laying down of collagen. The principal

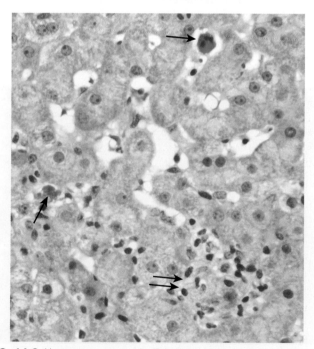

FIG. 14.3 Hepatocyte apoptosis. This biopsy from a patient with hepatitis due to chronic hepatitis C shows scattered apoptotic hepatocytes ("acidophil bodies"; *single arrows*) and a patchy inflammatory infiltrate (*double arrows*).

cell type involved in scar formation is the perisinusoidal hepatic stellate cell. These cells become activated and are converted into highly fibrogenic myofibroblasts, which lay down fibrous septa. Eventually, these fibrous septa encircle surviving, regenerating hepatocytes in late-stage chronic liver disease giving rise to *cirrhosis.*

Inflammation and immunologic reactions are involved in many forms of liver disease. Systemic inflammation alters the metabolic and biosynthetic activities of the liver, leading to increased secretion of acute-phase reactants such as C-reactive protein, serum amyloid A protein (a precursor of some forms of amyloid), and hepcidin, a key regulator of iron metabolism (Chapter 10). As we will discuss, adaptive immune cells play a critical role in viral hepatitis, with CD4+ and CD8+ T cells being particularly important in the eradication of virus-infected hepatocytes and in causing liver injury in chronic disease.

Liver Failure

The most severe clinical consequence of liver disease is liver failure. It occurs primarily in three clinical scenarios: acute, chronic, and acute-on-chronic liver failure.

Acute Liver Failure

Acute liver failure is defined as an acute liver illness that produces hepatic encephalopathy within 6 months of the initial diagnosis. In the United States, accidental or deliberate ingestion of acetaminophen accounts for almost 50% of cases of acute liver failure, while autoimmune hepatitis, other drugs and toxins, and acute hepatitis A and B infections account for the remainder of cases. In Asia, acute hepatitis B and E predominate as causes of acute liver failure.

> ### MORPHOLOGY
> The clinical syndrome of acute liver failure is reflected anatomically and histologically as **massive hepatic necrosis.** The liver is small and shrunken due to loss of parenchyma (Fig. 14.4A). Microscopically, there are large zones of destruction surrounding occasional islands of regenerating hepatocytes (Fig. 14.4B). Scarring is mostly absent because of the acute nature of the process.

Clinical Features. Acute liver failure manifests with nausea, vomiting, jaundice, and fatigue, which are followed by the onset of life-threatening encephalopathy, coagulation defects, and portal hypertension associated with ascites. Typically, transaminase levels in the serum are elevated into the thousands. The liver is initially enlarged by swelling and edema related to inflammation, but then as parenchyma is destroyed, the liver shrinks dramatically. Eventually, as hepatocytes are lost, serum transaminase values level off and then decline rapidly as their source disappears. Worsening jaundice, coagulopathy, and encephalopathy develop; with unabated progression, multiorgan failure ensues, potentially resulting in death. Manifestations of acute liver failure include the following:

- *Jaundice* and *icterus* (yellow discoloration of the skin and sclera, respectively) due to retention of bilirubin, and *cholestasis* due to systemic retention of bilirubin as well as other solutes eliminated in bile.
- *Hepatic encephalopathy,* with symptoms ranging from subtle behavioral abnormalities to confusion, stupor, coma, and death. Hepatic encephalopathy is believed to be caused by elevated ammonia levels, which correlate with impaired neuronal function and cerebral edema. The principal source of the ammonia is the

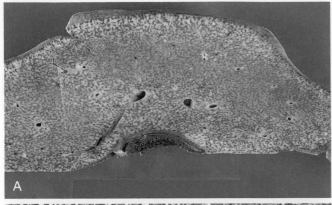

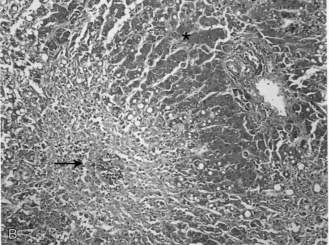

FIG. 14.4 Massive liver necrosis. (A) The liver is small (700 gm), bile-stained, soft, and congested. (B) Hepatocellular necrosis caused by acetaminophen overdose. Confluent necrosis is seen in the perivenular region (zone 3, *arrow*). There is little inflammation. Residual normal tissue is indicated by the *star*. (Courtesy of Dr. Matthew Yeh, University of Washington, Seattle, Washington.)

gastrointestinal tract, where it is produced by microorganisms and by enterocytes during glutamine metabolism. Normally, ammonia is transported in the portal vein to the liver, where it is metabolized in the urea cycle; in severe liver disease, this detoxification mechanism fails. Thus, ammonia enters the systemic circulation. In the CNS, the accumulated ammonia impairs neuronal function and causes cerebral edema. A typical neurologic sign is *asterixis*, a non-rhythmic, rapid, extension-flexion movement of the head and extremities, best seen as "flapping" of the hands when the arms are held in extension with dorsiflexed wrists.

- *Coagulopathy.* The liver produces a number of coagulation factors whose levels decline in liver failure, leading to easy bruising and bleeding. Paradoxically, *disseminated intravascular coagulation* (Chapter 10) may also occur due to failure of the damaged liver to remove activated coagulation factors.
- *Portal hypertension* arises when there is diminished flow through the portal venous system, which may occur because of obstruction at the prehepatic, intrahepatic, or posthepatic level. While it can occur in acute liver failure, portal hypertension is more commonly seen with chronic liver failure and is discussed later. In acute liver failure, the obstruction is usually intrahepatic, and

its major clinical consequences are *ascites* and *hepatic encephalopathy*. In chronic liver disease, portal hypertension develops over months to years, and its effects are more complex and widespread (see later).

- *Hepatorenal syndrome* is a form of renal failure occurring in individuals with acute or chronic liver failure in whom there is no intrinsic renal pathology to account for renal dysfunction. Liver failure results in the production of vasodilators such as nitric oxide that increase blood flow in the abdominal viscera with consequent decreased renal perfusion pressure and reduced glomerular filtration rate. In response to renal hypotension, the renal sympathetic nervous system is activated, as is the renin-angiotensin axis, both of which cause vasoconstriction of the afferent renal arterioles, further decreasing renal perfusion. The syndrome's onset begins with a decrease in urine output and rising blood urea nitrogen and creatinine levels (azotemia).

Chronic Liver Failure and Cirrhosis

Cirrhosis refers to the diffuse transformation of the liver into regenerative parenchymal nodules surrounded by fibrous bands (Fig. 14.5). It is the morphologic change most often associated with chronic liver disease. The leading causes of chronic liver failure worldwide include chronic hepatitis B, chronic hepatitis C, nonalcoholic fatty liver disease (NAFLD), and alcohol-related liver disease. While cirrhosis is a common feature of a number of chronic liver diseases, it is not a specific entity, and it is important to recognize that (1) not all chronic liver disease terminates in cirrhosis and (2) not all cirrhosis leads to end-stage liver disease. For example, chronic biliary tract diseases often do not lead to cirrhosis even at the end stage, whereas patients with treated autoimmune hepatitis or cured hepatitis C may have adequate liver function despite the presence of cirrhosis. Even in diseases that are likely to give rise to cirrhosis, the morphology and pathophysiology of cirrhosis in each may differ. Thus, while the term cirrhosis implies the presence of severe chronic disease, it is not a specific diagnosis and has variable prognostic implications. There are also some instances in which cirrhosis arises without any clear cause; the term cryptogenic cirrhosis is sometimes applied to such cases.

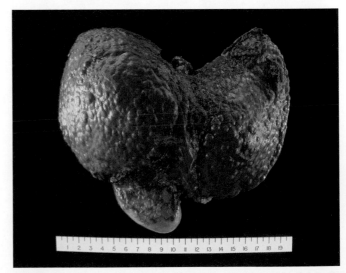

FIG. 14.5 Cirrhosis resulting from chronic viral hepatitis. Note the broad scars separating bulging regenerative nodules over the liver surface.

MORPHOLOGY

Cirrhosis is characterized by transformation of the entire liver into regenerative parenchymal nodules surrounded by fibrous bands. The nodular nature of the process is readily evident grossly (Fig. 14.5) and microscopically (Fig. 14.6A). The size of the nodules, the pattern of scarring (linking of portal tracts to each other vs. linking of portal tracts to central veins), the degree of parenchymal loss, and the frequency of vascular thrombosis (particularly of the portal vein) vary between diseases and even, in some cases, between individuals with the same disease.

As mentioned earlier, stem cell activation and differentiation give rise to ductlike structures, the so-called ductular reactions. **In chronic liver disease, ductular reactions increase with disease progression and are usually most prominent in cirrhosis.**

Regression of fibrosis and even of fully established cirrhosis may follow disease remission or cure. Scars become thinner and more densely compacted, and eventually start to fragment (see Fig. 14.6B). As fibrous septa break apart, adjacent nodules of regenerating parenchyma coalesce into larger islands. All cirrhotic livers show elements of both progression and regression, with the balance being dictated by the severity and persistence of the underlying disease.

Clinical Features. About 40% of individuals with cirrhosis are asymptomatic until the most advanced stages of the disease. Even at late stages, they present with nonspecific clinical manifestations, such as anorexia, weight loss, weakness, and eventually signs and symptoms of liver failure discussed earlier. Jaundice, encephalopathy, and coagulopathy may result from chronic liver disease, much the same as in acute liver failure. However, there are some significant additional features:

- Chronic severe jaundice can lead to *pruritus* (itching), which may be so severe that patients scratch their skin raw and risk repeated bouts of potentially life-threatening infection. Pruritus is also seen in other disorders associated with cholestasis, suggesting that it is related to the accumulation of bile salts in the body; its precise pathogenesis is unknown.

- *Portal hypertension* is more frequent and manifests in more complex ways in chronic liver failure than in acute liver failure (Fig. 14.7). **It stems from increased vascular resistance coupled with increased portal blood flow.** The increased resistance to portal flow is at the level of the sinusoids and is caused by contraction of vascular smooth muscle cells and myofibroblasts, and disruption of blood flow by scarring and the formation of parenchymal nodules. Increase in portal venous blood flow is due to arterial vasodilation. The increased splanchnic arterial blood flow in turn leads to increased venous efflux into the portal venous system.

- *Portosystemic shunts* develop due to sustained portal hypertension. These shunts are produced principally by dilation of collateral vessels. Most notably, venous bypasses develop wherever the systemic and the portal circulations share common capillary beds; the most clinically important of these are *esophagogastric varices* (Chapter 13), which arise in about 40% of individuals with advanced-stage liver disease and may be the source of massive, frequently fatal hematemesis, particularly when there is associated coagulopathy.

- *Ascites* is the accumulation of fluid in the peritoneal cavity. About 85% of cases of ascites are caused by portal hypertension due to cirrhosis. The fluid is a transudate, having less than 3 gm/dL of protein (largely albumin), and a serum-to-ascites albumin gradient of ≥1.1 gm/dL.

- Long-standing portal hypertension may cause *congestive splenomegaly*. The degree of splenic enlargement varies widely, and the splenic weight may reach as much as 1000 gm (five to six times normal), but it is not necessarily correlated with other features of portal hypertension. Splenomegaly may secondarily induce hematologic abnormalities such as thrombocytopenia or even pancytopenia, due to destruction of blood elements by the increased numbers of splenic macrophages. This condition is sometimes referred to as *hypersplenism*.

- *Hyperestrogenemia* due to impaired estrogen metabolism in male patients with chronic liver failure can give rise to *palmar erythema* (a reflection of local vasodilatation) and *spider angiomas* of the

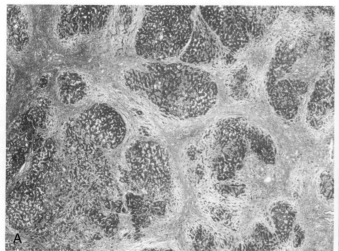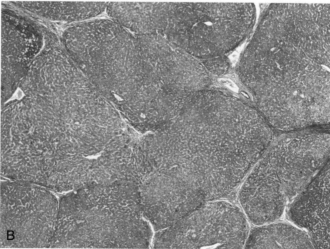

FIG. 14.6 Alcohol-related cirrhosis in a patient who was actively drinking (A) and following long-term abstinence (B). (A) Thick bands of collagen separate rounded cirrhotic nodules. (B) After 1 year of abstinence, most scars are gone (Masson trichrome stain). (Courtesy of Drs. Hongfa Zhu and Isabel Fiel, Mount Sinai School of Medicine, New York, New York.)

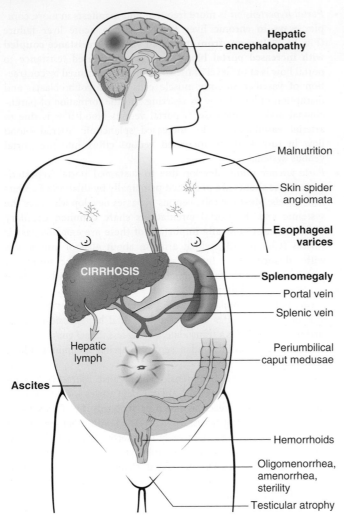

Hepatic
encephalopathy

Malnutrition

Skin spider
angiomata

**Esophageal
varices**

CIRRHOSIS

Splenomegaly

Portal vein

Splenic vein

Hepatic
lymph

Periumbilical
caput medusae

Ascites

Hemorrhoids

Oligomenorrhea,
amenorrhea,
sterility

Testicular atrophy

FIG. 14.7 Major clinical consequences of portal hypertension in the setting of cirrhosis.

skin. Such male hyperestrogenemia also leads to *hypogonadism* and *gynecomastia.*

- Most chronic liver diseases predispose to development of *hepatocellular carcinoma* (discussed later).

The course and severity of chronic liver disease with cirrhosis vary widely from patient to patient. Even in those uncommon instances in which cirrhosis regresses following disease remission, portal hypertension may persist due to the presence of irreversible shunts. The most common causes of death are liver failure (as in acute liver disease) and hepatocellular carcinoma. Clinical and laboratory findings are the main criteria used to gauge prognosis and disease progression.

Acute On-Chronic Liver Failure

After years of stable, well-compensated, chronic liver disease, some individuals suddenly develop signs of acute liver failure. Hepatic insults that cause sudden decompensation of patients with chronic liver disease include hepatitis D superinfection in those with chronic hepatitis B; emergence of resistance to medical therapy in those with viral hepatitis; and systemic disorders, such as sepsis, acute cardiac failure, or a superimposed toxic injury that tips a well-compensated patient with cirrhosis into liver failure.

INFECTIOUS DISORDERS

Viral Hepatitis

The terminology for acute and chronic viral hepatitis can be confusing, because the same word, *hepatitis,* is used to describe several different entities; careful attention to context can clarify its meaning in each situation. Firstly, *hepatitis* is applied to diseases caused by viruses (hepatitis A, B, C, D, and E virus) that are *hepatotropic,* that is, have a specific tropism for the liver. Secondly, *hepatitis* is applied to patterns of acute and chronic hepatic injuries produced by other viruses (such as Epstein-Barr virus [EBV], cytomegalovirus [CMV], and yellow fever) as well as autoimmune reactions, drugs, and toxins. In this section, we will focus on the main features of hepatotropic viruses, which are summarized in Table 14.2, and we will then discuss the clinicopathologic characteristics of acute and chronic viral hepatitis.

Hepatitis A Virus

HAV infection is usually benign and self-limited, does not cause chronic hepatitis, and rarely (in about 0.1% of cases) produces fulminant hepatitis. HAV has an incubation period of 2 to 6 weeks. It is typically cleared by the host immune response, so it does not establish a carrier state. The infection occurs throughout the world and is endemic in countries with poor healthcare infrastructure. Acute HAV tends to cause a febrile illness associated with jaundice and nonspecific symptoms such as fatigue and loss of appetite. Overall, HAV accounts for about 25% of acute hepatitis worldwide. It does not cause chronic hepatitis.

HAV is a nonenveloped, positive-strand RNA picornavirus that occupies its own genus, *Hepatovirus*. It is spread by ingestion of contaminated water and food and is shed in the stool for 2 to 3 weeks before and 1 week after the onset of jaundice. Thus, close personal contact with an infected individual or fecal-oral contamination accounts for most cases and explains outbreaks in institutional settings such as schools and nurseries, as well as waterborne epidemics in places where people live in overcrowded, unsanitary conditions. HAV can also be detected in serum and saliva of infected individuals.

In high-income countries, sporadic infections may be contracted by the consumption of raw or steamed shellfish that have concentrated the virus from seawater contaminated with human sewage. Infected workers in the food industry are another source of outbreaks. HAV itself does not seem to be cytopathic. The cellular immune response, particularly that involving cytotoxic CD8+ T cells, plays a key role in HAV-mediated hepatocellular injury.

Because HAV viremia is transient, bloodborne transmission is very rare; therefore, donated blood is not specifically screened for this virus. IgM antibody against HAV appears in the blood at the onset of symptoms and is a reliable marker of acute infection (Fig. 14.8). Fecal shedding of the virus ends as the IgM titer rises. The IgM response usually declines in a few months followed by the appearance of IgG anti-HAV that persists for years, often conferring lifelong immunity. The HAV vaccine, available since 1995, is effective in preventing infection. Hepatitis A rates have declined by more than 95% since the introduction of the vaccine; there are now about 2800 cases annually in the United States.

Hepatitis B Virus

The outcome of HBV infection varies widely and includes: (1) acute hepatitis with recovery and clearance of the virus; (2) nonprogressive chronic hepatitis; (3) progressive chronic disease ending in cirrhosis; (4) fulminant hepatitis with massive liver necrosis; or (5) an asymptomatic "healthy" carrier state. HBV-induced chronic liver

Table 14.2 The Hepatitis Viruses

Virus	Hepatitis A (HAV)	Hepatitis B (HBV)	Hepatitis C (HCV)	Hepatitis D (HDV)	Hepatitis E (HEV)
Viral genome	ssRNA	Partially dsDNA	ssRNA	Circular defective ssRNA	ssRNA
Viral family	Hepatovirus; related to picornavirus	Hepadnavirus	Flaviviridae	Subviral particle in Deltaviridae family	Hepeviridae family, *Hepevirus* genus
Route of transmission	Fecal-oral (contaminated food or water)	Parenteral, sexual contact, perinatal	Parenteral; intranasal cocaine use is a risk factor	Parenteral	Fecal-oral
Incubation period	2–6 weeks	2–26 weeks (mean 8 weeks)	4–26 weeks (mean 9 weeks)	Same as HBV	4–5 weeks
Frequency of chronic liver disease	Never	5%–10%	>80%	10% (coinfection); 90%–100% for superinfection	In immunocompromised hosts only
Diagnosis	Detection of serum IgM antibodies	Detection of HBsAg or antibody to HBcAg; PCR for HBV DNA	ELISA for antibody detection; PCR for HCV RNA	Detection of IgM and IgG antibodies, HDV RNA in serum, or HDAg in liver biopsy	Detection of serum IgM and IgG antibodies; PCR for HEV RNA

dsDNA, Double-stranded DNA; *ELISA*, enzyme-linked immunosorbent assay; *HBcAg*, hepatitis B core antigen; *HBsAg*, hepatitis B surface antigen; *HDAg*, hepatitis D antigen; *ssRNA*, single-stranded RNA.

From Washington K: Inflammatory and infectious diseases of the liver. In Iacobuzio-Donahue CA, Montgomery EA, editors: *Gastrointestinal and Liver Pathology*, Philadelphia, 2005, Churchill Livingstone.

disease is also an important precursor for the development of hepatocellular carcinoma.

Liver disease due to HBV infection is an enormous global health problem. One-third of the world's population (2 billion individuals) has been infected with HBV, and 250 million individuals have chronic infections. Seventy-five percent of chronic carriers live in Asia and the Western Pacific rim. The global prevalence of chronic hepatitis B infection varies from greater than 8% in parts of Africa to less than 2% in Western Europe, North America, and Australia. In Africa the prevalence is highest in West Africa.

The mode of transmission of HBV also varies with the geographic locale. In high-prevalence regions of the world, perinatal transmission during childbirth accounts for 90% of cases. In areas with intermediate prevalence, horizontal transmission, especially in early childhood, dominates. Spread among children usually occurs through minor breaks in the skin or mucous membranes following physical contact with infected individuals. In low-prevalence areas, unprotected sex and intravenous substance use are the chief modes of spread. Transfusion-related spread has been reduced greatly by screening of donated blood for HBsAg and by stopping the practice of paying blood donors. Vaccination induces a protective antibody response in 95% of individuals.

HBV is a member of *Hepadnaviridae*, a family of DNA viruses that cause hepatitis in multiple animal species. The HBV genome is a partially double-stranded, 3200-nucleotide, circular DNA with four open reading frames, which encode the following proteins:

- *Nucleocapsid "core" protein* (HBcAg, hepatitis B core antigen) and a longer polypeptide with a precore and core region, designated HBeAg (hepatitis B e antigen). The precore region directs the secretion of the HBeAg polypeptide into blood, whereas HBcAg remains in hepatocytes, where it participates in the assembly of virions.
- *Envelope glycoproteins* (HBsAg, hepatitis B surface antigen). Infected hepatocytes synthesize and secrete massive quantities of noninfective envelope glycoproteins (mainly small HBsAg).
- A *polymerase (Pol)* with both DNA polymerase activity and reverse transcriptase activity, which enables genomic replication to occur through a unique DNA → RNA → DNA cycle via an intermediate RNA template. This unusual polymerase is the target of drugs used to treat hepatitis B infection (described later).

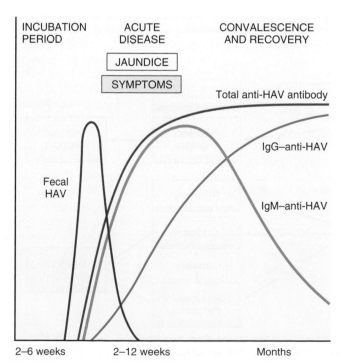

FIG. 14.8 Temporal changes in serologic markers in acute hepatitis A infection. *HAV*, Hepatitis A virus; *IgG*, immunoglobulin G; *IgM*, immunoglobulin M.

- *HBx protein,* which is required for virus replication and may act as a transcriptional transactivator for viral genes and a wide variety of host genes. It has been implicated in the pathogenesis of HBV-associated liver cancer.

HBV has a long incubation period (2—26 weeks). Unlike HAV, HBV remains in the blood during active episodes of acute and chronic hepatitis. Approximately 65% of adults with newly acquired HBV have mild or no symptoms and do not develop jaundice (acute anicteric hepatitis). The remaining 25% have nonspecific constitutional symptoms such as anorexia, fever, jaundice, and right upper quadrant pain (acute icteric hepatitis). Fulminant hepatitis and chronic hepatitis are uncommon, occurring in approximately 0.1% to 0.5% and 5% to 10%, respectively, of individuals who are acutely infected.

In most cases, the infection is self-limited and resolves without treatment, but chronic disease develops in 5% to 10% of individuals who are infected. **The risk of chronic infection is inversely related to age and is greatest (approximately 90%) in infants who are exposed to the virus through transmission from their mothers at birth.** Chronic hepatitis may progress to cirrhosis, and a subset develop hepatocellular carcinoma. The approximate frequencies of various clinical outcomes of HBV infection are depicted in Fig. 14.9.

The host immune response is the main determinant of the outcome of the infection. Innate immune mechanisms, particularly the production of interferon (IFN)-α, protect the host during initial phases of the infection, and a strong response by virus-specific CD4+ and CD8+ interferon γ—producing cells is associated with the resolution of acute infection. Like HAV, HBV is generally not directly hepatotoxic, and most hepatocyte injury is caused by CD8+ cytotoxic T cells attacking infected cells.

The course of the disease can be followed clinically by monitoring certain serum markers (Fig. 14.10).

- HBsAg appears before the onset of symptoms, peaks during symptomatic disease, and then usually declines to undetectable levels in 12 weeks (though it may occasionally persist for as long as 24 weeks). By contrast, HBsAg persists in cases that progress to chronicity.

- Anti-HBs antibody appears after the acute disease is over and is usually not detected until a few weeks to several months after HBsAg disappears. Anti-HBs antibodies may persist for life and confer protection, which is the rationale for HBsAg-containing vaccines. By contrast, anti-HBs antibodies are not produced in cases that progress to chronic liver disease
- HBeAg and HBV DNA appear in serum soon after HBsAg and signify ongoing viral replication. Persistence of HBeAg is an indicator of progression to chronic hepatitis. The appearance of anti-HBe antibodies implies that an acute infection has peaked and is waning.
- IgM anti-HBc becomes detectable in serum shortly before the onset of symptoms, concurrent with the onset of elevated serum aminotransferase levels (indicative of hepatocyte destruction). Over a period of months, the IgM anti-HBc antibody is replaced by IgG anti-HBc.

Treatment of chronic hepatitis B with HBV polymerase inhibitors and IFN-α can slow disease progression, reduce liver damage, and prevent liver cirrhosis or liver cancer but does not eliminate the infection.

Hepatitis C Virus

HCV is a major cause of chronic liver disease, with approximately 170 million individuals affected worldwide. Approximately 2.7 million Americans have chronic HCV infection. HCV is a blood-borne infection. Notably, there has been a decrease in the annual incidence of infection from a mid-1980s peak of over 230,000 new infections per year to 17,000 new infections per year currently, due primarily to a reduction in transfusion-associated cases as a result of effective screening procedures. It is worrisome that these gains made may not be sustained. There is a recent increase in new HCV infections primarily due to the ongoing opioid epidemic and the associated injection drug use. Until recently, the number of patients with chronic infection appeared likely to continue to increase, but new therapies (discussed later) are improving the outlook.

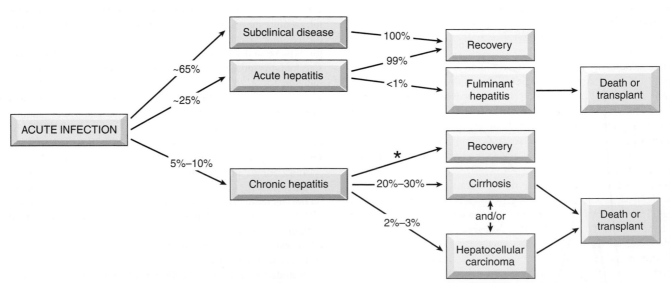

FIG. 14.9 Potential outcomes of hepatitis B infection in adults, with their approximate frequencies in the United States. *Spontaneous HBsAg clearance occurs during chronic HBV infection at an estimated annual incidence of 1% to 2% in Western countries. As mentioned in the text, fulminant hepatitis and acute hepatic failure are used interchangeably.

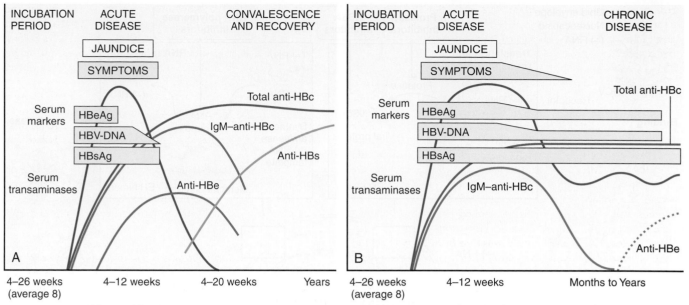

FIG. 14.10 Temporal changes in serologic markers for hepatitis B viral infection. (A) Acute infection with resolution. (B) Progression to chronic infection. Total anti-HBc includes both IgM and IgG anti-HBc antibodies. Note in some cases of chronic HBV infection, serum transaminases may become normal.

The risk factors for HCV infection are as follows:

- Intravenous substance use
- Needlestick injury
- Perinatal transmission of HCV at the time of birth occurs in about 5% to 6% of infants born to HCV infected women.

Currently, transmission of HCV by blood transfusion is close to zero in the United States; the risk for acquiring HCV by needlestick is about six times higher than that for HIV (1.8 vs. 0.3%). The efficiency of HCV transmission by sexual intercourse is low, as is transmission by household contacts. One-third of individuals have no identifiable risk factors, an enduring mystery.

HCV is a member of the *Flaviviridae* family. Just as with HIV, an understanding of viral replication and assembly has facilitated the development of highly effective anti-HCV drugs (described below). HCV is an enveloped, single-stranded RNA virus with a genome encoding a single polyprotein that is processed by several proteases into 10 functional proteins. Included among these proteins is a protease that is needed for complete processing of the polyprotein; NS5A, which is essential for assembly of HCV into mature virions; and a RNA polymerase that is necessary for replication of the viral genome (Fig. 14.11). Because of the inability of the host immune response to eliminate HCV and the low fidelity of the HCV RNA polymerase, new genetic variants develop at a rapid pace. This has led to the appearance of seven major HCV genotypes worldwide, each with one or more "subspecies." Infections in most individuals are due to a virus of a single genotype, but new genetic variants are generated in the host while viral replication persists. As a result, each patient usually comes to be infected with a population of divergent but closely related HCV variants known as *quasispecies*.

The incubation period for HCV ranges from 4 to 26 weeks, with a mean of 9 weeks. In about 85% of individuals, the acute infection is asymptomatic and goes unrecognized. HCV RNA is detectable in blood for 1 to 3 weeks, coincident with elevations in serum transaminases (Fig. 14.12). The clinical course of acute HCV hepatitis is milder than that of HBV; severe acute hepatitis is rare.

Persistent infection and chronic hepatitis are the hallmarks of HCV infection, despite the generally asymptomatic nature of the acute illness. In contrast to HBV, chronic disease occurs in the majority of individuals infected with HCV (80%–90%), and cirrhosis eventually occurs in approximately 20% over a period of 20 to 30 years. The mechanisms leading to chronicity are not well understood. Older age, male gender, alcohol use, immunosuppressive drugs, hepatitis B/HIV coinfection, and diseases associated with insulin resistance, including obesity, type 2 diabetes, and metabolic syndrome, have been associated with progression. Those who develop cirrhosis are at risk for development of hepatocellular carcinoma. Although the overall risk is small, in the United States, HCV is responsible for about one-third of cases of liver cancer.

In chronic HCV infection, circulating HCV RNA persists in 90% of patients despite the presence of neutralizing antibodies (see Fig. 14.12B). Hence, testing for HCV RNA is done to confirm the diagnosis of chronic HCV infection. A characteristic clinical feature of chronic HCV infection is episodic elevations in serum aminotransferases separated by periods of normal or near-normal enzyme levels. However, even patients infected by HCV who have normal transaminases are at high risk for developing permanent liver damage, and anyone with detectable serum HCV RNA needs treatment and long-term medical follow-up.

Fortunately, **recent years have seen dramatic improvements in treatment of HCV infection that stem from development of drugs that specifically target the viral protease, RNA polymerase, and NS5A protein, all of which are required for production of virus** (see Fig. 14.11). Combination therapy with these drugs (a strategy akin to

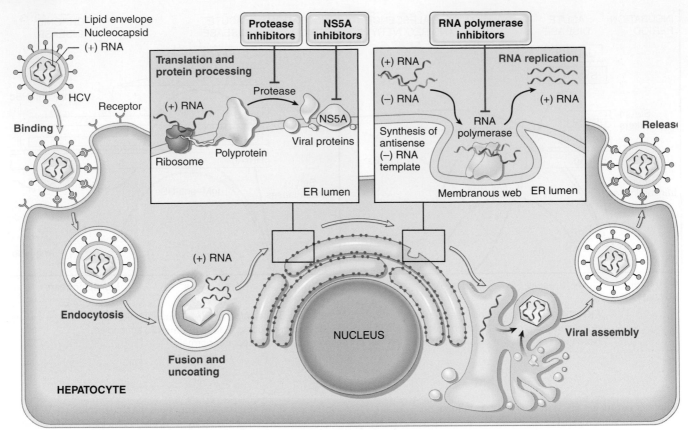

FIG. 14.11 Life cycle of hepatitis C virus (HCV). Viral entry, replication, assembly, and release are shown. Steps that can be effectively targeted with antiviral drugs are emphasized. Following viral entry and release of genetic material inside the host cell, HCV polyprotein is translated in rough endoplasmic reticulum (ER). During polyprotein processing, viral RNA replication takes place in "membranous webs," which are ER-derived double-membrane vesicles. Final steps involve viral assembly and release from the host cell. *NS5A*, Nonstructural protein 5A; *RNA*, ribonucleic acid.

triple drug therapy for HIV) is remarkably effective. The goal of current treatment is to eradicate HCV, which is defined by the absence of detectable HCV RNA in the blood after treatment is stopped. Currently, over 95% of HCV infections are curable.

Hepatitis D Virus

Also called *delta agent*, HDV is a unique RNA virus that is dependent for its life cycle on HBV. Infection with HDV arises in the following settings:

- *Coinfection* occurs following exposure to serum containing both HDV and HBV. Coinfection can result in a clinical syndrome that is indistinguishable from acute hepatitis B. It is self-limited and is usually followed by clearance of both viruses. However, there is a higher rate of acute hepatic failure in individuals who use intravenous drugs.
- *Superinfection* occurs when a chronic carrier of HBV is exposed to a new inoculum of HDV. This results in disease 30 to 50 days later, presenting either as severe acute hepatitis in a previously asymptomatic HBV carrier, or as an exacerbation of chronic hepatitis B infection. Chronic HDV infection occurs in more than 80% of superinfections and may have two phases: (1) an acute phase with active HDV replication and suppression of HBV associated with high transaminase levels and (2) a chronic phase in which HDV replication decreases, HBV replication increases, and transaminase levels fluctuate.

HDV infection occurs worldwide and affects an estimated 15 million individuals (about 5% of the 300 million individuals infected by HBV). Its prevalence varies, being highest in the Amazon basin, Africa, the Middle East, and Southern Italy, and lowest in Southeast Asia and China. In most higher-income countries, it is largely restricted to individuals who use intravenous drugs and those who have had multiple blood transfusions. Coinfection with HDV and HBV increases the risk of progression to cirrhosis and HCC.

HDV RNA is detectable in the blood and liver at the time of onset of acute symptomatic disease. Anti-HDV IgM is a reliable indicator of recent HDV exposure but is frequently short-lived. Acute coinfection by HDV and HBV is associated with the presence of IgM against HDAg and HBcAg (denoting new infection with hepatitis B). When chronic hepatitis arises from HDV superinfection, HBsAg is present in serum, and anti-HDV antibodies (IgG and IgM) persist for months or longer. Because of its dependency on HBV, HDV infection is prevented by vaccination against HBV.

Hepatitis E Virus

HEV is an enterically transmitted, waterborne infection that usually produces a self-limiting disease. The virus typically infects young to middle-aged adults. HEV is a zoonotic disease with animal reservoirs that include monkeys, cats, pigs, and dogs. Epidemics have been reported in Asia and the Indian subcontinent, sub-Saharan Africa, and Mexico, and sporadic cases are seen in the United States, Canada, and

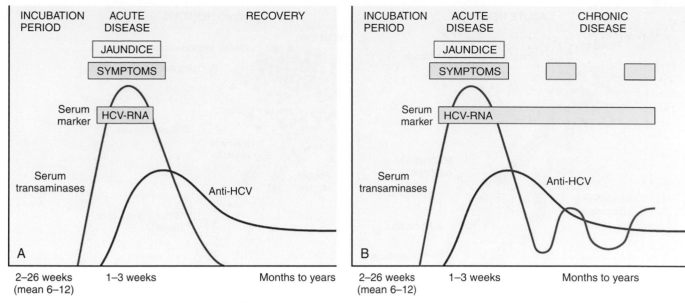

FIG. 14.12 Temporal changes in serologic markers in hepatitis C infection. (A) Acute infection with resolution; (B) progression to chronic infection.

Europe, particularly where pig farming is common, and in travelers returning from regions of high incidence. Of greater importance, HEV infection accounts for 30% to 60% of cases of sporadic acute hepatitis in India, exceeding the frequency of HAV. **A characteristic feature of HEV infection is the high mortality rate among pregnant women, approaching 20%.** In most cases, HEV is not associated with chronic liver disease or persistent viremia. The average incubation period following exposure is 4 to 5 weeks.

HEV is an unenveloped, positive-stranded RNA virus in the Hepeviridae family (*Hepevirus* genus). Virions are shed in stool during the acute illness. Before the onset of clinical illness, HEV RNA and HEV virions can be detected by PCR in stool and serum. The onset of rising serum aminotransferases, clinical illness, and elevated IgM anti-HEV titers are virtually simultaneous. Symptoms resolve in 2 to 4 weeks, during which time the IgM titers fall and anti-HEV IgG titers rise.

Clinicopathologic Syndromes of Viral Hepatitis

As already discussed, infection with hepatitis viruses produces a wide range of outcomes. Acute infection by each of the hepatotropic viruses may be symptomatic or asymptomatic. HAV and HEV do not cause chronic hepatitis, and only a small number of adults infected with HBV develop chronic hepatitis. By contrast, HCV commonly causes chronic infections. Fulminant hepatitis is unusual and is seen primarily with HAV, HBV, or HDV infections. HEV can cause acute liver failure in pregnant women. Although HBV and HCV are responsible for most cases of chronic hepatitis, there are many other causes of similar clinicopathologic presentations, including autoimmune hepatitis and drug- and toxin-induced hepatitis (discussed later). Therefore, serologic and molecular studies are essential for the diagnosis of viral hepatitis and for distinguishing the various types.

Major features of the main clinicopathologic syndromes associated with hepatitis viruses are as follows:
- *Acute asymptomatic infection with recovery.* Patients in this group are identified incidentally because of elevated serum transaminases or the presence of antiviral antibodies. HAV and HBV infections, particularly in childhood, are frequently subclinical.

- *Acute symptomatic infection with recovery.* Acute disease follows a similar course for all viruses and consists of (1) an incubation period of variable length (see Table 14.2); (2) a symptomatic preicteric phase; (3) a symptomatic icteric phase; and (4) convalescence. Peak infectivity occurs during the last asymptomatic days of the incubation period and the early days of acute symptoms.
- *Acute liver failure.* Viral hepatitis is responsible for about 10% of cases of acute hepatic failure. HAV is the most common cause worldwide, but HBV is more common in Asia and the Mediterranean. Survival for more than 1 week may permit recovery to occur via replication of residual hepatocytes.
- *Chronic hepatitis* is defined as symptomatic, biochemical, or serologic evidence of continuing or relapsing hepatic disease for more than 6 months. In some patients, the only signs of chronic disease are elevations of serum transaminases. Laboratory studies may reveal impaired liver functions such as prolongation of the prothrombin time and hyperbilirubinemia. Occasionally, in cases of HBV and HCV, immune complex disease develops that results in vasculitis (Chapter 8) and glomerulonephritis (Chapter 12). Cryoglobulinemia is found in about 35% of individuals with chronic hepatitis C.
- *Carrier state.* A "carrier" is an individual who harbors and can transmit an organism but has no symptoms. Carriers include (1) individuals who harbor the virus but have no liver disease and (2) individuals who harbor the virus and have asymptomatic nonprogressive liver damage. In both cases, particularly the latter, affected individuals constitute reservoirs of infection. HBV infection acquired early in life in endemic areas (such as Southeast Asia, China, and sub-Saharan Africa) gives rise to a carrier state in more than 90% of cases, whereas in nonendemic regions the carrier state is rare.

Because of their similar transmission modes and overlapping risk factors, coinfection of HIV and hepatitis viruses is a common clinical problem. In the United States, 10% of individuals who are infected with HIV are coinfected with HBV and 25% with HCV, and, when untreated, chronic HBV and HCV infection are important causes of morbidity and mortality in these individuals. However, in adequately

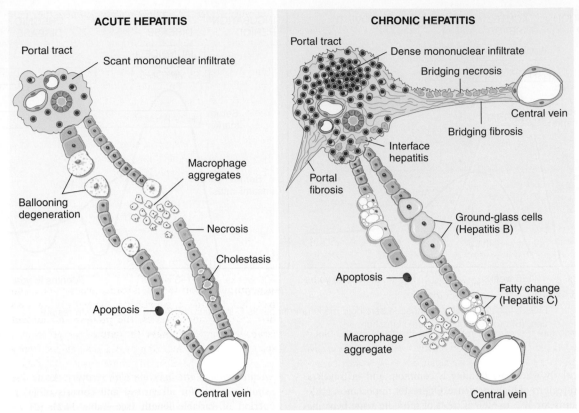

FIG. 14.13 Morphologic features of acute and chronic hepatitis. There is very little portal mononuclear infiltration in acute hepatitis (or sometimes none at all), while in chronic hepatitis portal infiltrates are dense and prominent—the defining feature of chronic hepatitis. Bridging necrosis and fibrosis are shown only for chronic hepatitis, but bridging necrosis may also occur in more severe acute hepatitis. Ductular reactions in chronic hepatitis are minimal in early stages of scarring but become extensive in late-stage disease.

treated immunocompetent patients with HIV, the severity and progression of HBV and HCV infection and response to anti–hepatitis virus therapy resembles that seen in individuals who are not infected with HIV.

MORPHOLOGY

The morphologic changes in acute and chronic viral hepatitis are shared among the hepatotropic viruses and can be mimicked by drug reactions or autoimmune hepatitis. They are depicted schematically in Fig. 14.13.

In **acute viral hepatitis,** the liver may be normal in size, enlarged (due to inflammation), or shrunken (massive liver necrosis due to acute liver failure; see Fig. 14.4). Microscopically, there is a portal and lobular inflammatory infiltrate comprising predominantly lymphocytes variably admixed with plasma cells and eosinophils. The hepatocyte injury may result in necrosis or apoptosis (see Figs. 14.2 and 14.3). Necrosis of groups of hepatocytes (i.e., confluent necrosis) may be seen in severe cases and can progress to necrosis of the entire lobule (i.e., panlobular or panacinar necrosis) or to connect vascular structures (i.e., bridging necrosis). Liver failure can develop with massive hepatic necrosis.

In **chronic viral hepatitis,** the defining histologic feature is portal lymphocytic or lymphoplasmacytic inflammation with fibrosis. The inflammatory cells often cross the limiting plate and injure periportal hepatocytes (interface activity). This may be accompanied by a variable degree of lobular inflammation. Fibrosis develops with increasing liver damage, manifesting

initially as portal and periportal fibrosis. Fibrous septa develop and lead to portoportal bridging fibrosis, and eventually cirrhosis.

Certain histologic features point to specific viral etiologies in chronic hepatitis. In chronic hepatitis B, **"ground-glass" hepatocytes** (cells with endoplasmic reticulum swollen by HBsAg) are a diagnostic hallmark, and the presence of viral antigen in these cells can be confirmed by immunostaining (Fig. 14.14). Liver biopsies involved by chronic hepatitis C commonly show large lymphoid aggregates (Fig. 14.15). Often, hepatitis C is associated with **fatty change** in scattered hepatocytes. Bile duct injury is also prominent in some cases of hepatitis C and may mimic the histologic changes seen in primary biliary cholangitis (see later); clinical parameters easily distinguish these two diseases, however.

Bacterial, Parasitic, and Helminthic Infections

A multitude of organisms can infect the liver and biliary tree, including bacteria, fungi, helminths and other parasites, and protozoa. Infectious organisms can reach the liver through several pathways:

- *Ascending infection,* via the gut and biliary tract (ascending cholangitis)
- *Vascular seeding,* most often through the portal system via the gastrointestinal tract
- *Direct invasion,* from an adjacent source (e.g., bacterial cholecystitis)
- *Penetrating injury*

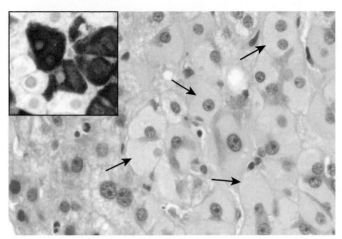

FIG. 14.14 Ground-glass hepatocytes *(arrows)* in chronic hepatitis B, caused by accumulation of hepatitis B surface antigen. Hematoxylineosin staining shows the presence of abundant, finely granular pink cytoplasmic inclusions; immunostaining *(inset)* with a specific antibody confirms the presence of surface antigen *(brown)*.

Bacteria that may establish an infection in the liver via the blood include *Staphylococcus aureus* in toxic shock syndrome, *Salmonella typhi* in typhoid fever, and *Treponema pallidum* in secondary or tertiary syphilis. Ascending infections are most common in the setting of partial or complete biliary tract obstruction and are typically caused by gut flora, which can grow in the ducts. Whatever the source of the bacteria, pyogenic organisms can cause intrahepatic abscesses, producing fever, right upper quadrant pain, and tender hepatomegaly. Although antibiotic therapy may sterilize small abscesses, surgical drainage is often necessary for larger lesions. More commonly, extrahepatic bacterial infections, particularly sepsis, induce mild hepatic inflammation and varying degrees of hepatocellular cholestasis indirectly, without establishing an infectious nidus in the liver.

Other nonbacterial infectious agents cause liver disease with important or unusual pathogenic features that merit specific comment. These include the following:

- *Schistosomiasis,* most commonly found in Asia, Africa, and South America. Adult worms in the gut produce numerous eggs, some

of which enter the portal circulation, where they lodge and induce a granulomatous reaction associated with marked fibrosis.

- *Entamoeba histolytica,* an important cause of dysentery (Chapter 13), sometimes ascends to the liver through the portal circulation and produces secondary foci of infection that can progress to large necrotic areas called amebic liver abscesses. Amebic abscesses are more common in the right lobe of the liver. The abscess cavity contains necrotic liver cells, but unlike pyogenic abscesses, neutrophils are absent.
- *Liver fluke infection,* most common in Southeast Asia, is associated with a high rate of cholangiocarcinoma. Responsible organisms include *Fasciola hepatica, Opisthorchis* species, and *Clonorchis sinensis.*
- *Echinococcal infections* may cause the formation of intrahepatic hydatid cysts that produce symptoms due to pressure on surrounding structures or following rupture.

AUTOIMMUNE HEPATITIS

Autoimmune hepatitis is a chronic, progressive disorder with features that include a genetic predisposition, an association with other autoimmune diseases, the presence of autoantibodies, and therapeutic responsiveness to immunosuppression. Autoimmune hepatitis has a wide range of presentations ranging from asymptomatic disease detected by elevated transaminases to acute and chronic hepatitis. There is a female predominance (78%). It is classified into two types, based on the patterns of circulating antibodies:

- *Type 1* is characterized by the presence of antinuclear antibodies (ANAs), which are most common but not specific; antismooth muscle antibodies (ASMAs), which are present in 65% of cases; and anti−soluble liver antigen/liver-pancreas antigen (anti-SLA/LP) antibodies, present in 25% to 35% of cases. The latter are also present in type 2 autoimmune hepatitis.
- *Type 2,* usually seen in children and teenagers, is characterized by anti−liver kidney microsome-1 antibodies (anti-LKM-1); anti−liver cytosol-1 (anti-LC1) antibodies; and anti-SLA/LP.

In a small subset of patients, there may be features that overlap with those of primary biliary cholangitis or primary sclerosing cholangitis. Cirrhosis is common in patients with autoimmune hepatitis; up to 30% of patients with adult-onset disease have cirrhosis at the time of diagnosis.

> ### MORPHOLOGY
>
> Autoimmune hepatitis shares patterns of injury with acute or chronic viral hepatitis. The following features are typical of autoimmune hepatitis (eFig. 14.1):
>
> - **Necrosis and inflammation,** indicated by extensive interface hepatitis or foci of confluent (perivenular or bridging) necrosis or parenchymal collapse
> - **Plasma cell predominance** in the mononuclear inflammatory infiltrates
> - **Hepatocyte "rosettes"** comprising a circular arrangement of regenerating hepatocytes around a dilated canaliculus

Immunosuppressive therapy is usually effective, leading to remission in 90% of patients including those who have cirrhosis at diagnosis. End-stage disease is an indication for liver transplantation. The 10-year survival rate after liver transplant is 75%, but recurrence in the transplanted organ occurs in 20% of cases.

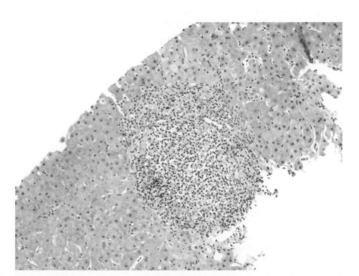

FIG. 14.15 Chronic viral hepatitis due to HCV, showing characteristic portal tract expansion by a dense lymphoid infiltrate.

DRUG- AND TOXIN-INDUCED LIVER INJURY

As the major drug metabolizing and detoxifying organ in the body, the liver is subject to injury from an enormous array of therapeutic and environmental chemicals. Injury may result from direct toxicity, occur through hepatic conversion of a xenobiotic compound to an active toxin, or be produced by immune mechanisms in which the drug or its metabolite chemically bond with a cellular protein and convert it into an immunogen. A diagnosis of drug- or toxin-induced liver injury may be made on the basis of a temporal association of liver damage with drug or toxin exposure, recovery (usually) upon removal of the inciting agent, and exclusion of other potential causes. **Exposure to a toxin or therapeutic agent should always be included in the differential diagnosis of any form of liver disease.**

Principles of drug and toxic injury are discussed in Chapter 7. Here it suffices to note that drug reactions may be *predictable* (intrinsic) or *unpredictable* (idiosyncratic). Predictable drug or toxin reactions affect all individuals in a dose-dependent fashion. Unpredictable reactions depend on host-specific factors, such as a propensity to mount an immune response to the drug or toxin or to metabolize the responsible agent in an unusual fashion. Both classes of injury may be immediate or take weeks to months to develop (Table 14.3).

- A classic, predictable hepatotoxin is *acetaminophen,* now the most common cause of acute liver failure necessitating transplantation in

the United States. The toxic agent is not acetaminophen itself but rather toxic metabolites produced by the cytochrome P-450 system. Since these enzymes are more active in the central zone of the lobule, necrosis of perivenular hepatocytes is a typical feature of drug-induced liver injury. Eventually necrosis can involve the entire lobule.

- Examples of drugs that can cause *idiosyncratic reactions* include chlorpromazine, an agent that causes cholestasis in patients who are slow to metabolize it, and halothane and its derivatives, which can cause a fatal immune-mediated hepatitis after repeated exposure.

ALCOHOL-RELATED AND NONALCOHOLIC FATTY LIVER DISEASE

Alcohol is a well-known cause of fatty liver disease in adults and can manifest histologically as steatosis, steatohepatitis, and cirrhosis. In recent years, it has become evident that another entity, so-called nonalcoholic fatty liver disease (NAFLD), which is associated with insulin resistance and the metabolic syndrome, can mimic the entire spectrum of hepatic changes associated with excessive alcohol use. Since the morphologic changes of alcohol-related liver disease and NAFLD are indistinguishable, they are discussed together, followed by the pathogenesis and distinctive clinical features of each entity.

Table 14.3 Patterns of Injury in Drug- and Toxin-Induced Hepatic Injury

Pattern of Injury	Morphologic Findings	Examples of Associated Agents
Cholestatic	Bland hepatocellular cholestasis, without inflammation	Contraceptive and anabolic steroids, antibiotics, antiretroviral therapy
Cholestatic hepatitis	Cholestasis with lobular necroinflammatory activity; may show bile duct destruction	Antibiotics, phenothiazines, statins
Hepatocellular necrosis	Spotty hepatocyte necrosis	Methyldopa, phenytoin
	Massive necrosis	Acetaminophen, halothane
	Chronic hepatitis	Isoniazid
Fatty liver disease	Large and small droplet fat	Ethanol, corticosteroids, methotrexate, total parenteral nutrition
	"Microvesicular steatosis" (diffuse small droplet fat)	Valproate, tetracycline, aspirin (Reye syndrome), antiretroviral therapy
	Steatohepatitis with Mallory hyaline	Ethanol, amiodarone, irinotecan
Fibrosis and cirrhosis	Periportal and pericellular fibrosis	Alcohol, methotrexate, enalapril, vitamin A and other retinoids
Granulomas	Noncaseating epithelioid granulomas	Sulfonamides, amiodarone, isoniazid
	Fibrin ring granulomas: granulomas with fibrin surrounding a central lipid vacuole	Allopurinol
Vascular lesions	Sinusoidal obstruction syndrome (veno-occlusive disease): obliteration of central veins	High-dose chemotherapy, bush teas
	Budd-Chiari syndrome	Oral contraceptives
	Peliosis hepatis: blood-filled cavities, not lined by endothelial cells	Anabolic steroids, tamoxifen
Neoplasms	Hepatocellular adenoma	Oral contraceptives, anabolic steroids
	Hepatocellular carcinoma	Alcohol, Thorotrast
	Cholangiocarcinoma	Thorotrast
	Angiosarcoma	Thorotrast, vinyl chloride

Modified from Washington K: Metabolic and toxic conditions of the liver. In Iacobuzio-Donahue CA, Montgomery EA, editors: *Gastrointestinal and Liver Pathology,* Philadelphia, 2005, Churchill Livingstone.

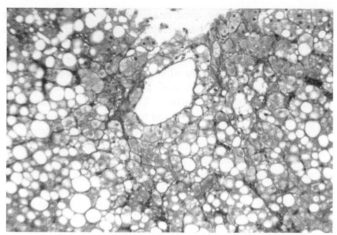

FIG. 14.16 Fatty liver disease associated with chronic alcohol use. A mix of small and large fat droplets (seen as clear vacuoles) is prominent. Some fibrosis *(stained blue)* is present in a characteristic perisinusoidal "chicken wire fence" pattern (Masson trichrome stain). (Courtesy of Dr. Elizabeth Brunt, Washington University, St. Louis, Missouri.)

MORPHOLOGY

Three types of liver alterations are observed in fatty liver disease: steatosis (fatty change), steatohepatitis, and fibrosis.

Hepatocellular steatosis. Fat accumulation typically begins in centrilobular hepatocytes. The lipid droplets range from small (microvesicular) to large (macrovesicular); the largest fill and expand the cell and displace the nucleus. As steatosis becomes more extensive, the lipid accumulation spreads outward from the central vein to hepatocytes in the midlobule and then the periportal regions (Fig. 14.16). Macroscopically, fatty livers with widespread steatosis are large (weighing 4–6 kg or more), soft, yellow, and greasy. In general, fatty change is completely reversible if there is abstention from further intake of alcohol.

Steatohepatitis. These changes typically are more pronounced with alcohol use than in NAFLD but can be seen in either (Fig. 14.17):

- **Hepatocyte ballooning.** Single or scattered foci of cells undergo swelling and necrosis; as with steatosis, these features are most prominent in the centrilobular regions.
- **Mallory hyaline bodies.** These consist of tangled skeins of intermediate filaments (including ubiquitinylated keratins 8 and 18) and are visible as eosinophilic cytoplasmic inclusions in degenerating hepatocytes (Fig. 14.17B).
- **Neutrophil infiltration.** Neutrophilic infiltration may permeate the lobule and accumulate around degenerating hepatocytes, particularly those containing Mallory hyaline bodies. Lymphocytes and macrophages also may be seen in portal tracts or parenchyma.

Steatofibrosis. Fatty liver disease of all kinds has a distinctive pattern of scarring. Like other changes, fibrosis appears first in the centrilobular region as **central vein sclerosis.** Perisinusoidal scarring appears next in the space of Disse of the centrilobular region and then spreads outward, encircling individual or small clusters of hepatocytes in a **chicken-wire fence pattern** (see Fig. 14.16). Tendrils of fibrosis eventually link to portal tracts and then condense to create **central portal fibrous septa.** As these become more prominent, the liver takes on a nodular, cirrhotic appearance. Because the underlying cause persists in most cases, the continual subdivision of established nodules by new perisinusoidal scarring leads to a classic **micronodular cirrhosis.** Early in the course, the liver is yellow-tan, fatty, and enlarged, but with persistent damage over the course of years, the liver is transformed into a brown, shrunken organ composed of cirrhotic nodules that are usually less than 0.3 cm in diameter—smaller than is typical for most forms of chronic viral hepatitis. The end-stage cirrhotic liver may enter a "burned-out" phase devoid of fatty change and other typical features. A majority of cases of **cryptogenic cirrhosis,** without clear etiology, are now recognized as "burned-out" NAFLD.

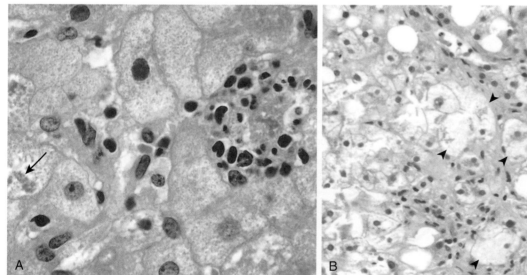
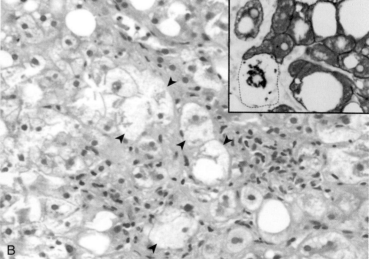

FIG. 14.17 Hepatocyte injury in fatty liver disease associated with chronic alcohol use. (A) Clustered inflammatory cells marking the site of a necrotic hepatocyte. A Mallory hyaline body is present in another hepatocyte *(arrow)*. (B) "Ballooned" hepatocytes *(arrowheads)* associated with clusters of inflammatory cells. The inset stained for keratins 8 and 18 *(brown)* shows a ballooned cell *(dotted line)* in which keratins have been ubiquitinated and have collapsed into an immunoreactive Mallory hyaline body, leaving the cytoplasm "empty." (Courtesy of Dr. Elizabeth Brunt, Washington University, St. Louis, Missouri.)

Alcohol-Related Liver Disease

Excessive ethanol consumption causes more than 60% of cases of chronic liver disease in Western countries and accounts for 40% to 50% of deaths resulting from cirrhosis. Among the most important adverse effects of chronic alcohol consumption are the overlapping forms of alcohol-related fatty liver disease already discussed: (1) hepatic steatosis, (2) steatohepatitis, and (3) fibrosis and cirrhosis, collectively referred to as *alcohol-related liver disease* (Fig. 14.18).

Between 90% and 100% of individuals who chronically consume excess alcohol develop fatty liver (i.e., hepatic steatosis), and of those, 10% to 35% develop steatohepatitis, whereas only 8% to 20% of this population develop cirrhosis. Steatosis, steatohepatitis, and fibrosis may develop sequentially or independently, so they do not necessarily represent a sequential continuum of changes. Hepatocellular carcinoma arises in 10% to 20% of patients with cirrhosis secondary to excess alcohol use.

Pathogenesis. Short-term ingestion of as much as 80 gm of ethanol per day (5–6 beers or 8–9 ounces of 80-proof liquor) generally produces mild reversible hepatic changes, such as fatty liver. Chronic intake of 40 to 80 gm/day is considered a borderline risk factor for severe injury. The risk of severe hepatic injury becomes significant with intake of 80 gm or more of ethanol per day. However, only 10% to 15% of individuals who chronically consume excess alcohol develop cirrhosis. In the absence of a clear understanding of the factors that influence liver damage, it is difficult to state what constitutes a safe level of alcohol consumption. For reasons that may relate to decreased gastric metabolism of ethanol and differences in body composition, women are more susceptible than men to hepatic

injury. It seems that how often one drinks may affect the risk for liver disease development. For example, binge drinking causes more liver injury than that associated with steady, lower-level consumption.

Hepatocellular steatosis is caused by alcohol through several mechanisms. First, metabolism of ethanol by alcohol dehydrogenase and acetaldehyde dehydrogenase generates large amounts of nicotinamide-adenine dinucleotide (NADH), which shunts fatty acid precursors away from catabolism and toward lipid biosynthesis. Second, ethanol impairs the assembly and secretion of lipoproteins. The net effect is to cause the accumulation of intracellular lipids.

The cause of *steatohepatitis* secondary to alcohol is uncertain, but it may stem from one or more of the following toxic byproducts of ethanol and its metabolites:

- *Acetaldehyde* (a major metabolite of ethanol) induces lipid peroxidation and acetaldehyde-protein adduct formation, which may disrupt cytoskeleton and membrane function.
- *Alcohol* directly affects mitochondrial function and membrane fluidity.
- *Reactive oxygen species* generated during oxidation of ethanol by the microsomal ethanol oxidizing system react with and damage membranes and proteins. Reactive oxygen species are also produced by neutrophils, which infiltrate areas of hepatocyte necrosis.

Because generation of acetaldehyde and free radicals is maximal in the centrilobular region, this region is most susceptible to alcohol-induced injury. Pericellular and sinusoidal fibrosis develop first in this area of the lobule. Concurrent viral hepatitis, particularly hepatitis C, is a major accelerator of alcohol-related liver disease.

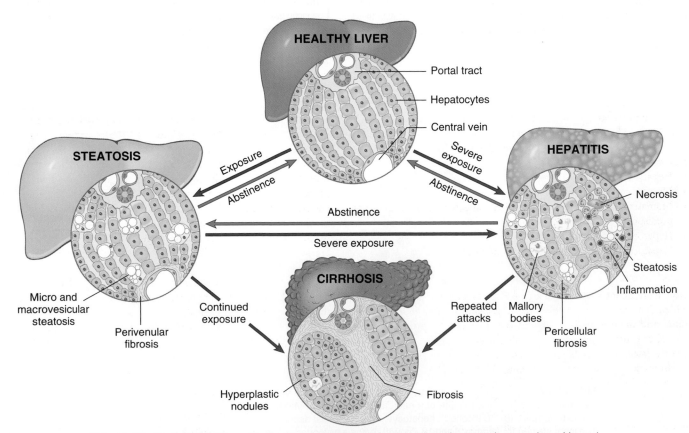

FIG. 14.18 Alcohol-related liver disease. The interrelationships among hepatic steatosis, steatohepatitis, and alcohol-related cirrhosis are shown and key morphologic features are listed. As discussed in the text, steatosis, steatohepatitis, and steatofibrosis may all develop independently and not along a continuum.

For unknown reasons, *cirrhosis* develops in only a small fraction of people who chronically drink excess alcohol. With complete abstinence, at least partial regression of scarring occurs, and by parenchymal regeneration the micronodular liver transforms into a macronodular cirrhotic organ (see Fig. 14.6); rarely, there is complete regression of cirrhosis.

Clinical Features. Steatosis may be innocuous or give rise to hepatomegaly with mild elevations of serum bilirubin and alkaline phosphatase. Severe hepatic compromise is unusual. Alcohol cessation and an adequate diet are sufficient treatment.

It is estimated that 15 to 20 years of excessive drinking are necessary to develop *cirrhosis,* but *steatohepatitis* can occur after just weeks or months of heavy alcohol use. The onset of steatohepatitis is typically acute and often follows an episode of particularly heavy drinking. Symptoms and laboratory abnormalities range from minimal to severe. Most patients present with malaise, anorexia, weight loss, upper abdominal discomfort, tender hepatomegaly, and fever. Typical laboratory findings include hyperbilirubinemia, elevated serum alkaline phosphatase levels, and neutrophilic leukocytosis. Serum alanine and aspartate aminotransferases are elevated but usually remain below 500 U/mL. In contrast to other chronic liver diseases, in which serum ALT tends to be higher than serum AST, in alcohol-related liver disease serum AST tends to be higher than serum ALT levels by a ratio of 2 : 1 or greater. The outlook is unpredictable; each bout of alcohol-related hepatitis carries a 10% to 20% risk for death. With repeated bouts, cirrhosis appears in about one-third of patients within a few years.

The manifestations of alcohol-related cirrhosis are similar to those of other forms of cirrhosis. In addition, when ethanol becomes the major source of calories in the diet, other nutrients are displaced, leading to malnutrition and vitamin deficiencies (e.g., thiamine, folate). Compounding these effects is impaired digestive function, primarily related to chronic gastric and intestinal mucosal damage and pancreatitis.

The long-term outlook for alcohol-related liver disease is variable. The most important part of treatment is abstinence from alcohol. The 5-year survival rate approaches 90% in those who abstain and who are free of jaundice, ascites, and hematemesis but drops to 50% to 60% in individuals who continue to imbibe. Among those with end-stage alcohol-related liver disease, the immediate causes of death are as follows:

- Hepatic failure
- Massive gastrointestinal hemorrhage
- Intercurrent infection (to which affected individuals are predisposed)
- Hepatorenal syndrome
- Hepatocellular carcinoma (3%—6% of cases)

Nonalcoholic Fatty Liver Disease

Nonalcoholic fatty liver disease (NAFLD) is a common condition in which fatty liver disease develops in association with insulin resistance and the metabolic syndrome (Chapter 18). The liver can show any of the three types of changes that occur in alcohol-related liver disease (steatosis, steatohepatitis, and cirrhosis), though on average inflammation is less prominent (eFig. 14.2). The term *nonalcoholic steatohepatitis (NASH)* is used to describe overt clinical features of liver injury, such as elevated transaminases, and the histologic features of hepatitis already discussed. Since systemic metabolic dysfunction underlies NAFLD, the term metabolic-associated fatty liver disease (MAFLD) has been proposed. In addition to insulin resistance and the metabolic syndrome, NAFLD is characterized by the following:

- *Type 2 diabetes* (or family history of the condition)
- *Obesity,* primarily central obesity
- *Dyslipidemia* (hypertriglyceridemia, low high-density lipoprotein cholesterol, high low-density lipoprotein cholesterol)
- *Hypertension*

Pathogenesis. **The key initiating events in NAFLD appear to be the development of obesity and insulin resistance** (Fig. 14.19). The latter leads to increased release of free fatty acids from adipocytes due to overactivity of lipoprotein lipase. This is associated with reduced production of the hormone adiponectin from adipocytes, which decreases oxidation of free fatty acids by skeletal muscle and increases free fatty acid uptake into hepatocytes, where the fatty acids are stored as triglycerides. In addition, hepatocytes in patients with NASH show evidence of inflammasome activation, possibly due to direct or indirect effects of particular lipids, leading to local release of the proinflammatory cytokine IL-1. Other products of lipid metabolism appear to be directly toxic to hepatocytes; proposed mechanisms include increased production of reactive oxygen species, induction of ER stress, and disruption of mitochondrial function. Alterations in the gut microbiome and increased gut-derived endotoxin production may also play a role in liver inflammation and injury. Hepatocyte injury resulting from these various insults causes stellate cell activation, collagen deposition, and hepatic fibrosis, which along with ongoing hepatocyte damage lead to full-blown NASH.

Clinical Features. NAFLD is the most common cause of incidental elevation of serum transaminases. The AST to ALT ratio is typically less than one (unlike alcohol-related fatty liver disease, which usually has a ratio greater than two). Most individuals with steatosis are asymptomatic; patients with active steatohepatitis or fibrosis may also be asymptomatic, while others have fatigue, malaise, right upper quadrant discomfort, or more severe symptoms of chronic liver disease. Liver biopsy is required to identify NASH and distinguish it from uncomplicated NAFLD. Fortunately, the frequency of progression from steatosis to active steatohepatitis and then from active steatohepatitis to cirrhosis is low. Nevertheless, NAFLD is considered to be a significant contributor to the pathogenesis of "cryptogenic" cirrhosis. Because they share common risk factors, the incidence of coronary artery disease is also increased in patients with NAFLD. One of the worrisome complications of NASH is development of hepatocellular carcinoma (see Fig. 14.19). With successful treatment of hepatitis C, the proportion of liver cancers arising in the setting of NASH is increasing and is likely to overtake HCV as a risk factor for HCC in the United States.

Current therapy is directed toward weight reduction and reversal of insulin resistance. Lifestyle modifications such as diet and exercise appear to be the most effective form of treatment. In selected cases bariatric surgery can help.

Pediatric NAFLD is becoming an increasing problem as obesity and metabolic syndrome approach epidemic proportions. In children, the appearance of the histologic lesions is somewhat different: inflammation and scarring tend to be more prominent in the portal tracts and periportal regions, and mononuclear infiltrates rather than neutrophilic infiltrates predominate.

INHERITED METABOLIC LIVER DISEASES

Although there are many inherited metabolic liver diseases, only some relatively common, pathogenically interesting entities are discussed here: hereditary hemochromatosis, Wilson disease, and α_1-antitrypsin (α_1AT) deficiency.

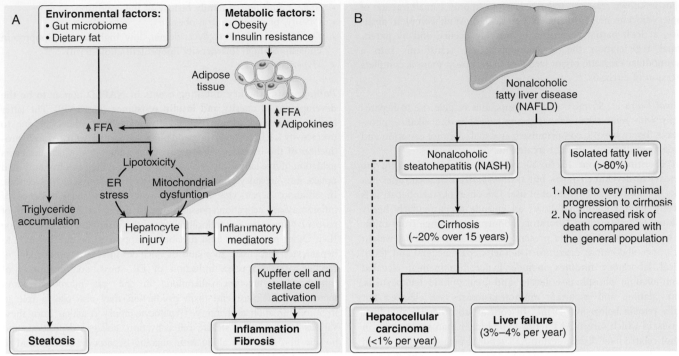

FIG. 14.19 (A) Pathogenesis of nonalcoholic fatty liver disease (NAFLD). (B) Natural history of NAFLD. Isolated fatty liver disease shows minimal risk for progression to cirrhosis or increased mortality, while nonalcoholic steatohepatitis shows increased overall mortality as well as increased risk for cirrhosis and hepatocellular carcinoma. *ER*, Endoplasmic reticulum; *FFA*, free fatty acid.

Hemochromatosis

Hemochromatosis is caused by excessive absorption of iron, which is deposited in organs such as the liver and pancreas, as well as in the heart, joints, and endocrine organs. It results most commonly from an inherited disorder, *hereditary hemochromatosis.*

As discussed in Chapter 10, the total body iron pool ranges from 3 to 4 gm in healthy adults; about 0.5 gm is stored in hepatocytes. In severe hemochromatosis, total iron may exceed 50 gm, one-third of which accumulates in the liver. Fully developed cases exhibit (1) micronodular cirrhosis; (2) diabetes (up to 80% of patients); and (3) abnormal skin pigmentation (up to 80% of patients).

Pathogenesis. Because there is no regulated iron excretion from the body, the total body content of iron is tightly regulated by intestinal absorption. As discussed in Chapter 10, hepcidin, encoded by the *HAMP* gene, is a circulating peptide hormone that acts as a key negative regulator of intestinal iron uptake. HFE, HJV, and TFR2 are membrane proteins expressed on hepatocytes. In a manner that is still poorly understood, HFE, HJV, and TFR2 (a transferrin receptor) function together as a sensor for iron, such that when iron is plentiful, signals are transmitted that stimulate the expression of *HAMP* transcripts and the secretion of hepcidin. Hepcidin in turn circulates to the gut and binds to ferroportin on enterocytes, leading to its internalization and degradation, thereby reducing the efflux of iron from enterocytes. **Diverse loss-of-function mutations in the components of this negative feedback loop lead to increased iron absorption and hemochromatosis** (Fig. 14.20). The most common genetic alterations underlying hereditary hemochromatosis are as follows:

- *HFE* (for *Hereditary Fe* [iron]) is the most frequently mutated gene in patients with hereditary hemochromatosis. It encodes an HLA

class I–like molecule that regulates the synthesis of hepcidin in hepatocytes. Loss-of-function mutations of the *HFE* gene reduce hepcidin levels and are present in over 70% of patients diagnosed with hereditary hemochromatosis.

- Less commonly, hereditary hemochromatosis is caused by mutations in genes encoding proteins that are directly involved in iron trafficking, such as the receptor for transferrin (the plasma transport molecule for iron) or ferroportin (a transmembrane iron transporter). With these mutations, the associated clinical condition is milder in some cases and more severe in others, sometimes resulting in disease that manifests in young adults or even during childhood.

An acquired form of hemochromatosis (*secondary hemochromatosis*) may develop in patients who receive multiple blood transfusions or have chronic ineffective erythropoiesis, as occurs in β-thalassemia and certain myeloid neoplasms. Ineffective erythropoiesis is marked by the premature death of red cell progenitors in the bone marrow, causing anemia that triggers increased production of erythropoietin from the kidney. This leads to an expansion of early red cell progenitors, which release a hormone called *erythroferrone* that suppresses hepcidin production. If uncorrected, the inevitable result is hemochromatosis.

Whatever the underlying defect, the net result is an increase in intestinal absorption of dietary iron, leading to an accumulation of 0.5 to 1 gm of iron per year, with disease developing after iron stores reach about 20 gm. Excessive iron appears to be directly toxic to host tissues. Mechanisms of liver injury include the following:

- *Lipid peroxidation* via iron-catalyzed free radical reactions
- *Stimulation of collagen formation* by activation of hepatic stellate cells

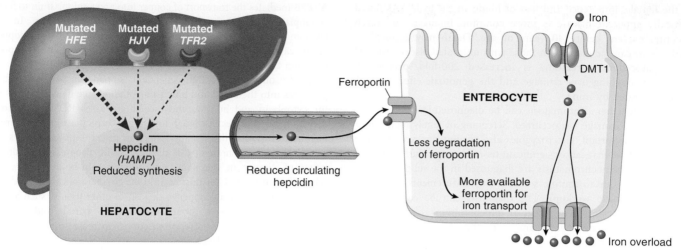

FIG. 14.20 Pathogenesis of hemochromatosis. Following iron uptake into enterocytes mediated by divalent metal transporter 1 (DMT1), iron secretion into the plasma depends on a second transporter, ferroportin. Hepcidin negatively regulates this process by binding ferroportin and stimulating its proteolytic degradation. Hepcidin production is regulated by an "iron sensor" in the liver that requires multiple factors, including HFE, HJV, and TFR2. Defects in any of these factors or hepcidin itself (encoded by the *HAMP* gene) result in increased iron uptake and hemochromatosis. *DMT1,* Divalent metal transporter 1; *HAMP,* hepcidin antimicrobial peptide; *HFE,* high Fe; *HJV,* hemojuvelin; *TFR2,* transferrin receptor 2.

- *DNA damage by reactive oxygen species,* leading to lethal cell injury or predisposition to hepatocellular cancer

The deleterious effects of iron on cells that are not fatally injured are reversible, and removal of excess iron with therapy promotes recovery of tissue function.

MORPHOLOGY

The morphologic changes in severe hemochromatosis are characterized principally by (1) **tissue deposition of hemosiderin** in the following organs (in decreasing order of severity): liver, pancreas, myocardium, pituitary gland, adrenal gland, thyroid and parathyroid glands, joints, and skin; (2) **cirrhosis;** and (3) **pancreatic fibrosis.** In the liver, iron becomes evident first as golden-yellow hemosiderin granules in the cytoplasm of periportal hepatocytes, which can be histochemically stained with Prussian blue (Fig. 14.21). With increasing iron load, there is progressive deposition in the rest of the lobule, the bile duct epithelium, and Kupffer cells. At this stage, the liver is typically slightly enlarged and chocolate brown. Fibrous septa develop slowly, linking portal tracts to each other and leading ultimately to **cirrhosis** in an intensely pigmented (very dark brown to black) liver.

The **pancreas** also becomes pigmented, acquires diffuse interstitial fibrosis, and may show parenchymal atrophy. Hemosiderin is found in the acinar and the islet cells and sometimes in the interstitial fibrous stroma. The **heart** is often enlarged, with hemosiderin granules within the myocardial fibers. The pigmentation may induce a striking brown coloration to the myocardium. A delicate interstitial fibrosis may appear. Although darkening of the natural skin color is partially attributable to hemosiderin deposition in dermal macrophages and fibroblasts, most of the coloration results from increased epidermal melanin production. The combination of these pigments gives the skin a grayish tinge. With hemosiderin deposition in the joint synovial linings, an acute synovitis may develop. There is also excessive deposition of calcium pyrophosphate, which damages the articular cartilage and sometimes produces disabling polyarthritis, referred to as *pseudogout.* With the onset of cirrhosis, the testes may become atrophic.

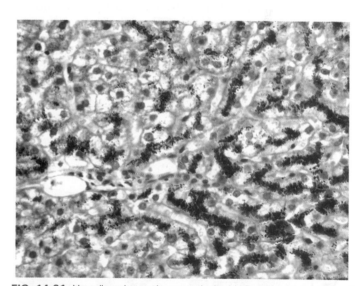

FIG. 14.21 Hereditary hemochromatosis. In this Prussian blue—stained section, hepatocellular iron appears blue. The parenchymal architecture is normal at this stage of disease, even with such abundant iron.

Clinical Features. Symptoms usually appear earlier in men than in women since menstrual bleeding limits the accumulation of iron until menopause. This results in a male-to-female ratio of clinically significant iron overload of approximately 5:1 to 7:1. In the most common form (due to *HFE* mutations), symptoms usually appear in the fifth and sixth decades of life in men and later in women.

The principal manifestations include hepatomegaly, abdominal pain, changes in skin pigmentation (particularly in sun-exposed areas of light skinned individuals), glucose intolerance or diabetes due to destruction of pancreatic islets, cardiac dysfunction (e.g., arrhythmias, cardiomyopathy), and atypical arthritis. In some patients, the presenting complaint is hypogonadism (e.g., amenorrhea in the female, impotence and loss of libido in the male). As noted, clinically apparent disease is more common in males and rarely becomes evident before 40 years of age. Death may result from cirrhosis or cardiac disease. In those with untreated disease, the risk for hepatocellular carcinoma is increased 200-fold, presumably because of ongoing liver damage and the genotoxic effects of oxidants generated by iron.

Fortunately, hemochromatosis can be diagnosed long before irreversible tissue damage has occurred. Screening of family members of probands is important. Heterozygotes also accumulate excessive iron, but not to a level that causes significant tissue damage. Currently, most patients with hemochromatosis are diagnosed in the subclinical, pre-cirrhotic stage due to routine serum iron measurements (as part of another diagnostic workup). The diagnosis can be confirmed by sequencing the *HFE* gene. Regular phlebotomy results in steady removal of excess tissue iron, and, with this simple treatment, life expectancy is normal.

Wilson Disease

Wilson disease is an autosomal recessive disorder caused by loss-of-function mutations of the *ATP7B* gene, which results in impaired copper excretion into bile and a failure to incorporate copper into ceruloplasmin (Fig. 14.22). This disorder is marked by the accumulation of toxic levels of copper in many tissues and organs, principally the liver, brain, and eye. Normally, 40% to 60% of ingested copper (2–5 mg/day) is absorbed in the duodenum and proximal small intestine, where it is transported in a complex with albumin and histidine to the liver. Within hepatocytes copper binds to ATP7B, a copper-transporting transmembrane protein that is found predominantly in the trans-Golgi network and in lysosomes. In the trans-Golgi network,

ATP7B mediates the transport of copper into apoceruloplasmin to form ceruloplasmin, which is then secreted into the bloodstream. In the lysosomes, ATP7B transports nonceruloplasmin-bound hepatic copper to bile canaliculi for excretion through bile, the major route of copper excretion from the body.

In Wilson disease ATP7B-dependent copper transport out of hepatocytes into the blood and bile is impaired. Hence it accumulates in the cytoplasm and in lysosomes, which increases ROS production, damaging hepatocytes. Although low serum ceruloplasmin levels are a hallmark of Wilson disease, the reduction in ceruloplasmin plays no role in the pathogenesis of this disorder. With progressive accumulation of copper in the liver, nonceruloplasmin-bound copper is released from injured hepatocytes into the circulation, causing red cell hemolysis and allowing copper to deposit in other tissues, such as the brain, corneas, kidneys, bones, joints, and parathyroid glands. Concomitantly, urinary excretion of copper increases markedly from its normal minuscule levels.

MORPHOLOGY

The liver often bears the brunt of injury. The hepatic changes are variable, ranging from relatively minor to severe, and mimic many other disease processes. There may be mild to moderate **fatty change (steatosis)** associated with focal hepatocyte necrosis. **Acute, fulminant hepatitis** can mimic acute viral hepatitis. **Chronic hepatitis** in Wilson disease exhibits moderate to severe inflammation and hepatocyte necrosis, areas of fatty change, and features of steatohepatitis (hepatocyte ballooning with prominent Mallory hyaline bodies). In advanced cases, **cirrhosis** may be seen. Copper deposition in hepatocytes can be demonstrated by special stains (eFig. 14.3).

Toxic injury to the brain primarily affects the basal ganglia. Nearly all patients with neurologic involvement develop eye lesions called **Kayser-Fleischer rings,** green to brown deposits of copper in the Descemet membrane in the limbus of the cornea.

Clinical Features. The age at onset and the clinical presentation of Wilson disease are extremely variable. Symptoms usually appear between 6 and 40 years of age. Acute or chronic liver disease are common presenting features. Neuropsychiatric manifestations are the initial features in most of the remaining cases and stem from deposition of copper in the basal ganglia.

The diagnosis of Wilson disease is based on low levels of serum ceruloplasmin, an increase in hepatic copper content (the most sensitive test), and increased urinary excretion of copper (the most specific test). Hepatic copper content in excess of 250 μg per gram dry weight of liver is considered diagnostic but is only about 80% sensitive. In those with lower liver copper levels, the diagnosis depends on other abnormalities, such as elevated urinary copper, low serum ceruloplasmin, and the presence of Kayser-Fleischer rings. Unlike hereditary hemochromatosis, where the limited number of genetic variants makes genetic testing fairly simple, the large number of different causative mutations in *ATP7B7* complicates the use of DNA sequencing as a diagnostic test. Serum copper levels are also of no diagnostic value, as they may be low, normal, or elevated, depending on the stage of the liver disease.

Early recognition and long-term copper chelation therapy (with D-penicillamine or trientine) or zinc-based therapy (which inhibits copper uptake in the gut) has dramatically altered the usual progressive course. Individuals with hepatitis or advanced cirrhosis require liver transplantation, which can be curative.

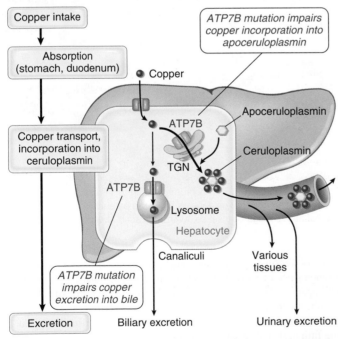

FIG. 14.22 Copper metabolism and consequences of mutation affecting ATP7B, the copper transporting hepatic protein. In Wilson disease failure of copper transport out of the hepatocytes into the blood in the form of ceruloplasmin and into bile cause accumulation of copper in the liver with resultant hepatocyte injury and eventual release of copper into the bloodstream with toxic injury to other tissues. *TGN,* Trans-Golgi network.

α_1-Antitrypsin Deficiency

α1-Antitrypsin deficiency is an autosomal recessive disorder caused by mutations that lead to misfolding of α_1AT and loss of α_1AT function. The major function of α_1AT is to inhibit proteases, particularly neutrophil elastase, cathepsin G, and proteinase 3, which are released from neutrophils at sites of inflammation. α_1AT deficiency leads to unopposed activation of neutrophil proteases (e.g., elastase), which destroy elastic fibers in alveolar walls, resulting in pulmonary emphysema (Chapter 11).

α_1AT is a plasma glycoprotein synthesized predominantly by hepatocytes. At least 75 α_1AT variants have been identified and denoted alphabetically. The general notation is "Pi" for "protease inhibitor" and an alphabetic letter for each of the two alleles. The most common genotype, homozygous for the M allele, is called PiMM, occurring in 90% of individuals (the "wild-type").

The most common clinically significant mutation is PiZ; PiZZ homozygotes have circulating α_1AT levels that are only 10% of the level in unaffected individuals. These individuals are at high risk for developing clinical disease. Variant alleles are codominant, and, consequently, PiMZ heterozygotes have intermediate plasma levels of α_1AT. Due to early presentation of the liver disease, α_1AT deficiency is the most commonly diagnosed genetic hepatic disorder in infants and children.

Pathogenesis. **Liver disease results from the accumulation of misfolded variant α_1AT protein within hepatocytes, leading to endoplasmic reticulum stress and the unfolded protein response, which ultimately leads to apoptosis of hepatocytes.** The PiZ polypeptide is prone to misfolding and aggregation due to a single amino acid glutamine-to-lysine substitution at residue 342 (E342K). It is worth emphasizing that the liver damage is caused by protein misfolding, whereas lung damage is due to loss of α_1AT function and consequent excessive protease activity. Although all individuals with the PiZZ genotype accumulate α_1AT in hepatocytes, only 10% to 15% develop overt clinical liver disease; thus, other genetic or environmental factors must play a role in the development of liver disease.

> ### MORPHOLOGY
>
> α_1-Antitrypsin deficiency is characterized by the presence of round-to-oval cytoplasmic **globular inclusions** in hepatocytes that are strongly periodic acid–Schiff (PAS) positive and diastase resistant (Fig. 14.23). Periportal hepatocytes are most affected in early or mild forms of the disease, with central lobular hepatocytes being affected later or in more severe disease. Other pathologic features vary, ranging from hepatitis to fibrosis to full-blown cirrhosis.

Clinical Features. Hepatitis with cholestatic jaundice appears in 10% to 20% of newborns with α_1AT deficiency. In adolescence, presenting symptoms may be related to hepatitis or cirrhosis. Attacks of hepatitis may subside with apparent complete recovery, or they may become chronic and lead progressively to cirrhosis. Alternatively, the disease may remain silent until cirrhosis appears in middle to later adult life. Hepatocellular carcinoma develops in 2% to 3% of adults with PiZZ, usually in the setting of cirrhosis. The only definitive treatment for severe hepatic disease is liver transplantation. In patients with pulmonary disease, avoidance of cigarette smoking is crucial, because smoking results in accumulation of neutrophils and release of elastase in the lung that is not inactivated because of lack of α_1AT.

CHOLESTATIC DISORDERS

Hepatic bile serves two major functions: (1) the emulsification of dietary fat in the lumen of the gut through the detergent action of bile salts, enabling the absorption of lipids, and (2) the elimination of bilirubin, excess cholesterol, xenobiotics, trace metals like copper, and other waste products that are insufficiently water soluble to be excreted in urine. Processes that interfere with excretion of bile lead to *jaundice (icterus)* due to retention of bilirubin, and to *cholestasis* (discussed later).

Jaundice may occur in settings of increased bilirubin production (e.g., extravascular red cell hemolysis), hepatocyte dysfunction (e.g., hepatitis), or obstruction of the flow of bile (e.g., an impacted gallstone), any of which can disturb the equilibrium between bilirubin production and clearance (summarized in Table 14.4).

Table 14.4 Major Causes of Jaundice

Predominantly Unconjugated Hyperbilirubinemia
Excess Production of Bilirubin
Hemolytic anemias
Resorption of blood from internal hemorrhage (e.g., alimentary tract bleeding, hematomas)
Ineffective erythropoiesis (e.g., pernicious anemia, thalassemia)
Reduced Hepatic Uptake
Drug interference with membrane carrier systems
Impaired Bilirubin Conjugation
Physiologic jaundice of the newborn
Diffuse hepatocellular disease (e.g., viral or drug-induced hepatitis, cirrhosis)
Predominantly Conjugated Hyperbilirubinemia
Decreased Hepatocellular Excretion
Drug-induced canalicular membrane dysfunction (e.g., oral contraceptives, cyclosporine)
Hepatocellular damage or toxicity (e.g., viral or drug-induced hepatitis, total parenteral nutrition, systemic infection)
Impaired Intrahepatic or Extrahepatic Bile Flow
Inflammatory destruction of intrahepatic bile ducts (e.g., primary biliary cirrhosis, primary sclerosing cholangitis, graft-versus-host disease, liver transplantation)
Gallstones
External compression (e.g., carcinoma of the pancreas)

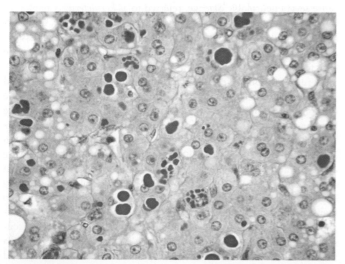

FIG. 14.23 α_1-Antitrypsin deficiency. Periodic acid–Schiff (PAS) stain after diastase digestion of the liver highlights the characteristic magenta cytoplasmic globules.

Bilirubin and Bile Formation

The metabolism of bilirubin by the liver occurs in steps illustrated in Fig. 14.24 as follows:

- Bilirubin is the end product of heme degradation. Approximately 85% of daily production (0.2–0.3 gm) is derived from the breakdown of senescent red cells by macrophages in the spleen, liver, and bone marrow. The remainder is derived from the turnover of hepatic heme or hemoproteins (e.g., the P-450 cytochromes) and from destruction of red cell precursors in the bone marrow (Chapter 10). Whatever the source, intracellular heme oxygenase converts heme to biliverdin (step 1 in Fig. 14.24), which is immediately reduced to bilirubin by biliverdin reductase.
- Bilirubin thus formed is released and binds to serum albumin (step 2), which is critical since bilirubin is virtually insoluble in aqueous solutions at physiologic pH and also highly toxic to tissues.

- Albumin carries bilirubin to the liver, where bilirubin is taken up into hepatocytes (step 3).
- In the liver, bilirubin is conjugated with one or two molecules of glucuronic acid by bilirubin uridine diphosphate (UDP)–glucuronyltransferase (UGT1A1, step 4) in the endoplasmic reticulum. Water-soluble, nontoxic bilirubin glucuronides are then excreted into the bile.
- Most bilirubin glucuronides are deconjugated in the gut lumen by bacterial β-glucuronidases and degraded to colorless urobilinogens (step 5). The urobilinogens and the residue of intact pigment are largely excreted in feces. Approximately 20% of the urobilinogens formed are reabsorbed in the ileum and colon, returned to the liver, and reexcreted into bile. A small amount of reabsorbed urobilinogen is excreted in the urine.

Two-thirds of the organic materials in bile are bile salts, which are formed by the conjugation of bile acids with taurine or glycine. Bile acids, the major catabolic products of cholesterol, are a family of water-soluble sterols with carboxylated side chains. The primary human bile acids are cholic acid and chenodeoxycholic acid. Bile acids are highly effective detergents. Their primary physiologic role is to solubilize water-insoluble lipids secreted by hepatocytes into bile and to solubilize dietary lipids in the gut lumen. Ninety-five percent of secreted bile acids, conjugated or unconjugated, are reabsorbed from the gut lumen and recirculate to the liver (*enterohepatic circulation*), thus helping to maintain a large endogenous pool of bile acids for digestive and excretory purposes.

Pathophysiology of Jaundice

Both unconjugated bilirubin and conjugated bilirubin (bilirubin glucuronides) may accumulate systemically. As discussed earlier, unconjugated bilirubin is virtually insoluble and tightly bound to albumin. As a result, it cannot be excreted in the urine, even when blood levels are high. Normally, a very small amount of unconjugated bilirubin is present as a free anion in plasma. If unconjugated bilirubin levels rise, this unbound fraction may diffuse into tissues, particularly the brain in infants, and produce toxic injury. The unbound plasma fraction increases in severe hemolytic disease. Hence, hemolytic disease of the newborn (erythroblastosis fetalis) may lead to accumulation of unconjugated bilirubin in the brain, which can cause severe neurologic damage, referred to as *kernicterus* (Chapter 4). By contrast, conjugated bilirubin is water soluble, nontoxic, and only loosely bound to albumin. Because of its solubility and weak association with albumin, excess conjugated bilirubin in plasma can be excreted in urine.

Serum bilirubin levels in the healthy adult vary between 0.3 and 1.2 mg/dL. Normally, the rate of bilirubin production is equal to the rate of hepatic uptake, conjugation, and biliary excretion. Jaundice becomes evident when there is imbalance between bilirubin production and excretion such that the serum bilirubin levels rise above 2 to 2.5 mg/dL; levels as high as 30 to 40 mg/dL can occur with severe disease. Causes of conjugated and unconjugated hyperbilirubinemia differ; therefore, measurement of both forms is of value in evaluating a patient with jaundice. Excess bilirubin production (e.g., due to hemolytic anemia or ineffective erythropoiesis) or defective conjugation (due to immaturity or hereditary causes) leads to the accumulation of unconjugated bilirubin. Conjugated hyperbilirubinemia most often results from hepatocellular disease, bile duct injury, and biliary obstruction.

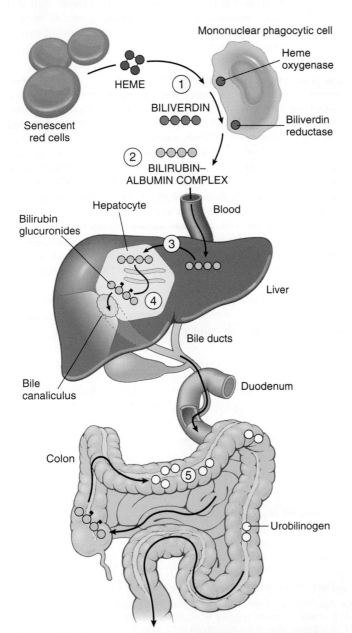

FIG. 14.24 Bilirubin metabolism and elimination. See text for details.

Defects in Hepatocellular Bilirubin Metabolism

Neonatal Jaundice

Because the hepatic machinery for conjugating and excreting bilirubin does not fully mature until about 2 weeks of age, almost every newborn develops transient, mild unconjugated hyperbilirubinemia, termed *neonatal jaundice* or *physiologic jaundice of the newborn*. This may be exacerbated by breastfeeding due to the action of bilirubin-deconjugating enzymes in breast milk. Phototherapy with blue light (which converts bilirubin to a soluble isomer that is readily excreted in the urine) is sufficient to keep the levels of bilirubin within a safe range until the hepatic processes for conjugation mature sufficiently. Nevertheless, sustained jaundice in the newborn is abnormal and is discussed later under Neonatal Cholestasis.

Hereditary Hyperbilirubinemias

Jaundice may also result from inborn errors of metabolism, including the following:

- *Gilbert syndrome* is a common (4%—16% of various populations) autosomal recessive condition that manifests as fluctuating unconjugated hyperbilirubinemia of variable severity. The usual cause is mildly decreased hepatic levels of glucuronosyltransferase due to a mutation in the promoter of the gene, *UGT1A1* that leads to decreased expression. Gilbert syndrome is not associated with any morbidity. By contrast, other mutations in *UGT1A1* that lead to severe glucuronosyltransferase deficiency causes a rare autosomal recessive disorder called *Crigler-Najjar syndrome type 1*, which is fatal in infancy.
- *Dubin-Johnson syndrome* is an autosomal recessive disorder caused by a defect in the transport protein responsible for hepatocellular excretion of bilirubin glucuronides across the canalicular membrane. Affected individuals exhibit conjugated hyperbilirubinemia. The only clinical manifestations are a darkly pigmented liver (from polymerized epinephrine metabolites, not bilirubin) and hepatomegaly.

Cholestasis

Cholestasis is a condition caused by extrahepatic or intrahepatic obstruction of bile channels or by defects in hepatocyte bile secretion. Patients may have yellow discoloration of the skin (jaundice) and sclera (icterus), pruritus, skin xanthomas (focal accumulation of cholesterol), or symptoms related to intestinal malabsorption, including nutritional deficiencies of the fat-soluble vitamins A, D, E, or K. Characteristic laboratory findings are elevated serum alkaline phosphatase and γ-glutamyl transpeptidase (GGT), enzymes that are present on the apical membranes of hepatocytes and cholangiocytes.

MORPHOLOGY

The morphologic features of cholestasis depend on its severity, duration, and underlying cause. Common to both obstructive and nonobstructive cholestasis is the **accumulation of bile pigment within the hepatic parenchyma** (Fig. 14.25). Elongated green-brown plugs of bile are visible in dilated bile canaliculi. Rupture of canaliculi leads to extravasation of bile, which is quickly phagocytosed by Kupffer cells. Droplets of bile pigment also accumulate within hepatocytes, which can take on a fine, foamy appearance referred to as *feathery degeneration*. Occasional apoptotic hepatocytes may also be seen.

Bile Duct Obstruction and Ascending Cholangitis

The most common cause of bile duct obstruction in adults is extrahepatic cholelithiasis (i.e., gallstones, discussed later), followed by obstruction by tumors and postsurgical strictures. Obstructive conditions in children include biliary atresia, cystic fibrosis, choledochal cysts (a cystic anomaly of the extrahepatic biliary tree), and syndromes in which there are insufficient intrahepatic bile ducts (paucity of bile duct syndromes). The initial morphologic features of cholestasis have been discussed and are entirely reversible with correction of the obstruction. Prolonged obstruction can lead to biliary cirrhosis, discussed later.

Ascending cholangitis (secondary bacterial infection of the biliary tree) may complicate duct obstruction. Enteric organisms such as coliforms and enterococci are common culprits. Cholangitis usually presents with fever, chills, abdominal pain, and jaundice. The most severe form of cholangitis is *suppurative cholangitis*, in which purulent bile fills and distends bile ducts. Since sepsis rather than cholestasis tends to dominate this potentially grave process, prompt diagnostic evaluation and intervention are imperative.

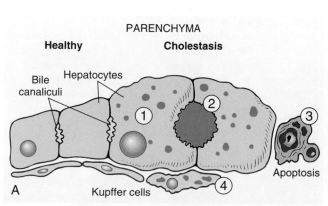

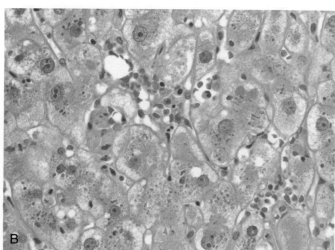

FIG. 14.25 Cholestasis. (A) Morphologic features of cholestasis *(right)* and comparison with normal liver *(left)*. Cholestatic hepatocytes *(1)* are enlarged and are associated with dilated canalicular spaces *(2)*. Apoptotic cells *(3)* may be seen, and Kupffer cells *(4)* frequently contain regurgitated bile pigments. (B) Cholestasis, showing the characteristic accumulation of bile pigments in the cytoplasm.

Because extrahepatic biliary obstruction is frequently amenable to surgical treatment, correct and prompt diagnosis is critical. By contrast, cholestasis due to diseases of the intrahepatic biliary tree or hepatocellular secretory failure (collectively termed *intrahepatic cholestasis*) is not improved by surgery (short of transplantation), and the patient's condition may be worsened by an operative procedure. Thus, it is important to establish the underlying basis for jaundice and cholestasis.

MORPHOLOGY

Acute biliary obstruction, either intrahepatic or extrahepatic, causes distention of upstream bile ducts, which often become dilated. In addition, **ductular reactions** (see earlier) appear at the portal-parenchymal interface along with stromal edema and neutrophils. The hallmark of superimposed infection **(ascending cholangitis)** is the influx of periductular neutrophils into the bile duct epithelium and lumen (Fig. 14.26).

Left uncorrected, the inflammation and ductular reactions resulting from **chronic biliary obstruction** initiate periportal fibrosis, eventually producing **secondary** or **obstructive biliary cirrhosis** (Fig. 14.27). Cholestatic features in the parenchyma may be prominent. These take the form of extensive **feathery degeneration of periportal hepatocytes,** a type of cytoplasmic swelling often associated with **Mallory hyaline bodies,** and **bile infarcts** caused by the detergent effects of extravasated bile.

Neonatal Cholestasis

Prolonged conjugated hyperbilirubinemia in the neonate, termed *neonatal cholestasis* (as opposed to the previously discussed neonatal jaundice), affects approximately 1 in 2500 live births. The major conditions causing it are (1) cholangiopathies, primarily *biliary atresia* (discussed later), and (2) a variety of disorders causing conjugated hyperbilirubinemia in the neonate, collectively referred to as *neonatal hepatitis*, described next.

Neonatal Hepatitis

Neonatal hepatitis is not a specific entity, nor does it necessarily have an inflammatory basis. Rather it is an indication to conduct a diligent search for recognizable toxic, metabolic, genetic, and infectious liver diseases, as

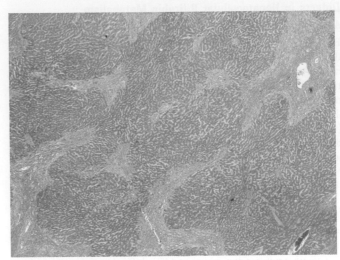

FIG. 14.27 Cirrhosis secondary to chronic biliary obstruction.

greater than 85% of cases have identifiable causes. The remaining 10% to 15% of cases are referred to as "idiopathic neonatal hepatitis."

Differentiation of biliary atresia from nonobstructive neonatal cholestasis is very important, since definitive treatment of biliary atresia requires surgical intervention, whereas surgery may adversely affect a child with other disorders. Fortunately, the two entities can be distinguished on the basis of clinical data in about 90% of cases. In 10% of cases, liver biopsy may be necessary to discriminate idiopathic neonatal hepatitis from a treatable cholangiopathy. Affected infants have jaundice, dark urine, light or acholic stools, and hepatomegaly. Variable degrees of hepatic synthetic dysfunction may be identified, such as hypoprothrombinemia.

MORPHOLOGY

The morphologic features of idiopathic neonatal hepatitis (Fig. 14.28) include striking **giant-cell transformation of hepatocytes,** associated with lobular disarray, focal liver cell apoptosis, and prominent hepatocellular and canalicular cholestasis. In some cases, this parenchymal pattern of injury is also accompanied by ductular reaction and fibrosis of portal tracts.

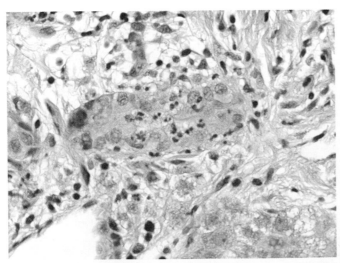

FIG. 14.26 Acute large-duct obstruction with ascending cholangitis. Superimposed on features of duct obstruction (stromal edema) is an infiltrate of neutrophils involving the bile duct, the hallmark of ascending cholangitis.

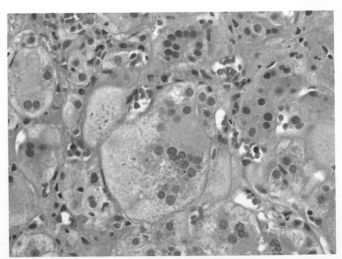

FIG. 14.28 Idiopathic neonatal hepatitis. Note the multinucleated giant hepatocytes.

Biliary Atresia

Biliary atresia is defined as a complete or partial obstruction of the extrahepatic biliary tree that occurs within the first 3 months of life. It underlies approximately one-third of cases of neonatal cholestasis and is the most frequent cause of death from liver disease in early childhood. Approximately 50% to 60% of children referred for liver transplantation have biliary atresia.

Pathogenesis. Two major forms of biliary atresia are recognized based on the presumed timing of luminal obliteration.

- The *fetal form* accounts for as many as 20% of cases and is commonly associated with other developmental anomalies involving the thoracic and abdominal organs, including malrotation of abdominal viscera, interrupted inferior vena cava, polysplenia, and congenital heart disease.
- Much more common is the *perinatal form* of biliary atresia, in which an apparently normally developed biliary tree is injured and obstructed following birth. The etiology of perinatal biliary atresia is unknown; viral infection and toxic exposures are considered prime suspects.

MORPHOLOGY

The salient features of biliary atresia include **inflammation and fibrosing stricture of the hepatic or common bile ducts;** in some individuals, periductular inflammation also extends into the intrahepatic bile ducts, leading to progressive destruction of the intrahepatic biliary tree as well. When biliary atresia is unrecognized or uncorrected, cirrhosis develops within 3 to 6 months of birth.

There is considerable variability in the pattern of biliary atresia. When the disease is limited to the common duct or right and/or left hepatic bile ducts with patent intrahepatic branches, the disease is surgically correctable (Kasai procedure). Unfortunately, in 90% of patients the obstruction also involves bile ducts at or above the porta hepatis. These cases are not correctable, since there are no patent bile ducts amenable to surgical anastomosis.

Clinical Features. Infants with biliary atresia present with neonatal cholestasis. There is a slight female predominance. Initially stools are normal, but they become acholic as the disease progresses. Ascending cholangitis and/or intrahepatic progression of the disease may impede attempts at surgical resection of the obstruction and bypass of the biliary tree. Transplantation of a donor liver and its accompanying bile ducts is the main hope for saving these young patients. Without surgical intervention, death usually occurs within 2 years of birth.

Autoimmune Cholangiopathies

Autoimmune cholangiopathies comprise two distinct immunologically mediated disorders that involve intrahepatic bile ducts: primary biliary cholangitis and primary sclerosing cholangitis. The salient features of these are listed in Table 14.5.

Primary Biliary Cholangitis

Primary biliary cholangitis (PBC) is an autoimmune disease whose principal feature is nonsuppurative, inflammatory destruction of small- and medium-sized intrahepatic bile ducts. Large intrahepatic ducts and the extrahepatic biliary tree are not involved. Previously, this disease was known as primary biliary cirrhosis, but most patients do not progress to cirrhosis, hence the name primary biliary cholangitis is preferred.

PBC is primarily a disease of middle-age women, with a female-to-male ratio of 9 : 1. Its peak incidence is between 40 and 50 years of age. The disease is most prevalent in northern European countries (England and Scotland) and the northern United States (Minnesota), where the prevalence is as high as 400 per 1 million. Recent increases in incidence and prevalence along with geographic clustering suggest that both environmental and genetic factors are important in its pathogenesis. Family members of patients with PBC have an increased risk for developing the disease.

Pathogenesis. **PBC is thought to be an autoimmune disorder resulting from T lymphocyte—mediated destruction of small interlobular bile ducts.** The retention of bile salts due to bile duct injury leads to secondary hepatocellular injury that can eventually progress to cirrhosis. As with other autoimmune diseases, the triggers that initiate PBC are unknown. **Antimitochondrial antibodies are present in 90% to 95% of patients.** Although they are highly characteristic of PBC, their role in the pathogenesis is unclear, as 5% of patients with otherwise typical PBC are antimitochondrial antibody (AMA)-negative. Moreover, antibody titers do not correlate with disease severity or disease progression, and they are not predictive of response to therapy.

Table 14.5 Main Features of Primary Biliary Cholangitis and Primary Sclerosing Cholangitis

Parameter	Primary Biliary Cholangitis	Primary Sclerosing Cholangitis
Age	Median age 50 years	Median age 30 years
Sex	90% female	70% male
Clinical course	Progressive	Unpredictable, but progressive—may progress to cholangiocarcinoma
Associated conditions	Sjögren syndrome (70%)	Inflammatory bowel disease (70%)
	Scleroderma (5%)	Autoimmune pancreatitis
	Thyroid disease (20%)	IgG4 related fibrosing diseases
Serology	95% AMA-positive	0%–5% AMA-positive (low titer)
	20% ANA-positive	6% ANA-positive
	40% ANCA-positive	65% ANCA-positive
Radiology	Normal	Strictures and beading of large bile ducts; pruning of smaller ducts
Duct lesion	Florid duct lesions and loss of small ducts only	Inflammatory destruction of extrahepatic and large intrahepatic ducts; fibrotic obliteration of medium and small intrahepatic ducts

AMA, Antimitochondrial antibody; *ANA,* antinuclear antibody; *ANCA,* antineutrophil cytoplasmic antibody.

MORPHOLOGY

Interlobular bile ducts are actively destroyed by lymphoplasmacytic inflammation with or without granulomas (often called the *florid duct lesion*) (Fig. 14.29). Some biopsy specimens, however, do not have active lesions and show only the absence of bile ducts in portal tracts. The disease is quite patchy in distribution: it is common to see a single bile duct under immune attack in one level of a biopsy specimen, while other nearby ducts are unaffected. **Ductular reactions** follow on this duct injury, and these in turn participate in the development of **portal-portal septal fibrosis.**

In the absence of treatment, the disease follows one of two paths to end-stage disease. In the first, more common pathway, there is increasingly widespread duct loss, slowly leading to established cirrhosis and eventually to profound cholestasis. Alternatively, some patients eventually develop prominent portal hypertension rather than severe cholestasis. Fortunately, both of these outcomes are now rarely seen.

Clinical Features. **Most patients are diagnosed in the early stages of disease following a workup triggered by the identification of an elevated serum alkaline phosphatase level or severe itching.** Hypercholesterolemia is common. The disease is confirmed by liver biopsy, which is considered diagnostic if a florid duct lesion is present. Symptom onset is insidious, with patients typically noticing slowly increasing fatigue and pruritus.

In recent years, treatment with oral ursodeoxycholic acid has dramatically improved outcomes and slowed disease progression. The mechanism of action remains unclear but is presumably related to the ability of ursodeoxycholate to enter the bile acid pool and alter the biochemical composition of bile.

With time, even with treatment, secondary features may emerge, including skin hyperpigmentation, xanthelasmas, steatorrhea, and vitamin D malabsorption–related osteomalacia and/or osteoporosis. Individuals with PBC may also have extrahepatic manifestations of autoimmunity, including the sicca complex of dry eyes and mouth (Sjögren syndrome), systemic sclerosis, thyroiditis, rheumatoid arthritis, Raynaud phenomenon, and celiac disease. Liver transplantation is the best treatment for individuals with advanced liver disease.

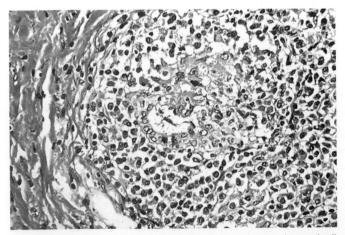

FIG. 14.29 Primary biliary cholangitis. A portal tract is markedly expanded by an infiltrate of lymphocytes and plasma cells. Note the granulomatous reaction to the bile duct undergoing destruction (the "florid duct lesion").

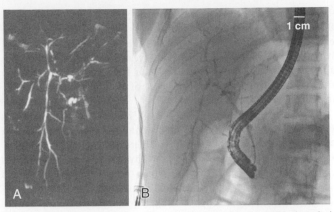

FIG. 14.30 Imaging studies of a patient with primary sclerosing cholangitis. (A) Magnetic resonance cholangiography of the bile ducts shows focal dilation in some ducts *(bright, broad areas)* and stricturing of others *(thinning or absence)*. (B) Endoscopic retrograde cholangiography of the same patient shows nearly identical features as in (A). (Courtesy of Dr. M. Edwyn Harrison, MD, Mayo Clinic, Scottsdale, Arizona.)

Primary Sclerosing Cholangitis

Primary sclerosing cholangitis (PSC) is characterized by inflammation and obliterative fibrosis of intrahepatic and extrahepatic bile ducts, leading to dilation of preserved segments. Irregular biliary strictures and dilations cause the characteristic "beading" of the intrahepatic and extrahepatic biliary tree seen by MRI (Fig. 14.30). Inflammatory bowel disease (Chapter 13), most commonly ulcerative colitis, coexists in approximately 70% of individuals with PSC. Conversely, the prevalence of PSC in individuals with ulcerative colitis is about 4%. Like inflammatory bowel disease, PSC tends to occur in the third through fifth decades of life. It has a 2:1 male predominance (see Table 14.5).

Pathogenesis. Several features of PSC suggest immunologically mediated injury to bile ducts. T cells in the periductal stroma. The presence of autoantibodies, an association with HLA-B8 and other MHC alleles, and clinical linkage to ulcerative colitis all support an immune etiology. First-degree relatives of patients with PSC are at increased risk for developing the disease, suggesting that genetic factors contribute. Several autoantibodies are present in PSC. Approximately 75% of patients have antismooth muscle antibodies and antinuclear antibodies. In addition, antibodies directed against cytoplasmic and nuclear antigens of neutrophils (ANCA) are found in up to 80% of affected adults. In one model, it is proposed that T cells activated in the damaged mucosa of patients with ulcerative colitis migrate to the liver, where they cross-react with a bile duct antigen and initiate an autoimmune assault on bile ducts.

MORPHOLOGY

Morphologic changes differ between large ducts (intrahepatic and extrahepatic) and smaller intrahepatic ducts. **Large duct inflammation** resembles that seen in ulcerative colitis, taking the form of neutrophils infiltrating into the epithelium superimposed on a chronic inflammatory background. Inflamed areas develop strictures as scarring narrows the lumen. The **smaller ducts,** however, often have little inflammation and show a striking **circumferential "onion skin" fibrosis** around an atrophic duct lumen (Fig. 14.31), which is eventually obliterated, leaving a "tombstone" scar. As the disease progresses, the liver becomes markedly cholestatic, culminating in cirrhosis. Biliary intraepithelial neoplasia often appears in the setting of chronic inflammation, and it may progress to cholangiocarcinoma, which is usually fatal.

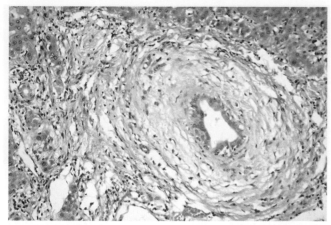

FIG. 14.31 Primary sclerosing cholangitis. A bile duct undergoing degeneration is entrapped in a dense, "onion-skin" concentric scar.

Clinical Features. Patients may come to attention because of persistent elevation of serum alkaline phosphatase, particularly in those with ulcerative colitis who are being routinely screened. Alternatively, progressive fatigue, pruritus, and jaundice may develop. Acute bouts of ascending cholangitis may also signal the presence or progression of PSC. Chronic pancreatitis and chronic cholecystitis due to involvement of the pancreatic ducts and gallbladder are also seen. In some patients, sclerosing cholangitis is associated with autoimmune pancreatitis. In such cases, PSC may be a manifestation of IgG4-related chronic disease (Chapter 5). The gold standard for diagnosis of PSC is the characteristic "beading" seen in the large intrahepatic and extrahepatic biliary tree by MRI (see Fig. 14.30).

PSC follows a protracted course; severely afflicted patients have symptoms typical of chronic cholestatic liver disease, including steatorrhea. In contrast to PBC, there is no satisfactory medical treatment. Without liver transplantation, median survival is 10 to 12 years after diagnosis. Progression to cholangiocarcinoma may occur.

CIRCULATORY DISORDERS

Hepatic circulatory disorders can be grouped according to whether the disorder leads to abnormalities in the inflow, flow-through, or outflow of blood (Fig. 14.32).

Impaired Blood Flow Into the Liver

Hepatic Artery Compromise

Liver infarcts are rare due to the double blood supply to the liver. Nonetheless, thrombosis or obstruction of an intrahepatic branch of the hepatic artery by embolism (Fig. 14.33), neoplasia, or an inflammatory process such as polyarteritis nodosa (Chapter 8) may produce an infarct, which may be pale, or hemorrhagic if suffused with blood from the portal circulation. Blockage of the main hepatic artery may not produce ischemic necrosis of the organ, particularly if the liver is otherwise healthy, as retrograde arterial flow through accessory vessels and the portal venous supply are usually sufficient to keep the liver parenchyma viable.

Portal Vein Obstruction and Thrombosis

Blockage of the extrahepatic portal vein may cause only vague symptoms or may be a catastrophic and potentially lethal event; most cases fall somewhere in between. Occlusive disease of the portal vein

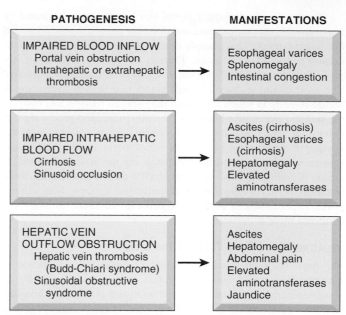

PATHOGENESIS	MANIFESTATIONS
IMPAIRED BLOOD INFLOW Portal vein obstruction Intrahepatic or extrahepatic thrombosis	Esophageal varices Splenomegaly Intestinal congestion
IMPAIRED INTRAHEPATIC BLOOD FLOW Cirrhosis Sinusoid occlusion	Ascites (cirrhosis) Esophageal varices (cirrhosis) Hepatomegaly Elevated aminotransferases
HEPATIC VEIN OUTFLOW OBSTRUCTION Hepatic vein thrombosis (Budd-Chiari syndrome) Sinusoidal obstructive syndrome	Ascites Hepatomegaly Abdominal pain Elevated aminotransferases Jaundice

FIG. 14.32 Hepatic circulatory disorders. Forms and clinical manifestations of compromised hepatic blood flow.

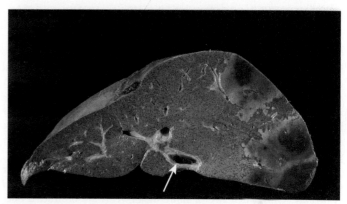

FIG. 14.33 Liver infarct. A thrombus is lodged in a peripheral branch of the hepatic artery *(arrow)* and compresses the adjacent portal vein; the distal hepatic tissue has hemorrhagic margin.

or its major branches typically produces abdominal pain and manifestations of portal hypertension, principally esophageal varices that are prone to rupture. Ascites is not common (because the block is presinusoidal), but, when present, is often massive and intractable.

Extrahepatic portal vein obstruction may be idiopathic (approximately one-third of cases) or may arise from a number of conditions. Some of the most common settings for its development include the following:

- *Cirrhosis,* which is associated with portal vein thrombosis in 25% of patients, some of whom have additional risk factors
- *Hypercoagulable states,* including myeloproliferative diseases such as polycythemia vera (Chapter 10), inherited thrombophilias such as factor V Leiden (Chapter 4), and miscellaneous hypercoagulable conditions such as paroxysmal nocturnal hemoglobinuria and antiphospholipid antibody syndrome
- *Inflammatory processes* involving the splenic vein or portal vein, such as in pancreatitis and intraabdominal sepsis
- *Trauma,* surgical or otherwise

Obstruction of intrahepatic portal vein branches may be caused by acute thrombosis. Such thrombosis does not cause ischemic infarction but instead results in a sharply demarcated area of red-blue discoloration called *infarct of Zahn*. There is no necrosis, only severe hepatocellular atrophy and marked congestion of distended sinusoids. The most common cause of small portal vein branch obstruction is *schistosomiasis*, in which the eggs of the parasites lodge in and obstruct the smallest portal vein branches. The other disorders producing this pattern of injury are collectively referred to as *obliterative portal venopathy*, which often presents as noncirrhotic portal hypertension. Causes of obliterative portal venopathy are not well understood. It occurs in both untreated and treated HIV disease and may in some instances be a complication of antiretroviral therapy. Noncirrhotic portal hypertension is particularly common in India, although the incidence there is declining.

Impaired Blood Flow Through the Liver

The most common intrahepatic cause of blood flow obstruction is cirrhosis, as discussed earlier. In addition, physical occlusion of the sinusoids occurs in *sickle cell disease, disseminated intravascular coagulation, eclampsia,* and *intrasinusoidal metastasis* of solid tumors. If severe, all of these disorders may produce sufficient obstruction of blood flow to cause massive necrosis of hepatocytes and fulminant hepatic failure.

Hepatic Venous Outflow Obstruction

Hepatic Vein Thrombosis

Occlusive events can occur in any caliber of hepatic vein branches. Occlusion of the smallest intrahepatic branches is known as *sinusoidal obstruction syndrome* (formally known as *veno-occlusive disease*). A rare but well-known cause of this syndrome is consumption of pyrrolizidine alkaloid–containing Jamaican bush tea; more commonly hepatic vein thrombosis occurs following allogeneic hematopoietic stem cell transplantation, usually within the first 3 weeks, or in cancer patients receiving chemotherapy.

The obstruction of the major hepatic veins produces liver enlargement, pain, and ascites, a condition known as *Budd-Chiari syndrome*. Only when two or more major veins are obstructed does intrahepatic blood pressure rise to the point of causing hepatic damage. Hepatic vein thrombosis is associated with the same hypercoagulable states as portal vein thrombosis and includes intraabdominal cancers, particularly hepatocellular carcinoma. As is often the case in those affected by various thrombotic disorders, Budd-Chiari syndrome frequently occurs in patients with several risk factors, such as pregnancy or oral contraceptive use combined with an underlying thrombophilic disorder.

> #### MORPHOLOGY
>
> In Budd-Chiari syndrome, the liver is swollen and red-purple and has a tense capsule (Fig. 14.34). There may be areas of hemorrhagic collapse alternating with areas of preserved or regenerating parenchyma, depending on which small and large hepatic veins are obstructed. Microscopically, the affected hepatic parenchyma reveals severe centrilobular congestion and necrosis. Centrilobular fibrosis develops in instances in which the thrombosis is more slowly developing. The major veins may contain fresh occlusive thrombi or, in chronic cases, organized adherent thrombi.

The mortality of untreated acute hepatic vein thrombosis is high. The condition is rare and treatments are largely empiric. They include

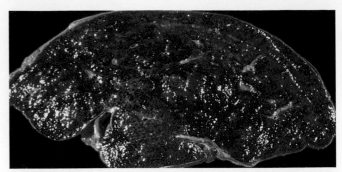

FIG. 14.34 Budd-Chiari syndrome. Thrombosis of the major hepatic veins has caused severe hepatic congestion.

anticoagulation to prevent clot propagation; angioplasty to restore the patency of occluded veins; thrombolysis; and creation of portovenous shunts, using either interventional radiologic approaches or surgery, in order to decompress the liver. The chronic form is far less lethal, and more than two-thirds of patients are alive after 5 years.

Passive Congestion and Centrilobular Necrosis

These hepatic manifestations of systemic circulatory compromise—passive congestion and centrilobular necrosis—are considered together because they represent a morphologic continuum. Both changes are commonly seen at autopsy, as there is an element of preterminal circulatory failure in virtually every nontraumatic death.

> #### MORPHOLOGY
>
> Passive congestion of the liver results from right-sided cardiac decompensation. The liver is slightly enlarged, tense, and cyanotic, with rounded edges. Microscopically there is congestion of **centrilobular sinusoids.** With time, centrilobular hepatocytes become atrophic, resulting in markedly attenuated liver cell plates. Left-sided cardiac failure or shock may lead to hepatic hypoperfusion and hypoxia, causing ischemic coagulative necrosis of hepatocytes in the central region of the lobule **(centrilobular necrosis).**
>
> The combination of hypoperfusion and retrograde congestion acts synergistically to cause **centrilobular hemorrhagic necrosis.** The liver takes on a variegated mottled appearance, reflecting hemorrhage and necrosis in the centrilobular regions (Fig. 14.35A). This finding is known as **nutmeg liver** due to its resemblance to the cut surface of a nutmeg. There is typically a sharp demarcation between viable periportal and necrotic or atrophic pericentral regions that are suffused with blood (see Fig. 14.35B). Uncommonly, with sustained chronic severe congestive heart failure, centrilobular fibrosis **(cardiac sclerosis),** or even cirrhosis, develops.

NODULES AND TUMORS

Hepatic masses come to attention for a variety of reasons. They may generate epigastric fullness and discomfort or be detected by routine physical examination or radiographic studies for other indications. Hepatic masses include nodular hyperplasias and true neoplasms.

Focal Nodular Hyperplasia

The term *focal nodular hyperplasia* (FNH) refers to solitary or multiple hyperplastic hepatocellular nodules that may develop in the noncirrhotic liver. FNH is thought to result from abnormally low vascular perfusion of a part of the liver, causing scarring and compensatory

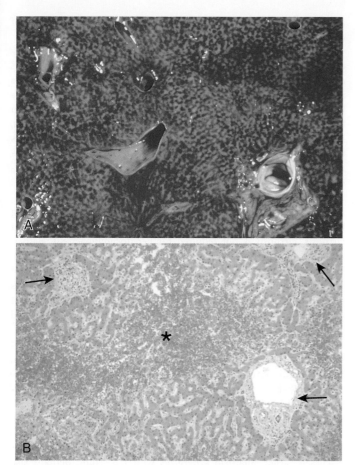

FIG. 14.35 Passive congestion ("nutmeg liver"). (A) The cut liver section, in which major blood vessels are visible, is notable for a variegated mottled red appearance, representing congestion and hemorrhage in the centrilobular regions of the parenchyma. (B) On microscopic examination, the centrilobular region *(asterisk)* is suffused with red blood cells, and atrophied hepatocytes are not easily seen. Portal tracts *(arrows)* and the periportal parenchyma are intact.

hyperperfusion, resulting in hyperplasia of surviving hepatocytes. The blood vessels in the center of the nodules are atypical and the likely basis of the hypoperfusion. It is possible that FNH is the result of a primary congenital vascular anomaly; supporting this idea, it is frequently associated with two congenital disorders of blood vessels, hereditary hemorrhagic telangiectasia and hepatic hemangioma.

MORPHOLOGY

Focal nodular hyperplasia appears as a well-demarcated, poorly encapsulated nodule that may be many centimeters in diameter (Fig. 14.36A). It presents as a mass lesion in an otherwise normal liver, most frequently in young to middle-age adults. Typically, there is a central gray-white, depressed stellate scar from which fibrous septa radiate to the periphery (Fig. 14.36B).

Microscopically, the central scar contains large abnormal vessels and ductular reactions along the spokes of the scar.

Benign Neoplasms

Cavernous Hemangioma

This is the most common benign liver tumor (Chapter 8). The chief clinical significance of cavernous hemangiomas is that they must be distinguished radiographically or intraoperatively from metastatic tumors.

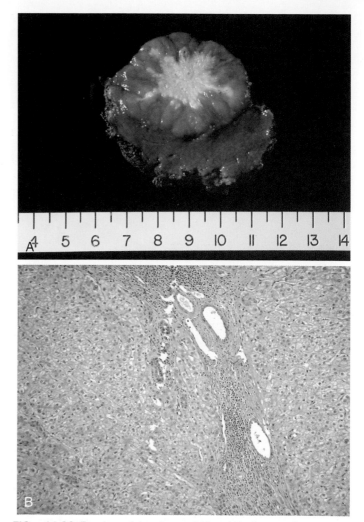

FIG. 14.36 Focal nodular hyperplasia. (A) Resected specimen showing lobulated contours and a central stellate scar. (B) Low-power photomicrograph showing a broad fibrous scar with mixed hepatic arterial and bile duct elements and chronic inflammation within hepatic parenchyma that lacks normal architecture due to hepatocyte regeneration.

Hepatocellular Adenoma

Hepatocellular adenoma (Fig. 14.37) is a benign tumor that usually arises in a noncirrhotic liver in reproductive-age women. In the past, hepatic adenoma was commonly associated with oral contraceptive use, but this cause has become less common with reduced estrogen doses; the major association now is with obesity and metabolic syndrome. Estrogens may stimulate the growth of established tumors. Driver mutations in several cancer genes have been described, including gain-of-function mutations in β-catenin. The morphology ranges from sheets of normal-appearing hepatocytes to tumors with significant cytologic atypia. They are usually asymptomatic but may cause local pain and, when large, are prone to rupture, resulting in intraabdominal bleeding. With accumulation of mutations, adenomas may undergo malignant transformation, particularly those with mutations of β-catenin. They may be detected incidentally as a hepatic mass on abdominal imaging or when they cause symptoms. The most common symptom is pain, which may be caused by pressure placed on the liver capsule by the expanding mass or hemorrhagic necrosis of the tumor as it outstrips its blood supply. Rupture of hepatocellular adenoma may lead to life-threatening intraabdominal bleeding.

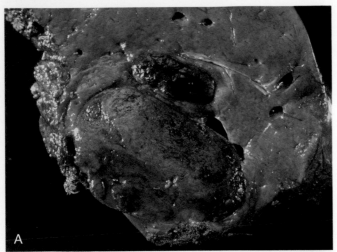

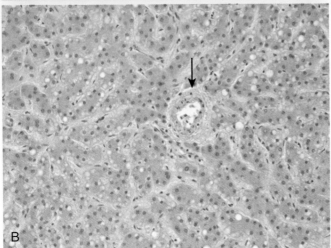

FIG. 14.37 Hepatic adenoma. (A) Resected specimen of the liver mass. (B) Microscopic view showing cords of hepatocytes, with an arterial vascular supply *(arrow)* and no portal tracts.

Malignant Neoplasms

Malignant tumors occurring in the liver can be primary or metastatic. The latter are far more common. Our discussion is focused on primary hepatic tumors. Most primary liver cancers arise from hepatocytes and are termed *hepatocellular carcinoma (HCC)*. Much less common are cancers of bile duct origin, *cholangiocarcinomas*. Other types of primary liver cancers, such as *hepatoblastoma* (a childhood hepatocellular tumor) and *angiosarcoma*, are too rare to merit further discussion here.

Hepatocellular Carcinoma (HCC)

Globally, HCC, also erroneously known as *hepatoma,* accounts for approximately 5% of all cancers, but its incidence varies widely in different parts of the world. More than 85% of cases occur in countries with high rates of chronic HBV infection. The incidence of HCC is highest in Asia (southeast China, Korea, Taiwan) and sub-Saharan Africa, areas in which HBV is transmitted vertically and, as already discussed, the carrier state starts in infancy. Moreover, many of these populations are exposed to aflatoxin, which when combined with HBV infection increases the risk for HCC dramatically. The peak incidence of HCC in these areas is between 20 and 40 years of age

and, in almost 50% of cases, the tumor appears in the absence of cirrhosis.

In Western counties, the incidence of HCC is rapidly rising, largely due to the increased prevalence of hepatitis C. The number of new HCC cases tripled in the United States in recent decades, but its incidence is still 8-fold to 30-fold lower than in countries with endemic HBV. It is hoped that new, effective treatments for hepatitis C infection will stem the rising tide of HCC in the United States. In Western populations, HCC rarely manifests before 60 years of age, and in almost 90% of cases the tumors emerge after cirrhosis becomes established. There is a pronounced male predominance throughout the world, about 3 : 1 in low-incidence areas and as high as 8 : 1 in high-incidence areas.

Pathogenesis. **Chronic liver diseases are the most common setting for emergence of HCC.** While usually identified in a background of cirrhosis, cirrhosis is not required for hepatocarcinogenesis. Rather, progression to cirrhosis and liver carcinogenesis are driven by chronic liver injury and take place in parallel. Viruses and other inducers of chronic hepatocyte injury and inflammation are not themselves oncogenic. It is believed that chronic inflammation, with its attendant growth factors and cytokines, promotes the proliferation of normal cells and predisposes to acquisition of mutations (Chapter 6).

The most important underlying factors in hepatocarcinogenesis are viral infections (HBV, HCV), toxic injuries (aflatoxin, alcohol), and increasingly NAFLD. Thus, where HBV and HCV are endemic, there is a very high incidence of HCC. Coinfection further increases risk. *Aflatoxin* is a mycotoxin produced by *Aspergillus* species that contaminates staple food crops in Africa and Asia. Aflatoxin metabolites are present in the urine of individuals who consume these foods, as are aflatoxin-albumin adducts in serum. As discussed earlier, aflatoxin synergizes with HBV (and perhaps also with HCV) to increase risk further.

Other HCC risk factors all share the ability to cause chronic liver injury associated with varying degrees of inflammation. These factors include:

- *Alcohol consumption,* which synergistically increases risk with HBV, HCV, and possibly cigarette smoking
- *Inherited disorders,* particularly hereditary hemochromatosis and α_1AT deficiency, and, to a lesser degree, Wilson disease
- *Metabolic syndrome* and its attendant obesity, diabetes, and NAFLD, all of which increase the risk for HCC. These are becoming increasingly important risk factors. It is expected that in the coming years, NAFLD will overtake HCV as a risk factor for HCC in the United States.

As with all cancers, HCC is induced by acquired mutations in oncogenes and tumor suppressor genes. No single sequence of molecular or genetic alterations leads to emergence of HCC. Among the most common are activating mutations in the β-catenin gene (40% of tumors), mutations in the *TERT* (telomerase transcriptase) gene promoter that upregulate telomerase activity (50% to 60% of tumors), and inactivating mutations in *TP53* (up to 60% of tumors). The latter are strongly associated with exposure to aflatoxin, which appears in many cases to be directly responsible for the causative *TP53* mutations.

HCC often appears to arise from premalignant precursor lesions. *Hepatic adenoma* has already been discussed, some of which carry β-catenin—activating mutations. Some HCC arise in dysplastic *nodules* (Fig. 14.38). *Low-grade dysplastic nodules* may or may not undergo transformation to higher-grade lesions, but they indicate a higher risk for HCC. *High-grade dysplastic nodules* are probably the most important precursor of HCC in viral hepatitis and alcohol-related liver

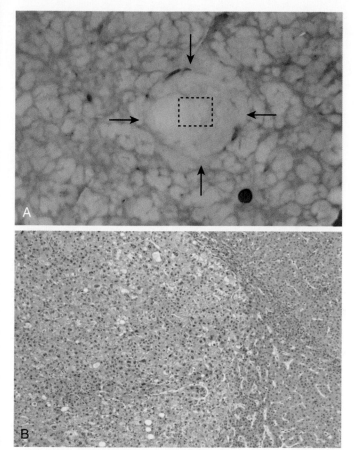

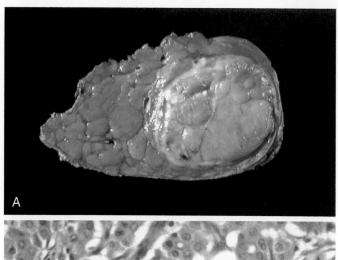

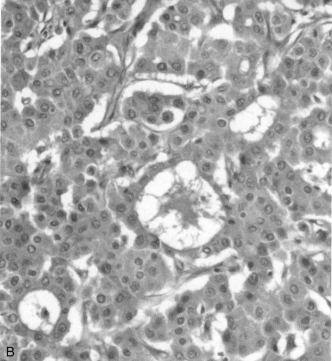

FIG. 14.38 (A) Hepatitis C—related cirrhosis with a distinct large dysplastic nodule *(arrows)*. Nodule-in-nodule growth suggests an evolving cancer. (B) Histologically the region within the box in (A) shows a well-differentiated hepatocellular carcinoma *(right side)* and a sub-nodule of moderately differentiated hepatocellular carcinoma within it *(center, left)*. (Courtesy of Dr. Masamichi Kojiro, Kurume University, Kurume, Japan.)

FIG. 14.39 Hepatocellular carcinoma. (A) Liver removed at autopsy showing a unifocal, massive neoplasm replacing most of the right hepatic lobe in a noncirrhotic liver. (B) Malignant hepatocytes growing in distorted versions of normal architecture: large pseudoacinar spaces, essentially malformed, dilated bile canaliculi, and thickened hepatocyte trabeculae.

disease. Overt HCC is often found in high-grade dysplastic nodules in biopsy or resection specimens (Fig. 14.38B).

MORPHOLOGY

HCC may appear grossly as (1) a unifocal (usually large) mass (Fig. 14.39, eFig. 14.4); **(2) multifocal, widely distributed nodules of variable size; or (3) a diffusely infiltrative cancer,** permeating widely and sometimes involving the entire liver. Sometimes HCCs arise within dysplastic nodules (Fig. 14.38B), eventually overgrowing these precursor lesions. Intrahepatic metastases by either vascular invasion or direct extension become more likely once tumors reach 3 cm in size. These metastases are usually small, satellite tumor nodules around a larger primary mass. Vascular invasion is the most likely route for extrahepatic metastasis, especially by the hepatic venous system in advanced cases. Occasionally, long, snakelike masses of tumor invade the portal vein (causing portal hypertension) or inferior vena cava; in the latter instance, the tumor may extend all the way up into the right ventricle. Lymph node metastases are less common.

HCCs range from well differentiated to highly anaplastic lesions. Well-differentiated HCCs are composed of cells that resemble normal hepatocytes and grow as thick trabeculae resembling liver cell plates or in pseudoglandular patterns that recapitulate poorly formed, ectatic bile canaliculi (see Fig. 14.39).

Clinical Features. The clinical manifestations of HCC are varied and in Western populations are often masked by symptoms related to underlying cirrhosis or chronic hepatitis. In areas of high incidence, such as tropical Africa where aflatoxin exposure is common, patients usually have no clinical history of liver disease (although cirrhosis may be detected at autopsy). In both populations, most patients have ill-defined upper abdominal pain, malaise, fatigue, weight loss, and sometimes awareness of an abdominal mass or abdominal fullness. Jaundice, fever, and gastrointestinal or esophageal variceal bleeding are occasional findings.

Laboratory studies may provide clues but are rarely conclusive. Elevated serum levels of α-fetoprotein are found in 50% of individuals with advanced HCC, but this is neither a sensitive nor a specific marker. Imaging studies, such as ultrasonography, computed tomography, and magnetic resonance imaging, are better tests for detection of small tumors. As HCC grow and progress, their increasing arterialization can be identified by imaging studies. The appearance is so characteristic that tissue biopsy may not be necessary for diagnosis.

The natural history of HCC involves progressive enlargement of the primary mass until it disturbs hepatic function or it metastasizes, most commonly to the lungs. Death usually occurs from (1) cachexia; (2) gastrointestinal or esophageal variceal bleeding; (3) liver failure with hepatic coma; or rarely (4) rupture of the tumor with fatal hemorrhage. The 5-year survival of large tumors is extremely low, and the majority of patients die within 2 years of diagnosis.

With implementation of screening procedures and advances in imaging, the detection of HCCs less than 2 cm in diameter has increased in countries where these are available. Small tumors can be removed surgically or ablated (e.g., through embolization, microwave radiation or freezing) with good outcomes. When relatively small HCCs arise in the setting of advanced (cirrhotic) liver disease, liver transplantation is a better option and may be curative. Radiofrequency ablation and chemoembolization are used for local control of unresectable tumors. The kinase inhibitor sorafenib can prolong the life of individuals with advanced-stage HCC.

Cholangiocarcinoma

Cholangiocarcinoma (CCA), the second most common primary malignant tumor of the liver after HCC, arises from intrahepatic and extrahepatic bile ducts. It accounts for 3% of gastrointestinal cancers in the United States, where there are approximately 2000 to 3000 new cases each year. However, in some regions of southeast Asia, such as northeastern Thailand, Laos, and Cambodia, where infestation with liver flukes is endemic, cholangiocarcinoma is much more common, occurring at rates 30 to 40 times higher than in areas of Asia without liver fluke infestation. Between 50% and 60% of all cholangiocarcinomas are perihilar *(Klatskin tumors),* and 20% to 30% are distal tumors, arising in the common bile duct where it lies posterior to the duodenum. The remaining 10% are intrahepatic.

All risk factors for cholangiocarcinoma cause chronic inflammation and cholestasis, which presumably promote somatic mutations or epigenetic alterations in cholangiocytes. The risk factors include infestation by liver flukes (particularly *Opisthorchis* and *Clonorchis* species), chronic inflammatory disease of the large bile ducts (such as primary sclerosing cholangitis), hepatolithiasis (intrahepatic gallstones), and fibropolycystic liver disease. As with HCC, rates of cholangiocarcinoma are also elevated in patients with hepatitis B and C and NAFLD. The prognosis is extremely poor, regardless of the site of origin: survival rates are about 15% at 2 years after diagnosis for extrahepatic tumors. For intrahepatic tumors, which are often detected at an advanced stage, the median time to death from time of diagnosis is 6 months, even following surgical treatment.

MORPHOLOGY

Extrahepatic cholangiocarcinomas are generally small lesions at the time of diagnosis, as they cause obstruction of the biliary tract early in their course. Most tumors are firm, gray nodules within the bile duct wall, which may be diffusely infiltrative. **Intrahepatic cholangiocarcinomas** occur in noncirrhotic livers (Fig. 14.40A) and may track along the intrahepatic portal tract system or produce a single large tumor.

Cholangiocarcinomas are typical mucin-producing adenocarcinomas. Most are well to moderately differentiated, growing as glandular or tubular structures lined by malignant epithelial cells (Fig. 14.40B). They typically incite marked desmoplasia. Lymphovascular invasion and perineural invasion are both common and often lead to extensive intrahepatic and extrahepatic metastases.

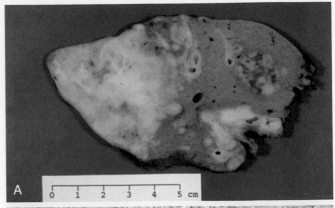

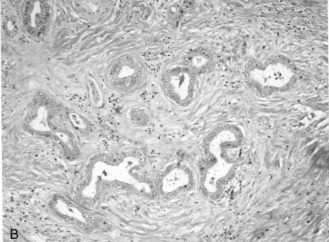

FIG. 14.40 Cholangiocarcinoma. (A) Multifocal cholangiocarcinoma in a liver from a patient with infestation by the liver fluke *Clonorchis sinensis* (flukes not visible). (B) Invasive malignant glands in a reactive, sclerotic stroma. (A, Courtesy of Dr. Wilson M.S. Tsui, Caritas Medical Centre, Hong Kong.)

GALLBLADDER

CHOLELITHIASIS (GALLSTONE DISEASE)

Gallstones afflict 10% to 20% of adults residing in the United States, Canada, and Europe, 20% to 40% in Latin American countries, and only 3% to 4% in Asian countries. In the United States, about 1 million new cases of gallstones are diagnosed annually, and two-thirds of affected individuals undergo surgery, resulting in the removal of as much as 25 to 50 tons of stones per year! There are two main types of gallstones: *cholesterol stones,* containing crystalline cholesterol monohydrate (80% of stones in United States, Canada, Europe), and *pigment stones,* made of bilirubin calcium salts. Cholesterol gallstones are more prevalent in the United States and Western Europe (90%) and uncommon in low income countries. The prevalence rates of cholesterol gallstones approach 50% in Native Americans of the Pima, Hopi, and Navajo groups. Pigment gallstones, the predominant type of gallstone in non-Western populations, arise primarily in individuals with diseases that lead to chronic red cell hemolysis.

Prevalence and Risk Factors. The major risk factors for gallstones are listed in Table 14.6. Some elaboration on these risk factors follows:
- *Age and sex.* In up to 80% of individuals with gallstones, the only identifiable risk factors are age and sex. The prevalence of

Table 14.6 Risk Factors for Gallstones

Cholesterol Stones
Advancing age
Female sex hormones
Female sex
Oral contraceptives
Pregnancy
Obesity and insulin resistance
Rapid weight reduction
Gallbladder stasis
Inborn disorders of bile acid metabolism
Dyslipidemia syndromes

Pigment Stones
Chronic hemolysis (e.g., sickle cell anemia, hereditary spherocytosis)
Biliary infection
Gastrointestinal disorders: ileal disease (e.g., Crohn disease), ileal resection or bypass, cystic fibrosis with pancreatic insufficiency

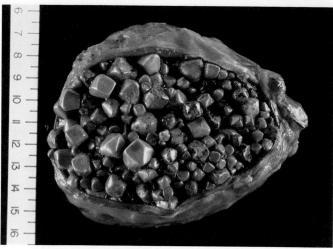

FIG. 14.41 Cholesterol gallstones. The wall of the gallbladder is thickened and fibrotic due to chronic cholecystitis.

gallstones increases throughout life. In the United States, less than 5% to 6% of the population younger than 40 years of age have stones, in contrast with 25% to 30% of those older than 80 years of age. The prevalence in women of all ages is about twice as high as in men.

- *Heredity.* A positive family history imparts increased risk, as do a variety of inborn errors of metabolism, such as those associated with impaired bile salt synthesis and secretion. Studies of twins suggest that approximately 25% of the risk of cholelithiasis is determined by an underlying genetic predisposition.
- *Environment.* Estrogens increase hepatic cholesterol uptake and synthesis, leading to excess biliary secretion of cholesterol. These effects explain the increased risk for gallstone disease with oral contraceptive use and with pregnancy. Obesity, metabolic syndrome, and rapid weight loss are also strongly associated with increased biliary cholesterol secretion and risk for gallstone disease.
- *Gallbladder hypomotility.* Any setting in which gallbladder motility is reduced predisposes to gallstones, such as pregnancy, rapid weight loss, and spinal cord injury. In most cases, however, gallbladder hypomotility is without obvious cause.

Pathogenesis. Pathogenesis of the two main forms of gallstones differs and so will be discussed separately:

- *Cholesterol stones.* Bile formation is the only significant pathway for elimination of excess cholesterol from the body, either as free cholesterol or as bile salts. Cholesterol is rendered water soluble by aggregation with bile salts and lecithins. When cholesterol concentrations exceed the solubilizing capacity of bile (supersaturation), cholesterol can no longer remain dispersed and crystallizes out of solution. Cholesterol gallstone formation is enhanced by *hypomobility of the gallbladder* (stasis), which promotes crystal nucleation, and by *mucus hypersecretion,* which traps crystals, thereby enhancing their aggregation into stones.
- *Pigment stones* are made up of insoluble calcium bilirubinate salts. They form when bile contains a high concentration of unconjugated bilirubin, as may occur in patients with chronic red cell hemolysis or with certain infections of the biliary tract, such as liver flukes. Cirrhosis and Crohn disease are also associated with pigment gallstones. In cirrhosis, reduced bile salt synthesis hinders solubilization of bilirubin. In Crohn disease, there is increased

concentration of bilirubin likely due to altered enterohepatic cycling of bilirubin.

MORPHOLOGY

Cholesterol stones arise exclusively in the gallbladder and consist of 50% to 100% cholesterol. Pure cholesterol stones are pale yellow; increasing proportions of calcium carbonate, phosphates, and bilirubin impart gray-white to black discoloration (Fig. 14.41). They are ovoid and firm; they can occur singly, but most often are several, with faceted surfaces resulting from their apposition (eFig. 14.5). Most cholesterol stones are radiolucent, although as many as 20% may contain sufficient calcium carbonate to be radiopaque.

Pigment stones may arise anywhere in the biliary tree and are classified into black and brown stones. In general, black pigment stones are found in sterile gallbladder bile, while brown stones are found in infected intrahepatic or extrahepatic ducts. The stones contain calcium salts of unconjugated bilirubin and lesser amounts of other calcium salts, mucin glycoproteins, and cholesterol. Black stones are usually small, numerous, and fragile to the touch (Fig. 14.42). Brown stones tend to be single or few in number and to have a soft, greasy, soaplike consistency due to the presence of fatty acid salts released from biliary lecithins by bacterial phospholipases. Because of calcium carbonates and phosphates, 50% to 75% of black stones are radiopaque. Brown stones, which contain calcium soaps, are radiolucent.

Clinical Features. Gallstones may be asymptomatic for decades, and 70% to 80% of individuals with gallstones never develop symptoms. In a minority of individuals, however, the clinical manifestations are striking: there is usually right upper quadrant or epigastric pain, often excruciating, which may be constant or, less commonly, spasmodic. Such "biliary colic" is caused by gallbladder or biliary tree obstruction or by inflammation of the gallbladder itself.

Pain often follows a fatty meal that induces gallbladder contraction, which presses a stone against the gallbladder outlet, leading to increased pressure and eventually pain. More severe complications include empyema, perforation, fistulas, inflammation of the biliary tree, cholestasis, and pancreatitis. The larger the stone, the less likely it is to enter the cystic or common ducts to produce obstruction; thus,

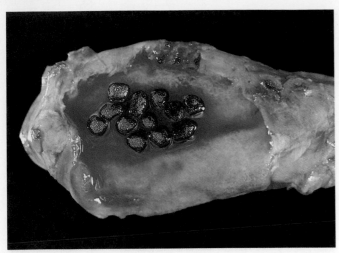

FIG. 14.42 Pigment gallstones. Several faceted black gallstones are present in this otherwise unremarkable gallbladder from a patient with a mechanical mitral valve prosthesis, leading to chronic hemolysis.

the very small stones, or "gravel," are more dangerous. Occasionally a large stone may erode directly into an adjacent loop of small bowel, generating intestinal obstruction (*gallstone ileus*). Gallstones are also an important risk factor for carcinoma of the gallbladder (discussed later).

CHOLECYSTITIS

Inflammation of the gallbladder may be acute, chronic, or acute superimposed on chronic and almost always occurs in association with gallstones. In the United States, cholecystitis is one of the most common indications for abdominal surgery. Its epidemiologic distribution closely parallels that of gallstones.

Acute Calculous Cholecystitis

Acute inflammation of a gallbladder that contains stones is termed *acute calculous cholecystitis* **and is precipitated in 90% of cases by obstruction of the gallbladder neck or cystic duct by a stone.** It is the most common major complication of gallstones and the most frequent indication for emergency cholecystectomy. Manifestations of obstruction may appear with remarkable suddenness and constitute a surgical emergency. In some cases, however, symptoms may be mild and resolve without intervention.

Acute calculous cholecystitis initially results from chemical irritation and inflammation of the gallbladder wall due to obstruction of bile outflow. Gallbladder injury in the setting of bile obstruction stems from several sources: phospholipases derived from the mucosa hydrolyze biliary lecithin to lysolecithin, which is toxic to the mucosa; the normally protective glycoprotein mucous layer is disrupted, exposing the mucosal epithelium to the detergent action of bile salts; prostaglandins released within the wall of the distended gallbladder enhance mucosal and mural inflammation; and distention and increased intraluminal pressure may compromise blood flow to the mucosa, leading to ischemia. All of these effects occur in the absence of bacterial infection, which may be superimposed later.

Acute Acalculous Cholecystitis

Between 5% and 12% of gallbladders removed for acute cholecystitis contain no gallstones. Acute acalculous cholecystitis is thought to result from gallbladder stasis and ischemia leading to a local

inflammatory response. Most cases occur in seriously ill patients. Some of the most common predisposing insults are as follows:

- *Major surgery*
- *Severe trauma* (e.g., from motor vehicle crashes)
- *Severe burns*
- *Sepsis*

The mortality rate from acute acalculous cholecystitis is high because of the associated conditions.

Chronic Cholecystitis

Chronic cholecystitis may become evident after repeated bouts of acute cholecystitis, but in most instances, it develops without an antecedent history of acute attacks. Like acute cholecystitis, it is almost always associated with gallstones. However, gallstones do not seem to be an essential part of the initiation of inflammation or the development of pain, because chronic acalculous cholecystitis causes symptoms and morphologic alterations similar to those seen in the calculous form. Rather, supersaturation of bile appears to predispose to both chronic inflammation and, in most instances, stone formation. Microorganisms, usually *E. coli* and enterococci, can be cultured from the bile in about one-third of cases.

> **MORPHOLOGY**
>
> In **acute cholecystitis,** the gallbladder is usually enlarged and tense and has a bright red or blotchy, violaceous color, the latter imparted by subserosal hemorrhages. The serosa is frequently covered by a fibrinous or, in severe cases, a fibrinopurulent exudate. In 90% of cases, stones are present, often obstructing the neck of the gallbladder or the cystic duct. The gallbladder lumen is filled with cloudy or turbid bile that may contain fibrin, blood, and pus. When the contained exudate is mostly pus, the condition is referred to as **empyema of the gallbladder.** In mild cases, the gallbladder wall is thickened, edematous, and hyperemic. In more severe cases, the gallbladder wall is green-black and necrotic—a condition termed **gangrenous cholecystitis.** On histologic examination, the inflammatory reactions are not distinctive and consist of some combination of the usual patterns of acute inflammation (i.e., edema, leukocytic infiltration, vascular congestion, abscess formation, gangrenous necrosis).
>
> The morphologic changes in **chronic cholecystitis** are extremely variable and sometimes subtle. The gallbladder may be contracted, of normal size, or enlarged. There is marked subepithelial and subserosal fibrosis. In the absence of superimposed acute cholecystitis, collections of lymphocytes in the wall are the only sign of inflammation (Fig. 14.43A). Outpouchings of mucosal epithelium through the wall of the gallbladder (**Rokitansky-Aschoff sinuses**) may be quite prominent (Fig. 14.43B).

Clinical Features. Acute calculous cholecystitis usually presents with steady, severe, upper abdominal pain that often radiates to the right shoulder. Fever, nausea, leukocytosis, and extreme weakness are commonly present. The right subcostal region is markedly painful and rigid as a result of abdominal muscle spasm; occasionally a tender, distended gallbladder can be palpated. Mild attacks usually subside spontaneously over 1 to 10 days; however, recurrence is common. Approximately 25% of symptomatic patients are sufficiently ill to require surgical intervention.

The diagnosis of acute cholecystitis is usually based on the detection of gallstones by ultrasonography, typically accompanied by evidence of a thickened gallbladder wall. Attention to this disorder is important because of the potential for serious complications including:

- *Bacterial superinfection* leading to cholangitis or sepsis

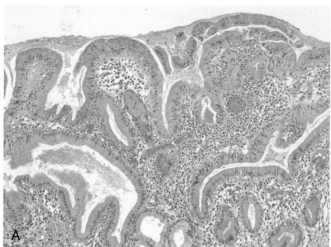
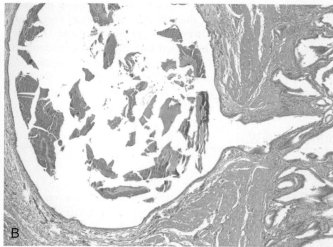

FIG. 14.43 Chronic cholecystitis. (A) The gallbladder mucosa is infiltrated by chronic inflammatory cells. (B) A Rokitansky-Aschoff sinus containing a fragmented bile pigment stone.

- *Gallbladder perforation* leading to local abscess formation or diffuse peritonitis
- *Biliary enteric (cholecystoenteric) fistula*, with drainage of bile into adjacent organs, entry of air and bacteria into the biliary tree, and potentially gallstone-induced intestinal obstruction (ileus)

Symptoms arising from *acute acalculous cholecystitis* are usually obscured by another serious medical or surgical condition, which sets the stage for the development of cholecystitis. The diagnosis therefore rests on a high index of suspicion. *Chronic cholecystitis* lacks the striking manifestations of the acute forms and is usually characterized by recurrent attacks of epigastric or right upper quadrant pain. Nausea, vomiting, and intolerance for fatty foods are frequent accompaniments. Chronic cholecystitis is a pathologic diagnosis based on examination of the resected gallbladder. Beyond signs and symptoms mentioned above, its principal importance may lie in the association of gallstones and chronic inflammation with carcinoma of the gallbladder (discussed next).

CARCINOMA OF THE GALLBLADDER

Carcinoma of the gallbladder is the most common malignancy of the extrahepatic biliary tract. It is slightly more common in women and occurs most frequently in the seventh decade of life. Approximately 5000 cases are diagnosed annually in the United States. Only rarely is it discovered at a resectable stage, and the mean 5-year survival rate has remained unchanged at about 5% to 12% over many years. Risk factors for development of gallbladder cancers include:

- *Gallstones* are present in 95% of cases of gallbladder carcinoma and are thus the most important risk factor associated with this tumor. Presumably, gallbladders containing stones develop cancer as a result of chronic inflammation, a known enabler of malignancy in several organs (Chapter 6).
- *Carcinogenic derivatives of bile acids* are also suspected to play a role.
- *Primary sclerosing cholangitis* may predispose to the occurrence of gallbladder cancer.

MORPHOLOGY

Carcinomas of the gallbladder show two patterns of growth: **infiltrating** and **exophytic.** The infiltrating pattern is more common and usually appears as a poorly defined area of diffuse wall thickening and induration. The exophytic pattern grows into the lumen as an irregular, exophytic mass, that at the same time invades the underlying wall (Fig. 14.44). Most carcinomas of the gallbladder are adenocarcinomas. About 5% are squamous cell carcinomas or have adenosquamous differentiation.

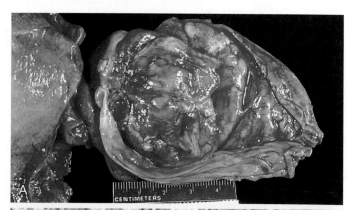
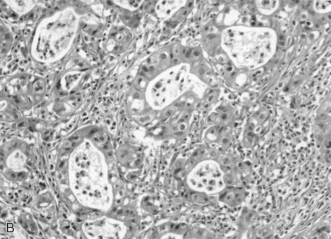

FIG. 14.44 Gallbladder adenocarcinoma. (A) The opened gallbladder contains a large, exophytic tumor that virtually fills the lumen. (B) Microscopically, the tumor shows glandular differentiation along with inflammation.

Clinical Features. Preoperative diagnosis of carcinoma of the gallbladder is the exception rather than the rule, occurring in fewer than 20% of patients. Presenting symptoms are insidious and typically indistinguishable from those associated with cholelithiasis: abdominal pain, jaundice, anorexia, nausea, and vomiting. There is no satisfactory treatment of gallbladder cancer due to the advanced stage at the time of diagnosis. Only 10% of cases are diagnosed at a stage that is early enough to attempt curative surgery.

■ RAPID REVIEW

Liver Failure

- Liver failure may follow acute injury or chronic injury, or it may occur as an acute insult superimposed on otherwise well-compensated chronic liver disease.
- The causes of acute liver failure are the following:
  - Drugs—acetaminophen
  - Hepatitis A, B, C, D, and E
  - Autoimmune hepatitis
  - Wilson disease, Budd-Chiari syndrome
- Potentially fatal sequelae of liver failure include coagulopathy, encephalopathy, portal hypertension and ascites, hepatorenal syndrome, and portopulmonary hypertension.

Viral Hepatitis

- Clinically hepatitis viruses have the following features:
  - Hepatitis A and E cause acute but not chronic hepatitis.
  - Hepatitis B, C, D have the potential to cause chronic disease.
  - Hepatitis B can be transmitted by blood, birthing, and by sexual intercourse.
  - Hepatitis C is the single virus that is more often chronic than not (almost never detected acutely; 85% or more of patients develop chronic hepatitis, 20% of whom develop cirrhosis).
  - Hepatitis D, the delta agent, is a defective virus, requiring hepatitis B coinfection for its own capacity to infect and replicate.
  - Hepatitis E is endemic in equatorial regions and frequently epidemic. High mortality rate in pregnant women.
- The inflammatory cells that cause hepatocyte injury in both acute and chronic viral hepatitis are mainly cytotoxic T cells.
- Diagnosis is based on detection of viral antigens and specific antibodies in the blood.
- Patients with long-standing HBV or HCV infections are at increased risk for development of hepatocellular carcinoma.

Autoimmune Hepatitis

- Diagnosis is based on a combination of four features: autoantibodies, elevated serum IgG, pathologic findings, and exclusion of viral/drug etiologies.
- The most common autoantibodies in type 1 autoimmune hepatitis are antinuclear antibodies (ANAs) and antismooth muscle antibodies (ASMAs), while type 2 autoimmune hepatitis is characterized by anti-LKM1 (liver kidney microsome type 1) autoantibodies.
- Autoimmune hepatitis can have varied presentations: asymptomatic liver enzyme elevation, acute liver failure, chronic hepatitis, and cirrhosis.
- Typical histologic features of autoimmune hepatitis include hepatocyte necrosis, variable inflammation, and numerous plasma cells.

Alcohol-Related Liver Disease

- Alcohol-related liver disease is a chronic disorder that can give rise to steatosis, steatohepatitis, progressive fibrosis, and marked derangement of vascular perfusion leading eventually to cirrhosis.
- Consumption of 80 g/day of alcohol is considered to be the threshold for development of alcohol-related liver disease but may be lower in women.
- It may take 10 to 15 years of chronic excess drinking for development of cirrhosis, which occurs only in a small proportion of these individuals.
- The pathologic effects of alcohol on hepatocytes include changes in lipid metabolism related to altered redox potential, injury caused by ROS generated by metabolism of alcohol by the P450 system, and protein adducts formed by acetaldehyde, a major metabolite of alcohol.

Nonalcoholic Fatty Liver Disease

- Nonalcoholic fatty liver disease (NAFLD) is associated with the metabolic syndrome, obesity, type 2 diabetes, and dyslipidemia and/or hypertension.
- NAFLD may show all the changes associated with alcohol-related liver disease: steatosis, nonalcoholic steatohepatitis (NASH), and cirrhosis, although the features of steatohepatitis (such as hepatocyte ballooning, Mallory hyaline bodies, and neutrophilic infiltration) are often less prominent than they are in alcohol-related injury.
- NAFLD is a risk factor for development of hepatocellular carcinoma.
- Pediatric NAFLD is increasingly being recognized as the obesity epidemic spreads to pediatric age groups, although its histologic pattern differs somewhat from that seen in adults.

Inherited Metabolic Liver Disease

- Hemochromatosis is most commonly caused by mutations in the *HFE* gene and less commonly by mutations in other genes, all of which result in decreased hepcidin levels or function and increased intestinal iron uptake. It is characterized by accumulation of iron in the liver, pancreas, and other tissues.
- Wilson disease is caused by loss-of-function mutations in the metal ion transporter ATP7B, which results in accumulation of copper in the liver, brain (particularly basal ganglia), and eyes (Kayser-Fleischer rings). Wilson disease effects on the liver are protean, ranging from acute massive hepatic necrosis, to fatty liver disease, to chronic hepatitis and cirrhosis.
- α_1AT deficiency is a disease in which mutations in α_1AT lead to its misfolding, causing liver toxicity and a functional deficit of α_1AT in the plasma. This deficiency places affected individuals at high risk for emphysema, particularly individuals who smoke, due to the unopposed effects of proteases released from neutrophils.

Cholestatic Diseases

- Cholestasis occurs with impaired excretion of bile, leading to jaundice and accumulation of bile pigment in the hepatic parenchyma. Causes include mechanical or inflammatory obstruction or destruction of the bile ducts or metabolic defects in hepatocyte bile secretion.
- Large bile duct obstruction is most commonly associated with gallstones and malignancies involving the head of the pancreas. Chronic obstruction can lead to cirrhosis.

- Neonatal cholestasis is not a specific entity; it is variously associated with cholangiopathies such as *biliary atresia* and a variety of disorders causing conjugated hyperbilirubinemia in the neonate, collectively referred to as *neonatal hepatitis*.
- Primary biliary cholangitis is an autoimmune disease with progressive, inflammatory, often granulomatous, destruction of small to medium intrahepatic bile ducts. It most often occurs in middle-age women and is associated with antimitochondrial antibodies and often with other autoimmune diseases, such as Sjögren syndrome and Hashimoto thyroiditis.
- Primary sclerosing cholangitis is an autoimmune disease with progressive inflammatory and sclerosing destruction of intrahepatic and extrahepatic bile ducts of all sizes. Diagnosis is made by radiologic imaging of the biliary tree. It most often occurs in younger men and has a strong association with inflammatory bowel disease, particularly ulcerative colitis.

Circulatory Disorders

- Circulatory disorders of the liver can be caused by impaired blood inflow, defects in intrahepatic blood flow, and obstruction of blood outflow.
- Portal vein obstruction by intrahepatic or extrahepatic thrombosis may cause portal hypertension, esophageal varices, and ascites.
- The most common cause of impaired intrahepatic blood flow is cirrhosis.
- Obstructions of blood outflow include hepatic vein thrombosis (Budd-Chiari syndrome) and sinusoidal obstruction syndrome (*veno-occlusive disease*).
- Right-sided cardiac failure causes passive venous congestion of the liver characterized by centrilobular congestion and if cardiac failure is severe, then centrilobular hemorrhagic necrosis. Grossly, seen as nutmeg liver.

Liver Tumors

- The liver is the most common site of metastatic cancers from primary tumors of the colon, lung, and breast.
- Hepatic adenomas are benign tumors of hepatocytes. Most can be subclassified on the basis of molecular changes with varying degrees of malignant potential. They are associated with use of oral contraceptives and androgens.

- The two main types of malignant tumors are hepatocellular carcinomas (HCCs) and cholangiocarcinomas; HCCs are much more common.
  - HCC is a common tumor in regions of Asia and Africa, and its incidence is increasing in the United States.
  - The main etiologic agents for HCC are hepatitis B and C, alcohol-related cirrhosis, nonalcoholic fatty liver disease, hemochromatosis, and exposure to aflatoxins. In the United States, Canada, and Europe, about 90% of HCCs develop in cirrhotic livers; in Asia, almost 50% of cases develop in noncirrhotic livers.
  - The chronic inflammation and cellular regeneration associated with liver cell injury are predisposing factors for the development of carcinomas.
  - HCC may be unifocal or multifocal, tends to invade blood vessels, and recapitulates normal liver architecture to varying degrees. They are associated with mutations in the beta-catenin gene and the telomerase gene.
  - Cholangiocarcinoma is a tumor of intrahepatic or extrahepatic bile ducts that is relatively common in areas where liver flukes, such as *Opisthorchis* and *Clonorchis* species, are endemic.

Gallbladder Diseases

- Gallbladder diseases include cholelithiasis, acute and chronic cholecystitis, and gallbladder carcinoma.
- Gallstone formation is a common condition in the United States, Canada, and Europe. The great majority of the gallstones are cholesterol stones caused by supersaturation of cholesterol in bile. Pigmented stones containing bilirubin and calcium are most common in Asian countries due to the higher incidence of chronic hemolytic disorders and liver fluke infestations in these locales.
- Risk factors for the development of cholesterol stones are advancing age, female sex, estrogen use, obesity, and heredity.
- Cholecystitis almost always occurs in association with cholelithiasis, although in about 10% of cases it occurs in the absence of gallstones.
- Acute calculous cholecystitis is the most common reason for emergency cholecystectomy.
- Gallbladder carcinoma is almost always associated with gallstones. Because of the advanced stage at diagnosis, it has a very poor prognosis.

■ Laboratory Tests[a]

Test	Reference Values	Pathophysiology/Clinical Relevance
α_1-antitrypsin (AAT), serum	100–190 mg/dL	Alpha-1 antitrypsin (AAT) is produced by hepatocytes and inhibits neutrophil serine proteases, most notably neutrophil elastase. AAT deficiency is caused by mutations that result in misfolding of the protein and its accumulation in the liver. Consequent low serum levels of AAT in lung alveolar cells render them vulnerable to destructive proteases, thereby increasing risk for emphysema. AAT serum measurements and protease inhibitor (Pi) genotyping are important parts of the diagnostic workup for symptomatic patients. PiZZ type is the most common clinically relevant form with loss of up to 90% serum AAT.
Alanine aminotransferase (ALT) Aspartate aminotransferase (AST), serum	ALT: Males: 7–55 U/L Females: 7–45 U/L AST: Males: 8–48 U/L Females: 8–43 U/L	ALT and AST are enzymes normally present in the cytoplasm of hepatocytes. AST is also present in mitochondria. With plasma membrane injury, both are released into the blood. ALT is more specific for liver injury and remains elevated longer than AST. In inflammatory liver diseases, ALT levels are usually equal to or higher than that of AST, resulting in an ALT : AST ratio of more than 1. Compared to ALT, AST is elevated to a greater extent in liver diseases secondary to alcohol-related injury because alcohol causes mitochondrial damage; typically, the AST: ALT ratio is >2 : 1. In end-stage cirrhosis both enzymes may be low due to loss of hepatocytes.

Alkaline phosphatase (AP), serum	Varies with age and sex Adult males: 40–129 U/L Adult females: 35–104 U/L	AP is an enzyme from the cellular membrane. The major isoenzymes are liver, bone, and placental. In nonpregnant adults, the liver isoenzyme is predominant. Intestinal AP increases after meals. AP is a sensitive marker for biliary disease (e.g., biliary obstruction, primary sclerosing cholangitis) or metastasis to the liver. Other causes of increased AP include chronic inflammatory conditions (e.g., sarcoidosis, ulcerative colitis), sepsis and, in older patients, Paget disease.
Alphafetoprotein (AFP), serum	<8.4 ng/mL	AFP is synthesized during development by embryonic hepatocytes and fetal yolk sac cells and after birth by some tumors. It is increased in ~70% of patients with hepatocellular carcinoma (HCC); the assay lacks sensitivity and specificity for diagnosis of HCC but is useful in monitoring response to treatment and detecting recurrences. AFP is increased in certain germ cell tumors of the ovary and testis and in maternal serum in the setting of open neural tube defects (e.g., anencephaly, spina bifida).
Antismooth muscle antibody (ASMA), serum	Negative	ASMAs are associated with autoimmune hepatitis (AIH), though their role in pathogenesis is unknown. ASMAs are positive in approximately 50% of patients with type I autoimmune hepatitis. ANAs may also be present in AIH but ASMA is more specific than ANA for AIH. ASMA (and ANA) levels may fluctuate during treatment and may disappear with corticosteroid therapy. Antibody titer does not predict outcome.
Bilirubin (total, direct and indirect), serum	Total bilirubin Varies with age Adults: ≤1.2 mg/dL Direct 0.0–0.3 mg/dL	Bilirubin is the principal pigment in bile and 80% is derived from breakdown of aged red blood cells; the remaining 20% is derived from destruction of heme-containing proteins (e.g., myoglobin, cytochromes) and from heme catabolism. Total bilirubin is the sum of direct (conjugated) bilirubin, which is water soluble and excreted in urine, and indirect (unconjugated) bilirubin, which is not water soluble. Conjugated hyperbilirubinemia results in dark urine and is indicative of hepatobiliary disease. Unconjugated hyperbilirubinemia may be due to increased production (e.g., hemolytic anemia), impaired hepatic uptake, or decreased conjugation. Neonates are at risk for kernicterus (brain injury due to hyperbilirubinemia caused by hemolytic disease of the newborn).
Ceruloplasmin, serum	Varies with age and sex Adult males: 19.0–31.0 mg/dL Adult females: 20.0–51.0 mg/dL	Ceruloplasmin is an acute-phase reactant synthesized by the liver and is the primary (95%) copper-carrying protein in the blood. In Wilson disease, a mutation in the *ATP7B* gene results in decreased copper transport into bile, decreased incorporation into ceruloplasmin, and decreased ceruloplasmin secretion into blood. The resulting copper accumulation in tissues, particularly the liver, brain, and eye, causes toxic injury. Pathologic effects of excess copper include cirrhosis, neuropsychiatric symptoms, hematuria/proteinuria, and Kayser-Fleischer rings in the limbus of cornea.
Gamma-glutamyltranspeptidase (GGT), serum	Adult males: 8–61 U/L Adult females: 5–36 U/L	GGT is present in multiple tissues including liver, kidney, and pancreas. The highest levels of GGT elevations are seen in intra- and posthepatic biliary obstruction; moderate levels are less specific and can be seen in all types of liver disease (e.g., alcohol-related hepatitis) and with some medications (e.g., anticonvulsants, oral contraceptives). Combined elevations of alkaline phosphatase and GGT suggest biliary tract disease.
Hepatitis Tests		
Hepatitis A virus (HAV) IgM antibody, serum	Negative	IgM antibodies directed against HAV (IgM anti-HAV) are produced at the onset of symptoms or a few days before the onset; levels decline after 3–6 months and become undetectable. The presence of IgM anti-HAV is used to diagnose acute infection with HAV.
Hepatitis A virus IgG antibody, serum	Negative	IgG antibodies directed against HAV (IgG anti-HAV) are produced at the onset of clinical symptoms. These antibodies persist and provide immunity for the patient's lifetime. IgG anti-HAV are produced by either acute infection with hepatitis A or through immunization.
Hepatitis A virus polymerase chain reaction (PCR), serum	Negative	PCR can be used to detect HAV RNA during the viremic period, shortly after infection until ALT levels decline. This test is not as commonly used as serologic tests for diagnosis but is useful in assessing outbreaks or response to therapy.

Hepatitis B virus (HBV) core antibody, IgM, serum	Negative	Antibodies to the hepatitis B core (HBc-Ab or Anti-HBc) are produced only when the patient has been naturally infected with hepatitis B. Anti-HBc IgM is produced during acute infection and decreases after a few months, regardless of whether the infection is acute and resolves or remains chronic. A positive test for IgM indicates recent infection. Anti-HBc IgM may be the only serologic test that is positive once HBV surface antigen declines and before the appearance of HBV surface antibody ("serologic window period").
Hepatitis B virus e-antibody (HBeAb), serum	Negative	HBeAb is seen in patients recovering from acute hepatitis and is typically present before the HBsAg to HBsAb conversion. As HBeAb increases, HBeAg decreases. HBeAb is a sign of resolving acute hepatitis. HBeAb are produced in patients who have been naturally infected with hepatitis B and are absent in individuals who have been vaccinated.
Hepatitis B virus surface antibody (HBsAb), serum	Negative	Levels typically increase with resolution of acute hepatitis and falling HBsAg; however, in some patients, HBsAb is not detectable for months after HBsAg disappears; in such patients, diagnosis can be confirmed by detecting IgM against the HB core protein. HBsAb is present in naturally infected individuals as well as immunized persons.
Hepatitis B virus surface antigen (HBsAg), serum	Negative	HBsAg is the first serologic marker to be detectable, even before a patient is symptomatic, typically 6 to 16 weeks after HBV infection. With resolution of acute hepatitis, HBsAg disappears about 12 weeks after symptom onset.
Hepatitis B virus (HBV) core (HBc) total antibodies, serum	Negative	Antibodies to HBc can be detected soon after symptom onset and after antibodies to HBV surface antigen are present. Initial antibodies are IgM, followed by IgG. Total Anti-HBc antibody is a measure of both IgM and IgG.
Hepatitis B virus (HBV) DNA PCR, serum	Negative	HBV DNA is detectable by 30 days after infection, about 3 weeks before HBsAg appears, peaks with acute hepatitis, and slowly declines with resolution of infection. Although serologic methods are the primary means of diagnosis in acute HBV infection, HBV DNA PCR is useful for the diagnosis of early infection, prior to appearance of HBsAg; differentiating between active and inactive HBV infection; and monitoring response to anti-HBV treatment.
Hepatitis B virus (HBV) e-antigen (HBe-Ag), serum	Negative	The hepatitis B e-antigen (HBeAg) is a secretory protein that is seen with active viral replication. HBeAg can be detected soon after HBV surface antigen appears. Persistence of HBeAg is an indicator of progression to chronic hepatitis. The appearance of anti-HBe antibodies implies that an acute infection has peaked and is resolving.
Hepatitis C virus (HCV) antibody screen, serum	Negative	IgG antibodies to HCV are generally not detectable for the first 2 months after infection but are usually seen by 6 months. Delay is more common in individuals who are immunocompromised. Antibodies do not confer protection from the virus. Though typically persistent, they can be lost over time.
Hepatitis C virus (HCV) RNA, RT-PCR, serum	Undetected	HCV RNA is detectable 1–3 weeks after infection (1–1.5 months before HCV antibodies are seen) and can be reported either qualitatively or quantitatively (via real time RT-PCR). In chronic HCV infection, circulating HCV RNA persists in 90% of patients despite the presence of neutralizing antibodies.
Hepatitis D virus (HDV) total antibodies, serum	Negative	IgM anti-HDV appears 2 to 3 weeks after infection and is a reliable indicator of recent HDV exposure but is frequently short lived. Acute coinfection by HDV and HBV is associated with the presence of IgM against HDAg and HBcAg (denoting new infection with hepatitis B). When chronic hepatitis arises from HDV superinfection, HBsAg is present in serum, and anti-HDV antibodies (IgG and IgM) persist for months or longer.
Hepatitis E virus (HEV) IgG and IgM antibody, serum	Negative	IgM antibodies are detectable early and disappear within 4 to 5 months. IgG antibodies appear almost immediately after the IgM response; it is not clear how long they persist.

[a]Helpful review of this table by Dr. Anjana Pillai, Department of Medicine, University of Chicago is acknowledged.

References values from https://www.mayocliniclabs.com/ by permission of Mayo Foundation for Medical Education and Research. All rights reserved.

Adapted from Deyrup AT, D'Ambrosio D, Muir J, et al. Essential Laboratory Tests for Medical Education. *Acad Pathol.* 2022;9. doi: 10.1016/j.acpath.2022.100046.

Pancreas

The pancreas is a transversely oriented retroperitoneal organ extending from the so-called "C loop" of the duodenum to the hilum of the spleen. Although the pancreas does not have well-defined anatomic subdivisions, adjacent vessels and ligaments serve to demarcate the organ into a head, body, and tail.

The pancreas is really two organs packaged into one. The first, the islets of Langerhans, which make up 1% to 2% of the pancreas and are scattered throughout, serve critical endocrine functions. The second, the exocrine portion, makes up the bulk of the organ and is a major source of enzymes that are essential for digestion. Diseases affecting the pancreas can be the source of significant morbidity and mortality. Unfortunately, the retroperitoneal location of the pancreas and the generally nonspecific signs and symptoms associated with disorders of the exocrine portion allow many pancreatic diseases to remain undiagnosed for extended periods of time; thus, recognition of pancreatic disorders requires a high degree of suspicion.

The *exocrine pancreas* is composed of *acinar cells* and the ductules and ducts that convey their secretions to the duodenum. The acinar cells are responsible for the synthesis of digestive enzymes, which are synthesized as inactive proenzymes that are stored in *zymogen granules*. When acinar cells are stimulated to secrete the enzymes, the granules fuse with the apical plasma membrane and release their contents into the central acinar lumen. These secretions are transported to the duodenum through a series of anastomosing ducts.

The epithelial cells lining the ducts are also active participants in pancreatic secretion. The cuboidal cells that line the smaller ductules secrete bicarbonate-rich fluid, while the columnar cells lining the larger ducts produce mucin. Ductal epithelial cells also express the *cystic fibrosis transmembrane conductance regulator (CFTR)*; aberrant function of this membrane protein affects the biochemical, in particular bicarbonate, content and viscosity of pancreatic secretions. CFTR dysfunction has a fundamental role in the pathophysiology of pancreatic disease in individuals with cystic fibrosis (Chapter 4).

As discussed later, autodigestion of the pancreas (e.g., in pancreatitis) can be a catastrophic event. A number of "fail-safe"

mechanisms have evolved to minimize the risk for occurrence of this phenomenon:

- A majority of pancreatic enzymes are synthesized as inactive proenzymes and sequestered in membrane-bound zymogen granules, as mentioned earlier.
- *Proenzymes are typically activated by trypsin*, which itself is activated (from trypsinogen) by duodenal enteropeptidase (enterokinase) in the small bowel. Hence, the pancreatic enzymes are activated in the duodenum.
- Trypsin inhibitors (e.g., SPINK1, also known as *pancreatic secretory trypsin inhibitor*) are also secreted by acinar and ductal cells.
- In addition, trypsin cleaves and inactivates itself, a negative feedback mechanism that normally puts a limit on local levels of activated trypsin. Hence, trypsin is not activated within the pancreas itself, and neither are the pancreatic enzymes.
- Acinar cells are remarkably resistant to the action of activated enzymes such as trypsin, chymotrypsin, and phospholipase A_2.

Diseases of the exocrine pancreas include cystic fibrosis, congenital anomalies, acute and chronic pancreatitis, and neoplasms. Cystic fibrosis is discussed in detail in Chapter 4; the other pathologic processes are discussed in this chapter.

CONGENITAL ANOMALIES

Congenital anomalies of the pancreas are uncommon. The most significant are briefly described below:

- *Pancreas divisum* (Fig. 15.1) is the most common congenital anomaly of the pancreas, with an incidence of 3% to 10%. In most individuals, the main pancreatic duct (the duct of Wirsung) joins the common bile duct just proximal to the papilla of Vater, and the accessory pancreatic duct (the duct of Santorini) drains into the duodenum through a separate minor papilla. Pancreas divisum is caused by a failure of fusion of the fetal duct systems of the dorsal and ventral pancreatic primordia. As a result, the bulk of the pancreas (formed by the dorsal pancreatic primordium) drains into the duodenum through the small-caliber minor papilla. The duct of Wirsung in individuals with divisum drains only a small portion of the head of the gland through the papilla of Vater. More than 95% of individuals are asymptomatic. The remaining

The contributions to this chapter by Dr. Anirban Maitra, University of Texas, MD Anderson Cancer Center, Houston, Texas, in previous editions of this book are gratefully acknowledged.

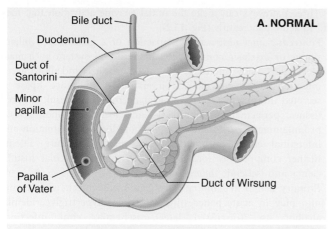

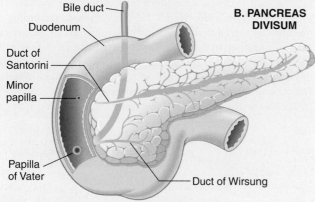

FIG. 15.1 Pancreatic ductal anatomy in (A) normal pancreas and (B) pancreatic divisum.

5% develop acute or chronic pancreatitis, possibly related to inadequate drainage of pancreatic secretions through the minor papilla.
- *Annular pancreas* is a relatively uncommon variant of pancreatic fusion in which a ring of pancreatic tissue completely encircles the duodenum. It can manifest with signs and symptoms of duodenal obstruction such as gastric distention and vomiting.
- *Ectopic pancreas* is aberrantly situated pancreatic tissue, which occurs in about 2% of the population. Common sites are the stomach and duodenum, followed by the jejunum, Meckel diverticulum, and ileum. These embryologic rests are typically small (ranging from millimeters to centimeters in diameter) and are located in the submucosa; they are composed of normal pancreatic acini with occasional islets. Though usually incidental and asymptomatic, ectopic pancreas may become inflamed, leading to pain, or—rarely—can cause mucosal bleeding. Approximately 2% of pancreatic neuroendocrine tumors (Chapter 18) arise in ectopic pancreatic tissue.
- *Congenital cysts* result from anomalous development of the pancreatic ducts. In *polycystic disease,* the kidneys, liver, and pancreas may all contain cysts (Chapter 12). Congenital cysts are generally unilocular and range from microscopic to 5 cm in diameter. They are lined by uniform cuboidal or flattened epithelium and are enclosed in a thin, fibrous capsule. These benign cysts contain clear *serous* fluid—an important point of distinction from pancreatic cystic neoplasms, which are often *mucinous* (discussed later).

PANCREATITIS

Inflammatory disorders of the pancreas are divided into acute and chronic forms. In *acute pancreatitis,* function can return to normal if the underlying cause of inflammation is removed. By contrast, *chronic pancreatitis* causes irreversible destruction of exocrine pancreas.

Acute Pancreatitis

Acute pancreatitis is a reversible inflammatory disorder that varies in severity, from focal edema and fat necrosis to widespread hemorrhagic necrosis. It is a relatively common and serious condition, with an annual incidence of 33 to 74 per 100,000 globally. In the Western world the incidence is 5 to 35 per 100,000. Overall mortality is about 5%. The incidence of acute pancreatitis is increasing due to the obesity epidemic and related increase in gallstone disease.

Etiology and Pathogenesis. The most common cause of acute pancreatitis in the United States is the impaction of gallstones within the common bile duct, impeding the flow of pancreatic enzymes through the ampulla of Vater ("gallstone pancreatitis"); this is closely followed by pancreatitis secondary to excessive alcohol intake. **Overall, gallstones and chronic excessive alcohol use account for close to 80% of acute pancreatitis cases,** with the remainder caused by a multitude of factors (Table 15.1). These include the following:
- *Nongallstone-related obstruction* of the pancreatic ducts (e.g., due to pancreatic cancer or other periampullary neoplasms, pancreas divisum, particulate solids that have precipitated from bile ("biliary sludge"), or parasites, particularly *Ascaris lumbricoides* and *Clonorchis sinensis*
- *Metabolic disorders,* in particular hypertriglyceridemia, hyperparathyroidism, and other hypercalcemic states. Hypertriglyceridemia (above 1000 mg/dL) has been reported to cause 5% to 10% of cases of acute pancreatitis.
- *Medications,* including anticonvulsants, cancer chemotherapeutic agents, thiazide diuretics, estrogens, and many others
- *Infections* with mumps virus or coxsackievirus, which can directly infect pancreatic exocrine cells

Of note, 10% to 20% of cases of acute pancreatitis have no identifiable cause *(idiopathic pancreatitis),* although a growing body of

Table 15.1 Etiologic Factors in Acute Pancreatitis

Metabolic
Alcohol use disorder[a]
Hypertriglyceridemia
Hypercalcemia
Drugs (e.g., azathioprine)
Genetic
Mutations in the cationic trypsinogen *(PRSS1)* and trypsin inhibitor *(SPINK1)* genes
Mechanical
Gallstones[a]
Trauma
Iatrogenic injury
Perioperative injury
Endoscopic procedures with dye injection
Vascular
Shock
Atheroembolism
Polyarteritis nodosa
Infectious
Mumps
Coxsackievirus

[a]Most common causes in the United States.

evidence suggests that many have an underlying genetic basis. For example, a subset of these patients with so-called *idiopathic pancreatitis* has underlying germline mutations affecting various genes: the autosomal dominant form is caused most often by mutations in the gene encoding trypsin, and most autosomal recessive disease is caused by mutations in CFTR. In those caused by mutations in the *CFTR* gene the symptoms are restricted to the pancreas (Chapter 4).

Acute pancreatitis is caused by autodigestion of the pancreas by intraacinar activation of pancreatic enzymes. Study of hereditary forms of acute pancreatitis has revealed the key role of premature activation of trypsin in this process. The feature shared by most forms of hereditary pancreatitis is a defect that increases or sustains the activity of trypsin such as mutations in the *PRSS1* gene, which encodes trypsinogen, the proenzyme of pancreatic trypsin. The pathogenic mutations alter the site through which trypsin cleaves and inactivates itself, abrogating an important negative feedback mechanism. This modification leads not only to the hyperactivation of trypsin but also to the activation of many other digestive enzymes that require trypsin cleavage for their activation. The released enzymes can inflict damage on blood vessels, causing hemorrhage within the pancreatic substance. Trypsin also converts prekallikrein to its activated form, thus initiating the kinin system, and, by activation of factor XII (Hageman factor), also sets in motion the clotting and complement systems (Chapter 3).

Three pathways can incite the initial enzyme activation that may lead to acute pancreatitis (Fig. 15.2):

- *Pancreatic duct obstruction.* Impaction of a gallstone or biliary sludge or extrinsic compression of the ductal system by a mass blocks ductal flow, increases intraductal pressure, and allows accumulation of an enzyme-rich interstitial fluid. Since lipase is secreted in an active form, local fat necrosis may result. Injured tissues, periacinar myofibroblasts, and leukocytes then release proinflammatory cytokines that promote local inflammation and interstitial edema through a leaky microvasculature. Edema further compromises local blood flow, causing vascular insufficiency and ischemic injury to acinar cells.
- *Primary acinar cell injury.* This pathogenic mechanism comes into play in acute pancreatitis caused by hypertriglyceridemia, alcohol use (discussed later), ischemia, viral infections (e.g., mumps), drugs, and direct trauma to the pancreas. The toxicity of triglycerides is not fully understood. According to one view large triglyceride-rich chylomicrons retard capillary circulation, leading to ischemic injury to pancreatic acinar cells. Injured cells release lipase into the interstitium, causing hydrolysis of triglycerides and local release of toxic free fatty acids release.
- *Defective intracellular transport of proenzymes within acinar cells.* In healthy acinar cells, digestive enzymes intended for zymogen

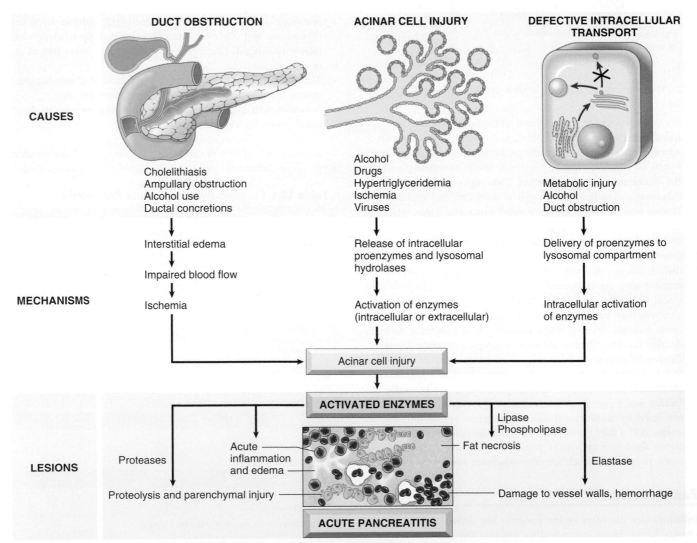

FIG. 15.2 Proposed pathogenesis of acute pancreatitis.

granules (and eventually extracellular release), and hydrolytic enzymes destined for lysosomes are transported in discrete pathways after synthesis in the endoplasmic reticulum. However, in at least some animal models of metabolic injury, pancreatic proenzymes and lysosomal hydrolases become packaged together. This results in proenzyme activation, lysosomal rupture (action of phospholipases), and local release of activated enzymes. A similar series of events is very likely in human acute pancreatitis, although definitive proof is lacking.

Alcohol consumption may cause pancreatitis by several mechanisms (see Fig. 15.2). Alcohol transiently increases pancreatic exocrine secretion and contraction of the sphincter of Oddi (the muscle regulating the flow of pancreatic secretions through the papilla of Vater). Alcohol also has direct toxic effects, including induction of oxidative stress in acinar cells, which leads to membrane damage; alcohol may also lead to delivery of proenzymes to lysosomal compartment with subsequent intracellular activation of trypsin and other digestive enzymes (discussed earlier). Finally, chronic alcohol ingestion results in the secretion of protein-rich pancreatic fluid, which leads to the deposition of inspissated protein plugs and obstruction of small pancreatic ducts.

MORPHOLOGY

The basic alterations in acute pancreatitis are **(1) microvascular leakage causing edema; (2) necrosis of fat by lipases; (3) an acute inflammatory reaction; (4) proteolytic destruction of pancreatic parenchyma and blood vessels leading to interstitial hemorrhage.**

In mild forms, there is interstitial edema and focal areas of fat necrosis in the pancreas and peripancreatic fat (Fig. 15.3A). Fat necrosis results from enzymatic destruction of fat cells; the released fatty acids combine with calcium to form insoluble salts that precipitate in situ.

In more severe forms, such as **acute necrotizing pancreatitis,** the damage also involves acinar and ductal cells, the islets of Langerhans, and blood vessels (eFig. 15.1). Macroscopically, the pancreas exhibits red-black hemorrhagic areas interspersed with foci of yellow-white, chalky **fat necrosis** (Fig. 15.3B). Fat necrosis can also occur in extrapancreatic fat, including the omentum and bowel mesentery, and even outside the abdominal cavity (e.g., in subcutaneous fat). In most cases, the peritoneum contains a serous, slightly turbid, brown-tinged fluid with globules of fat (derived from enzymatically digested adipose tissue). In the most severe form, **hemorrhagic pancreatitis,** extensive parenchymal necrosis is accompanied by diffuse hemorrhage within the substance of the gland (eFig. 15.2).

Clinical Features. **Abdominal pain is the cardinal manifestation of acute pancreatitis.** Its severity varies from mild and uncomfortable to severe and incapacitating. Acute pancreatitis is diagnosed primarily by the presence of elevated plasma levels of lipase and amylase and the exclusion of other causes of abdominal pain. In 80% of cases, acute pancreatitis is mild and self-limiting; the remaining 20% develop severe disease.

Full-blown acute pancreatitis is a medical emergency of the first order. Affected individuals usually experience the sudden calamitous onset of an "acute abdomen" with pain, guarding, and the ominous absence of bowel sounds. Characteristically, the pain is constant, intense, and referred to the upper back; it must be differentiated from similar pain due to perforated peptic ulcer, biliary colic, acute

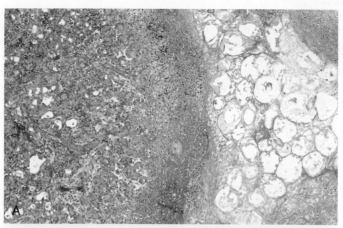

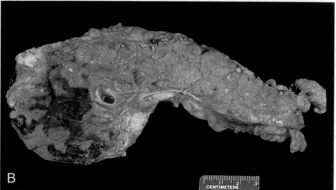

FIG. 15.3 Acute pancreatitis. (A) The microscopic field shows a region of fat necrosis *(right)* and focal pancreatic parenchymal necrosis *(center).* (B) The pancreas has been sectioned longitudinally to reveal dark areas of hemorrhage in the pancreatic substance and a focal area of pale fat necrosis in the peripancreatic fat *(upper left).*

cholecystitis with rupture, and occlusion of mesenteric vessels with infarction of the bowel.

The manifestations of severe acute pancreatitis are attributable to systemic release of digestive enzymes and explosive activation of the inflammatory response. The initial clinical evaluation may reveal leukocytosis, disseminated intravascular coagulation (Chapter 10), acute respiratory distress syndrome secondary to diffuse alveolar damage (Chapter 11), and diffuse fat necrosis. Peripheral vascular collapse (shock) can rapidly ensue as a result of increased microvascular permeability and consequent hypovolemia, compounded by endotoxemia (from breakdown of the barriers between gastrointestinal flora and the bloodstream) and renal failure due to acute tubular injury (Chapter 12).

Laboratory findings include elevation of serum lipase and amylase, both of which increase 4 to 12 hours after onset of pain. **Serum lipase is the most specific and sensitive marker of acute pancreatitis, as serum amylase has a short half-life and may return to normal in 3 to 5 days, whereas lipase levels remain elevated for 8 to 14 days.** Hypocalcemia can result from precipitation of calcium in areas of fat necrosis; if persistent, it is a poor prognostic sign. The enlarged inflamed pancreas can be visualized by computed tomography (CT) or magnetic resonance imaging (MRI).

The crux of the management is supportive therapy (e.g., maintaining blood pressure and alleviating pain) and "resting" the pancreas by total restriction of oral food and fluids. In 40% to 60% of cases of acute necrotizing pancreatitis, the necrotic debris becomes infected, usually by gram-negative organisms from the alimentary tract, further complicating the clinical course. Although most individuals with acute pancreatitis eventually recover, in a minority, the systemic release of digestive enzymes may lead to serious consequences, such as the systemic inflammatory response syndrome with shock and disseminated intravascular coagulation (Chapter 3), acute respiratory distress syndrome (Chapter 11), and systemic fat necrosis. In such cases, acute pancreatitis is a dire medical emergency. In patients who survive, sequelae include sterile or infected *pancreatic "abscesses"* or *pancreatic pseudocysts.*

Pancreatic Pseudocysts

A pseudocyst is an encapsulated collection of fluid that may occur in the pancreas, but more commonly is outside the pancreas. It arises weeks after a bout of acute pancreatitis, when liquefied areas of necrotic tissue become walled off by inflammatory and fibrous tissue that lacks an epithelial lining (hence a "pseudo," or false, cyst) (Fig. 15.4). The cyst contents are rich in pancreatic enzymes and a laboratory assessment of the cyst aspirate can be diagnostic. Pseudocysts are usually solitary; they are commonly attached to the surface of the gland and involve peripancreatic tissues such as the lesser omental sac or the retroperitoneum between the stomach and transverse colon or liver. They can range in diameter from 2 cm to 30 cm. Pseudocysts account for approximately 75% of all pancreatic cysts. Most resolve spontaneously, but some persist and may lead to complications such as infection, compression, obstruction of adjacent structures, rupture, and hemorrhage.

Chronic Pancreatitis

Chronic pancreatitis is characterized by long-standing inflammation that leads to irreversible destruction of the exocrine pancreas, followed eventually by loss of the islets of Langerhans. Of note, recurrent bouts of acute pancreatitis regardless of etiology can evolve over time into chronic pancreatitis. The prevalence of chronic pancreatitis is difficult to determine but probably ranges between 0.04% and 5% of the U.S. population and 9 to 62 per 100,000 globally.

Pathogenesis. Acute and chronic pancreatitis share similar pathogenic mechanisms. By far **the most common cause of chronic pancreatitis is chronic excessive alcohol consumption,** especially among middle-aged men. How alcohol triggers chronic pancreatic injury and inflammation is not known; it may alter the activation of digestive enzymes, increase the production of oxygen-derived free radicals, or exert direct toxic effects on acinar cells. Other predisposing factors include functional or anatomic duct obstruction.

Autoimmune pancreatitis is a pathogenically distinct form of chronic pancreatitis that is associated with the presence of IgG4-secreting plasma cells in the pancreas. Autoimmune pancreatitis is one manifestation of IgG4-related disease (Chapter 5), which may involve multiple tissues. Recognizing this entity is important because it responds to anti-B cell and steroid therapy.

As many as 40% of individuals with chronic pancreatitis have no recognizable predisposing factors. It is increasingly being recognized that many "idiopathic" cases are associated with germline mutations in *CFTR, PRRS1,* and *SPINK1* genes, the very same genes that are often found to be mutated in familial acute pancreatitis. As discussed earlier, mutations in *PRRS1* (encoding trypsinogen) and *SPINK1* (encoding a trypsin inhibitor) both allow excessive activation of trypsin.

MORPHOLOGY

On gross evaluation, the gland is hard, sometimes with extremely dilated ducts and visible calcific concretions. Microscopically, chronic pancreatitis is characterized by **parenchymal fibrosis, reduced number and size of acini, and variable dilation of the pancreatic ducts;** initially there is a relative sparing of the islets of Langerhans (Fig. 15.5A). **Acinar loss** is a constant feature, usually with a chronic inflammatory infiltrate around remaining lobules and ducts. The ductal epithelium may be atrophied or hyperplastic or exhibit squamous metaplasia, and ductal concretions may be noted (Fig. 15.5B). The remaining islets of Langerhans become embedded in the sclerotic tissue and may fuse and appear enlarged; eventually they also disappear (eFig. 15.3).

Autoimmune pancreatitis is characterized by striking infiltration of the pancreas by lymphocytes and plasma cells, many of which are positive for IgG4, accompanied by a "swirling" fibrosis and venulitis **(lymphoplasmacytic sclerosing pancreatitis).**

Clinical Features. Abdominal pain is the most common symptom of chronic pancreatitis. It can also manifest as repeated bouts of jaundice, vague indigestion, or persistent or recurrent abdominal and back pain, or it may be entirely silent until exocrine pancreatic insufficiency and diabetes develop (the latter as a consequence of islet destruction).

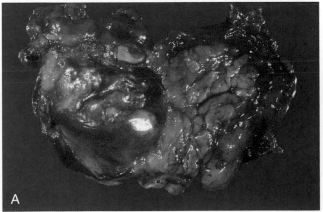
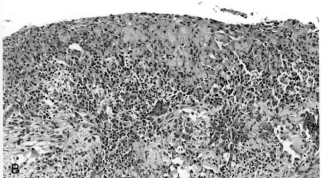

FIG. 15.4 Pancreatic pseudocyst. (A) Cross-section revealing a poorly defined cyst with a necrotic brownish wall. (B) Histologically, the cyst lacks an epithelial lining and instead is lined by fibrin and granulation tissue, with typical changes of chronic inflammation.

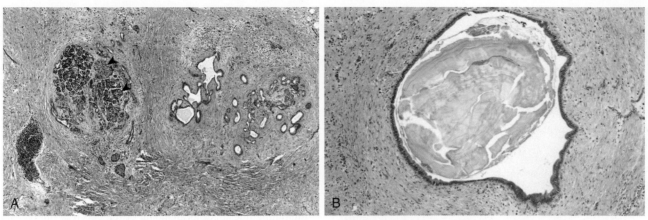

FIG. 15.5 Chronic pancreatitis. (A) Extensive fibrosis and atrophy have left only residual islets *(arrowheads)* and ducts *(right),* with a sprinkling of chronic inflammatory cells and acinar tissue. (B) A higher-power view demonstrating a dilated duct with inspissated eosinophilic concretions in a patient with alcohol-related chronic pancreatitis.

Attacks can be precipitated by excessive alcohol use, overeating (which increases demand on pancreatic secretions), or opiates or other drugs that increase the muscle tone of the sphincter of Oddi.

The diagnosis of chronic pancreatitis requires a high degree of clinical suspicion. With extensive fibrosis, acinar destruction may be so advanced that enzyme elevations are absent. Weight loss and hypoalbuminemic edema from malabsorption caused by pancreatic exocrine insufficiency can also point to the disease. Deficiency of fat-soluble vitamins, particularly vitamin D, can cause osteopenia. A helpful finding is visualization of calcifications within the pancreas by CT or ultrasonography.

Although chronic pancreatitis is usually not acutely life threatening, the long-term outlook is poor, with a 50% mortality rate over 20 to 25 years. *Pancreatic pseudocysts* (discussed earlier) develop in about 10% of patients. The most serious long-term complication of chronic pancreatitis is pancreatic cancer. Patients with hereditary pancreatitis associated with *PRSS1* mutations have a 40% lifetime risk of developing pancreatic cancer; the risk of pancreatic cancer is only modestly elevated in other forms of chronic pancreatitis.

PANCREATIC NEOPLASMS

Pancreatic exocrine neoplasms can be cystic or solid. Some tumors are benign, while others are among the most lethal of all malignancies.

Cystic Neoplasms

Cystic neoplasms are diverse tumors that range from harmless benign cysts to invasive, potentially lethal, cancers. Approximately 5% to 15% of all pancreatic cysts are neoplastic; these constitute less than 5% of all pancreatic neoplasms. There are three variants of cystic neoplasms. Some, such as serous cystic neoplasms, are almost always benign, whereas others, such as intraductal papillary mucinous neoplasms (IPMN) and mucinous cystic neoplasms, are precancerous. Most cystic neoplasms are detected incidentally when abdominal imaging is done for other reasons. IPMNs account for 38% of lesions, mucinous cystic neoplasms for 23%, and serous cystic tumors for 16%. Each of these is described next.

Serous Cystadenomas

These tumors are composed of glycogen-rich cuboidal cells surrounding small cysts containing clear, straw-colored fluid (Fig. 15.6).

The cysts are small (1—3 mm) and can be solitary, multiple, or present as a honeycomb of microcystic lesions. They typically manifest in the seventh decade of life with nonspecific symptoms such as abdominal

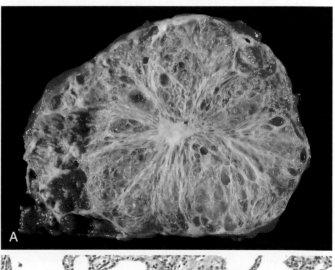

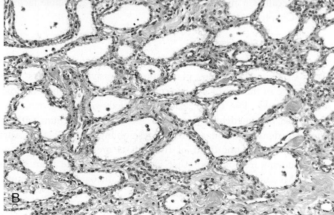

FIG. 15.6 Serous cystadenoma. (A) Cross-section through a serous cystadenoma. The lesion consists of honeycomb of microcystic lesions, only a thin rim of normal pancreatic parenchyma remains. The cysts are relatively small and contain clear, straw-colored fluid. (B) The cysts are lined by cuboidal epithelium without atypia.

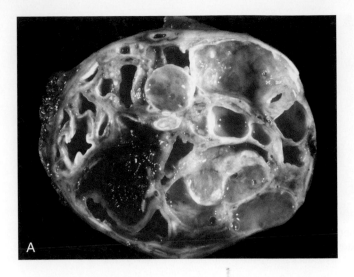

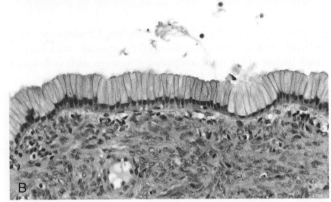

FIG. 15.7 Mucinous cystic neoplasm. (A) Cross-section through a mucinous multiloculated cyst in the tail of the pancreas. The cysts are large and filled with tenacious mucin. (B) The cysts are lined by columnar mucinous epithelium, with a densely cellular "ovarian" stroma.

pain; the female-to-male ratio is 2 : 1. They are almost uniformly benign, and surgical resection is curative in the vast majority of patients. Most serous cystadenomas carry somatic loss-of-function mutations of the von Hippel-Lindau *(VHL)* tumor suppressor gene, which you will recall is a negative regulator of hypoxia-inducible factor-α (HIFα) (Chapter 12).

Mucinous Cystic Neoplasms

In contrast to serous cysts, close to 95% of mucinous cystic neoplasms arise in women, and they are precursors to invasive carcinomas. They usually arise in the tail of the pancreas and present as painless, slow-growing masses. The cystic spaces are filled with thick, tenacious mucin, and are lined by a columnar mucinous epithelium with an associated densely cellular stroma resembling that of the ovary (Fig. 15.7). Up to one-third of these cysts are associated with an invasive adenocarcinoma, another important difference from serous tumors. Mucinous cystic neoplasms harbor oncogenic *KRAS* mutations in approximately half of cases.

Intraductal Papillary Mucinous Neoplasms

In contrast with mucinous cystic neoplasms, IPMNs occur more frequently in men than in women and more commonly involve the head of the pancreas. IPMNs arise in the main pancreatic ducts, or one of its major branch ducts, and lack the cellular stroma seen in

mucinous cystic neoplasms (Fig. 15.8). As with mucinous cystic neoplasms, IPMNs can progress to an invasive cancer: 70% of those affecting the main duct incur the risk of developing an invasive cancer, whereas the risk is smaller in branch duct lesions. In particular, "colloid" carcinomas of the pancreas, which are adenocarcinomas associated with abundant extracellular mucin production, nearly always arise through malignant transformation of an IPMN. Up to 80% of IPMNs harbor *KRAS* mutations, and two-thirds have oncogenic mutations of *GNAS*, which encodes the alpha subunit of a stimulatory G protein, G_s (Chapter 18). Constitutive activation of this G protein elevates levels of the second messenger cyclic AMP, activating certain kinases that promote cell proliferation.

Pancreatic Carcinoma

Infiltrating ductal adenocarcinoma of the pancreas (more commonly referred to as *pancreatic cancer*) is the third leading cause of cancer deaths in the United States, exceeded only by lung and colon cancers. Although it is substantially less common than the other two malignancies, pancreatic carcinoma is near the top of the list of killers because it carries one of the highest mortality rates. Close to 60,000 Americans were diagnosed with pancreatic cancer in 2021, and virtually all will die in a short period after diagnosis; the 5-year survival rate is a dismal 8%. The global rate is 8 to 14 per 100,000 with 6.92 per 100,000 dying.

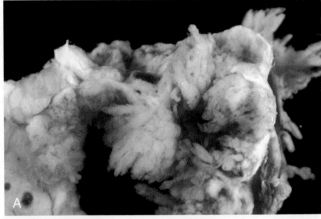

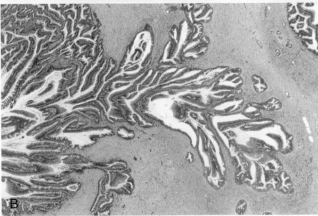

FIG. 15.8 Intraductal papillary mucinous neoplasm. (A) Cross-section through the head of the pancreas showing a prominent papillary neoplasm distending the main pancreatic duct. (B) The papillary mucinous neoplasm involves the main pancreatic duct *(left)* and is extending down into the smaller ducts and ductules *(right)*.

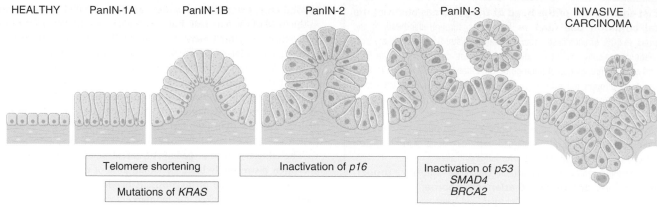

HEALTHY   PanIN-1A   PanIN-1B   PanIN-2   PanIN-3   INVASIVE CARCINOMA

Telomere shortening

Mutations of *KRAS*

Inactivation of *p16*

Inactivation of *p53*
SMAD4
BRCA2

FIG. 15.9* Progression model for the development of pancreatic cancer. It is postulated that telomere shortening and mutations of the *KRAS* oncogene occur at early stages of carcinogenesis, inactivation of the *p16* tumor suppressor gene occurs at intermediate stages, and inactivation of the *TP53, SMAD4,* and *BRCA2* tumor suppressor genes occurs at late stages. Note that while there is a general temporal sequence of changes, the accumulation of multiple mutations is more important than their occurrence in a specific order. *PanIN,* Pancreatic intraepithelial neoplasm. The numbers following the labels on the top refer to stages in the development of PanINs. *Stages refers to stages of development of the cancer, not clinical staging. (Modified from Maitra A, Hruban RH: Pancreatic cancer, *Annu Rev Pathol Mech Dis* 3:157, 2008.)

Pathogenesis. Like all cancers, pancreatic cancer arises as a consequence of inherited and acquired mutations in cancer-associated genes. In a pattern analogous to that seen in the multistep progression of colon cancer (Chapters 6 and 13), there is a progressive accumulation of genetic changes in pancreatic epithelium as it proceeds from nonneoplastic, to noninvasive precursor lesions, to invasive carcinoma (Fig. 15.9). While both intraductal papillary mucinous neoplasms (IPMNs) and mucinous cystic neoplasms can progress to invasive adenocarcinoma, **the most common antecedent lesions of pancreatic cancer arise in small ducts and ductules and are called pancreatic intraepithelial neoplasias (PanINs).** Evidence in favor of the precursor relationship of PanINs to frank malignancy includes the observations that these microscopic lesions are often found adjacent to infiltrating carcinomas and the two share a number of genetic alterations. Moreover, the epithelial cells in PanINs show dramatic telomere shortening, potentially predisposing these lesions to pathogenic chromosomal abnormalities that may contribute to acquisition of the full spectrum of cancer hallmarks. It should be noted that while most pancreatic cancers arise from PanINs, the vast majority of PanINs do not progress to frank malignancy.

The recent sequencing of the pancreatic cancer genome has confirmed that **four genes are most commonly affected by somatic mutations in this neoplasm: *KRAS, CDKN2A/p16, SMAD4,* and *TP53*:**

• *KRAS is the most frequently altered oncogene in pancreatic cancer;* it is activated by a point mutation in greater than 90% of cases. These mutations impair the intrinsic GTPase activity of the KRAS protein so that it is constitutively active. In turn, KRAS activates a number of intracellular signaling pathways that promote carcinogenesis (Chapter 6).

• *CDKN2A is inactivated in 30% of cases.* This complex locus encodes two tumor suppressor proteins (Chapter 6): p16/INK4a, a cyclin-dependent kinase inhibitor that antagonizes cell cycle progression, and ARF, a protein that augments the function of the p53 tumor suppressor protein.

• *The SMAD4 tumor suppressor gene is inactivated in 55% of pancreatic cancers* and only rarely in other tumors; it codes for a protein

that plays an important role in signal transduction downstream of the transforming growth factor-β receptor.

• *Inactivation of the TP53 tumor suppressor gene occurs in 70% to 75% of pancreatic cancers.* Its gene product, p53, acts both to enforce cell-cycle checkpoints and as an inducer of apoptosis or senescence (Chapter 6). *BRCA2* is also mutated late in a subset of pancreatic cancers.

Pancreatic cancer is primarily a disease of older adults, with 80% of cases occurring between 60 and 80 years of age. The strongest environmental influence is smoking, which doubles the risk. Long-standing chronic pancreatitis and diabetes are also associated with a modestly increased risk for pancreatic cancer. In addition to being risk factors for pancreatic cancer, chronic pancreatitis and diabetes may be manifestations of pancreatic cancer. Thus, for example, tumors arising in the head of the pancreas often cause chronic pancreatitis in the distal parenchyma, while diabetes caused by duct obstruction and subsequent pancreatitis may be the manifestation of an underlying neoplasm. In fact, approximately 1% of the older adult population with new-onset diabetes harbors an unsuspected pancreatic cancer. Familial clustering of pancreatic cancer has been reported, and a growing number of inherited genetic defects are now recognized that increase pancreatic cancer risk. Included in these are germline mutations of the familial breast/ovarian cancer gene *BRCA2* and mismatch repair genes, both seen in approximately 10% of cases.

MORPHOLOGY

Approximately 60% of pancreatic cancers arise in the head of the gland, 15% in the body, and 5% in the tail; in the remaining 20%, the neoplasm diffusely involves the entire organ. Carcinomas of the pancreas are usually hard, gray-white, stellate, poorly defined masses (Fig. 15.10A).

Two features are characteristic of pancreatic cancer: It is highly invasive (even "early" invasive pancreatic cancers invade peripancreatic tissues extensively), and it elicits an intense host reaction in the form of dense fibrosis **(desmoplastic response).**

Most carcinomas of the head of the pancreas obstruct the distal common bile duct as it courses through the head of the pancreas. In 50% of such cases, there is marked distention of the biliary tree, and patients typically exhibit jaundice. By contrast, carcinomas of the body and tail of the pancreas do not impinge on the biliary tract. Pancreatic cancers often extend through the retroperitoneal space, entrapping adjacent nerves (thus, accounting for the pain), and occasionally invade the spleen, adrenal glands, vertebral column, transverse colon, and stomach. Peripancreatic, gastric, mesenteric, omental, and portahepatic lymph nodes are frequently involved, and the liver is often enlarged with metastatic deposits. Distant metastases may occur, principally to the lungs and bones.

On microscopic examination, pancreatic carcinoma is usually a **moderately to poorly differentiated adenocarcinoma,** forming abortive glands with mucin secretion or cell clusters and exhibiting an aggressive, deeply infiltrative growth pattern (Fig. 15.10B). Dense stromal fibrosis accompanies tumor invasion, and there is a tendency for perineural invasion within and beyond the organ. Lymphatic invasion is also commonly seen.

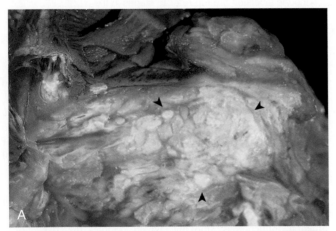

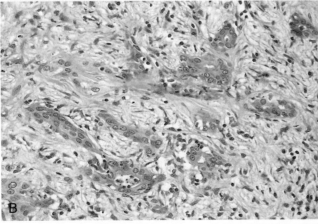

FIG. 15.10 Carcinoma of the pancreas. (A) Cross-section through the head of the pancreas and adjacent common bile duct showing both an ill-defined mass in the pancreatic substance *(arrowheads)* and the green discoloration of the duct resulting from total obstruction of bile flow. (B) Poorly formed glands are present in a densely fibrotic (desmoplastic) stroma within the pancreatic substance.

Clinical Features. **Carcinomas of the pancreas typically remain silent until their extension impinges on some other structure.** Pain is usually the first symptom, but by that point these cancers are often beyond cure. *Obstructive jaundice* can be associated with carcinoma in the head of the pancreas, but it rarely draws attention to the cancer sufficiently early for timely intervention. Weight loss, anorexia, and generalized malaise and weakness are manifestations of advanced disease. *Migratory thrombophlebitis (Trousseau syndrome)* occurs in about 10% of patients and is attributable to the elaboration of platelet-aggregating factors and procoagulants from the tumor or its necrotic products (Chapter 6). As previously stated, new-onset diabetes is the first manifestation of pancreatic cancer in some patients.

The clinical course of pancreatic carcinoma is rapidly progressive and often distressingly brief. Less than 20% of pancreatic cancers are resectable at the time of diagnosis. It has long been recognized that there is a profound need for biomarkers capable of detecting early, potentially curable, pancreatic cancers. Although serum levels of many enzymes and antigens (e.g., carcinoembryonic and CA19-9 antigens) are elevated, these markers are neither specific nor sensitive enough to be useful for screening. Several imaging techniques, such as endoscopic ultrasonography and high-resolution CT scans, are helpful for investigation in cases of suspected cancer but are not practical screening tests.

■ RAPID REVIEW

Pancreatitis

- *Acute pancreatitis* is characterized by inflammation and reversible parenchymal damage that ranges from focal edema and fat necrosis to widespread parenchymal necrosis and hemorrhage; the clinical presentation varies widely, from mild abdominal pain to rapidly fatal vascular collapse.
- *Chronic pancreatitis* is characterized by irreversible parenchymal damage and scar formation; clinical presentations include chronic malabsorption (due to pancreatic exocrine insufficiency) and diabetes (due to islet cell loss).
- Both entities share similar pathogenic mechanisms, and indeed recurrent acute pancreatitis can result in chronic pancreatitis. *Ductal obstruction by gallstones* and *chronic alcohol excess* are the most common causes in both forms. Inappropriate activation of pancreatic digestive enzymes (due to mutations in genes encoding trypsinogen or trypsin inhibitors) and primary acinar injury (due to toxins, infections, ischemia, or trauma) also cause pancreatitis. In some cases mutation in *CFTR* underlies pancreatitis.

Pancreatic Neoplasms

- Virtually all serous cystic neoplasms are benign; mucinous cystic neoplasms and intraductal papillary mucinous neoplasms are curable but incur a higher risk of developing cancer.
- Pancreatic cancer probably arises from noninvasive precursor lesions (most commonly, PanINs), developing by progressive accumulation of mutations of oncogenes (e.g., *KRAS*) and tumor suppressor genes (e.g., *CDKN2A/p16, TP53,* and *SMAD4*).
- Typically, these neoplasms are ductal adenocarcinomas that produce an intense desmoplastic response.
- Most pancreatic cancers are diagnosed at an advanced stage, accounting for the high mortality rate.
- Obstructive jaundice is a feature of carcinoma of the head of the pancreas; many patients also experience debilitating pain.
- Carcinomas of the tail of the pancreas are often not detected until late in their course.

■ **Laboratory Tests**

Test	Normal Value	Pathophysiology/Clinical Relevance
Amylase, serum	28–100 U/L	Amylase hydrolyzes complex carbohydrates and is primarily secreted by the salivary glands and the pancreas. Its level increases with gland inflammation or duct obstruction. Amylase level is increased in acute pancreatitis, pancreatic pseudocyst, and pancreatic duct obstruction (e.g., choledocholithiasis, pancreatic cancer). In acute pancreatitis, amylase levels increase rapidly (4–12 hours of symptom onset) but decline to normal in 3–5 days. Serum lipase level is currently the preferred test for the diagnosis of acute pancreatitis (see below). Amylase levels are decreased in pancreatic insufficiency and chronic pancreatitis.
Lipase, serum	13–60 U/L	Lipase is a digestive enzyme produced in pancreatic acinar cells and secreted into the duodenum to digest lipids. With acinar cell injury (e.g., acute pancreatitis), lipase is released into the pancreas, where it contributes to local tissue damage, including acute inflammation, autodigestion of pancreatic parenchyma, fat necrosis, and vascular damage. In acute pancreatitis, serum lipase is elevated, typically >3 times the upper limit of normal. The rise occurs within 4–8 hours and levels may remain elevated for up to 14 days. It is a more sensitive and specific test for acute pancreatitis. The degree of lipase elevation does not correlate with the severity of pancreatitis.

References values from https://www.mayocliniclabs.com/ by permission of Mayo Foundation for Medical Education and Research. All rights reserved.

Adapted from Deyrup AT, D'Ambrosio D, Muir J, et al. Essential Laboratory Tests for Medical Education. *Acad Pathol.* 2022;9. doi: 10.1016/j.acpath.2022.100046.

16

Male Genital System and Lower Urinary Tract

PENIS

Malformations

Among the most common malformations of the penis are those in which the distal urethral orifice is abnormally located, either on the ventral *(hypospadias)* or dorsal *(epispadias)* aspect of the penis. The anomalous orifice may be constricted, resulting in urinary tract obstruction and an increased risk for urinary tract infections. Hypospadias occurs in 1 in 300 live male births and may be associated with other congenital anomalies, such as inguinal hernia and undescended testis.

Inflammatory Lesions

Balanitis and *balanoposthitis* refer to local inflammation of the glans penis and of the overlying prepuce, respectively, due to infection. Among the more common agents are *Candida albicans;* anaerobic bacteria, including *Gardnerella;* and pyogenic bacteria. Most cases occur because of poor hygiene in uncircumcised males, which leads to the accumulation of desquamated epithelial cells, sweat, and debris, termed *smegma,* that acts as a local irritant and nidus for infection. *Phimosis* is a condition in which the prepuce cannot be retracted easily over the glans penis, usually due to scarring secondary to balanoposthitis, though it may also be a congenital anomaly.

The contributions to this chapter by Dr. Jonathan I. Epstein and Dr. Tamara L. Lotan, Department of Pathology, Johns Hopkins University School of Medicine, Baltimore, Maryland, in several previous editions of this book are gratefully acknowledged. The editors also appreciate the contributions to the current chapter by Dr. George Jabboure Netto, Department of Pathology, University of Alabama at Birmingham.

Neoplasms

The vast majority (more than 95%) of penile malignancies are squamous cell carcinomas. These are very rare in the United States, Europe, and other higher-resource countries; however, in lower-resource countries, penile carcinoma accounts for 10% to 20% of cancers in men. Most cases occur in uncircumcised patients older than 40 years of age. Low-income status, poor hygiene habits, smoking, chronic inflammation, and human papillomavirus (HPV) infection are risk factors.

Squamous cell carcinoma precursor of the penis (penile intraepithelial neoplasm [PeIN]) most commonly affects the penile shaft and scrotum of older men and appears grossly as a solitary plaque. Histologic examination reveals dysplastic cells throughout the epidermis without invasion of the underlying stroma (Fig. 16.1). Ten percent of patients subsequently develop invasive squamous cell carcinoma.

Invasive squamous cell carcinoma of the penis typically appears as a gray, crusted, papular lesion on the glans penis or prepuce. Infiltration of the underlying connective tissue produces an indurated, ulcerated lesion with irregular margins (Fig. 16.2). It is associated with HPV-16 and HPV-18 (high-risk types) infections. Histologically, the tumor is most often a typical keratinizing squamous cell carcinoma. The prognosis is related to the stage of the tumor. Patients with metastasis to multiple (3 or greater) or bilateral inguinal lymph nodes or to pelvic lymph nodes have a poor prognosis. *Verrucous carcinoma,* a non-HPV—related variant of squamous cell carcinoma, is characterized by papillary architecture, virtually no cytologic atypia, and rounded, pushing deep margins; such tumors are locally invasive but do not metastasize.

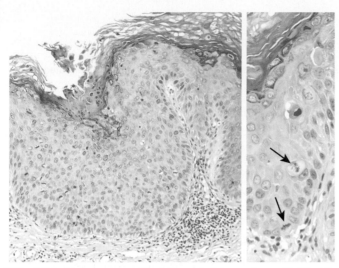

FIG. 16.1 High grade penile intraepithelial neoplasm (PeIN). The epithelium above the intact basement membrane shows delayed maturation and disorganization *(left)*. Higher magnification *(right)* shows several mitotic figures *(arrows)*, one above the basal layer.

SCROTUM, TESTIS, AND EPIDIDYMIS

Several inflammatory processes may affect the skin of the scrotum, including local fungal infections and systemic dermatoses, such as psoriasis (Chapter 22). Neoplasms of the scrotal sac are unusual; *squamous cell carcinoma* is the most common of these. Scrotal enlargement may be due to accumulation of fluid in the tunica vaginalis: *hydrocele* (serous fluid), which may be idiopathic or in response to adjacent infections or tumors; *hematocele* (blood) secondary to trauma or torsion; and *chylocele* (lymphatic fluid), which may be secondary to filariasis. The clear fluid of a hydrocele allows light to pass through (transluminescence), allowing distinction from other fluids and tumors of the testis.

Cryptorchidism and Testicular Atrophy

Cryptorchidism is a complete or partial failure of the intra-abdominal testes to descend into the scrotal sac. It is associated

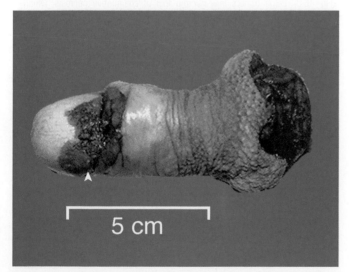

FIG. 16.2 Carcinoma of the penis. The glans penis is deformed by an ulcerated, infiltrative mass. (From Klatt EC: *Robbins and Cotran Atlas of Pathology*, ed 4, Fig. 12.6, Philadelphia, 2021, Elsevier.)

with testicular dysfunction and an increased risk of testicular cancer. Cryptorchidism is found in approximately 1% of 1-year-old boys. Normally, the testes descend from the abdominal cavity into the pelvis by the third month of gestation and then through the inguinal canals into the scrotum during the last 2 months of intrauterine life. The diagnosis of cryptorchidism is only established with certainty after 1 year of age, particularly in premature infants, because testicular descent into the scrotum is not always complete at birth. The condition is bilateral in approximately 25% of affected patients. Because undescended testes become atrophic, bilateral cryptorchidism results in sterility. Even unilateral cryptorchidism may be associated with atrophy of the contralateral descended gonad.

In addition to infertility, failure of testicular descent is associated with an increased risk for testicular cancer. Patients with unilateral cryptorchidism are also at increased risk for the development of cancer in the contralateral, normally descended testis, suggesting that an intrinsic abnormality, rather than simple failure of descent, underlies both the increased cancer risk and the aforementioned increased risk of testicular atrophy and sterility. Cryptorchid testes are small and firm. The histologic changes in the malpositioned testis begin as early as 2 years of age and include thickening of the basement membrane, loss of spermatogonia, increased interstitial stroma, and relative prominence of Leydig cells. *Germ cell neoplasia in situ* (discussed later) may be present in cryptorchid testes and is a likely precursor of subsequent germ cell tumors. Current recommendations are for surgical repositioning (orchiopexy), to be performed at 6 to 12 months of age.

Inflammatory Lesions

Inflammatory lesions of the testis are more common in the epididymis than in the testis proper. Sexually transmitted infectious disorders are discussed later in the chapter. Other causes of testicular inflammation include nonspecific epididymitis and orchitis, mumps, and tuberculosis.

- *Nonspecific epididymitis* and *orchitis* usually begin as a primary urinary tract infection that spreads to the testis through the vas deferens or the lymphatics of the spermatic cord. The involved testis is swollen and tender, and histologic examination reveals numerous neutrophils.
- *Mumps infection* involving the testes is rare in children but occurs in 20% to 30% of postpubertal males; typically, acute interstitial orchitis develops 1 week after the onset of swelling of the parotid glands. Sterility is a rare complication.
- *Testicular tuberculosis* is the most common cause of testicular granulomatous inflammation. It generally begins as an epididymitis, with secondary involvement of the testis. Histologic findings are identical to those seen in active tuberculosis elsewhere. Other causes of granulamatous inflammation include autoimmune orchitis, which sometimes develops after injury and release of normally sequestered testicular antigens.

Vascular Disturbances

Torsion, or twisting of the spermatic cord, typically results in obstruction of testicular venous drainage while the thick-walled and more resilient arteries remain patent. If untreated, this results in intense vascular engorgement and infarction (eFig. 16.1). There are two types of testicular torsion: *neonatal torsion,* which occurs either in utero or shortly after birth and has no associated anatomic defect, and *"adult" torsion.* The latter results from a bilateral anatomic defect in anchoring of the testis in the scrotal sac that leads to their increased

Table 16.1 Summary of Testicular Tumors

Tumor	Peak Patient Age (years)	Morphology	Tumor Marker(s)
Seminoma	40–50	Sheets of uniform polygonal cells with clear cytoplasm; lymphocytes in the stroma	10% of patients have elevated hCG
Embryonal carcinoma	20–30	Poorly differentiated, pleomorphic cells in cords, sheets, or papillary formation; most contain some yolk sac and choriocarcinoma cells	AFP may be elevated
Spermatocytic tumor	50–60	Small, medium, and large polygonal cells; no inflammatory infiltrate	Negative
Yolk sac tumor	3	Poorly differentiated flattened, cuboidal, or columnar cells	90% of patients have elevated AFP
Choriocarcinoma	20–30	Cytotrophoblast and syncytiotrophoblast without villus formation	100% of patients have elevated hCG
Teratoma	All ages	Tissues from all three germ cell layers with varying degrees of differentiation	20%–25% have elevated AFP
Mixed tumor	15–30	Variable, depending on mixture; commonly teratoma and embryonal carcinoma	AFP and hCG are variably elevated, depending on mixture

AFP, Alphafetoprotein; *hCG*, human chorionic gonadotropin.

mobility. Adult torsion typically occurs in adolescence and manifests with the sudden onset of testicular pain.

Torsion constitutes one of the few urologic emergencies. If the testis can be manually untwisted within 6 hours of onset, it remains viable. Contralateral *orchiopexy* is performed to prevent recurrence in the unaffected testis.

Testicular Neoplasms

Ninety-five percent of testicular tumors arise from germ cells, and almost all are malignant. By contrast, sex cord-stromal tumors derived from Sertoli or Leydig cells are uncommon and usually benign. The focus of the remainder of this discussion is on testicular germ cell tumors.

Pathogenesis. The cause of testicular neoplasms is poorly understood; both genetic and environmental factors contribute to their development. Incidence is lowest in Africa and Asia but has increased worldwide over recent decades. Family history is important, as fathers and sons of affected patients have a 4-fold increased risk and brothers of males with germ cell tumors have an 8- to 10-fold increased risk. As discussed earlier, cryptorchidism is associated with an increased risk for cancer in the undescended testis, as well as in the contralateral descended testis. In keeping with this, a history of cryptorchidism is present in approximately 10% of cases of testicular cancer. Intersex syndromes, including androgen insensitivity syndrome and gonadal dysgenesis, are also associated with an increased frequency of testicular cancer. The development of cancer in one testis is associated with a markedly increased risk for neoplasia in the contralateral testis. Extra copies of the short arm of chromosome 12, usually due to the presence of an isochromosome 12 [i(12p)], are found in virtually all germ cell tumors; it is not known which genes in this chromosomal segment are linked to tumorigenesis. Oncogenic mutations in *KIT* are found in up to 25% of tumors.

Most testicular tumors in postpubertal males arise from a precursor lesion called *germ cell neoplasia in situ*. This lesion is present in conditions associated with a high risk for developing germ cell tumors (e.g., cryptorchidism) and exhibits the same abnormality of

chromosome 12 when associated with fully developed germ cell tumors. Germ cell neoplasia in situ is often found in testicular tissue adjacent to germ cell tumors. Recall that in many other organs (e.g., pancreas, colon, prostate), precursor lesions are also found adjacent to cancers.

Testicular germ cell tumors are subclassified into seminoma and nonseminomatous tumors (Table 16.1). Seminoma is most common, accounting for about 50% of testicular germ cell neoplasms. They are histologically identical to tumors called *dysgerminomas*, which occur in the ovary, and *germinomas*, which occur in the central nervous system and other extragonadal sites.

MORPHOLOGY

Germ cell tumors may be composed of a single (~60% of cases) or multiple histologic types. **Seminoma** presents as a soft, well-demarcated, gray-white tumor that bulges from the cut surface of the affected testis (Fig. 16.3). Large tumors may contain foci of coagulative necrosis, usually

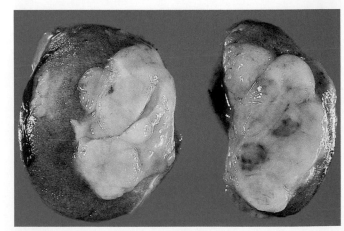

FIG. 16.3 Seminoma of the testis appearing as a well-circumscribed, pale, fleshy, homogeneous mass. (From Fletcher CD: *Diagnostic Histopathology of Tumors*, ed 5, Fig. 14B.7, Philadelphia, 2021, Elsevier.)

without hemorrhage. It is composed of **large uniform cells with distinct cell borders, clear glycogen-rich cytoplasm, round nuclei, and conspicuous nucleoli** (Fig. 16.4). The cells often are arrayed in small lobules with intervening fibrous septa. A lymphocytic infiltrate is usually present. Seminoma may also elicit a granulomatous reaction. In approximately 15% of cases, syncytiotrophoblasts are present; these cells are the source of the minimally elevated serum human choriogonadotropin (hCG) that is seen in 10% to 15% of patients with stage I disease, increasing to 30% to 50% in disseminated disease. Their presence has no bearing on prognosis, and the levels of hCG are usually much lower than in choriocarcinoma, described later.

Spermatocytic tumor (previously called spermatocytic seminoma) is uncommon, representing 1% to 2% of all testicular germ cell neoplasms. In contrast to other germ cell tumors, affected individuals are generally older (usually more than 65 years old). This slow-growing tumor does not metastasize and when treated by surgical resection has an excellent prognosis. The polygonal cells bear some morphologic resemblance to seminoma, but the origin and pathogenesis of spermatocytic tumor are quite distinct: it is not associated with germ cell neoplasia in situ, lacks isochromosome 12p, and is characteristically associated with gain of chromosome 9q.

Embryonal carcinoma presents as ill-defined, invasive masses containing foci of hemorrhage and necrosis (Fig. 16.5). The primary lesions may be small, even in patients with systemic metastases. **The tumor cells are large and have basophilic cytoplasm, indistinct cell borders, large nuclei, and prominent nucleoli.** The neoplastic cells may be arranged in undifferentiated, solid sheets or may form primitive glandular structures and irregular papillae (Fig. 16.6). In most cases, cells characteristic of other germ cell tumors (e.g., yolk sac tumor, teratoma, choriocarcinoma) are admixed with the embryonal areas. Pure embryonal carcinomas account for only 2% to 3% of all testicular germ cell tumors.

Yolk sac tumor is the most common primary testicular neoplasm in children younger than 3 years of age; in this age group, it has a very good prognosis. By contrast, postpubertal yolk sac tumor is rarely "pure" and more frequently occurs in combination with embryonal carcinoma or other germ cell components. Tumors are composed of low cuboidal to columnar epithelial cells that form microcysts, lacelike (reticular) patterns, sheets, glands, and papillae (Fig. 16.7). A distinctive feature is the presence of structures resembling primitive glomeruli, so-called **Schiller-Duval bodies**. These tumors often have eosinophilic hyaline globules containing α_1-antitrypsin and alphafetoprotein (AFP), which can be demonstrated by immunohistochemical techniques.

Choriocarcinoma is a highly malignant tumor in which the neoplastic germ cells differentiate into cells resembling placental **trophoblasts.** The primary tumors are often small and nonpalpable, even in patients with extensive metastatic disease. The tumor is composed of sheets of small cuboidal **cytotrophoblast-like cells** that are irregularly intermingled with or capped by large, eosinophilic **syncytiotrophoblast-like cells** containing multiple dark, pleomorphic nuclei (Fig. 16.8). Hemorrhage and necrosis are extremely common. hCG can be identified in the syncytiotrophoblastic cells by immunohistochemical staining.

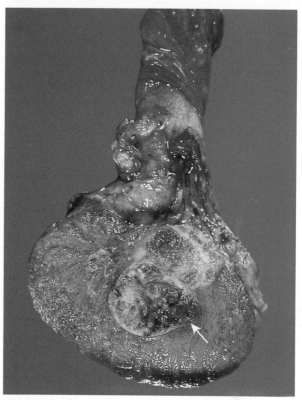

FIG. 16.5 Embryonal carcinoma. In contrast with the seminoma in Fig. 16.3, this tumor is hemorrhagic *(arrow)*. (From Fletcher CD: *Diagnostic Histopathology of Tumors*, ed 5, Fig. 14B.20, Philadelphia, 2021, Elsevier.)

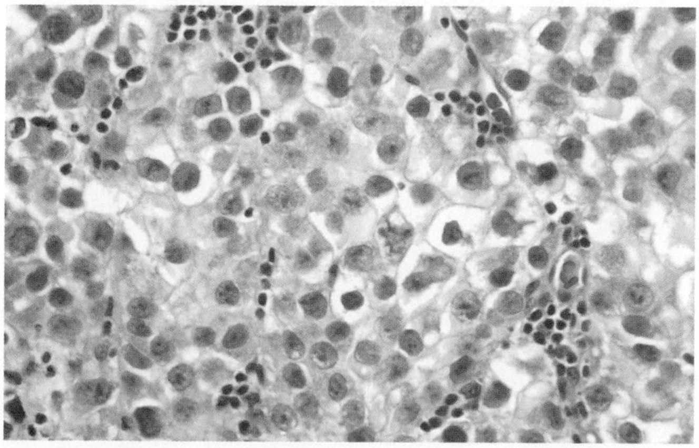

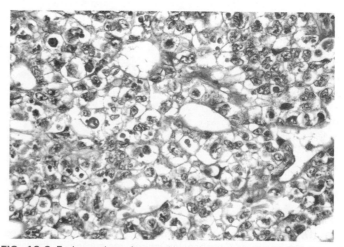

FIG. 16.4 Seminoma of the testis. Microscopic examination reveals large cells with distinct cell borders, pale nuclei, prominent nucleoli, and a sparse lymphocytic infiltrate.

FIG. 16.6 Embryonal carcinoma. Note the sheets of undifferentiated cells and primitive glandlike structures. The nuclei are large and hyperchromatic.

Teratoma is a tumor in which the neoplastic germ cells differentiate along multiple somatic cell lineages. They may occur at any age from infancy to adulthood. Pure teratoma is fairly common in infants and children and is referred to as the "prepubertal type." Among germ cell tumors, teratomas are second in frequency in infants and children only to yolk sac tumors. In adults, pure teratomas are rare, constituting 2% to 3% of germ cell tumors; more often teratomas are found mixed with other tumor types such as embryonal carcinoma or yolk sac tumor. The presence of a variety of tissues imparts a heterogeneous appearance, with solid, sometimes cartilaginous, and cystic areas (eFig. 16.2). Microscopically, there are collections of differentiated cells or organoid structures, such as neural tissue, muscle bundles, islands of cartilage, squamous epithelium lining epidermal-like surfaces with or without skin adnexal structures, structures reminiscent of thyroid gland, bronchial epithelium, and bits of intestinal wall or brain substance, embedded in a fibrous or myxoid stroma (Fig. 16.9). Elements may be mature (resembling various tissues within the adult) or immature (sharing histologic features with fetal or embryonal tissues). Prepubertal teratomas are not associated with germ cell neoplasia in situ or isochromosome 12p and pursue a benign course. Only a minor fraction of teratomas occurring in adults share these features, and postpubertal adult teratomas are generally taken to be malignant, regardless of the presence of immature elements.

Rarely, nongerm cell cancers may arise in teratoma, a phenomenon referred to as **teratoma with somatic-type malignancy.** Examples of such neoplasms include squamous cell carcinoma, adenocarcinoma, and various sarcomas. These nongerm cell malignancies do not respond to therapies that are effective against metastatic germ cell tumors (discussed later); thus, the only hope for cure in such cases is surgical resection.

Clinical Features. Patients with testicular germ cell neoplasms present most frequently with a painless testicular mass that (unlike enlargements caused by hydroceles) is nontranslucent. Biopsy of a testicular neoplasm is associated with a risk for tumor spillage, which would necessitate excision of the scrotal skin in addition to orchiectomy. Consequently, the standard management of a solid testicular mass is radical orchiectomy, based on the presumption of malignancy. Some tumors, especially nonseminomatous germ cell neoplasms, may

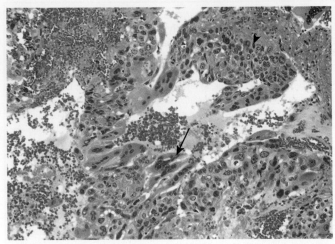

FIG. 16.8 Choriocarcinoma. Both cytotrophoblastic cells with single central nuclei *(arrowhead, upper-right)* and syncytiotrophoblastic cells with multiple dark nuclei embedded in eosinophilic cytoplasm *(arrow, middle)* are present. Hemorrhage and necrosis are prominent.

metastasize by the time of diagnosis in the absence of a palpable testicular lesion.

Seminoma and nonseminomatous tumors differ in their behavior and clinical course.

- *Seminoma* often remains confined to the testis for long periods and may reach considerable size before diagnosis. Metastases are most commonly encountered in the iliac and paraaortic lymph nodes. Hematogenous metastases occur late in the course of the disease.
- *Nonseminomatous germ cell neoplasms* tend to metastasize earlier, by lymphatic as well as hematogenous routes. Hematogenous metastases are most common in the liver and lungs. The histology of metastases and distant recurrences may differ from that of the testicular lesion.

Assay of *tumor markers* secreted by germ cell tumors is important for two reasons: (1) these markers (summarized in Table 16.1, along with salient clinical and morphologic features) are helpful diagnostically and (2) they are valuable in following the response of tumors to

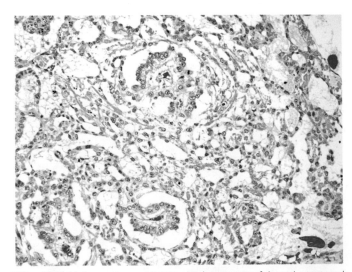

FIG. 16.7 Yolk sac tumor demonstrating areas of loosely textured, microcystic tissue and papillary structures resembling a developing glomerulus (Schiller-Duval bodies).

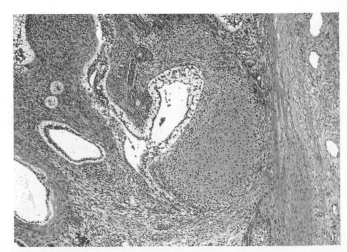

FIG. 16.9 Teratoma of the testis, consisting of a disorganized collection of glands, cartilage, smooth muscle, and immature stroma.

therapy after the diagnosis is established. hCG is always elevated in patients with choriocarcinoma and, as noted, may be minimally elevated in individuals with other germ cell tumors containing syncytiotrophoblastic cells. Increased AFP in the setting of a testicular neoplasm indicates a yolk sac tumor component and can also be seen in some embryonal carcinomas and teratomas. Serum levels of lactate dehydrogenase (LDH) correlate with the tumor burden.

The therapy and prognosis of testicular tumors depend largely on the clinical and pathologic stage and the histologic type. Seminoma, which is radiosensitive and chemosensitive, has the best prognosis. More than 95% of patients with stage I and II seminoma are cured by orchiectomy with or without chemotherapy or radiotherapy. In patients with nonseminomatous germ cell tumors, approximately 90% achieve complete remission with aggressive chemotherapy, and most can be cured. Pure embryonal carcinoma behaves more aggressively than mixed germ cell tumors. Pure choriocarcinoma and mixed germ cell tumors with predominantly choriocarcinoma have a poor prognosis.

PROSTATE

The prostate can be divided into biologically distinct regions, the most important of which are the peripheral and transition zones (Fig. 16.10). The types of proliferative lesions are different in each region. For example, most hyperplastic lesions arise in the inner transition zone, while most carcinomas (70%–80%) arise in the peripheral zones. As a result, carcinomas can be detected by rectal examination, whereas hyperplasias are more likely to come to attention due to symptoms of urinary obstruction. The normal prostate contains glands with two cell layers, a flat basal cell layer and an overlying columnar secretory cell layer. Surrounding prostatic stroma contains a mixture of smooth muscle and fibrous tissue. The prostate is involved by infectious, inflammatory, hyperplastic, and neoplastic disorders, of which prostate cancer is by far the most important clinically.

Prostatitis

There are three main types of prostatitis: (1) *acute bacterial prostatitis*, caused by the same organisms that cause other acute urinary tract infections; (2) *chronic bacterial prostatitis*, also caused by common uropathogens; and (3) *chronic abacterial prostatitis*, often referred to clinically as *pelvic pain syndrome*. The latter is the most common form of prostatitis.

The diagnosis of prostatitis is not typically based on biopsy, since the histologic findings are nonspecific and biopsy of an infected prostate can result in sepsis. The exception is *granulomatous prostatitis*, which may produce prostatic induration, leading to biopsy to rule out prostate cancer. In the United States, the most common cause of granulomatous prostatitis is instillation of bacille Calmette-Guérin (BCG) within the bladder for treatment of superficial bladder cancer (see later). Fungal granulomatous prostatitis is typically seen only in patients who are immunocompromised. *Nonspecific granulomatous prostatitis* is relatively common and stems from a foreign-body reaction to fluids that leak into tissue from ruptured prostatic ducts and acini.

Clinical Features. Acute bacterial prostatitis presents with sudden onset of fever, chills, dysuria, perineal pain, and bladder outlet obstruction; it may be complicated by sepsis. If acute prostatitis is suspected, digital rectal examination is contraindicated, as pressure on the exquisitely tender prostate can cause bacteremia; diagnosis can be established by urine culture and clinical features. *Chronic bacterial prostatitis* is usually associated with recurrent urinary tract infections interspersed with asymptomatic periods. Presenting manifestations include low back pain, dysuria, and perineal and suprapubic discomfort. Diagnosis depends on the demonstration of leukocytosis in expressed prostatic secretions and positive bacterial cultures. Both acute and chronic bacterial prostatitis are treated with antibiotics. *Chronic abacterial prostatitis* is indistinguishable from chronic bacterial prostatitis in terms of signs and symptoms, but lacks a history of recurrent urinary tract infection. Expressed prostatic secretions contain more than 10 leukocytes per high-power field (indicating presence of inflammation), but bacterial cultures are uniformly negative. The etiology is uncertain, and it is a diagnosis of exclusion. Therapy for chronic pelvic pain syndrome is empirical and depends on the nature of the symptoms.

Benign Prostatic Hyperplasia

Benign prostatic hyperplasia (BPH) results from stromal and glandular proliferation and is the most common benign prostatic disease in men older than 50 years. Its frequency rises progressively with age, reaching 90% by the eighth decade of life. Enlargement of the prostate in men with BPH is an important cause of urinary obstruction.

Pathogenesis. **Although the cause of BPH is incompletely understood, excessive androgen-dependent growth of stromal and glandular elements has a central role.** BPH does not occur in males who are castrated before the onset of puberty or in males with genetic diseases that block androgen activity. Dihydrotestosterone (DHT), the androgen that is the ultimate mediator of prostatic growth, is 10 times more potent than testosterone and is synthesized in the prostate from circulating testosterone by the action of the enzyme 5α-reductase, type 2. DHT binds to nuclear androgen receptors (which also bind testosterone) and thereby regulates the expression of genes that support the growth and survival of prostatic epithelium and stromal cells.

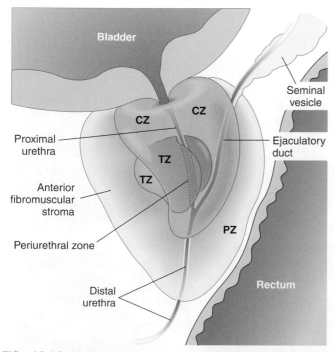

FIG. 16.10 Adult prostate. The normal prostate contains several distinct regions, including a central zone *(CZ)*, a peripheral zone *(PZ)*, a transitional zone *(TZ)*, and a periurethral zone. Most carcinomas arise from the peripheral glands of the organ, whereas nodular hyperplasia arises from more centrally situated glands.

It is believed that DHT-induced growth factors act by increasing the proliferation of stromal cells and decreasing the death of epithelial cells. With aging, testosterone levels decline while estrogen levels remain unchanged and may increase due to peripheral conversion of androgens; estrogens may act synergistically with DHT to drive growth of epithelial and stromal cells, both of which express estrogen receptors.

MORPHOLOGY

In BPH the weight of the enlarged prostate often increases 3- to 5-fold (60 to 100 g) or greater. BPH affects the transition zone and thus often encroaches on the urethra, compressing it to a slitlike orifice. On cross-section, **hyperplastic nodules** are seen that vary in color and consistency depending on their cellular content (Fig. 16.11A). The nodules may appear solid or contain cystic spaces, the latter corresponding to dilated glands.

Microscopically, the hyperplastic nodules are composed of variable proportions of proliferating glandular elements and fibromuscular stroma (Fig. 16.11B). The hyperplastic glands are lined by tall, columnar epithelial cells and a peripheral layer of flattened basal cells (Fig. 16.11C). This is a point of distinction from malignant glands in prostatic carcinoma (discussed next). The glandular lumina often contain laminated proteinaceous secretory material known as corpora amylacea (eFig. 16.3).

Clinical Features. **The main symptoms of BPH are due to urinary obstruction caused by prostatic enlargement and stromal smooth muscle–mediated contraction.** The increased resistance to urinary outflow leads to bladder hypertrophy and distention, accompanied by incomplete emptying of the bladder and presence of residual urine (eFig. 16.4). The reservoir of residual urine provides a culture medium for bacteria, a common source of infection. Patients experience increased urinary frequency, nocturia, difficulty in starting and stopping the stream of urine, overflow dribbling, and dysuria (painful micturition) and have an increased risk of developing bacterial infections of the bladder and kidney. Complete urinary obstruction can result in painful distention of the bladder and, without appropriate treatment, hydronephrosis (Chapter 12). Symptomatic BPH is usually managed medically with α-adrenergic blockers (which relax prostatic smooth muscle by blocking α₁-adrenergic receptors) and 5α-reductase inhibitors (which inhibit the formation of DHT from testosterone). Various surgical techniques (e.g., transurethral resection of the prostate, high-intensity focused ultrasound [HIFU], laser therapy, hyperthermia, transurethral electrovaporization, and radiofrequency ablation) are reserved for symptomatic cases that are recalcitrant to medical therapy.

Carcinoma of the Prostate

Adenocarcinoma of the prostate is the most common form of cancer in men, estimated to account for 21% of male cancer cases in the United States in 2022. Prostate cancer is the second leading cause of cancer-related death in men, surpassed only by lung cancer. It is largely a disease of aging. Based on autopsy studies, the incidence of prostate cancer increases from 20% in men in their 50s to approximately 70% in men between the ages of 70 and 80 years. There is a wide variation in the natural history of prostate cancer, from aggressive and rapidly fatal to more common indolent disease of little clinical significance. In the United States, African American men die from prostate cancer at a rate more than double that of European American men. The causes of this disparity are not understood though unequal access to screening and treatment make a major contribution.

Pathogenesis. Clinical and experimental observations suggest that androgens, heredity, environmental factors, and acquired somatic mutations have roles in the pathogenesis and progression of prostate cancer.

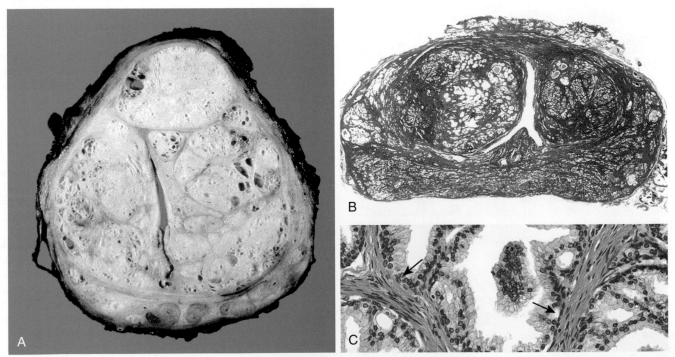

FIG. 16.11 Benign prostatic hyperplasia (BPH). (A) Well-defined nodules of BPH compress the urethra into a slitlike lumen. (B) Low-power photomicrograph demonstrates nodules of hyperplastic glands on both sides of the urethra. In other cases of nodular hyperplasia, the nodularity is caused predominantly by stromal, rather than glandular, proliferation. (C) Higher-power photomicrograph demonstrates the morphology of the hyperplastic glands, which are large and have papillary infoldings. Unlike prostatic adenocarcinoma, basal cells are present *(arrows)*.

- *Androgens* are of central importance. The dependence on androgens extends to established cancers, which often regress for a time in response to surgical or chemical castration. Most tumors eventually become resistant to androgen blockade by acquiring androgen receptor gene amplifications (which increase sensitivity to lower androgen levels) or mutations that allow ligand-independent androgen receptor activation. Other mutations or epigenetic changes can activate alternative signaling pathways and bypass the need for androgen receptor signaling.

- *Heredity* also contributes, as men with first-degree relatives affected by the disease have a 2-fold increased risk, and numerous germline variants that are associated with increased risk have been identified. Variants in regulatory regions that influence the expression of *MYC* and mutations that disrupt proteins involved in homologous recombination (e.g., BRCA2) and DNA mismatch repair increase risk of early onset, aggressive disease. Clinical features and incidence vary by population.

- *Environmental exposures* to carcinogens, estrogens, and oxidants are hypothesized to damage prostatic epithelium, setting the stage for acquisition of genetic and epigenetic changes that lead to cancer development. A Western diet that includes charred red meats and animal fats is associated with increased risk of prostate cancer based on epidemiologic and animal studies.

- *Acquired genetic aberrations,* as in other cancers, are the actual drivers of cellular transformation. The most common genetic alteration is a chromosomal rearrangement that juxtaposes the coding sequence of an ETS family transcription factor gene next to the *TMPRSS2* promoter. This translocation places the ETS oncogene under the control of the androgen-regulated *TMPRSS2* promoter, leading to its overexpression in an androgen-dependent fashion. Amplification of *MYC* and deletion of *PTEN* accelerate cell growth and may contribute to resistance to antiandrogen therapy. In late-stage disease, loss of *TP53* (by deletion or mutation) and deletions of *RB* are common, as are amplifications of the androgen receptor gene. Epigenetic events that modify gene expression are also common in prostate cancer. One frequent early event is epigenetic silencing by DNA methylation of the *GSTP1* (glutathione-S transferase Pi 1) gene whose product is involved in the detoxification of xenobiotic compounds. This functional deficit may enhance the genotoxic effect of environmental carcinogens. Other genes silenced by epigenetic modifications in a subset of prostate cancers include genes involved in cell cycle regulation (*RB, CDKN2A*), maintenance of genomic stability (*MLH1, MSH2*), and Wnt signaling (*APC*).

MORPHOLOGY

In approximately 70% of cases, carcinoma of the prostate arises in the peripheral zone of the gland, classically in a posterior location, where it may be palpable on rectal examination. On cross-section, the neoplastic tissue is gritty and firm to palpation, but it is sometimes extremely difficult to discern. Advanced lesions appear as firm, gray-white lesions with ill-defined margins that infiltrate the adjacent gland (Fig. 16.12).

Most prostate cancers are **moderately differentiated adenocarcinomas** that produce well-defined glands. The glands are typically smaller than benign glands (Fig. 16.13A) and are lined by a single uniform layer of cuboidal or low columnar epithelium, lacking the basal cell layer seen in benign glands involved by BPH. Furthermore, malignant glands are crowded and usually lack the branching and papillary infoldings seen in benign glands. Nuclei are enlarged and often contain one or more prominent nucleoli

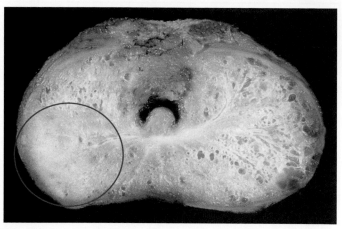

FIG. 16.12 Adenocarcinoma of the prostate. Carcinomatous tissue is seen on the posterior aspect *(circled, lower left)*. Note the solid appearance of the cancer, in contrast with the spongy appearance of the benign peripheral zone on the contralateral side.

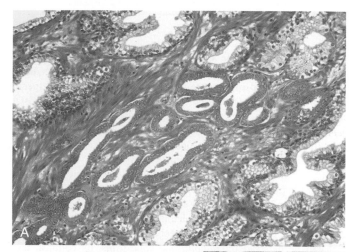

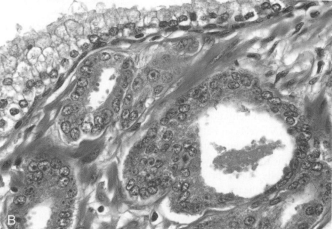

FIG. 16.13 (A) Adenocarcinoma of the prostate demonstrating small glands crowded in between larger benign glands. (B) Higher magnification shows several small malignant glands with enlarged nuclei, prominent nucleoli, and dark cytoplasm, as compared with the larger, benign gland *(top)*.

(Fig. 16.13B). Some variation in nuclear size and shape is usual, but, in general, pleomorphism is not marked. Mitotic figures are uncommon. With increasing grade, irregular or ragged glandular structures, cribriform glands, sheets of cells, or infiltrating individual cells are present. In approximately 80% of cases, prostatic tissue removed for carcinoma also harbors presumptive precursor lesions, referred to as *high-grade prostatic intraepithelial neoplasia (HGPIN)*. Notably, many of the molecular changes seen in invasive cancers are also seen in HGPIN.

Grading is based on the Gleason system, which stratifies prostate cancer into five grades on the basis of glandular patterns of growth. Grade 1 represents the most well-differentiated tumors, similar to benign prostatic tissue (Fig 16.14A), while grade 5 tumors do not form glands and infiltrate the stroma in cords, sheets, and solid nests (Fig. 16.14C). Other grades fall between these extremes (Fig. 16.14B). Most tumors contain more than one pattern; in such instances, a primary grade is assigned to the dominant pattern, and a secondary grade is assigned to the second-most frequent pattern. The two numeric grades are then added to obtain a combined Gleason score. The majority of potentially treatable cancers detected on needle biopsy as a result of screening have Gleason scores of 6 or 7. Tumors with Gleason scores of 8 through 10 tend to be advanced cancers that are less likely to be cured. Presently, Gleason scores are combined into five Grade Groups, each with a different prognosis. Pathologic staging of prostatic cancer is used in combination with the grade to stratify management of prostate cancer.

Clinical Features. **In the United States, most prostate cancers are small, nonpalpable, asymptomatic lesions discovered on needle biopsy performed to investigate an elevated serum prostate-specific antigen (PSA) level** (discussed later). Some 70% to 80% of prostate cancers arise in the outer (peripheral) glands, and a subset of these may be palpable as irregular hard nodules on digital rectal examination. Because of the peripheral location, prostate cancer is less likely than BPH to cause urethral obstruction in its initial stages. Locally advanced cancers often infiltrate the seminal vesicles and periurethral zones of the prostate and may invade the adjacent soft tissues, the wall of the urinary bladder, or (less commonly) the rectum. Bone metastases, particularly to the axial skeleton (eFig. 16.5), are frequent late in the disease and typically cause osteoblastic (bone-producing) lesions that can be detected on *radionuclide bone scans*. By contrast, most other cancers that spread to the bones cause lytic lesions.

Measurement of serum PSA levels is widely used to assist with the diagnosis and management of prostate cancer but is controversial. PSA is a product of prostatic epithelium and is normally secreted in the semen. As a screening test for prostate cancer, PSA measurement has suboptimal sensitivity and specificity since levels may be elevated in a variety of benign conditions (e.g., prostatitis, or following instrumentation of the prostate); MRI in the setting of elevated PSA levels can help identify nonpalpable cancers. Conversely, 20% to 40% of patients with organ-confined prostate cancer have PSA values below the cutoffs that identify individuals likely to have prostate cancer. Finally, many prostate cancers are so indolent that they are clinically insignificant, and detection of such cancers by PSA screening may lead to overtreatment, with its associated morbidity and economic costs. Large studies have shown that PSA screening has little or no impact on reducing prostate cancer mortality. Because of these concerns, PSA assays are of uncertain value as screening tests. By contrast, once cancer is diagnosed, serial measurements of PSA are of great value in assessing the response to therapy. For example, an elevated

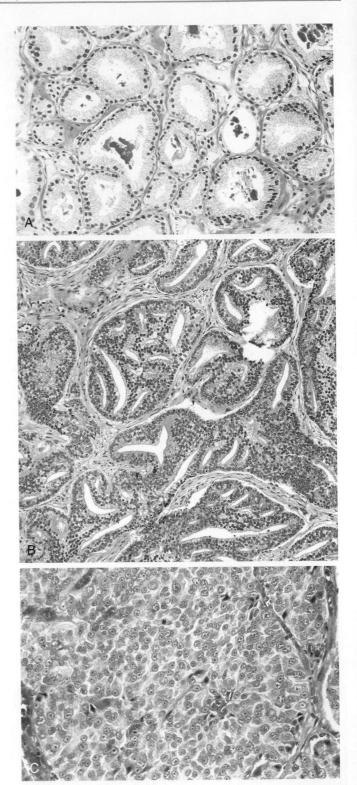

FIG. 16.14 Gleason grading of prostate cancer. (A) Low-grade prostate adenocarcinoma (Gleason score 1 + 1 = 2) consisting of back-to-back uniform-sized malignant glands lined by a single layer of epithelial cells. (B) A focus of Gleason grade 4 prostatic adenocarcinoma displays large cribriform glands with multiple cellular bridges crossing the central lumina. (C) Grade group 5 adenocarcinoma (Gleason score 5 + 5 = 10) composed of sheets of malignant cells with no identifiable gland formation. (B, Courtesy of ExpertPath, copyright Elsevier.)

PSA level after radical prostatectomy or radiotherapy for localized disease is indicative of recurrent or disseminated disease.

Patients with prostate cancer can be treated with surgery or radiation, with or without hormonal manipulation. More than 90% of patients who receive such therapy can expect to live for 15 years. The prognosis following radical prostatectomy is based on the pathologic stage, margin status, and Gleason grade. Since the growth and survival of prostate cancer cells depend on androgens, androgen deprivation is a key therapeutic component. It is usually achieved by administration of synthetic agonists of luteinizing hormone-releasing hormone (LHRH), thereby regulating production of LH, which is required for testosterone production. Although, LHRH agonists, like the body's own LHRH, initially stimulate the release of LH, the continued presence of high levels of LHRH causes the pituitary gland to stop producing luteinizing hormone. As a result, the testicles are not stimulated to produce androgens. Although antiandrogen therapy induces remissions, androgen-independent clones almost invariably emerge and can lead to disease progression and death.

LOWER URINARY TRACT

The renal pelvis, ureter, bladder, and urethra are lined by specialized multilayer transitional epithelium called urothelium. Beneath the mucosa are the lamina propria and, deeper yet, the muscularis propria (detrusor muscle), which makes up the bladder wall. Clinically significant disorders involving these organs include congenital anomalies, infectious and other inflammatory diseases, and neoplasms.

Ureter

Disorders of the ureter are uncommon and include congenital disorders, neoplasms, and reactive conditions. A few merit brief mention.
- *Ureteropelvic junction* (UPJ) obstruction, a congenital disorder, is the most frequent cause of hydronephrosis in infants and children. It is much more common in boys than in girls.
- *Malignant tumors* of the ureter are pathologically similar to those arising in the renal pelvis, calyces, and bladder (discussed later). Most are urothelial carcinomas.
- *Retroperitoneal fibrosis* is an uncommon cause of ureteral narrowing or obstruction characterized by a fibrous proliferative inflammatory process that encases the retroperitoneal structures and causes hydronephrosis. The disorder occurs in middle to old age and is more common in men than in women. A subset of these cases occurs in association with IgG4-related disease, characterized by fibroinflammatory lesions rich in IgG4-secreting plasma cells (Chapter 5). Other cases are associated with malignant disease (e.g., lymphomas, urinary tract carcinomas), radiation, prior surgery, and exposures to drugs (e.g., ergot derivatives, adrenergic blockers, TNF inhibitors). Most cases, however, have no obvious cause and are considered primary, or idiopathic (Ormond disease).

Urinary Bladder
Nonneoplastic Conditions

Diverticula are pouchlike invaginations of the bladder wall that vary from less than 1 cm to 10 cm in diameter and may be congenital or acquired as a consequence of persistent urethral obstruction (e.g., benign prostatic hyperplasia). Although most diverticula are small and asymptomatic, they sometimes lead to urinary stasis predisposing to recurrent urinary tract infections and bladder stone formation.

Cystitis takes many forms.
- *Bacterial cystitis* is common, particularly in women because their shorter urethra allows colonization by enteric bacteria. The most common etiologic agents are coliform bacteria, followed by *Proteus, Klebsiella,* and *Enterobacter.*

- *Hemorrhagic cystitis* may occur in patients receiving cytotoxic antitumor drugs, such as cyclophosphamide, and sometimes complicates adenovirus infection.
- *Malakoplakia* is a distinctive chronic inflammatory reaction that arises in the setting of chronic bacterial infection, mostly by *E. coli* or occasionally *Proteus* species. It appears to stem from acquired defects in phagocyte function. Consequently, undigested bacterial products accumulate within distended phagosomes, where they may form laminated mineralized concretions *(Michaelis-Gutmann bodies)* due to deposition of calcium salts.

In areas in which schistosomiasis is endemic, chronic cystitis leads to squamous metaplasia of the bladder and an increased incidence of squamous cell carcinoma.

Neoplasms

Bladder cancer is the ninth most common cancer type worldwide and is responsible for significant morbidity and mortality. Carcinoma of the bladder is more common in men, in higher-resource countries, and in urban populations. About 80% of patients are between 50 and 80 years of age. The vast majority of bladder cancers (about 90% in the United States) are urothelial carcinomas. Squamous cell carcinoma represents about 2% to 5% of bladder cancers in the United States but is much more common in countries where urinary schistosomiasis is endemic, such as East Africa and the Middle East. Adenocarcinomas of the bladder are rare.

Pathogenesis. **Environmental factors are important in the pathogenesis of urothelial carcinoma and include cigarette smoking, various occupational carcinogens, radiation therapy, and prolonged exposure to cyclophosphamide.** A family history of bladder cancer is a known risk factor. Transitional epithelium lining the bladder can undergo various forms of metaplasia. For example, as a response to injury, the urothelium often undergoes squamous metaplasia, which is a precursor to dysplastic lesions and in situ and invasive squamous cell carcinoma. One trigger of this sequence is schistosomiasis, an important risk factor for squamous carcinoma of the bladder in areas where this infection is endemic. Cancers occurring in this setting arise in a background of chronic inflammation, which predisposes to neoplasia (Chapter 6).

There are two major molecular pathways of tumor progression.
- *Superficial papillary tumors* often have gain-of-function alterations that increase signaling through growth factor receptor pathways (e.g., amplifications of the *FGFR3* tyrosine kinase receptor gene and activating mutations in the genes encoding RAS and PI3-kinase). These tumors frequently recur but muscle invasion only occurs in about 20% of cases, usually associated with *TP53* mutations.
- *Carcinoma in situ* develops from flat (i.e., not papillary) lesions with mutations that disrupt the function of p53 and RB. Additional genetic and epigenetic changes lead to muscular invasion.

MORPHOLOGY

The appearance of urothelial tumors varies from purely papillary to nodular or flat. Papillary lesions are red, elevated excrescences ranging in size from less than 1 cm in diameter to large masses up to 5 cm in diameter (eFig. 16.6). Multiple discrete tumors are often present.

Two distinct **precursor lesions** of invasive urothelial carcinoma are recognized (Fig. 16.15). The most common is a noninvasive papillary tumor (Fig. 16.16). The other precursor is carcinoma in situ (CIS). In about one-half of patients with invasive bladder cancer, no precursor lesion is found; in such cases, it is presumed that the precursor lesion was overgrown by the high-grade invasive component.

The most important prognostic factor in noninvasive papillary urothelial neoplasms is their grade, which is based on both architectural and cytologic features. The grading system subclassifies tumors as follows: (1) **papilloma**; (2) **papillary urothelial neoplasm of low malignant potential (PUNLMP)**; (3) **low-grade papillary urothelial carcinoma**; and (4) **high-grade papillary urothelial carcinoma** (Fig. 16.17).

CIS is defined by the presence of overtly malignant-appearing cells within a flat urothelium (Fig. 16.18). A common feature shared with high-grade papillary urothelial carcinoma is a lack of cohesiveness, which leads to shedding of malignant cells into the urine, where they can be identified by cytology. CIS is commonly multifocal and sometimes involves most of the bladder surface or extends into the ureters and urethra. Without treatment, 50% to 75% of CIS cases progress to invasive cancer.

Invasive papillary urothelial cancer (usually of high grade) may superficially extend into the lamina propria or penetrate more deeply into underlying muscle (eFig. 16.7). **The extent of invasion and spread (staging) at the time of initial diagnosis is the most important prognostic factor.**

Squamous cell carcinoma of the bladder typically shows extensive keratinization and is nearly always associated with chronic bladder irritation and infection. Adenocarcinomas of the bladder are histologically identical to adenocarcinomas seen in the gastrointestinal tract. Some arise from urachal remnants in the dome of the bladder or in association with intestinal metaplasia, an uncommon alteration that is also associated with chronic inflammation from a variety of causes.

Clinical Features. Bladder tumors most commonly present with *painless hematuria.* Patients with urothelial tumors, whatever their grade, have a tendency to develop new tumors after excision, and recurrences may exhibit a higher grade. The risk for recurrence is related to several factors, including tumor size, stage, grade, multifocality, mitotic index, and associated CIS in the surrounding mucosa. Recurrent tumors may arise at sites other than that of the original lesion, yet are clonally related, apparently arising from shedding and implantation of cells from the original tumor at a distant site. **Whereas high-grade papillary urothelial carcinomas are frequently invasive,**

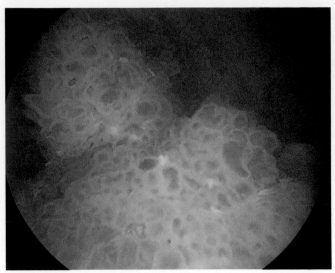

FIG. 16.16 Cystoscopic appearance of a papillary urothelial tumor, resembling coral, within the bladder.

lower-grade papillary urothelial neoplasms often recur but infrequently invade.

Treatment of bladder cancer depends on tumor grade and stage, the key variable being whether the tumor is muscle invasive or not. For

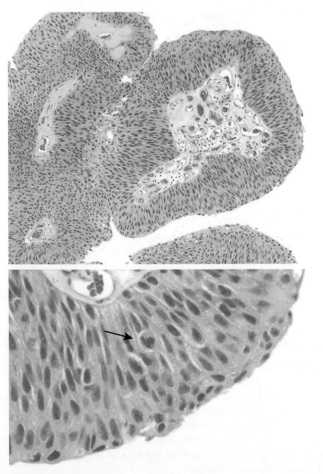

FIG. 16.17 Noninvasive low-grade papillary urothelial carcinoma. Higher magnification *(bottom)* shows slightly irregular nuclei with scattered mitotic figures *(arrow)*.

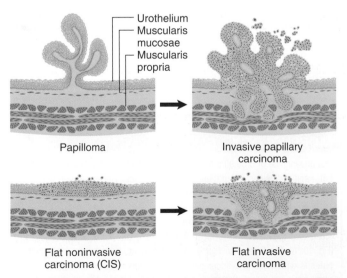

Urothelium
Muscularis mucosae
Muscularis propria

Papilloma

Invasive papillary carcinoma

Flat noninvasive carcinoma (CIS)

Flat invasive carcinoma

FIG. 16.15 Morphologic patterns of urothelial neoplasia. *CIS*, Carcinoma in situ.

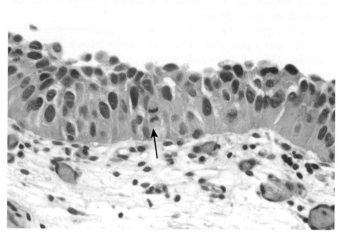

FIG. 16.18 Carcinoma in situ *(CIS)* with enlarged hyperchromatic nuclei and a mitotic figure *(arrow).*

small, localized papillary tumors that are not high grade, transurethral resection is both diagnostic and therapeutic. Patients with tumors that are at high risk for recurrence or progression are treated with intravesical instillation of an attenuated strain of *Mycobacterium bovis* called bacillus Calmette-Guérin (BCG), which elicits a localized delayed hypersensitivity reaction that destroys the tumor. Patients are closely monitored for tumor recurrence with periodic cystoscopy and urine cytologic studies. Radical cystectomy is primary therapy for

muscle-invasive bladder carcinoma and may be combined with radiation therapy and chemotherapy, as appropriate. Most metastatic tumors respond poorly to chemotherapy. A subset (roughly 30%) of metastatic bladder carcinomas respond to immune checkpoint inhibitors, sometimes dramatically, providing hope for this group of patients.

SEXUALLY TRANSMITTED INFECTIONS

A variety of infectious pathogens can be transmitted through sexual contact (Table 16.2) Behavioral factors associated with an increased risk of acquiring a sexually transmitted infection (STI) include (1) lower age at first sexual intercourse; (2) multiple sexual partners; (3) partners with multiple other partners; and (4) inconsistent condom use. Without ready access to healthcare for STI assessment and treatment, infections may persist, thereby increasing risk of transmission.

The various pathogens that cause STIs differ in many ways, but some general features should be noted.

- *STIs may become established locally and then spread from the urethra, vagina, cervix, rectum, or oral pharynx.* Transmission of STIs often occurs from asymptomatic people who do not realize that they have an infection.
- *Infection with one STI-associated organism increases the risk for others,* due to common risk factors as well as epithelial injury caused by infection.
- *The microbes that cause STIs can be spread from a pregnant woman and cause severe damage to the fetus or child.*

Table 16.2 Classification of Important Sexually Transmitted Diseases

	Associated Disease(s)—Distribution by Sex		
Pathogen	Males	Both	Females
Viruses			
Herpes simplex virus		Primary and recurrent herpes, neonatal herpes	
Hepatitis B virus		Hepatitis	
Human papillomavirus	Penile cancer	Condyloma acuminatum, anal cancer, oropharyngeal carcinoma	Cervical dysplasia and cancer, vulvar cancer
Human immunodeficiency virus		Acquired immunodeficiency syndrome	
Chlamydiae			
Chlamydia trachomatis	Urethritis, epididymitis, proctitis	Lymphogranuloma venereum	Urethral syndrome, cervicitis, bartholinitis, salpingitis, and sequelae
Mollicutes			
Ureaplasma urealyticum	Urethritis		Cervicitis
Bacteria			
Neisseria gonorrhoeae	Epididymitis, prostatitis, urethral stricture	Urethritis, proctitis, pharyngitis, disseminated gonococcal infection	Cervicitis, endometritis, bartholinitis, salpingitis, and sequelae (infertility, ectopic pregnancy, recurrent salpingitis)
Treponema pallidum		Syphilis	
Haemophilus ducreyi		Chancroid	
Calymmatobacterium granulomatis		Granuloma inguinale	
Protozoa			
Trichomonas vaginalis	Urethritis, balanitis		Vaginitis

Syphilis

Syphilis is a chronic STI caused by the spirochete *Treponema pallidum*. Despite public health measures and availability of effective treatment, its incidence has increased steadily since 2001. Rates of syphilis are significantly higher among marginalized communities with inadequate health care. Men are more commonly affected: 86% of primary and secondary syphilis cases occur in men, particularly men who have unprotected sex with men; however, since 2013, the incidence has also increased dramatically in women as has the rate of congenital syphilis. Syphilis is also more common in patients who are infected with HIV, in whom syphilis is more likely to progress to organ involvement and neurosyphilis.

Pathogenesis. **The usual source of infection is contact with a cutaneous or mucosal lesion in a sexual partner in the early (primary or secondary) stages of syphilis.** The organism is transmitted from such lesions during sexual activity through minute breaks in the skin or mucous membranes of the uninfected partner. In congenital cases, *T. pallidum* is transmitted across the placenta from mother to fetus, particularly during the early stages of maternal infection.

Once introduced into the body, the organisms rapidly disseminate to distant sites through lymphatics and the blood, even before the appearance of lesions at the primary inoculation site.

Syphilis is divided into three stages, with distinct clinical and pathologic manifestations (Fig. 16.19).

- *Primary syphilis.* Several weeks after infection (mean, 21 days), a primary lesion, termed a *chancre,* appears at the site of spirochete entry. Spirochetes are plentiful within the chancre and spread from there throughout the body by hematologic and lymphatic dissemination. The host mounts an immune response that fails to eradicate the organisms.
- *Secondary syphilis.* The chancre of *primary syphilis* resolves spontaneously over a period of 4 to 6 weeks and is followed in approximately 25% of untreated patients by the development of secondary syphilis. The manifestations of secondary syphilis, discussed in detail later, include mucocutaneous lesions, which are highly infectious, and generalized lymphadenopathy. Like the chancre, the lesions of secondary syphilis resolve even without antimicrobial therapy, at which point patients are said to be in *early latent-phase syphilis.*
- *Tertiary syphilis.* Patients who remain untreated next enter an asymptomatic, *late latent* phase of the illness, defined as being more than 1 year after the initial infection. In about one-third of patients, new symptoms develop over the next 5 to 20 years. This late symptomatic phase or tertiary syphilis is marked by the development of lesions in the cardiovascular system, central nervous system, or, less frequently, other organs. Spirochetes are much more difficult to demonstrate during the later stages of disease, and patients are accordingly much less likely to be infectious than are those in the primary or secondary stages of disease.

T. pallidum may also be transmitted across the placenta from an infected mother to the fetus at any time during pregnancy, which leads to the development of *congenital syphilis.* The likelihood of transmission is greatest during the early (primary and secondary) stages of disease, when spirochetes are most numerous. The stigmata of congenital syphilis do not develop until after the fourth month of pregnancy. Because the manifestations of maternal disease may be subtle, routine serologic testing for syphilis is performed in all

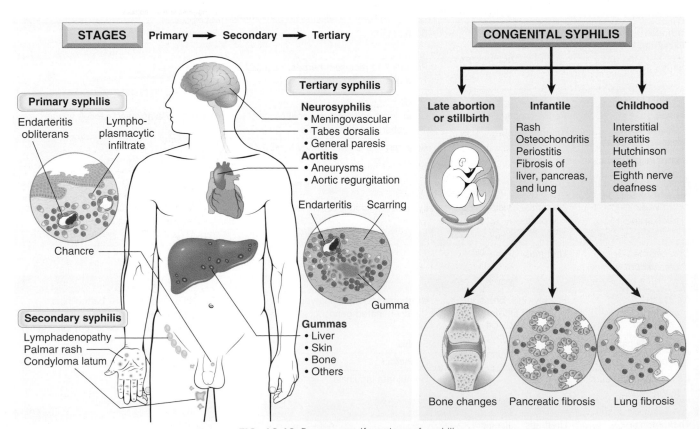

FIG. 16.19 Protean manifestations of syphilis.

pregnancies. Intrauterine death and perinatal death each occurs in approximately 25% of cases of untreated congenital syphilis.

MORPHOLOGY

The pathognomonic microscopic lesion of syphilis is a proliferative endarteritis with an accompanying inflammatory infiltrate rich in plasma cells that can be seen in all stages. Endarteritis has a central role in tissue injury at all sites involved by syphilis, but its pathogenesis is not understood; there is no evidence that the spirochetes directly infect and damage blood vessels. Instead, it is thought that the host immune response is responsible for the endothelial cell activation and proliferation that are the hallmark of the endarteritis, which eventually leads to perivascular fibrosis and luminal narrowing.

In primary syphilis, a **chancre** occurs on the penis or scrotum of 70% of men and on the vulva or cervix of 50% of women. The chancre is a slightly elevated, firm, reddened papule, up to several centimeters in diameter, that erodes to create a clean-based, shallow ulcer. The contiguous induration creates a buttonlike mass directly adjacent to the eroded skin ("hard chancre") (Fig. 16.20A). Regional lymph nodes are often slightly enlarged and firm. Microscopic examination of the ulcer reveals the typical lymphocytic and plasmacytic inflammatory infiltrate and inflammation and endarteritis (Fig. 16.20B). Spirochetes are readily demonstrable in histologic sections of early lesions with the use of immunohistochemical stains specific for spirochetes. Within approximately 2 months of resolution of the chancre, the lesions of secondary syphilis appear: generalized lymphadenopathy and widespread **mucocutaneous lesions** that involve the oral cavity and palmar and plantar surfaces. The rash frequently consists of discrete red-brown macules less than 5 mm in diameter but may be scaly or pustular. In moist skin areas, such as the anogenital region, inner thighs, and axillae, broad-based, elevated lesions termed **condylomata lata** may appear (not to be confused with condyloma acuminata caused by HPV) (Chapter 17). Histologic examination of mucocutaneous lesions during the secondary phase of the disease reveals the characteristic proliferative endarteritis and, with special stains or immunohistochemistry, spirochetes, which are often abundant. Lymphadenopathy is most common in the neck and inguinal areas. Histologic examination of enlarged nodes demonstrates hyperplasia of germinal centers accompanied by increased numbers of plasma cells or, less commonly, granulomas or neutrophils. Infrequent manifestations of secondary syphilis include hepatitis, renal disease, eye disease (iritis), and gastrointestinal symptoms.

Lesions associated with **tertiary syphilis** are divided into three major categories, which may occur singly or in combination: cardiovascular syphilis, neurosyphilis, and so-called "benign" tertiary syphilis. Cardiovascular syphilis takes the form of **syphilitic aortitis** due to endarteritis of the vasa vasorum (Chapter 8). **Neurosyphilis** occurs with increased frequency in patients with concomitant HIV infection (Chapter 21). Benign tertiary syphilis is characterized by the formation of **gummas,** white-gray, rubbery lesions that occur singly or multiply and vary in size from microscopic lesions to large tumorlike masses. They may occur in most organs but are particularly common in skin, subcutaneous tissue, bone, and joints. On microscopic examination, the gumma contains a central zone of coagulative necrosis surrounded by dense fibrous tissue with a mixed inflammatory infiltrate composed of lymphocytes, plasma cells, activated macrophages (epithelioid cells), and occasional giant cells, suggestive of a delayed hypersensitivity reaction. Spirochetes are only rarely demonstrable.

Manifestations of **congenital syphilis** include stillbirth, early congenital syphilis (onset before 2 years of age), and late congenital syphilis (onset after 2 years of age).

- **Early congenital syphilis** usually manifests at birth or within the first few months of life. Affected infants present with nasal discharge, hepatomegaly, jaundice, skeletal abnormalities, generalized lymphadenopathy, and mucocutaneous lesions similar to those seen in secondary syphilis in adults.

- **Late congenital syphilis** is characterized by a distinctive **triad of interstitial keratitis, Hutchinson teeth, and eighth-nerve deafness.** Hutchinson teeth are small, peg-shaped incisors, often with notches in the enamel. Eighth-nerve deafness and optic nerve atrophy develop secondary to meningovascular syphilis. Additional manifestations include anterior bowing of the shins ("saber shins"), frontal bossing of the skull, saddle nose deformity, and intellectual disability.

Clinical Features. *T. pallidum* is highly sensitive to antibiotics such as penicillin, a short course of which is sufficient to treat all stages of the disease. Serology is the mainstay of diagnosis. Serologic tests for syphilis include nontreponemal antibody tests and antitreponemal

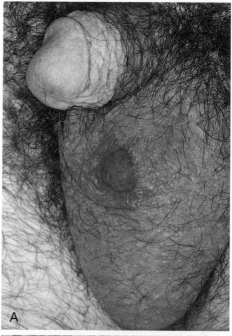

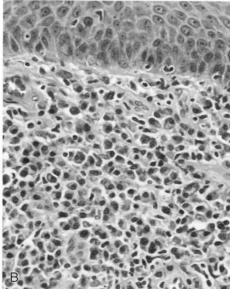

FIG. 16.20 (A) Syphilitic chancre of the scrotum. Such lesions are typically painless despite the presence of ulceration, and they heal spontaneously. (B) Histologic features of the chancre include a diffuse plasma cell infiltrate beneath squamous epithelium of skin.

antibody tests. Nontreponemal tests include the rapid plasma reagin (RPR) and venereal disease research laboratory (VDRL) tests, which detect antibodies to cardiolipin, an antigen that is present in both host tissues and the treponemal cell wall. Anticardiolipin antibodies in patients with lupus can result in a false-positive syphilis test. By contrast, treponemal antibody tests measure antibodies that specifically react with *T. pallidum.*

The interpretation of these tests is complex because of differences in the antibody responses they measure and imperfections in the tests.

- Both treponemal and nontreponemal antibody tests are only moderately sensitive (~70% to 85%) for primary syphilis.
- Both types of test are very sensitive (>95%) for secondary syphilis.
- Treponemal tests are very sensitive for tertiary and latent syphilis. By contrast, nontreponemal antibody titers fall with time, and so are somewhat less sensitive for tertiary or latent syphilis.
- Nontreponemal antibody levels fall with successful treatment of syphilis; therefore changes in the titers detected in these tests can be used to monitor therapy. Treponemal tests, which are nonquantitative, remain positive, even after successful therapy.
- Both types of tests can be used for initial screening for syphilis, but positive results should be confirmed using a test of the other type (e.g., confirm nontreponemal positive test results with a treponemal test and vice versa).

Confirmatory testing is needed because false-positive results can occur in both types of tests. Causes of false-positive results in these tests include pregnancy, autoimmune diseases (e.g., systemic lupus erythematosus), and infections other than syphilis.

Gonorrhea

Gonorrhea is a sexually transmitted infection caused by *Neisseria gonorrhoeae.* It is second only to *Chlamydia trachomatis* among bacterial STIs. Infection requires direct contact with the mucosa of an infected individual, usually during sexual activity. The bacteria initially attach to mucosal epithelium, particularly of the columnar or transitional type, using a variety of membrane-associated adhesion molecules and structures called *pili.* The organism then penetrates through the epithelial cells to invade the deeper tissues of the host.

Infection in men causes urethritis. In women, *N. gonorrhoeae* infection is often asymptomatic and may go unnoticed. The effects of untreated, asymptomatic gonorrhea in women are particularly serious, as ascending infection may lead to pelvic inflammatory disease, a cause of infertility and ectopic pregnancy (Chapter 17). Coinfection with other STIs is common, particularly *Chlamydia trachomatis,* which shares a similar clinical course with gonorrhea (described later). Infection is diagnosed by culture and PCR tests. Gonorrhea is treated with specific antibiotics; however, resistance to some of these treatments is emerging.

MORPHOLOGY

N. gonorrhoeae provokes an intense, suppurative inflammatory reaction. In males, this manifests most often as a purulent urethral discharge, associated with an edematous, congested urethral meatus. Gram-negative diplococci, many within the cytoplasm of neutrophils, are readily identified in Gram stains of the purulent exudate (Fig. 16.21). Ascending infection may result in acute prostatitis, epididymitis (Fig. 16.22), or orchitis. Abscesses may complicate severe cases. Urethral and endocervical exudates tend to be less conspicuous in females, although acute inflammation of adjacent structures, such as the Bartholin glands, is fairly common. Ascending infection involving the uterus, fallopian tubes, and ovaries results in acute salpingitis, sometimes complicated by tuboovarian abscesses. The acute inflammatory

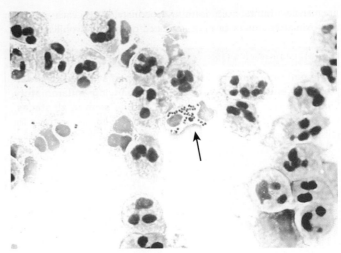

FIG. 16.21 *Neisseria gonorrhoeae.* Gram stain of urethral discharge demonstrates characteristic gram-negative, intracellular diplococci (*arrow*). (Courtesy of Dr. Rita Gander, Department of Pathology, University of Texas Southwestern Medical School, Dallas, Texas.)

process is followed by the development of granulation tissue and scarring, with resultant strictures and other permanent deformities of the involved structures, giving rise to **pelvic inflammatory disease** (Chapter 19).

Clinical Features. In most males who are infected with gonorrhea, *dysuria, urinary frequency,* and a *mucopurulent urethral exudate* develop within 2 to 14 days of the time of initial infection; however, infection may be asymptomatic. Treatment with appropriate antimicrobial therapy eradicates the organism and symptoms resolve promptly. Untreated infections may progress to involve the prostate, seminal vesicles, epididymis, and testis. In untreated cases, chronic urethral stricture, permanent sterility, and development of a chronic carrier state may occur.

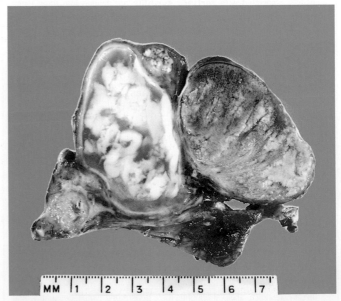

FIG. 16.22 Acute epididymitis caused by gonococcal infection. The epididymis is involved by an abscess. Normal testis is seen on the *right.*

Among females, acute infections acquired by vaginal intercourse may be asymptomatic or may be associated with *dysuria, lower pelvic pain, and vaginal discharge*. Untreated cases may be complicated by acute inflammation of the fallopian tubes (salpingitis) and ovaries *(pelvic inflammatory disease)*. Scarring of the fallopian tubes may occur, with resultant infertility and an increased risk for ectopic pregnancy. Gonococcal infection of the upper genital tract may spread to the peritoneal cavity, where the exudate may extend up the right paracolic gutter to the dome of the liver, resulting in gonococcal perihepatitis. Depending on sexual practices, other sites of primary infection in both males and females include the oropharynx and the anorectal area, with resultant acute pharyngitis and proctitis, respectively.

Disseminated infection of adults and adolescents is uncommon and usually presents as septic arthritis accompanied by a hemorrhagic papular and pustular rash. Strains that cause disseminated infection are usually resistant to the lytic action of complement, but rare patients with inherited complement deficiencies are susceptible to systemic spread regardless of the infecting strain. Gonococcal infection may be transmitted to infants during passage through the birth canal, resulting in conjunctivitis that can cause blindness. The eye infection, which is preventable by instillation of silver nitrate or antibiotics in the newborn's eyes, remains an important cause of blindness in some lower-resource nations.

Nucleic acid amplification testing is the preferred diagnostic modality due to its accuracy, rapid turnaround time, and its ability to be performed on patient-collected specimens. Culture permits determination of antibiotic sensitivity but is less sensitive than molecular testing and requires about 48 hours.

Nongonococcal Urethritis and Cervicitis

Nongonococcal urethritis (NGU) and cervicitis are the most common forms of STI, and genital infection by *C. trachomatis* is the most common bacterial STI worldwide. *Mycoplasma genitalium* is the second most common cause of NGU; other implicated organisms include *Trichomonas vaginalis* and *Ureaplasma urealyticum*. The causative agents vary geographically and in patient populations based on sexual practices. In nearly 50% of cases, no pathogen is identified. As discussed earlier, gonorrhea infection is frequently associated with chlamydial infection.

C. trachomatis is a small gram-negative bacterium that is an obligate intracellular pathogen. It exists in two forms. The infectious form, the *elementary body*, is capable of at least limited survival in the extracellular environment. The elementary body is taken up by host cells, primarily through a process of receptor-mediated endocytosis. Once inside the cell, the elementary body differentiates into a metabolically active form, termed the *reticulate body*. Using the energy sources of the host cell, the reticulate body replicates and ultimately forms new infectious elementary bodies, which have a tropism for columnar epithelial cells.

The clinical features of *C. trachomatis* infections are similar to those caused by *N. gonorrhoeae*. Patients may develop epididymitis, prostatitis, pelvic inflammatory disease, pharyngitis, conjunctivitis, perihepatic inflammation, and proctitis. *C. trachomatis* urethritis may be asymptomatic in both men and women and so may go untreated. The infection may be transmitted to newborns during vaginal birth; conjunctivitis is the most common manifestation, followed by pneumonia. *C. trachomatis* also causes lymphogranuloma venereum (LGV), discussed in the next section.

The morphologic and clinical features of chlamydial infection, with the exception of lymphogranuloma venereum, are virtually identical to those of gonorrhea. The primary infection is characterized by a watery to mucopurulent discharge with a predominance of neutrophils. Diagnosis is based on nucleic acid amplification tests performed on genital swabs or urine specimens. *C. trachomatis* appears to be the most common cause of *reactive arthritis,* which can also be seen in infections with other bacteria such as *Campylobacter jejuni* and *Shigella flexnari* (Chapter 19). Rarely, arthritis occurs in conjunction with urethritis/cervicitis and conjunctivitis.

Lymphogranuloma Venereum

Lymphogranuloma venereum (LGV) is a chronic, ulcerative disease caused by strains of *C. trachomatis* that are distinct from those causing nongonococcal urethritis or cervicitis (discussed earlier). Although previously considered an endemic disease of the tropics and subtropics, LGV is increasingly of concern beyond these geographic regions as a cause of inguinal lymphadenopathy and proctitis, spread primarily through unprotected intercourse in men who have sex with men. LGV infection has a strong correlation with HIV coinfection.

MORPHOLOGY

LGV may present as nonspecific urethritis or papular or ulcerative lesions involving the lower genitalia. Subsequently, the draining lymph nodes become swollen and tender; they may coalesce and rupture, resulting in fistulous tracts. If not treated, the infection can cause fibrosis and strictures in the anogenital tract. Rectal strictures are particularly common in women. Histologically, the lesions contain a **mixed granulomatous and neutrophilic inflammatory response.** Variable numbers of chlamydial inclusions may be seen in the cytoplasm of epithelial cells or inflammatory cells with special staining methods. Lymph node involvement is characterized by a granulomatous inflammatory reaction associated with irregularly shaped foci of necrosis and neutrophilic infiltration **(stellate abscesses)** (eFig. 16.8). With time, the inflammatory reaction gives rise to extensive fibrosis that can cause local lymphatic obstruction and strictures, producing **lymphedema.**

Clinical Features. The diagnosis of LGV is difficult because of its varied clinical presentation. As with other chlamydial infections, nucleic acid amplification tests have the highest sensitivity and specificity. Serologic testing is not specific and cannot distinguish prior from current infection.

Chancroid (Soft Chancre)

Chancroid is an acute, ulcerative infection caused by *Haemophilus ducreyi*, a gram-negative coccobacillus. The disease is most common in lower-resource countries in the tropics and subtropics; underdiagnosis is likely since testing for *H. ducreyi* is not routine. Furthermore, isolating the organism is challenging and PCR-based tests are not widely available. Due to skin ulceration, chancroid is an important cofactor for HIV infection.

MORPHOLOGY

The primary lesion of chancroid is a papule on the external genitalia that rapidly breaks down to produce an **ulcer**. Unlike syphilis, lesions are painful, may be multiple, and are not indurated. On microscopic examination, there is a superficial zone of neutrophilic debris and fibrin, with an underlying zone of granulation tissue, areas of necrosis, and thrombosed vessels. A dense, lymphoplasmacytic inflammatory infiltrate is present beneath the granulation tissue. Secondarily involved draining lymph nodes also exhibit necrotizing inflammation that frequently progresses to abscess formation, leading to draining ulcers.

Clinical Features. The primary lesion of chancroid appears within 4 to 7 days of inoculation. In male patients, the primary lesion is usually on the penis; in female patients, most lesions occur in the vagina or periurethral area. Over the course of several days, the surface of the primary lesion erodes to produce an irregular ulcer that may be painful. The regional lymph nodes, particularly in the inguinal region, become enlarged and tender in about 50% of cases within 1 to 2 weeks of the primary inoculation. Definitive diagnosis requires the identification of *H. ducreyi* on special culture media; even with appropriate media, sensitivity is less than 80%. Nucleic acid amplification and PCR tests have been developed; they are not widely available outside research laboratories.

Trichomoniasis

Trichomonas vaginalis is a large, flagellated protozoan that is usually transmitted by sexual contact. The trophozoite form adheres to the mucosa, where it causes superficial lesions. It is a frequent cause of vaginitis associated with pruritus and a profuse, frothy, yellow vaginal discharge. Urethral colonization may cause urinary frequency and dysuria. 70% of infected individuals are asymptomatic though, without treatment, many women do eventually develop symptoms. Infection during pregnancy can cause premature rupture of membranes and preterm delivery. In men, *T. vaginalis* infection may manifest as urethritis. The organism is usually demonstrable by microscopy of wet mounts from vaginal scrapings. Laboratory testing for chlamydia and gonorrhea is usually performed when trichomoniasis is suspected.

Genital Herpes Simplex

Genital herpes infection is a common STI. Both herpes simplex virus type 1 (HSV-1) and herpes simplex virus type 2 (HSV-2) can cause anogenital or oral infections; while most cases of genital herpes are due to HSV-2, an increasing number of cases are secondary to HSV-1 infection. According to the CDC, about one in eight persons between the ages of 14 and 49 is infected with HSV-2 in the United States, though there is regional variation. HSV is transmitted when the virus comes into contact with a mucosal surface or broken skin of a susceptible host. Because the virus is readily inactivated at room temperature, transmission requires direct contact with a person who is infected. As with other STIs, the risk for infection is related to the number of sexual partners. HSV-2 infection, particularly when recent, increases risk for HIV infection in part because of mucosal ulceration.

MORPHOLOGY

The initial lesions of genital HSV infection are **painful, erythematous vesicles** on the mucosa or skin of the lower genitalia and adjacent extragenital sites. Histologic changes include the presence of **intraepithelial vesicles** accompanied by necrotic cellular debris, neutrophils, and cells harboring characteristic intranuclear viral inclusions. The classic **Cowdry type A inclusion** is a light purple, homogeneous intranuclear structure surrounded by a clear halo (eFig. 16.9). Infected cells commonly fuse to form **multinucleate syncytia.** The inclusions stain with antibodies to HSV, permitting a rapid, specific diagnosis of HSV infection in histologic sections or smears.

Clinical Features. As discussed earlier, both HSV-1 and HSV-2 can cause genital or oral infection, and both produce indistinguishable primary or recurrent mucocutaneous lesions. Primary infection with HSV-2 is often asymptomatic. Signs and symptoms when present may last for several weeks and include painful vesicular lesions, dysuria, urethral discharge, draining lymph node enlargement and tenderness, and systemic manifestations, such as fever, muscle aches, and headache. HSV is actively shed during this period, and shedding continues until the mucosal lesions have completely healed. Asymptomatic viral shedding can occur as long as 3 months after diagnosis. Recurrences are milder and of shorter duration than in the primary episode. Diagnosis is most often made by viral culture or nucleic acid amplification testing of fluid from vesicular lesions.

In immunocompetent adults, genital herpes is rarely life threatening. However, HSV can pose a threat to patients who are immunocompromised, in whom fatal, disseminated disease may develop. Also potentially life threatening is *neonatal herpes infection,* which is typically acquired during passage through the birth canal of mothers with either primary or recurrent genital HSV infection. Its incidence has risen in parallel with the rise in genital HSV infection. For prognostic and therapeutic considerations, the manifestations of neonatal herpes infections are categorized as (1) localized involvement of skin, eyes, and mouth (SEM); (2) CNS involvement with or without SEM; and (3) disseminated disease (e.g., to liver and lungs). Mortality is highest with disseminated disease, which has a 1-year mortality rate of approximately 30%. About 70% of infants with CNS involvement have subsequent neurodevelopmental abnormalities.

Human Papillomavirus Infection

HPV causes a number of squamous proliferations in the genital tract, including condyloma acuminatum, as well as several precancerous lesions that can undergo transformation to carcinomas. The latter most commonly involve the cervix (Chapter 17) but also occur in the penis, vulva, oropharyngeal tonsil, and conjunctiva. *Condylomata acuminata,* also known as *anogenital warts,* are caused by HPV types 6 and 11. These lesions occur on the penis as well as on the female genitalia. They should not be confused with the condylomata lata of secondary syphilis. Genital HPV infection may be transmitted to neonates during vaginal delivery. HPV vaccines offer protection against both low-risk (types 6 and 11) and high-risk (types 16 and 18) HPV and therefore protect against development of anogenital warts as well as HPV-associated cancers.

MORPHOLOGY

In males, condylomata acuminata usually occur on the coronal sulcus or inner surface of the prepuce, where they range in size from small, sessile lesions to large, papillary proliferations measuring several centimeters in diameter (Fig. 16.23). In females, they commonly occur on the vulva. Examples of the microscopic appearance of these lesions are presented in Chapter 17.

■ RAPID REVIEW

Lesions of the Penis

- Squamous cell carcinoma and its precursor lesions are the most important penile lesions. Many are associated with HPV infection.
- Squamous cell carcinoma occurs on the glans or shaft of the penis as an ulcerated infiltrative lesion that may spread to inguinal nodes and infrequently to distant sites. Most cases occur in uncircumcised males.
- Other important penile disorders include congenital abnormalities involving the position of the urethra (epispadias, hypospadias) and inflammatory disorders (balanitis, phimosis).

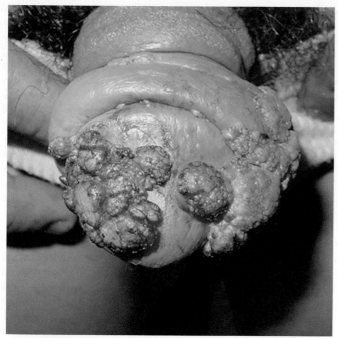

FIG. 16.23 Condyloma acuminatum. Multiple condylomatous lesions involve the glans, coronal sulcus, and foreskin. (From Amin MB, Tickoo SK: *Diagnostic Pathology: Genitourinary*, ed 3, St. Louis, 2023, Elsevier.)

Cryptorchidism

- *Cryptorchidism* refers to incomplete descent of the testis from the abdomen to the scrotum and is present in about 1% of 1-year-old male infants.
- Bilateral or, in some cases, even unilateral cryptorchidism is associated with tubular atrophy and sterility in both testes.
- The cryptorchid testis carries a higher risk for testicular cancer, which arises from foci of germ cell neoplasia in situ within the atrophic tubules. Early orchiopexy reduces the risk for sterility and cancer.

Testicular Tumors

- Testicular neoplasms are the most common cause of painless testicular enlargement. They occur with increased frequency in association with undescended testes and with testicular dysgenesis.
- Germ cells are the source of 95% of testicular tumors, and the remainder arise from Sertoli or Leydig cells. Germ cell tumors may be composed of a single "pure" histologic pattern (60% of cases) or mixed patterns.
- The most common histologic patterns of germ cell tumors are seminoma, embryonal carcinoma, yolk sac tumor, choriocarcinoma, and teratoma. Mixed tumors contain more than one element, most commonly embryonal carcinoma, teratoma, and yolk sac tumor.
- Clinically, testicular germ cell tumors are divided into two groups: seminoma and nonseminomatous tumors. Seminoma remains confined to the testis for a long time and spreads mainly to paraaortic nodes; distant spread is rare, and prognosis is better than nonseminomatous tumors. Nonseminomatous tumors tend to spread earlier, by both lymphatics and blood vessels.
- hCG is produced by syncytiotrophoblasts and is always elevated in patients with choriocarcinomas and those with seminomas

containing syncytiotrophoblasts. AFP is elevated when there is a yolk sac tumor component.

Prostatitis

- Bacterial prostatitis may be acute or chronic; the responsible organism usually is *E. coli* or another gram-negative rod.
- Chronic pelvic pain syndrome (chronic abacterial prostatitis), despite shared symptomatology with chronic bacterial prostatitis, is of unknown etiology and difficult to treat.
- Granulomatous prostatitis may be either infectious (e.g., following treatment with BCG) or noninfectious (foreign-body reaction to leaked fluids from ruptured prostatic ducts and acini).

Benign Prostatic Hyperplasia

- BPH is characterized by benign proliferations of stromal and glandular elements. Dihydrotestosterone (DHT), an androgen derived from testosterone, is the major hormonal stimulus for proliferation.
- BPH originates in the periurethral transition zone. The hyperplastic nodules exhibit variable proportions of stroma and glands. Hyperplastic glands are lined by two cell layers, an inner columnar layer and an outer layer composed of flattened basal cells.
- Clinical findings result from urinary tract obstruction caused by prostatic enlargement and contraction of smooth muscle elements in the stroma; they include hesitancy, urgency, nocturia, and poor urinary stream. Chronic obstruction predisposes to recurrent urinary tract infections.

Carcinoma of the Prostate

- Carcinoma of the prostate is a common cancer of men older than 50 years of age.
- Prostate carcinomas range from indolent lesions that never cause harm to aggressive fatal tumors.
- The most common acquired mutations in prostatic carcinomas create *TPRSS2-ETS* fusion genes or act to enhance PI3K/AKT signaling, which promotes tumor cell growth and survival.
- Carcinomas of the prostate arise most commonly in the outer, peripheral zone of the gland and may be palpable by rectal examination.
- Grading of prostate cancer by the Gleason system correlates with pathologic stage and prognosis.
- Serum PSA measurement is a controversial cancer screening test but has clear value in monitoring progressive or recurrent prostate cancer.
- Prostatic cancers are androgen dependent and hence treated with surgical or drug-induced castration, with or without radiation.

Bladder

- Nonneoplastic conditions of the bladder include diverticula and infections (cystitis).
- Inflammatory lesions of the bladder include bacterial cystitis, hemorrhagic cystitis, interstitial cystitis, and malakoplakia.
- The vast majority (95%–97% in the United States) of bladder cancers are urothelial; squamous cell carcinoma has a higher incidence in areas where urinary schistosomiasis is endemic.
- Risk factors for bladder cancer include cigarette smoking, various occupational carcinogens, and prior cyclophosphamide or radiation therapy.
- There are two distinct precursor lesions of invasive urothelial carcinoma: noninvasive papillary tumor and carcinoma in situ.
  - Noninvasive papillary tumor, including papilloma, papillary urothelial neoplasm of low malignant potential (PUNLMP),

low-grade papillary urothelial carcinoma, and high-grade papillary urothelial carcinoma, have gain-of-function mutations that increase signaling through growth factor receptor pathways (e.g., amplifications of *FGFR3*); progression is uncommon (~20%) and is associated with TP53 mutations.

- Carcinoma in situ is more likely to become muscle invasive; mutations that disrupt p53 and RB occur early in carcinogenesis.

Sexually Transmitted Infections

Syphilis

- Syphilis is caused by *T. pallidum* and has three stages.
  - Primary syphilis: A painless lesion called a *chancre* develops on the external genitalia along with regional lymph node enlargement.
  - Secondary syphilis: Generalized lymphadenopathy and mucocutaneous lesions that may be maculopapular or take the form of flat, raised lesions called *condylomata lata*. Both primary and secondary lesions contain bacteria and hence can transmit infections.
  - Tertiary syphilis: May cause proximal aortitis and aortic insufficiency; may involve the brain, meninges, and the spinal cord; or may cause focal granulomatous lesions called *gummas* in multiple organs. The lesions are usually sterile.
- Congenital syphilis is caused by maternal transmission of the spirochetes in utero or during vaginal birth, mostly during the primary and secondary stages of disease in the mother. It may lead to stillbirth or cause widespread tissue injury in the liver, spleen, lung, bones, and pancreas.
- Most syphilitic lesions demonstrate proliferative endarteritis and a plasma cell–rich inflammatory infiltrate. Gummas have a central area of necrosis surrounded by lymphoplasmacytic infiltrates, activated macrophages, and fibrosis.
- The diagnostic mainstay is serologic testing. Nontreponemal antibody tests (VDRL and RPR) are usually positive in early disease but may be negative in advanced disease. Treponeme-specific antibody test results become positive later in primary syphilis and remain positive indefinitely.

Gonorrhea

- Gonorrhea is a common STI affecting the genitourinary tract. Control of dissemination requires an effective complement-mediated immune response.
- Gonorrhea presents with dysuria and a milky, purulent urethral discharge, although a high percentage of cases, particularly in females, is asymptomatic.
- Uncontrolled infection in females can give rise to pelvic inflammatory disease, resulting in infertility and ectopic pregnancy.
- Coinfection with other STIs, especially *C. trachomatis,* is common.

- Gonorrhea can be transmitted to newborns during passage through the birth canal.
- Diagnosis can be made by culture of the exudates as well as by nucleic acid amplification techniques.

Nongonococcal Urethritis and Cervicitis

- NGU and cervicitis are the most common forms of STI. Most cases are caused by *C. trachomatis* and the rest by *T. vaginalis, M. genitalium,* and *U. urealyticum.*
- *C. trachomatis* is a gram-negative intracellular bacterium that causes a disease that is clinically indistinguishable from gonorrhea in both men and women. Diagnosis can be made by sensitive nucleic acid amplification tests in urine samples or vaginal swabs.
- *C. trachomatis* infection can cause reactive arthritis along with conjunctivitis and generalized mucocutaneous lesions.

Lymphogranuloma Venereum and Chancroid

- LGV is caused by *C. trachomatis* serotypes that are distinct from those that cause nongonococcal urethritis. LGV is associated with urethritis, ulcerative genital lesions, lymphadenopathy, and involvement of the rectum. The lesions show both acute and chronic inflammation; they progress to fibrosis, with consequent lymphedema and formation of rectal strictures. Diagnosis is made by nucleic acid amplification tests and serology.
- *H. ducreyi* infection causes an acute painful ulcerative genital infection called *chancroid.* Inguinal node involvement occurs in many cases and leads to their enlargement and ulceration. Ulcers show a superficial area of acute inflammation and necrosis, with an underlying zone of granulation tissue and mononuclear infiltrate. Diagnosis is possible by culture of the organism and PCR-based tests.

Herpes Simplex Virus and Human Papillomavirus Infections

- HSV-2 and, less commonly, HSV-1 can cause genital infections. Initial (primary) infection may be asymptomatic or cause painful, erythematous, intraepithelial vesicles on the mucosa and skin of external genitalia, along with painful regional lymph node enlargement.
- On histologic examination, the vesicles of HSV infection contain necrotic cells and fused multinucleate giant cells with intranuclear inclusions (Cowdry type A) that stain with antibodies to the virus.
- Neonatal herpes can be life threatening and occurs in children born to mothers with genital herpes. Affected infants may have generalized herpes, often associated with encephalitis and consequent high mortality.
- HPV causes many proliferative lesions of the genital mucosa, including nonneoplastic (condyloma acuminatum), precancerous lesions (e.g., carcinoma in situ of the cervix), and invasive squamous cell cancers of the cervix and penis. HPV vaccines protect against these lesions.

■ **Laboratory Tests**[a]

Test	Reference Values	Pathophysiology/Clinical Relevance
Alphafetoprotein (AFP), serum	<8.4 ng/mL	AFP is a glycoprotein normally expressed by embryonic hepatocytes and fetal yolk sac cells. Production drops after birth but rises again in patients with certain tumors. Serum AFP levels are increased in 90% of patients with hepatocellular carcinoma and in patients with certain germ cell tumors of the ovary and testis (e.g., yolk sac tumor, embryonal carcinoma, or mixed tumors with yolk sac component). AFP is also elevated in maternal serum in the setting of open neural tube defects (e.g., anencephaly, spina bifida).
Human chorionic gonadotropin (hCG), serum	Males and nonpregnant females: <5 mIU/mL Levels vary during pregnancy	hCG is a hormone comprised of α and β subunits. The α subunit is the same as that of FSH, LH, and TSH; therefore, most tests assess levels of the β subunit to increase sensitivity. During the first trimester, hCG synthesized by placental syncytiotrophoblastic cells stimulates the corpus luteum to secrete progesterone; subsequently, the placenta secretes progesterone and hCG levels fall. hCG may be secreted by multiple neoplasms including choriocarcinoma, seminomatous/nonseminomatous testicular tumors with syncytiotrophoblast differentiation, ovarian germ cell tumors, and gestational trophoblastic disease. hCG is clinically useful as a tumor marker for diagnosis and disease monitoring.
Nontreponemal syphilis tests (rapid plasma reagin [RPR], venereal disease research laboratory [VDRL], serum/cerebrospinal fluid [CSF])	Nonreactive	VDRL and RPR are nontreponemal serologic tests that measure antibodies to lipoprotein/cardiolipin antigens that are released from cells damaged by *Treponema pallidum*, the etiologic agent of syphilis. Titers decrease with time and following treatment, so these tests are most useful in the diagnosis of primary and secondary syphilis infection and in following response to therapy. Antibodies are detectable with both tests within a few weeks of development of the primary chancre, about 4–6 weeks after infection. Titers between different nontreponemal tests are not comparable, so the same test should be used to monitor response to treatment. Because the antibodies are not specific for syphilis, a treponemal test (e.g., *T. pallidum* IgG/IgM antibody test) is required for confirmation. Biologic false-positive results may be seen in systemic lupus erythematosus (SLE) due to formation of autoantibodies to lipoprotein/cardiolipin antigens. VDRL is useful in the diagnosis of neurosyphilis, but it has a high rate of false negatives hence only a positive test is useful.
Prostate specific antigen (PSA), serum	Total PSA 0–4 ng/mL	PSA, a protein produced by prostatic epithelium, can be used as a tumor marker in the diagnosis, staging, and treatment monitoring of prostate cancer. However, it is not specific for malignancy: PSA elevations can also be seen in prostatitis, benign prostatic hyperplasia, and after procedures and ejaculation. Therefore, definitive diagnosis of prostate cancer requires biopsy and pathologist examination. It is most useful in monitoring for disease recurrence after treatment.
Treponema pallidum IgG/IgM antibody, serum	Nonreactive	A test for IgG and IgM antibodies to *T. pallidum* is a specific test for the causative agent of syphilis. This test is particularly useful in diagnosing tertiary and latent syphilis. However, these antibodies persist after infection and can be seen in treated individuals. Therefore, a second method such as the nontreponemal RPR or VDRL tests can help establish how recent the infection is and whether or not the patient has received adequate treatment.

[a]The helpful review of this table by Dr. Gladell Paner, Department of Pathology, University of Chicago is greatly appreciated.

References values from https://www.mayocliniclabs.com/ by permission of Mayo Foundation for Medical Education and Research. All rights reserved.

Adapted from Deyrup AT, D'Ambrosio D, Muir J, et al. Essential Laboratory Tests for Medical Education. *Acad Pathol*. 2022;9. doi: 10.1016/j.acpath.2022.100046.

17

Female Genital System and Breast

OUTLINE

VULVA

The vulva is the external female genitalia and includes the hair-bearing skin (labia majora) and mucosa (labia minora). Disorders of the vulva most frequently are inflammatory; they are uncomfortable but not life threatening. By contrast malignant tumors of the vulva, although life threatening, are rare.

VULVITIS

One of the most common causes of vulvitis is reactive inflammation in response to an exogenous stimulus, which may be an allergen or an irritant. Scratching-induced trauma secondary to the associated intense pruritus often exacerbates the primary condition.

Allergic dermatitis and contact irritant dermatitis result from a reaction to additives in lotions and soaps, antiseptics, and chemical

The contributions to this chapter by Dr. Lora Hedrick Ellenson, Department of Pathology, Memorial Sloan Kettering Cancer Center, New York City, New York, and Dr. Susan C. Lester, Department of Pathology, Brigham and Women's Hospital, Harvard Medical School, Boston, Massachusetts, in the previous edition of this book are gratefully acknowledged. We also appreciate Dr. Lester's assistance in the current edition.

treatments on clothing, among others, and appear as well-defined erythematous weeping and crusting papules and plaques. Urine may be a cause of contact dermatitis in the elderly.

Vulvitis may also be caused by infections, which are often sexually transmitted. The most important infectious agents include human papillomavirus (HPV), the causative agent of condyloma acuminatum, vulvar intraepithelial neoplasia (VIN) and a subset of vulvar squamous carcinomas; herpes simplex virus (HSV-1 or HSV-2), the cause of genital herpes; *Neisseria gonorrhoeae,* a cause of suppurative infection of the vulvovaginal glands; and *Treponema pallidum,* which causes primary chancre at vulvar sites of inoculation. *Candida* is also a cause of vulvitis but is not sexually transmitted.

An important complication of vulvitis is obstruction of the excretory ducts of Bartholin glands. This blockage may result in painful dilation of the glands *(Bartholin cyst)* and abscess formation.

Nonneoplastic Epithelial Disorders

Lichen Sclerosus

Lichen sclerosus is characterized by thinning of the epidermis; disappearance of rete pegs; a zone of acellular, homogenized, dermal fibrosis; and a bandlike mononuclear inflammatory cell infiltrate (Fig. 17.1A). Clinically, it presents as smooth, white plaques *(leukoplakia)* or papules that in time may extend and coalesce. When the entire vulva is affected, the labia become atrophic and stiffened, and the vaginal orifice is constricted. Lichen sclerosus occurs in all age groups but most commonly affects postmenopausal women and prepubertal girls. The pathogenesis is uncertain, but the presence of activated T cells in the subepithelial inflammatory infiltrate and the increased frequency of autoimmune disorders in affected women suggest an autoimmune etiology. The risk of vulvar squamous cell carcinoma is slightly increased in women with lichen sclerosus, although it is not itself a premalignant lesion.

Squamous Cell Hyperplasia

Previously called hyperplastic dystrophy or lichen simplex chronicus, squamous cell hyperplasia is a nonspecific condition resulting from rubbing or scratching of the skin to relieve pruritus. Clinically it presents as *leukoplakia,* and histologic examination reveals thickening of the epidermis (acanthosis) and hyperkeratosis (Fig. 17.1B). Lymphocytic infiltration of the dermis is sometimes present. The hyperplastic epithelium may show mitotic activity but lacks cytologic atypia.

A variety of other benign dermatoses, such as psoriasis and lichen planus (Chapter 22), as well as malignant lesions of the vulva, such as squamous cell carcinoma in situ and invasive squamous cell carcinoma, may also present as leukoplakia. Thus, biopsy and microscopic examination are often needed to differentiate between these similar-appearing lesions.

TUMORS

Condylomas

***Condylomas* are warty lesions of the genitals that present in two distinctive forms, both of which are sexually transmitted.** *Condylomata lata,* uncommonly seen today, are flat, minimally elevated lesions that occur in secondary syphilis (Chapter 16). More common are *condylomata acuminata,* which are caused by low-risk HPV strains, mainly types 6 and 11; the lesions may be papillary and distinctly elevated or flat and rugose. They may occur anywhere on the anogenital surface as single or (more often) multiple lesions that are identical to those found on the penis and around the anus in males (Chapter 16). When located on the vulva, they range from a few millimeters to many centimeters in diameter and are red-pink to pink-brown (Fig. 17.2A). In darker skin, they may appear hyperpigmented. Histologically, they consist of papillary, exophytic cores of stroma covered by thickened squamous epithelium (eFig. 17.1) with characteristic viral cytopathic changes (koilocytic atypia), which consist of enlarged, wrinkled nuclei; hyperchromasia, and a cytoplasmic perinuclear halo (Fig. 17.2B). Vulvar condylomas do not progress to cancer. However, women with condyloma acuminata are at risk of having other HPV-related precancerous lesions of the vagina and cervix. HPV vaccines (described later) provide excellent protection against infection by low-risk HPV and genital warts.

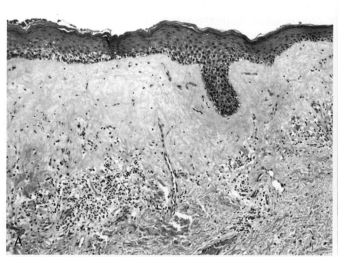
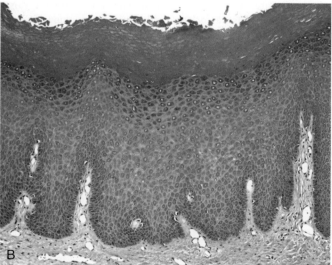

FIG. 17.1 Nonneoplastic vulvar epithelial disorders. (A) Lichen sclerosus. There is marked thinning of the epidermis, fibrosis of the superficial dermis, and chronic inflammatory cells in the deeper dermis. (B) Squamous cell hyperplasia displaying thickened epidermis and hyperkeratosis.

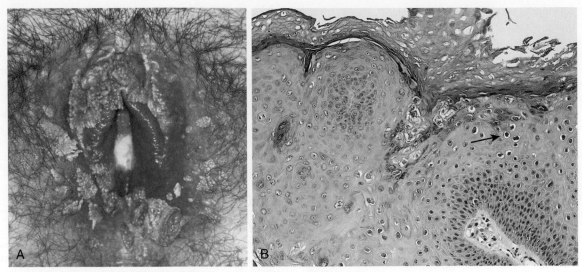

FIG. 17.2 (A) Numerous condylomas of the vulva. (B) Histopathologic features of condyloma acuminatum include acanthosis, hyperkeratosis, and human papillomavirus cytopathic effect (koilocytic atypia) characterized by atypical, enlarged, hyperchromatic nuclei with perinuclear halos (arrow).

Carcinoma of the Vulva

Carcinoma of the vulva represents about 3% of female genital tract cancers, occurring mostly in women older than age 60. Approximately 90% of carcinomas are squamous cell carcinomas; most of the other tumors are adenocarcinomas or basal cell carcinomas.

On the basis of etiology, pathogenesis, and histologic features, vulvar squamous cell carcinomas are divided into two groups. The less common form *(basaloid and warty carcinoma)* is related to high-risk HPV strains (especially HPV type 16) and occurs in women at an average age of 60 years, particularly in individuals who smoke. This form is often preceded by precancerous changes in the epithelium termed vulvar intraepithelial neoplasia (VIN). VIN progresses in many patients to greater degrees of atypia and eventually to carcinoma in situ; however, progression to invasive carcinoma is not inevitable and may take many years. The risk of progression to invasive carcinoma is higher in women who are older than 45 years of age or who are immunocompromised. The risk factors for VIN are the same as those associated with cervical squamous intra-epithelial lesions (see later), as both are related to HPV infection.

A second form of squamous carcinoma *(keratinizing squamous cell carcinoma)* occurs in older women (average age 75 years) with long-standing lichen sclerosus or squamous cell hyperplasia and is not related to HPV. It is preceded by differentiated vulvar intra-epithelial neoplasia (dVIN), characterized by abnormal keratinization and cytologic atypia confined to the basal layer. If left untreated, it may give rise to HPV-negative, well-differentiated, keratinizing squamous cell carcinoma. It is postulated that the chronic epithelial irritation and associated increase in cell turnover that occurs in lichen sclerosus or squamous cell hyperplasia contribute to the malignant phenotype, presumably by fostering the acquisition of driver mutations in oncogenes and tumor suppressor genes.

MORPHOLOGY

VIN and early vulvar carcinoma commonly presents as areas of **leukoplakia.** In about one-fourth of the cases, the lesions are pigmented due to the presence of melanin. With time, areas of leukoplakia are transformed into overt exophytic or ulcerated endophytic tumors. HPV-positive tumors are often multifocal and warty and tend to be poorly differentiated **squamous cell carcinomas,** whereas HPV-negative tumors are usually unifocal, well-differentiated keratinizing squamous cell carcinomas.

Both forms of vulvar carcinoma tend to remain confined to their site of origin for many years but ultimately invade and spread, usually first to regional lymph nodes. Ultimately, hematogenous spread to the lungs and other organs may occur. As with most carcinomas, outcome is dependent on tumor stage: the risk of metastasis correlates with the depth of invasion and tumor size.

Extramammary Paget Disease

Paget disease is an intraepidermal proliferation of atypical epithelial cells that can occur in the skin of the vulva or nipple of the breast (described later). In contrast to Paget disease of the nipple, which is always associated with an underlying ductal breast carcinoma, only a minority of cases of vulvar (extramammary) Paget disease have an underlying tumor. Instead, vulvar Paget cells most commonly appear to arise from multipotent cells found within the ducts of the vulvar skin.

Paget disease manifests as a red, scaly, crusted plaque that may mimic the appearance of dermatitis. On histologic examination, large cells with abundant pale, finely granular cytoplasm and occasional cytoplasmic vacuoles infiltrate the epidermis, singly and in groups (Fig. 17.3).

Intraepidermal Paget disease may persist for many years or even decades without invasion or metastases. Treatment consists of wide local excision. In the rare instances when invasion develops, the prognosis is poor.

VAGINA

In adults, the vagina is seldom a site of primary disease; more often, it is involved secondarily by cancer or infections arising in adjacent organs (e.g., cervix, bladder, rectum).

Congenital anomalies of the vagina are uncommon and include total absence of the vagina and a septate or double vagina (usually

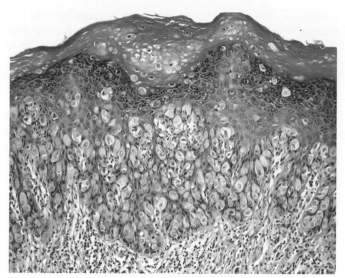

FIG. 17.3 Paget disease of the vulva. Large tumor cells with pale-pink cytoplasm are seen infiltrating the epidermis. Chronic inflammatory cells are present in the underlying dermis.

associated with a septate cervix and, sometimes, septate uterus), and lateral *Gartner duct cysts* arising from persistent wolffian duct rests.

VAGINITIS

Vaginitis secondary to infection is a common condition that is usually transient and is associated with a vaginal discharge (leukorrhea). Infectious agents include bacteria, fungi, and parasites. Many are normal commensals that become pathogenic only in the setting of diabetes, systemic antibiotic therapy (which disrupts normal microbial flora), immunodeficiency, pregnancy, or recent abortion. Frequent pathogenic organisms include *Candida albicans*, *Trichomonas vaginalis*, and *Gardnerella vaginalis*. *C. albicans* is part of the normal vaginal flora in about 20% of women; symptomatic infection almost always involves one of the predisposing influences listed above or superinfection by a new, more aggressive strain. Candidal vaginitis is characterized by a thick white discharge containing hyphal forms that can be identified on a Papanicolaou test (eFig. 17.2). Worldwide, *T. vaginalis* is the most common nonviral sexually transmitted infection. Infection is often asymptomatic but can produce a copious, watery, gray-green discharge in which parasites can be identified by microscopy (eFig. 17.3). *G. vaginalis* is a gram-negative coccobacillus that is implicated as the main cause of *bacterial vaginosis*. Patients present with a thin, malodorous discharge within which are found "clue cells," squamous cells covered with a shaggy coat of coccobacilli.

MALIGNANT NEOPLASMS

Squamous Cell Carcinoma

Vaginal carcinoma is extremely uncommon and arises from vaginal intraepithelial neoplasia (VAIN), a precursor lesion analogous to cervical squamous intraepithelial lesion (see later). Virtually all primary carcinomas of the vagina are squamous cell carcinomas associated with high-risk HPV infection. The greatest risk factor is a previous carcinoma of the cervix or vulva. Most often the invasive tumor affects the upper vagina, particularly the posterior wall at the junction with the ectocervix, and tends to spread to regional iliac nodes.

Embryonal Rhabdomyosarcoma

Also called *sarcoma botryoides,* this rare vaginal tumor composed of malignant embryonal rhabdomyoblasts is most frequently found in infants and children younger than 5 years of age. It may also be found in other sites, such as the urinary bladder and bile ducts. It is discussed further with other soft tissue tumors in Chapter 19.

CERVIX

The majority of cervical lesions are inflammatory (cervicitis). Cervical squamous cell carcinoma is one of the most common cancers in women worldwide.

CERVICITIS

Inflammatory conditions of the cervix are extremely common and may be associated with a purulent vaginal discharge. Cervicitis can be subclassified as infectious or noninfectious, although differentiation is difficult due to the presence of normal vaginal flora, including incidental vaginal aerobes and anaerobes, streptococci, staphylococci, enterococci, and *Escherichia coli* and *Candida* spp.

Sexually transmitted organisms, such as *Chlamydia trachomatis, Ureaplasma urealyticum, T. vaginalis, Neisseria gonorrhoeae,* HSV-2 (the agent of genital herpes), and certain types of HPV, can cause significant morbidity. *C. trachomatis* is by far the most common of these pathogens, accounting for as many as 40% of cases of cervicitis encountered in sexually transmitted disease clinics. Although less common, herpetic infections are noteworthy because maternal–infant transmission during childbirth may result in serious, sometimes fatal systemic herpetic infection in the newborn.

Cervicitis may come to attention on routine examination or due to leukorrhea. Treatment is usually empiric with antibiotics that are active against chlamydia and gonococcus. In some instances, nucleic acid amplification tests are used on vaginal fluid to identify the presence of these organisms as well as *Trichomonas vaginalis*.

Endocervical Polyp

Endocervical polyps are common benign exophytic growths that arise within the endocervical canal. They vary from small, sessile "bumps" to large polypoid masses that may protrude through the cervical os. Histologically, they consist of a fibrous stroma covered by mucus-secreting endocervical glands, often accompanied by inflammation. Their main significance is that they may be the source of irregular vaginal bleeding due to ulceration that arouses suspicion of an ominous lesion. However, these lesions have no malignant potential, and simple curettage or surgical excision is curative.

NEOPLASIA OF THE CERVIX

The vast majority of cervical tumors are carcinomas caused by oncogenic strains of HPV. The columnar mucus-secreting epithelium of the endocervix meets the squamous epithelial covering of the ectocervix at the squamocolumnar junction, the precise location of which varies with age and hormonal status. At puberty, the squamocolumnar junction undergoes eversion, and the columnar epithelium shifts outward to the ectocervical surface. The exposed columnar cells undergo squamous metaplasia, forming a region called the *transformation zone*. Immature squamous cells in this region are most susceptible to HPV, and this is where tumors most commonly arise (Fig. 17.4).

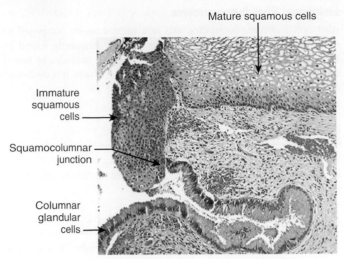

FIG. 17.4 Cervical transformation zone showing the transition from mature glycogenated squamous epithelium, to immature metaplastic squamous cells, to columnar endocervical glandular epithelium.

Pathogenesis. **High-risk HPVs are by far the most important factor in the development of cervical cancer.** HPVs are DNA viruses that are grouped into high and low oncogenic risk based on their genotypes. High-risk HPVs are also implicated in squamous cell carcinomas arising at many other sites, including the vagina, vulva, penis, anus, tonsil, and other oropharyngeal locations. Most HPV infections are transient and are eliminated within months by the host immune response. The duration of the infection is related to HPV type: infections with high-risk HPVs take longer to clear on average than infections with low-risk HPVs. Persistent infection increases the risk of development of cervical precursor lesions and subsequent carcinoma. Important risk factors for the development of cervical intraepithelial neoplasia (CIN) and invasive carcinoma are directly related to HPV exposure and include early age at first intercourse, multiple sexual partners, partner with multiple previous sexual partners, and persistent infection by high-risk strains of HPV.

The ability of HPV to act as a carcinogen depends on the viral E6 and E7 proteins, which interfere with the activity of the key tumor suppressor proteins, p53 and RB, respectively. Although HPV infects immature squamous cells, viral replication occurs in maturing squamous cells. Normally, these more mature cells are arrested in the G_1 phase of the cell cycle, but HPV infection prevents the growth arrest of these cells, an effect that is essential for replication of the viral genome and for productive shedding of virus. Two early viral proteins, E6 and E7, are prooncogenic: E6 binds to and mediates destruction of p53 and upregulates telomerase expression while E7 binds to the RB protein, displacing the E2F transcription factors that are normally sequestered by RB and promoting progression through the cell cycle (Chapter 6).

Two high-risk HPV viruses, types 16 and 18, account for approximately 70% of cases of cervical intraepithelial neoplasia (CIN) and cervical carcinoma (Fig. 17.5). These HPV types also show a propensity to integrate into the host cell genome, an event that is linked to progression. In low-risk HPV variants (e.g., types 6 and 11) associated with the development of condylomas of the lower genital tract, the E7 proteins bind RB with lower affinity and the E6 proteins fail to bind p53 altogether and instead appear to dysregulate growth and survival by interfering with the Notch signaling pathway.

Furthermore, low-risk HPV variants do not integrate into the host genome, remaining instead as free episomal viral DNA. Viral integration by high-risk HPVs appears to contribute to transformation in two ways: (1) integration always disrupts an HPV gene that negatively regulates E6 and E7, which leads to their increased expression, and (2) integration is associated with increased genomic instability, which may contribute to the acquisition of additional prooncogenic mutations.

Despite a high incidence of infection with one or more HPV types during the reproductive years, only a small number of individuals develop cancer. Thus, other factors, such as exposure to cocarcinogens (e.g., cigarette smoking) and host immune status, influence whether an HPV infection regresses or persists and eventually leads to cancer.

Squamous Intraepithelial Lesion (SIL) and Cervical Intraepithelial Neoplasia (CIN)

HPV-related carcinogenesis begins with the precancerous epithelial change termed SIL, which usually precedes the development of an overt cancer by many years, sometimes decades. In support of this idea, SIL peaks in incidence at about 30 years of age, whereas invasive carcinoma peaks at about 45 years of age.

The classification of cervical precursor lesions has evolved over time. Clinical management is based primarily on a two-tier system (low-grade SIL, LSIL; high-grade SIL, HSIL) that reflects the biology of the disease; however a three-tier system (CIN I, CIN II, and CIN III) plays a role in some treatment decisions.

- In the two-tier system, LSIL corresponds to CIN I and HSIL encompasses CIN II and III.

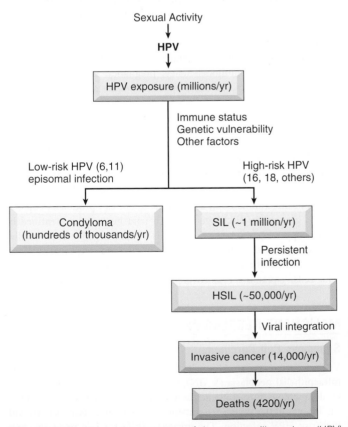

FIG. 17.5 Possible consequences of human papillomavirus (HPV) infection. Data are for the United States. Progression is associated with integration of virus and acquisition of additional mutations as discussed in the text. *HPV,* Human papillomavirus; *HSIL,* high-grade squamous intraepithelial lesion; *SIL,* squamous intraepithelial lesion.

Table 17.1 Natural History of Squamous Intraepithelial Lesions (SILs)

Lesion	Regress	Persist	Progress
LSIL (CIN I)	60%	30%	10% (to HSIL)
HSIL (CIN II, III)	30%	60%	10% (to carcinoma)[a]

HSIL, High-grade SIL; *LSIL,* low-grade SIL.
[a]Progression within 2 to 10 years.

- LSIL is far more common than HSIL. Most cases of LSIL regress spontaneously, but a small percentage progress to HSIL. In LSIL, there is a high level of viral replication and only mild alterations in the growth of the host cells. LSIL is not considered a premalignant lesion.
- HSIL demonstrates increased proliferation, arrested epithelial maturation, and lower levels of viral replication. It has a high risk for progression to carcinoma.

While HSIL is precancerous, in the majority of cases it does not progress to cancer, and some cases even regress. Risk factors for progression include cigarette smoking and immunocompromise, the latter suggesting that immune surveillance plays a role in preventing progression. Although the majority of HSILs develop from LSILs, approximately 20% of cases of HSIL develop de novo, independent of any known preexisting LSIL.

Because of the differences in the natural histories of these two groups of lesions (Table 17.1), optimal patient management depends on accurate diagnosis. Cervical precancerous lesions are associated with abnormalities in cytologic preparations that can be detected long before any abnormality is visible on gross inspection. Early detection of SIL is the rationale for the Papanicolaou (Pap) test, in which cells are scraped from the transformation zone and examined microscopically. The Pap test is the most successful cancer-screening test developed to date. Fifty years ago, carcinoma of the cervix was the leading cause of cancer death in women in the United States, but the death rate has declined by 75% to its present rank as the thirteenth cause of cancer mortality. By contrast, in countries with low-level screening with the Pap test, cervical cancer incidence remains high, with more than 85% of new cases being diagnosed in resource-limited countries. This disparity is also seen in cervical cancer mortality: the age-standardized mortality rate in lower- and middle-income countries is 12.4 per 100,000, compared to 5.2 per 100,000 in higher-income countries.

Testing for the presence of HPV DNA in cervical scrapes is a complementary molecular method of cervical cancer screening. HPV testing is highly sensitive for the identification of high-risk HPV types. It is most useful in women 30 years of age or older, since patients with a negative high-risk HPV test at this age are extremely unlikely to develop cervical neoplasia within the next 5 years. HPV testing of women younger than 30 years of age is less useful because of the high incidence of infection in this age group, lowering the predictive value of the HPV test for the presence of cervical neoplasia. Furthermore, while most women acquire HPV infections in their early 20s, these infections are usually cleared by the immune system and never progress to SIL, a process that occurs over many years.

Another important aspect of cervical cancer prevention is vaccination against high-risk HPV types. Vaccination is recommended for boys and girls by 11 to 12 years of age and young men and women up to 26 years of age. Vaccination of males is critical because of their role in the spread of HPV to women and the toll that HPV-related anal and oropharyngeal cancers take in men. The quadrivalent HPV vaccine for types 6, 11, 16, and 18, and the more recently introduced 9-valent vaccine, are very effective in preventing HPV infections and are expected to greatly lower the frequency of genital warts and cervical cancers associated with these HPV genotypes. The vaccines offer protection for up to 10 years; longer follow-up studies are pending. Despite its efficacy, vaccination does not supplant the need for routine cervical cancer screening—many at-risk women are already infected, and current vaccines protect against most but not all of the many oncogenic HPV genotypes.

MORPHOLOGY

Fig. 17.6 illustrates the spectrum of changes in SIL. LSIL (CIN I) is characterized by dysplastic changes in the lower third of the squamous epithelium and **koilocytotic change** in the superficial layers of the epithelium. In HSIL, immature squamous cells extend beyond the lower one-third of the epithelial thickness; involvement of the lower two-thirds corresponds to CIN II while in CIN III, these changes are seen in the full-thickness of the epithelium.

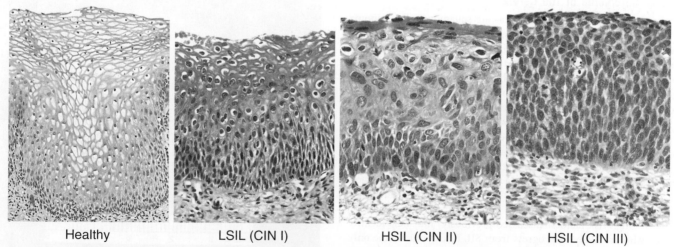

Healthy   LSIL (CIN I)   HSIL (CIN II)   HSIL (CIN III)

FIG. 17.6 Spectrum of squamous intraepithelial lesions (SILs) with healthy squamous epithelium for comparison: LSIL (CIN I) with koilocytotic atypia; HSIL (CIN II) with progressive atypia in all layers of the epithelium; and HSIL (CIN III) with diffuse atypia and loss of maturation *(far right image). CIN,* Cervical intraepithelial neoplasia; *HSIL,* high-grade squamous intraepithelial lesion; *LSIL,* low-grade squamous intraepithelial lesion.

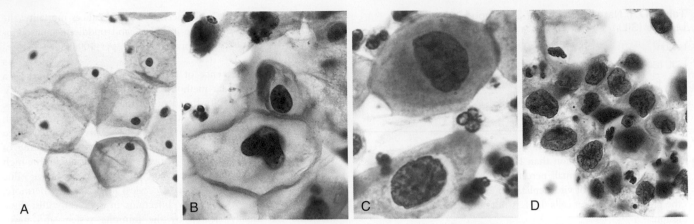

FIG. 17.7 Cytologic features of squamous intraepithelial lesion (SIL) in a Papanicolaou test. Superficial squamous cells may stain either red or blue. (A) Healthy exfoliated superficial squamous epithelial cells. (B) Low-grade squamous intraepithelial lesion (LSIL). (C and D) High-grade squamous intraepithelial lesions (HSILs). Note the reduction in cytoplasm and the increase in the nucleus-to-cytoplasm ratio as the grade of the lesion increases. This observation reflects the progressive loss of cellular differentiation on the surface of the cervical lesions from which these cells are exfoliated (see Fig. 17.6). (Courtesy of Dr. Edmund S. Cibas, Brigham and Women's Hospital, Boston, Massachusetts.)

There is variation in cell and nuclear size, heterogeneity of nuclear chromatin, and the presence of mitoses, some atypical, above the basal layer. With full thickness involvement, there is typically even greater variation in cell and nuclear size, chromatin heterogeneity, disorderly orientation of the cells, and abnormal mitoses. Koilocytic change is usually absent. These histologic features correlate with the cytologic appearances shown in Fig. 17.7.

Clinical Features. SIL is asymptomatic and comes to clinical attention through an abnormal Pap test result. Such cases are followed up by colposcopy, in which acetic acid identifies lesions for biopsy. Women with biopsy-documented LSIL are managed conservatively with careful observation, whereas HSILs and persistent LSIL are treated with surgical excision (cone biopsy). Follow-up tests and clinical examination are required in patients with HSIL, as these women remain at risk for HPV-associated cervical, vulvar, and vaginal cancers.

Invasive Carcinoma of the Cervix

The most common cervical carcinomas are squamous cell carcinoma (80%), followed by adenocarcinoma and mixed adenosquamous carcinoma (15%) and small cell neuroendocrine carcinoma (<5%), all caused by high-risk HPV. The proportion of adenocarcinoma has been increasing in recent decades due to the decreasing incidence of invasive squamous carcinoma and the limited ability of the Pap test to detect precancerous glandular lesions.

Squamous cell carcinoma incidence peaks at the age of about 45 years, some 10 to 15 years after the peak incidence of SIL. As already discussed, progression of SIL to invasive carcinoma is variable and unpredictable, and while HPV infection is necessary, it is not sufficient; dysregulation of oncogenes at the site of viral DNA insertion or accumulation of additional mutations acquired during increased cellular proliferation contribute to malignant transformation by HPV. Although risk factors (discussed previously) may help identify patients who are likely to progress from SIL to carcinoma, the only reliable way to monitor the disease course is with frequent physical examinations coupled with Pap tests and biopsy of suspicious lesions.

MORPHOLOGY

Invasive carcinomas of the cervix develop in the **transformation zone** and range from microscopic foci of stromal invasion to grossly conspicuous exophytic tumors (Fig. 17.8). Microscopically, the invasive tumors often consist of tongues and nests of squamous cells that produce a desmoplastic stromal response. Grading is based on the degree of squamous differentiation, which ranges from minimal to well-differentiated tumors that elaborate keratin pearls. Rare tumors with neuroendocrine differentiation resemble small cell carcinoma of the lung morphologically. Tumors encircling the cervix and penetrating into the underlying stroma produce a **barrel cervix,** which can be identified by direct palpation. Extension into the parametrial soft tissues can affix the uterus to the surrounding pelvic structures. The likelihood of spread to pelvic lymph nodes correlates with the depth of tumor invasion and the presence of tumor cells in vascular spaces. The risk of metastasis increases from less than 1% for tumors less than 3 mm in depth to more than 10% after invasion exceeds 3 mm.

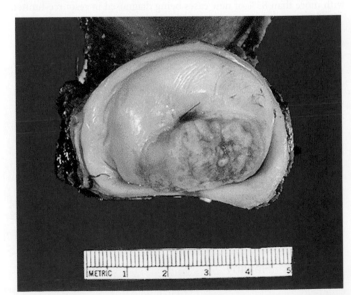

FIG. 17.8 Cervical os with invasive, exophytic cervical carcinoma. (From Klatt EC: *Robbins and Cotran Atlas of Pathology,* ed 4, Fig. 12.6, Philadelphia, 2021, Elsevier.)

Clinical Features. Invasive cervical cancer is most often diagnosed in patients who have never had a Pap test or who have not been screened for many years. Cervical cancer is often symptomatic, with patients coming to medical attention for unexpected vaginal bleeding, leukorrhea, dyspareunia (painful coitus), or dysuria. The primary treatment is hysterectomy and lymph node dissection; small microinvasive carcinomas may be treated with cone biopsy. Radiation and chemotherapy are of benefit when surgery alone is not curative. The prognosis for invasive carcinoma depends on the stage of the cancer at diagnosis and to some degree on histologic subtype, with small cell neuroendocrine tumors having a very poor prognosis.

UTERUS

The body (corpus) of the uterus is composed of the endometrium (glands and stroma) and the myometrium (smooth muscle). The more frequent and significant disorders of the uterus are considered here.

ENDOMETRITIS

Inflammation of the endometrium is classified as acute or chronic depending on whether a neutrophilic or a lymphoplasmacytic infiltrate predominates, respectively. *Acute endometritis* is uncommon and limited to bacterial infections that arise after delivery or miscarriage. The diagnosis of *chronic endometritis* generally requires the presence of plasma cells, as lymphocytes are present even in the healthy endometrium. Tuberculosis causes *granulomatous endometritis*, often associated with tuberculous salpingitis and peritonitis.

Endometritis is a component of pelvic inflammatory disease and is frequently a result of *N. gonorrhoeae* or *C. trachomatis* infection. In the United States, tuberculous endometritis is mainly seen in individuals who are immunocompromised. It is more common in countries where tuberculosis is endemic and should be considered in the differential diagnosis of pelvic inflammatory disease in recent emigrants from endemic areas. All forms of endometritis manifest with fever, abdominal pain, and menstrual abnormalities.

ADENOMYOSIS

Adenomyosis refers to the presence of endometrial tissue in the myometrium. Nests of endometrial stroma, glands, or both are found deep in the myometrium interposed between muscle bundles. The endometrial tissue induces reactive hypertrophy of the myometrium, resulting in an enlarged, globular uterus, often with a thickened uterine wall. Extensive adenomyosis may cause menorrhagia, dysmenorrhea, and pelvic pain, particularly just prior to menstruation, and can coexist with endometriosis.

ENDOMETRIOSIS

Endometriosis is defined by the presence of endometrial glands and stroma in a location outside the uterus. It occurs in as many as 10% of women in their reproductive years and in nearly half of women with infertility. It is frequently multifocal and often involves pelvic structures (e.g., ovaries, pouch of Douglas, uterine ligaments, fallopian tubes). Less frequently, distant areas of the peritoneal cavity, periumbilical tissues, or laparotomy scars are involved. There are three types of endometriosis: superficial peritoneal endometriosis, ovarian endometriosis, and deep infiltrating endometriosis. Risk of malignant transformation is mainly confined to deep infiltrating endometriosis.

Pathogenesis. The pathogenesis of endometriosis remains elusive. Proposed origins fall into two main categories: (1) those that propose an origin from the uterine endometrium and (2) those that propose an origin from cells outside the uterus that have the capacity to give rise to endometrial tissue. The leading theories are as follows:

- The *regurgitation theory* proposes that endometrial tissue implants at ectopic sites via retrograde flow of menstrual endometrium through the opening of the fallopian tube.
- The *benign metastasis theory* holds that endometrial tissue from the uterus can "spread" to distant sites (e.g., bone, lung, and brain) via blood vessels and lymphatic channels.
- The *metaplastic theory* suggests that endometrium arises directly from coelomic epithelium (mesothelium of pelvis or abdomen), from which the müllerian ducts and ultimately the endometrium originate during embryonic development. In addition, mesonephric remnants may undergo endometrial differentiation and give rise to ectopic endometrial tissue.
- The *extrauterine stem/progenitor cell theory* proposes that stem/progenitor cells from the bone marrow differentiate into endometrial tissue.

Studies reveal that endometrial implants are not just misplaced but have different characteristics than eutopic uterine endometrium (Fig. 17.9). Endometriotic tissue exhibits increased levels of proinflammatory and angiogenic factors, including prostaglandin E_2, vascular endothelial growth factor (VEGF), and matrix

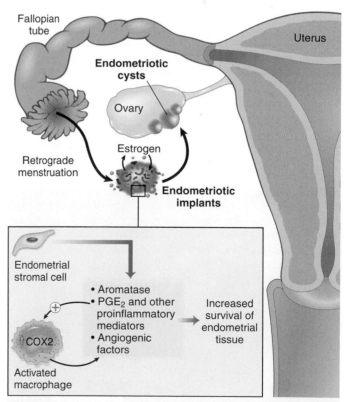

FIG. 17.9 Pathogenesis of endometriosis. Depicted is the interplay between factors expressed in endometriotic implants and activated macrophages that are hypothesized to play a role in the establishment and maintenance of endometriotic implants. *COX2*, Cyclooxygenase 2; *PGE₂*, prostaglandin E_2.

metalloproteinases (MMP), some of which are released by macrophages that are recruited to endometriotic implants by proinflammatory factors. Endometriotic stromal cells make high levels of aromatase, leading to increased local production of estrogen from androgens.

Clinical Features. Clinical signs and symptoms usually include severe dysmenorrhea, dyspareunia, and pelvic pain due to intrapelvic bleeding and periuterine adhesions. Menstrual irregularities are common, and infertility is the presenting issue for 30% to 40% of patients. Effective treatments include COX-2 inhibitors and aromatase inhibitors. Although uncommon, malignancies can develop within endometriotic tissue.

ABNORMAL UTERINE BLEEDING

Although abnormal uterine bleeding (e.g., menorrhagia [heavy menstrual bleeding], metrorrhagia [intermenstrual irregular bleeding], and postmenopausal bleeding) can arise in the setting of well-defined pathologic conditions, such as chronic endometritis, endometrial polyps, submucosal leiomyomas, or endometrial neoplasms, it most commonly stems from hormonal disturbances that produce *dysfunctional uterine bleeding* (Table 17.2). Dysfunctional uterine bleeding is a clinical term for uterine bleeding that lacks an underlying structural abnormality. The most common cause of dysfunctional uterine bleeding is anovulation (failure to ovulate). *Anovulatory cycles* result from hormonal imbalances and are most common at menarche and in the perimenopausal period due to fluctuations in the hypothalamus/pituitary/ovarian axis. Less common causes of anovulation include the following:

- *Endocrine disorders,* such as pituitary tumors that secrete prolactin, which disrupts gonadotropin releasing hormone (GnRH) secretion, thereby reducing levels of luteinizing hormone (LH) and follicle stimulating hormone (FSH)
- *Ovarian lesions,* such as a functioning ovarian tumor (granulosa cell tumors) or polycystic ovarian syndrome (see later)
- *Generalized metabolic disturbances,* such as obesity, malnutrition, or other chronic systemic disorders

Dysfunctional uterine bleeding may also result from an inadequate luteal phase *(luteal phase defect),* which is thought to stem from insufficient production of progesterone by the corpus luteum.

PROLIFERATIVE LESIONS OF THE ENDOMETRIUM AND MYOMETRIUM

The most common proliferative lesions of the uterine corpus are endometrial hyperplasia, endometrial carcinoma, endometrial polyps, and smooth muscle tumors. All tend to produce abnormal uterine bleeding as their earliest manifestation.

Endometrial Hyperplasia

An excess of estrogen relative to progestin, if sufficiently prolonged or marked, can induce exaggerated endometrial proliferation (hyperplasia), which is an important precursor of endometrial carcinoma. A common cause of estrogen excess is obesity, as adipose tissue converts steroid precursors into estrogens. Other causes of estrogen excess include prolonged administration of estrogenic steroids without counterbalancing progestin and estrogen-producing ovarian lesions (such as polycystic ovarian syndrome and granulosa-theca cell tumors of the ovary).

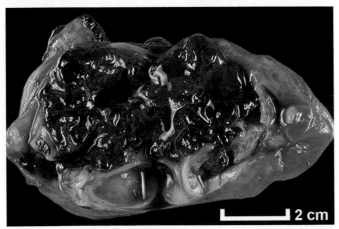

FIG. 17.10 Ovarian endometriosis. Sectioning of ovary shows multiple large and small endometriotic cysts with degenerated blood ("chocolate cyst"). (From Nucci MR, Parra-Herran C: *Gynecologic Pathology: A Volume in Foundations in Diagnostic Pathology Series,* ed 2, Fig. 13.25, Philadelphia, 2021, Elsevier.)

Table 17.2 Causes of Abnormal Uterine Bleeding by Age Group

Age Group	Cause(s)
Prepuberty	Precocious puberty (hypothalamic, pituitary, or ovarian origin)
Adolescence	Anovulatory cycle, coagulation disorders
Reproductive age	Complications of pregnancy (abortion, trophoblastic disease, ectopic pregnancy) Anatomic lesions (leiomyoma, adenomyosis, polyps, endometrial hyperplasia, carcinoma) Dysfunctional uterine bleeding Anovulatory cycle Ovulatory dysfunctional bleeding (e.g., inadequate luteal phase)
Perimenopause	Dysfunctional uterine bleeding Anovulatory cycle Anatomic lesions (carcinoma, hyperplasia, polyps)
Postmenopause	Anatomic lesions (carcinoma, hyperplasia, polyps) Endometrial atrophy

Endometrial hyperplasia takes two forms, hyperplasia without atypia and hyperplasia with atypia. Hyperplasia without atypia has a wide range of appearances, but the cardinal feature is an increased gland to stroma ratio (Fig. 17.11A). Hyperplasia with atypia additionally shows complex patterns of proliferating glands with nuclear atypia (Fig. 17.11B, C). It is now appreciated that endometrial hyperplasia with atypia is associated with acquired clonal mutations in cancer genes, particularly mutations in the tumor suppressor gene *PTEN*, a feature that is shared with endometrial carcinoma. For this reason, it is considered a precursor of carcinoma and is commonly referred to as endometrial intraepithelial neoplasia (EIN). Because of this association, when atypia is identified the specimen must be carefully evaluated to exclude invasive cancer. Hysterectomy is the treatment for patients no longer desiring fertility; in younger patients, treatment with high-dose progestins may be attempted to preserve the uterus. By contrast, hyperplasia without cellular atypia carries a low risk (between 1% and 3%) for progression to endometrial carcinoma.

Endometrial Carcinoma

In higher-income countries, endometrial carcinoma is the most frequent cancer occurring in the female genital tract. Endometrial carcinoma is broadly divided into two histologically and pathogenically distinct categories: endometrioid and serous carcinoma. There are other less common types of endometrial carcinoma, such as clear cell carcinoma and mixed Müllerian tumor (carcinosarcoma), but these are too rare to merit further discussion.

Pathogenesis. **Endometrioid cancers arise in association with estrogen excess in the setting of endometrial hyperplasia in perimenopausal women, whereas serous cancers arise in the setting of endometrial atrophy in older postmenopausal women.** The *endometrioid type* accounts for 80% of cases of endometrial carcinomas. Most are well differentiated and mimic proliferative endometrial glands, thus their name. They typically arise in the setting of endometrial hyperplasia with atypia and therefore are associated with conditions that lead to estrogen excess (e.g., obesity, estrogen-secreting ovarian tumors, and exposure to exogenous estrogens).

Mutations in mismatch repair genes and the tumor suppressor gene *PTEN* are early events in the stepwise development of endometrioid carcinoma. In most endometrioid carcinomas these mutations are acquired (somatic), but it is notable (and unsurprising) that women with germ line mutations in *PTEN* (Cowden syndrome) or DNA mismatch repair genes (Lynch syndrome) are at particularly high risk for developing this cancer. *TP53* mutations also occur in endometrioid carcinomas but are relatively uncommon, late events.

The *serous type* of endometrial carcinoma is less common but far more aggressive. It accounts for roughly 15% of tumors and is not associated with unopposed estrogen or endometrial hyperplasia. Nearly all cases of serous carcinoma have mutations in the *TP53* tumor suppressor gene, whereas mutations in DNA mismatch repair genes and in *PTEN* are rare. Serous tumors are preceded by a lesion called serous endometrial intraepithelial carcinoma (SEIC), in which *TP53* mutations are often detected, indicating a central role for altered p53 function in the development of this form of endometrial carcinoma, which shows significant morphologic and biologic overlap with ovarian serous carcinoma.

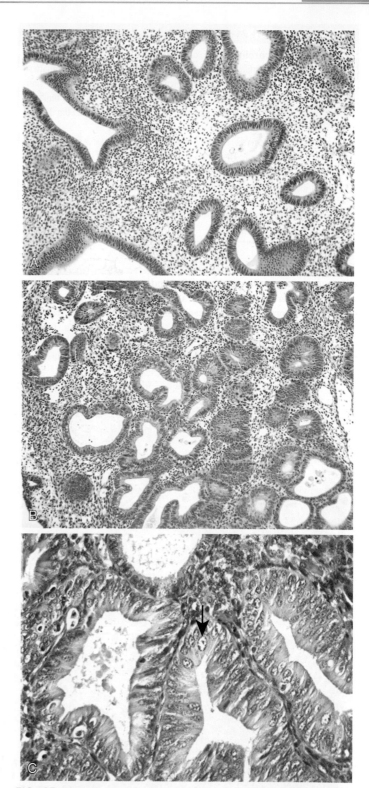

FIG. 17.11 Endometrial hyperplasia. (A) Hyperplasia without atypia, showing architectural abnormalities including mild glandular crowding and cystic gland dilation. (B) Hyperplasia with atypia, seen as glandular crowding and cellular atypia. (C) High magnification of atypical hyperplasia showing rounded, vesicular nuclei with prominent nucleoli *(arrow)*.

MORPHOLOGY

Endometrioid carcinomas closely resemble normal endometrium and may be exophytic or infiltrative (Fig. 17.12A, B). Most are well differentiated. Spread generally occurs by myometrial invasion followed by direct extension to adjacent structures and organs. They may also metastasize to regional lymph nodes. Endometrioid carcinomas are graded 1 to 3, based on the degree of differentiation.

Serous carcinomas typically grow in small tufts and papillae with marked cytologic atypia. They can also form glands that at times mimic endometrioid carcinoma; however, serous carcinomas exhibit much greater cytologic atypia and are by definition high grade. Immunohistochemistry often shows diffuse, strong staining for p53 (Fig. 17.12C, D), a finding that correlates with the presence of *TP53* mutations (mutant p53 accumulates and hence is more easily detected by staining).

Clinical Features. Carcinoma of the endometrium is uncommon in women younger than 40 years of age; the peak incidence is in post-menopausal women 55 to 65 years of age. Endometrial carcinomas typically manifest with irregular or postmenopausal bleeding. They are usually slow to metastasize, but if left untreated, eventually disseminate to regional nodes and more distant sites. With therapy, the 5-year survival rate for early stage endometrioid carcinoma is 90%, but survival drops precipitously in higher-stage tumors. Patients with serous carcinoma tend to be older (65 to 70 years of age) and in contrast with patients who have endometroid carcinoma, are less likely to be obese. The prognosis of serous carcinoma is strongly dependent on operative staging, but because of its aggressive behavior it often presents as high-stage disease and the overall prognosis is poor.

Endometrial Polyps

Endometrial polyps are usually sessile and range from 0.5 to 3 cm in diameter. Larger polyps may project from the endometrial mucosa into the uterine cavity. They are composed of endometrium that resembles the basalis, frequently with small muscular arteries and cystically dilated glands. The stromal cells are clonal and are the neoplastic component of the polyp. Although endometrial polyps may occur at any age, incidence increases with age. They may result in abnormal uterine bleeding, raising a suspicion of malignancy but malignant transformation is rare.

Uterine Leiomyoma

Uterine leiomyoma (commonly called *fibroid*) is one of the most common tumors in women. They are benign smooth muscle neoplasms that may occur singly, but more often are multiple. Estrogen

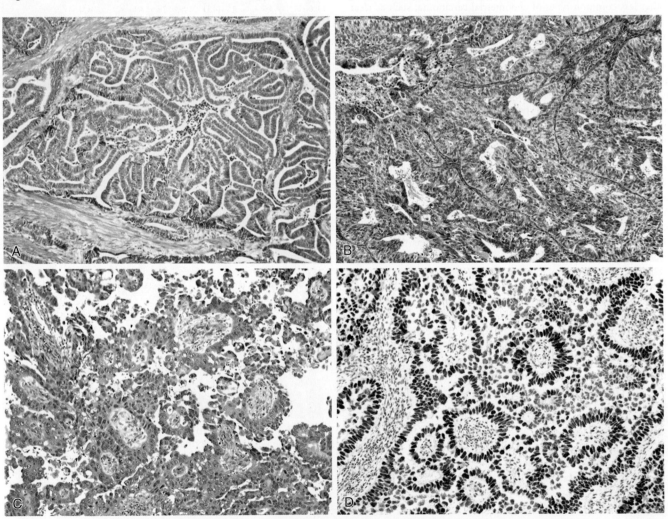

FIG. 17.12 Endometrial carcinoma. (A) Endometrioid type, grade 1, infiltrating myometrium and growing in a glandular pattern. (B) Endometrioid type, grade 3, has a predominantly solid growth pattern. (C) Serous carcinoma of the endometrium, with papilla formation and marked cytologic atypia. (D) Immunohistochemical staining shows accumulation of p53 in the malignant epithelial cells, a finding associated with *TP53* mutation.

and progesterone stimulate leiomyoma growth; hence, these tumors shrink after menopause. These tumors are associated with several different recurrent chromosomal abnormalities, including rearrangements of chromosomes 6 and 12 that are also found in a variety of other benign neoplasms, such as endometrial polyps and lipomas. Mutations in the *MED12* gene, which encodes a protein that regulates RNA polymerase II–mediated transcription, have been identified in up to 70% of leiomyomas. The mechanism by which *MED12* mutations contribute to the development of leiomyomas is not understood.

MORPHOLOGY

Leiomyomas are typically **sharply circumscribed,** firm gray-white masses with a characteristic **whorled cut surface.** When multiple, they are scattered throughout the uterus, ranging from small nodules to large tumors (Fig. 17.13) that may dwarf the uterus. Some are embedded within the myometrium (intramural), whereas others lie immediately beneath the endometrium (submucosal) or the serosa (subserosal). In the latter location, tumors may extend out on attenuated stalks and even become attached to surrounding organs, from which they may develop a blood supply (parasitic leiomyomas). Submucosal leiomyomas may ulcerate and cause abnormal uterine bleeding. On histologic examination, the tumors are characterized by **bundles of smooth muscle cells** similar in appearance to typical myometrium. Foci of fibrosis, calcification, and degenerative softening may be present.

Clinical Features. Leiomyomas of the uterus are often asymptomatic, being discovered incidentally on routine pelvic examination. In symptomatic cases, the most frequent presenting sign is menorrhagia, with or without metrorrhagia. Malignant transformation to leiomyosarcoma is extremely rare.

Leiomyosarcoma

These uncommon malignant neoplasms are thought to arise from the myometrium or endometrial stromal precursor cells. They are almost always solitary and most often occur in postmenopausal women, in contrast to leiomyomas, which are frequently multiple and usually arise before menopause. They have complex, highly variable karyotypes that frequently include chromosomal deletions. Like leiomyomas, they contain *MED12* mutations but in a smaller subset (30%).

MORPHOLOGY

Leiomyosarcomas are typically **soft, hemorrhagic, necrotic masses.** The histologic appearance varies widely, from tumors that closely resemble leiomyoma to wildly anaplastic neoplasms (eFig. 17.4). The diagnostic features of leiomyosarcoma include **tumor necrosis, cytologic atypia,** and **mitotic activity.** Because increased mitotic activity is sometimes seen in benign smooth muscle tumors, particularly in young women, an assessment of all three features is necessary to make a diagnosis of malignancy.

These tumors often recur following surgery and more than one-half eventually metastasize hematogenously to distant organs, such as the lungs, bone, and brain. Dissemination throughout the abdominal cavity is also encountered.

FALLOPIAN TUBES

The most common disorders affecting the fallopian tubes are infections and associated inflammatory conditions, followed in frequency by ectopic (tubal) pregnancy and endometriosis.

Inflammation of the fallopian tubes is almost always caused by infection. Suppurative salpingitis may be caused by any pyogenic organism; in some cases, more than one organism is involved. *N. gonorrhoeae* is the causative organism in more than 60% of cases, with *C. trachomatis* being responsible for many of the remaining cases. Tuberculous salpingitis is rare in the United States but is more common in parts of the world where tuberculosis is endemic; it is an important cause of infertility in these areas.

All forms of salpingitis may produce fever, lower abdominal or pelvic pain, and pelvic masses due to distention of the tubes with exudate, inflammatory debris or tuboovarian abscess (Fig. 17.14). Adhesions may form between the ovary and the tubes or the tubal plicae; the latter is associated with increased risk of tubal ectopic pregnancy (discussed later). Damage to or obstruction of the tubal lumina may result in permanent sterility.

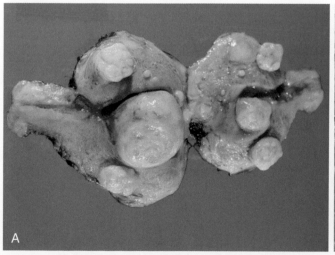
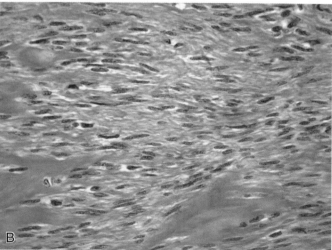

FIG. 17.13 Uterine leiomyomas. (A) The uterus is opened to show multiple submucosal, intramural, and subserosal tan-white tumors, each with a characteristic whorled appearance on cut section. (B) Microscopic appearance of leiomyoma shows bundles of bland smooth muscle cells.

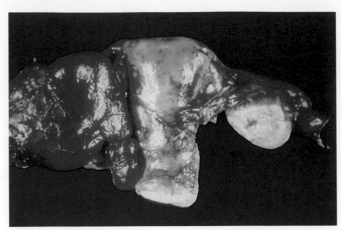

FIG. 17.14 Pelvic inflammatory disease, bilateral and asymmetric. The tube and ovary to the left of the uterus are totally obscured by a hemorrhagic inflammatory mass. The tube is adherent to the adjacent ovary on the other side.

Once believed to be uncommon, primary adenocarcinomas of the fallopian tube may be the site of origin for many high-grade serous carcinomas, long thought to arise in the ovary. Studies have identified the presence of serous tubal intraepithelial carcinoma (STIC) in the fimbriated ends of fallopian tubes. Like the precursor of uterine serous carcinoma, more than 90% of STICs have mutations in *TP53*. These lesions are found frequently in fallopian tubes removed prophylactically from women who carry mutations in *BRCA1* and *BRCA2* and less commonly in instances where tubes are removed from women without known genetic risk factors. This has led to the idea that sporadic "ovarian" serous carcinomas (discussed later) also originate in the fallopian tube. Because the fimbriated end of the fallopian tube is intimately associated with the ovary and has access to the peritoneal cavity, fallopian tube carcinoma frequently involves the ovary, omentum, and peritoneal cavity at presentation.

OVARIES

FOLLICLE AND LUTEAL CYSTS

Follicle and luteal cysts in the ovaries are so commonplace that they may be considered variants of normal physiology. These innocuous lesions originate from unruptured graafian follicles or from follicles that rupture and then immediately seal. Such cysts are often multiple and develop under the serosa of the ovary. They are typically small (1–1.5 cm in diameter) and are filled with clear serous fluid. Occasionally, they become sufficiently large (4–5 cm) to produce palpable masses and pelvic pain. When small, they are lined by granulosa cells or luteal cells, but as fluid accumulates pressure may cause atrophy of these cells. Sometimes these cysts rupture, producing intraperitoneal bleeding and symptoms of acute abdomen.

POLYCYSTIC OVARIAN SYNDROME

Polycystic ovarian syndrome (PCOS) is a complex endocrine disorder characterized by signs and symptoms of androgen excess and ovulatory dysfunction (e.g., menstrual abnormalities, hirsutism, polycystic ovaries, chronic anovulation, and decreased fertility). It is one of the most common endocrine/metabolic disorders of women and affects between 6% and 10% of women of reproductive age, typically first presenting at puberty. The etiology of PCOS remains incompletely understood but appears to involve both environmental and genetic factors. It is marked by a dysregulation of enzymes involved in androgen biosynthesis resulting in excessive androgen production, which is considered to be a central feature of this disorder. Patients are at increased risk for metabolic syndrome, type 2 diabetes, hypertension, cerebrovascular accidents, and endometrial hyperplasia and carcinoma.

The ovaries are usually twice the normal size and studded with subcortical cysts that are 0.5 to 1.5 cm in diameter (eFig. 17.5). Histologic examination shows a thickened, fibrotic ovarian capsule overlying cystic follicles lined by granulosa cells with a hyperplastic luteinized theca interna. There is a conspicuous absence of corpora lutea due to anovulation.

TUMORS OF THE OVARY

In the United States, ovarian cancer is the second most common gynecologic malignancy (following endometrial carcinoma) and the leading cause of gynecologic cancer death. Tumors of the ovary are remarkably varied, arising from any of the three cell types in the normal ovary: (1) multipotent surface/fallopian tube epithelium; (2) pluripotent germ cells; and (3) sex cord–stromal cells. Neoplasms of epithelial origin account for the great majority of ovarian tumors and, in their malignant forms, account for almost 90% of ovarian cancers (Table 17.3). Germ cell and sex cord–stromal cell tumors are much less frequent; although they constitute 20% to 30% of ovarian tumors, they collectively make up less than 10% of malignant tumors of the ovary.

Surface Epithelial Tumors

Most primary ovarian neoplasms arise from müllerian epithelium. The classification of these tumors is based on both differentiation and extent of proliferation of the epithelium. There are three major

Table 17.3 Frequency of Major Ovarian Tumors

Type	Percentage of Malignant Ovarian Tumors	Percentage That Are Bilateral
Serous	47	
Benign (60%)		25
Borderline (15%)		30
Malignant (25%)		65
Mucinous	3	
Benign (80%)		5
Borderline (10%)		10
Malignant (10%)		<5
Endometrioid carcinoma	20	20
Undifferentiated carcinoma	10	—
Granulosa cell tumor	5	5
Teratoma	1	
Benign (96%)		15
Malignant (4%)		Rare
Metastatic	5	>50
Others	3	—

histologic tumor types, serous, mucinous, and endometrioid, which may be benign, borderline, or malignant. About 80% of surface epithelial tumors are benign; they occur mostly in young women between 20 and 45 years of age, are frequently cystic and may have an accompanying stromal component. So-called borderline tumors (tumors of indeterminate malignancy) occur at slightly older ages and fall into an intermediate "gray-zone" category; although the majority behave in a benign manner, some recur, and a few progress to carcinoma. Malignant tumors are more common in women between 45 and 65 years of age and may be cystic (cystadenocarcinoma) or solid (carcinoma). On the basis of their derivation and pathogenesis, ovarian carcinomas can be further grouped into two types: types I and II (Fig. 17.15).

- *Type I carcinoma*: low-grade tumor that often arises in association with borderline tumors or endometriosis and includes low-grade serous, endometrioid, and mucinous tumors (see below).
- *Type II carcinoma*: most often high-grade serous carcinoma that arises from serous intraepithelial carcinoma.

Important risk factors for surface epithelial carcinomas include increasing age, early menarche/late menopause, nulliparity, family history, and germline mutations in certain tumor suppressor genes. Prolonged use of oral contraceptives reduces the risk, presumably due to suppression of ovulation. Around 5% to 10% of ovarian cancers are familial, and most of these are associated with mutations in the *BRCA1* or *BRCA2* tumor suppressor genes, which are also mutated in a subset of hereditary breast cancers (see later). The estimated risk of ovarian cancer in women bearing *BRCA1* or *BRCA2* mutations is 20% to 60% by 70 years of age. Such mutations are found in only 8% to 10% of sporadic ovarian cancers, while the majority arise through alternative molecular mechanisms (see later).

Serous Tumors

Serous tumors are the most common of the ovarian epithelial tumors and also make up the greatest fraction of malignant ovarian tumors.

About 70% are benign or borderline and 30% are malignant. Benign and borderline tumors are most common between 20 and 45 years of age. Serous carcinomas generally occur later in life except in familial cases.

Serous carcinomas may be low grade or high grade. The former arises from benign or borderline lesions and progresses slowly in a stepwise manner to become invasive carcinoma. Low-grade tumors arising in serous borderline tumors have mutations in the *KRAS*, *BRAF*, or *ERBB2* oncogenes and usually have wild-type *TP53* alleles. High-grade serous tumors develop rapidly. As already mentioned, many of these high-grade lesions arise in the fimbriated end of the fallopian tube via serous tubal intraepithelial carcinoma. *TP53* mutations are virtually ubiquitous in high-grade serous cancers, being present in over 95% of cases. Almost all ovarian carcinomas arising in women with *BRCA1* or *BRCA2* mutations are high-grade serous carcinomas with *TP53* mutations.

MORPHOLOGY

Most serous tumors are large, spherical to ovoid, cystic structures up to 30 to 40 cm in diameter. **About 25% of benign tumors are bilateral.** In benign tumors, the serosal covering is smooth and glistening. By contrast, the surface of adenocarcinoma often has nodular irregularities where tumor has invaded the serosa. Small cystic tumors may have a single cavity, but larger ones are frequently divided by multiple septa into multiloculated masses. The cystic spaces are usually filled with a clear, serous fluid. Protruding into the cystic cavities are papillary projections, which are more prominent in malignant tumors (Fig. 17.16).

On histologic examination, benign tumors contain a single layer of **columnar epithelial cells** that line the cyst or cysts (Fig. 17.17A). The cells are often ciliated. Concentric calcifications **(psammoma bodies)** are common in all types of serous tumors but are not specific for neoplasia. In high-grade carcinoma the cells are markedly atypical, the papillary formations are usually complex and multilayered, and, by definition, nests or sheets of malignant cells invade the ovarian stroma (Fig. 17.17C); low-grade carcinoma shows less cytologic atypia. Between clearly benign and obviously malignant forms lie **borderline tumors** (Fig. 17.17B), which exhibit less cytologic atypia and typically no stromal invasion; peritoneal implants are usually "noninvasive." Ovarian serous tumors, both low and high grade, have a propensity to spread to the peritoneal surfaces and omentum and are commonly associated with the presence of ascites.

Clinical Features. Prognosis is closely related to the histologic appearance of the tumor and the presence and extent of peritoneal disease. The 5-year survival rate for borderline and malignant tumors confined to the ovary is 100% and 70%, respectively, whereas the 5-year survival rate for the same tumors involving the peritoneum is about 90% and 25%, respectively. Because of their protracted course, borderline tumors may recur after many years, and 5-year survival is not synonymous with cure.

Mucinous Tumors

Mucinous tumors differ from serous tumors in two respects: the neoplastic epithelium consists of mucin-secreting cells, and mucinous tumors are less likely to be malignant. Overall, only 10% of mucinous tumors are malignant; another 10% are borderline, and 80% are benign. They occur principally in middle adult life and are rare before puberty and after menopause. Mutation of the *KRAS* proto-oncogene is a consistent genetic alteration in all mucinous tumors of the ovary.

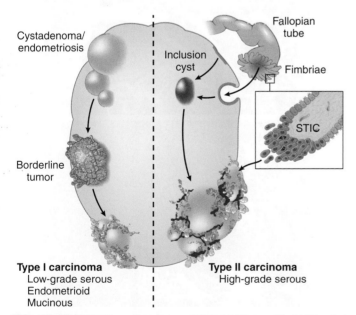

FIG. 17.15 Derivation of various ovarian neoplasms. Type I tumors progress from benign tumors through borderline tumors that may give rise to a low-grade carcinoma. Type II tumors arise from inclusion cysts/fallopian tube epithelium via intraepithelial precursors that are often not identified. They demonstrate high-grade features and are most commonly of serous histology. *STIC,* Serous tubal intraepithelial carcinoma.

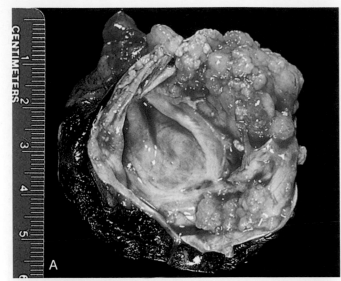

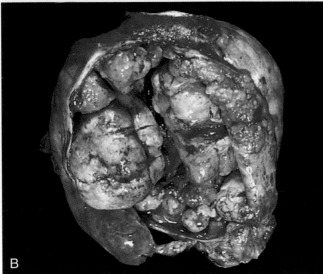

FIG. 17.16 Ovarian serous tumors. (A) Borderline serous tumor opened to display a cyst cavity lined by delicate papillary tumor growths. (B) Cystadenocarcinoma. The cyst is opened to show a large, bulky tumor mass. (Courtesy of Dr. Christopher Crum, Brigham and Women's Hospital, Boston, Massachusetts.)

MORPHOLOGY

On gross examination, mucinous tumors produce cystic masses that may be indistinguishable from serous tumors except for the mucinous nature of the cyst contents. However, they are more likely to be large and multicystic and to lack surface involvement (Fig. 17.18A). Mucin-producing epithelial cells line the cysts (Fig. 17.18B). Malignant tumors are characterized by solid areas of growth, stratification of lining cells, cytologic atypia, and stromal invasion.

Compared with serous tumors, mucinous tumors are much less likely to be bilateral. This feature is sometimes useful in differentiating mucinous tumors of the ovary from metastatic mucinous adenocarcinoma of gastrointestinal origin (the so-called "**Krukenberg tumor**"), which often involves the ovary bilaterally.

Ruptured ovarian mucinous tumors may seed the peritoneum; however, these deposits typically regress spontaneously. Stable implantation of mucinous tumor cells in the peritoneum with production of copious amounts of

mucin is called **pseudomyxoma peritonei;** in nearly all cases, however, this disorder is caused by metastases from the gastrointestinal tract, usually the appendix (Chapter 13).

Clinical Features. The prognosis of mucinous carcinoma is somewhat better than that of its serous counterpart, although stage rather than histologic type (serous versus mucinous) is the major determinant of outcome.

Endometrioid Tumors

These tumors may be solid or cystic; they sometimes develop in association with endometriosis. On microscopic examination, they are

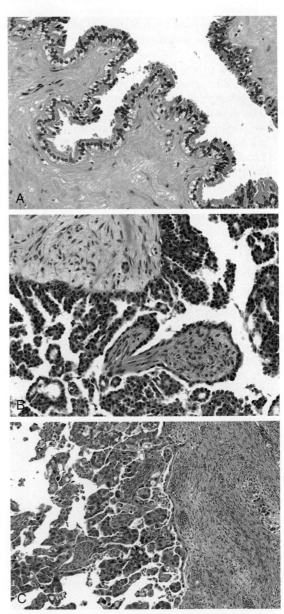

FIG. 17.17 Microscopic appearances of serous tumors of the ovary. (A) Serous cystadenoma revealing stromal papillae with a columnar epithelium. (B) Borderline serous tumor showing increased architectural complexity and epithelial cell stratification. (C) High-grade serous carcinoma of the ovary with invasion of underlying stroma. (© 2022 University of Michigan. Used with permission.)

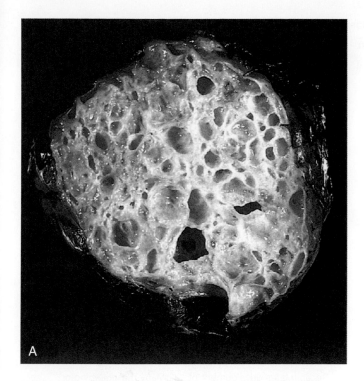

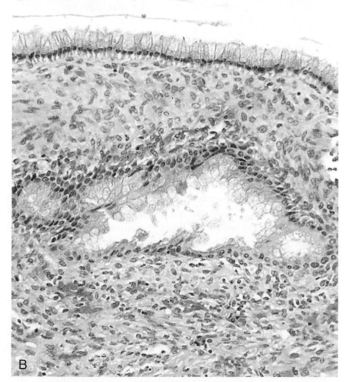

FIG. 17.18 Ovarian mucinous cystadenoma. (A) Mucinous cystadenoma with multicystic appearance and delicate septa. Note the presence of glistening mucin within the cysts. (B) Columnar cell lining of mucinous cystadenoma.

distinguished by the formation of tubular glands, similar to those of the endometrium, within the lining of cystic spaces. Although benign and borderline forms exist, endometrioid tumors are usually malignant. They are bilateral in about 20% of cases, and 15% to 20% of women with these ovarian tumors have a concomitant endometrial carcinoma.

Similar to endometrioid-type carcinoma of the endometrium, endometrioid carcinomas of the ovary frequently have mutations in the *PTEN* tumor suppressor gene and other genes that act to upregulate PI3K-AKT signaling.

Clear Cell Carcinoma

Clear cell tumors are a rare subtype of epithelial ovarian tumors. Benign and borderline clear cell tumors are exceedingly rare, and clear cell carcinomas are uncommon. They are composed of large epithelial cells with abundant clear cytoplasm, an appearance that resembles hypersecretory gestational endometrium. These tumors sometimes occur in association with endometriosis or endometrioid carcinoma of the ovary and are thought to be variants of endometrioid adenocarcinoma. In line with this idea, the most commonly mutated genes (*PIK3CA, ARID1A, KRAS, PTEN,* and *TP53*) are shared with endometrioid carcinoma. Clear cell carcinoma is treated like other types of ovarian carcinoma.

Other Ovarian Tumors

Many types of tumors of germ cell and sex cord–stromal origin also arise in the ovary, but only teratomas of germ cell origin are sufficiently common to merit further description. Table 17.4 presents some salient features of other neoplasms of germ cell and sex cord origin.

Teratomas

Teratomas constitute 15% to 20% of ovarian tumors. They are divided into three categories: (1) mature (benign); (2) immature (malignant); and (3) monodermal or highly specialized. More than 90% of these tumors are benign.

Mature (Benign) Teratomas. **Benign teratomas are marked by the presence of mature tissues derived from all three germ cell layers: ectoderm, endoderm, and mesoderm.** Most benign teratomas are cystic and are often referred to as *dermoid cysts* because they are almost always lined by skinlike structures. They are usually discovered in young women, either as ovarian masses or as incidental findings on abdominal imaging. About 90% are unilateral, with the right side more commonly affected. Rarely do they exceed 10 cm in diameter. On cut section, they are often filled with sebaceous secretion and matted hair (Fig. 17.19) that, when removed, reveal a hair-bearing epidermal lining. Sometimes there is a nodular projection from which teeth protrude. Foci of bone and cartilage, nests of bronchial or gastrointestinal epithelium, or other tissues may also be present.

Benign teratomas are prone to undergo torsion (10% to 15% of cases), which constitutes an acute surgical emergency. A rare paraneoplastic complication is *limbic encephalitis*, which may develop in women with teratomas containing mature neural tissue and often remits with tumor resection. This autoimmune disorder is also seen with certain other tumors, most commonly small cell carcinoma of the lung. Malignant transformation, usually to a squamous cell carcinoma, is seen in about 1% of cases.

Immature (Malignant) Teratomas. Immature (malignant) teratomas are rare tumors that differ from benign teratomas in that the component tissues resemble embryonal and immature fetal tissue. The tumor is found chiefly in prepubertal adolescents and young women, the mean age being 18 years. They are typically bulky and appear solid on cut section. On microscopic examination, there are variable amounts of immature neuroepithelium, cartilage, bone, or other immature elements (eFig. 17.6). The risk of metastasis correlates with the proportion of the tumor that comprises immature neuroepithelium.

Specialized Teratomas. A rare subtype of teratoma is composed entirely of specialized tissue. The most common example is *struma*

Table 17.4 Features of Ovarian Germ Cell and Sex Cord Neoplasms and Ovarian Metastases

Neoplasm	Peak Incidence	Usual Location	Morphologic Features	Behavior
Germ Cell Origin				
Dysgerminoma	Second to third decade of life; associated with gonadal dysgenesis	Unilateral in 80%–90%	Counterpart of testicular seminoma; sheets or cords of large cells with clear cytoplasm; stroma may contain lymphocytes and granulomas	Malignant but only one-third metastasize; radiosensitive; 80% cure rate
Choriocarcinoma	First 3 decades of life	Unilateral	Identical to placental tumor; two types of cells: cytotrophoblast and syncytiotrophoblast	Metastasizes early and widely; elaborate hCG; resistant to chemotherapy
Sex Cord Tumors				
Granulosa cell tumor	Most postmenopausal, but may occur at any age	Unilateral	Composed of mixture of cuboidal granulosa cells and spindled or plump lipid-laden theca cells. Granulosa elements may recapitulate ovarian follicles	May elaborate large amounts of estrogen; may be malignant (5%–25%)
Thecoma-fibroma	Any age	Unilateral	Plump yellow (lipid-laden) thecal cells admixed with fibroblasts	Most hormonally inactive; about 40% produce ascites and hydrothorax (Meigs syndrome); rarely malignant
Sertoli-Leydig cell tumor	All ages; peak 2nd to 3rd decades	Unilateral	Recapitulates development of testis with tubules or cords and plump pink Sertoli cells	Many masculinizing or defeminizing; rarely malignant
Metastases to Ovary				
	Older ages	Mostly bilateral	Anaplastic tumor cells, cords, glands, dispersed through fibrous background; mucin-secreting cells may be "signet ring"	Primaries are gastrointestinal tract (Krukenberg tumors), breast, and lung; associated with pseudomyxoma peritonei

hCG, Human chorionic gonadotropin.

ovarii, which consists entirely of mature thyroid tissue and may cause hyperthyroidism. These tumors appear as small, solid, unilateral brown ovarian masses. Other specialized teratomas include *ovarian carcinoid,* which in rare instances produces carcinoid syndrome.

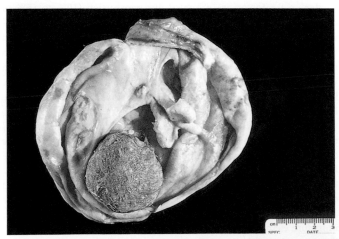

FIG. 17.19 Mature cystic teratoma (dermoid cyst) of the ovary. A ball of hair *(bottom)* and a mixture of tissues are evident. (Courtesy of Dr. Christopher Crum, Brigham and Women's Hospital, Boston, Massachusetts.)

Clinical Features. The management of ovarian neoplasms poses a formidable clinical challenge because tumors are typically at an advanced stage at diagnosis. All ovarian carcinomas produce similar clinical manifestations, most commonly lower abdominal pain and abdominal enlargement. Gastrointestinal complaints, urinary frequency, dysuria, pelvic pressure, and many other symptoms may appear. About 30% of all ovarian neoplasms are discovered incidentally on routine gynecologic examination. Larger masses may cause an increase in abdominal girth while smaller masses, particularly mature teratomas, may twist on their pedicles (torsion), producing severe abdominal pain. Metastatic seeding of malignant serous tumors often causes ascites, whereas the sex cord/stromal tumors may be functional and come to attention because they secrete hormones such as estrogens (granulosa cell tumors) and androgens (Leydig cell tumors). Granulosa cell tumors can present with vaginal bleeding due to endometrial hyperplasia.

Because most patients with ovarian carcinomas present with high-stage disease, the prognosis is generally poor. Current screening methods to detect early tumors are of minimal value due to limited specificity and sensitivity. One serum marker that has been studied, the protein CA-125, is elevated in 75% to 90% of women with epithelial ovarian cancer but is undetectable in up to 50% of women with cancer limited to the ovary; furthermore, it is often elevated in a variety of benign conditions and nonovarian cancers. Its greatest utility is in monitoring response to therapy after the diagnosis has been established.

DISEASES OF PREGNANCY

Diseases of pregnancy and pathologic conditions of the placenta are important contributors to morbidity and mortality for both mother and child. Discussed in this section are a limited number of disorders in which knowledge of the morphologic lesions contributes to an understanding of clinical disease.

PLACENTAL INFLAMMATIONS AND INFECTIONS

Infections may reach the placenta by two paths: (1) ascension through the birth canal or (2) hematogenous (transplacental) spread. Ascending infections are by far the most common and are virtually always bacterial; they are usually polymicrobial and include vaginal and enteric organisms. In many such instances, infection of the chorioamnion causes premature rupture of membranes and preterm delivery. On microscopic examination, the chorioamnion shows neutrophilic infiltration, edema, and congestion (acute chorioamnionitis). The infection may also extend to the umbilical cord and placental villi, resulting in acute vasculitis of the cord (funisitis).

Several hematogenous infections, classically components of the so-called TORCH group (toxoplasmosis and others [syphilis, tuberculosis, listeriosis], rubella, cytomegalovirus, herpes simplex), can affect the placenta. These infections give rise to chronic inflammatory cell infiltrates in the chorionic villi (chronic villitis) and may spread to the fetus, resulting in tissue injury (e.g., encephalitis, chorioretinitis) and chronic sequelae (e.g., intellectual disability, cardiac anomalies) (Chapter 4).

ECTOPIC PREGNANCY

Ectopic pregnancy refers to implantation of the embryo in an extrauterine site, most commonly the extrauterine portion of the fallopian tube (approximately 90% of cases). Other sites include the ovary, the abdominal cavity, and the intrauterine portion of the fallopian tube (cornual pregnancy). Ectopic pregnancies account for 2% of confirmed pregnancies. The most important predisposing condition is intraluminal fallopian tube scarring and narrowing/obstruction (chronic salpingitis) secondary to pelvic inflammatory disease. Other causes include intrauterine tumors, endometriosis, and peritubal scarring (due to appendicitis, previous surgery, etc.). Intrauterine contraceptive devices are associated with a 2-fold increase in ectopic pregnancy. Often, no anatomic cause is evident. Ovarian pregnancies ensue when the ovum is fertilized just as the follicle ruptures. Gestation within the abdominal cavity occurs when the fertilized egg drops out of the fimbriated end of the fallopian tube and implants on the peritoneum.

MORPHOLOGY

In all sites, early development of ectopic pregnancies proceeds typically, with formation of placental tissue, the amniotic sac, and decidual changes. With tubal pregnancies, the invading placenta eventually burrows through the wall of the fallopian tube, causing **intratubal hematoma (hematosalpinx), intraperitoneal hemorrhage,** or both. The tube is usually distended by freshly clotted blood containing bits of placental and fetal tissue. Histologic diagnosis depends on visualization of placental villi or, rarely, of the embryo.

Clinical Features. Until rupture occurs, an ectopic pregnancy may be indistinguishable from a typical pregnancy, with cessation of menstruation and elevation of serum and urinary placental hormones.

Rupture of an ectopic pregnancy may be catastrophic, with sudden onset of intense abdominal pain and signs of an acute abdomen, often followed by shock. Prompt surgical intervention is necessary to prevent death.

PREECLAMPSIA/ECLAMPSIA

Preeclampsia is a systemic syndrome caused by maternal endothelial dysfunction during pregnancy. It occurs in 3% to 5% of pregnant women and occurs more commonly in women pregnant for the first time. It usually presents in the last trimester with hypertension, edema, and proteinuria. Some affected women become seriously ill, developing convulsions; this particularly severe form of the disorder is termed *eclampsia*. Recognition and early treatment of preeclampsia have now made eclampsia, particularly fatal eclampsia, rare.

Pathogenesis. **While exact triggering events are unknown, a common feature is insufficient maternal blood flow to the placenta secondary to inadequate remodeling of the spiral arteries of the uteroplacental vascular bed.** In a typical pregnancy, the musculoelastic walls of the spiral arteries are invaded by trophoblasts, causing them to dilate into wide vascular sinusoids. In preeclampsia and eclampsia, this vascular remodeling is impaired, the musculoelastic walls are retained, and the channels remain narrow. Decreased uteroplacental blood flow appears to result in placental hypoxia, placental dysfunction, and the altered release of circulating factors that regulate angiogenesis, such as the antiangiogenic factors soluble FMS-like tyrosine kinase-1 and endoglin, which antagonize the effects of VEGF and TGF-β. These disturbances are hypothesized to result in endothelial cell dysfunction, vascular hyperreactivity, and end-organ microangiopathy.

The vascular dysfunction associated with preeclampsia and eclampsia may have several serious consequences, including:
- *Placental infarction,* stemming from chronic hypoperfusion
- *Hypertension,* resulting from reduced endothelial production of the vasodilators prostacyclin and prostaglandin E_2 and increased production of the vasoconstrictor thromboxane A_2
- *Hypercoagulability,* due to endothelial dysfunction, decreased release of antithrombotic factors (e.g., PGI_2), and increased elaboration of procoagulant factors
- *End-organ failure,* most notably of the kidney and liver, which occurs in patients with eclampsia. Approximately 10% of patients with severe preeclampsia develop the so-called "*HELLP syndrome,*" characterized by microangiopathic hemolytic anemia, elevated liver enzymes, and low platelets due to platelet consumption, and sometimes disseminated intravascular coagulation (DIC).

MORPHOLOGY

The morphologic changes are variable and correlate to some degree with the severity of the disorder. Placental abnormalities include:
- **Infarcts,** which can be a feature of a healthy pregnancy but are much more numerous with severe preeclampsia or eclampsia
- **Retroplacental hemorrhage**
- **Ischemic changes of placental villi** (increased production of syncytial epithelial knots, which are aggregates of syncytial nuclei at the surface of terminal villi)
- **Abnormal decidual vessels,** characterized by **fibrinoid necrosis** and focal accumulation of lipid-containing macrophages (**acute atherosis**)

Clinical Features. Preeclampsia most commonly starts after 34 weeks of gestation but begins earlier in women with hydatidiform mole or preexisting kidney disease, hypertension, or coagulopathies. If the condition evolves into eclampsia, renal function is impaired and blood pressure rises further. Convulsions and coma may occur. The most effective therapy is prompt delivery; however, in preterm pregnancies, the risks of early delivery must be balanced with the hazards of continued preeclampsia. Proteinuria and hypertension usually disappear within 1 to 2 weeks after delivery; in most instances, there are no lasting sequelae.

GESTATIONAL TROPHOBLASTIC DISEASE

Gestational trophoblastic disease encompasses a spectrum of tumors and tumorlike conditions characterized by proliferation of placental tissue, either villous or trophoblastic. The major disorders of this type are hydatidiform mole (complete and partial), invasive mole, choriocarcinoma, and placental site trophoblastic tumor (PSTT). All elaborate human chorionic gonadotropins (hCG) to varying degrees.

Hydatidiform Mole: Complete and Partial

Hydatidiform moles are important to recognize because they are associated with an increased risk of persistent trophoblastic disease (invasive mole) and choriocarcinoma. Moles are characterized histologically by cystic swelling of the chorionic villi and variable trophoblastic proliferation. They are usually diagnosed during early pregnancy (average 9 weeks) by pelvic sonography or excessively high elevations of hCG. Molar pregnancy can develop at any age, but the risk is higher at the two ends of reproductive life: teenagers and women between 40 and 50 years of age.

There are two distinctive subtypes of hydatidiform moles: *complete* and *partial.* Complete hydatidiform moles are not compatible with embryogenesis and rarely contain fetal parts. All the chorionic villi are abnormal and the chorionic epithelial cells are diploid (46,XX or, uncommonly, 46,XY). Partial hydatidiform mole is compatible with early embryo formation and therefore may contain fetal parts, has some normal chorionic villi, and is almost always triploid (e.g., 69,XXY) (Table 17.5). Both types of mole result from fertilization with an excess of paternal genetic material (eFig. 17.7). In a complete mole, the entire genetic content is supplied by two spermatozoa (or a diploid sperm), yielding diploid cells containing only paternal chromosomes, whereas in a partial mole, an egg is fertilized by two spermatozoa (or a diploid sperm), resulting in a triploid karyotype with a preponderance of paternal genes. Like complete moles, partial moles have an increased risk of persistent molar disease but differ in lacking an association with choriocarcinoma.

The incidence of complete hydatidiform mole is about 1 to 1.5 per 2000 pregnancies in the United States and other Western countries. Moles are most common before the age of 20 and after the age of 40 years, and a history of the condition increases the risk for molar disease in subsequent pregnancies. Although molar disease formerly was discovered at 12 to 14 weeks of pregnancy during investigation for a gestation that was "too large for dates," early monitoring of pregnancies by ultrasound has lowered the gestational age at detection. In complete moles, hCG levels are often much higher than expected for the apparent gestational age, sometimes exceeding 100,000 IU/L, whereas hCG levels may be elevated or within normal limits in partial mole due to a lower amount of trophoblastic proliferation. In both complete and partial moles, absence of fetal heart sounds is typical. Most moles are successfully removed by curettage, after which hCG levels are monitored for 6 months to 1 year to ensure that hCG levels decrease to nonpregnant levels.

> ### MORPHOLOGY
>
> In advanced cases, the uterine cavity is expanded by a delicate, friable mass of thin-walled, translucent cystic structures (Fig. 17.20). Fetal parts are rarely seen in complete moles but are common in partial moles. On microscopic examination, the **complete mole** shows hydropic swelling of poorly vascularized chorionic villi with a loose, myxomatous, edematous stroma. The chorionic epithelium typically shows a proliferation of both cytotrophoblasts and syncytiotrophoblasts (Fig. 17.21). In **partial moles,** villous edema involves only a subset of the villi, and the trophoblastic proliferation is focal and slight. In most cases of partial mole, some fetal cells are present, ranging from fetal red cells in placental villi to, in rare cases, a fully formed fetus.

Invasive Mole

Invasive moles are complete moles that are locally aggressive but lack the metastatic potential of choriocarcinoma. An invasive mole retains hydropic villi, which penetrate deeply or even perforate the uterine wall, possibly resulting in life-threatening hemorrhage. On microscopic examination, the villus epithelium shows proliferation of both trophoblastic and syncytiotrophoblast components.

Table 17.5 Features of Complete and Partial Hydatidiform Mole

Feature	Complete Mole	Partial Mole
Karyotype	Diploid	Triploid
Villous edema	All villi	Some villi
Trophoblast proliferation	Diffuse; circumferential	Focal; slight
Serum hCG	Elevated[a]	Less elevated[a]
Tissue hCG	++++	+
Risk of subsequent choriocarcinoma	2.5%	Rare

hCG, Human chorionic gonadotropin.

[a]For gestational age.

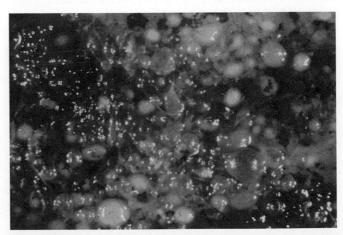

FIG. 17.20 Complete hydatidiform mole, consisting of numerous swollen (hydropic) villi.

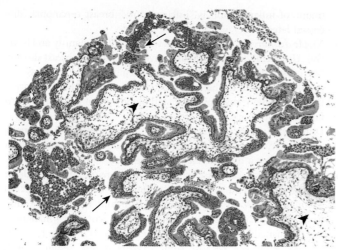

FIG. 17.21 Complete hydatidiform mole. In this microscopic image, distended hydropic villi *(arrowheads)* and proliferation of the chorionic epithelium *(arrows)* are evident.

Hydropic villi may embolize to distant organs, such as the lungs or brain, but these emboli do not grow and eventually regress spontaneously. Surgical removal of invasive mole is difficult due to deep infiltration of the myometrium. Curettage may be insufficient and if serum hCG remains elevated, further treatment is required; cure is possible in most cases with chemotherapy.

Gestational Choriocarcinoma

Choriocarcinoma, a very aggressive malignant tumor, arises from gestational chorionic epithelium or, rarely, from totipotential cells within the gonads. Gestational choriocarcinoma is an uncommon condition that arises in 1 in 20,000 to 30,000 pregnancies in the United States. It may be preceded by several conditions: 50% arise in complete hydatidiform moles, 25% in previous abortions, approximately 22% follow healthy pregnancies, and the remainder occur in ectopic pregnancies. In most cases, choriocarcinoma presents as a bloody, brownish discharge accompanied by a rising titer of hCG in blood and urine in the absence of uterine enlargement.

MORPHOLOGY

Choriocarcinoma usually appears as hemorrhagic, necrotic uterine mass; viable tumor may be minimal or seen only in metastatic foci. In contrast with hydatidiform mole and invasive mole, chorionic villi are not formed; instead, the tumor is composed of **anaplastic cuboidal cytotrophoblasts and syncytiotrophoblasts** (Fig. 17.22). Mitoses are abundant and sometimes abnormal. The tumor invades the underlying myometrium, frequently penetrates blood vessels, and in some cases extends out onto the uterine serosa and into adjacent structures.

Clinical Features. By the time a choriocarcinoma is discovered, widespread vascular spread has usually occurred to the lungs (50%), vagina (30%–40%), brain, liver, or kidneys. Lymphatic invasion is uncommon. Although extremely aggressive, placental choriocarcinoma is remarkably sensitive to chemotherapy. Nearly 100% of affected patients are cured, even those with distant metastases. By contrast, response to chemotherapy in choriocarcinomas that arise in the gonads (ovary or testis) is relatively poor.

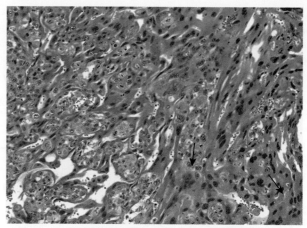

FIG. 17.22 Choriocarcinoma. This field contains both neoplastic cytotrophoblast and multinucleate syncytiotrophoblast *(arrows)*. (© 2022 - University of Michigan. Used with permission.)

Placental Site Trophoblastic Tumor

Placental site trophoblastic tumors comprise less than 2% of gestational trophoblastic neoplasms. They are neoplastic proliferations of extravillous trophoblasts, also called intermediate trophoblasts; these cells proliferate and migrate from the cytotrophoblast of the placenta and invade the maternal decidua and myometrium. They have features overlapping with cytotrophoblasts and syncytiotrophoblasts. Unlike syncytiotrophoblasts, intermediate trophoblasts do not produce hCG in large amounts, hence serum hCG levels are low. However, they do elaborate human placental lactogen (hPL). These diploid tumors, often with XX karyotype, usually arise a few months after pregnancy. An indolent clinical course is typical, with a generally favorable outcome if the tumor is confined to the endometrium and myometrium. Placental site trophoblastic tumors are not as sensitive to chemotherapy as are other trophoblastic tumors and the prognosis is poor once the tumor spreads to extrauterine sites.

▌BREAST

The functional unit of the breast is the lobule, which is supported by a specialized intralobular stroma. There are two layers of cells lining the breast lobules. The inner luminal epithelial cells produce milk during lactation. The basally located myoepithelial cells have a contractile function that aids in milk ejection and also help support the basement membrane. The ducts are conduits for milk to reach the nipple. The size of the breast is determined primarily by interlobular stroma, which increases during puberty and involutes with age. Each constituent is a source of both benign and malignant lesions (Fig. 17.23).

CLINICAL PRESENTATIONS OF BREAST DISEASE

The predominant symptoms and signs of diseases of the breast are pain, inflammatory changes, nipple discharge, diffuse nodularity, or a palpable mass (Fig. 17.24A). Most lesions (>90%) are benign and do not require treatment but must be investigated to exclude malignancy. The likelihood of cancer increases with age. Of women with cancer, about 45% have symptoms, whereas the remainder come to attention through screening tests (Fig. 17.24B).
- *Pain* (mastalgia or mastodynia) is a common symptom often related to menses, possibly due to cyclic edema and swelling.

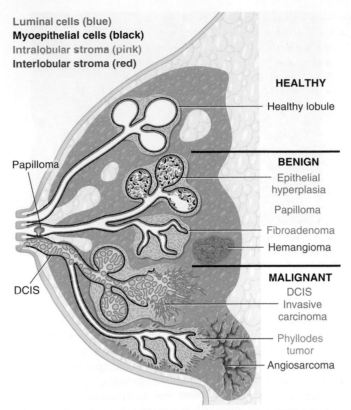

Luminal cells (blue)
Myoepithelial cells (black)
Intralobular stroma (pink)
Interlobular stroma (red)

HEALTHY
— Healthy lobule

BENIGN
— Epithelial hyperplasia
— Papilloma
— Fibroadenoma
— Hemangioma

MALIGNANT
— DCIS
— Invasive carcinoma
— Phyllodes tumor
— Angiosarcoma

Papilloma

DCIS

FIG. 17.23 Origins of breast disorders. Benign epithelial lesions include intraductal papillomas that grow in sinuses below the nipple and epithelial hyperplasia that arises in lobules. Malignant epithelial lesions are mainly breast carcinomas, which may remain in situ or invade into the breast and spread by metastasis. Specialized intralobular stromal *(pink)* cells may give rise to fibroadenomas and phyllodes tumors, whereas interlobular stroma *(red)* may give rise to a variety of rare benign and malignant tumors. *DCIS,* Ductal carcinoma in situ.

Localized pain is usually caused by a ruptured cyst or trauma to adipose tissue (fat necrosis). Although most painful masses are benign, in about 5% of cases the underlying cause is breast cancer.

- *Inflammation* causes erythema and edema involving all or part of a breast. This rare symptom is most often caused by infections, usually in the setting of lactation and breastfeeding. An important

mimic of inflammation is "inflammatory" breast carcinoma (discussed later).

- *Nipple discharge* is not worrisome when small in quantity and bilateral. Unilateral discharge is indicative of underlying breast disease. The most common benign lesion producing a nipple discharge is a papilloma arising in the large ducts below the nipple. Discharges that are spontaneous, unilateral, and bloody are of greatest concern for malignancy.

- Diffuse *nodularity* ("lumpiness") throughout the breast is usually physiologic. When pronounced, imaging studies may help to determine whether a discrete mass is present.

- *Palpable masses* can arise from proliferations of stromal cells or epithelial cells and are generally detected when they are 2 to 3 cm in size. Most (~95%) are benign and tend to be round to oval with circumscribed borders. By contrast, malignant tumors usually invade across tissue planes and have irregular borders. However, because some cancers mimic benign lesions by growing as circumscribed masses, all palpable masses require evaluation.

- *Gynecomastia* is the only common breast symptom in males. There is an increase in both stroma and epithelial cells resulting from an imbalance between estrogens, which stimulate breast tissue, and androgens, which counteract these effects.

Mammographic screening was introduced in the 1980s as a means to detect early, nonpalpable asymptomatic breast carcinomas before metastatic spread has occurred. The sensitivity and specificity of mammography increase with age; the likelihood that an abnormal mammographic finding is caused by malignancy increases from 10% at age 40 to more than 25% in women older than age 50. In the United States, most cancers in women more than 50 years of age are now detected by mammography. The principal mammographic signs of breast carcinoma are densities and calcifications.

INFLAMMATORY PROCESSES

Inflammatory diseases of the breast are rare and may be caused by infections, autoimmune disease, or foreign body–type reactions. Symptoms include erythema and edema, often accompanied by pain and focal tenderness. Because inflammatory diseases are rare, the possibility that the symptoms are caused by inflammatory carcinoma should always be considered (see later).

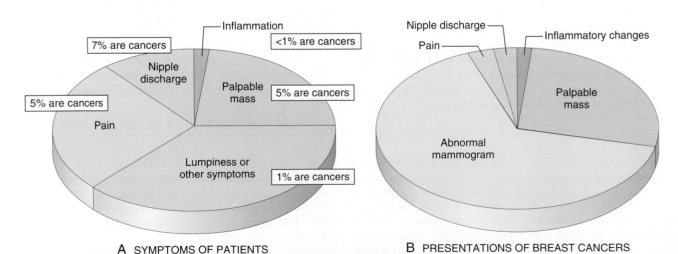

A SYMPTOMS OF PATIENTS

Inflammation
7% are cancers
Nipple discharge
<1% are cancers
Palpable mass
5% are cancers
5% are cancers
Pain
Lumpiness or other symptoms
1% are cancers

B PRESENTATIONS OF BREAST CANCERS

Nipple discharge
Pain
Inflammatory changes
Palpable mass
Abnormal mammogram

FIG. 17.24 Presenting symptoms of breast disease. (A) Common breast-related symptoms that bring patients to clinical attention. (B) Presentations of breast cancer.

Bacterial infections most commonly are lactational abscesses that occur during the first month of breastfeeding and are due to *Staphylococcus aureus* or, less commonly, streptococci. Most cases are treated adequately with antibiotics and continued expression of milk. Rarely, surgical incision and drainage are required. Abscesses outside the lactational period are rare and are often due to mixed anaerobic infections.

STROMAL NEOPLASMS

The two types of stroma in the breast, intralobular and interlobular, give rise to different types of neoplasms (see Fig. 17.23). Tumors derived from intralobular stroma have been divided into fibroadenomas and phyllodes tumors; the former are benign, while the latter may recur following excision and rarely pursue a malignant course. These two tumors share driver mutations in the same genes and appear to be part of a spectrum of related neoplasms. Interlobular stroma may be the source of the same types of tumors (e.g., lipomas and angiosarcomas) that occur in connective tissue elsewhere in the body.

MORPHOLOGY

Fibroadenomas are composed of both neoplastic stromal cells and a reactive proliferation of epithelial cells. As the fibroblasts proliferate, they push and distort the epithelial cells to form elongated, slitlike structures. The tumor mass is circumscribed and has low cellularity (Fig. 17.25A). By contrast, in **phyllodes tumors** the stromal cells tend to outgrow the epithelial cells, resulting in bulbous nodules of proliferating stromal cells that are covered by epithelium (Fig. 17.25B), the characteristic "phyllodes" (Greek for "leaflike") growth pattern. In high-grade phyllodes tumors, epithelium may be scant or absent, producing a sarcomatous appearance.

BENIGN EPITHELIAL LESIONS

Benign epithelial lesions are classified into three groups, each with a different risk for subsequent development of breast cancer: (1) *nonproliferative breast changes*; (2) *proliferative breast lesions*; and (3) *proliferative disease with atypia*. They are important to distinguish because they have different associations with breast cancer risk, as follows (Table 17.6):

- Nonproliferative changes are not associated with an increased risk
- Proliferative lesions without atypia are associated with a 1.5- to 2-fold increased risk
- Proliferative disease with atypia confers a 4- to 5-fold increased risk

Most come to clinical attention when detected by mammography or as incidental findings in surgical specimens.

MORPHOLOGY

Nonproliferative changes consist of three major morphologic patterns: cysts, fibrosis, and adenosis. The term "nonproliferative" refers to the single layers of epithelial cells seen in these lesions, in contrast to the multilayered hyperplastic epithelium seen in proliferative lesions. The most common nonproliferative breast lesions are **simple cysts** lined by a layer of luminal cells that often undergo apocrine metaplasia (Fig. 17.26A). Secretions may calcify and be detected by mammography. When cysts rupture, chronic inflammation and fibrosis in response to the spilled debris may produce palpable nodularity of the breast (so-called "fibrocystic changes"). In **adenosis** there is an increase in the number of acini per lobule. It is normal in pregnancy and may be found focally in nonpregnant women. **Proliferative lesions without atypia** include epithelial hyperplasia, sclerosing adenosis, complex sclerosing lesion, radial sclerosing lesion (radial scar), and papilloma (eFig. 17.8). Each is associated with varying degrees of epithelial cell proliferation. They are commonly detected as mammographic densities, calcifications, or incidental findings in biopsies performed for other reasons. **Proliferative disease with atypia** includes atypical ductal hyperplasia (ADH) and atypical lobular hyperplasia (ALH). The terms *ductal* and *lobular* are still used to describe subsets of both in situ and invasive carcinomas, but most evidence suggests all breast carcinomas arise from cells in the terminal duct lobular unit. ADH closely resembles ductal carcinoma in situ (DCIS) and ALH closely resembles lobular carcinoma in situ (LCIS); both are more limited in extent. The cells in ADH are uniform in appearance and form sharply marginated spaces or rigid bridges (Fig. 17.27A), whereas those of ALH are monomorphic with bland, round nuclei (Fig. 17.27B).

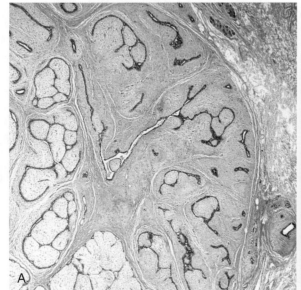
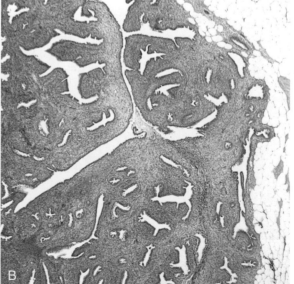

FIG. 17.25 Intralobular stromal neoplasms. (A) Fibroadenoma. This benign tumor has an expansile growth pattern with pushing circumscribed borders. (B) Phyllodes tumor. Proliferating stromal cells distort the glandular tissue, forming cleftlike spaces, and bulge into surrounding stroma.

Table 17.6 Epithelial Breast Lesions and Risk of Developing Invasive Carcinoma

Pathologic Lesions	Relative Risk (Absolute Lifetime Risk)[a]
Nonproliferative breast changes (mild hyperplasia, duct ectasia, cysts, apocrine metaplasia, adenosis, fibroadenoma without complex features)	1.0 (~3%)
Proliferative disease without atypia (moderate or florid hyperplasia, sclerosing adenosis, complex sclerosing lesion, fibroadenoma with complex features)	1.5–2 (~5%–7%)
Proliferative disease with atypia (atypical ductal hyperplasia, atypical lobular hyperplasia)	4–5 (~13%–17%)
Carcinoma in situ (lobular carcinoma in situ, ductal carcinoma in situ)	8–10 (~25%–30%)

[a]Relative risk is the likelihood of developing invasive carcinoma compared to women without any risk factors. Absolute lifetime risk is the percentage of women expected to develop invasive carcinoma in the absence of an intervention.

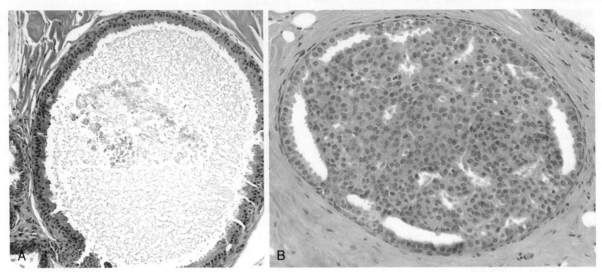

FIG. 17.26 Benign epithelial breast lesions. (A) Nonproliferative changes. This apocrine cyst, lined by cells with abundant granular cytoplasm, is a common feature of nonproliferative changes. (B) Epithelial hyperplasia. The lumen is filled with a heterogeneous mixed population of luminal and myoepithelial cell types.

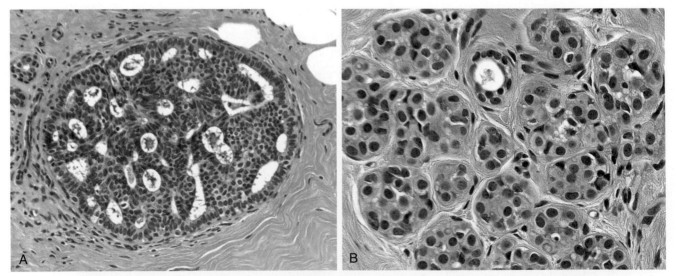

FIG. 17.27 Proliferative breast disease with atypia. (A) Atypical ductal hyperplasia. A duct is filled with a mixed population of cells consisting of oriented columnar cells at the periphery and more rounded cells within the central portion. Although some of the spaces are round and regular, the peripheral spaces are irregular and slitlike. These features are highly atypical but fall short of ductal carcinoma in situ. (B) Atypical lobular hyperplasia. A population of monomorphic small, round, loosely cohesive cells partially fills a lobule. Although the cells are morphologically identical to the cells of lobular carcinoma in situ, the extent of involvement is not sufficient for this diagnosis.

CARCINOMA

Breast carcinoma is the most common and deadly malignancy of women globally; each year, more than 2 million women are newly diagnosed, one-third of whom will die of the disease. The incidence of breast cancer is four to seven times higher in the United States and Europe than elsewhere; however, worldwide incidence and mortality is increasing rapidly, particularly in lower-income countries. The factors underlying this trend are thought to be social changes that increase breast cancer risk—specifically delayed childbearing, fewer pregnancies, and reduced breastfeeding—combined with longer lifespan and a lack of access to optimal health care.

The lifetime risk of breast cancer is 1 in 8 for women living to age 90 in the United States. It is estimated that in 2021, more than 280,000 women in the United States were diagnosed with invasive breast cancer, and more than 43,000 women died of the disease—a toll among cancers second only to lung cancer. Since the mid-1980s the mortality rate has dropped from 30% to less than 20%, a decrease attributed to both improved screening, which detects lower-stage cancers, and more effective systemic treatment.

Almost all breast malignancies are adenocarcinomas. They are divided into three major groups defined by the expression of three proteins, estrogen receptor (ER), progesterone receptor (PR), and HER2 (also known as ERBB2). In this chapter, the following terms are used to refer to these groups:

- Luminal (50%–65% of cancers): positive for ER and negative for HER2
- HER2 (10%–20% of cancers): positive for HER2 and positive or negative for ER
- Triple-negative (10%–20% of cancers): negative for ER, PR, and HER2

Luminal cancers with high expression of ER typically also express high levels of PR; such ER-positive/PR-positive tumors are usually well differentiated and slow growing. By contrast, luminal carcinomas with low ER and absent PR tend to lie at the other end of the spectrum, as they are typically poorly differentiated and have a high proliferative rate.

These three groups show striking differences in patient characteristics, pathologic features, treatment response, metastatic patterns, time to relapse, and outcome (Table 17.7). Within each group are additional histologic subtypes (discussed later), some of which also have clinical importance.

Epidemiology and Risk Factors

Breast cancer is rare in women younger than age 25 and increases in incidence rapidly after age 30. Triple negative and HER2 cancers have a relatively constant incidence after age 40 years. By contrast, luminal cancers show a marked increase in incidence with age. As a result, triple-negative and HER2-positive cancers comprise almost half of cancers in younger women and fewer than 20% of cancers in older women.

Breast cancer biology and outcomes vary with socially defined race, ethnicity, and socioeconomic status. Breast cancer rates are highest in higher-income countries and lowest in lower-income countries. According to the CDC, in the United States the rate of new breast cancer diagnoses is similar across socially defined races. However, age at diagnosis varies across socially defined races with the median age at diagnosis being highest for European Americans and lowest for Hispanic Americans. Triple-negative and HER2 cancers make up a greater proportion of cancers in African Americans. The reasons for this disparity are not known, though social factors such as parity and breast feeding likely contribute. By contrast, hormone receptor-positive/HER2-negative cancers are more common in European Americans. Although breast cancer incidence is similar for African American and European American women, the former are 42% more likely to die of their disease. Tumor biology plays a role in this disparity (i.e., tumors in this population are more likely to be triple negative); however, other factors such as lack of access to care (which may delay diagnosis until the disease is advanced) and inadequate treatment also contribute.

The most important risk factors are sex (99% of those affected are female), age, lifetime exposure to estrogen, genetic inheritance, and, to a lesser extent, environmental and lifestyle factors (Table 17.8). The major factors that decrease risk are early pregnancy (prior to 20 years of age) and prolonged breastfeeding.

Table 17.7 Summary of the Major Biologic Types of Breast Cancer

Feature	ER Positive/HER2 Negative: "Luminal"	HER2 Positive (ER Positive or Negative): "HER2"	Triple Negative (ER, PR, and HER2 Negative): "TNBC"
Overall frequency	50%–65%	20%	15%
Typical patient groups	Older women; men; cancers detected by screening; germline *BRCA2* mutation	Younger women; germline *TP53* mutation	Young women; germline *BRCA1* mutation carriers; African American women
Grade	Mainly grade 1 and 2	Mainly grade 2 and 3	Mainly grade 3
Complete response to chemotherapy	~10%	ER positive (15%), ER negative (~30%–60%)	~30%
Timing of relapse	Low rate over many years; late recurrence possible (>10 years after diagnosis); long survival possible with bone metastases	Bimodal with early and late (10 years) peaks	Early peak at <8 years, late recurrence rare, survival with metastases rare
Metastatic sites	Bone (70%–80%), viscera (25%–30%), brain (~10%)	Bone (70%), viscera (45%), brain (30%)	Bone (40%), viscera (35%), brain (25%)
Common somatic mutations	*PIK3CA* (29%–45%), *TP53* (12%–29%)	*TP53* (70%–80%), *PIK3CA* (~40%)	*TP53* (70%–80%), *PIK3CA* (9%)

PIK3CA encodes phosphoinositide 3-kinase (PI3K); *TNBC*, triple-negative breast cancer.

Table 17.8 Risk Factors for Developing Breast Cancer

Risk Factors	Relative Risk[a]
Female sex Increasing age Germline mutations of high penetrance Strong family history (>1 first-degree relative, young age, multiple cancers) Personal history of breast cancer High breast density	>4.0
Germline mutations of moderate penetrance High-dose radiation to chest at young age Family history (1 first-degree relative)	2.1–4.0
Early menarche (age <12 years) Late menopause (age >55 years) Late first pregnancy (age >35 years) Nulliparity Absence of breastfeeding Exogenous hormone therapy Postmenopausal obesity Physical inactivity High alcohol consumption	1.1–2.0

[a]Relative risk is the likelihood of developing invasive carcinoma compared to women without any risk factors.

Pathogenesis. The three major subtypes of breast cancer (luminal, HER2 positive, and triple negative) arise through largely distinct pathways that involve the stepwise acquisition of driver mutations in the epithelial cells of the duct/lobular system (Fig. 17.28). Both inherited and acquired driver mutations in cancer genes contribute to breast carcinogenesis. The major germline mutations conferring susceptibility to breast cancer affect genes that regulate genomic stability or that are involved in progrowth signaling pathways. *BRCA1* and *BRCA2* are classic tumor suppressor genes, in that cancer arises only when both alleles are inactivated or defective (Chapter 6). Both proteins have important functions in repair of double-stranded DNA breaks. The degree of penetrance, age of onset, and susceptibility to other types of cancers differ among the many *BRCA1* and *BRCA2* germline mutations that have been identified, but breast cancer risk in carriers is 45% to 75% by age 70 (compared to 12% in the general population). *BRCA2* mutations are primarily associated with ER-positive tumors, whereas *BRCA1* mutations show a strong association with triple-negative cancers (see Fig. 17.28). Other mutated genes associated with familial breast cancer include *TP53* and *PTEN*, a negative regulator of the PI3K-AKT pathway (Chapter 6). Mutations in other tumor suppressor genes associated with germline mutations, often as part of well-described syndromes, increase risk for breast cancer as well as other malignancies (Table 17.9).

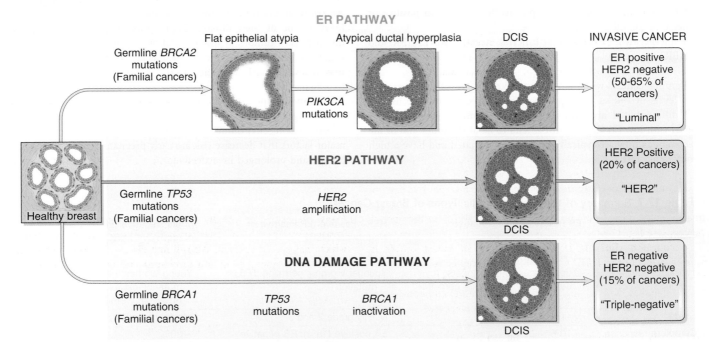

FIG. 17.28 Major pathways of ductal breast cancer development. The most common pathway *(yellow arrow)* leads to ER-positive cancers. Morphologically recognized precursor lesions include atypical ductal hyperplasia (ADH) and ductal carcinoma in situ (DCIS), both of which share certain genomic events with invasive ER-positive carcinomas, such as mutations of *PIK3CA* (the gene encoding PI3K). By gene expression profiling, these cancers are classified as "luminal." This is the type of cancer that arises most commonly in individuals with germline *BRCA2* mutations. Less common are cancers that overexpress HER2 because of gene amplification *(green arrow)*. These cancers may be positive or negative for ER; this is the most common type of cancer to arise in individuals with germline *TP53* mutations. The least common but molecularly most distinctive type of breast cancer is negative for ER and HER2 ("triple negative"; *blue arrow*). These cancers have loss of BRCA1 and p53 function and are genomically unstable; they are associated with germline *BRCA1* mutations.

Table 17.9 Most Common Single Gene Mutations Associated With Hereditary Susceptibility to Breast Cancer

Gene (Syndrome)	% of Single Gene Cancers[a]	Risk of Breast Cancer to Age 70[b]	Other Cancers	Comments
High Penetrance Germline Mutations				
BRCA1 (familial breast and ovarian cancer)	~55%	~40%–90%, females; 1%, males	Ovarian (~20%–40%), fallopian tube, pancreas, prostate, others	Majority of cancers are TNBC
BRCA2 (familial breast and ovarian cancer)	~35%	~30%–60%, females; 6%, males	Ovarian (~10%–20%), pancreas, prostate, others	Majority of cancers are ER positive. Biallelic mutations cause a form of Fanconi anemia.
TP53 (Li-Fraumeni)	<1%	~50%–60%, females; <1%, males	Sarcoma, leukemia, brain tumors, others	Majority of cancers are ER and HER2 positive
PTEN (Cowden)	<1%	~20%–80%, females; <1%, males	Thyroid, endometrium, others	Also associated with benign tumors
STK11 (Peutz-Jeghers)	<1%	~40%–60%, females	Ovarian, colon, pancreas, others	Also associated with benign colon polyps
CDH1 (hereditary diffuse gastric cancer)	<1%	~50%, females	Gastric signet ring cell carcinoma, colon	Majority of cancers are lobular in type
PALPB2 (hereditary breast cancer)	<1%	~30%–60%, females; <1%, males	Pancreas, prostate	Biallelic mutations cause a form of Fanconi anemia
Moderate Penetrance Germline Mutations				
ATM (ataxia-telangiectasia)	~5%	~15%–30%, females		Biallelic mutations cause ataxia-telangiectasia
CHEK2 (hereditary breast cancer)	~5%	~10%–30%, females	Prostate, thyroid, colon, kidney	Majority of cancers are ER positive

High penetrance germline mutations confer a >4-fold increased risk and represent 3%–7% of all breast cancers. Moderate penetrance germline mutations have a 2- to 4-fold increased risk and represent 5%–10% of breast cancers.

ER, Estrogen receptor; TNBC, triple-negative breast cancer.

[a]The percentage of all breast cancers that are associated with a germline mutation conferring an increased risk of breast cancer.

[b]Risk for specific patients can vary with the specific mutation and the presence of other gene mutations.

Somatic mutations in *BRCA1* and *BRCA2* are rare in sporadic cancers, but *BRCA1* is inactivated by methylation in up to 50% of triple-negative cancers. Somatic mutations in *TP53* are common in breast cancer, particularly triple-negative and HER2-positive tumors (see Table 17.7). Mutations that activate PI3K-AKT signaling are frequently found in sporadic ER-positive and HER2-positive breast cancers (see Fig. 17.28).

A common clinically important finding in breast cancer is amplification of the *HER2* gene. HER2 is a receptor tyrosine kinase that promotes cell proliferation and opposes apoptosis by stimulating the RAS- and PI3K-AKT signaling pathways. Cancers that overexpress HER2 are pathogenically distinct and highly proliferative.

Estrogens have an important role in breast cancer development, particularly after menopause. By binding to ER and stimulating the transcription of numerous target genes, estrogens promote the proliferation and survival of breast epithelial cells, a physiologic effect of estrogen during puberty, menstrual cycles, and pregnancy. The DNA replication caused by excessive estrogenic stimulation may be conducive to the accumulation of mutations. This may account for the association between the cumulative number of menstrual cycles and a woman's risk of developing breast cancer, as well as the strong association between luminal cancers and age. Clear measures of the importance of the prooncogenic effect of estrogen are found in the benefits of estrogen antagonists, which reduce the development of luminal cancers in women at high risk; the increased incidence of luminal cancers in women treated with postmenopausal hormone therapy; and the response of ER-positive cancers to treatment with estrogen antagonists.

Carcinoma In Situ

Breast cancer can be broadly divided into carcinoma in situ, a noninvasive cancer with no metastatic potential, and invasive carcinoma, which may spread and kill. We will first discuss the morphology and clinical implications of in situ carcinoma and then turn to invasive carcinoma.

MORPHOLOGY

There are two morphologic types of noninvasive breast carcinoma: ductal carcinoma in situ (DCIS) and lobular carcinoma in situ (LCIS). DCIS distorts lobules into ductlike spaces (Fig. 17.29A), whereas LCIS usually expands involved lobules with bland, monomorphic cells (Fig. 17.29B). By definition, both "respect" the basement membrane and do not invade into stroma or lymphovascular vessels. DCIS has a wide variety of histologic appearances. Nuclear appearances range from bland and monotonous (low nuclear grade) to pleomorphic (high nuclear grade). DCIS does not create a palpable mass and is almost always detected by mammography due to calcifications forming on membrane fragments in secretions or in central necrosis ("comedonecrosis") (Fig. 17.29C, D).

Paget disease of the nipple is caused by the extension of DCIS up the lactiferous ducts and into the contiguous skin of the nipple, producing a

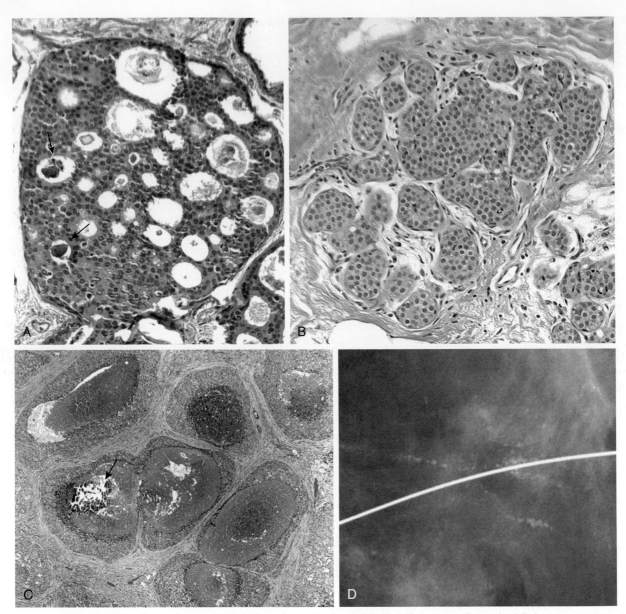

FIG. 17.29 In situ carcinoma. (A) Ductal carcinoma in situ (DCIS). Ductlike spaces distort the lobule; note calcified secretory material *(arrows)*. (B) Lobular carcinoma in situ (LCIS). Monomorphic cells fill the breast lobule. (C) DCIS, comedo type. High-grade proliferation associated with large central zones of necrosis and calcifications *(arrow)* fills several ducts. (D) Specimen radiograph reveals linear and branching calcifications within the ductal system of a breast involved by ductal carcinoma in situ.

unilateral crusting exudate over the nipple and areolar skin. The tumor cells are present singly and in clusters within the squamous epithelium of the nipple (eFig. 17.9), with an appearance similar to Paget disease of the vulva (see earlier). Unlike Paget disease of the vulva, which is not associated with an underlying malignancy, Paget disease of the nipple is often associated with invasive carcinoma.

Clinical Features. The current treatment of DCIS is surgical excision, usually followed by radiation, which results in greater than 95% survival at 20 years. Observation trials are underway to determine if such treatment is necessary for women with small, low-grade DCIS, who develop invasive cancer at a rate of only about 1% per year. When invasive cancer develops in the same breast quadrant, it tends to have a similar grade and expression of ER and HER2 as the associated DCIS. Patients with high-grade or extensive DCIS are believed to have a higher risk for progression to invasive carcinoma.

LCIS is almost always an incidental finding since it is rarely associated with calcifications or stromal reactions that produce mammographic densities. LCIS is a risk factor for developing invasive carcinoma in either breast, with a slightly higher risk to the ipsilateral breast. Invasive carcinoma develops at a rate of about 1% per year, similar to that observed for untreated DCIS. However, unlike DCIS, it is unclear if surgical removal of the identified lesion lowers risk. Approximately one-third of women with LCIS eventually develop invasive carcinoma. Current treatment options include close clinical and radiologic follow-up as well as risk reduction through treatment with antiestrogens.

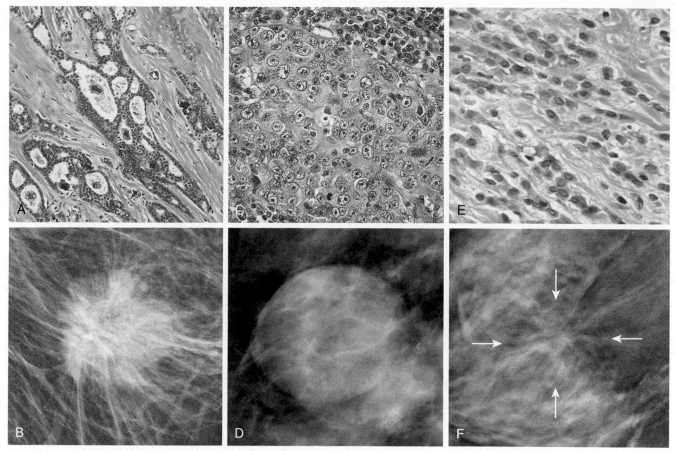

FIG. 17.30 Growth patterns of invasive breast carcinomas. (A) Most grow as tubules ("ductal" carcinoma) and stimulate a reactive desmoplastic stromal proliferation. In mammograms (B), these carcinomas appear as dense masses with spicular margins resulting from invasion of adjacent radiolucent breast tissue. (C) Uncommonly, carcinomas consist of sheets of tightly cohesive cells, as in this carcinoma with medullary features. (D) Such tumors may appear as well-circumscribed masses in mammograms, mimicking the appearance of a benign lesion. (E) Lobular carcinomas are composed of noncohesive tumor cells that invade as linear cords of cells and induce little stromal response. Accordingly, in mammograms (F) lobular carcinomas often appear as subtle, irregular masses *(arrows)*. (A, C from Fletcher CD: *Diagnostic Histopathology of Tumors*, ed 5, Figs. 16.61, 16.63, Philadelphia, 2021, Elsevier.)

Invasive (Infiltrating) Carcinoma

Invasive breast carcinoma has a wide variety of morphologic appearances. About one-third can be classified into special histologic types that merit discussion because they have important biologic and clinical associations.

MORPHOLOGY

The most common location of invasive tumors within the breast is in the upper outer quadrant (50%), followed by the central portion (20%). About 4% of women with breast cancer have bilateral primary tumors or sequential lesions in the same breast. The distinctive histologic patterns of the subtypes of invasive carcinoma are described first, followed by grading, which is used for all.

The majority (70% to 80%) of invasive breast cancers are carcinomas that are not classified further into a special type and are commonly referred to as **ductal carcinoma** (Fig. 17.30A). They are usually associated with DCIS. Their microscopic appearance varies from tumors with well-developed tubules and low-grade nuclei to tumors consisting of sheets of anaplastic cells. Most invasive ductal carcinomas produce a desmoplastic response (resulting in a

mammographic density; Fig. 17.30B), eventually leading to a hard, palpable irregular mass.

Another carcinoma of no special type is one with a **medullary pattern;** these account for about 5% of all breast cancers and are almost always triple negative. Over half of *BRCA1*-associated carcinomas have this appearance. These carcinomas typically grow as rounded masses that can be difficult to distinguish from benign tumors on imaging (Fig. 17.30D). They consist of sheets of large anaplastic cells associated with pronounced lymphocytic infiltrates composed predominantly of T cells (Fig. 17.30C).

Invasive lobular carcinoma consists of infiltrating cells that are morphologically similar to those seen in LCIS. These tumors comprise 10% to 15% of all breast carcinomas. The cells invade stroma individually and are often aligned in "single file" (Fig. 17.30E). The observed loss of cellular adhesion seen in atypical lobular hyperplasia, LCIS, and invasive lobular carcinoma is usually due to dysfunction of E-cadherin, a transmembrane protein that contributes to the cohesion of normal epithelial cells in the breast and other glandular tissues. Although most invasive lobular carcinomas manifest as palpable masses or mammographic densities, a significant subgroup invade without producing a desmoplastic response; such tumors may be clinically occult and difficult to detect by imaging (Fig. 17.30F). The pattern of metastasis of lobular carcinoma is unique among breast cancers, as they frequently spread to cerebrospinal fluid, serosal surfaces, gastrointestinal tract, ovary, uterus, and bone marrow. Almost all lobular carcinomas express hormone receptors, whereas HER2 overexpression is rare.

Inflammatory carcinoma is defined by its clinical presentation, rather than a specific morphology. Patients present with a swollen erythematous breast without a palpable mass (eFig. 17.10). The underlying invasive carcinoma is generally poorly differentiated and diffusely infiltrates and obstructs dermal lymphatic spaces, causing edema and skin thickening that mimics an inflammatory process (peau d'orange); however, there is no true inflammation. These tumors are usually of high grade and may be luminal, HER2, or triple-negative.

Mucinous (colloid) carcinoma is most commonly in the luminal group and produces abundant amounts of extracellular mucin. The tumors are soft and gelatinous due to the presence of mucin pools that create an expansile circumscribed mass.

Tubular carcinoma is another type of luminal cancer that is almost always detected on mammography as a small, irregular mass. The tumor cells are arranged in well-formed tubules and have low-grade nuclei. Lymph node metastases are rare, and the prognosis is excellent.

All types of invasive breast carcinoma are assigned a grade from 1 (low-grade) to 3 (high-grade) based on nuclear pleomorphism, tubule formation, and proliferation (eFig. 17.11). Low-grade nuclei are similar in appearance to the nuclei of normal cells. High-grade nuclei are enlarged and have irregular nuclear contours. Most low-grade carcinomas form well-defined tubules and may be difficult to distinguish from benign lesions, whereas high-grade carcinomas lose this capacity and invade as solid sheets or single cells.

Clinical Features. In unscreened populations (including young women, for whom screening is not indicated), most breast cancers are detected as a palpable mass. Almost all such carcinomas are invasive and are typically at least 2 to 3 cm in size. At least half of these cancers will already have spread to regional lymph nodes. In older, screened populations, approximately 60% of breast cancers are discovered before symptoms are present. About 20% are in situ carcinomas. Invasive carcinomas detected by screening in older women are smaller, and only 15% will have metastasized to lymph nodes.

Prognosis depends on tumor spread (i.e., anatomic stage) and tumor biology (e.g., ER and HER2 expression, tumor subtype, proliferation). Anatomic stage is based on the size/extent of the primary tumor (T), involvement of regional lymph nodes (N), and the presence of distant metastases (M). Tumor size is an independent prognostic factor and correlates with the risk of axillary lymph node metastasis. Local invasion of skin (ulceration or involvement of dermal lymphatics) or skeletal muscle is also associated with a worse prognosis.

The majority of cancers first metastasize to regional nodes, and nodal involvement is a very important prognostic factor. Lymphatic drainage goes to one or two sentinel lymph nodes in the axilla in most patients. If these nodes are not involved, the remaining axillary nodes are usually free of carcinoma. *Sentinel node biopsy* has become the standard for assessing nodal involvement, replacing more extensive lymph node dissections, which are associated with significant morbidity. Once distant metastases are present, cure is unlikely, although long-term remissions and palliation can be achieved, especially in women with ER-positive tumors. The most likely site and time of metastasis vary with the biologic type of cancer: triple-negative cancers and HER2 cancers are more likely to metastasize to the brain and viscera within the first 8 years, whereas ER-positive cancers most often metastasize to bones and are prone to late recurrences (see Table 17.7).

Additional prognostic factors are related to tumor biology and response to therapy.

- *Proliferation,* which is considered in tumor grading and measured by assessing mitotic count, is closely tied to responsiveness to cytotoxic chemotherapy. This is because rapidly growing cancer cells are more sensitive to agents that damage DNA or otherwise interfere with cell division.
- *Expression of estrogen and progesterone receptors* predicts response to antiestrogen therapy. The growth of hormone receptor–positive cancers can be inhibited for many years with therapy, and it is possible for patients to survive for long periods with distant metastases.
- *Special histologic types,* such as mucinous (colloid) and tubular carcinomas, tend to have a better prognosis. By contrast, inflammatory carcinoma has a particularly poor prognosis, with a 3-year survival of only 3% to 10%.
- *Gene expression profiling.* A number of proprietary assays that quantify mRNA levels in breast cancer cells have been developed. Most are heavily weighted toward inclusion of genes that are involved in proliferation. Currently, the greatest clinical value of these assays is to identify patients with slow-growing, antiestrogen-responsive cancers who can be spared the toxicity of chemotherapy.
- *Response to neoadjuvant chemotherapy.* Treating patients prior to surgery provides the opportunity to observe the tumor response to chemotherapy. A third or more of triple-negative and HER2 cancers regress completely (termed a pathologic complete response). By contrast, very few luminal cancers respond completely to chemotherapy.

Combining anatomic stage and biologic factors improves the prediction of outcomes. In recognition of this, the American Joint Committee on Cancer (AJCC) staging system combines anatomic stage with biologic features (ER, PR, HER2, grade, and for select cases, gene expression profiling) to create prognostic stage groups. For example, in some cases triple-negative cancer is moved to a higher stage in the prognostic staging system to reflect its more aggressive behavior.

The goals of breast cancer therapy are to control local disease and to prolong survival by treating known or potential distant metastases. Local control is achieved in the majority of patients with breast-conserving surgery ("lumpectomy") and radiation therapy. Mastectomy is generally only necessary for locally advanced disease or for women at high risk of a second primary cancer who wish to reduce the risk of recurrence.

Systemic targeted therapy is used to treat known or likely distant disease and to reduce local recurrences (Table 17.10). For ER-positive cancers, endocrine therapy with tamoxifen and aromatase inhibitors is a very effective option. Chemotherapy is used for highly proliferative carcinomas, regardless of molecular subtype. For HER2-positive cancers, targeted therapy with HER2 antagonists has markedly improved prognosis, though not all tumors respond and some develop resistance to HER2 antagonists. Triple-negative cancer remains a therapeutic challenge. Cytotoxic therapy combined with agents that are selectively active against cancers with defective homologous recombination results in complete or almost complete responses in about a third of cases. The genomic instability of these tumors leads to profound genetic

Table 17.10 Targeted Treatment of Breast Cancer

Target	Treatment
ER	Estrogen deprivation (oophorectomy, aromatase inhibitors) Blockage of ER (tamoxifen) Degradation of ER
Cyclin-dependent kinases 4 and 6 (CDK4/6)	Kinase inhibitors (palbociclib, abemaciclib, ribociclib)
HER2	Antibodies to HER2 Cytotoxic therapy linked to HER2 antibody Tyrosine kinase inhibitors Vaccines
Susceptibility to DNA damage from BRCA1/2 mutations that cause defects in HRR[a]	Chemotherapy with agents causing DNA damage requiring HRR (e.g., platinum agents) Inhibition of alternative DNA repair pathway (PARP inhibitors)
PI3K/AKT/mTOR pathway	Inhibition of proteins in the pathway
Immune checkpoint proteins	Blocking antibodies to PD-L1, PD-I, and other immune checkpoint proteins

ER, Estrogen receptor; *HRR*, homologous recombination repair; *PARP*, poly-ADP ribose polymerase.

[a]Mutations in *BRCA1* and *BRCA2* cause defects in HRR.

heterogeneity, increasing the likelihood of emergence of more aggressive, therapy-resistant subclones. However, genomic instability also may lead to expression of tumor neoantigens, and the use of immune checkpoint inhibitors is under evaluation in numerous clinical trials.

■ RAPID REVIEW

Vulva

Nonneoplastic Epithelial Disorders

- Lichen sclerosus is characterized by atrophic epithelium, subepithelial dermal fibrosis, and bandlike chronic inflammation. There is a slightly increased risk for development of squamous cell carcinoma.
- Squamous cell hyperplasia is characterized by thickened epithelium (hyperplasia), usually with a dermal inflammatory infiltrate.
- The lesions of lichen sclerosus and squamous cell hyperplasia must be biopsied to distinguish them definitively from other causes of leukoplakia, as well as squamous cell carcinoma of the vulva.

Tumors of the Vulva

- HPV-related vulvar squamous cell carcinomas are usually poorly differentiated lesions and sometimes are multifocal. They often evolve from vulvar intraepithelial neoplasia (VIN).
- Non–HPV-related vulvar squamous cell carcinomas occur in older women and are usually well differentiated and unifocal. They are often preceded by "differentiated" vulvar intraepithelial neoplasia (dVIN) associated with lichen sclerosus.
- Vulvar Paget disease is characterized by a red, scaly plaque caused by proliferation of epithelial cells within the epidermis; usually, there is no underlying carcinoma, unlike Paget disease of the nipple.

Cervix

Cervical Neoplasia

- Risk factors for cervical carcinoma are related to HPV exposure, such as early age at first intercourse, multiple sexual partners, and other factors including cigarette smoking and immunodeficiency.
- Nearly all cervical carcinomas are caused by HPV infections, particularly high-risk HPV types 16, 18, 31, and 33; the HPV vaccine is effective in preventing infection resulting from the HPV types most commonly associated with carcinoma.
- HPV expresses E6 and E7 proteins that inactivate the p53 and RB tumor suppressors, respectively, resulting in increased cell proliferation and suppression of DNA damage–induced apoptosis.
- In cervical cancer, high-risk HPV is integrated in the host genome, an event that increases the expression of E6 and E7 and contributes to progression to cancer.
- Low-grade squamous intraepithelial lesion (LSIL) and high-grade squamous intraepithelial lesion (HSIL) are precursor lesions for invasive carcinoma.
- The Pap test is a highly effective screening tool for the detection of SIL and carcinoma and has significantly reduced the incidence of cervical carcinoma. HPV testing is currently being used in conjunction with the Pap test.

Uterus

Nonneoplastic Disorders of Endometrium

- Adenomyosis refers to growth of endometrium, into the myometrium, often with uterine enlargement.
- Endometriosis refers to endometrial glands and stroma located outside the uterus and most often involves the pelvic or abdominal peritoneum. Rarely, distant sites such as the lymph nodes and the lungs are involved.
- The ectopic endometrium in endometriosis undergoes cyclic bleeding, a condition that is a common cause of dysmenorrhea and pelvic pain.
- Ectopic endometrium expresses increased level of inflammatory mediators and may be treated with COX-2 inhibitors.

Endometrial Hyperplasia and Endometrial Carcinoma

- Endometrial hyperplasia results from unopposed endogenous or exogenous estrogen.
- Risk factors for developing endometrial hyperplasia include anovulatory cycles, polycystic ovarian syndrome, estrogen-producing ovarian tumor, obesity, and estrogen therapy without counterbalancing progestin.
- Hyperplasia is classified based on the presence or absence of cytologic atypia, which determines the risk of developing endometrioid carcinoma.
- On the basis of clinical and molecular data, two major types of endometrial carcinoma are recognized:
  - *Endometrioid carcinoma* is associated with estrogen excess and endometrial hyperplasia. Early molecular changes include inactivation of DNA mismatch repair genes and the *PTEN* gene.
  - *Serous carcinoma* of the endometrium arises in older women and is usually associated with endometrial atrophy and a distinct precursor lesion, serous endometrial intraepithelial carcinoma. Mutations in the *TP53* gene are an early event, usually being present in serous endometrial intraepithelial carcinoma as well as invasive serous carcinoma.

- Stage is the major determinant of survival in both types. Serous tumors tend to manifest more frequently with extrauterine extension and therefore have a worse prognosis than endometrioid carcinomas.

Fallopian Tubes

- Inflammation of the fallopian tubes (salpingitis) is most commonly due to *Neisseria gonorrhoeae* (60%) and *Chlamydia trachomatis*.
- Primary adenocarcinoma of the fallopian tube may be the origin of many high-grade serous carcinomas of the ovary.

Ovary
Ovarian Tumors

- Tumors may arise from epithelium, sex cord–stromal cells, or germ cells.
- Epithelial tumors are the most common malignant ovarian tumor and are more common in women older than 40 years of age.
- The major types of epithelial tumors are serous, mucinous, and endometrioid. Each has benign, malignant, and borderline counterparts. Serous and endometroid tumors are more likely to be malignant; mucinous tumors are typically benign.
- Serous carcinoma is most common and many arise in the distal fallopian tube rather than the ovary.
- Sex cord–stromal tumors may display differentiation toward granulosa, Sertoli, Leydig, or ovarian stromal cell type. Depending on differentiation, they may produce estrogens or androgens.
- Germ cell tumors (mostly cystic teratomas) are the most common ovarian tumor in young women; the vast majority are benign.
- Germ cell tumors may differentiate toward oogonia (dysgerminoma), primitive embryonal tissue (embryonal carcinoma), yolk sac (endodermal sinus tumor), placental tissue (choriocarcinoma), or multiple tissue types (teratoma).

Diseases of Pregnancy
Ectopic Pregnancy

- Ectopic pregnancy is defined as implantation of the fertilized ovum outside of the uterine corpus. Approximately 1% of pregnancies implant ectopically; the most common site is the fallopian tube.
- Chronic salpingitis with scarring is a major risk factor for tubal ectopic pregnancy.
- Rupture of an ectopic pregnancy is a medical emergency that, if left untreated, may result in exsanguination and death.

Gestational Trophoblastic Disease

- Molar disease is a result of an abnormal contribution of paternal chromosomes to the conceptus.
- Partial moles are triploid and have two sets of paternal chromosomes. They are typically accompanied by fetal tissue. There is a low rate of persistent disease.

- Complete moles are diploid and all chromosomes are paternal. Only rarely are embryonic or fetal tissues associated with a complete mole.
- Among complete moles, 10% to 15% are associated with persistent disease that usually takes the form of an invasive mole. Only about 2.5% of complete moles progress to choriocarcinoma.
- Gestational choriocarcinoma is a highly invasive and frequently metastatic tumor that, in contrast with ovarian choriocarcinoma, is responsive to chemotherapy and curable in most cases.
- Placental site trophoblastic tumor is an indolent tumor of intermediate trophoblasts that produces human placental lactogen. It can be cured surgically, but once it spreads it does not respond well to chemotherapy.

Breast
Clinical Presentations of Breast Disease

- Symptoms affecting the breasts are evaluated primarily to determine if malignancy is present.
- Regardless of the symptom, the underlying cause is benign in the majority of cases.
- Breast cancer is most commonly detected by palpation of a mass in younger women and in unscreened populations and by mammographic screening in older women.

Breast Carcinoma

- The lifetime risk of developing breast cancer for an American woman is 1 in 8.
- A majority (75%) of breast cancers are diagnosed after the age of 50.
- The major risk factors for developing breast cancer are related to hormonal factors and inherited susceptibility.
- About 12% of all breast cancers are caused by germline mutations; *BRCA1* and *BRCA2* genes account for one-half of the cases associated with single-gene mutations.
- Ductal carcinoma in situ (DCIS) is a precursor to invasive ductal carcinoma and is most often found on mammographic screening as calcifications. When carcinoma develops in a woman with a previous diagnosis of untreated DCIS, it is usually an invasive ductal carcinoma in the same breast.
- Lobular carcinoma in situ (LCIS) is a marker of increased risk and a precursor lesion. When carcinoma develops in a woman with a previous diagnosis of LCIS, two-thirds are in the same breast and one-third are in the contralateral breast.
- Invasive carcinomas are classified according to histologic type and biologic type (ER positive/HER2 negative, HER2 positive, and ER/PR/HER2 negative [triple negative]). The biologic types of cancer have important differences in patient characteristics, grade, mutation profile, metastatic pattern, response to therapy, time to recurrence, and prognosis.
- Prognosis is dependent on the biologic type of tumor, stage, and availability of treatment modalities.

Laboratory Tests[a]

Test	Reference Values	Pathophysiology/Clinical Correlations
Alphafetoprotein (AFP), serum	<8.4 ng/mL	AFP is a glycoprotein normally expressed by embryonic hepatocytes and fetal yolk sac cells. Production drops after birth but rises again in patients with certain tumors. Serum AFP levels are increased in 90% of patients with hepatocellular carcinoma and in patients with certain germ cell tumors of the ovary and testis (e.g., yolk sac tumor, embryonal carcinoma). AFP is also elevated in maternal serum in the setting of open neural tube defects (e.g., anencephaly, spina bifida).
Androstenedione, serum	Varies with age, sex, and sexual development Adult males: 40–150 ng/dL Adult females: 30–200 ng/dL	Androstenedione is a steroid hormone produced from cholesterol in the testes, adrenal cortex, and ovaries. Androstenedione production in the adrenal glands is controlled by adrenocorticotropic hormone (ACTH). Androstenedione is a precursor of testosterone and is increased in hirsutism, polycystic ovarian syndrome (PCOS), virilizing adrenal tumors, precocious puberty, Cushing disease, ectopic ACTH-producing tumors, and congenital adrenal hyperplasia.
Cancer antigen 19-9 (CA19-9), serum	<35 U/mL	CA19-9 is a cell-surface glycoprotein complex that is primarily produced by ductal cells in the gastrointestinal tract. Most frequently monitored in pancreatic cancer, levels can also be elevated in both benign and malignant gynecologic disease. CA 19-9 levels are not helpful in differentiating between benign and malignant adnexal masses but may provide useful prognostic data for both endometrial and ovarian cancer.
Cancer antigen 125 (CA-125), serum	<46 U/mL	CA-125 is a glycoprotein that is normally expressed on cells derived from coelomic epithelium (e.g., fallopian tube, ovary, colon). Serum CA-125 is increased in advanced epithelial ovarian cancer and can be used to assess the presence of residual disease following debulking surgery or to monitor for recurrence. CA-125 is not specific for ovarian carcinoma, since it can also be elevated with pregnancy, nonmalignant pathology such as endometriosis and pelvic inflammatory disease, and other nongynecologic cancers.
Estradiol, serum	Varies with age, sex, and sexual development (i.e., Tanner stage) Adult males: 10–40 pg/mL Adult females (premenopausal): 15–350 pg/mL Adult females (postmenopausal): <10 pg/mL	Estrone (E1), estradiol (E2), and estriol (E3) are three endogenously produced estrogens that are responsible for the development and regulation of the female reproductive system and secondary sex characteristics. Estradiol is the dominant estrogen hormone present in nonpregnant, premenopausal females. It is produced in the ovarian follicles and regulates the menstrual cycle. Estradiol levels are used to evaluate fertility, monitor ovulation, and evaluate oligomenorrhea and menopausal status.
Estrogen receptor (ER), progesterone receptor (PR), HER2 testing in breast cancers	ER/PR: Positive: >1% tumor cells immunoreactive for ER or PR HER2: Positive by IHC: Intense membrane staining in >10% of tumor cells Positive by ISH: Varies depending on probe used	All newly diagnosed invasive breast carcinomas are tested for ER, PR, and HER2 to categorize tumors into subtypes that correlate with clinical behavior. HER2 is a receptor tyrosine kinase that belongs to the epidermal growth factor receptor family; overexpression is usually due to gene amplification. The majority of breast cancers (50% to 65%) are ER+/PR+/HER2 negative; these tumors respond well to estrogen antagonists and typically have a good prognosis. Tumors with amplified HER2 often benefit from anti-HER2 therapy (about 20% of breast cancers). Tumors that are negative for ER, PR, and HER2 are referred to as triple-negative breast cancer and comprise about 15% of breast cancers.
Estrone, serum	Varies with age, sex, and sexual development (i.e., Tanner stage) Adult males: 10–60 pg/mL Adult females (premenopausal): 17–200 pg/mL Adult females (postmenopausal): <10 pg/mL	Estrone (E1) is the dominant form of estrogen during menopause and is principally derived from peripheral aromatization of androstenedione in adipose tissue and adrenal gland. Estrone acts as a precursor to estradiol, which is more potent than estrone, and conversion back and forth occurs. E1 levels are used in conjunction with other steroid hormones to evaluate delayed/precocious puberty (females > males), in evaluation of sex steroid disorders (e.g., 17 alpha-hydroxylase deficiency), and in fracture risk assessment and hormone therapy monitoring in postmenopausal women. Levels may be increased in the setting of hyperthyroidism, cirrhosis, Turner syndrome, estrogen- or androgen-producing tumors, and polycystic ovarian syndrome (PCOS).

Follicle-stimulating hormone (FSH), serum	Varies with age, sex, menstrual cycle, and sexual development (i.e., Tanner stage)
	Adult males: 1.2–15.8 IU/L
	Adult females:
	Premenopausal:
	  Follicular: 2.9–14.6 IU/L
	  Midcycle: 4.7–23.2 IU/L
	  Luteal: 1.4–8.9 IU/L
	Postmenopausal: 16.0–157.0 IU/L
		FSH is a gonadotropin released by the anterior pituitary that stimulates the growth of ovarian follicles. The mid-menstrual cycle surge in FSH and luteinizing hormone (LH) culminates in ovulation. FSH assays are useful in assessing fertility, evaluating menstrual irregularities, predicting ovulation, and investigating pituitary disorders. FSH and LH are elevated in primary gonadal failure, precocious puberty, and menopause.

High-risk HPV (hrHPV) test, site varies	Absence of high-risk HPV types	hrHPV tests look for the presence of certain HPV types that are more likely to lead to cervical carcinoma. Pap and hrHPV tests may be used alone or in combination, depending on patient age and which professional guideline is being followed.
Human chorionic gonadotropin (hCG), serum	Males and nonpregnant females: <5 mIU/mL Levels vary during pregnancy	hCG is a hormone comprising α and β subunits. The α subunit is the same as that of FSH, LH, and TSH; therefore, most tests assess levels of the β subunit to increase sensitivity. During the first trimester, hCG synthesized by placental syncytiotrophoblastic cells stimulates the corpus luteum to secrete progesterone; subsequently, the placenta secretes progesterone and hCG levels fall. hCG may be secreted by multiple neoplasms including choriocarcinoma, seminomatous/nonseminomatous testicular tumors, ovarian germ cell tumors, and gestational trophoblastic disease. hCG measured in urine or blood can be used to detect early pregnancies; blood levels of hCG are used to help distinguish between normally developing pregnancies, miscarriage, and ectopic pregnancies. hCG is clinically useful as a tumor marker for diagnosis and disease monitoring.

Luteinizing hormone (LH), serum	Males: 1.3–9.6 IU/L
	Females:
	Premenopausal:
	  Follicular: 1.9–14.6 IU/L
	  Mid-cycle: 12.2–118.0 IU/L
	  Luteal: 0.7–12.9 IU/L
	Postmenopausal: 5.3–65.4 IU/L
		LH is a hormone cosecreted with FSH. LH is measured in the workup of hypogonadism and is low if failure is central (pituitary or hypothalamus) and elevated if failure is primary to the ovaries or testes. LH is measured to predict ovulation and in the workup of menstrual irregularities and infertility.

Pap test cytology, cervix	Absence of squamous cells with morphologic features consistent with HPV infection	Most invasive cervical cancers are squamous cell carcinoma; persistent infection with high-risk HPV is usually necessary but not sufficient for the development of squamous cell carcinoma. The goal of the Pap test is to identify precursor lesions likely to progress to cervical carcinoma. Pap tests assess the morphologic features of cells, particularly the degree of dysplasia, sampled from the ectocervix and endocervix. Screening recommendations evolve over time and referral to the most recent guidelines is strongly recommended.

Progesterone, serum	Adult females (nonpregnant):
	  Follicular phase: ≤0.89 ng/mL
	  Ovulation: ≤12 ng/mL
	  Luteal phase: 1.8–24 ng/mL
	Pregnancy:
	  1st trimester: 11–44 ng/mL
	  2nd trimester: 25–83 ng/mL
	  3rd trimester: 58–214 ng/mL
	Postmenopausal: ≤0.20 ng/mL
		Progesterone is produced by the corpus luteum, the placenta during pregnancy, and the adrenal cortex. During the luteal phase of the menstrual cycle, progesterone helps prepare the endometrium for embryo implantation by promoting endometrial gland secretions and the development of spiral arteries. Measurement of a midluteal progesterone level can be used to determine whether ovulation has occurred. In the absence of fertilization, the corpus luteum regresses, which causes progesterone levels to drop, and menses occur as the uterine lining sheds.

Total testosterone, serum	Adult males: 240–950 ng/dL Adult females: 8–60 ng/dL	In females, testosterone is produced in the ovaries and adrenal glands, and through peripheral conversion of precursor hormones. Excess testosterone in females can result in signs of hyperandrogenism including acne, hirsutism, and male-pattern hair loss. Hyperandrogenism can be caused by polycystic ovarian syndrome (PCOS), nonclassical congenital adrenal hyperplasia, and other less common endocrine disorders, such as ovarian hyperthecosis and ovarian and adrenal neoplasms. Testing for total testosterone and free testosterone can be performed when evaluating signs of hyperandrogenism and menstrual abnormalities and to help make a diagnosis of PCOS. Total testosterone >150 ng/dL in female patients requires further evaluation for androgen-secreting tumors.

Molecular Tests of Relevance

Analyte	Method	Clinical Relevance
BRCA1 and *BRCA2*	Targeted DNA sequencing or Next-Gen sequencing panels	*BRCA1* (chromosome 17q21) and *BRCA2* (chromosome 13q12.3) are tumor suppressor genes that play a role in repair of double-stranded DNA breaks. *BRCA1* and *BRCA2* mutations are seen in hereditary breast and ovarian cancers as well as several other tumor types including carcinomas of the prostate and pancreas. *BRCA1* mutations are associated with triple-negative breast cancer while the majority of breast cancers with *BRCA2* mutations are ER-positive. PARP (polyadenosine diphosphate-ribose polymerase) inhibitors can be used in the treatment of some *BRCA* mutation-associated breast and ovarian cancers.
PIK3CA	Targeted DNA sequencing or Next-Gen sequencing panels	PIK3CA encodes phosphoinositide-3 kinase (PI3K). Activating mutations of the gene are seen in approximately 40% of hormone receptor-positive/HER2-negative breast carcinomas. PI3K inhibitors can be used in the treatment of some breast carcinomas.

[a]The editing of this table by Dr. Julie Chor, Department of Obstetrics and Gynecology, University of Chicago, and Hannah Caldwell (medical student IV) is gratefully acknowledged.

References values from https://www.mayocliniclabs.com/ by permission of Mayo Foundation for Medical Education and Research. All rights reserved.

Adapted from Deyrup AT, D'Ambrosio D, Muir J, et al. Essential Laboratory Tests for Medical Education. *Acad Pathol.* 2022;9. doi: 10.1016/j.acpath.2022.100046.

Endocrine System

OUTLINE

Endocrine organs (also called *glands*) secrete *hormones* that act on other tissues to maintain the body's metabolic homeostasis and to mediate responses to the metabolic demands of acute stresses. Secretion of most hormones is regulated by so-called trophic hormones that are produced in response to particular metabolic needs. Production of a hormone often downregulates the activity of the gland that secretes the stimulating trophic hormone, a process known as *feedback inhibition*.

Hormones can be classified into several categories, based on their mechanisms of action:

The contributions to this chapter by Dr. Anirban Maitra, Professor of Pathology and Translational Molecular Pathology, The University of Texas, MD Anderson Cancer Center, Houston, Texas, in several previous editions of this book are gratefully acknowledged.

- *Hormones that act by binding to cell surface receptors* include (1) peptide hormones, such as *growth hormone* and *insulin,* and (2) small molecules, such as *epinephrine.* Binding of these hormones to cell surface receptors leads to an increase in intracellular second messengers, such as cyclic adenosine monophosphate (cAMP), inositol 1,4,5-trisphosphate (IP3), and ionized calcium. These second messengers activate intracellular signaling pathways that regulate the transcription of genes whose products mediate the functions of the hormone.
- *Hormones that act by binding to intracellular receptors:* Lipid-soluble hormones diffuse through the plasma membrane and interact with receptors in the cytosol or the nucleus. The resulting hormone-receptor complexes then bind to regulatory elements in DNA, thereby altering the expression of specific target genes. Hormones of this type include *steroids* (e.g., estrogen, androgens, glucocorticoids) and *thyroxine.*

Endocrine diseases are generally caused by (1) *underproduction or overproduction* of hormones, with associated biochemical and clinical consequences; (2) *end-organ resistance* to the effects of a hormone; or (3) *neoplasms,* which may be nonfunctional or may be associated with overproduction or underproduction of hormones. The diagnosis and management of endocrine diseases rely heavily on biochemical measurements of the levels of hormones, their regulators, and other metabolites.

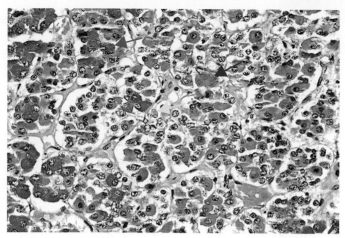

FIG. 18.1 Normal anterior pituitary gland. The gland is populated by several distinct cell types that express different peptide hormones, which impart different staining characteristics. In tissue sections stained with hematoxylin and eosin (H&E), the blue-staining (basophilic) cells *(blue arrow)* are thyrotrophs, gonadotrophs, and corticotrophs; the red-staining (eosinophilic, or acidophilic) cells *(red arrow)* are somatotrophs and lactotrophs; and the nonstaining cells (chromophobes) *(yellow arrow)* may have secreted and thus lost their hormones or are immature cells incapable of hormone production. The functions of the hormones produced by these cells are described in the text.

PITUITARY

The pituitary gland is a small, bean-shaped structure that lies at the base of the brain within the confines of the sella turcica. It is intimately related to the hypothalamus, with which it is connected by a stalk composed of axons extending from the hypothalamus and a rich venous plexus. The pituitary is composed of two morphologically and functionally distinct components: the anterior lobe *(adenohypophysis)* and the posterior lobe *(neurohypophysis).* Diseases of the pituitary affect either the anterior lobe or the posterior lobe.

The anterior pituitary produces trophic hormones that stimulate the production of hormones from the thyroid, adrenal, gonads, as well as tissues such as the breast. The anterior pituitary is composed of epithelial cells derived embryologically from the developing oral cavity. In routine histologic sections, a colorful array of cells containing basophilic cytoplasm, eosinophilic cytoplasm, or poorly staining (chromophobic) cytoplasm is present (Fig. 18.1). The staining properties of these cells are related to the synthesis of different polypeptide hormones.
- *Somatotrophs* produce growth hormone (GH).
- *Mammosomatotrophs* produce GH and prolactin (PRL).
- *Lactotrophs* produce PRL.
- *Corticotrophs* produce adrenocorticotropic hormone (ACTH), pro-opiomelanocortin (POMC), and melanocyte-stimulating hormone (MSH).
- *Thyrotrophs* produce thyroid-stimulating hormone (TSH).
- *Gonadotrophs* produce follicle-stimulating hormone (FSH) and luteinizing hormone (LH). In women, FSH stimulates the formation of graafian follicles in the ovary, and LH induces ovulation and the formation of corpora lutea in the ovary. The same two hormones also regulate spermatogenesis and testosterone production in males.

The release of these pituitary hormones is under the control of factors produced in the hypothalamus; while most hypothalamic factors are stimulatory and promote pituitary hormone release, others (e.g., somatostatin and dopamine) are inhibitory (Fig. 18.2). Rarely, signs and symptoms of pituitary disease may be caused by overproduction or underproduction of hypothalamic factors, rather than a primary pituitary abnormality.

The posterior pituitary produces two peptide hormones, antidiuretic hormone (ADH) and oxytocin, that are synthesized in the hypothalamus, stored in the posterior pituitary, and released rapidly into the circulation when needed. The posterior pituitary is composed of modified glial cells (termed pituicytes) and axonal processes extending from the hypothalamus through the pituitary stalk to the posterior lobe. ADH is produced in response to increased plasma osmotic pressure and other stimuli such as exercise and certain emotional states. It acts on the collecting tubules of the kidney to promote the resorption of water. Oxytocin stimulates the contraction of smooth muscle in the pregnant uterus and surrounding the lactiferous ducts of the mammary glands.

CLINICAL MANIFESTATIONS OF PITUITARY DISEASES

Symptoms and signs of pituitary disease fall into the following categories:
- *Local mass effects:* Because of the close proximity of the optic nerves and chiasm to the sella, expanding pituitary lesions often compress decussating fibers in the optic chiasm. This can give rise to visual field abnormalities, most commonly defects in the lateral (temporal) visual fields—so-called *bitemporal hemianopsia.* Like any expanding intracranial mass, pituitary tumors may produce signs and symptoms of elevated intracranial pressure, including headache, nausea, and vomiting. On occasion, acute hemorrhage into a pituitary neoplasm is associated with sudden enlargement of the lesion and loss of consciousness, a situation termed *pituitary apoplexy.* Acute pituitary apoplexy may be rapidly fatal and is a neurosurgical emergency.

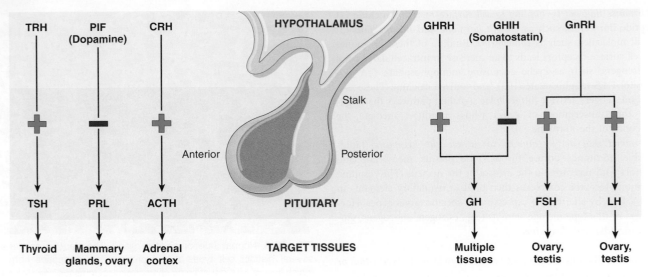

FIG. 18.2 The hypothalamic-pituitary axis. The hypothalamus regulates the secretion of hormones from the adenohypophysis (anterior pituitary gland) by releasing stimulatory (plus signs) and inhibitory factors (minus signs). These in turn modulate the release of six hormones from the anterior pituitary: adrenocorticotropic hormone (ACTH or corticotropin); follicle-stimulating hormone (FSH); growth hormone (GH, or somatotropin); luteinizing hormone (LH); prolactin (PRL); and thyroid-stimulating hormone (TSH, or thyrotropin). *CRH*, Corticotropin-releasing hormone; *GHIH*, growth hormone-inhibiting hormone; *GHRH*, growth hormone-releasing hormone; *GnRH*, gonadotropin-releasing hormone; *PIF*, prolactin-inhibiting factor; *TRH*, thyrotropin-releasing hormone.

- *Hyperpituitarism* arises from excessive secretion of trophic hormones. It most often results from an *anterior pituitary adenoma* but may also be caused by other pituitary and extrapituitary lesions. The symptoms and signs of hyperpituitarism reflect the specific hormones that are produced in excess and are discussed in the context of individual pituitary adenomas.
- *Hypopituitarism* is caused by deficiency of trophic hormones and results from destructive processes that may damage the pituitary, including ischemic injury, surgery, radiation, inflammatory reactions, and nonfunctional pituitary adenomas (described later).

ANTERIOR PITUITARY TUMORS

Anterior pituitary adenomas have been renamed *pituitary neuroendocrine tumors,* which is a more accurate term, but we will continue to refer to them as adenomas because this name is firmly entrenched in clinical practice and the medical literature. They are the most common type of pituitary tumors, produce hormones that cause endocrine abnormalities, or are nonfunctional and produce mass effects. We discuss first the general features of pituitary adenomas, then specific tumors.

General Features of Pituitary Adenomas

The most common cause of hyperpituitarism is a hormone-producing adenoma arising in the anterior lobe. Other, less common, causes include hyperplasia and carcinoma of the anterior pituitary, secretion of hormones by some extrapituitary tumors, and certain hypothalamic disorders. Some salient features of pituitary adenomas are as follows:

- *Pituitary adenomas are classified on the basis of hormone(s) produced by the neoplastic cells,* which are detected by immunohistochemical stains performed on tissue sections (Table 18.1).
- Pituitary adenomas can be *functional* (hormone producing), *nonfunctioning* (not producing hormone), or *silent* (detectable hormone production in cells without manifestations of hormone excess). Both functional and nonfunctioning pituitary adenomas are usually composed of a single cell type and the functional ones produce a single hormone, but there are exceptions, as some pituitary adenomas secrete two different hormones (growth hormone and prolactin being the most common combination).
- Pituitary adenomas are designated *microadenomas* if they are less than 1 cm in diameter and *macroadenomas* if they exceed 1 cm in diameter.
- Nonfunctioning adenomas are likely to come to clinical attention at a later stage and are, therefore, more likely to be macroadenomas. Because of their larger size, nonfunctioning adenomas may encroach upon and destroy adjacent anterior pituitary parenchyma, leading to hypopituitarism.

The peak incidence of pituitary adenomas is in the 35- to 60-year age group. Autopsy studies show that these tumors are present in more than 10% of the population, but nearly all are clinically silent.

Pathogenesis. As with other neoplasms, pituitary adenomas are caused by mutations in cancer genes. These are most commonly acquired somatic mutations but may also be germline mutations associated with an inherited predisposition to pituitary neoplasms.

- **G-protein mutations are among the most common genetic alterations in pituitary adenomas.** G-proteins transmit signals from cell surface receptors (e.g., growth hormone—releasing hormone [GHRH] receptor) that may be stimulatory or inhibitory; the stimulatory form is called G_s (eFig. 18.1). They are heterotrimeric proteins composed of α, β, and γ subunits. In its inactive state, the α-subunit of G_s, called $G_s\alpha$, binds guanosine diphosphate (GDP), which is replaced by guanosine triphosphate (GTP) upon receptor engagement. The GTP-bound form activates second messengers such as cAMP that promote cell proliferation and hormone synthesis and secretion in many endocrine cell types. Normally, $G_s\alpha$ activation is

Table 18.1 Classification of Pituitary Adenomas

Pituitary Cell Type	Hormone	Associated Adenoma	Syndrome[a]
Lactotroph	Prolactin	Lactotroph adenoma	Galactorrhea and amenorrhea (in females) Sexual dysfunction, infertility
Somatotroph	GH	Somatotroph adenoma	Gigantism (children) Acromegaly (adults)
Mammosomatotroph	Prolactin, GH	Mammosomatotroph adenoma	Combined features of GH and prolactin excess
Corticotroph	ACTH and other POMC-derived peptides	Corticotroph adenoma	Cushing syndrome, hyperpigmentation (light-skinned individuals)
Thyrotroph	TSH	Thyrotroph adenoma	Hyperthyroidism
Gonadotroph	FSH, LH	Gonadotroph adenoma	Ovarian hyperstimulation, menstrual irregularities in women Testicular enlargement in males Precocious puberty in adolescents

ACTH, Adrenocorticotrophic hormone; *FSH,* follicle-stimulating hormone; *GH,* growth hormone; *LH,* luteinizing hormone; *POMC,* proopiomelanocortin; *TSH,* thyroid-stimulating hormone.

[a]These syndromes are confined to functional adenomas. Nonfunctional (silent) adenomas in each category express the corresponding hormone(s) within the neoplastic cells, as determined by special immunohistochemical staining on tissues, but do not produce the associated clinical syndrome, and typically present with mass effects and hypopituitarism due to destruction of normal pituitary parenchyma.

Adapted from Asa SL, Essat S: The pathogenesis of pituitary tumors. *Annu Rev Pathol* 4:97, 2009.

transient due to an intrinsic GTPase activity in the α-subunit, which hydrolyzes GTP into GDP. Mutations of the gene encoding $G_s\alpha$, called *GNAS*, abrogate this GTPase activity, leading to constitutive activation of $G_s\alpha$. *GNAS* mutations occur in ~40% of somatotroph adenomas and a minority of corticotroph adenomas, but not in thyrotroph, lactotroph, and gonadotroph adenomas.

- Activating mutations of *ubiquitin-specific protease 8 (USP8)* occur in 30% to 60% of corticotroph adenomas. The encoded protein is an enzyme that removes ubiquitin residues from proteins such as epidermal growth factor receptor (EGFR), preventing their proteasome-dependent degradation. Excessive function of USP8 thus enhances the activity of EGFR and other progrowth signaling pathways in pituitary adenomas.

- *Approximately 5% of pituitary adenomas arise as a result of an inherited predisposition.* The genes that are mutated in these cases (including *MEN1* and *CDKN1B*) normally regulate transcription and the cell cycle. Somatic mutations of such genes are rarely encountered in sporadic pituitary adenomas.

- *Molecular abnormalities associated with aggressive behavior include aberrations in known oncogenes and tumor suppressor genes,* such as overexpression of cyclin D1, mutations of *TP53*, and epigenetic silencing of the retinoblastoma gene *(RB).* In addition, activating mutations of the *RAS* oncogene are observed in rare *pituitary carcinomas,* more precisely known as pituitary neuroendocrine carcinoma. The functions of these genes are discussed in Chapter 6.

MORPHOLOGY

The typical pituitary adenoma is a well-circumscribed, soft lesion. Small tumors may be confined to the sella turcica, while larger lesions may compress the optic chiasm and adjacent structures (Fig. 18.3A), erode the sella turcica and anterior clinoid processes, and extend into the cavernous and sphenoidal sinuses. In as many as 30% of cases, adenomas are not encapsulated and infiltrate adjacent bone, dura, and rarely brain. Foci of hemorrhage and/or necrosis are common in larger adenomas.

Pituitary adenomas are composed of uniform, polygonal cells arrayed in sheets, cords, or papillae. Supporting connective tissue, or reticulin, is sparse. The nuclei

of the neoplastic cells may be uniform or pleomorphic. **Cellular monomorphism and the absence of a significant reticulin network distinguish pituitary adenomas from nonneoplastic anterior pituitary parenchyma** (Fig. 18.3B). Mitotic activity is usually scanty. The cytoplasm of the constituent cells may be acidophilic, basophilic, or chromophobic, depending on the type and amount of secretory product within the cell. The functional status of the adenoma cannot be predicted from its histologic appearance.

Functioning Adenomas and Hyperpituitarism

Adenomas arising from different pituitary cells produce hormones characteristic of that cell type and cause clinical syndromes that reflect the activity of the hormones.

Lactotroph Adenomas

Prolactin-secreting lactotroph adenomas are the most common type of hyperfunctioning pituitary adenoma, accounting for 30% to 50% of cases; they cause hyperprolactinemia, which suppresses the function of the gonads. They range in size from microadenomas to large, expansile tumors associated with mass effects. Prolactin is demonstrable within the cytoplasm of the neoplastic cells by immunohistochemical techniques.

Prolactin secretion by lactotroph adenomas is highly efficient, such that even microadenomas can secrete sufficient hormone to induce symptoms, typically consisting of amenorrhea, galactorrhea, loss of libido, and infertility. Because manifestations of hyperprolactinemia (e.g., amenorrhea) are more apparent in premenopausal women, prolactinomas are diagnosed at an earlier stage in women of reproductive age. By contrast, the effects of hyperprolactinemia are subtle in men and older women, in whom the tumor may reach a large size before coming to clinical attention. Hyperprolactinemia is also a feature of other conditions, including pregnancy, high-dose estrogen therapy, renal failure, hypothyroidism, hypothalamic lesions, and drugs that inhibit dopamine reuptake. In addition, any mass in the suprasellar compartment may disturb

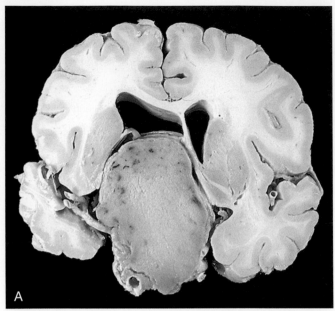

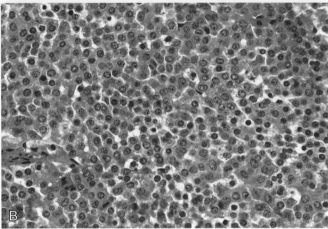

FIG. 18.3 Pituitary adenoma. (A) This large, nonfunctioning adenoma has grown beyond the confines of the sella turcica and distorts the overlying brain. Nonfunctioning adenomas tend to be larger at the time of diagnosis than those that secrete a hormone. (B) The adenoma consists of monomorphic cells with scant interspersed reticulin. (Contrast with the normal pituitary, Fig. 18.1.)

the normal inhibitory influence of the hypothalamus on prolactin secretion, resulting in hyperprolactinemia—a mechanism known as the *stalk effect.* Thus, mild elevations of serum prolactin (<200 μg/L) in a patient with a pituitary adenoma do not necessarily indicate a prolactin-secreting neoplasm.

Somatotroph Adenomas

Growth hormone—secreting somatotroph adenomas are the second most common type of functioning pituitary adenoma, accounting for about 10% of cases, and cause gigantism in children or acromegaly in adults. Because the manifestations of excess growth hormone may be subtle, somatotroph cell adenomas may be quite large by the time they come to clinical attention. On microscopic examination, growth hormone—producing adenomas are composed of densely or sparsely granulated cells, and immunohistochemical staining demonstrates growth hormone within the cytoplasm of the neoplastic

cells. Small amounts of immunoreactive prolactin are often present as well.

Persistent growth hormone excess stimulates the hepatic secretion of insulin-like growth factor 1 (IGF-1), which acts in conjunction with growth hormone to induce overgrowth of bones and muscles. When a growth hormone—secreting adenoma develops before the epiphyses close in prepubertal children, excessive levels of growth hormone and IGF-1 result in *gigantism.* This condition is characterized by a generalized increase in body size, with disproportionately long arms and legs. When elevated levels of growth hormone and IGF-1 persist or develop after closure of the epiphyses, affected individuals develop *acromegaly,* in which growth is most conspicuous in soft tissues, skin, viscera, and the bones of the face, hands, and feet. Enlargement of the jaw results in its protrusion *(prognathism),* broadening of the lower face, and separation of the teeth. The hands and feet are enlarged, and the fingers are broad and thickened. In most instances, gigantism is accompanied by evidence of acromegaly. These changes may develop slowly over decades before being recognized; hence, the adenoma may be quite large before it is detected.

Persistent growth hormone excess is also associated with metabolic abnormalities, the most important of which is diabetes. This arises because of growth hormone—induced peripheral insulin resistance, which attenuates the body's response to elevated glucose levels (see discussion of diabetes later). Failure to suppress growth hormone production in response to an oral load of glucose is one of the most sensitive tests for acromegaly. Other manifestations of growth hormone excess include gonadal dysfunction, generalized muscle weakness, hypertension, arthritis, congestive heart failure, and an increased risk for gastrointestinal cancers.

Corticotroph Adenomas

Excess production of ACTH by functioning corticotroph adenomas leads to adrenal hypersecretion of cortisol, causing Cushing disease. This is the most common cause of hypercortisolism. The disorder caused by excessive endogenous cortisol production from all causes (not only pituitary adenomas) is known as *Cushing syndrome* and is discussed later with diseases of the adrenal gland.

Corticotroph adenomas account for about 5% of pituitary adenomas. Most are small (microadenomas) at the time of diagnosis. They contain glycosylated ACTH protein, which stains positively with periodic acid—Schiff (PAS) stain and by immunohistochemistry. Large, clinically aggressive corticotroph cell adenomas may develop after surgical removal of the adrenal glands for treatment of Cushing syndrome. In most instances this condition, known as *Nelson syndrome,* results from loss of the inhibitory effect of adrenal corticosteroids on a preexisting corticotroph microadenoma; patients present with mass effects of the pituitary tumor. Patients with Cushing syndrome often have hyperpigmented skin due to increased production of melanocyte stimulating hormone (MSH), which is derived by proteolytic cleavage from the same precursor molecule (proopiomelanocortin) as ACTH.

Other Anterior Pituitary Neoplasms

Other pituitary adenomas are associated with hormonal disorders not considered part of hyperpituitarism or are nonfunctional and do not produce hormonal disturbances.

- *Gonadotroph adenomas* produce hormones *(luteinizing hormone [LH]* and *follicle-stimulating hormone [FSH])* that act on reproductive organs (gonads). These adenomas are usually clinically silent and are detected when the tumors become sufficiently large to produce mass effects. The neoplastic cells typically demonstrate immunoreactivity for the common gonadotropin α-subunit and the specific β-FSH and β-LH subunits; FSH secretion usually dominates.

- *Thyrotroph (thyroid-stimulating hormone [TSH]—producing) adenomas* account for about 1% of all pituitary adenomas and are a rare cause of hyperthyroidism.
- *Nonfunctioning pituitary adenomas* are a heterogeneous group that constitutes 25% to 30% of pituitary tumors. The typical presentation is due to mass effects. These lesions may also impinge on normal anterior pituitary cells and produce hypopituitarism, which may appear acutely due to hemorrhage within the tumor or may be gradual because of progressive enlargement of the adenoma.
- *Pituitary carcinomas are exceedingly rare.* These tumors usually extend beyond the sella and metastasize.

HYPOPITUITARISM

Clinically significant hypopituitarism most often results from pituitary lesions, but may also be caused by disorders that interfere with the delivery of pituitary hormone—releasing factors from the hypothalamus, such as hypothalamic tumors. Hypopituitarism accompanied by evidence of posterior pituitary dysfunction in the form of diabetes insipidus (discussed later) is almost always of hypothalamic origin. Anterior pituitary hypofunction is caused by the following:

- *Tumors and other mass lesions* (especially nonfunctioning pituitary adenomas)
- *Ischemic necrosis of the anterior pituitary.* Postpartum necrosis of the anterior pituitary, called *Sheehan syndrome,* is the most common form of clinically significant necrosis of the anterior pituitary. During pregnancy, the anterior pituitary enlarges secondary to an increase in the size and number of prolactin-secreting cells, but the blood supply from the low-pressure hypophyseal portal venous system does not increase proportionately. The enlarged gland is thus vulnerable to ischemic injury, especially in the setting of obstetric hemorrhage or hypotension. By contrast, the posterior pituitary receives its blood directly from arterial branches and is much less susceptible to ischemic injury. Pituitary necrosis may also occur in the setting of disseminated intravascular coagulation, sickle cell anemia, elevated intracranial pressure, traumatic injury, shock of any origin, and complication of checkpoint blockade therapy for cancer.
- *Iatrogenic causes* include ablation of the pituitary by surgery or radiation.
- Other, less common, causes of anterior pituitary hypofunction include inflammatory lesions such as sarcoidosis or tuberculosis, trauma, and metastatic tumors involving the pituitary.
- Mutations affecting transcription factors involved in development or function of the pituitary are rare genetic causes of hypopituitarism.

The clinical manifestations of anterior pituitary hypofunction depend on the specific hormones that are deficient. In children, growth failure may occur as a result of growth hormone deficiency. Gonadotropin or gonadotropin-releasing hormone (GnRH) deficiency leads to amenorrhea and infertility in women and to decreased libido, impotence, and loss of pubic and axillary hair. TSH and ACTH deficiencies result in hypothyroidism and hypoadrenalism, respectively (discussed later). Prolactin deficiency results in failure of postpartum lactation. The anterior pituitary is also a rich source of MSH, synthesized from the same precursor molecule

that produces ACTH; therefore, one of the manifestations of hypopituitarism is skin pallor due to loss of the stimulatory effects of MSH on melanocytes.

POSTERIOR PITUITARY DISORDERS

The clinically important posterior pituitary disorders involve antidiuretic hormone (ADH) under- or overproduction.

- **ADH deficiency causes diabetes insipidus, characterized by excessive urination (polyuria) due to an inability of the kidney to resorb water properly from the urine.** Diabetes insipidus can result from head trauma, neoplasms, inflammatory disorders, and surgical procedures involving the hypothalamus or pituitary. The condition may also arise spontaneously *(idiopathic).* Diabetes insipidus from ADH deficiency is designated *central,* to differentiate it from *nephrogenic* diabetes insipidus, which is caused by renal tubular unresponsiveness to circulating ADH. The manifestations of both diseases are similar and include the excretion of large volumes of dilute urine with a low specific gravity and increased serum sodium and osmolality. Excessive renal loss of water results in thirst and polydipsia. Patients who can drink water generally compensate for urinary losses, but patients who are obtunded, bedridden, or otherwise limited in their ability to obtain water may develop life-threatening dehydration.
- **The syndrome of inappropriate ADH (SIADH) secretion is typically associated with ADH overproduction, which causes excessive renal resorption of water.** Causes of SIADH include the secretion of ectopic ADH by malignant neoplasms (particularly small cell carcinomas of the lung), nonneoplastic diseases of the lung, and local injury to the hypothalamus or neurohypophysis. The manifestations of SIADH are dominated by hyponatremia, cerebral edema, and resultant neurologic dysfunction. Although total body water is increased, blood volume remains normal, and peripheral edema does not develop.

THYROID

The thyroid gland consists of two lobes connected by a thin isthmus, usually located below and anterior to the larynx. Each lobe is divided into lobules, each containing 20 to 40 evenly dispersed follicles. The follicles are lined by cuboidal to low columnar epithelial cells that synthesize thyroglobulin, the iodinated precursor protein of active thyroid hormone. Thyroglobulin is stored in the lumen of follicles as a homogeneous suspension called *colloid.* In response to trophic factors from the hypothalamus, TSH (also called *thyrotropin*) is released by thyrotrophs in the anterior pituitary into the circulation. TSH binds to its receptor on thyroid follicular epithelial cells, activating a stimulatory G-protein, and this signaling pathway induces the synthesis and release of thyroid hormone. Thyroid follicular epithelial cells convert thyroglobulin into *thyroxine* (T_4) and lesser amounts of *triiodothyronine* (T_3). T_4 and T_3 are released into the systemic circulation, where most of these peptides are bound to circulating plasma proteins for transport to peripheral tissues. The binding proteins maintain the serum unbound (free) T_3 and T_4 concentrations within narrow limits while ensuring that the hormones are readily available to the tissues. In the periphery, the majority of free T_4 is deiodinated to T_3; the latter binds to thyroid hormone nuclear receptors in target cells with 10-fold greater affinity than T_4 and has proportionately greater activity. Thyroid hormone binds to its nuclear thyroid hormone receptor (TR) in a wide range of cell types. The hormone-receptor complex regulates the transcription of numerous cellular genes, leading to diverse effects, including increased carbohydrate and lipid catabolism and protein synthesis. The net result of these processes is an increase in the basal metabolic rate.

Recognition of diseases of the thyroid is important because most are amenable to medical or surgical management. Such diseases include conditions associated with excessive release of thyroid hormones (hyperthyroidism), thyroid hormone deficiency (hypothyroidism), and mass lesions of the thyroid.

HYPERTHYROIDISM

Elevated circulating levels of thyroid hormones cause a hypermetabolic state called thyrotoxicosis. Because it usually results from hyperfunction of the thyroid gland, it is often referred to as *hyperthyroidism*.

Pathogenesis. The three most common causes of hyperthyroidism are:

- *Graves disease,* a form of autoimmune thyroid disease associated with diffuse hyperplasia of the thyroid (about 85% of cases)
- *Hyperfunctioning ("toxic") multinodular goiter*
- *Hyperfunctional ("toxic") adenoma of the thyroid*

Excessive release of thyroid hormones may also be seen transiently in some forms of thyroiditis and rarely as a result of TSH-producing pituitary adenomas.

Clinical Features. The clinical manifestations of thyrotoxicosis are attributable to the hypermetabolic state induced by thyroid hormone and overactivity of the autonomic nervous system.

- *Constitutional symptoms:* The skin is soft, warm, and flushed because of increased blood flow and peripheral vasodilation to increase heat loss; heat intolerance and excessive sweating are common. Increased sympathetic activity and hypermetabolism result in weight loss despite increased appetite.
- *Gastrointestinal:* Stimulation of the gut results in rapid transit time (hypermotility), which can cause diarrhea, malabsorption, and steatorrhea.
- *Cardiac:* Palpitations and tachycardia are common due to increases in cardiac contractility and peripheral oxygen requirements. Older adult patients with preexisting heart disease may develop congestive heart failure.
- *Neuromuscular:* Patients frequently experience anxiety, tremor, and irritability due to sympathetic overactivity. Nearly 50% develop proximal muscle weakness *(thyroid myopathy).*
- *Ocular changes* often call attention to hyperthyroidism. A wide, staring gaze and lid lag are present due to sympathetic overstimulation of the superior tarsal muscle, which raises the upper eyelid.
- *Thyroid storm* designates the abrupt onset of severe hyperthyroidism. It occurs most often in patients with Graves disease and probably results from an acute elevation in catecholamine levels, as might be encountered during infection, surgery, cessation of antithyroid medication, or any form of stress. Thyroid storm is a medical emergency; a significant number of untreated patients die of cardiac arrhythmias.
- *Apathetic hyperthyroidism* refers to thyrotoxicosis occurring in older adults, in whom the typical features of thyroid hormone excess are often blunted. The underlying thyroid disease is usually detected during laboratory workup for unexplained weight loss or worsening cardiovascular disease.

The diagnosis of hyperthyroidism is based on clinical features and laboratory data. *The measurement of serum TSH is the single most useful screening test for hyperthyroidism,* because in the majority of cases TSH levels are decreased, even at the earliest stages when the disease may still be subclinical. In rare cases of secondary hyperthyroidism caused by pituitary or hypothalamic lesions, TSH levels are normal or elevated. A low TSH value is usually associated with increased circulating levels of free T_4, but occasionally, increased levels of T_3 (T_3 toxicosis) are observed instead. In such cases, free T_4 levels may be decreased, and direct measurement of serum T_3 may be useful. Once the diagnosis of thyrotoxicosis has been confirmed by TSH and free thyroid hormone assays, measurement of radioactive iodine uptake by the thyroid gland can be valuable in determining the etiology. For example, such scans may show diffusely increased uptake in Graves disease, increased uptake in a solitary nodule in toxic adenoma, or decreased uptake in thyroiditis.

HYPOTHYROIDISM

Hypothyroidism is caused by deficient thyroid hormone production. It may be the result of intrinsic abnormalities in the thyroid (primary) or pituitary defects (secondary) (Table 18.2).

Pathogenesis. Primary hypothyroidism has *congenital, autoimmune,* and *iatrogenic* causes.

- *Genetic variants* that perturb thyroid development (thyroid dysgenesis) or the synthesis of thyroid hormone (dyshormonogenetic goiter) cause congenital hypothyroidism.
- *Endemic deficiency of dietary iodine* is typically manifested by hypothyroidism early in childhood and hence has been called congenital, but it is not caused by genetic defects. It is the most common cause of hypothyroidism worldwide, affecting about 2 billion people.

Table 18.2 Causes of Hypothyroidism

Causes	Mechanisms
Primary	
Surgery, radiation exposure	Loss of thyroid tissue
Thyroiditis	Inflammatory destruction of follicles
Iodine deficiency	Decreased synthesis of thyroid hormone
Drugs (lithium, iodides)	Interference with thyroid hormone synthesis
Dyshormonogenetic goiter (rare)	Congenital defect in thyroid hormone synthesis
Genetic defects in thyroid development (rare)	Defective development of thyroid glands
Thyroid hormone resistance (rare)	Mutations in thyroid hormone receptor
Secondary (Central)	
Pituitary failure (rare)	Defective TSH production
Hypothalamic failure (rare)	Defective TSH production

- *Autoimmune thyroid disease* is a common cause of hypothyroidism in regions of the world where dietary iodine is sufficient. The majority of cases of autoimmune hypothyroidism are due to Hashimoto thyroiditis (discussed later).
- *Iatrogenic hypothyroidism* may be caused by surgical or radiation-induced ablation of the thyroid, or arise as an adverse effect of certain drugs.

Clinical Features. The manifestations of hypothyroidism vary depending on the age of onset.

- *Congenital iodine deficiency* refers to hypothyroidism developing in infancy or early childhood. In the past, this disorder was fairly common in areas of the world with endemic dietary iodine deficiency, including mountainous regions such as the Himalayas and the Andes. It is now much less frequent because of the widespread supplementation of dietary salt with iodine. Enzyme defects that interfere with thyroid hormone synthesis are a rare cause of sporadic cases. Clinical features of congenital iodine deficiency include impaired development of the skeletal system and central nervous system, severe mental disability, short stature, coarse facial features, a protruding tongue, and umbilical hernia. The severity of the mental impairment is influenced by the time of onset of the deficient state in utero. In early stages of pregnancy before the fetal thyroid develops, the fetus is dependent on maternal T_3 and T_4, which readily cross the placenta. Maternal hypothyroidism during this critical period may lead to severe fetal mental disability. By contrast, reduction in maternal thyroid hormones later in pregnancy, after the fetal thyroid has developed, has no effect on brain development.
- Hypothyroidism in older children and adults results in a condition known as *myxedema*. The initial symptoms include generalized fatigue, apathy, mental sluggishness, which may mimic depression, constipation, and decreased sweating. The skin is cool and pale due to decreased blood flow. Reduced cardiac output contributes to shortness of breath and decreased exercise capacity. Thyroid hormones regulate the transcription of several sarcolemmal genes that encode proteins that are critical for maintaining efficient cardiac output. In addition, hypothyroidism promotes an increase in total cholesterol and low-density lipoprotein (LDL) levels, which may contribute to the development of atherosclerosis and cardiovascular disease. Histologically, there is an accumulation of matrix substances, such as glycosaminoglycans and hyaluronic acid, in skin, subcutaneous tissue, and viscera. This results in nonpitting

edema, broadening and coarsening of facial features, enlargement of the tongue, and deepening of the voice.

The diagnosis of hypothyroidism is based on laboratory evaluation. As in the case of hyperthyroidism, *measurement of serum TSH is the most sensitive screening test.* Serum TSH levels are increased in primary hypothyroidism because of a loss of feedback inhibition of thyrotropin-releasing hormone (TRH) and TSH production by the hypothalamus and pituitary, respectively. By contrast, TSH levels are not increased when hypothyroidism is caused by primary hypothalamic or pituitary disease. Serum T_4 is decreased in patients with hypothyroidism of any origin.

AUTOIMMUNE THYROID DISEASE

Autoimmunity causes a variety of thyroid diseases, which are collectively referred to as *autoimmune thyroid disease*. These disorders include thyroiditis and antibody-mediated disturbances in thyroid function that are not necessarily associated with inflammation (e.g., Graves disease).

Thyroiditis encompasses a diverse group of disorders characterized by some form of thyroid inflammation. This discussion focuses on the three most common and clinically significant subtypes: (1) Hashimoto (chronic lymphocytic) thyroiditis; (2) subacute granulomatous (de Quervain) thyroiditis; and (3) painless thyroiditis (Table 18.3).

Hashimoto (Chronic Lymphocytic) Thyroiditis

Hashimoto thyroiditis is the most common cause of hypothyroidism in areas of the world where iodine levels are sufficient. It is most prevalent between 45 and 65 years of age and is much more common in women (female to male ratio of 10:1 to 20:1).

Pathogenesis. **Hashimoto thyroiditis is an autoimmune disease in which the thyroid is destroyed by an immune response against thyroid antigens.** The disease process is marked by the progressive depletion of thyroid epithelial cells associated with lymphocytic infiltrates and fibrosis. Circulating autoantibodies against thyroid antigens are present in nearly all patients. Several immunologic mechanisms may contribute to thyroid cell damage, although their relative contributions are undefined (Fig. 18.4):

- *CD8+ cytotoxic T cells* specific for thyroid antigens kill thyroid epithelial cells.
- *Cytokine-mediated cell death.* Activation of CD4+ T cells leads to the production of inflammatory cytokines such as interferon-γ in

Table 18.3 Thyroiditis

	Hashimoto (Chronic Lymphocytic) Thyroiditis	Subacute Granulomatous (de Quervain) Thyroiditis	Painless Thyroiditis	Reidel Thyroiditis
Pathogenesis	Autoimmune response against thyroid antigens; destruction of the gland by CTLs and cytokine-mediated inflammation	Postulated to be viral infection or host response to a virus	Presumed autoimmune	IgG4-related disease
Histologic features	Prominent mononuclear inflammation, often with germinal centers; atrophic thyroid epithelium	Disrupted follicles; inflammation	Lymphocytic inflammation, sometimes with germinal centers	Extensive fibrosis with scattered lymphoplasmacytic infiltrate with IgG4-positive B cells
Clinical features	Painless diffuse enlargement of the thyroid; progressive hypothyroidism	Acute onset of neck pain, fever, variable thyroid enlargement, transient hypothyroidism	Painless neck mass, features of transient hyperthyroidism	Hard, fixed thyroid mass, usually euthyroid

CTLs, Cytotoxic T lymphocytes.

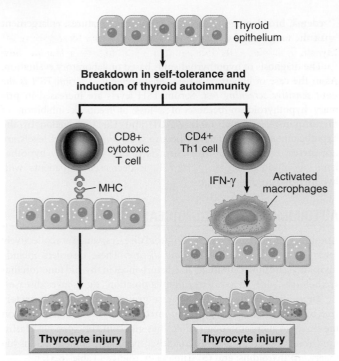

FIG. 18.4 Pathogenesis of Hashimoto thyroiditis. Breakdown of immune tolerance to thyroid autoantigens results in progressive autoimmune destruction of thyrocytes by infiltrating cytotoxic T cells, locally released cytokines, and other mechanisms (not shown). *IFN-γ*, Interferon gamma; *MHC*, major histocompatibility complex.

the thyroid gland, with resultant recruitment and activation of macrophages, which damage follicles.

- In the past it was believed that a contributing mechanism is binding of *antithyroid antibodies* (antithyroglobulin and antithyroid peroxidase antibodies), followed by antibody-dependent cell—mediated cytotoxicity (Chapter 5). It is also possible that antithyroid antibodies damage follicular cells by complement-dependent mechanisms. However, it is unclear if these antibodies are the cause or consequence of thyroid injury.

As with other autoimmune diseases, Hashimoto thyroiditis appears to have a genetic component, based on a concordance rate of about 40% in monozygotic twins and the presence of antithyroid antibodies in approximately 50% of asymptomatic siblings of affected patients. Increased susceptibility to the disease is associated with polymorphisms in immune regulation—associated genes, including the cytotoxic T lymphocyte—associated antigen-4 gene *(CTLA4)*, which codes for an inhibitor of T-cell responses (Chapter 5).

MORPHOLOGY

The thyroid is usually diffusely and symmetrically enlarged. Microscopic examination reveals widespread infiltration of the parenchyma by a **mononuclear inflammatory infiltrate** containing lymphocytes, plasma cells, and macrophages with well-developed **germinal centers** (Fig. 18.5). The thyroid follicles are atrophic and are lined in many areas by epithelial cells with abundant eosinophilic, granular cytoplasm, termed **Hürthle**, or **oxyphil, cells,** a metaplastic response to ongoing injury. On ultrastructural examination, Hürthle cells are characterized by numerous prominent mitochondria, which account for their appearance. Interstitial connective tissue is increased and may be abundant.

Clinical Features. Hashimoto thyroiditis comes to clinical attention as painless, diffuse enlargement of the thyroid, usually associated with some degree of hypothyroidism that develops slowly, often in a middle-aged woman. Hypothyroidism may be preceded by transient thyrotoxicosis caused by disruption of thyroid follicles, resulting in release of thyroid hormones *(hashitoxicosis)*. During this phase, free T_4 and T_3 concentrations are elevated, TSH is diminished, and radioactive iodine uptake is decreased. As hypothyroidism supervenes, T_4 and T_3 levels progressively fall, accompanied by a compensatory increase in TSH. Patients with Hashimoto thyroiditis often have other autoimmune diseases and are at increased risk for the development of B-cell non-Hodgkin lymphomas (Chapter 10), which typically arise within the thyroid gland. The relationship between Hashimoto disease and thyroid epithelial cancers remains controversial, with some morphologic and molecular studies suggesting an increased predisposition to papillary carcinomas.

Subacute Granulomatous (de Quervain) Thyroiditis

Subacute granulomatous thyroiditis, also known as *de Quervain thyroiditis,* is much less common than Hashimoto disease. It most often presents between 30 and 50 years of age and, like other forms of thyroiditis, occurs more frequently in women than in men. Subacute thyroiditis is believed to be caused by a viral infection or an inflammatory process triggered by viral infections. A majority of patients have a history of an upper respiratory infection shortly before the onset of thyroiditis. Unlike in Hashimoto thyroiditis, the immune response in subacute granulomatous thyroiditis is not self-perpetuating, so the process spontaneously remits.

MORPHOLOGY

The gland is firm, with an intact capsule, and may be unilaterally or bilaterally enlarged. Histologic examination reveals disruption of thyroid follicles, colloid extravasation, and infiltrating neutrophils, which are replaced over time by lymphocytes, plasma cells, and macrophages. The extravasated colloid provokes an exuberant granulomatous reaction with giant cells, some containing fragments of colloid (Fig. 18.6). Healing occurs by resolution of inflammation and fibrosis.

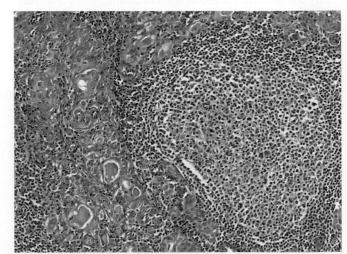

FIG. 18.5 Hashimoto thyroiditis. Lymphocytes densely infiltrate the thyroid parenchyma. A germinal center is present. (© 2022 University of Michigan. Used with permission.)

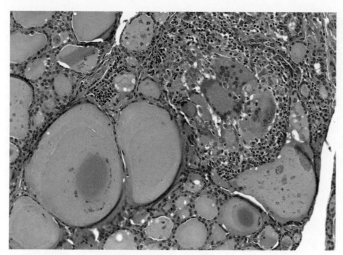

FIG. 18.6 Granulomatous thyroiditis. There is partial destruction of follicles with a mononuclear lymphocytic infiltrate and granulomatous inflammation. (© 2022 University of Michigan. Used with permission.)

Clinical Features. The onset is often acute and is characterized by neck pain (particularly with swallowing), fever, malaise, and variable enlargement of the thyroid. Transient hyperthyroidism may occur, as in other forms of thyroiditis. The leukocyte count and erythrocyte sedimentation rate are increased. With progressive gland destruction, a transient hypothyroid phase may ensue. The condition is typically self-limited, with most patients returning to a euthyroid state within 6 to 8 weeks.

Other Forms of Thyroiditis

Painless Thyroiditis. This disorder is also called subacute lymphocytic thyroiditis; in a subset of patients, the onset follows pregnancy *(postpartum thyroiditis).* It is considered a variant of Hashimoto thyroiditis and shares with it an autoimmune etiology. Circulating antithyroid antibodies are found in a majority of patients. It affects mostly middle-aged women, who present with a painless neck mass or features of thyroid hormone excess. The initial phase of thyrotoxicosis (which is likely secondary to thyroid tissue damage) is followed by return to a euthyroid state within a few months. In a minority of affected individuals, the condition eventually progresses to hypothyroidism. There may be mild symmetric enlargement of the thyroid. The histologic features consist of lymphocytic infiltration and hyperplastic germinal centers within the thyroid parenchyma.

Riedel thyroiditis. This rare disorder is a manifestation of IgG4-related disease (Chapter 5). It is characterized by lymphoplasmacytic infiltrates and extensive fibrosis involving the thyroid and contiguous neck structures, encroaching on parathyroid glands or the recurrent laryngeal nerve. Clinical evaluation demonstrates a hard and fixed thyroid mass, simulating a malignant thyroid neoplasm. It may be associated with idiopathic fibrosis in other sites in the body, such as the retroperitoneum. About one-third of patients may be hypothyroid.

Graves Disease

Graves disease is an autoantibody-mediated disorder and the most common cause of endogenous hyperthyroidism. The disease has a peak incidence between 20 and 40 years of age, with women being affected up to seven times more often than men. It is estimated to affect 1.5% to 2% of women in the United States.

Pathogenesis. **Many manifestations of Graves disease are caused by autoantibodies against the TSH receptor that bind to and stimulate thyroid follicular cells independent of endogenous trophic hormones.** Multiple autoantibodies are produced in Graves disease, the most common being *thyrotropin (TSH) receptor antibody.* This IgG antibody binds to the TSH receptor and mimics the action of TSH, with consequent increased production and release of thyroid hormones. Almost all individuals with Graves disease have detectable amounts of this autoantibody. Other TSH receptor–binding antibodies, including some that block TSH binding, have been detected. The coexistence of stimulating and inhibiting immunoglobulins in the serum of the same patient is not unusual and may explain why some patients have intercurrent episodes of hypothyroidism. Why patients develop autoimmune reactions against their TSH receptor is not known. As in other autoimmune diseases, there is a genetic component, reflected in an increased incidence in monozygotic twins and associations with genes involved in immune responses and regulation, such as particular *HLA* alleles and *CTLA4.*

Autoimmunity may be involved in the development of the *infiltrative ophthalmopathy* characteristic of Graves disease. The TSH receptor is expressed not only in the thyroid but also on ocular fibroblasts and fat cells. Activated CD4+ T cells secrete cytokines that increase production of extracellular matrix proteins, which accumulate in the retroorbital space and cause the ophthalmopathy.

MORPHOLOGY

The thyroid gland is symmetrically enlarged due to **diffuse hypertrophy and hyperplasia** of thyroid follicular epithelial cells. The gland is usually smooth and soft, and the capsule is intact (Fig. 18.7). On microscopic examination, the follicular epithelial cells in untreated cases are tall and more crowded than usual. This crowding often results in formation of small papillae that project into the follicle lumen. Such papillae lack fibrovascular cores, in contrast with those of papillary carcinoma. The colloid within the follicular lumen is pale, with scalloped margins. Lymphoid infiltrates, consisting predominantly of T cells, with fewer B cells and mature plasma cells, are present throughout the interstitium; scattered germinal centers are typically also present.

Changes in extrathyroidal tissues include generalized lymphoid hyperplasia. In individuals with ophthalmopathy, the tissues of the orbit are edematous because of the presence of mucopolysaccharides. In addition, there is infiltration by lymphocytes, mostly T cells, and fibrosis. Orbital muscles are initially edematous but may undergo fibrosis late in the course of the disease. Dermopathy, if present, is characterized by thickening of the dermis, as a result of deposition of glycosaminoglycans and lymphocyte infiltration.

Clinical Features. The clinical manifestations of Graves disease include those common to all forms of thyrotoxicosis (discussed earlier) and others that are unique, such as diffuse hyperplasia of the thyroid, ophthalmopathy, and dermopathy. The degree of thyrotoxicosis varies and is sometimes less conspicuous than other manifestations of the disease. Increased blood flow through the hyperactive gland can produce an audible bruit. The ophthalmopathy of Graves disease results in abnormal protrusion of the eyeball *(exophthalmos)* with a wide, staring gaze and lid lag (Fig. 18.8). The exophthalmos may persist or progress despite successful treatment of the thyrotoxicosis, sometimes resulting in corneal injury. The extraocular muscles are often weak. The infiltrative dermopathy most commonly involves the skin overlying the shins, where it manifests as scaly thickening and induration of the skin *(pretibial myxedema).* The skin lesions may be

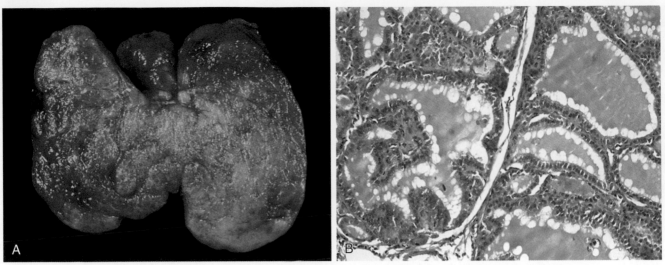

FIG. 18.7 Graves disease. (A) There is diffuse symmetric enlargement of the gland and a beefy deep red parenchyma. (B) Diffusely hyperplastic thyroid with follicles lined by tall, columnar epithelium. The crowded, enlarged epithelial cells project into the lumens of the follicles. These cells actively resorb the colloid in the centers of the follicles, resulting in the scalloped appearance of the edges of the colloid. (A, Used with permission from American Registry of Pathology. Published as Figure 5-2, in Medeiros, L. Jeffrey et al. Tumors of the Lymph Node and Spleen, AFIP Atlas of Tumor Pathology. Series 4, Fascicle 25. American Registry of Pathology, 2017.)

slightly pigmented papules or nodules and often have an orange peel texture. Laboratory findings include elevated serum free T_4 and T_3 and decreased serum TSH. Because of persistent stimulation of thyroid follicles by autoantibodies, radioactive iodine uptake is diffusely increased.

Autoimmune thyroid diseases thus span a continuum, in which Hashimoto thyroiditis, manifesting as hypothyroidism, lies at one extreme, and Graves disease, characterized by hyperfunction of the thyroid, occupies the other. These distinctions may blur, however. Sometimes, hyperthyroidism supervenes on preexisting Hashimoto thyroiditis, while at other times individuals with Graves disease spontaneously develop thyroid hypofunction. Occasionally, Hashimoto thyroiditis and Graves disease may even coexist within an affected family. Not surprisingly, there is also histologic overlap between these autoimmune disorders (most characteristically, prominent lymphocytic infiltrates and germinal center formation in the thyroid gland). In both disorders, the frequency of other autoimmune diseases, such as systemic lupus erythematosus, pernicious anemia, type 1 diabetes, and Addison disease, is increased.

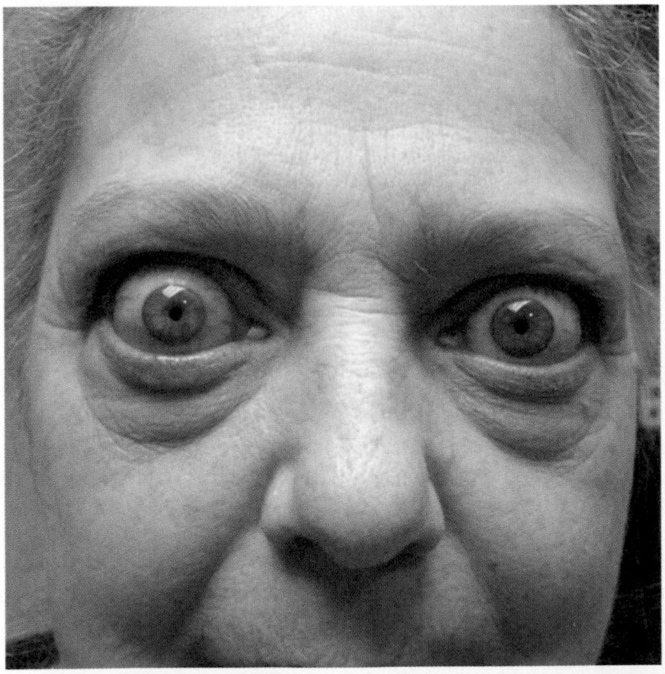

DIFFUSE AND MULTINODULAR GOITER

Enlargement of the thyroid, or goiter, is caused by reduced synthesis of thyroid hormone, most often the result of dietary iodine deficiency. Because iodine is required for the synthesis of thyroid hormones, its deficiency leads to impaired hormone production. This in turn results in a compensatory rise in the serum TSH, which drives the hypertrophy and hyperplasia of thyroid follicular cells and, ultimately, diffuse enlargement of the thyroid gland (*diffuse goiter*). Over time, recurrent episodes of hyperplasia and involution produce irregular enlargement of the gland (*multinodular goiter*). The degree of thyroid enlargement is proportional to the level and duration of thyroid hormone deficiency. These compensatory changes overcome the hormone deficiency and maintain a euthyroid metabolic state in a high percentage of affected individuals. However, if the underlying disorder is severe (e.g., a congenital biosynthetic defect), the compensatory responses may be inadequate, resulting in *goitrous hypothyroidism*.

Pathogenesis. Goiters may be endemic or sporadic.
- *Endemic goiter* occurs in geographic areas where the diet is deficient in iodine. The designation *endemic* is used when goiters are present in more than 10% of the population in a given region.

FIG. 18.8 Graves ophthalmopathy. Protruding eyes in a patient with Graves disease. (Courtesy K. B. Krantz, MD. https://app.expertpath.com/document/graves-disease-diffuse-hyperplasia/e4eecfb6-ca6d-4451-9bf8-0460bd95e1a5?searchTerm=graves.)

With increased availability of dietary iodine supplementation, the frequency and severity of endemic goiter have declined significantly.

- *Sporadic goiter* occurs less frequently than endemic goiter. The condition is more common in females than in males, with a peak incidence in puberty or young adulthood, when there is an increased physiologic demand for thyroxine. Sporadic goiter may be caused by several conditions, including the excessive ingestion of substances that interfere with thyroid hormone synthesis, such as calcium and vegetables belonging to the *Brassicaceae* (also called *Cruciferae*) family (e.g., cabbage, cauliflower). In other instances, goiter may result from inherited enzyme defects that interfere with thyroid hormone synthesis (*dyshormonogenetic goiter*). In most cases, however, the cause of sporadic goiter is unknown.

MORPHOLOGY

In **diffuse goiters**, the follicles are lined by crowded columnar cells, which may pile up and form projections similar to those seen in Graves disease. If dietary iodine subsequently increases, or if the demands for thyroid hormone decrease, the follicular epithelium involutes to form an enlarged, colloid-rich gland (**colloid goiter**). The cut surface of the thyroid in such cases is usually brown, glassy-appearing, and translucent. On microscopic examination, the follicular epithelium may be hyperplastic in the early stages of disease or flattened and cuboidal during periods of involution.

Virtually all long-standing diffuse goiters convert to **multinodular goiters**. Multinodular goiters are lobulated, asymmetrically enlarged, and may attain a massive size. On the cut surface, irregular nodules containing variable amounts of brown, gelatinous colloid are evident (Fig. 18.9A). Older lesions often show areas of fibrosis, hemorrhage, calcification, and cystic change. The microscopic appearance includes colloid-rich follicles lined by flattened, inactive epithelium (Fig. 18.9B) and areas of **follicular hyperplasia,** accompanied by degenerative changes.

Clinical Features. The dominant clinical features of goiter are those caused by the mass effects of the enlarged gland. In addition to the cosmetic issue of a large neck mass, goiters may also cause airway obstruction, dysphagia, and compression of large vessels in the neck and upper thorax (superior vena cava syndrome, Chapter 8).

Typically, multinodular goiters are hormonally silent, but a minority (approximately 10% over 10 years) manifest with thyrotoxicosis secondary to the development of autonomous nodules that produce thyroid hormone independent of TSH stimulation. This condition, known as *toxic multinodular goiter* or *Plummer syndrome,* lacks the infiltrative ophthalmopathy and dermopathy of Graves disease—associated thyrotoxicosis. The incidence of malignancy in long-standing multinodular goiters is low (<5%) but not zero, and concern for malignancy arises with goiters that suddenly increase in size or produce new symptoms (e.g., hoarseness).

THYROID NEOPLASMS

Thyroid tumors range from circumscribed, benign adenomas to highly aggressive, anaplastic carcinomas. Thyroid carcinoma is always a concern in patients who present with thyroid nodules. The majority of solitary nodules of the thyroid are either benign adenomas or localized, nonneoplastic conditions (e.g., a dominant nodule in multinodular goiter, simple cysts, or foci of thyroiditis). By contrast, carcinomas of the thyroid are uncommon, accounting for less than 1% of solitary thyroid nodules. Several clinical criteria provide a clue to the nature of a given thyroid nodule:

- Solitary nodules, nodules in children and younger patients (<30 years of age), and nodules in males are more likely to be malignant.
- A history of radiation exposure is associated with an increased incidence of thyroid malignancy.
- Hormonally inactive nodules that do not take up radioactive iodine in imaging studies (cold nodules) are more likely to be malignant.

Such associations, however, are of little significance in the evaluation of a given patient. Ultimately, morphologic evaluation of a thyroid nodule by fine-needle aspiration, combined with the histologic study of surgically resected thyroid tissue, provide the most definitive information about the nature of thyroid nodules.

Thyroid Adenomas

Adenomas of the thyroid are typically discrete, solitary masses derived from follicular epithelium and hence are known as follicular adenomas. On clinical and morphologic grounds, they may be difficult to distinguish from a dominant nodule in multinodular goiter or from less common follicular carcinomas. Although the vast

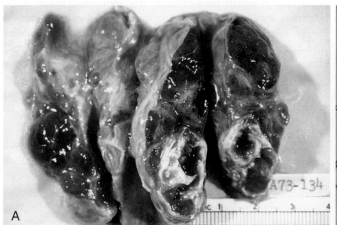 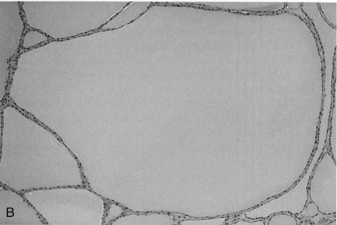

FIG. 18.9 Multinodular goiter. (A) The coarsely nodular gland contains areas of fibrosis and cystic change. (B) The enlarged thyroid follicles are lined with inactive, flattened epithelial cells and filled with abundant stored pink colloid. (B, From Klatt EC: *Robbins and Cotran Atlas of Pathology,* ed 4, Fig. 15.21, Philadelphia, 2021, Elsevier.)

majority of adenomas are nonfunctional, a small proportion produce thyroid hormones *(toxic adenomas),* causing clinically apparent thyrotoxicosis. In general, follicular adenomas are not forerunners to carcinomas; however, shared genetic alterations raise the possibility that a subset of follicular carcinomas may arise in preexisting adenomas.

Pathogenesis. **The most common genetic abnormality in toxic adenomas are somatic mutations that lead to constitutive activation of the TSH receptor signaling pathway.** Gain-of-function mutations—most often in the gene encoding the TSH receptor itself *(TSHR)* and, less commonly, in the α-subunit of G$_s$ *(GNAS)*—stimulate thyrocytes to proliferate and secrete thyroid hormone independent of TSH stimulation (thyroid autonomy), resulting in hyperthyroidism. Overall, somatic mutations in the TSH receptor signaling pathway are present in slightly over half of toxic adenomas. Such mutations are also observed in a subset of autonomous nodules present in toxic multinodular goiters, discussed earlier.

Nonfunctioning follicular adenomas are characterized by a variety of genetic aberrations, including mutations in *RAS* (<20%) and *PTEN* that are also seen in follicular carcinoma.

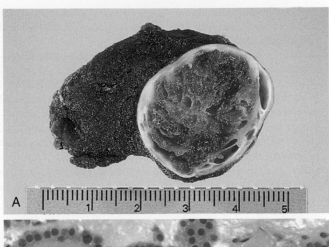

MORPHOLOGY

The typical thyroid adenoma is a **solitary,** spherical lesion that compresses the adjacent nonneoplastic thyroid. The neoplastic cells are demarcated from the adjacent parenchyma by a **well-defined, intact capsule** (Fig. 18.10A). On microscopic examination, the cells are arranged in uniform follicles that contain colloid and show little variation in cell size, shape, or nuclear morphology; mitotic figures are rare (Fig. 18.10B). Occasionally, the neoplastic cells acquire brightly eosinophilic granular cytoplasm (oxyphil or Hürthle cell change). The hallmark of all follicular adenomas is the presence of an intact capsule encircling the entire tumor. **Careful evaluation of the integrity of the capsule is therefore critical in distinguishing follicular adenomas from follicular carcinoma,** which demonstrates capsular and/or vascular invasion (discussed later).

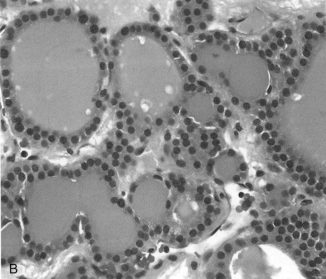

FIG. 18.10 Follicular adenoma of the thyroid. (A) A solitary, well-circumscribed nodule is visible in this gross specimen. (B) The photomicrograph shows well-differentiated follicles resembling those of normal thyroid parenchyma.

Clinical Features. Most adenomas of the thyroid manifest as painless nodules, often discovered during a routine physical examination. Larger masses may produce local symptoms such as difficulty in swallowing. Individuals with toxic adenomas may present with features of thyrotoxicosis. After injection of radioactive iodine, nonfunctional adenomas take up less iodine than the normal thyroid parenchyma. On radionuclide scanning, therefore, these appear as *cold nodules* relative to the adjacent normal thyroid gland. Toxic adenomas, however, appear as *warm* or *hot nodules* in the scan. As many as 10% of cold nodules eventually prove to be malignant. By contrast, malignancy is uncommon in hot nodules. Ultrasonography and fine-needle aspiration biopsy are essential in the preoperative evaluation of suspected adenomas. Because of the need for evaluating capsular integrity to exclude malignancy, suspected adenomas of the thyroid are removed surgically. Thyroid adenomas carry an excellent prognosis and do not recur.

Thyroid Carcinomas

The detection of small, clinically asymptomatic cancerous nodules of the thyroid gland has increased dramatically in the United States over the last few years, largely due to the increasing use of thyroid ultrasound and other imaging studies. Nonetheless, deaths from thyroid cancer have remained relatively stable during this period,

underscoring the favorable outcome for incidentally detected thyroid carcinomas (and also raising questions about the value of their detection). A female predominance has been noted among patients who develop thyroid carcinoma in the early and middle adult years. By contrast, cases seen in childhood and late adult life are distributed equally between males and females. Most thyroid carcinomas (except medullary carcinomas) are derived from the thyroid follicular epithelium, and of these, nearly all are well-differentiated lesions. The major subtypes of thyroid carcinoma and their relative frequencies are as follows:

- *Papillary thyroid carcinoma* (more than 85% of cases)
- *Follicular thyroid carcinoma* (5% to 15% of cases)
- *Anaplastic (undifferentiated) thyroid carcinoma* (<5% of cases)
- *Medullary thyroid carcinoma* (5% of cases)

Because of the unique clinical and biologic features of each type of thyroid carcinoma, these are described separately. Presented next is an overview of the molecular pathogenesis of each type of thyroid cancer.

Pathogenesis. Each major type of thyroid cancer has a distinct molecular pathogenesis. Genetic alterations in the three follicular cell–derived malignancies result in constitutive activation of signaling pathways that are normally activated by binding of growth factors to their receptor tyrosine kinases, thus promoting carcinogenesis (Fig. 18.11).

- *Papillary thyroid carcinoma.* **Activation of the MAP kinase pathway is a feature of most papillary carcinomas.** The most common mechanisms of unregulated MAPK signaling are (1) translocations that result in gene fusions of *RET* or *NTRK* (10%–20%); (2) point mutations in *BRAF* (40%–65%); and (3) oncogenic mutations of *RAS* (10%–30%). Since chromosomal rearrangements of the *RET* or *NTRK1* genes and mutations of *BRAF* and *RAS* have redundant effects, these molecular abnormalities are mutually exclusive.

  A major risk factor for papillary thyroid cancer is exposure to ionizing radiation, particularly during the first 2 decades of life. In keeping with this finding, there was a marked increase in the incidence of papillary carcinomas among children exposed to ionizing radiation after the Chernobyl nuclear disaster in 1986.

- *Follicular thyroid carcinoma.* **Follicular thyroid carcinomas frequently harbor mutations in *RAS* or in components of the PI3K/AKT signaling pathway.** Both gain-of-function mutations in *PIK3CA*, which encodes PI3K, and loss-of-function mutations in *PTEN*, a negative regulator of PI3K, are seen. *RAS* and *PIK3CA* mutations are also found in benign follicular adenomas and anaplastic carcinomas (see next), suggesting a shared histogenesis. Up to one-half of follicular carcinomas have a unique (2;3)(q13;p25) translocation that creates a fusion gene composed of *PAX8*, a paired homeobox gene that is important in thyroid

development, and the peroxisome proliferator–activated receptor gene *(PPARG)*, whose product is a nuclear hormone receptor implicated in terminal differentiation of thyroid epithelial cells.

Deficiency of dietary iodine (and, by extension, an association with goiter) is linked with a higher frequency of follicular carcinomas; the underlying mechanism is unknown.

- *Anaplastic thyroid carcinoma.* **These highly aggressive tumors can arise de novo or, more commonly, by progression of a well-differentiated papillary or follicular carcinoma.** Molecular alterations present in anaplastic carcinomas include those also seen in well-differentiated carcinomas (e.g., *RAS* or *PIK3CA* mutations), as well as additional mutations that are specific to anaplastic carcinoma. The most common of these unique mutations are loss-of-function mutations in *TP53*, which are believed to have an important role in the development of anaplastic carcinomas.

- *Medullary thyroid carcinoma.* **In contrast with the subtypes described earlier, these neoplasms arise from the parafollicular C cells**, rather than the follicular epithelium. Familial medullary thyroid carcinomas occur in *multiple endocrine neoplasia type 2* (MEN-2) (see later) and are associated with germline *RET* mutations that lead to constitutive activation of the RET tyrosine kinase receptor. Acquired *RET* mutations are also seen in approximately one-half of nonfamilial (sporadic) medullary thyroid cancers.

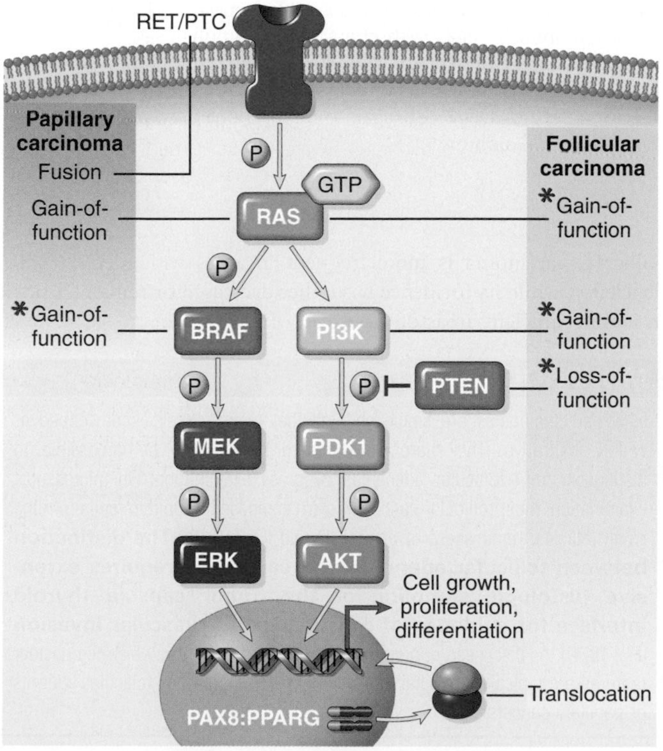

Papillary Thyroid Carcinoma

These account for the vast majority of thyroid carcinomas associated with previous exposure to ionizing radiation.

FIG. 18.11 Genetic alterations in follicular cell–derived malignancies of the thyroid. The most common mutations in MAP-kinase and PI3K/AKT signaling pathways are indicated by *asterisks*.

MORPHOLOGY

Papillary thyroid carcinomas are solitary or multifocal lesions. Tumors may be well circumscribed and encapsulated or may infiltrate the adjacent parenchyma and have ill-defined margins. Papillary foci may be visible on the cut surface, pointing to the diagnosis (Fig. 18.12A). The microscopic hallmarks of papillary neoplasms include the following:

- Branching **papillae** having a fibrovascular stalk covered by a single to multiple layers of cuboidal epithelial cells (Fig. 18.12B). In most cases, the epithelium covering the papillae has well-differentiated, uniform orderly cuboidal cells, but pleomorphic or even anaplastic morphologies may be seen.
- Nuclei with finely dispersed chromatin, which imparts an optically clear or empty appearance, giving rise to the designation **ground-glass nuclei** (Fig. 18.12C). In addition, invaginations of the cytoplasm often give the appearance of intranuclear inclusions ("pseudo-inclusions") or intranuclear grooves (Fig. 18.12D). **These nuclear features are sufficient for the diagnosis of papillary thyroid carcinoma,** even in the absence of papillary architecture.
- Concentrically calcified structures termed **psammoma bodies** are often present within the lesion, usually within the cores of papillae. These structures are almost never found in follicular and medullary carcinomas.
- Foci of lymphatic invasion by tumor are often present, but involvement of blood vessels is uncommon, particularly in smaller lesions. Metastases to adjacent cervical lymph nodes occur in up to one-half of cases.

There are over a dozen variants of papillary thyroid carcinoma, the most common of which is the so-called **encapsulated follicular variant,** which has the characteristic nuclear features of papillary carcinoma and an almost totally follicular architecture. Up to a third of these tumors contain the translocation that creates a *PAX8-PPARG* fusion gene, which is typical of follicular carcinomas, discussed earlier.

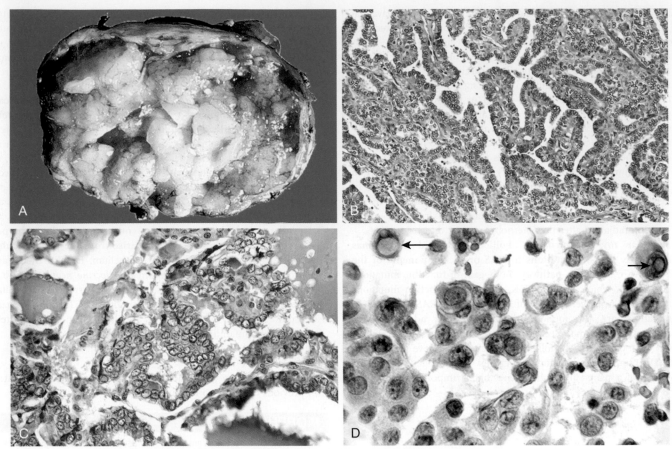

FIG. 18.12 Papillary thyroid carcinoma. (A to C) A papillary carcinoma with grossly discernible papillary structures. In this particular example, well-formed papillae (B) are lined by cells with characteristic empty-appearing nuclei (C), sometimes called *Orphan Annie eye nuclei*, based on a cartoon character from the 1920s. (D) Cells obtained by fine-needle aspiration of a papillary carcinoma. Characteristic intranuclear inclusions are visible in some of the aspirated cells *(arrows)*. (Courtesy of Dr. S. Gokasalan, Department of Pathology, University of Texas Southwestern Medical School, Dallas, Texas.)

Clinical Features. Papillary thyroid carcinomas are nonfunctional, so they manifest most often as a painless mass in the neck, either within the thyroid or as a metastasis in a cervical lymph node. A preoperative diagnosis based on the characteristic nuclear features can usually be established by fine-needle aspiration. Papillary thyroid carcinomas are indolent lesions, with 10-year survival rates in excess of 95%. The presence of isolated cervical node metastases does not have a significant influence on prognosis. In a minority of patients, hematogenous metastases are present at the time of diagnosis, most commonly to the lung. The long-term survival of patients with papillary thyroid cancer is dependent on several factors, including age (in general, the prognosis is less favorable among patients older than 40 years of age), extension outside the thyroid gland, and presence of distant metastases (stage).

Some follicular variants of papillary thyroid carcinoma show capsular invasion, whereas others lack evidence of invasion and have essentially no potential for malignant behavior.

Follicular Thyroid Carcinoma

Follicular thyroid carcinomas are more common in women than in men (ratio of 3 : 1) and manifest at an older age than papillary thyroid carcinomas, with a peak incidence between 40 and 60 years of age.

Follicular carcinoma is more frequent in areas with dietary iodine deficiency, while its incidence has either decreased or remained stable in iodine-sufficient areas of the world.

MORPHOLOGY

Follicular carcinomas are single nodules that may be well circumscribed or widely infiltrative. The sharply demarcated lesions may be impossible to distinguish from follicular adenomas by gross examination. On microscopic examination, most follicular carcinomas are composed of uniform cells forming small follicles, reminiscent of normal thyroid (Fig. 18.13). **The distinction between follicular adenoma and carcinoma requires extensive histologic sampling of the tumor capsule—thyroid interface for evidence of capsular and/or vascular invasion** (Fig. 18.14). As discussed earlier, invasive follicular lesions in which the nuclear features are typical of papillary carcinomas are regarded as follicular variants of papillary cancers.

Clinical Features. Follicular thyroid carcinomas manifest most frequently as solitary cold thyroid nodules. In rare cases, they may be hyperfunctional. These neoplasms tend to metastasize through the

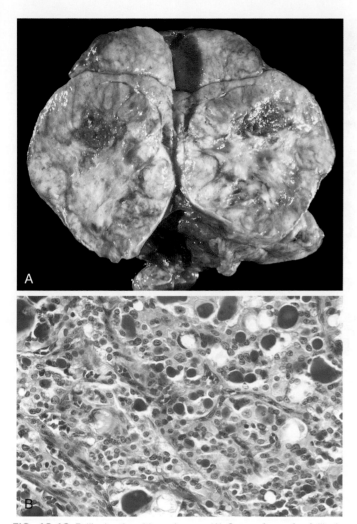

FIG. 18.13 Follicular thyroid carcinoma. (A) Cut surface of a follicular carcinoma with substantial replacement of the lobe of the thyroid. The tumor has a light-tan appearance and contains small foci of hemorrhage. (B) A few of the glandular lumens contain recognizable colloid.

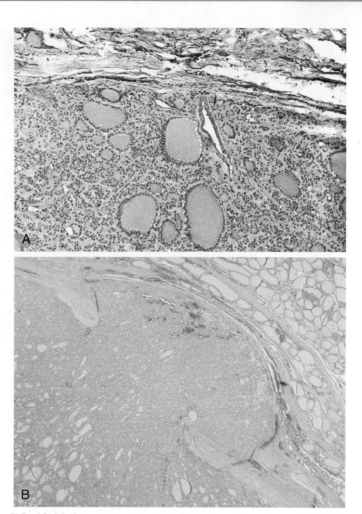

FIG. 18.14 Capsular invasion in follicular thyroid carcinoma. Evaluating the integrity of the capsule is critical in distinguishing follicular adenoma from follicular carcinoma. (A) In adenoma, a fibrous capsule surrounds the neoplastic follicles and no capsular invasion is seen; compressed normal thyroid parenchyma is usually present external to the capsule *(top)*. (B) By contrast, follicular carcinoma demonstrates capsular invasion that may be minimal, as in this case, or widespread, with extension into local structures of the neck.

bloodstream to the lungs, bone, and liver. In contrast with papillary carcinomas, regional lymph node metastases are uncommon. As many as one-half of patients with widely invasive carcinomas die from disease within 10 years, while less than 10% with minimally invasive follicular carcinomas die within the same time span. Follicular carcinomas are treated with surgical excision. Well-differentiated metastases may take up radioactive iodine, which can be used to identify and also ablate such lesions.

Anaplastic Thyroid Carcinoma

Anaplastic thyroid carcinomas are undifferentiated tumors of the thyroid follicular epithelium. They are aggressive, with a mortality rate approaching 100%. Patients with anaplastic carcinoma are older than those with other types of thyroid cancer, with a mean age of 65 years. Approximately one-fourth of patients with anaplastic thyroid carcinomas have a history of a well-differentiated thyroid carcinoma, and another one-fourth harbor a concurrent well-differentiated tumor in the resected specimen.

> **MORPHOLOGY**
>
> Anaplastic thyroid carcinomas manifest as bulky masses that typically grow rapidly beyond the thyroid capsule into adjacent neck structures. On microscopic examination, these neoplasms are composed of highly anaplastic cells, which may be large and pleomorphic or spindle-shaped and, in some cases, a mixture of the two cell types (Fig. 18.15).
>
> Foci of papillary or follicular differentiation may be present in some tumors, suggesting origin from a better-differentiated carcinoma.

Clinical Features. Anaplastic thyroid carcinomas grow rapidly despite therapy. Metastases to distant sites are common, but in most cases death occurs in less than 1 year as a result of aggressive local growth and compromise of vital structures in the neck.

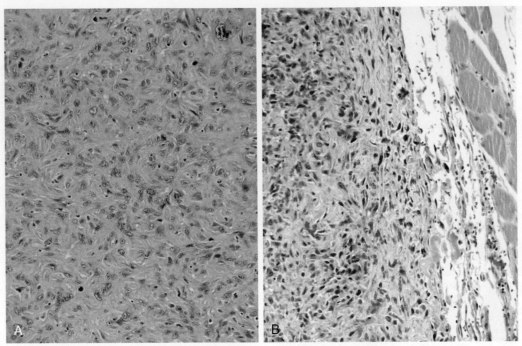

FIG. 18.15 Anaplastic thyroid carcinoma. (A) Highly pleomorphic epithelioid and spindle cells with desmoplasia. (B) Spindle cells infiltrating into adjacent skeletal muscle on the right. (From Klatt EC: *Robbins and Cotran Atlas of Pathology*, ed 4, Fig. 15.31, Philadelphia, 2021, Elsevier.)

Medullary Thyroid Carcinoma

Medullary thyroid carcinoma is a neuroendocrine tumor derived from the parafollicular cells, or C cells, of the thyroid. Like normal C cells, medullary carcinomas secrete calcitonin, measurement of which plays an important role in the diagnosis and postoperative follow-up of patients. In some cases, the tumor cells elaborate other polypeptide hormones such as somatostatin, serotonin, and vasoactive intestinal peptide. Medullary carcinomas arise sporadically in about 70% of cases. The remaining 30% are familial, occurring in the setting of multiple endocrine neoplasia (MEN) syndrome 2A or 2B or familial medullary thyroid carcinoma without an associated MEN syndrome, all of which are associated with germline *RET* mutations. Sporadic medullary carcinomas, as well as familial cases without an associated MEN syndrome, occur in adults, with a peak incidence in the fifth and sixth decades. Cases associated with MEN-2A or MEN-2B, by contrast, tend to occur in younger patients, including children.

MORPHOLOGY

Medullary thyroid carcinoma may arise as a solitary nodule or as multiple lesions involving both lobes of the thyroid. **Familial cases tend to be bilateral and multicentric.** Larger lesions often contain areas of necrosis and hemorrhage and may extend through the capsule of the thyroid (Fig. 18.16A). On microscopic examination, medullary carcinomas are composed of polygonal to spindle-shaped cells, which may form nests, trabeculae, and even glandlike structures. **Amyloid deposits,** derived from altered calcitonin molecules, are present in the stroma in many cases (Fig. 18.16B) and are a distinctive feature. Calcitonin is readily demonstrable both within the tumor cells and in the amyloid by immunohistochemical

methods. A characteristic feature of familial medullary carcinoma is the presence of **multicentric C-cell hyperplasia** in the surrounding thyroid parenchyma, a finding usually not seen in sporadic lesions. Foci of C-cell hyperplasia are believed to represent the precursor lesions from which medullary carcinoma arises.

Clinical Features. In sporadic cases, medullary thyroid carcinoma manifests most often as a mass in the neck, sometimes associated with compression effects such as dysphagia or hoarseness. In some instances, the initial manifestations are caused by the secretion of a peptide hormone (e.g., diarrhea caused by the secretion of vasoactive intestinal peptide). Screening of the patient's relatives for elevated calcitonin levels or *RET* mutations permits early detection of tumors in familial cases. As discussed later, members of MEN-2 kindreds carrying *RET* mutations are offered prophylactic thyroidectomies to preempt the development of medullary carcinoma; often, the only histologic finding in the resected thyroid of these asymptomatic carriers is the presence of C-cell hyperplasia or small (<1 cm) *micromedullary carcinomas*.

PARATHYROID GLANDS

The parathyroid glands are derived developmentally from the third and fourth pharyngeal pouches. They are most commonly located in close proximity to the upper and lower poles of each thyroid lobe but may be found anywhere along the pathway of descent of the pharyngeal pouches, including the carotid sheath, the thymus, and elsewhere in the anterior mediastinum. Most of the gland is composed

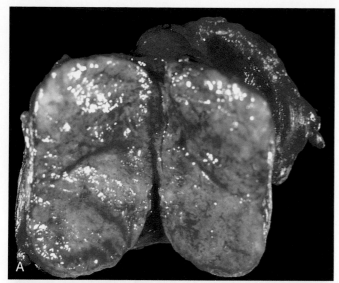

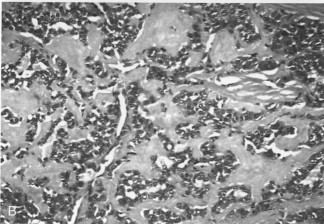

FIG. 18.16 Medullary thyroid carcinoma. (A) Bisected solid mass without a fibrous capsule. (B) Abundant amyloid, visible as homogeneous pink extracellular material. (Courtesy of the late Dr. Joseph Corson, Brigham and Women's Hospital, Boston.)

of *chief cells*, which have secretory granules containing *parathyroid hormone (PTH)*. *Oxyphil cells* are found throughout the normal parathyroid, either singly or in small clusters. They are slightly larger than chief cells, have acidophilic cytoplasm, and are tightly packed with mitochondria.

Parathyroid hormone regulates calcium homeostasis. The activity of the parathyroid glands is controlled by the level of free, ionized calcium in the blood, rather than by trophic hormones secreted by the hypothalamus and pituitary. Normally, decreased levels of free calcium stimulate the synthesis and secretion of PTH, which has several effects on its target tissues, the kidneys and the bones:

- *Increased renal tubular reabsorption of calcium*
- *Increased urinary phosphate excretion,* thereby lowering serum phosphate levels and raising free calcium levels (since phosphate binds to ionized calcium)
- *Increased conversion of vitamin D to its active dihydroxy form in the kidneys,* which in turn augments gastrointestinal calcium absorption
- *Enhanced osteoclastic activity* (i.e., bone resorption, thus releasing ionized calcium), mediated indirectly by promoting the differentiation of osteoclast progenitor cells into mature osteoclasts by

stimulating the production of receptor activator of NF-κB ligand (RANKL) and inhibiting the expression of osteoprotegerin (Chapter 19)

The net result of these activities is an increase in the level of free calcium in the blood, which inhibits PTH secretion from chief cells. Abnormalities of the parathyroids include both hyperfunction and hypofunction. Tumors of the parathyroid glands, unlike thyroid tumors, usually come to attention because of excessive secretion of PTH rather than mass effects.

HYPERPARATHYROIDISM

Hyperparathyroidism occurs in two major forms, *primary* and *secondary,* and, less commonly, as *tertiary* hyperparathyroidism. The first condition is caused by autonomous overproduction of PTH, while the latter two conditions typically occur as secondary phenomena in patients with chronic renal insufficiency.

Primary Hyperparathyroidism

Primary hyperparathyroidism is a common endocrine disorder and an important cause of hypercalcemia. There was a dramatic increase in the detection of cases in the latter half of the 20th century, mainly due to routine measurement of serum calcium levels in hospitalized patients. The frequency of occurrence of the various parathyroid lesions underlying primary hyperparathyroidism is as follows:

- Adenoma—85% to 95%
- Primary hyperplasia (diffuse or nodular)—5% to 10%
- Parathyroid carcinoma—1%

Pathogenesis. Abnormalities in two genes are commonly associated with parathyroid tumors:

- *Cyclin D1 gene rearrangements.* Cyclin D1 is a positive regulator of the cell cycle (Chapter 6). Between 10% and 20% of adenomas have an acquired inversion on chromosome 11 that positions the gene that encodes cyclin D1 (normally on 11q) adjacent to genomic elements that regulate the *PTH* gene (on 11p). These elements drive abnormal expression of cyclin D1 and the proliferation of PTH-producing cells. Cyclin D1 is also overexpressed in approximately 40% of parathyroid adenomas without the gene inversion, indicating the existence of additional mechanisms that dysregulate cyclin D1.
- *MEN1 mutations.* Approximately 30% to 35% of sporadic parathyroid tumors have mutations in both copies of the *MEN1* tumor suppressor gene (see later). The spectrum of *MEN1* mutations in sporadic tumors is virtually identical to that in familial parathyroid adenomas.

MORPHOLOGY

Morphologic changes in primary hyperparathyroidism are seen in the parathyroid glands and in organs affected by hypercalcemia. In 75% to 80% of cases, one of the parathyroid glands harbors a solitary **adenoma.** The typical parathyroid adenoma is a well-circumscribed, soft, tan nodule invested by a delicate capsule. **By definition, parathyroid adenomas are confined to a single gland.** The other glands are normal in size or somewhat shrunken, as a result of feedback inhibition by elevated serum calcium. Most parathyroid adenomas weigh between 0.5 and 5 gm. On microscopic examination, parathyroid adenomas are composed predominantly of chief cells (Fig. 18.17). A rim of compressed, nonneoplastic parathyroid tissue, generally separated by a fibrous capsule, often surrounds the adenoma.

The chief cells of the adenoma are larger and show greater variability in nuclear size than normal chief cells. Cells with bizarre and pleomorphic nuclei are often seen (so-called "**endocrine atypia**") and are not a sign of malignancy. Mitotic figures are rare. In contrast with the normal parathyroid parenchyma, adipose tissue is inconspicuous within adenomas.

Primary parathyroid hyperplasia is typically a multi-glandular process; however, in some cases only one or two glands are enlarged, complicating the distinction from adenoma. Microscopically, the most common finding is chief cell hyperplasia, which may involve the glands in a diffuse or multinodular pattern. As in the case of adenomas, stromal fat is inconspicuous within hyperplastic glands.

Parathyroid carcinomas may be circumscribed lesions that are difficult to distinguish from adenomas. These tumors enlarge one gland and consist of gray-white, irregular masses that sometimes exceed 10 gm in weight. The cells are usually uniform and resemble normal parathyroid cells. They are arrayed in nodular or trabecular patterns. The tumor mass is usually enclosed by a dense, fibrous capsule. There is agreement that **diagnosis of carcinoma based on cytologic detail is unreliable; invasion of surrounding tissues and metastasis are the only definitive criteria.** Local recurrence occurs in one-third of cases, and more distant dissemination occurs in another one-third.

In primary hyperparathyroidism, morphologic changes are also seen in other organs:

- **Skeletal changes** include increased osteoclastic activity, which results in erosion of bone matrix and mobilization of calcium salts, particularly in the metaphyses of long tubular bones. Bone resorption is accompanied by increased osteoblastic activity and the formation of new bone trabeculae. In more severe cases, the cortex is thinned and the bone marrow contains increased amounts of fibrous tissue accompanied by foci of hemorrhage and cysts (**osteitis fibrosa cystica**) (Chapter 19). Aggregates of osteoclasts, reactive giant cells, and hemorrhagic debris occasionally form masses that may be mistaken for neoplasms (**brown tumors** of hyperparathyroidism).
- **Renal changes.** PTH-induced hypercalcemia favors the formation of urinary tract calcium stones (**nephrolithiasis**) as well as calcification of the renal interstitium and tubules (**nephrocalcinosis**).
- **Metastatic calcification** secondary to hypercalcemia may also be seen in other sites, including the stomach, lungs, myocardium, and blood vessels.

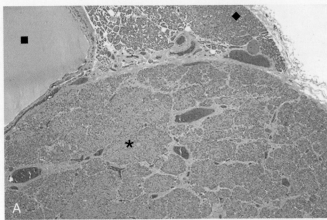
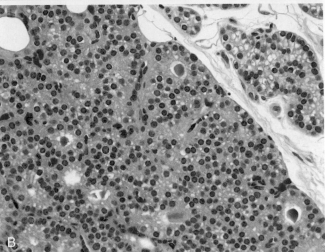

FIG. 18.17 Parathyroid adenoma. (A) Adjacent to this parathyroid adenoma *(asterisk)* is a rim of normal parathyroid, with a pink oxyphil cell nodule *(diamond)* at the upper right, and a small benign parathyroid cyst *(square)*, an incidental finding filled with pink proteinaceous fluid, at the upper left. (B) High-power detail shows minimal variation in nuclear size and occasional follicle formation. (A, From Klatt EC: *Robbins and Cotran Atlas of Pathology*, ed 4, Fig. 15.34, Philadelphia, 2021, Elsevier. B, Courtesy of Dr. Nicole Cipriani, Department of Pathology, University of Chicago, Chicago, Illinois.)

Clinical Features. Primary hyperparathyroidism is usually a disease of adults and is more frequent in women than in men (4:1). The most common manifestation is an increase in serum ionized calcium. In fact, primary hyperparathyroidism is the most common cause of clinically silent hypercalcemia. Other conditions may also produce hypercalcemia (Table 18.4). The most common cause of clinically apparent hypercalcemia in adults is cancer, in which it may be part of a paraneoplastic syndrome caused by secretion of PTH-like polypeptides (PTHrP) from tumor cells or may stem from osteolytic bone metastases (Chapter 6). Hypercalcemia in sarcoidosis results from increased synthesis of 1,25-dihydroxyvitamin D3 by macrophages. The prognosis for patients with malignancy-associated hypercalcemia is poor because it is typically associated with advanced cancers. In individuals with hypercalcemia caused by parathyroid hyperfunction, serum PTH is inappropriately elevated, whereas serum PTH is low to undetectable in those with hypercalcemia caused by nonparathyroid diseases, including malignancy. Other laboratory alterations referable to PTH excess include hypophosphatemia and increased urinary excretion of both calcium and phosphate.

Table 18.4 Causes of Hypercalcemia

Increased PTH	Decreased PTH

Hyperparathyroidism
   Primary (adenoma >
      hyperplasia)[a]
   Secondary[b]
   Tertiary[b]
Familial hypocalciuric
   hypercalcemia
	Hypercalcemia of malignancy
	   Osteolytic metastases
	   PTH-rP—mediated
	Vitamin D toxicity
	Immobilization
	Drugs (thiazide diuretics)
	Granulomatous diseases
	   (sarcoidosis)

PTH, Parathyroid hormone; *PTHrP,* PTH-related protein.

[a]Primary hyperparathyroidism is the most common cause of hypercalcemia overall.

[b]Secondary and tertiary hyperparathyroidism are most commonly associated with progressive renal failure.

The symptoms of primary hyperparathyroidism include pain secondary to urinary tract obstruction by stones, formerly a common presentation, and fractures of bones weakened by osteoporosis or osteitis fibrosa cystica. Additional signs and symptoms that may be encountered in some cases include the following:

- *Gastrointestinal disturbances,* including constipation, nausea, peptic ulcers, pancreatitis, and gallstones
- *Central nervous system alterations,* including depression, lethargy, and seizures
- *Neuromuscular abnormalities,* including weakness and hypotonia
- *Polyuria* and secondary polydipsia

Although some of these alterations (e.g., polyuria and muscle weakness) are clearly related to hypercalcemia, the pathophysiology of many of the other manifestations of the disorder remains poorly understood. Because serum calcium is now routinely screened in most patients, hyperparathyroidism is usually detected early in its course. Hence, many of the classic clinical manifestations, particularly those referable to bone and renal disease, are seen much less frequently.

Secondary Hyperparathyroidism

Secondary hyperparathyroidism is caused by chronic depression of serum calcium levels, usually as a result of renal failure, leading to compensatory overactivity of the parathyroids. The mechanisms by which chronic renal failure induces secondary hyperparathyroidism are complex and not fully understood. Chronic renal insufficiency is associated with decreased phosphate excretion, which in turn results in hyperphosphatemia. The elevated serum phosphate levels directly depress serum calcium levels. In addition, loss of renal α_1-hydroxylase activity, which is required for the synthesis of the active form of vitamin D, reduces the intestinal absorption of calcium (Chapter 7). These alterations cause chronic hypocalcemia, which stimulates the production of PTH from the parathyroid glands.

MORPHOLOGY

The parathyroid glands in secondary hyperparathyroidism are hyperplastic. As in primary hyperplasia, the degree of glandular enlargement is not necessarily symmetric. On microscopic examination, the hyperplastic glands contain an increased number of chief cells, or cells with more abundant, clear cytoplasm **(water-clear cells)**, in a diffuse or multinodular distribution. Fat cells are decreased in number. **Bone changes** similar to those seen in primary hyperparathyroidism may be present. **Metastatic calcification** may be seen in many tissues.

Clinical Features. The clinical manifestations of secondary hyperparathyroidism are usually dominated by those related to chronic renal failure. Bone abnormalities *(renal osteodystrophy)* and other changes associated with PTH excess are, in general, less severe than those seen in primary hyperparathyroidism. Free serum calcium remains near normal because of the compensatory increase in PTH levels, but the concomitant rise in phosphate levels promotes metastatic calcification. The metastatic calcification of blood vessels may occasionally result in significant ischemic damage to skin and other organs—a process referred to as *calciphylaxis.* In a minority of patients, parathyroid activity may become autonomous and excessive, with resultant hypercalcemia—a process sometimes termed *tertiary hyperparathyroidism.* Parathyroidectomy may be necessary to control hyperparathyroidism in such patients.

HYPOPARATHYROIDISM

Hypoparathyroidism is far less common than hyperparathyroidism. The major causes of hypoparathyroidism include the following:

- *Surgical ablation:* The most common cause is inadvertent removal of parathyroids during thyroidectomy or other surgical neck dissections.
- *Congenital absence:* This occurs in conjunction with thymic aplasia (Di George syndrome) and cardiac defects, secondary to deletions on chromosome 22q11.2 (Chapter 4).
- *Autoimmune hypoparathyroidism:* Parathyroids may be affected in the autoimmune polyglandular syndrome, which is caused by mutations in the autoimmune regulator *(AIRE)* gene and is discussed later, in the context of autoimmune adrenalitis.

The major clinical manifestations of hypoparathyroidism are secondary to hypocalcemia. Acute cases (as may occur after surgical ablation) manifest as increased neuromuscular irritability (e.g., tingling, muscle spasms, facial grimacing, and sustained carpopedal spasm or tetany), cardiac arrhythmias, and, on occasion, increased intracranial pressure and seizures. Manifestations of chronic hypoparathyroidism include cataracts, calcification of the cerebral basal ganglia, and dental abnormalities.

ENDOCRINE PANCREAS

The endocrine pancreas consists of the islets of Langerhans, which contain four major cell types.

- The *beta cell produces insulin,* which regulates glucose utilization in tissues and reduces blood glucose levels, as will be detailed in the discussion of diabetes.
- The *alpha cell secretes glucagon,* which raises glucose levels through its glycogenolytic activity in the liver.
- The *delta cell secretes somatostatin,* which suppresses both insulin and glucagon release.
- *PP cell secretes pancreatic polypeptide,* which exerts several gastrointestinal effects, such as stimulation of secretion of gastric and intestinal enzymes and inhibition of intestinal motility.

The most important disease of the endocrine pancreas is diabetes, caused by deficient production or action of insulin.

DIABETES

Diabetes is a group of metabolic disorders characterized by hyperglycemia. Hyperglycemia in diabetes is due to defects in insulin secretion, insulin action, or, most commonly, both. The chronic hyperglycemia and attendant metabolic abnormalities of diabetes often cause damage in multiple organ systems, especially the kidneys, eyes, nerves, and blood vessels. **In the United States, diabetes is the leading cause of end-stage renal disease, adult-onset blindness, and nontraumatic lower-extremity amputations.**

According to the American Diabetes Association, in 2019, over 37 million children and adults, or 11% of the population, in the United States, had diabetes, nearly one-fourth of whom were unaware that they had hyperglycemia. Approximately 1.4 million new cases of diabetes are diagnosed each year in the United States. The two major forms of the disease are type 1 diabetes (T1D, a minority of cases) and type 2 diabetes (T2D, the vast majority). Increasingly sedentary lifestyles and poor eating habits have contributed to increases in T2D and obesity in recent years in the United States and other parts of the world that have adopted a Western diet.

Diagnosis

Blood glucose is normally maintained in a narrow range, usually 70 to 120 mg/dL. According to the American Diabetes Association (ADA) and the World Health Organization (WHO), **diagnostic criteria for diabetes include the following:**

- A fasting plasma glucose ≥126 mg/dL or
- A random plasma glucose ≥200 mg/dL (in a patient with classic hyperglycemic signs, discussed later) or
- A 2-hour plasma glucose ≥200 mg/dL during an oral glucose tolerance test with a loading dose of 75 gm or
- A glycated hemoglobin (HbA1c) level ≥6.5% (glycated hemoglobin is further discussed under clinical features of diabetes)

All tests, except the random blood glucose test in a patient with classic hyperglycemic signs, must be repeated and confirmed on a separate day. Of note, many acute conditions associated with stress, such as severe infections, burns, or trauma, can lead to transient hyperglycemia due to secretion of hormones such as catecholamines and cortisol that oppose the effects of insulin. The diagnosis of diabetes thus requires persistent hyperglycemia following resolution of the acute illness.

Prediabetes, a state of dysglycemia that often precedes the development of T2D, is defined as:

- A fasting plasma glucose between 100 and 125 mg/dL ("impaired fasting glucose") or
- A 2-hour plasma glucose between 140 and 199 mg/dL during an oral glucose tolerance test or
- HbA1c level between 5.7% and 6.4%

As many as one-fourth of individuals with impaired glucose tolerance will develop overt T2D in the following 5 years. The risk is highest in those with obesity and a positive family history. In addition, individuals with prediabetes have an elevated risk of cardiovascular disease.

Classification

Although all forms of diabetes share hyperglycemia as a common feature, the underlying causes of hyperglycemia vary widely. Previous classification schemes of diabetes were based on age at onset of the disease or on the mode of therapy; by contrast, the current classification is based on pathogenesis (Table 18.5). Almost all cases of diabetes fall into one of two broad classes:

- *Type 1 diabetes (T1D)* is an autoimmune disease characterized by immunologically mediated destruction of pancreatic β cells and a resulting absolute deficiency of insulin. It accounts for 5% to 10% of cases of diabetes and is the most common type diagnosed in patients younger than 20 years of age. Previously, it was called insulin-dependent diabetes; however, that is no longer considered a distinguishing feature because type 2 diabetes may also require insulin treatment.
- *Type 2 diabetes (T2D)* is caused by a combination of peripheral resistance to insulin action and an inadequate secretory response by pancreatic β cells ("relative insulin deficiency"). Ninety to ninety-five percent of patients with diabetes have T2D, and many of them are overweight. This disease was previously called adult-onset diabetes; however, due to the increasing prevalence of T2D

in children and adolescents as obesity rates in this population increase, this term is no longer used.

The important similarities and differences between T1D and T2D are summarized in Table 18.6.

A variety of monogenic and secondary causes (see later) are responsible for the remaining cases. When combined, monogenic and secondary forms of diabetes account for more than 10% of diabetes (which together make them more common than type 1 diabetes). Although the major types of diabetes arise by different pathogenic mechanisms, the long-term complications in kidneys, eyes, nerves, and blood vessels are the same because they are all related to hyperglycemia, and these long-term effects are the principal causes of morbidity and death.

Table 18.5 Classification of Diabetes

Type 1 Diabetes (β-Cell Destruction, Usually Leading to Absolute Insulin Deficiency)
Immune-mediated
Idiopathic (autoantibody-negative)
Type 2 Diabetes (Combination of Insulin Resistance and β-Cell Dysfunction)
Other Types
Genetic Defects of β-Cell Function
Monogenic diabetes (maturity-onset diabetes of the young [MODY]) caused by mutations in various genes involved in β-cell development and function
Neonatal diabetes caused by mutations in genes involved in β-cell development and insulin production
Maternally inherited diabetes and deafness (MIDD) due to mitochondrial DNA mutations
Disorders of the Exocrine Pancreas ("Pancreatogenic" Diabetes)
Chronic pancreatitis
Pancreatectomy/trauma
Pancreatic cancer
Cystic fibrosis
Hemochromatosis
Fibrocalculous pancreatopathy
Endocrinopathies
Acromegaly
Cushing syndrome
Hyperthyroidism
Pheochromocytoma
Glucagonoma
Drugs
Glucocorticoids
Thyroid hormone
Interferon-α
Protease inhibitors
β-adrenergic agonists
Genetic Syndromes Associated With Diabetes
Down syndrome
Klinefelter syndrome
Turner syndrome
Gestational Diabetes Mellitus

Modified from American Diabetes Association: Diagnosis and classification of diabetes mellitus, *Diabetes Care* 37(Suppl 1):S81–S90, 2014.

Table 18.6 Features of Type 1 and Type 2 Diabetes

Type 1 Diabetes	Type 2 Diabetes
Clinical	
Onset usually in childhood and adolescence	Onset usually in adulthood; increasing incidence in childhood and adolescence
Nonobese, may lose weight preceding diagnosis	Obese (80%)
Progressive decrease in insulin levels	Increased blood insulin (early); normal or moderate decrease in insulin late
Circulating islet autoantibodies	No islet autoantibodies
Diabetic ketoacidosis in absence of insulin therapy	Nonketotic hyperosmolar coma
Genetics	
Major linkage to MHC class I and II genes; also linked to polymorphisms in CTLA4 and PTPN22	No HLA linkage; linkage to candidate diabetogenic and obesity-related genes
Pathogenesis	
Breakdown in self-tolerance to islet antigens	Insulin resistance in peripheral tissues, inadequate insulin secretion by β cells
	Multiple obesity-associated factors (circulating nonesterified fatty acids, inflammatory mediators, adipocytokines) linked to insulin resistance
Pathology	
Autoimmune "insulitis"	Amyloid deposition in islets (late)
β-cell depletion, islet atrophy	Mild β-cell depletion

HLA, Human leukocyte antigen; *MHC,* major histocompatibility complex.

Pathogenesis of Diabetes

Normal Insulin Physiology and Glucose Homeostasis

Before discussing the pathogenesis of the two major types of diabetes, we briefly review normal insulin physiology and glucose metabolism.

Normal glucose homeostasis is tightly regulated by three interrelated processes: (1) glucose production in the liver; (2) glucose uptake and utilization by peripheral tissues, chiefly skeletal muscle; and (3) the actions of insulin and counterregulatory hormones (especially glucagon).

The principal function of insulin is to increase the rate of glucose transport into certain cells in the body (Fig. 18.18). Following a meal, when blood glucose levels increase, insulin levels rise and glucagon levels decrease. Insulin promotes glucose uptake and utilization mainly into striated (skeletal) muscle. In muscle cells, glucose is either stored as glycogen or oxidized to generate adenosine triphosphate (ATP) and metabolic intermediates needed for cell growth. Insulin also promotes amino acid uptake and protein synthesis while inhibiting protein degradation. Thus, the metabolic effects of insulin are anabolic, with increased synthesis and reduced degradation of glycogen, lipid, and protein. In addition to these metabolic effects, insulin has several mitogenic functions, including initiation of DNA synthesis in certain cells and stimulation of their growth and

differentiation. Although less dependent on insulin, brain and adipose tissues also extract a significant amount of glucose from the circulation. In adipose tissue, glucose is metabolized to lipids, which are stored as fat. In addition to promoting lipid synthesis (lipogenesis), insulin also inhibits lipid degradation (lipolysis) in adipocytes.

Insulin reduces the production of glucose from the liver. Insulin and glucagon have opposing regulatory effects on glucose homeostasis. During fasting states, low insulin and high glucagon levels facilitate hepatic gluconeogenesis and glycogenolysis (glycogen breakdown) while decreasing glycogen synthesis, thereby preventing hypoglycemia. Thus, fasting plasma glucose levels are determined primarily by hepatic glucose output.

The most important stimulus that triggers insulin release from pancreatic β cells is glucose. Oral intake of food increases blood glucose, which is taken up into β cells and metabolized to generate ATP. There is a concomitant increase in intracellular calcium, which stimulates the release of insulin from β-cell granules and the synthesis of insulin. Food intake also leads to secretion of multiple hormones, notably the *incretins* produced by cells in the intestines. These hormones stimulate insulin secretion from pancreatic β cells, and also reduce glucagon secretion and delay gastric emptying, which promotes satiety. The incretin effect is significantly blunted in patients with T2D; restoring incretin function can lead to improved glycemic control and weight loss (by restoring satiety). These observations have resulted in the development of new classes of drugs for patients with T2D that mimic incretins or enhance the levels of endogenous incretins by delaying their degradation.

In peripheral tissues (skeletal muscle and adipose tissue), secreted insulin binds to the *insulin receptor,* triggering a number of intracellular responses that promote glucose uptake and postprandial glucose utilization, thereby maintaining glucose homeostasis. Abnormalities at various points along this complex signaling cascade, from synthesis

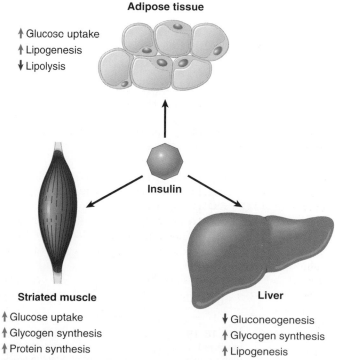

Adipose tissue

↑ Glucose uptake
↑ Lipogenesis
↓ Lipolysis

Insulin

Striated muscle

↑ Glucose uptake
↑ Glycogen synthesis
↑ Protein synthesis

Liver

↓ Gluconeogenesis
↑ Glycogen synthesis
↑ Lipogenesis

FIG. 18.18 Metabolic actions of insulin in striated muscle, adipose tissue, and liver.

and release of insulin by β cells to insulin receptor interactions in peripheral tissues, can result in the diabetic phenotype.

Pathogenesis of Type 1 Diabetes. **Type 1 diabetes is an autoimmune disease in which islet destruction is caused primarily by immune effector cells reacting against β-cell antigens.** Although the clinical onset of T1D is abrupt, the autoimmune attack on β cells usually starts years before the disease becomes evident (Fig. 18.19). The classic manifestations of the disease occur late in its course, after more than 90% of the β cells have been destroyed.

As with all autoimmune diseases, the pathogenesis of T1D involves genetic susceptibility and environmental factors. Genome-wide association studies have identified over 20 susceptibility loci for T1D. Of these, the strongest association is with class II MHC (HLA-DR) genes. Between 90% and 95% of Americans of European descent with T1D have HLA-DR3, or DR4, or both, in contrast with about 40% of unaffected subjects; 40% to 50% of patients are DR3/DR4 heterozygotes, in contrast with 5% of unaffected individuals. Of note, however, most people who inherit these HLA alleles do not develop diabetes, indicating that while these genes may predispose to the disease, they do not cause it. Several non-HLA alleles also increase susceptibility to T1D, including polymorphisms within the gene encoding insulin itself, as well as *CTLA4* and *PTPN22*. As discussed in Chapter 5, CTLA-4 is an inhibitory receptor of T cells and PTPN-22 is a protein tyrosine phosphatase; both are thought to inhibit T-cell responses. Therefore, polymorphisms that diminish their functional activity are expected to promote excessive T-cell activation. T1D-associated polymorphisms in the insulin gene may reduce its expression in the thymus, leading to a failure to eliminate developing T cells specific for this self protein (Chapter 5).

Environmental factors, especially infections, such as coxsackievirus infection of the pancreas, have also been implicated in T1D, as have changes in the microbiome, but their role in the development of T1D is unclear. Some infections may also protect from the disease, by as yet undefined mechanisms.

The fundamental immune abnormality in type 1 diabetes is a failure of self-tolerance in T cells specific for β-cell antigens. This failure of tolerance may result from some combination of defective deletion of self-reactive T cells in the thymus and abnormalities of regulatory T cells that normally dampen effector T-cell responses (Chapter 5). The destruction of islet cells is mediated primarily by T cells reacting against islet antigens (type IV hypersensitivity, Chapter 5). In the rare cases in which the pancreatic lesions have been examined early in the disease process, the islets show necrosis of β cells and lymphocytic infiltration (so-called "insulitis," described later). Although autoantibodies against a variety of β-cell antigens, including insulin and the β-cell enzyme glutamic acid decarboxylase, are detected in the blood of 70% to 80% of patients, even prior to disease onset, it is not clear if these antibodies contribute to β-cell destruction.

Pathogenesis of Type 2 Diabetes. Type 2 diabetes is a complex disease that involves interactions of genetic and environmental factors. Unlike T1D, it is not an autoimmune disease. **The two defects that characterize T2D are: (1) a decreased ability of peripheral tissues to respond to insulin (insulin resistance) and (2) β-cell dysfunction that is manifested as inadequate insulin secretion in the presence of insulin resistance and hyperglycemia** (Fig. 18.20). Environmental factors, such as a sedentary lifestyle and dietary habits, unequivocally play a role (see below). Genetic factors are also involved, as evidenced by a concordance rate of 80% to 90% in monozygotic twins, which is greater than that for type 1 diabetes (approximately 50% concordance rates in twins). Additional evidence for a genetic basis has emerged from recent large-scale genome-wide association studies, which have identified dozens of susceptibility loci called *diabetogenic genes*. It is not clearly established how these genes contribute to diabetes. Unlike T1D, however, the disease is not linked to genes involved in immune tolerance and regulation (e.g., *HLA, CTLA4*).

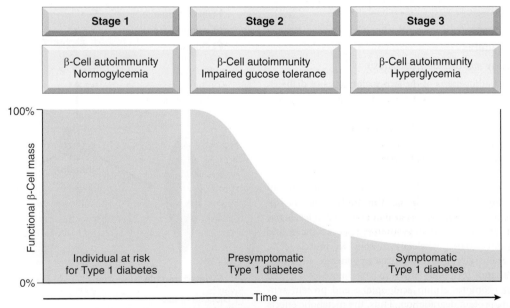

FIG. 18.19 Stages in the development of type 1 diabetes. The hypothetical β-cell mass is plotted against age. In stage 1, β-cell autoimmunity is evidenced by the presence of two or more antiislet autoantibodies. (Modified with permission from Insel RA, et al: Staging presymptomatic type 1 diabetes. *Diabetes Care* 38:1864–1974, 2015.)

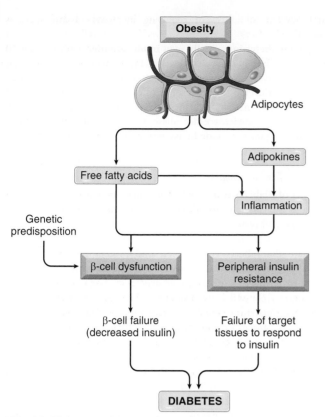

FIG. 18.20 Development of type 2 diabetes. Insulin resistance associated with obesity and β-cell failure together result in diabetes. *FFAs,* Free fatty acids. (Modified from Kasuga M: Insulin resistance and pancreatic β-cell failure. *J Clin Invest* 116:1756, 2006.)

Insulin Resistance

Insulin resistance is defined as the failure of target tissues to respond normally to insulin. The liver, skeletal muscle, and adipose tissue are the major tissues where insulin resistance contributes to hyperglycemia, as follows:

- Failure to inhibit endogenous glucose production (gluconeogenesis) in the liver, which leads to high fasting blood glucose levels
- Abnormally low glucose uptake and glycogen synthesis in skeletal muscle following a meal, which results in a high postprandial blood glucose level
- Failure to inhibit hormone-sensitive lipase in adipose tissue, leading to excess circulating free fatty acids (FFAs), which, as will be discussed, exacerbates the state of insulin resistance

β-Cell Dysfunction

β-cell dysfunction is an essential component in the development of overt diabetes. β-cell function increases early in the disease process in most patients with T2D, mainly as a compensatory measure to counter insulin resistance and maintain euglycemia. Eventually, however, β cells are unable to cope with the long-term demands of peripheral insulin resistance, resulting in a state of relative insulin deficiency.

Several mechanisms have been implicated in causing β-cell dysfunction in T2D, including the following:

- Polymorphisms in genes that control insulin secretion are associated with an increased lifetime risk for T2D.
- Excess free fatty acids compromise β-cell function and attenuate insulin release (*lipotoxicity*)

- Chronic hyperglycemia (*glucotoxicity*)
- Abnormal *incretin effect,* leading to reduced secretion of hormones that promote insulin release (discussed earlier)
- Amyloid replacement of islets, present in more than 90% of diabetic islets (described later). It is unclear if the amyloid actually causes β-cell loss.

Obesity

The most important factor in the development of insulin resistance is obesity. The association of obesity with T2D has been recognized for decades. Central obesity (abdominal fat) is more likely to be associated with insulin resistance than is peripheral (gluteal/subcutaneous) obesity. Insulin resistance is present even with simple obesity unaccompanied by hyperglycemia, indicating a fundamental abnormality of insulin signaling in states of fat excess. The term *metabolic syndrome* has been applied to a constellation of findings dominated by visceral obesity accompanied by insulin resistance, glucose intolerance, and cardiovascular risk factors such as hypertension and abnormal lipid profiles. Individuals with metabolic syndrome are at high risk for the development of T2D.

Obesity can have an adverse impact on insulin sensitivity in numerous ways (see Fig. 18.20):

- *Free fatty acids (FFAs).* Cross-sectional studies have demonstrated an inverse correlation between fasting plasma FFAs and insulin sensitivity. The level of intracellular triglycerides is often markedly increased in muscle and liver in individuals who are obese, presumably because excess circulating FFAs are taken up into these organs. Central adipose tissue is more "lipolytic" than peripheral adipose tissue, which might explain the particularly deleterious consequences of the central pattern of fat distribution. Intracellular triglycerides and products of fatty acid metabolism inhibit insulin signaling and result in an acquired state of insulin resistance.
- *Adipokines.* Adipose tissue is not merely a passive storage depot for fat; it is also an endocrine organ that releases soluble mediators in response to changes in metabolic state. A variety of proteins secreted into the systemic circulation by adipose tissue have been identified that are known collectively as *adipokines* (or *adipose cytokines*). Some of these cause insulin resistance and others (such as leptin and adiponectin) decrease blood glucose, in part by increasing the insulin sensitivity of peripheral tissues (Chapter 7). Adiponectin levels are decreased in obesity, which contributes to insulin resistance.

Inflammation

Over the past several years, inflammation has emerged as an important contributor to the pathogenesis of T2D. It is now known that a permissive inflammatory milieu (mediated by proinflammatory cytokines that are secreted in response to excess nutrients such as FFAs) results in both peripheral insulin resistance and β-cell dysfunction (discussed later). Excess FFAs within macrophages and β cells can activate the inflammasome, a multiprotein cytoplasmic complex that leads to secretion of the cytokine interleukin-1 (IL-1, Chapter 5). IL-1 stimulates the secretion of additional proinflammatory cytokines from macrophages and other cells, and IL-1 as well as other cytokines promote insulin resistance in peripheral tissues and may inhibit the function of β cells.

Monogenic Forms of Diabetes

Monogenic forms of diabetes (see Table 18.5) are uncommon and are the result of loss-of-function mutations in a single gene. Monogenic diabetes can be classified based on age of onset into *congenital early onset diabetes* (manifesting in neonates) and *maturity onset diabetes of the young* (MODY), which develops beyond the neonatal period but usually before 25 years of age. Some of the causes of congenital diabetes include mutations of the insulin gene itself and mutations in mitochondrial DNA that lead to a syndrome of maternally inherited diabetes and bilateral deafness. Rare loss-of-function insulin receptor mutations can cause severe insulin resistance, accompanied by hyperinsulinemia (due to lack of feedback inhibition) and congenital diabetes. By contrast, MODY is caused by mutations in genes encoding proteins involved in β-cell development and function and resembles T2D in many of its clinical features. Hence, the diagnosis of MODY is often missed, and the underlying pathogenic mutation is not identified.

Other Subtypes of Diabetes

In addition to types 1 and 2 and monogenic forms of diabetes, there are other uncommon subtypes of diabetes. Secondary diabetes associated with various endocrinopathies (e.g., Cushing syndrome or growth hormone excess) is described in relevant portions of this chapter. Here, we will briefly discuss pregnancy-associated (gestational) diabetes and diabetes arising as a result of a variety of chronic exocrine pancreatic diseases (pancreatogenic diabetes).

- *Gestational diabetes.* Approximately 5% of pregnancies occurring in the United States are complicated by hyperglycemia. Pregnancy is a diabetogenic state in which the prevailing hormonal milieu favors insulin resistance. In some euglycemic women who are pregnant, this can give rise to gestational diabetes. Women with pregestational diabetes (where hyperglycemia is already present in the periconception period) have an increased risk for stillbirth and congenital malformations in the fetus (Chapter 4). Therefore, tight glycemic control is necessary early in pregnancy to prevent congenital defects, and through the later trimesters of pregnancy to prevent fetal overgrowth (macrosomia). The latter occurs because maternal hyperglycemia can induce compensatory secretion of insulin-like growth factors in the fetus. Most pregnant women who develop gestational diabetes require insulin for glycemic control. Gestational diabetes typically resolves following delivery; however, there is an elevated risk for developing outright diabetes within the next 10 years, which is highest in the first 5 years after pregnancy. Subsequently, the risk of diabetes reverts to baseline.
- *Pancreatogenic diabetes* is hyperglycemia occurring due to damage to the exocrine pancreas that encroaches upon and injures islets (see Table 18.5). The underlying causes include cystic fibrosis, chronic pancreatitis, and pancreatic adenocarcinoma. Approximately 1% of new-onset diabetes in older adults is actually a manifestation of an occult pancreatic adenocarcinoma (Chapter 15).

Clinical Features of Diabetes

It is difficult to discuss with brevity the diverse clinical presentations of diabetes. We will describe the affected populations for each of the two major subtypes, followed by a discussion of the acute and chronic complications and clinical manifestations.

Type 1 diabetes may arise at any age, most often in childhood or young adulthood. In the initial 1 to 2 years after onset of overt T1D, the requirement for insulin administration may be minimal because residual β-cells produce adequate insulin. Eventually, the β-cell reserve is exhausted and exogenous insulin becomes essential to control hyperglycemia. Although β-cell destruction is a gradual process, the transition from impaired glucose tolerance to overt diabetes may be abrupt, incited by an event requiring increased insulin such as infection.

Type 2 diabetes is typically seen in obese patients older than 40 years of age, but it may also develop in younger adults and even children, especially if they are obese. It should, however, be noted that T2D can develop in the absence of overt obesity; it is estimated that 10% of patients in high-income countries and even more in lower-income countries are not obese, based on body mass indices. Often, the diagnosis is made in asymptomatic individuals by routine blood tests.

The Classic Triad of Diabetes

The onset of diabetes is marked by polyuria, polydipsia, polyphagia (known as the classic triad of diabetes), and, in severe cases of T1D, ketoacidosis, all resulting from metabolic derangements (Fig. 18.21). Since insulin is an anabolic hormone, its deficiency results in a catabolic state that affects glucose, fat, and protein metabolism. The assimilation of glucose into muscle and adipose tissue is sharply diminished. Storage of glycogen in liver and muscle decreases, and reserves are depleted by glycogenolysis. The resultant *hyperglycemia* exceeds the renal threshold for reabsorption, and glycosuria ensues. The glycosuria induces osmotic diuresis and thus *polyuria*, causing the loss of water and electrolytes. Renal water loss combined with hyperosmolarity due to increased levels of glucose in the blood depletes intracellular water, triggering osmoreceptors in the brain and producing intense thirst *(polydipsia)*. Insulin deficiency leads to the catabolism of proteins and fats. Gluconeogenic amino acids produced by proteolysis are taken up by the liver and used as building blocks for glucose. The catabolism of proteins and fats induces a negative energy balance, which in turn leads to increased appetite *(polyphagia)*, thus completing the classic triad. Despite the increased appetite, catabolic effects dominate, resulting in weight loss and muscle weakness. The combination of polyphagia and weight loss is paradoxical and should always raise the possibility of diabetes.

Acute Metabolic Complications of Diabetes

Diabetic ketoacidosis is a severe acute metabolic complication of diabetes, usually T1D. It is caused by severe hyperglycemia (plasma glucose in the range of 500 to 700 mg/dL) in the setting of insulin deficiency, usually due to the patient not taking insulin. It may also be triggered by stresses such as significant deviations from normal dietary intake, unusual physical activity, or infection. These cause the release of the catecholamine epinephrine, which exacerbates functional insulin deficiency by blocking insulin action and stimulating the secretion of the counterregulatory hormone glucagon. The consequent hyperglycemia causes an osmotic diuresis and dehydration. Insulin deficiency also leads to activation of hormone-sensitive lipase, which leads to excessive breakdown of adipose stores and increased FFAs. These FFAs are oxidized by the liver to produce ketones. In times of starvation, ketogenesis is an adaptive phenomenon that generates an energy source for vital organs (e.g., the brain). The rate at which ketones are formed may exceed the rate at which they can be used by peripheral tissues, leading to ketonemia and ketonuria. The accumulating ketones decrease blood pH, resulting in metabolic acidosis. This is exacerbated if the urinary excretion of ketones is compromised by dehydration.

The clinical manifestations of diabetic ketoacidosis include fatigue, nausea and vomiting, severe abdominal pain, a characteristic fruity odor, and deep, labored breathing (also known as *Kussmaul breathing*). Persistence of the ketotic state eventually leads to depressed consciousness and coma. Reversal of ketoacidosis requires

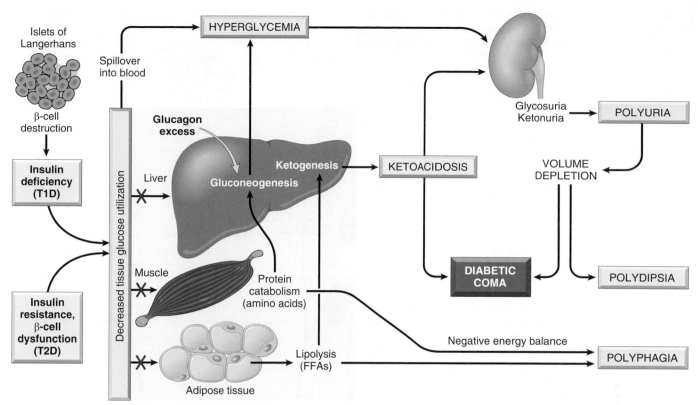

FIG. 18.21 Sequence of metabolic derangements leading to clinical manifestations of type 1 diabetes. An absolute insulin deficiency leads to a catabolic state, eventuating in ketoacidosis and severe volume depletion. These derangements bring about sufficient central nervous system compromise to cause coma and, eventually, death if left untreated. *FFAs*, Free fatty acids.

administration of insulin, correction of metabolic acidosis, and treatment of any underlying precipitating factors, such as infection.

Hyperosmolar hyperglycemic nonketotic syndrome is a dangerous condition resulting from very high blood glucose levels. It can affect both types of diabetics, but it usually occurs amongst people with T2D. There is severe dehydration resulting from sustained osmotic diuresis. Typically, it develops in older adult diabetics who are unable to maintain adequate water intake due to stroke or infections. Untreated patients develop coma. The hyperglycemia is usually very severe with blood glucose ranging from 600 to 1200 mg/dL.

In patients being treated with insulin, the most common acute complication is hypoglycemia. Causes include missing a meal, excessive physical exertion, excessive insulin administration, or inappropriate dosing when antidiabetic agents such as sulfonylureas are incorporated into the treatment plan. The signs and symptoms of hypoglycemia include dizziness, confusion, sweating, palpitations, and tachycardia; if hypoglycemia persists, loss of consciousness may occur. Rapid reversal of hypoglycemia through oral or intravenous glucose intake is critical to prevent permanent neurologic damage.

Chronic Complications of Diabetes

Morbidity associated with long-standing diabetes of any type results mainly from the chronic complications of hyperglycemia and the resulting damage of large- and medium-sized muscular arteries (diabetic macrovascular disease) and small vessels (diabetic microvascular disease). Macrovascular disease causes accelerated atherosclerosis, resulting in increased myocardial infarction, stroke, and lower-extremity ischemia. The effects of microvascular disease are most profound in the retina, kidneys, and peripheral nerves, resulting in diabetic retinopathy, nephropathy, and neuropathy, respectively (Fig. 18.22). There is much variability between patients in the time of onset of these complications, their severity, and the particular organs involved. Tight control of hyperglycemia may delay or prevent their onset.

Pathogenesis. **Persistent hyperglycemia (glucotoxicity) seems to be responsible for the long-term complications of diabetes.** Persistent hyperglycemia has deleterious effects on multiple tissues, by several mechanisms.

- *Advanced glycation end products (AGEs).* AGEs are formed as a result of nonenzymatic reactions between intracellular glucose-derived precursors (e.g., glyoxal, methylglyoxal, and 3-deoxyglucosone) and the amino groups of proteins. The rate of AGE formation is accelerated by hyperglycemia. AGEs bind to a specific receptor (RAGE), which is expressed on inflammatory cells (macrophages and T cells), endothelium, and vascular smooth muscle. The detrimental effects of AGE signaling within the vascular compartment include the following:
  - Release of *cytokines and growth factors*, including transforming growth factor-β (TGF-β), which leads to deposition of excess basement membrane material, and vascular endothelial growth factor (VEGF), implicated in diabetic retinopathy.
  - Generation of *reactive oxygen species (ROS)* in endothelial cells
  - Increased *procoagulant activity* of endothelial cells and macrophages

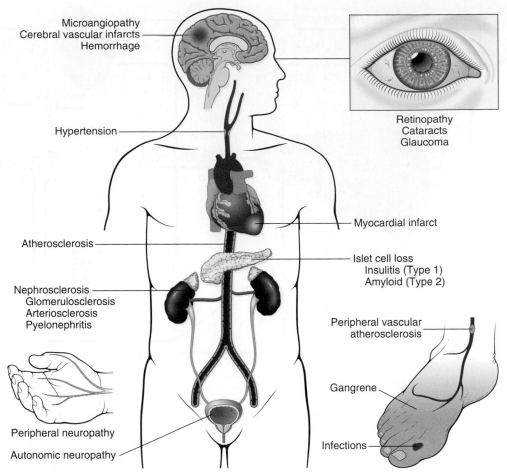

FIG. 18.22 Long-term complications of diabetes.

- Enhanced *proliferation of vascular smooth muscle cells and synthesis of extracellular matrix*

  In addition to receptor-mediated effects, AGEs can directly cross-link extracellular matrix proteins. These cross-linked proteins can trap other plasma or interstitial proteins; for example, low-density lipoprotein (LDL) gets trapped within AGE-modified large-vessel walls, accelerating atherosclerosis (Chapter 8), while albumin can be trapped within capillary walls, accounting in part for the basement membrane thickening that is characteristic of diabetic microangiopathy (discussed later). All these effects contribute to the vascular lesions associated with diabetes.

- *Activation of protein kinase C.* Activation of protein kinase C (PKC) by calcium ions and the second messenger diacylglycerol (DAG) is an important signal transduction pathway. Intracellular hyperglycemia can stimulate the de novo synthesis of DAG from glycolytic intermediates and hence cause activation of PKC. The downstream effects of PKC activation are numerous and include production of proangiogenic molecules such as VEGF, implicated in the neovascularization seen in diabetic retinopathy, and profibrogenic molecules such as TGF-β, leading to increased deposition of extracellular matrix and basement membrane material.

- *Disturbances in metabolic pathways.* In some tissues that do not require insulin for glucose transport (e.g., nerves, lens, kidneys, blood vessels), hyperglycemia leads to an increase in intracellular glucose that is then metabolized by the enzyme aldose reductase to sorbitol, a polyol, and eventually to fructose, in a reaction that uses NADPH (the reduced form of nicotinamide dinucleotide phosphate) as a cofactor. NADPH is also required by the enzyme glutathione reductase in a reaction that regenerates reduced glutathione (GSH). As described in Chapter 1, GSH is one of the important antioxidant mechanisms in the cell, and reductions in GSH increase cellular susceptibility to *oxidative stress*. In the face of sustained hyperglycemia, progressive depletion of intracellular NADPH compromises GSH regeneration, increasing oxidative stress.

MORPHOLOGY

The most important morphologic changes are related to the many chronic complications of diabetes. These changes are seen in both T1D and T2D.

Pancreas

Lesions in the pancreas are variable. One or more of the following alterations may be present:

- **Reduction in the number and size of islets.** This change is most often seen in T1D, particularly in rapidly advancing disease. Most of the islets are small, inconspicuous, and hard to detect.
- **Leukocytic infiltrates in the islets (insulitis) are seen in T1D** and are composed principally of T lymphocytes (Fig. 18.23A).
- **Amyloid deposition within islets is seen in T2D.** It begins in and around capillaries and between cells. At advanced stages, the islets may be virtually obliterated (Fig. 18.23B); fibrosis may also be observed.

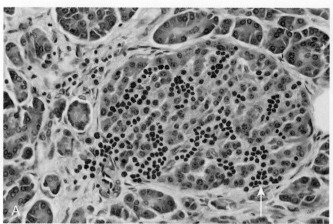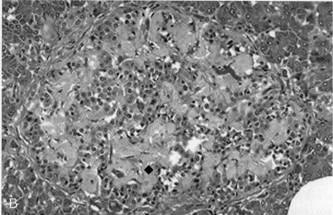

FIG. 18.23 Morphologic alterations in the islets in diabetes. (A) Autoimmune insulitis in type 1 diabetes. The *arrow* points to inflammation surrounding islet of Langerhans, while the surrounding acinar structures are normal. (B) Amyloid in islets in type 2 diabetes. This islet contains deposits of pink hyaline *(diamond)* material (amyloid) around many of the islet cells. (From Klatt EC: *Robbins and Cotran Atlas of Pathology*, ed 4, Figs. 9.18, 9.19, Philadelphia, 2021, Elsevier.)

- An increase in the number and size of islets, especially in the nondiabetic newborns of mothers with diabetes. Presumably, fetal islets undergo hyperplasia in response to the maternal hyperglycemia.

Diabetic Macrovascular Disease

The hallmark of diabetic macrovascular disease is **accelerated atherosclerosis** affecting the aorta and large- and medium-sized arteries. Except for its greater severity and earlier onset, atherosclerosis in patients with and without diabetes is indistinguishable (Chapter 8). **Myocardial infarction, caused by atherosclerosis of the coronary arteries, is the most common cause of death in patients with diabetes.** It is almost as common in women as in men. By contrast, myocardial infarction is infrequent in nondiabetic women of reproductive age. **Gangrene of the lower extremities,** as a result of advanced vascular disease, is about 100 times more common in individuals with diabetes than in the general population. The larger renal arteries are also subject to severe atherosclerosis, but the most damaging effect of diabetes on the kidneys is on the glomeruli and the microcirculation, as discussed later.

Hyaline arteriolosclerosis, the vascular lesion associated with hypertension (Chapters 8 and 12), is both more prevalent and more severe in patients with diabetes than in unaffected individuals, but it is not specific for diabetes and may be seen in older adults without diabetes or hypertension. It is characterized by an amorphous, hyaline thickening of the wall of the arterioles that narrows the lumen (Fig. 18.24). In patients with diabetes, its severity is related to the duration of the disease and the presence or absence of hypertension.

Diabetic Microangiopathy

One of the most consistent morphologic features of diabetes is **diffuse thickening of basement membranes.** The thickening is most evident in the capillaries of the skin, skeletal muscle, retina, renal glomeruli, and renal medulla. However, it may also be seen in nonvascular structures such as renal tubules (Fig. 18.25), the Bowman capsule, peripheral nerves, and placenta. By light and electron microscopy, the basal lamina separating parenchymal or endothelial cells from the surrounding tissue is markedly thickened by concentric layers of hyaline material composed predominantly of type IV collagen. Despite the increase in the thickness of basement membranes, diabetic capillaries are leaky, leading to extravasation of plasma proteins. **The microangiopathy underlies the development of diabetic**

nephropathy, retinopathy, and some forms of neuropathy. A similar microangiopathy can be found in elderly nondiabetic patients, but it is rarely as severe as that seen in individuals with long-standing diabetes.

Diabetic Nephropathy

The kidneys are prime targets of diabetes (see also Chapter 12). The lesions include (1) glomerular lesions; (2) renal vascular lesions, principally arteriolosclerosis; and (3) pyelonephritis, including necrotizing papillitis.

The most important **glomerular lesions** are capillary basement membrane thickening, diffuse mesangial sclerosis, and nodular glomerulosclerosis. The glomerular capillary basement membranes are thickened along their entire length. This change can be detected by electron microscopy within a few years of the onset of diabetes, sometimes preceding any change in renal function (Fig. 18.26).

Diffuse mesangial sclerosis refers to an increase in mesangial matrix associated with mesangial cell proliferation and basement membrane

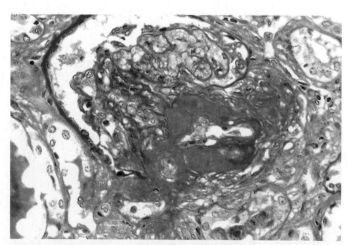

FIG. 18.24 Severe renal hyaline arteriolosclerosis in a periodic acid–Schiff stained specimen. Note the markedly thickened, tortuous afferent arteriole. The amorphous nature of the thickened vascular wall is evident. (Courtesy of Dr. M.A. Venkatachalam, Department of Pathology, University of Texas Health Science Center, San Antonio, Texas.)

thickening. It is found in most individuals with disease of more than 10 years' duration and is more common in older patients and those with hypertension. When glomerulosclerosis is severe, patients develop the nephrotic syndrome, characterized by proteinuria, hypoalbuminemia, and edema (Chapter 12).

Nodular glomerulosclerosis (Kimmelstiel-Wilson lesion) is a distinctive glomerular lesion characterized by ball-like deposits of a laminated matrix in the periphery of the glomerulus (Fig. 18.27). It is encountered in approximately 15% to 30% of individuals with long-term diabetes and is a major contributor to renal dysfunction. In contrast to diffuse mesangial sclerosis, the nodular form of glomerulosclerosis is virtually pathognomonic of diabetes.

Renal atherosclerosis and arteriolosclerosis constitute part of the macrovascular disease seen in diabetics. The kidney is one of the most frequently and severely affected organs; the changes in the arteries and arterioles are similar to those found throughout the body. Hyaline arteriolosclerosis affects not only the afferent but also the efferent arterioles; the latter is virtually unique to individuals with diabetes. The vascular compromise and glomerulosclerosis induce sufficient ischemia to cause diffuse scarring of the kidneys, manifested by a finely granular cortical surface (nephrosclerosis) (Fig. 18.28).

Pyelonephritis is an acute or chronic inflammation of the kidneys that usually begins in the interstitial tissue and then spreads to involve the tubules. Both the acute and chronic forms of this disease occur in nondiabetics as well as in patients with diabetes but are more severe in the latter population. One special pattern of acute pyelonephritis, **necrotizing papillitis** (or papillary necrosis, Chapter 12), is much more prevalent in patients with diabetes than in nondiabetics.

Ocular Complications of Diabetes

Visual impairment, sometimes even total blindness, is one of the most feared consequences of long-standing diabetes. Diabetic retinopathy is discussed in Chapter 21, in the section on diseases of the eye.

Diabetic Neuropathy

The most frequent nervous system lesion caused by diabetes is a peripheral, symmetric neuropathy of the lower extremities affecting motor and sensory function, particularly the latter (Chapter 20). The neurologic changes may be the result of microangiopathy and increased permeability of the capillaries that supply the nerves, as well as direct axonal damage.

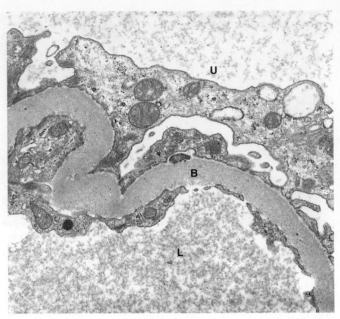

FIG. 18.26 Diabetic nephropathy showing markedly thickened glomerular basement membrane. *B,* Glomerular basement membrane; *L,* glomerular capillary lumen; *U,* urinary space. (Courtesy of Dr. Michael Kashgarian, Department of Pathology, Yale University School of Medicine, New Haven, Connecticut.)

Clinical Features of Chronic Diabetes

As the previous discussion has emphasized, T1D and T2D are distinct pathophysiologic entities with the common manifestation of hyperglycemia. Table 18.6 summarizes some of the clinical, genetic, and histopathologic features that distinguish the two diseases. Nonetheless, as previously stated, the long-term sequelae of both types, arising as a result of uncontrolled or poorly controlled hyperglycemia, are similar and are responsible for much of the morbidity and mortality in patients with diabetes. In most instances, these complications occur approximately 15 to 20 years after the onset of hyperglycemia. The major chronic complications of the disease are described next.

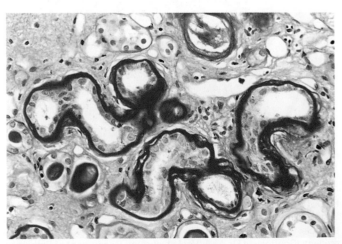

FIG. 18.25 Thickening of tubular basement membranes in the kidney from a patient with diabetes (periodic acid–Schiff stain).

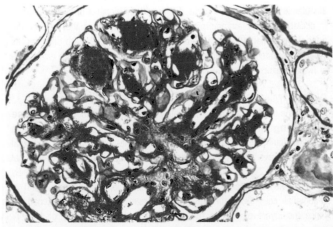

FIG. 18.27 Diabetic nephropathy. Nodular glomerulosclerosis in a renal specimen (PAS stain) from a patient with long-standing diabetes. (Courtesy of Dr. Lisa Yerian, Department of Pathology, University of Chicago, Chicago, Illinois.)

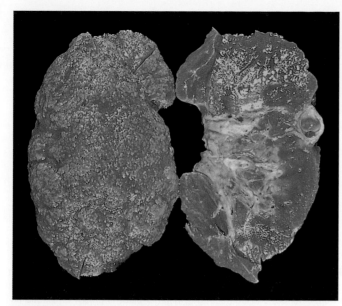

FIG. 18.28 Nephrosclerosis in a patient with long-standing diabetes. The bisected kidney demonstrates diffuse granular transformation of the surface *(left)* and marked thinning of the cortex *(right)*. Additional features include some irregular depressions, the result of pyelonephritis, and an incidental cortical cyst *(far right)*.

- *Macrovascular complications*, such as myocardial infarction, renal vascular insufficiency, and cerebrovascular accidents, are the most common causes of mortality in long-standing diabetes. Patients with diabetes have a two to four times greater incidence of coronary artery disease, and a fourfold higher risk of death from cardiovascular complications, than nondiabetics. Diabetes is often accompanied by underlying conditions that favor the development of adverse cardiovascular events, including hypertension and dyslipidemia (see earlier discussion on metabolic syndrome).
- *Diabetic nephropathy* is a leading cause of end-stage renal disease in the United States, and renal failure is second only to myocardial infarction as a cause of death in affected patients. The earliest manifestation of diabetic nephropathy is the appearance of small amounts of albumin in the urine (>30 mg but <3.5 g/day). Without treatment, approximately 80% of patients with T1D and 20% to 40% of those with T2D will develop overt nephrotic syndrome (protein excretion of >3.5 g/day; Chapter 12) over 10 to 15 years, usually accompanied by hypertension. The progression from overt nephropathy to end-stage renal disease is variable and is evidenced by a progressive drop in glomerular filtration rate. By 20 years after diagnosis, more than 75% of individuals with T1D and about 20% of those with T2D with overt nephropathy will develop end-stage renal disease, which requires dialysis or renal transplantation.
- *Visual impairment* is one of the most feared consequences of long-standing diabetes. Diabetes is the leading cause of acquired blindness in adults in the United States. Approximately 60% to 80% of patients develop some form of diabetic retinopathy within 15 to 20 years after diagnosis. Because the fundamental lesion of retinopathy—neovascularization—is attributable to hypoxia-induced overexpression of VEGF in the retina, current treatment includes intravitreous injection of antiangiogenic agents (Chapter 21).

- *Diabetic neuropathy* can produce a variety of clinical syndromes affecting the central nervous system, peripheral sensorimotor nerves, and autonomic nervous system. The characteristic polyneuropathy usually affects the lower extremities initially, but, over time, the upper extremities may be involved as well. Other forms include autonomic neuropathy, which produces disturbances in bowel and bladder function and sometimes sexual impotence, and diabetic mononeuropathy, which may manifest as sudden footdrop, wristdrop, or isolated cranial nerve palsies.
- Patients with diabetes have an increased susceptibility to infections of the skin, tuberculosis, pneumonia, and pyelonephritis. Infections cause about 5% of diabetes-related deaths. In an individual with diabetic neuropathy, a trivial infection in a toe may be the first event in a long succession of complications (gangrene, bacteremia, pneumonia) that may ultimately lead to death.

The chronic complications and associated morbidity and mortality are mitigated by strict glycemic control. For patients with T1D, insulin replacement therapy is the mainstay of treatment, while nonpharmacologic approaches such as dietary restrictions and exercise (which improves insulin sensitivity) are often the initial treatment for T2D. Most patients with T2D eventually require therapeutic intervention to reduce hyperglycemia. Glycemic control is assessed clinically by measuring the percentage of glycated hemoglobin, also known as *HbA1C*, which is formed by nonenzymatic addition of glucose moieties to hemoglobin in red cells. HbA1C is a measure of glycemic control over long periods of time (2–3 months) and is less affected by day-to-day variations than is blood glucose. The American Diabetes Association recommends maintaining HbA1C levels at less than 7% to reduce the risk for long-term complications. In addition, patients with diabetes need to maintain LDL and HDL cholesterol and triglycerides at optimal levels to reduce the risk for macrovascular complications. The adoption of a healthy and active lifestyle remains one of the best defenses against this modern-day scourge.

PANCREATIC NEUROENDOCRINE TUMORS

Pancreatic neuroendocrine tumors (PanNETs), also known as *islet cell tumors*, are rare in comparison with tumors of the exocrine pancreas (Chapter 15), accounting for only 2% of all pancreatic neoplasms. PanNETs are most common in adults and may be single or multifocal; when they are malignant, the liver is the most common site of metastases. The tumors often secrete pancreatic hormones, but some are nonfunctional. The latter are typically larger at the time of diagnosis, since they come to clinical attention later in their natural history than functional PanNETs, which often present with symptoms related to excessive hormone production. These tumors frequently have mutations in the tumor suppressor genes *MEN1* and *PTEN*, or inactivating mutations in *ATRX*, loss of function of which leads to maintenance of telomeres through a mechanism referred to as alternative lengthening of telomeres.

Insulinoma

β-cell tumors (insulinomas) are the most common type of PanNET and elaborate sufficient insulin to induce attacks of severe hypoglycemia that manifest as confusion, stupor, and loss of consciousness. These attacks are precipitated by fasting or exercise and are promptly relieved by feeding or parenteral administration of glucose. Most insulinomas are cured by surgical resection.

The majority of insulinomas are identified while they are small (<2 cm in diameter) and localized to the pancreas. Most are solitary lesions, although multifocal tumors or tumors ectopic to the pancreas may be encountered. Malignancy in insulinomas occurs in less than 10% of cases and is diagnosed on the basis of local invasion or metastases. On histologic examination, the benign tumors look remarkably like giant islets, with preservation of the regular cords of monotonous cells. Malignant lesions also tend to be well differentiated and may be deceptively encapsulated. **Deposition of amyloid** is a characteristic feature of many insulinomas (Fig. 18.29).

Gastrinoma

Marked hypersecretion of gastrin is usually caused by a gastrin-producing tumor *(gastrinoma)*. *Zollinger-Ellison syndrome* refers to the association of these tumors with hypersecretion of gastrin, which stimulates gastric acid secretion. This in turn leads to the development of peptic ulcers, which are seen in 90% to 95% of patients. The duodenal and gastric ulcers are often multiple; although they are identical to those found in peptic ulcer disease (Chapter 13), they are often unresponsive to usual therapy. In addition, ulcers may occur in unusual locations such as the jejunum; when intractable jejunal ulcers are found, Zollinger-Ellison syndrome should be suspected. More than one-half of affected patients have diarrhea; in 30%, it is the presenting manifestation. In approximately 25% of patients, gastrinomas arise in conjunction with other endocrine tumors, such as in the MEN-1 syndrome (discussed later).

Gastrinomas may arise in the pancreas, the peripancreatic region, or the wall of the duodenum. **Over one-half of gastrin-producing tumors are locally invasive or have already metastasized at the time of diagnosis.** MEN-1—associated gastrinomas are frequently multifocal, while sporadic gastrinomas are usually single. As with insulin-secreting tumors of the pancreas, gastrin-producing tumors are histologically bland and rarely exhibit marked anaplasia.

ADRENAL GLANDS

The adrenal glands are paired endocrine organs consisting of two regions, the cortex and the medulla, which differ in their development, structure, and function. The *cortex* consists of three layers of distinct cell types. Beneath the capsule of the adrenal gland is the narrow layer of zona glomerulosa. An equally narrow zona reticularis abuts the medulla. Intervening is the broad zona fasciculata, which makes up about 75% of the cortex.

The adrenal cortex synthesizes three different types of steroids:
- *Glucocorticoids* (principally cortisol), synthesized primarily in the zona fasciculata, with a small contribution from the zona reticularis
- *Mineralocorticoids,* the most important being aldosterone, produced in the zona glomerulosa
- *Sex steroids* (estrogens and androgens), produced largely in the zona reticularis

The adrenal *medulla* is composed of chromaffin cells, so named because of their brown-black color after exposure to potassium dichromate. They synthesize and secrete catecholamines in response to

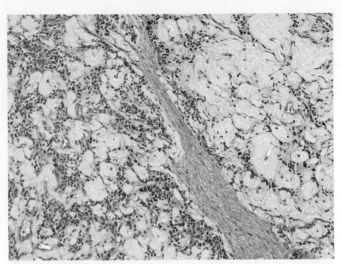

FIG. 18.29 Pancreatic neuroendocrine tumor (PanNET), also called *islet cell tumor.* The neoplastic cells are present in clusters, are monotonous in appearance, and demonstrate minimal pleomorphism or mitotic activity. There is abundant deposition of pale pink amyloid, characteristic of an insulinoma. A fibrous trabeculum is also seen.

signals from preganglionic nerve fibers in the sympathetic nervous system. Similar collections of cells are distributed throughout the body in the extraadrenal paraganglion system.

We first discuss disorders of the adrenal cortex and then of the medulla. Diseases of the adrenal cortex can be divided into those associated with cortical hyperfunction or hypofunction.

ADRENOCORTICAL HYPERFUNCTION: HYPERADRENALISM

There are three distinctive hyperadrenal clinical syndromes, each caused by abnormal production of one or more of the hormones produced by the three layers of the cortex:
- *Cushing syndrome,* characterized by an excess of cortisol
- *Hyperaldosteronism,* caused by an excess of mineralocorticoid
- *Adrenogenital* or *virilizing syndromes,* caused by an excess of androgens

The clinical features of some of these syndromes overlap because of the shared functions of adrenal steroids.

Hypercortisolism: Cushing Syndrome

Hypercortisolism (Cushing syndrome) is caused by elevated glucocorticoid levels. In clinical practice, most cases of Cushing syndrome are due to administration of exogenous glucocorticoids (iatrogenic). The remaining cases are endogenous; the three most common disorders are as follows (Fig. 18.30):
- Primary hypothalamic-pituitary diseases associated with hypersecretion of ACTH
- Secretion of ectopic ACTH by nonpituitary neoplasms
- Primary adrenocortical neoplasms (adenoma or carcinoma) and, rarely, primary cortical hyperplasia

Primary hypothalamic-pituitary disease associated with hypersecretion of ACTH, also known as *Cushing disease,* accounts for approximately 70% of cases of endogenous hypercortisolism. The prevalence of this disorder is about four times higher in women than

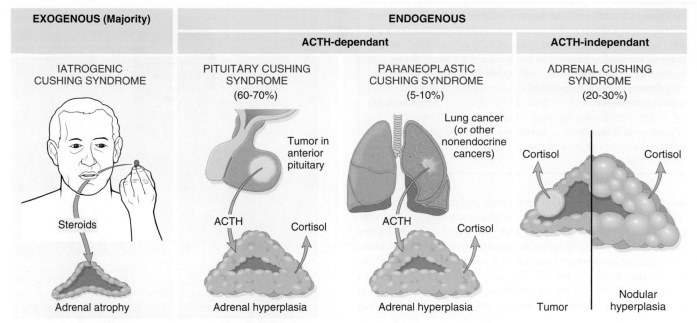

EXOGENOUS (Majority)	ENDOGENOUS		
	ACTH-dependant		ACTH-independant
IATROGENIC CUSHING SYNDROME	PITUITARY CUSHING SYNDROME (60-70%)	PARANEOPLASTIC CUSHING SYNDROME (5-10%)	ADRENAL CUSHING SYNDROME (20-30%)

FIG. 18.30 Causes of Cushing syndrome: The three endogenous forms, as well as the more common exogenous (iatrogenic) form. *ACTH,* Adrenocorticotropic hormone.

in men, and it occurs most frequently in the 20- to 40-year age group. In nearly all cases, the pituitary gland contains an ACTH-producing adenoma. These are usually too small to produce mass effects, but exceptions occur. Rarely, the cause is *corticotroph cell hyperplasia* without a discrete adenoma. Corticotroph cell hyperplasia may be primary or, much less commonly, secondary to excessive ACTH release by a hypothalamic corticotropin-releasing hormone (CRH)—producing tumor. The adrenal glands in patients with Cushing disease show variable degrees of bilateral nodular cortical hyperplasia (discussed later), secondary to the elevated levels of ACTH *(ACTH-dependent Cushing syndrome)*, leading to hypercortisolism.

Secretion of ectopic ACTH by nonpituitary tumors accounts for 10% to 15% of cases of Cushing syndrome. In many instances the responsible tumor is a *small cell carcinoma of the lung,* although other neoplasms, including carcinoid, medullary thyroid carcinoma, and PanNET, have been associated with this paraneoplastic syndrome. Alternatively, occasional neuroendocrine neoplasms produce ectopic CRH, which, in turn, causes ACTH secretion and hypercortisolism. In either case, the adrenal glands again undergo bilateral cortical hyperplasia secondary to elevated ACTH.

Primary adrenal neoplasms, such as adrenal adenoma and carcinoma, and, rarely, *primary cortical hyperplasia,* are responsible for 15% to 20% of cases of endogenous Cushing syndrome, also designated *ACTH-independent Cushing syndrome* because the tumors or hyperplastic glands function autonomously. The biochemical hallmark of adrenal Cushing syndrome is elevated serum levels of cortisol and low levels of ACTH.

MORPHOLOGY

The main lesions of hypercortisolism are found in the pituitary and adrenal glands. The **pituitary** changes vary according to the cause. The most common alteration, resulting from high levels of endogenous or exogenous glucocorticoids, is **Crooke hyaline change**, marked by replacement of the normal granular, basophilic cytoplasm of the ACTH-producing cells in the anterior pituitary by homogeneous, lightly basophilic material. This alteration is

the result of accumulation of intermediate keratin filaments in the cytoplasm. In pituitary Cushing disease, an adenoma is also present (described earlier).

Morphologic changes in the adrenal glands depend on the cause of the hypercortisolism and include: (1) cortical atrophy; (2) diffuse hyperplasia; (3) macronodular or micronodular hyperplasia; or (4) an adenoma or carcinoma.

In patients in whom the syndrome results from exogenous glucocorticoids, suppression of endogenous ACTH results in bilateral **cortical atrophy,** specifically of the zona fasciculata and zona reticularis (Fig. 18.31). The zona glomerulosa is of normal thickness in such cases, because this portion of the cortex is not ACTH-dependent. In cases of endogenous hypercortisolism, by contrast, the adrenals are either hyperplastic or contain a cortical neoplasm.

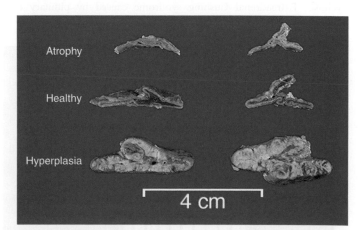

FIG. 18.31 Adrenal cortical atrophy and hyperplasia. In atrophy, the glands are shrunken *(top row)* compared to normal glands *(middle).* In diffuse hyperplasia *(bottom row),* the adrenal cortex is yellow and thickened, and a subtle nodularity is evident. The atrophic gland was from a patient treated for a prolonged period with steroids, and the hyperplastic gland from a patient with ACTH-dependent Cushing syndrome. *ACTH,* Adrenocorticotropic hormone. (From Klatt EC: *Robbins and Cotran Atlas of Pathology,* ed 4, Fig. 15.40, Philadelphia, 2021, Elsevier.)

Diffuse adrenal cortical hyperplasia is found in patients with ACTH-dependent Cushing syndrome (see Fig. 18.31). Both glands are enlarged, either subtly or markedly, each weighing up to 30 g. The adrenal cortex is thickened and variably nodular. The yellow color of the glands derives from the presence of **lipid-rich** cells, which appear vacuolated microscopically.

In **primary cortical hyperplasia,** the cortex is replaced almost entirely by **macronodules** or 1- to 3-mm darkly pigmented **micronodules** (Fig. 18.32). The pigment is lipofuscin, a product of aging (Chapter 1).

Functional adenomas or carcinomas of the adrenal cortex are not morphologically distinct from nonfunctioning adrenal neoplasms and are discussed later.

Clinical Features. The signs and symptoms of Cushing syndrome are an exaggeration of the known actions of glucocorticoids. Cushing syndrome usually develops gradually and, like many other endocrine abnormalities, may be quite subtle in its early stages. This is particularly true of Cushing syndrome associated with small cell carcinoma of the lung, as the rapid course of the underlying disease precludes development of the full-blown syndrome. Early manifestations of Cushing syndrome include hypertension and weight gain. With time, the more characteristic centripetal redistribution of adipose tissue becomes apparent, with resultant truncal obesity, rounded facies, and accumulation of fat in the posterior neck and back. Hypercortisolism causes selective atrophy of fast-twitch (type II) myofibers, with resultant decreased muscle mass and proximal limb weakness. Glucocorticoids induce gluconeogenesis and inhibit the uptake of glucose by cells, resulting in secondary diabetes with its attendant hyperglycemia, glycosuria, and polydipsia. The catabolic effects of glucocorticoids cause loss of collagen. Thus, the skin is thin, fragile, and easily bruised; cutaneous striae are particularly common in the abdominal area (Fig. 18.33). Cortisol has diverse effects on calcium metabolism, including reduced renal absorption and increased urinary loss, that lead to resorption of bone, osteoporosis, and increased susceptibility to fractures. Because glucocorticoids suppress the immune response, patients with Cushing syndrome are also at increased risk for a variety of infections. Additional manifestations include hirsutism and menstrual abnormalities, as well as a number of psychiatric symptoms including mood swings, depression, and frank psychosis. Extraadrenal Cushing syndrome caused by pituitary or

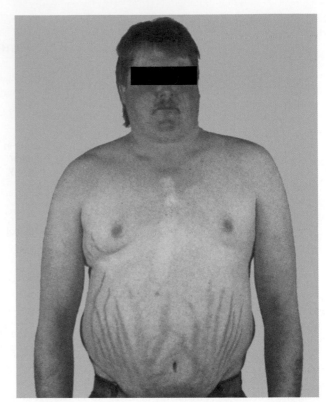

FIG. 18.33 A patient with Cushing syndrome. Characteristic features include central obesity, "moon facies," and abdominal striae. (Reproduced with permission from Lloyd RV, et al: *Atlas of Nontumor Pathology: Endocrine Diseases*, Washington, DC, 2002, American Registry of Pathology.)

ectopic ACTH secretion is usually associated with increased skin pigmentation secondary to the concomitant secretion of melanocyte-stimulating hormone.

In pituitary and ectopic Cushing syndrome, ACTH levels are elevated and the levels of corticosteroids excreted in the urine are increased. By contrast, ACTH levels are low in Cushing syndrome

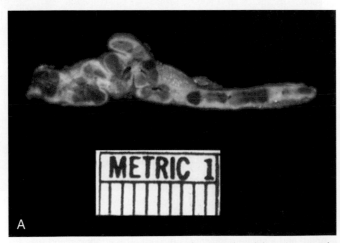

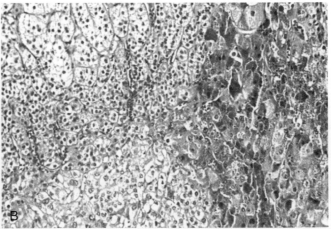

FIG. 18.32 Primary pigmented nodular adrenocortical hyperplasia. (A) Prominent pigmented nodules in the enlarged adrenal. (B) On histologic examination, the nodules are composed of cells containing lipofuscin pigment, seen in the right part of the field. (Photographs courtesy of Dr. Aidan Carney, Department of Medicine, Mayo Clinic, Rochester, Minnesota.)

secondary to adrenal tumors or caused by administration of corticosteroids.

Hyperaldosteronism

Hyperaldosteronism is the generic term for a group of closely related conditions characterized by chronic excessive aldosterone secretion. Hyperaldosteronism may be primary, or it may be secondary to an extraadrenal cause.

Primary hyperaldosteronism refers to autonomous overproduction of aldosterone with resultant suppression of the renin-angiotensin system and decreased plasma renin. Normally, aldosterone production is regulated by renin but in this disease it is usually renin-independent. The causes of primary hyperaldosteronism are as follows (Fig. 18.34).

- *Bilateral idiopathic hyperaldosteronism,* characterized by bilateral nodular hyperplasia of the adrenal glands of unknown cause. This is the most common form of primary hyperaldosteronism, accounting for about 60% of cases.
- *Adrenocortical neoplasm,* most commonly an aldosterone-producing adenoma or, rarely, an adrenocortical carcinoma. In approximately 35% of cases, primary hyperaldosteronism is caused by a solitary aldosterone-secreting adenoma, a condition referred to as *Conn syndrome.*
- *Familial hyperaldosteronism,* which results from a rare genetic defect that leads to overactivity of the aldosterone synthase gene, *CYP11B2.*

In *secondary hyperaldosteronism,* aldosterone release occurs in response to activation of the renin-angiotensin system. This condition is characterized by increased levels of plasma renin and is encountered in association with the following:

- *Decreased renal perfusion* (e.g., arteriolar nephrosclerosis, renal artery stenosis)
- *Arterial hypovolemia and edema* (e.g., congestive heart failure, cirrhosis, nephrotic syndrome)
- *Pregnancy* (estrogen increases the plasma renin substrate)

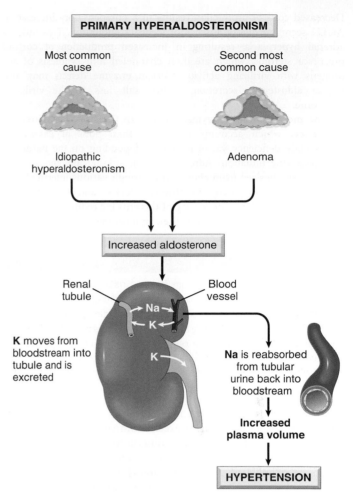

PRIMARY HYPERALDOSTERONISM

Most common cause — Idiopathic hyperaldosteronism

Second most common cause — Adenoma

Increased aldosterone

Renal tubule — Na, K — Blood vessel

K moves from bloodstream into tubule and is excreted

Na is reabsorbed from tubular urine back into bloodstream

Increased plasma volume

HYPERTENSION

FIG. 18.34 The major causes of primary hyperaldosteronism and its principal effects on the kidney.

MORPHOLOGY

Bilateral idiopathic hyperplasia is marked by diffuse or focal hyperplasia of cells resembling those of the normal zona glomerulosa.

Aldosterone-producing adenomas are almost always solitary, small (<2 cm in diameter), well-circumscribed lesions. They are bright yellow on cut section and are composed of lipid-laden cortical cells more closely resembling fasciculata cells than glomerulosa cells (the normal source of aldosterone). The cells tend to be uniform in size and shape; occasionally there is some nuclear and cellular pleomorphism. In patients who have been treated with the antihypertensive agent spironolactone, eosinophilic, laminated cytoplasmic inclusions can be seen (eFig. 18.2). In contrast with cortical adenomas associated with Cushing syndrome, those associated with hyperaldosteronism do not usually suppress ACTH secretion. Therefore, the adjacent adrenal cortex and that of the contralateral gland are not atrophic.

Clinical Features. The most important clinical consequence of hyperaldosteronism is *hypertension,* resulting mainly from sodium retention and increased blood volume. With an estimated prevalence rate of 5% to 10% among hypertensive individuals, primary hyperaldosteronism is the most common cause of secondary hypertension. The long-term effects of hyperaldosteronism-induced hypertension are the same as those of primary hypertension (Chapter 8) and include heart failure, myocardial infarction, arrhythmias, and stroke. Hypokalemia resulting from renal potassium loss can cause a variety of neuromuscular manifestations, including weakness, paresthesias, visual disturbances, and tetany. Previously, hypokalemia was a cardinal feature of primary hyperaldosteronism, but now nearly 50% of newly diagnosed patients are normokalemic, largely due to early detection.

Adrenogenital Syndromes

Adrenogenital syndromes are a group of disorders caused by androgen excess, which may stem from several etiologies, including primary gonadal disorders and several primary adrenal disorders. The adrenal cortex secretes two compounds—dehydroepiandrosterone and androstenedione—that are converted to testosterone in peripheral tissues and have androgenic effects. Unlike gonadal androgens, adrenal androgen formation is regulated by ACTH; thus, excessive secretion can present as an isolated syndrome or in combination with features of Cushing syndrome. The adrenal causes of androgen excess include *adrenocortical neoplasms* and *congenital adrenal hyperplasia.* Adrenocortical neoplasms with symptoms of androgen excess (*virilization*) are more likely to be carcinomas than adenomas.

Congenital adrenal hyperplasia (CAH) is a heterogeneous autosomal recessive condition caused by deficiencies of enzymes involved in adrenal steroid biosynthesis, particularly cortisol.

Decreased cortisol production results in a compensatory increase in ACTH secretion due to absence of feedback inhibition. This induces adrenal hyperplasia, resulting in increased production of cortisol precursor steroids, which are then channeled into synthesis of androgens with virilizing activity. Certain enzyme defects may also impair aldosterone secretion, adding salt loss to the virilizing syndrome.

The most common enzymatic defect in CAH is 21-hydroxylase deficiency, which accounts for more than 90% of cases. 21-hydroxylase deficiency varies in degree depending on the nature of the underlying mutation. Adrenal cortisol, aldosterone, and sex steroids are synthesized from cholesterol through various intermediates. 21-hydroxylase is required for synthesis of cortisol and aldosterone but not sex steroids. Thus, a deficiency of this enzyme reduces cortisol and aldosterone synthesis and shunts the common precursors into the sex steroid pathway (eFig. 18.3).

MORPHOLOGY

In all cases of CAH, the adrenals are **hyperplastic bilaterally,** sometimes to 10 to 15 times their normal weight. The adrenal cortex is thickened and nodular, and, on the cut section, the widened cortex appears brown due to lipid depletion. The proliferating cells are mostly compact, eosinophilic cells intermixed with lipid-laden clear cells. Hyperplasia of corticotroph (ACTH-producing) cells is present in the anterior pituitary in most patients.

Clinical Features. The clinical manifestations of CAH include abnormalities related to androgen excess, with or without aldosterone and glucocorticoid deficiency. Depending on the nature and severity of the enzyme defect, the onset of symptoms may occur in the perinatal period, later childhood, or (less commonly) adulthood.

In 21-hydroxylase deficiency, excessive androgenic activity causes signs of masculinization in females, ranging from clitoral hypertrophy and pseudohermaphroditism in infants to oligomenorrhea, hirsutism, and acne in postpubertal girls. In males, androgen excess is associated with enlargement of the external genitalia and other evidence of precocious puberty in young patients. Most men with CAH are fertile but some have failure of Leydig cell development and oligospermia. In approximately one-third of individuals with 21-hydroxylase deficiency, the enzyme defect is sufficiently severe to produce aldosterone deficiency, with resultant salt (sodium) wasting. Concomitant cortisol deficiency places individuals with CAH at risk for acute adrenal insufficiency (discussed later).

CAH should be suspected in any neonate with ambiguous genitalia. Severe enzyme deficiency in infancy can be life-threatening due to vomiting, dehydration, and salt wasting. In milder variants, women may present with delayed menarche, oligomenorrhea, or hirsutism; in all cases, an androgen-producing ovarian neoplasm must be excluded. Treatment of CAH with exogenous glucocorticoids provides adequate levels of glucocorticoids and also suppresses ACTH levels, thereby decreasing the steroid hormone synthesis responsible for many of the clinical findings. Mineralocorticoid supplementation is required in the salt-wasting variants of CAH.

ADRENOCORTICAL INSUFFICIENCY

Adrenocortical insufficiency, or hypofunction, may be caused by either primary adrenal disease (primary hypoadrenalism) or ACTH deficiency (secondary hypoadrenalism). Primary adrenocortical insufficiency may be *acute (adrenal crisis)* or *chronic (Addison disease).*

Acute Adrenocortical Insufficiency

Acute adrenal insufficiency is the result of several disorders. *Massive adrenal hemorrhage* may cause acute adrenocortical insufficiency by extensive cortical destruction. This may occur in patients on anticoagulant therapy, in postoperative patients who develop disseminated intravascular coagulation, and in patients experiencing overwhelming sepsis; in the latter setting, it is known as the *Waterhouse-Friderichsen syndrome* (Fig. 18.35). This catastrophic syndrome is classically associated with *Neisseria meningitidis* septicemia but can also be caused by other infections. Waterhouse-Friderichsen syndrome can occur at any age but is somewhat more common in children. The basis for the adrenal hemorrhage is uncertain but may be attributable to direct bacterial seeding of small vessels in the adrenal, the development of disseminated intravascular coagulation (Chapter 3), or sepsis-induced enothelial injury. Individuals with chronic adrenocortical insufficiency may develop an acute crisis after a stress that taxes their already limited physiologic reserves. Because of the inability of their atrophic adrenals to produce glucocorticoid hormones, patients who are maintained on exogenous corticosteroids may experience a similar adrenal crisis if there is rapid withdrawal of steroids or failure to increase steroid doses in response to an acute stress.

Chronic Adrenocortical Insufficiency: Addison Disease

Addison disease, or chronic adrenocortical insufficiency, is an uncommon disorder resulting from progressive destruction of the adrenal cortex. More than 90% of cases are attributable to one of four disorders: autoimmune adrenalitis, tuberculosis, acquired immune deficiency syndrome (AIDS), or metastatic cancer.

- *Autoimmune adrenalitis* accounts for 70% to 90% of cases in countries where infectious causes are rare. Autoimmune adrenalitis may be isolated or may be accompanied by autoimmune disease involving other endocrine organs as well. Among these autoimmune polyglandular syndromes (APS), the best defined is APS1, caused by mutations in the autoimmune regulator *(AIRE)* gene on chromosome 21. It is characterized by

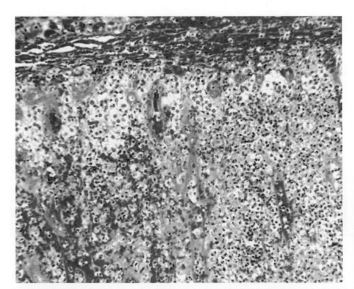

FIG. 18.35 Waterhouse-Friderichsen syndrome. Bilateral adrenal hemorrhage in an infant with overwhelming sepsis, resulting in acute adrenal insufficiency. At autopsy, the adrenal glands were grossly hemorrhagic and shrunken; in this photomicrograph, little residual cortical architecture is discernible.

autoimmune destruction of endocrine organs, mainly the adrenal and parathyroid glands, often with mucocutaneous candidiasis and abnormalities of the skin, dental enamel, and nails. The AIRE protein is involved in the expression of tissue antigens in the thymus and the elimination of T cells specific for these antigens (Chapter 5). Individuals with APS1 also develop autoantibodies against IL-17, which is the principal effector cytokine secreted by Th17 T cells (Chapter 5). Because this cytokine is crucial for defense against fungal infections, its antibody-mediated depletion or blocking leads to chronic mucocutaneous candidiasis.

- *Infections,* particularly tuberculosis and some fungal infections, may cause chronic adrenocortical insufficiency. Tuberculous adrenalitis, which once accounted for as many as 90% of cases of Addison disease, has become less common with improved therapy. With the resurgence of tuberculosis in the setting of HIV infection and immunodeficiency, this cause of adrenal deficiency must be considered clinically. When present, tuberculous adrenalitis is usually associated with active infection in other sites, particularly the lungs and genitourinary tract. Among fungi, disseminated infections by *Histoplasma capsulatum* and *Coccidioides immitis* may involve the adrenal glands and cause chronic adrenocortical insufficiency. Patients with AIDS are at risk for the development of adrenal insufficiency from several other infectious (e.g., cytomegalovirus, *Mycobacterium avium-intracellulare*).

- *Metastatic neoplasms* involving the adrenals are another cause of adrenal insufficiency. The adrenals are a fairly common site for metastases in patients with disseminated carcinomas, which sometimes destroy sufficient adrenal cortex to produce a degree of adrenal insufficiency. Carcinomas of the lung and breast are the source of the majority of metastases in the adrenals.

Secondary Adrenocortical Insufficiency

Any disorder of the hypothalamus and pituitary that reduces the output of ACTH, such as metastatic cancer, infection, infarction, or irradiation, leads to a syndrome of hypoadrenalism having many similarities to Addison disease. ACTH deficiency may occur alone or may be a component of panhypopituitarism, with multiple pituitary hormone deficiencies. Secondary adrenocortical insufficiency is characterized by low serum ACTH and a prompt rise in plasma cortisol levels in response to ACTH administration. This is in contrast to patients with primary adrenal disease, in whom destruction of the adrenal cortex prevents a response to exogenously administered ACTH.

MORPHOLOGY

The appearance of the adrenal glands varies with the cause of the adrenocortical insufficiency. **Primary autoimmune adrenalitis** is characterized by irregularly shrunken glands, which may be exceedingly difficult to identify within the suprarenal adipose tissue. On histologic examination, the cortex contains only scattered residual cortical cells in a collapsed network of connective tissue. A variable lymphoid infiltrate is present in the cortex and may extend into the subjacent medulla, which is otherwise preserved. In **tuberculosis or fungal diseases,** the adrenal architecture may be effaced by a granulomatous inflammatory reaction identical to that encountered in other sites of infection. When hypoadrenalism is caused by **metastatic carcinoma,** the adrenals are enlarged, and their normal architecture is distorted and replaced by infiltrating tumor cells. In **secondary hypoadrenalism**, the adrenals are reduced to small, flattened structures that usually retain their yellow color because of a small amount of residual lipid. A uniform, thin rim of atrophic yellow cortex surrounds a

central, normal medulla. Histologic evaluation reveals atrophy of cortical cells with loss of cytoplasmic lipid, particularly in the zona fasciculata and zona reticularis.

Clinical Features. Clinical manifestations of adrenocortical insufficiency typically do not appear until at least 90% of the adrenal cortex has been damaged. Early symptoms often include progressive weakness and easy fatigability, which may be dismissed as nonspecific complaints. Gastrointestinal disturbances are common and include anorexia, nausea, vomiting, weight loss, and diarrhea. There are clinical differences between primary and secondary hypoadrenalism. In patients with primary adrenal disease, increased levels of melanocyte stimulating hormone, which is derived from the same precursor polypeptide as ACTH, results in hyperpigmentation of the skin and mucosal surfaces. The face, axillae, nipples, areolae, and perineum are particularly common sites of hyperpigmentation. By contrast, hyperpigmentation is not seen in patients with secondary adrenocortical insufficiency because melanocyte stimulating hormone levels are not increased. Decreased aldosterone levels in patients with primary adrenal insufficiency results in potassium retention and sodium loss, with consequent hyperkalemia, hyponatremia, volume depletion, and hypotension, whereas secondary hypoadrenalism is characterized by deficient cortisol and androgen output and normal or near-normal aldosterone levels. Hypoglycemia may occasionally occur as a result of glucocorticoid deficiency and impaired gluconeogenesis. It is more common in infants and children than adults. Stresses such as infections, trauma, or surgical procedures in affected patients may precipitate an acute adrenal crisis, manifested by intractable vomiting, abdominal pain, hypotension, coma, and vascular collapse. Death follows rapidly unless corticosteroids are replaced immediately.

ADRENOCORTICAL NEOPLASMS

Functional adrenal neoplasms may be responsible for any of the various forms of hyperadrenalism. Adenomas are most commonly associated with hyperaldosteronism and Cushing syndrome, whereas a neoplasm causing virilization is more likely to be a carcinoma. Not all adrenocortical neoplasms, however, elaborate steroid hormones. Determination of whether a cortical neoplasm is functional is based on clinical evaluation and measurement of hormones or hormone metabolites in the laboratory.

MORPHOLOGY

Adrenocortical adenomas are yellow tumors surrounded by thin or well-developed capsules. Most are small, 1 to 2 cm in diameter and weigh less than 30 gm (Fig. 18.36A). On microscopic examination, they are composed of cells similar to those encountered in the normal zona fasciculata (Fig. 18.36B). Most are not hyperfunctional and these are often encountered as incidental findings at the time of autopsy or during abdominal imaging for an unrelated cause.

Adrenocortical carcinomas are rare neoplasms that may occur at any age, including in childhood. They are usually large, nonencapsulated masses, frequently exceeding 200 to 300 gm in weight, that replace the adrenal gland. On the cut surface, they are typically variegated, poorly demarcated lesions containing areas of necrosis, hemorrhage, and cystic change (Fig. 18.37A). Microscopic examination usually shows well-differentiated tumor cells resembling those seen in cortical adenomas or, alternatively, bizarre, pleomorphic cells, which may be difficult to distinguish

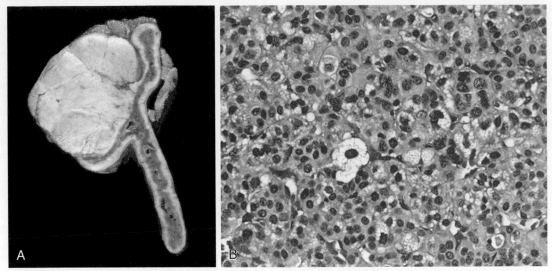

FIG. 18.36 Adrenocortical adenoma. (A) Adenoma is distinguished from nodular hyperplasia by its solitary, circumscribed nature. Its functional status cannot be predicted from its gross or microscopic appearance. (B) The neoplastic cells are vacuolated because of the presence of intracytoplasmic lipid. There is mild nuclear pleomorphism. Mitotic activity and necrosis are not seen.

from those of an undifferentiated carcinoma metastatic to the adrenal gland (Fig. 18.37B). Adrenal cancers have a strong tendency to invade the adrenal vein, vena cava, and lymphatics. Metastases to regional and periaortic nodes are common, as is distant hematogenous spread to the lungs and other viscera. The median patient survival is about 2 years. Of note, **carcinomas metastatic to the adrenal cortex are significantly more frequent than primary adrenocortical carcinoma.** With functioning tumors, both benign and malignant, the adjacent adrenal cortex and that of the contralateral adrenal gland are atrophic, as a result of suppression of endogenous ACTH by high cortisol levels.

TUMORS OF THE ADRENAL MEDULLA

The most important diseases of the adrenal medulla are neoplasms, which include tumors derived from chromaffin cells (pheochromocytoma) and neuronal tumors (including neuroblastoma and more mature ganglion cell tumor).

Pheochromocytoma

Pheochromocytomas are neoplasms of chromaffin cells, which, like their nonneoplastic counterparts, synthesize and release catecholamines and, in some cases, other peptide hormones. These tumors are of special importance because, although uncommon, they (like aldosterone-secreting adenomas) give rise to a surgically correctable form of hypertension.

Pheochromocytomas have historically followed the "10 percent rule":

- *10% are extraadrenal,* occurring in sites such as the organ of Zuckerkandl (located at the bifurcation of the aorta or at the origin of the inferior mesenteric artery) and the carotid body, where they are called *paragangliomas.*
- *10% are bilateral;* this proportion may rise to 50% in cases associated with familial syndromes.
- *10% are malignant.* Malignancy is more common in tumors arising in extraadrenal sites (up to 20% of the tumors).

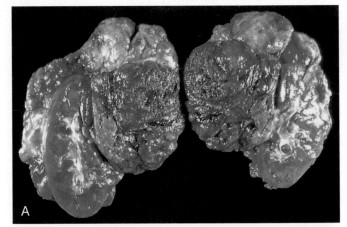

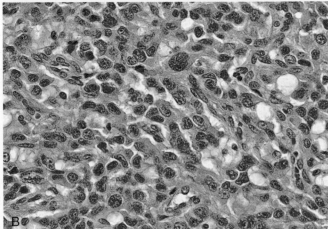

FIG. 18.37 Adrenal carcinoma. (A) The tumor is hemorrhagic and necrotic; it dwarfs the kidney, compressing the upper pole. (B) Histology shows anaplastic, pleomorphic cells. (© 2022 University of Michigan. Used with permission.)

- *10% are not associated with hypertension.* The frequency of these tumors in normotensive patients is increasing because they may be detected during imaging carried out for other reasons.

The 10% rule has been modified to apply only to familial cases.

Pathogenesis. Pheochromocytomas and paragangliomas are genetically heterogeneous, with driver mutations in at least a dozen different genes. The encoded proteins promote carcinogenesis by several mechanisms: RET, which causes type 2 MEN syndromes (described later), and NF1, which causes type 1 neurofibromatosis (Chapter 21), enhance signaling through growth factor receptor pathways; VHL, which causes von Hippel-Lindau disease (Chapters 12 and 21), subunits of the succinate dehydrogenase complex, and EPAS1 all lead to increased activity of hypoxia-inducible factors (HIFs) (see Chapter 6).

MORPHOLOGY

Pheochromocytomas range in size from small, circumscribed lesions confined to the adrenal gland to large, hemorrhagic masses weighing several kilograms. On the cut surface, smaller pheochromocytomas are yellow-tan, well-defined lesions that compress the adjacent adrenal gland (Fig. 18.38A). Larger lesions tend to be hemorrhagic, necrotic, and cystic and typically efface the adrenal gland. Incubation of the fresh tissue with potassium dichromate solution turns the tumor dark brown because it reacts with catecholamines.

On microscopic examination, pheochromocytomas are composed of polygonal to spindle-shaped chromaffin cells and their supporting cells, compartmentalized into small nests by a rich vascular network (Fig. 18.38B). The cytoplasm of the neoplastic cells often has a finely granular appearance because of the presence of granules containing catecholamines, which can be highlighted by silver stains. Electron microscopy reveals variable numbers of membrane-bound, electron-dense granules, which contain catecholamines and sometimes other peptides. The nuclei of the neoplastic cells are often quite pleomorphic. Both capsular and vascular invasion, as well as cellular pleomorphism, may be encountered in benign lesions. Therefore, **the definitive diagnosis of malignancy in pheochromocytomas is based on the presence of metastases.** These may involve regional lymph nodes as well as more distant sites, including the liver, lung, and bone.

Clinical Features. Catecholamines (dopamine, epinephrine, and norepinephrine) mediate the functions of the sympathetic nervous system; hence, their release from pheochromocytoma mimics sympathetic nervous hyperactivity. The dominant clinical manifestation is *hypertension,* observed in the majority of patients. Most patients present with chronic, sustained elevation in blood pressure. Approximately two-thirds also demonstrate paroxysmal hypertensive episodes. These consist of abrupt, precipitous elevations in blood pressure associated with tachycardia, palpitations, headache, sweating, tremor, and a sense of apprehension. There may also be pain in the abdomen or chest, nausea, and vomiting. The paroxysms are induced by the sudden release of catecholamines and may acutely precipitate congestive heart failure, pulmonary edema, myocardial infarction, ventricular fibrillation, and cerebrovascular accidents. Other frequent symptoms are headache and generalized sweating. In some cases, pheochromocytomas secrete other hormones such as ACTH and somatostatin and may therefore be associated with clinical features related to the effects of these hormones. The laboratory diagnosis is based on demonstration of increased urinary excretion of free

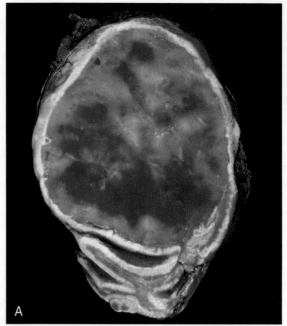

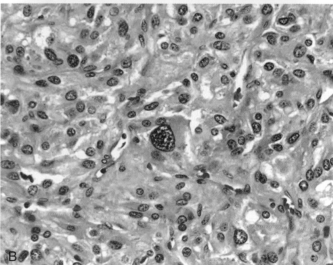

FIG. 18.38 Pheochromocytoma. (A) The tumor is enclosed within an attenuated cortex and demonstrates areas of hemorrhage. The residual adrenal gland is seen below. (B) Photomicrograph of pheochromocytoma, demonstrating characteristic nests of cells with abundant cytoplasm. Granules containing catecholamine are not visible in this preparation. It is common to find bizarre cells (such as the one in the center of this image) even in benign tumors.

catecholamines and their metabolites, such as vanillylmandelic acid and metanephrines. Isolated benign pheochromocytomas are treated with surgical excision. When excision is not feasible, long-term medical treatment for hypertension may be required.

Neuroblastoma and Other Neuronal Neoplasms

Neuroblastoma is the most common extracranial solid tumor of childhood. These neoplasms occur most commonly during the first 5 years of life, sometimes during infancy. A majority of these tumors arise in the adrenal medulla or the retroperitoneal sympathetic ganglia, but they may occur anywhere in the sympathetic nervous system and occasionally within the brain. Most neuroblastomas are sporadic, although familial cases also occur. These tumors are discussed in Chapter 4 along with other pediatric neoplasms.

MULTIPLE ENDOCRINE NEOPLASIA (MEN) SYNDROMES

MEN syndromes are autosomal dominant disorders characterized by proliferative lesions (hyperplasias, adenomas, and carcinomas) in multiple endocrine organs. Like other inherited cancer disorders (Chapter 6), endocrine tumors arising in the context of MEN syndromes have features that are distinct from their sporadic counterparts:

- Tumors occur at a younger age.
- Tumors arise in multiple endocrine organs, either synchronously (at the same time) or metachronously (at different times).
- Even in one organ, the tumors are often multifocal.
- Tumors are usually preceded by an asymptomatic stage of endocrine hyperplasia involving the cell of origin (e.g., in MEN-2, the parenchyma adjacent to medullary thyroid carcinoma virtually always demonstrates C-cell hyperplasia).
- Tumors are usually more aggressive and recur in a higher proportion of cases.

MULTIPLE ENDOCRINE NEOPLASIA TYPE 1

MEN-1 syndrome is caused by germline mutations in the *MEN1* tumor suppressor gene, which encodes a protein called menin. Menin is a component of several different transcription factor complexes, and loss of menin function leads to deregulation of the corresponding binding partners, promoting uncontrolled transcriptional activity and neoplasia. Organs most commonly involved are the parathyroid, the pancreas, and the pituitary.

- *Parathyroid. Primary hyperparathyroidism* is the most common manifestation of MEN-1 (80%–95% of patients) and is the presenting disorder in most patients, appearing in almost all by 40 to 50 years of age. Parathyroid abnormalities include hyperplasias and adenomas.
- *Pancreas.* Endocrine tumors of the pancreas are the leading cause of death in MEN-1. These tumors are usually aggressive and present with metastatic disease. Pancreatic endocrine tumors are often functional (i.e., secrete hormones). Zollinger-Ellison syndrome, associated with gastrinoma, and hypoglycemia, associated with insulinoma, are common endocrine manifestations.
- *Pituitary.* The most frequent pituitary tumor in patients with MEN-1 syndrome is a prolactin-secreting macroadenoma. In some cases, acromegaly develops in association with somatotropin-secreting tumors.
- Other tumors in these patients include duodenal gastrinomas, thyroid and adrenocortical adenomas, and lipomas, all of which occur more frequently than in the general population.

MULTIPLE ENDOCRINE NEOPLASIA TYPE 2

MEN-2 syndrome encompasses two phenotypically distinct disorders, MEN-2A and MEN-2B, that share the same molecular pathogenesis, activating mutations of the *RET* proto-oncogene. The phenotypic differences are related to different classes of *RET* mutations, which appear to account for the variable features in the two subtypes.

Multiple Endocrine Neoplasia Type 2A

Organs commonly involved in MEN-2A include the following:

- *Thyroid:* Medullary carcinoma of the thyroid develops in virtually all untreated patients, usually during the first two decades of life. The tumors are commonly multifocal and C-cell hyperplasia can be found in the adjacent "normal" thyroid. *Familial medullary thyroid cancer* is seen in a variant of MEN-2A, without the other characteristic manifestations listed below. Relative to MEN-2A and -2B, familial medullary carcinoma typically occurs at an older age and follows a more indolent course.
- *Adrenal medulla:* Adrenal *pheochromocytomas* develop in 50% of the patients; no more than 10% of these tumors are malignant.
- *Parathyroid:* Approximately 10% to 20% of patients develop *parathyroid gland hyperplasia* leading to primary hyperparathyroidism.

Multiple Endocrine Neoplasia Type 2B

A particular mutation that results in a single amino acid substitution in RET, that is distinct from the mutations seen in MEN-2A is responsible for virtually all cases of MEN-2B (which is now often referred to as MEN-3). Patients develop *medullary thyroid carcinomas,* which are usually multifocal and more aggressive than in MEN-2A, and *pheochromocytomas.* MEN-2B has the following distinctive features:

- *Primary hyperparathyroidism does not develop.*
- *Extraendocrine manifestations,* including ganglioneuromas of mucosal sites (e.g., gastrointestinal tract, lips, tongue) and a marfanoid habitus, in which overly long bones of the axial skeleton give an appearance resembling that in Marfan syndrome (Chapter 4).

Before the advent of genetic testing, relatives of patients with MEN-2 syndrome were screened with annual biochemical assays for calcitonin, which lacked sensitivity. Now, routine genetic testing identifies *RET* mutation carriers earlier and more reliably in MEN-2 kindreds. All individuals carrying germline *RET* mutations are advised to have prophylactic thyroidectomy to prevent the inevitable development of medullary carcinomas.

Two other recently described MEN syndromes are MEN-4 and MEN-5. MEN-4 is characterized by inactivating germline mutations in the *CDKN1B* gene. Phenotypically, it mimics MEN-1. Germline mutation in the *MAX* tumor suppressor gene causes the MEN-5 syndrome. Patients with MEN-5 often develop bilateral pheochromocytomas and other tumors. Unlike MEN-2, medullary thyroid carcinomas and C-cell hyperplasia are not seen in MEN-5.

■ RAPID REVIEW

Pituitary

Pituitary Adenoma (Neuroendocrine Tumor)

- The most common cause of hyperpituitarism is an anterior lobe pituitary adenoma.
- Pituitary adenomas can be macroadenomas (>1 cm in diameter) or microadenomas (<1 cm in diameter); on clinical evaluation they can be functional or nonfunctional.
- Macroadenomas may lead to mass effects, including visual disturbances.
- Functioning adenomas are associated with distinct endocrine signs and symptoms that reflect the hormones produced in excess.
  - *Lactotroph (prolactin-producing) adenoma:* amenorrhea, galactorrhea, loss of libido, infertility

- *Somatotroph (growth hormone-producing) adenoma:* gigantism (children), acromegaly (adults), and impaired glucose tolerance and diabetes
- *Corticotroph (ACTH and melanocyte stimulating hormone-producing) adenoma:* Cushing syndrome, hyperpigmentation
- Mutation of the *GNAS* gene, which results in constitutive activation of a stimulatory G protein, is one of the more common genetic alterations.
- The two distinctive morphologic features of most adenomas are their cellular monomorphism and absence of a reticulin network.

Other Pituitary Disorders

- *Hypopituitarism* (deficiency of anterior pituitary hormones) is rare and most often caused by encroachment by tumors or ischemic necrosis (postpartum, called *Sheehan syndrome*).
- The most common disorder of the posterior pituitary is *diabetes insipidus,* caused by deficiency of ADH, which leads to water loss in the urine.

Thyroid
Thyroiditis

- Hashimoto (chronic lymphocytic) thyroiditis is the most common cause of hypothyroidism in regions where dietary iodine levels are sufficient.
- Hashimoto thyroiditis is an autoimmune disease characterized by progressive destruction of thyroid parenchyma, Hürthle cell change, lymphoplasmacytic infiltrates, and germinal centers with or without extensive fibrosis.
- Multiple autoimmune mechanisms account for thyroid injury in Hashimoto disease, including cytotoxicity mediated by CD8+ T cells, cytokines (IFN-γ), and antithyroid antibodies.
- Subacute granulomatous (de Quervain) thyroiditis is a self-limited disease, probably secondary to a viral infection, characterized by pain and the presence of granulomatous inflammation in the thyroid.
- Painless (subacute lymphocytic) thyroiditis is a self-limited disease that often occurs after a pregnancy (postpartum thyroiditis), is typically painless, and is characterized by lymphocytic inflammation in the thyroid.

Graves Disease

- Graves disease, the most common cause of endogenous hyperthyroidism, is characterized by the triad of thyrotoxicosis, ophthalmopathy, and dermopathy.
- Graves disease is an autoimmune disorder caused by autoantibodies to the TSH receptor that mimic TSH by activating TSH receptors on thyroid epithelial cells.
- The thyroid in Graves disease is characterized by diffuse hypertrophy and hyperplasia of follicles and lymphoid infiltrates; glycosaminoglycan deposition and lymphoid infiltrates are responsible for the ophthalmopathy and dermopathy.
- Laboratory features include elevations in serum free T_3 and T_4 and decreased serum TSH.

Thyroid Neoplasms

- Most thyroid neoplasms manifest as *solitary thyroid nodules,* but only 1% of thyroid nodules are neoplastic.

- *Follicular adenoma* is the most common benign neoplasm, and *papillary carcinoma* is the most common malignancy.
- Multiple genetic pathways are involved in thyroid carcinogenesis. Some of the driver mutations that are characteristic of thyroid cancers include *PAX8/PPARG* fusion (in follicular carcinoma), chromosomal rearrangements involving the *RET* oncogene (in papillary carcinoma), and point mutations of *RET* (in medullary carcinoma).
- *Follicular adenoma and carcinoma* are composed of well-differentiated follicular epithelial cells; the latter are distinguished by the presence of capsular and/or vascular invasion.
- *Papillary carcinoma* is recognized by nuclear features (ground-glass nuclei, pseudoinclusions), even in the absence of papillae. This neoplasm typically metastasizes by way of the lymphatics, but the prognosis is excellent.
- *Anaplastic carcinoma* is thought to arise from follicular or papillary carcinoma through loss of *TP53* function. It is highly aggressive and uniformly lethal.
- *Medullary thyroid carcinoma* arises from parafollicular C cells and can be sporadic (70%) or familial (30%). Multicentricity and C-cell hyperplasia are features of familial cases. Amyloid deposits composed of calcitonin are a characteristic histologic finding.

Parathyroid Glands
Hyperparathyroidism

- Primary hyperparathyroidism is the most common cause of asymptomatic hypercalcemia.
- In a majority of cases, primary hyperparathyroidism is caused by a sporadic parathyroid adenoma and, less commonly, by parathyroid hyperplasia.
- Parathyroid adenomas are solitary, while hyperplasia is typically a multiglandular process.
- Skeletal manifestations of hyperparathyroidism include bone resorption, osteitis fibrosa cystica, and brown tumors. Renal changes include nephrolithiasis (stones) and nephrocalcinosis.
- Most cases of hyperparathyroidism are clinically silent because of early detection of hypercalcemia during routine blood testing.
- Secondary hyperparathyroidism is caused by chronic hypocalcemia, most often secondary to renal failure, and resultant parathyroid gland hyperplasia.
- Malignancies are the most important cause of symptomatic hypercalcemia, which results from osteolytic metastases or tumor-derived PTH-related protein.

Endocrine Pancreas
Diabetes: Pathogenesis and Long-Term Complications

- Type 1 diabetes is an autoimmune disease characterized by progressive destruction of islet β cells, leading to absolute insulin deficiency. Both autoreactive T cells and autoantibodies are involved.
- Type 2 diabetes is caused by insulin resistance and β-cell dysfunction, resulting in relative insulin deficiency. Autoimmunity is not involved.
- Obesity has an important relationship with insulin resistance (and hence type 2 diabetes), mediated by various factors, including excess free fatty acids, aberrant levels of adipokines, and an altered inflammatory milieu within adipose tissue.

- Monogenic forms of diabetes are uncommon and are caused by single-gene defects that result in primary β-cell dysfunction or lead to abnormalities of insulin–insulin receptor signaling.
- The long-term complications of diabetes are similar in all types and affect mainly blood vessels and the kidneys, nerves, and eyes. The development of these complications is attributed to three underlying mechanisms: formation of advanced glycation end products, activation of protein kinase C, and disturbances in polyol pathways leading to oxidative stress.

Pancreatic Neuroendocrine Tumors (PanNETs)

- Insulinoma is the most common type of PanNET. It is usually benign but elaborates sufficient insulin to induce attacks of hypoglycemia.
- Gastrinoma may arise in the pancreas, the peripancreatic region, or the wall of the duodenum. It produces gastrin, which increases secretion of gastric acid and promotes peptic ulcers.

Adrenal Glands
Hypercortisolism (Cushing Syndrome)

- The most common cause of hypercortisolism is exogenous administration of steroids.
- Endogenous hypercortisolism is most often secondary to an ACTH-producing pituitary microadenoma *(Cushing disease)*, followed by primary adrenal neoplasms *(ACTH-independent hypercortisolism)* and paraneoplastic ACTH production by tumors (e.g., small cell lung cancer).
- The morphologic features in the adrenal gland include bilateral cortical atrophy (in exogenous steroid-induced disease), bilateral diffuse or nodular hyperplasia (most common finding in endogenous Cushing syndrome), or an adrenocortical neoplasm.

Adrenogenital Syndromes

- The adrenal cortex can secrete excess androgens in either of two settings: adrenocortical neoplasms (usually virilizing carcinomas) or congenital adrenal hyperplasia (CAH).
- CAH encompasses a group of autosomal recessive disorders characterized by defects in steroid biosynthesis, usually cortisol; the most common subtype is caused by deficiency of the enzyme 21-hydroxylase.

- Reduction in cortisol production causes a compensatory increase in ACTH secretion, which in turn stimulates androgen production. Androgens have virilizing effects, including masculinization in females (ambiguous genitalia, oligomenorrhea, hirsutism), precocious puberty in males, and, in some instances, salt (sodium) wasting and hypotension.
- Bilateral hyperplasia of the adrenal cortex is characteristic.

Adrenocortical Insufficiency (Hypoadrenalism)

- Primary adrenocortical insufficiency can be acute *(Waterhouse-Friderichsen syndrome)* or chronic *(Addison disease)*.
- Chronic adrenal insufficiency in the Western world is most often secondary to autoimmune adrenalitis, which may occur in the context of autoimmune polyendocrine syndromes.
- Tuberculosis and infections due to opportunistic pathogens associated with the human immunodeficiency virus and tumors metastatic to the adrenals are the other important causes of chronic hypoadrenalism.
- Patients typically present with fatigue, weakness, and gastrointestinal disturbances. Primary adrenocortical insufficiency is also characterized by high melanocyte stimulating hormone levels leading to skin hyperpigmentation.

Adrenal Medulla

- Pheochromocytomas are tumors of catecholamine-producing cells that cause hypertension. Similar tumors arising outside the adrenals are called paragangliomas.

MEN Syndromes

- MEN-1 is caused by germline mutations in the *MEN1* gene, which encodes a transcriptional regulator (menin). Patients develop tumors of the parathyroids (adenomas), pancreas (endocrine tumors), pituitary (lactotroph adenomas), and other endocrine organs.
- MEN-2 is caused by mutations in the *RET* oncogene. Two variants are caused by different mutations. MEN-2A presents with tumors of the thyroid (medullary carcinoma), adrenal medulla (pheochromocytoma), and parathyroids (adenomas), whereas MEN-2B (also called MEN-3) presents with tumors of the thyroid and adrenal glands, ganglioneuromas at mucosal sites, and developmental disorders of the skeleton.

■ Laboratory Tests[a]

Test	Reference Values	Pathophysiology/Clinical Relevance
Adrenocorticotropic hormone (ACTH), plasma	7.2 to 63 pg/mL a.m. draws	Corticotropin-releasing hormone (CRH) from the hypothalamus induces ACTH synthesis in the adenohypophysis. ACTH stimulates cortisol and androgen secretion by the adrenal gland. Elevated cortisol levels can be seen with exogenous corticosteroid administration and in Cushing disease (pituitary ACTH-secreting tumor), Cushing syndrome, ectopic ACTH-secreting tumor, and adrenal hyperplasia. A dexamethasone suppression test can help distinguish Cushing disease from other causes of hypercortisolism. Important causes of hypocortisolism include primary and secondary adrenal insufficiency and congenital adrenal hyperplasia.

Aldosterone, serum	Adults: ≤21 ng/dL	Aldosterone is the main mineralocorticoid produced by the adrenal cortex. Aldosterone stimulates sodium transport in the distal renal tubules and is a key regulator of blood pressure and blood volume. Conditions that increase aldosterone include adrenal adenoma, adrenal hyperplasia, and excessive activation of the renin-angiotensin-aldosterone system (e.g., renin-producing tumor, renal artery stenosis, arterial hypovolemia and edema). Aldosterone deficiency can be seen with low renin (such as in renal disease) or with high renin (from primary adrenal insufficiency).
Androstenedione, serum	Varies with age, sex, and sexual development Adult males: 40–150 ng/dL Adult females: 30–200 ng/dL	Androstenedione is a steroid hormone produced from cholesterol in the testes, adrenal cortex, and ovaries. Androstenedione production in the adrenal glands is controlled by adrenocorticotropic hormone (ACTH); in the gonads it is controlled by luteinizing hormone (LH) and follicle-stimulating hormone (FSH). Androstenedione is a precursor of testosterone and is increased in hirsutism, polycystic ovarian syndrome (PCOS), virilizing adrenal tumors, precocious puberty, Cushing disease, ectopic ACTH-producing tumors, and congenital adrenal hyperplasia.
Calcitonin, serum	Adult males: ≤14.3 pg/mL Adult females: ≤7.6 pg/mL	Calcitonin is secreted by parafollicular cells (C cells) of the thyroid gland in response to elevated ionized calcium concentration. Calcitonin inhibits the action of parathyroid hormone and inhibits bone resorption by directly binding to osteoclasts. Calcitonin lowers serum calcium and phosphorus levels. Calcitonin can be elevated in patients with medullary thyroid carcinoma.

Calcium, serum	Ionized (free) calcium
	    Adults: 4.57–5.43 mg/dL
	Total: calcium
	    Adults: 8.6–10.0 mg/dL
		Calcium binds to negatively charged sites on proteins and is affected by pH. Alkalosis leads to an increase in negative charge and binding and thus a decrease in free calcium. Acidosis leads to a decrease in negative charge and binding and thus an increase in free calcium. Decreased ionized calcium levels stimulate the parathyroid glands to secrete parathyroid hormone (PTH), which leads renal tubular cells to increase calcium absorption and drives osteoclasts to release calcium from bone. PTH also increases intestinal absorption of calcium. Hypercalcemia can be seen in primary hyperparathyroidism (increased PTH secretion) or in malignancy (secretion of PTH-related proteins or by bone destruction from metastases). Other causes of hypercalcemia include drugs/supplements, endocrine disorders, granulomatous diseases, and syndromic diseases (e.g., multiple endocrine neoplasia). Common causes of hypocalcemia include chronic renal failure and hypomagnesemia (impairs PTH secretion and causes PTH end-organ resistance).

Copeptin proAVP (arginine vasopressin), plasma	Nonwater deprived, nonfasting adults: <13.1 pmol/L Water deprived, fasting adults: <15.2 pmol/L	Neurosecretory cells in the hypothalamus secrete a preprohormone that is composed of AVP (also known as antidiuretic hormone, ADH), copeptin, and neurophysin II, and the three components are transported to the posterior pituitary. In response to decreased intravascular volume and increased plasma osmolarity/sodium concentration, AVP stimulates water reabsorption in the distal renal tubules. When there is inadequate ADH, most commonly due to damage to the hypothalamus or pituitary stalk, diabetes insipidus results with consequent polyuria, polydipsia, and hypernatremia. Syndrome of inappropriate antidiuretic hormone (SIADH) is when there is an inappropriate release of ADH leading to hyponatremia. This can occur in CNS disorders, in lung disease, or from a paraneoplastic syndrome caused by ectopic ADH secretion (e.g., small-cell carcinoma of the lung). AVP has a short half-life in plasma, which makes analysis challenging; however, copeptin, which is secreted in equimolar amounts as AVP, has a longer half-life and, therefore, is used as a surrogate marker for AVP.
Cortisol (free), serum	0.121–1.065 μg/dL (morning collection)	Cortisol is the major endogenous glucocorticoid and is a key regulator of the stress response and glucose metabolism. Cortisol levels are regulated by adrenocorticotropic hormone (ACTH) from the pituitary gland in response to cyclic release of corticotropin-releasing hormone (CRH) from the hypothalamus. Levels of ACTH and cortisol peak in the morning and trough in the late evening. Conditions that increase cortisol are known as hypercortisolism (Cushing syndrome). Hypocortisolism can be due to damage/disease of the adrenal glands or pituitary glands. Use of glucocorticoid medications cause suppression of the CRH-ACTH-adrenal axis, causing reduction in endogenous cortisol production until medications are withdrawn.

Dehydroepiandrosterone sulfate (DHEAS), serum	Varies with age	DHEA is the major adrenal androgen and is a precursor for sex steroids; the majority is secreted as a conjugate to sulfate, DHEAS. DHEA and DHEAS test results can be used interchangeably in most clinical situations. Elevated DHEAS levels can cause symptoms or signs of hyperandrogenism in women, though men are usually asymptomatic. DHEA/DHEAS are typically assessed in investigations of adrenal androgen production, such as the assessment of (1) hyperplasia, (2) adrenal tumors, (3) adrenarche (sexual maturation), (4) delayed puberty, and (5) hirsutism.
Glucose, serum	≥1 year old: 70–140 mg/dL	Physiologic glucose levels are primarily maintained by insulin and glucagon. Hyperglycemia may be due to either insufficient insulin (e.g., type I diabetes) or peripheral insulin resistance (e.g., type II diabetes). Measurement of serum glucose is useful in the diagnosis and management of diabetes. Hemoglobin A1c provides a longer-term assessment of glucose control and is thus complementary to day-to-day glucose levels. Hypoglycemia, usually in the setting of excess insulin dose, can be life threatening.
Growth hormone (GH; somatotropin), serum	Adult males: 0.01–0.97 ng/mL Adult females: 0.01–3.61 ng/mL	GH secretion from somatotroph cells in the anterior pituitary is stimulated by ghrelin (stomach) and GH releasing hormone (GHRH) (hypothalamus) and inhibited by somatostatin (hypothalamus). GH and insulin-like growth factor 1 (IGF-1) inhibit GH secretion. GH induces growth in most tissues and organs, but its effect is most pronounced on cartilage and bone. GH levels increase in childhood, are at their peak during puberty, and decrease with increasing age. Low levels of GH in infancy or early childhood can cause dwarfism, and elevated levels causes gigantism in children (before physis closure) or acromegaly once the growth plate has closed. GH is released in a pulsatile fashion such that random GH levels are of little diagnostic value. GH stimulation tests use drugs (e.g., L-dopa, clonidine) to stimulate GH secretion.
Growth hormone releasing hormone (GHRH), serum	Baseline ranges: 5–18 pg/mL	GHRH stimulates synthesis and secretion of growth hormone (GH) by the anterior pituitary. GHRH is secreted in a pulsatile fashion, with a bolus at the onset of sleep. Hypothalamic somatostatin suppresses release of both GH and GHRH. GHRH synthesis is inhibited by negative feedback by GH and IGF-1. Excess GHRH may be due to hypothalamic tumors or as a paraneoplastic syndrome (e.g., well-differentiated neuroendocrine tumors such as bronchial carcinoids). Excess GHRH can cause gigantism or acromegaly. Decreased GHRH can result in dwarfism.
Hemoglobin A1c (HbA1c, glycated hemoglobin), blood	4.0%–5.6%	When glucose attaches nonenzymatically to hemoglobin, a glycated hemoglobin (HbA1c) is formed. This process occurs continually and therefore reflects mean plasma glucose levels over the course of the red cell's life span of 8–12 weeks. Patients with high average blood concentrations of glucose (e.g., in the setting of diabetes) will have higher HbA1c levels than those with unimpaired glucose metabolism. HbA1c is the key laboratory test for monitoring long-term glucose control. HbA1c is also a diagnostic test for diabetes: HbA1c of 6.5% or higher on two different days is diagnostic of diabetes. HbA1c can also identify patients who may become diabetic (prediabetes): values of 5.7%–6.4% are associated with increased risk of diabetes. HbA1c may be falsely low in conditions associated with rapid red cell turnover (e.g., chronic hemolysis, patients treated with erythropoietin). HbA1c may be falsely high when red cell turnover is low (e.g., vitamin B_{12} deficiency).

Metanephrines, plasma free or 24-hour urine	Plasma:
	  <0.050 nmol/L
	Urine:
	  Normotensive adult males:
	    261 µg/24 hours
	  Normotensive adult females:
	    180 µg/24 hours
	  Hypertensive adults:
	    <400 µg/24 hours
		Metanephrines are the main metabolites of norepinephrine and epinephrine, two hormones that are secreted by pheochromocytomas and other tumors of neural crest origin. Measurement of metanephrines is more accurate than directly measuring epinephrine or norepinephrine. Measurement of plasma free metanephrines has very high sensitivity for pheochromocytoma and paraganglioma. Elevated metanephrine levels are suggestive of neural crest tumors but should be confirmed by a second test (24-hour urine metanephrines). 24-hour collection is preferred given episodic secretion of catecholamines.

Parathyroid hormone (PTH), serum	15–65 pg/mL	PTH is synthesized and secreted by the chief cells of parathyroid glands. It plays a crucial role in maintaining calcium homeostasis by acting directly on bone and kidney, and indirectly on the intestine through 1,25-dihydroxyvitamin D. PTH promotes osteoclastic bone resorption and calcium and phosphate release. In the kidney, PTH stimulates calcium reabsorption, increases conversion of vitamin D to its active dihydroxy form, and inhibits phosphate reabsorption. These actions increase the plasma concentration of free calcium and decrease plasma phosphate concentration. Determination of PTH is useful in the differential diagnosis of both hypercalcemia and hypocalcemia.

		In hypercalcemia due to primary hyperparathyroidism (adenoma, hyperplasia), patients have increased PTH levels. In hypercalcemia due to other causes (e.g., PTHrP in malignancy), PTH is typically low. Secondary hyperparathyroidism is compensatory oversecretion of PTH due to abnormally low serum calcium (e.g., in renal failure, gastrointestinal malabsorption, vitamin D deficiency). The most common causes of hypoparathyroidism are parathyroidectomy or thyroidectomy with accidental removal of parathyroids.
Parathyroid hormone–related peptide (PTHrP), plasma	≤4.2 pmol/L	PTHrP is secreted by certain malignant tumors (e.g., breast carcinoma, squamous cell carcinoma of the lung and head and neck) and binds to the parathyroid hormone receptor to stimulate calcium resorption in bone and calcium reabsorption in the kidney. In paraneoplastic hypercalcemia, parathyroid hormone levels are generally low or undetectable due to feedback inhibition. Successful treatment of the underlying malignancy usually results in decreased levels of PTHrP and calcium and subsequent increases in parathyroid hormone levels.
T3 (triiodothyronine), total, serum	80–200 ng/dL	T3 (triiodothyronine) is the more physiologically active form of thyroid hormone. Only a small percentage of thyroid hormone is released as T3; the rest is thyroxine (T4). T4 is deiodinated to T3 once in circulation. Several tests may be used to evaluate T3 including total T3 and free T3 (measures unbound T3). T3 levels are assessed in conjunction with TSH and total and free T4 to evaluate thyroid function and to assess treatment for thyroid disease. T3 and free T3 are not routinely used for this purpose, since total and free T4 are sufficient in most cases. T3 is used to evaluate thyrotoxicosis.
T4 (thyroxine), free, serum	0.9–1.7 ng/dL	Thyroxine (T4) is synthesized in the thyroid gland and metabolized peripherally to triiodothyronine (T3). The majority of T4 is bound to thyroid binding globulin; free T4 is the active form. Although only about 0.05% of circulating T4 is unbound to binding proteins ("free"), measurement of free T4 provides an accurate assessment of thyroid status in most patient populations. Total T4, free T4, and TSH are often used together to evaluate thyroid function. Low free T4 is seen in hypothyroidism; high free T4 is seen in hyperthyroidism. Free T4 should be assessed in conjunction with TSH. A common algorithm is TSH measurement, which reflexes to free T4 if TSH concentration is abnormal.
Thyroid peroxidase antibody, serum	<9.0 IU/mL	Thyroid peroxidase (TPO) catalyzes iodination of thyroglobulin to form monoiodotyrosine and diiodotyrosine, precursors of thyroid hormone. Antibodies against TPO are common in autoimmune thyroid disease, though they are also present in 5%–20% of the general population. Anti-TPO antibodies are sensitive tests for autoimmune thyroid disease (e.g., Hashimoto thyroiditis, Graves disease) but are not specific within this class of disorders. The highest anti TPO levels are generally seen with Hashimoto thyroiditis.
Thyroid-stimulating hormone (TSH), serum	Adults: 0.3–4.2 mIU/L	TSH (thyrotropin) is produced by the anterior pituitary with feedback inhibition by thyroid hormones. It interacts with cell receptors on the thyroid follicular cells to stimulate cell division, cell hypertrophy, and increased synthesis of thyroid hormones (thyroxine and triiodothyronine). TSH is the primary screen for primary hypothyroidism and primary hyperthyroidism. If TSH is low, free T4 and T3 are added to determine the extent of hyperthyroidism, and if TSH is high, free T4 is performed to assess the degree of hypothyroidism. For patients with primary hypothyroidism who are treated with levothyroxine, TSH alone is a sufficient screening test. For patients with central hypothyroidism (hypothyroidism caused by hypothalamic or pituitary disease), free T4 is low or low-normal and the TSH may be low or normal.
Thyrotropin (TSH) receptor antibody, serum	≤1.75 IU/L	In Graves disease, TSH receptor antibodies (also called thyroid-stimulating immunoglobulins) bind to and activate the TSH receptor without feedback inhibition, causing thyrotoxicosis. TSH receptor antibodies that block the receptor may also be seen, and it is thought that the balance between blocking vs. activating antibodies may contribute to disease severity in Graves disease. TSH receptor antibody testing is useful when Graves disease is suspected clinically but thyroid function tests are normal and in patients for whom radioisotope testing is contraindicated (e.g., people who are pregnant). TSH receptor antibodies may persist even with successful therapy (ablation or surgery); since they are IgG antibodies, they can cross the placenta and cause neonatal thyrotoxicosis.

[a]The assistance of Dr. Katie O'Sullivan, Department of Medicine, University of Chicago, in editing this table is greatly appreciated.

References values from https://www.mayocliniclabs.com/ by permission of Mayo Foundation for Medical Education and Research. All rights reserved.

Adapted from Deyrup AT, D'Ambrosio D, Muir J, et al. Essential Laboratory Tests for Medical Education. *Acad Pathol.* 2022;9. doi: 10.1016/j.acpath.2022.100046.

Bones, Joints, and Soft Tissue Tumors

OUTLINE

BONE

STRUCTURE AND FUNCTION OF BONE

Bone provides mechanical support for the body, transmits forces generated by muscles, protects viscera, provides a niche for blood cell progenitors, and is intimately involved in calcium and phosphate homeostasis. It is produced and maintained by specialized cells that elaborate and remodel the calcified matrix that makes up most of the substance of bone.

Bone Matrix

Bone matrix consists of an organic component called osteoid (35%) and a mineral component (65%), within which are embedded a variety of cells that maintain bone homeostasis. Osteoid consists

The contributions to this chapter by Dr. Andrew Horvai, Department of Pathology, University of California, San Francisco in the previous edition of this book are gratefully acknowledged.

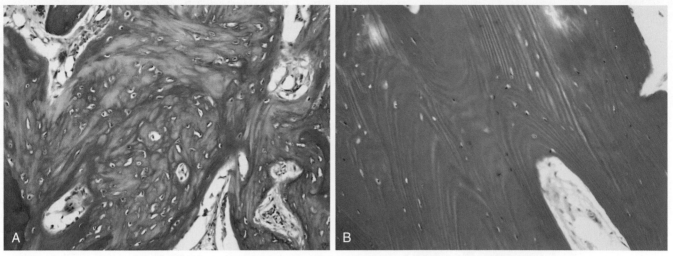

FIG. 19.1 Woven bone (A) is more cellular and disorganized than lamellar bone (B).

predominantly of type I collagen and smaller amounts of glycosaminoglycans and other proteins. The mineral component of bone that is responsible for its hardness is the inorganic moiety *hydroxyapatite*. Bone matrix is synthesized in two forms, woven and lamellar bone (Fig. 19.1). Woven bone is produced rapidly during fetal development and repair of fractures but has a haphazard arrangement of collagen fibers that impart less structural stability than the parallel collagen fibers found in lamellar bone. In an adult, the presence of woven bone is always abnormal, as it indicates ongoing repair of damaged bone.

Bone Cells

Embedded within the bone matrix are a variety of bone cells:

- *Osteoblasts,* located on the surface of the matrix, synthesize and assemble bone matrix and regulate its mineralization (Fig. 19.2A). They are derived from mesenchymal stem cells that are located under the periosteum in developing bone and in the medullary space later in life.
- *Osteocytes* are derived from osteoblasts and are located within the bone; they are interconnected by an intricate network of tunnels (canaliculi) containing cytoplasmic processes. Osteocytes help control calcium and phosphate levels and detect and respond to mechanical forces by altering the remodeling of bone.
- *Osteoclasts,* located on the surface of bone, are specialized multinucleate macrophages derived from circulating monocytes. Osteoclasts attach to proteins found in bone matrix and create a sealed extracellular trench (resorption pit) into which they secrete acid and neutral proteases (predominantly matrix metalloproteases [MMPs]), leading to bone resorption (Fig. 19.2B).

Bone Development

During embryogenesis, long bones develop from cartilage precursors by the process of endochondral ossification. A cartilage mold *(anlage)* is synthesized by mesenchymal precursor cells. At approximately 8 weeks of gestation the central portion of the anlage is resorbed, creating the medullary canal. Simultaneously at midshaft *(diaphysis)* osteoblasts begin to deposit the cortex beneath the periosteum, producing the *primary center of ossification* and initiating radial bone growth. At each end of the bone *(epiphysis),* endochondral ossification proceeds in a centrifugal fashion *(secondary center of ossification).* Eventually, a plate of cartilage becomes entrapped

between the two expanding centers of ossification, forming the *physis* or *growth plate* (Fig. 19.3). The chondrocytes within the growth plate sequentially proliferate, hypertrophy, and undergo apoptosis. In the

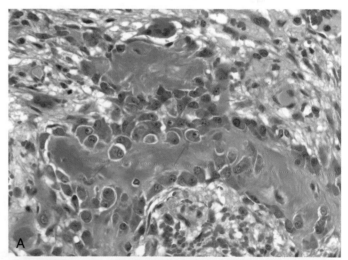

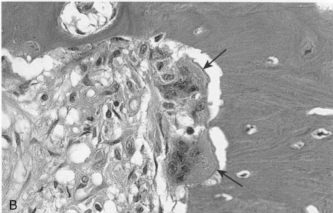

FIG. 19.2 (A) Active osteoblasts *(yellow arrows)* synthesizing bone matrix. (B) Two osteoclasts *(red arrows)* resorbing bone.

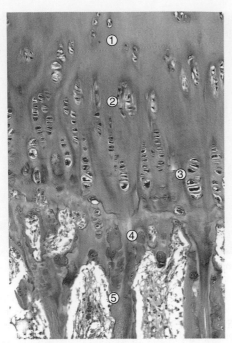

FIG. 19.3 Active growth plate with ongoing endochondral ossification. *1,* Reserve zone. *2,* Zone of proliferation. *3,* Zone of hypertrophy. *4,* Zone of apoptosis and mineralization. *5,* Primary spongiosa.

region of apoptosis, the matrix mineralizes and is invaded by capillaries, providing the nutrients for osteoblasts, which synthesize osteoid. This process produces longitudinal bone growth.

Flat bones develop by a different process called intramembranous ossification. Bones of the cranium, for example, are formed by osteoblasts directly from a fibrous layer of tissue, without cartilage anlagen. The enlargement of flat bones is achieved by deposition of new bone on a preexisting surface.

Bone Homeostasis and Remodeling

The adult skeleton is constantly turning over in a tightly regulated process known as remodeling through coupled osteoblast and osteoclast activity, which together constitute the bone multicellular unit (BMU).

Remodeling is regulated by cell–cell interactions and cytokines (Fig. 19.4). An important signaling pathway that controls remodeling involves three factors: (1) the transmembrane receptor activator of NF-κB (RANK), which is expressed on osteoclast precursors; (2) RANK ligand (RANKL), which is expressed on osteoblasts and marrow stromal cells; and (3) osteoprotegerin (OPG), a secreted "decoy" receptor made by osteoblasts that can block RANK interaction with RANKL. RANK signaling activates the transcription factor NF-κB, which is essential for the generation and survival of osteoclasts. Other important factors regulating remodeling include monocyte-colony stimulating factor (M-CSF), produced by osteoblasts, and WNT proteins, which are produced by various cells and trigger the production of OPG. The importance of these pathways is proven by rare but informative germline mutations in the *OPG, RANK,* and *RANKL* genes that cause severe disturbances of bone metabolism.

The balance between bone formation and resorption is modulated by RANK and WNT signaling. For example, because OPG and RANKL oppose one another, bone resorption or formation is favored by increasing or decreasing the RANK-to-OPG ratio, respectively. Systemic factors that influence this balance include hormones, vitamin D, inflammatory cytokines (e.g., IL-1), and growth factors (e.g., bone morphogenetic proteins [BMPs]). Through complex mechanisms, parathyroid hormone (PTH), IL-1, and glucocorticoids promote osteoclast differentiation and bone turnover. By contrast, BMPs and sex hormones (estrogen, testosterone) generally block osteoclast differentiation or activity by favoring OPG expression.

Peak bone mass is achieved in early adulthood after the cessation of skeletal growth. This set point is determined by many factors, including polymorphisms in the vitamin D receptor gene, nutrition, and physical activity. Beginning in the fourth decade, resorption exceeds formation, resulting in a decline in skeletal mass.

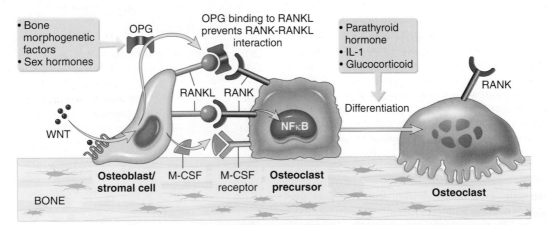

FIG. 19.4 Paracrine mechanisms that regulate osteoclast formation and function. Osteoclasts are derived from monocytes, the same cells that differentiate into macrophages. Osteoblast/stromal cell membrane-associated RANKL binds to its receptor RANK located on the cell surface of osteoclast precursors. Signals transduced by RANK and macrophage colony-stimulating factor (M-CSF) receptor cause the precursor cells to differentiate into functional osteoclasts. By contrast, WNT protein binding triggers stromal cells/osteoblasts to secrete osteoprotegerin (OPG), a "decoy" receptor that prevents RANKL from binding the RANK receptor. Consequently, OPG prevents bone resorption by inhibiting osteoclast differentiation. *IL-1,* Interleukin-1; *NFκB,* nuclear factor kappa-B; *RANK,* receptor activator of nuclear factor kappa-B; *RANKL,* receptor activator of nuclear factor kappa-B ligand.

DEVELOPMENTAL DISORDERS OF BONE AND CARTILAGE

Developmental abnormalities of the skeleton frequently result from germline mutations and become apparent during the early stages of bone formation. The spectrum of developmental disorders of bone is broad, and there is no standard approach to their classification. Here, we categorize the major diseases according to their pathogenesis.

Developmental disorders may be caused by localized abnormalities in the migration and condensation of mesenchyme (dysostosis) or global disorganization of bone and/or cartilage (dysplasia). More than 350 skeletal dysostoses and dysplasias, most of them extremely rare, have been described. The most common dysostoses include complete absence of a bone or a digit (aplasia), extra bones or digits (supernumerary digit), and abnormal fusion of bones (e.g., syndactyly, craniosynostosis). Mutations in homeobox genes, genes encoding cytokines, and cytokine receptors are common causes of dysostoses. By contrast, dysplasias arise from mutations in genes that control development or remodeling of the entire skeleton (discussed below). It is important to note that as used in bone biology the term dysplasia refers to an abnormal pattern of growth rather than a premalignant lesion (Chapter 6).

Achondroplasia

Achondroplasia, the most common skeletal dysplasia and a major cause of dwarfism, is an autosomal dominant disorder characterized by reduced endochondral cartilage growth. The disease is caused by gain-of-function mutations in fibroblast growth factor receptor 3 (FGFR3). FGFR3 typically inhibits endochondral growth; in achondroplasia, the receptor is constitutively active, causing a pathologic suppression of growth. Approximately 90% of cases stem from new mutations, almost all of which occur in the paternal allele. Affected individuals have shortened proximal extremities, a trunk of relatively typical length, and an enlarged head with a bulging forehead and conspicuous depression of the root of the nose. The skeletal abnormalities are usually not associated with changes in longevity or intelligence.

Thanatophoric Dysplasia

Thanatophoric dysplasia, the most common lethal form of dwarfism, is due to diminished proliferation of chondrocytes and disorganization in the zone of proliferation. Like achondroplasia, it is also caused by gain-of-function mutations in FGFR3, but in thanatophoric dysplasia the mutations cause even greater increases in signaling activity. Thanatophoric dysplasia occurs in about 1 of every 20,000 live births. Affected individuals have shortening of the limbs, frontal bossing, relative macrocephaly, a small chest cavity, and a bell-shaped abdomen. The underdeveloped thoracic cavity leads to respiratory insufficiency and affected individuals usually die at birth or soon thereafter.

Osteogenesis Imperfecta

Osteogenesis imperfecta (OI), the most common inherited disorder of connective tissue, is a phenotypically diverse disorder caused by mutations that impair the synthesis of type I collagen. OI principally affects bone and other tissues rich in type I collagen (e.g., joints, eyes, ears, skin, and teeth). It is genetically heterogeneous, but usually results from an autosomal dominant mutation in the genes that encode either the α1 or α2 chains of type I collagen. These mutations cause misfolding of collagen polypeptides, which interferes with the assembly of wild-type collagen chains (a dominant negative loss of function).

The fundamental abnormality in OI is synthesis of too little bone, resulting in extreme skeletal fragility. Other findings include blue sclerae, as the decreased collagen content of the sclerae allows visualization of the underlying choroid, which imparts a bluish color; hearing loss related to a sensorineural deficit and impeded conduction due to abnormalities in the bones of the middle ear; and small, misshapen, blue-yellow teeth, secondary to dentin deficiency.

OI is separated into multiple clinical subtypes that vary widely in severity; while some phenotypes are uniformly fatal in utero or during the perinatal period, other variants are associated with a normal life span despite a susceptibility to fractures, particularly during childhood.

Osteopetrosis

Osteopetrosis, also known as marble bone disease, refers to a group of rare genetic diseases that are characterized by reduced bone resorption and diffuse symmetric skeletal sclerosis resulting from impaired formation or function of osteoclasts. Although the term osteopetrosis refers to the stonelike quality of the bones, the bones are abnormally brittle and fracture easily.

Osteopetrosis is classified into variants based on both the mode of inheritance and the severity of clinical findings. Most mutations interfere with the process of acidification of the osteoclast resorption pit, which is required for the dissolution of calcium hydroxyapatite.

Autosomal dominant osteopetrosis is typically the mildest type of the disorder. It may not be detected until adolescence or adulthood, when it is discovered on radiographic studies done to evaluate repeated fractures. These individuals may also have mild cranial nerve deficits and anemia. The involved bones lack a medullary canal and the ends of long bones are bulbous (Erlenmeyer flask deformity) and misshapen. The neural foramina are small and compress exiting nerves. The primary spongiosa, which is normally removed during growth, persists and fills the medullary cavity, leaving no room for hematopoietic marrow resulting in anemia.

Severe infantile osteopetrosis is autosomal recessive and is often fatal due to leukopenia, despite extensive extramedullary hematopoiesis that can lead to prominent hepatosplenomegaly.

METABOLIC DISORDERS OF BONE

Osteopenia and Osteoporosis

Osteopenia refers to decreased bone mass, while osteoporosis is defined as osteopenia that is severe enough to significantly increase the risk of fracture. Radiographically, osteoporosis is diagnosed when bone mass is at least 2.5 standard deviations below mean peak bone mass, whereas osteopenia is 1 to 2.5 standard deviations below the mean. The disorder may be localized to a certain bone or region (e.g., disuse osteoporosis of a limb) or generalized, involving the entire skeleton. Although osteoporosis can be secondary to endocrine disorders (e.g., hyperthyroidism), gastrointestinal disorders (e.g., malnutrition), or drugs (e.g., corticosteroids), most osteoporosis is primary.

The most common forms of osteoporosis are the senile and postmenopausal types. The following discussion relates largely to these forms of osteoporosis.

Pathogenesis. Peak bone mass is achieved during young adulthood. The height of this peak is influenced by hereditary factors, especially polymorphisms in the genes that affect bone metabolism (discussed later). Physical activity, muscle strength, diet, and hormonal state also contribute. After maximal skeletal mass is attained, bone turnover

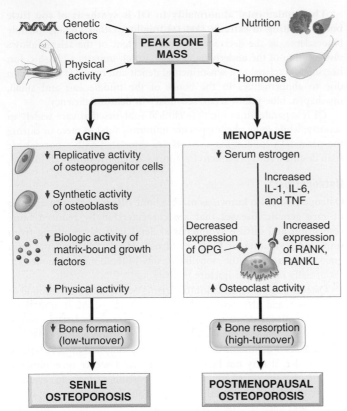

FIG. 19.5 Pathophysiology of postmenopausal and senile osteoporosis (see text). *IL,* Interleukin; *OPG,* osteoprotegerin; *RANK,* receptor activator of nuclear factor kappa-B; *RANKL,* receptor activator of nuclear factor kappa-B ligand; *TNF,* tumor necrosis factor.

leads to an average loss of 0.7% of bone mass per year. Several factors underlie the pathogenesis of osteoporosis (Fig. 19.5):

- *Age-related changes.* Compared to younger individuals, osteoblasts from older individuals have reduced proliferative and biosynthetic potential and reduced response to growth factors, resulting in a diminished capacity to make bone. This form of osteoporosis, known as *senile osteoporosis,* is considered *low-turnover* osteoporosis.
- *Reduced physical activity.* The decreased physical activity associated with aging results in reduced bone mass. Osteocytes respond to mechanical load by stimulating or inhibiting osteoblasts and osteoclasts to remodel normal bone, as evidenced by localized bone loss in an immobilized or paralyzed extremity or increased bone density in athletes. The type of exercise is important, as load magnitude influences bone density more than the number of load cycles. Thus, resistance exercises such as weight training are more effective stimuli for increasing bone mass than repetitive endurance activities such as bicycling.
- *Genetic factors.* Single gene defects account for only a small fraction of osteoporosis cases. Polymorphisms in certain genes have been linked to osteoporosis by genome-wide association studies. These include sequence variants in *RANK, RANKL,* and *OPG,* all of which encode key osteoclast regulators; the HLA locus (for unknown reasons); and the estrogen receptor gene.
- *Calcium nutritional state.* Adolescents (particularly girls) tend to have low dietary calcium intake, a factor that restricts peak bone mass. Calcium deficiency, increased PTH concentrations, and reduced levels of vitamin D may also play a role in the development of senile osteoporosis.
- *Hormonal influences.* Estrogen promotes bone density through a variety of mechanisms including inhibiting the apoptosis of osteoblasts, stimulating the apoptosis of osteoclasts, and suppressing RANKL production. In the decade after menopause, up to 2% of cortical bone and 9% of cancellous bone may be lost each year. *Estrogen deficiency* plays the major role in this process, and close to 40% of postmenopausal women are affected by osteoporosis. Although decreased estrogen increases both bone formation and resorption, the latter dominates, resulting in *high-turnover* osteoporosis. Estrogen loss also induces increased secretion of inflammatory cytokines, such as IL-6, TNF, and IL-1, by innate immune cells in the blood and marrow through unknown mechanisms (see Fig. 19.5). These cytokines increase RANKL and decrease OPG, stimulating osteoclast recruitment and activity.

MORPHOLOGY

The hallmark of osteoporosis is a decreased quantity of histologically normal bone. The entire skeleton is affected in postmenopausal and senile osteoporosis, but certain bones tend to be more severely affected. In postmenopausal osteoporosis, the increase in osteoclast activity affects mainly bones or portions of bones with increased surface area, such as the cancellous compartment of vertebral bodies (Fig. 19.6). The trabecular plates become perforated and thinned and lose their interconnections (Fig. 19.7), leading to progressive microfractures and eventual vertebral collapse.

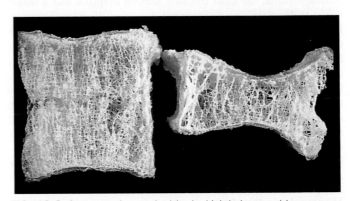

FIG. 19.6 Osteoporotic vertebral body *(right)* shortened by compression fractures compared with a healthy vertebral body *(left).* Note that the osteoporotic vertebra has a characteristic loss of horizontal trabeculae and thickened vertical trabeculae.

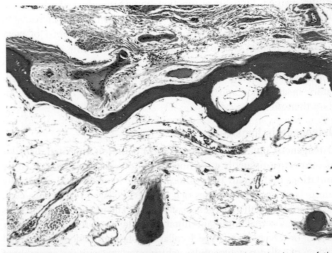

FIG. 19.7 In advanced osteoporosis, both the trabecular bone of the medulla *(bottom)* and the cortical bone *(top)* are markedly thinned.

Clinical Features. The clinical manifestations of osteoporosis depend on the bones that are involved. Vertebral fractures in the thoracic and lumbar regions are painful, and, when multiple, can cause significant loss of height and various deformities, including lumbar *lordosis* and *kyphoscoliosis.* Immobility following fractures of the femoral neck, pelvis, or spine results in complications such as pulmonary embolism and pneumonia, accounting for 40,000 to 50,000 deaths per year.

Osteoporosis cannot be reliably detected in plain radiographs until 30% to 40% of the bone mass has been lost, and measurement of blood levels of calcium, phosphorus, and alkaline phosphatase are not diagnostic. Osteoporosis is thus a difficult condition to screen for in asymptomatic people. The best estimates of bone loss are specialized radiographic imaging techniques, such as dual-energy x-ray absorptiometry and quantitative computed tomography, both of which measure bone density.

The prevention and treatment of senile and postmenopausal osteoporosis include exercise, appropriate calcium and vitamin D intake, and pharmacologic agents that decrease bone resorption (e.g., bisphosphonates). Denosumab, an anti-RANKL antibody that blocks osteoclast activation, is another effective therapy for postmenopausal osteoporosis. Menopausal hormone therapy with estrogen receptor agonists can slow bone loss, but complications, particularly deep venous thrombosis, stroke, and an increased risk of breast cancer, have limited the use of estrogen in the treatment of osteoporosis.

Rickets and Osteomalacia

Both rickets and osteomalacia are manifestations of vitamin D deficiency or its abnormal metabolism (Chapter 7). *Rickets* refers to the disorder in children, in whom it interferes with the deposition of bone in the growth plates. *Osteomalacia* is the adult counterpart, in which bone formed during remodeling is undermineralized, causing a predisposition to fractures. The fundamental defect is an impairment of mineralization and a consequent accumulation of unmineralized matrix.

Hyperparathyroidism

Excess production and activity of parathyroid hormone (PTH) cause increased osteoclast activity, bone resorption, and osteopenia. Although the entire skeleton is affected, osteopenia in some bones (e.g., phalanges) is more conspicuous radiographically. Isolated hyperparathyroidism peaks in middle adulthood and slightly earlier if presenting as a component of multiple endocrine neoplasia syndromes (MEN-1 and MEN-2A) (Chapter 18).

Pathogenesis. As discussed in Chapter 18, PTH plays a central role in calcium homeostasis through the following effects:

- *Osteoclast activation*, increased bone resorption, and calcium mobilization by increased RANKL expression on osteoblasts
- Increased *resorption of calcium* by the renal tubules
- Increased urinary *excretion of phosphates*
- Increased *synthesis of active vitamin D*, $1,25(OH)_2$-D, by the action of renal alpha-1 hydroxylase, which in turn enhances calcium absorption from the gut and mobilizes bone calcium by inducing RANKL on osteoblasts

The net result of these actions is an elevation in serum calcium, which, under normal circumstances, inhibits further PTH production. Excessive or inappropriate levels of PTH may stem from autonomous parathyroid secretion *(primary hyperparathyroidism)* or may occur in the setting of underlying renal disease *(secondary hyperparathyroidism)* (Chapter 18). PTH is directly responsible for the bone changes seen in primary hyperparathyroidism. Abnormalities stemming from chronic renal insufficiency that contribute to bone disease in secondary hyperparathyroidism include inadequate $1,25(OH)_2$-D synthesis, hyperphosphatemia, and metabolic acidosis.

MORPHOLOGY

Symptomatic, untreated primary hyperparathyroidism manifests with three interrelated skeletal abnormalities: osteoporosis, brown tumors, and osteitis fibrosa cystica. **Osteoporosis** is generalized but is most severe in the phalanges, vertebrae, and proximal femur. Osteoclasts may tunnel into and dissect centrally along the length of the trabeculae, creating a railroad track appearance that is referred to as *dissecting osteitis* (Fig. 19.8), a misnomer, as this is not an inflammatory lesion. The marrow spaces around the affected surfaces are replaced by fibrovascular tissue. Radiographs show a decrease in bone density.

Bone loss predisposes to microfractures and secondary hemorrhages that elicit an influx of macrophages and an ingrowth of reparative fibrous tissue, creating a mass of reactive tissue known as a **brown tumor.** The brown color is the result of the vascularity, hemorrhage, and hemosiderin. These lesions often undergo cystic degeneration. The combination of increased osteoclast activity, peritrabecular fibrosis, and cystic brown tumors is the hallmark of severe hyperparathyroidism and is known as **generalized osteitis fibrosa cystica.**

Clinical Features. As bone mass decreases, affected patients are increasingly susceptible to fractures, bone deformation, and joint problems. Osteitis fibrosa cystica is now rarely encountered because hyperparathyroidism is usually diagnosed on routine blood tests (that include serum calcium) and treated at an early stage. In symptomatic patients, restoration of PTH levels to normal by surgical removal of parathyroid glands can completely reverse the bone changes. Secondary hyperparathyroidism is usually not as severe or as prolonged as primary hyperparathyroidism; hence, the skeletal abnormalities tend to be milder. Asymptomatic cases that are increasingly recognized by routine blood testing are followed by measurement of serum calcium, creatinine, and bone mineral density.

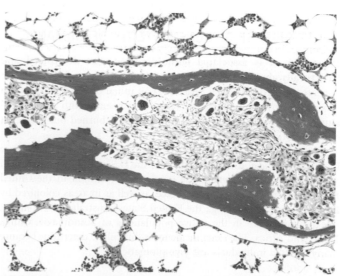

FIG. 19.8 Hyperparathyroidism with osteoclasts boring into the center of the trabecula (dissecting osteitis).

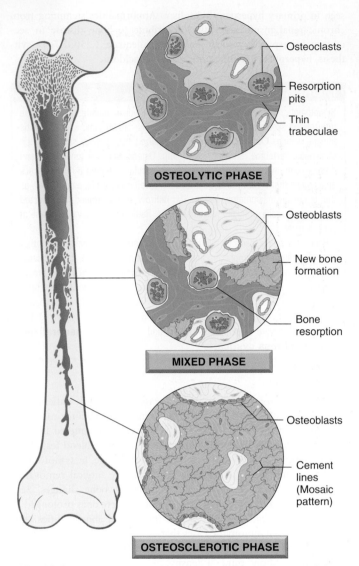

FIG. 19.9 Diagrammatic representation of Paget disease of bone demonstrating the three phases in the evolution of the disease.

OSTEOLYTIC PHASE
- Osteoclasts
- Resorption pits
- Thin trabeculae

MIXED PHASE
- Osteoblasts
- New bone formation
- Bone resorption

OSTEOSCLEROTIC PHASE
- Osteoblasts
- Cement lines (Mosaic pattern)

PAGET DISEASE OF BONE (OSTEITIS DEFORMANS)

Paget disease is associated with increased, but disordered and structurally abnormal, bone formation. This unique skeletal disease appears in three sequential phases: (1) an initial osteolytic stage; (2) a mixed osteoclastic—osteoblastic stage, which ends with a predominance of osteoblastic activity; and (3) a final burned-out quiescent osteosclerotic stage (Fig. 19.9).

Paget disease usually begins in late adulthood and its incidence increases with age. An estimated 1% of the U.S. population older than age 40 is affected. Paget disease is relatively common in the United Kingdom, central Europe, and Greece, as well as in areas colonized by European immigrants (e.g., the United States, Australia). By contrast, the disease is rare in the native populations of Scandinavia, China, Japan, and Africa. The exact incidence is difficult to determine because many affected individuals are asymptomatic.

Pathogenesis. Current evidence suggests both genetic and environmental factors are involved in Paget disease. Approximately 50% of

familial Paget disease cases and 10% of sporadic cases have mutations in *SQSTM1*, a gene that encodes a protein known as sequestosome-1. Mutations in *SQSTM1* appear to lead to increased NF-κB activity, which in turn increases osteoclast activity. Activating mutations in *RANK* and inactivating mutations in *OPG* account for some cases of juvenile Paget disease. The geographic distribution is suggestive of involvement of some unknown environmental factor. In vitro studies have raised the possibility that chronic infection of osteoclast precursors by measles or other RNA viruses may also play a role.

MORPHOLOGY

Paget disease shows remarkable histologic variation over time and from site to site. The initial lytic phase is characterized by numerous large osteoclasts and resorption pits. The osteoclasts may have 100 or more nuclei. Osteoclasts persist in the mixed phase, but many of the bone surfaces are also lined by prominent osteoblasts. The hallmark, seen in the sclerotic phase, is a **mosaic pattern of lamellar bone** (Fig. 19.10). The jigsaw puzzle—like appearance is produced by unusually **prominent cement lines,** which join haphazardly oriented units of lamellar bone. In the sclerotic phase, the bone is thickened but lacks structural stability, making it vulnerable to deformation and fracture.

Clinical Features. Paget disease is *monostotic* (about 15% of cases) or *polyostotic* (about 85%). The axial skeleton or proximal femur is involved in up to 80% of cases. Most cases are asymptomatic and are discovered as an incidental radiographic finding. Pain localized to the affected bone is a common symptom and may be due to microfractures or compression of spinal and cranial nerve roots by overgrown bone. Enlargement of the craniofacial skeleton may produce *leontiasis ossea* (lion face) and a cranium so heavy that is difficult for the person to hold the head erect. The weakened pagetic bone may lead to invagination of the skull base (*platybasia*) and compression of the posterior fossa. Weight bearing causes anterior bowing of the femurs and tibias (eFig. 19.1) and distorts the femoral heads, resulting in the development of severe *secondary osteoarthritis*. *Chalk stick—type fractures* are another frequent complication and usually occur in the long bones of the lower extremities. Compression fractures of the spine result in kyphosis and spinal cord injury. Rarely, the

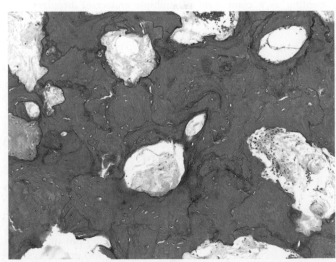

FIG. 19.10 Mosaic pattern of lamellar bone pathognomonic of Paget disease.

hypervascularity of pagetic bone warms the overlying skin, and in severe polyostotic disease increased blood flow can act as an arteriovenous shunt, occasionally leading to high-output heart failure or exacerbation of underlying cardiac disease. Many affected individuals have elevated serum alkaline phosphatase levels; serum calcium and phosphate levels are normal.

A variety of tumors develop in pagetic bone. Secondary osteosarcoma occurs in less than 1% of all individuals with Paget disease but affects 5% to 10% of those with severe polyostotic disease, in whom it is rapidly fatal. In the absence of malignant transformation, Paget disease is usually not a serious or life-threatening disease. Most affected individuals have mild symptoms that are readily suppressed by treatment with antiresorptive agents such as calcitonin and bisphosphonates, which act by reducing osteoclast activity.

FRACTURES

A fracture is defined as loss of bone integrity resulting from mechanical injury and/or diminished bone strength. Fractures are the most common pathologic conditions affecting bone. The following descriptors are used to describe fracture types:

- *Simple:* the overlying skin is intact
- *Compound:* the bone communicates with the skin surface
- *Comminuted:* the bone is fragmented
- *Displaced:* the ends of the bone at the fracture site are not aligned
- *Stress:* a slowly developing fracture that follows a period of increased physical activity in which the bone is subjected to repetitive loads
- *Greenstick:* extending only partially through the bone, common in infants and young children whose bones are soft
- *Pathologic:* involving bone weakened by an underlying disease process, such as a tumor

Healing of Fractures

At the time of fracture, rupture of blood vessels produces a hematoma that fills the fracture gap and surrounds the area of bone injury (Fig. 19.11). The clotted blood seals off the fracture site and creates a fibrin scaffold that guides the influx of inflammatory cells and the ingrowth of fibroblasts and new capillaries. Simultaneously, degranulated platelets and migrating inflammatory cells release PDGF, TGF-β, FGF, and other factors that activate osteoprogenitor cells in the periosteum, medullary cavity, and surrounding soft tissues and stimulate osteoclastic and osteoblastic activity. By the end of the first week, a mass of predominantly uncalcified tissue—called the *soft callus* or *procallus*—bridges the ends of the fractured bones. By approximately 2 weeks, the soft callus is converted to a *bony callus* by the deposition of woven bone by osteoblasts. In some cases, the activated mesenchymal cells in the soft tissues and bone surrounding the fracture line also differentiate into chondrocytes to make fibrocartilage and hyaline cartilage. The newly formed cartilage along the fracture line undergoes endochondral ossification, forming a contiguous network of bone with newly deposited bone trabeculae in the medulla and beneath the periosteum. In this fashion, the fractured ends are bridged (see Fig. 19.11).

As the callus matures and is subjected to weight-bearing forces, portions that are not physically stressed are resorbed. This remodeling reduces the size of the callus until the shape and outline of the fractured bone are reestablished as *lamellar bone*. The healing process is complete with restoration of the medullary cavity.

The healing of a fracture may be impeded by a number of factors.

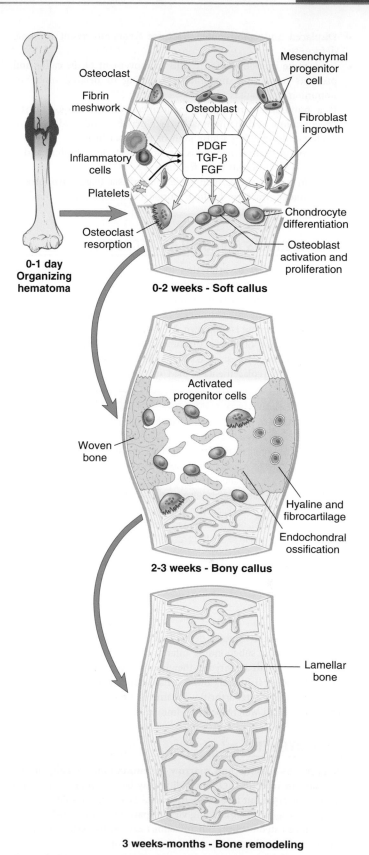

FIG. 19.11 The reaction to a fracture begins with an organizing hematoma. Within 2 weeks, the two ends of the bone are bridged by a fibrin meshwork in which osteoclasts, osteoblasts, and chondrocytes differentiate from precursors. These cells produce cartilage and bone matrix, which, with adequate immobilization, remodels into normal lamellar bone. *FGF,* Fibroblast growth factor; *PDGF,* platelet-derived growth factor; *TGF-β,* transforming growth factor-β.

- Displaced and comminuted fractures frequently result in some deformity.
- Inadequate immobilization results in movement of the callus and prevents its normal maturation, resulting in delayed union or nonunion.
- If a nonunion persists, the malformed callus undergoes cystic degeneration, and the luminal surface may become lined by synoviallike cells, creating a false joint or pseudoarthrosis.
- Infection of the fracture site is a serious obstacle to healing and is especially common in open fractures.
- Malnutrition, diabetes, and skeletal dysplasia (e.g., osteoporosis) also hinder fracture healing; surgical immobilization may be needed in such settings.

OSTEONECROSIS (AVASCULAR NECROSIS)

Osteonecrosis refers to infarction (ischemic necrosis) of bone and marrow. A diverse set of conditions predispose to bone ischemia, including vascular injury (e.g., trauma, vasculitis), drugs (e.g., corticosteroids), systemic disease (e.g., sickle cell crisis), and radiation. In about 25% of cases, the cause is unknown. Mechanisms of disease include mechanical disruption of vessels, thrombotic occlusion, and extravascular compression. Osteonecrosis peaks in middle adulthood and accounts for about 10% of hip replacements in the United States.

> ### MORPHOLOGY
>
> Bone infarcts may be medullary or subchondral. Regardless of etiology, medullary infarcts involve the trabecular bone and marrow but spare the cortex, which is protected by collateral blood flow from the periosteum. In subchondral infarcts, a triangular or wedge-shaped segment of tissue with the subchondral bone plate as its base undergoes necrosis. The overlying articular cartilage remains viable due to nutrients in the synovial fluid. Dead bone is recognized histologically by the presence of empty lacunae lacking osteocytes. The remaining viable trabeculae act as scaffolding for deposition of new bone, while osteoclasts resorb necrotic trabeculae. Because the pace of repair in subchondral infarcts is slow, there is collapse of the necrotic bone, with fracture and sloughing of the articular cartilage. (Fig. 19.12).

Clinical Features. Symptoms depend on the location and extent of the infarct. Typically, subchondral infarcts cause pain that is initially associated only with activity but then becomes constant. As mentioned above, subchondral infarcts often collapse and therefore may lead to severe, secondary osteoarthritis. Treatment ranges from conservative measures (limited weight bearing, immobilization) to surgery.

OSTEOMYELITIS

Osteomyelitis is bone and marrow inflammation, virtually always secondary to infection. Osteomyelitis may be a complication of any systemic infection but frequently manifests as a primary solitary focus. All types of organisms, including viruses, parasites, fungi, and bacteria, can produce osteomyelitis, but infections caused by certain pyogenic bacteria and mycobacteria are the most common.

Pyogenic Osteomyelitis

Pyogenic osteomyelitis is almost always caused by bacterial infection. Organisms may reach the bone by (1) hematogenous spread; (2) extension from a contiguous site; and (3) direct implantation after

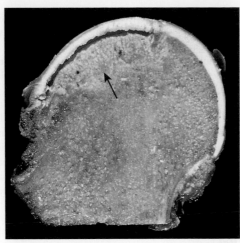

FIG. 19.12 Femoral head with a subchondral, wedge-shaped pale yellow area of osteonecrosis *(arrow)*. The space between the overlying articular cartilage and bone is caused by trabecular compression fractures.

compound fractures or orthopedic procedures. In otherwise healthy children, most osteomyelitis is hematogenous in origin and is more common in the long bones. In adults, osteomyelitis is most often a complication of open fractures, surgical procedures, or diabetes, the latter particularly predisposing to infections of the feet.

The etiologic agent varies depending on the anatomic location and clinical setting (e.g., diabetic foot, surgical site). Overall, *Staphylococcus aureus* is the most common pathogen identified in culture-positive pyogenic osteomyelitis. Staphylococcal cell wall proteins bind to bone matrix components, such as collagen, which facilitates adherence to bone. In the neonatal period, group B streptococci and *E. coli* are likely pathogens, whereas in older children gram-positive organisms such as *S. aureus* are the most likely cause. Mixed bacterial infections are common in the setting of direct spread, surgery, or open fractures. In patients with sickle cell anemia, areas of bone necrosis, which are susceptible to bacterial seeding, and loss of splenic function increases the risk of developing osteomyelitis, *Salmonella* and other gram-negative organisms being the most frequent culprits. Culture samples should be obtained from bone specimens whenever possible to increase the chances of identifying a causative organism. No specific organism is identified in nearly 50% of patients.

> ### MORPHOLOGY
>
> Changes associated with osteomyelitis depend on the stage (acute, subacute, or chronic) and location of the infection. In the acute phase, bacteria proliferate and induce a neutrophilic inflammatory reaction. Necrosis of bone cells and marrow ensues within the first 48 hours. The bacteria and inflammation spread longitudinally and radially throughout the Haversian systems to reach the periosteum. In children, the periosteum is loosely attached to the cortex and may be detached by the inflammatory infiltrate, leading to the formation of a subperiosteal abscess that may dissect along the bone surface. Lifting of the periosteum further impairs the blood supply to the affected region, contributing to the necrosis. Rupture of the periosteum may produce a soft tissue abscess that tracks to the skin, creating a draining sinus. Epiphyseal infection may spread through the articular surface or along capsular and tendoligamentous insertions into a joint, producing septic or suppurative arthritis, which can cause destruction of the articular cartilage and permanent disability.

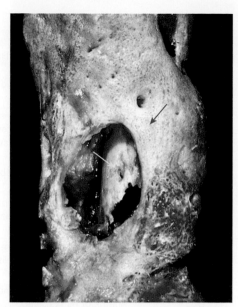

FIG. 19.13 Resected femur in a patient with draining osteomyelitis. The drainage tract in the subperiosteal shell of viable new bone (involucrum, *yellow arrow*) shows the original cortex (sequestrum, *red arrow*), which is necrotic.

> After the first week, chronic inflammatory cells release cytokines that stimulate osteoclastic bone resorption, ingrowth of fibrous tissue, and the deposition of reactive bone at the periphery. The dead bone is known as a **sequestrum.** The newly deposited bone can form a shell of living tissue, known as an **involucrum,** around the segment of devitalized infected bone (Fig. 19.13). The histologic findings of chronic osteomyelitis are more variable but typically involve marrow fibrosis, sequestrum, and an inflammatory infiltrate of lymphocytes and plasma cells.

Clinical Features. Hematogenous osteomyelitis may present acutely as a systemic illness with malaise, fever, chills, leukocytosis, and throbbing pain over the affected region. In other instances, the presentation is subtle, with only unexplained fever (infants) or localized pain (adults). Plain radiographs characteristically show a lytic focus of bone destruction and associated reactive bone; MRI is more specific and sensitive for identifying the changes of osteomyelitis. Biopsy and microbial cultures are required to identify the pathogen in most instances. The combination of antibiotics and surgical drainage is usually curative.

In 5% to 25% of cases, acute osteomyelitis fails to resolve, particularly in the setting of delayed diagnosis, weakened host defenses, extensive bone necrosis, or inadequate antibiotic therapy or surgical debridement. The course of such chronic infections may be punctuated by spontaneous acute flare-ups, sometimes after years of dormancy. Complications of chronic osteomyelitis include pathologic fracture, secondary (reactive) amyloidosis, endocarditis, sepsis, and the development of squamous cell carcinoma in draining sinus tracts or sarcoma in the infected bone.

Mycobacterial Osteomyelitis

Mycobacterial osteomyelitis, historically a problem in lower-income countries, has risen in incidence worldwide due to increases in immigration and in the number of patients who are immunocompromised.

Overall, approximately 1% to 3% of individuals with pulmonary or extrapulmonary tuberculosis develop osseous infection.

The organisms are usually bloodborne and originate from a focus of active visceral disease elsewhere. Direct extension (e.g., from a pulmonary focus into a rib or from tracheobronchial nodes into adjacent vertebrae) may also occur. The bone infection may persist for years before being recognized. Typically, affected individuals present with localized pain, low-grade fevers, chills, and weight loss. Infection is usually unifocal except in individuals who are immunocompromised. The principal histologic feature, the presence of caseating granulomas, is typical of tuberculosis at other sites. Mycobacterial osteomyelitis tends to be more destructive and resistant to control than pyogenic osteomyelitis.

The spine is involved in 40% of cases of mycobacterial osteomyelitis *(Pott disease)*. Infection breaks through intervertebral discs to affect multiple vertebrae and extends into the soft tissues where it may give rise to a psoas abscess (eFig. 19.2). Destruction of discs and vertebrae frequently results in permanent compression fractures that produce scoliosis or kyphosis and neurologic deficits secondary to spinal cord and nerve compression.

BONE TUMORS AND TUMORLIKE LESIONS

The rarity of primary bone tumors and the disfiguring surgery often required to treat bone malignancies make this group of disorders especially challenging. About 2400 primary bone sarcomas are diagnosed annually in the United States. Therapy aims to optimize survival while maintaining the function of affected body parts. The predilection of specific types of tumors for certain age groups and particular anatomic sites provides diagnostic clues. For example, osteosarcoma peaks during adolescence and most frequently involves the knee, whereas chondrosarcoma affects older adults and arises most often in the pelvis and proximal extremities.

Bone tumors may present in a variety of ways: benign lesions are often asymptomatic incidental findings while other tumors cause pain or are identified as a slow-growing mass or pathologic fracture. Radiographic imaging defines the location and extent of the tumor and can detect features that narrow the differential diagnosis, but biopsy is necessary for definitive diagnosis in almost all cases.

Bone tumors are classified according to the normal cell types they recapitulate or the matrix they produce (Table 19.1). Lesions that do not have normal tissue counterparts are grouped according to their clinicopathologic features. Benign tumors greatly outnumber malignant tumors and occur with greatest frequency within the first three decades of life. In older adults, a bone tumor is more likely to be malignant.

Bone-Forming Tumors

Tumors in this category produce unmineralized osteoid or mineralized woven bone.

Osteoid Osteoma and Osteoblastoma

Osteoid osteoma and osteoblastoma are benign bone-producing tumors that have similar histologic features but differ clinically and radiographically. By definition, osteoid osteomas are less than 2 cm in diameter. They are most common in young men. About 50% of cases involve the cortex of the femur or tibia. A thick rim of reactive cortical bone may be the only radiographic clue. Despite their small size, they present with severe nocturnal pain that is probably caused by prostaglandin E_2 produced by osteoblasts and is relieved by aspirin and other nonsteroidal antiinflammatory drugs. Osteoblastomas are

Table 19.1 Classification of Selected Primary Bone Tumors

Category	Behavior	Tumor Type	Common Locations	Age (yr)	Morphology
Cartilage forming	Benign	Osteochondroma	Metaphysis of long bones	10–30	Bony excrescence with cartilage cap
		Chondroma	Small bones of hands and feet	30–50	Circumscribed intramedullary hyaline cartilage nodule
	Malignant	Chondrosarcoma (conventional)	Pelvis, shoulder	40–60	Extends from medullary canal through cortex into soft tissue, chondrocytes with increased cellularity and atypia
Bone forming	Benign	Osteoid osteoma	Metaphysis of long bones	10–20	Cortical, interlacing microtrabeculae of woven bone
		Osteoblastoma	Vertebral column	10–20	Posterior elements of vertebra, histology similar to osteoid osteoma
	Malignant	Osteosarcoma	Metaphysis of distal femur, proximal tibia	10–20	Extends from medullary canal to lift periosteum, malignant cells producing woven bone
Unknown origin	Benign	Giant cell tumor	Epiphysis of long bones	20–40	Destroys medullary canal and cortex, sheets of osteoclasts
		Aneurysmal bone cyst	Proximal tibia, distal femur, vertebra	10–20	Hemorrhagic spaces separated by cellular, fibrous septa
	Malignant	Ewing sarcoma	Diaphysis of long bones	10–20	Sheets of primitive small round cells

Adapted from Unni KK, Inwards CY: *Dahlin's Bone Tumors,* ed 6, Philadelphia, 2010, Lippincott-Williams & Wilkins; by permission of Mayo Foundation.

larger than 2 cm and more frequently involve the posterior components of the vertebrae (laminae and pedicles). Any associated pain is unresponsive to aspirin and the tumor usually does not induce a marked bony reaction. Osteoid osteoma can be treated by radiofrequency ablation, whereas osteoblastoma is usually curetted or removed by en bloc excision.

> **MORPHOLOGY**
>
> Osteoid osteoma and osteoblastoma are round-to-oval masses of hemorrhagic gritty tan tissue. They are well circumscribed and composed of delicate interconnecting trabeculae of woven bone that are rimmed by a single layer of osteoblasts (Fig. 19.14). The stroma surrounding the neoplastic bone consists of loose connective tissue with abundant dilated and congested capillaries. The relatively small size, well-defined margins, and benign cytologic features of the neoplastic osteoblasts help distinguish these tumors from osteosarcoma.

Osteosarcoma

Osteosarcoma is a malignant tumor that produces osteoid matrix or mineralized bone. Excluding hematopoietic tumors, osteosarcoma is the most common primary malignant tumor of bone. The age distribution is bimodal, with about 75% occurring before 20 years of age, while a second smaller peak occurs in older adults in the setting of predisposing factors *(secondary osteosarcomas)* such as Paget disease, bone infarcts, and previous radiation. Men are more commonly affected than women (1.6 : 1). Although any bone can be involved, in adolescents tumors usually arise in the metaphyseal region of the long bones; almost 50% are near the knee in the distal femur or proximal tibia.

Osteosarcomas present as painful, progressively enlarging masses. A pathologic fracture may be the first indication. Typically, radiologic imaging reveals a large, destructive, mixed lytic and sclerotic mass with infiltrative margins (Fig. 19.15). The tumor frequently breaks through the cortex and lifts the periosteum, resulting in a triangular wedge of reactive subperiosteal bone formation *(Codman triangle).* This finding is indicative of an aggressive tumor but is not pathognomonic of osteosarcoma.

Pathogenesis. The peak incidence of osteosarcoma is during the adolescent growth spurt. The tumor occurs most frequently near the

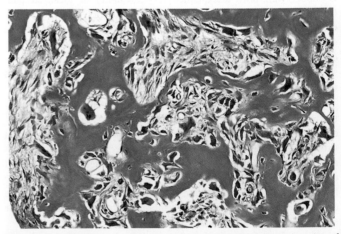

FIG. 19.14 Osteoid osteoma composed of anastomosing trabeculae of woven bone rimmed by osteoblasts and embedded in a hypocellular fibrovascular connective tissue stroma. (From Fletcher CD: *Diagnostic Histopathology of Tumors,* ed 5, Fig. 25.44B, Philadelphia, 2021, Elsevier.)

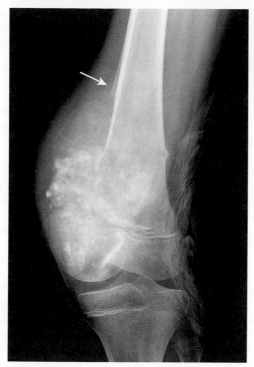

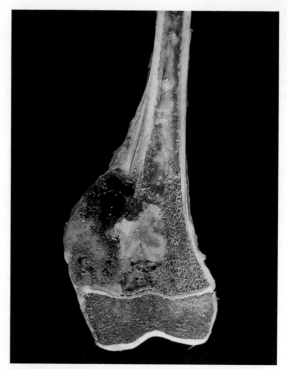

FIG. 19.15 Distal femur osteosarcoma with prominent bone formation extending into the soft tissue. The periosteum, which has been lifted, has laid down a triangular shell of reactive bone known as Codman triangle *(arrow)*. (From Czerniak B: *Dorfman and Czerniak's Bone Tumors,* ed 2, Fig. 5-15A, Philadelphia, 2016, Elsevier.)

FIG. 19.16 Osteosarcoma of distal femur. There is extensive cortical disruption and subperiosteal expansion. Tumor is confined to the metaphyseal side of the cartilaginous growth plate. Hemorrhagic area represents biopsy site. (From Czerniak B: *Dorfman and Czerniak's Bone Tumors,* ed 2, Fig. 5-17A, Philadelphia, 2016, Elsevier.)

growth plate of rapidly growing bones, where increased proliferation may predispose to mutations that drive oncogenesis. Osteosarcomas are characterized by complex karyotypes with numerous chromosomal aberrations and with mutations in well-known tumor suppressor genes and oncogenes (Chapter 6), including the following:

- *RB* mutations are present in up to 70% of sporadic osteosarcomas; germline *RB* mutations increase risk of osteosarcoma 1000-fold.
- *TP53* is mutated in the germline of patients with Li-Fraumeni syndrome, who have a greatly increased incidence of osteosarcoma. Mutations affecting the *TP53* gene are common in sporadic tumors.
- *MDM2* and *CDK4*, which inhibit p53 and RB function, respectively, are overexpressed in many low-grade osteosarcomas.
- *CDKN2A* (also known as *INK4a*), which encodes two tumor suppressors (p16 and p14), is inactivated in many osteosarcomas.
- *MYC* amplification is seen in up to half of cases and may be associated with a particularly poor prognosis.

MORPHOLOGY

Osteosarcomas are bulky tumors that are gritty and tan-white, often with areas of hemorrhage, and tend to destroy the surrounding cortices and invade into soft tissue (Fig. 19.16). Extensive intramedullary spread infiltrates and replaces the marrow. Infrequently, the tumor penetrates the epiphyseal plate and enters the adjacent joint.

The tumor cells demonstrate pleomorphism, large hyperchromatic nuclei, bizarre tumor giant cells, and abundant mitoses including abnormal (e.g., tripolar) forms. Extensive necrosis and intravascular invasion are also common. **Diagnosis of osteosarcoma requires the presence of malignant tumor cells producing unmineralized osteoid or mineralized bone** (Fig. 19.17), which is typically fine and lacelike but can also appear as broad sheets or primitive trabeculae.

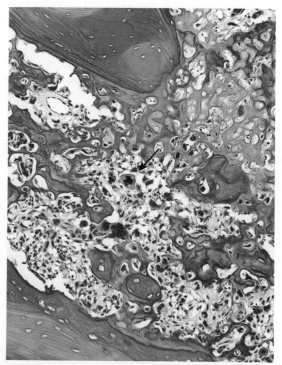

FIG. 19.17 Lacelike osteoid produced by pleomorphic malignant tumor cells bridges preexisting lamellar bone in an osteosarcoma. Note the abnormal mitotic figure *(arrow)*. (From Czerniak B: *Dorfman and Czerniak's Bone Tumors,* ed 2, Fig. 5-24D, Philadelphia, 2016, Elsevier.)

Clinical Features. All osteosarcomas are assumed to have occult metastases at the time of diagnosis. As a result, treatment generally includes neoadjuvant chemotherapy, surgery, and postoperative adjuvant chemotherapy. Chemotherapy has greatly improved osteosarcoma prognosis, with 5-year survival reaching 70% in individuals without overt metastases at initial diagnosis. Osteosarcoma metastasizes hematogenously to the lungs, bones, brain, and other sites. The outcome for those with clinically evident metastases, recurrent disease, or secondary osteosarcoma remains guarded, with a 5-year survival rate less than 20%.

Cartilage-Forming Tumors

These tumors are characterized by the formation of hyaline cartilage. Benign cartilaginous tumors are much more common than malignant ones.

Osteochondroma

Osteochondroma, or exostosis, is a benign, cartilage-capped tumor that arises from the bone surface. It may be sessile or pedunculated with a bony stalk. About 85% are solitary. The remainder are seen as part of the *multiple hereditary exostosis syndrome* (see later). Solitary osteochondromas are usually first diagnosed in late adolescence and early adulthood, whereas multiple osteochondromas present during childhood. Men are affected three times more often than women. Osteochondromas develop in bones of endochondral origin and arise from the metaphysis near the growth plate of long tubular bones, especially near the knee (Fig. 19.18). They are slow-growing masses that can be painful if they impinge on a nerve or if the stalk is fractured. In many cases they are detected incidentally. In multiple hereditary exostoses, the underlying bones may be bowed and shortened, reflecting an associated disturbance in epiphyseal growth.

Pathogenesis. Hereditary exostoses are associated with germline loss-of-function mutations in either the *EXT1* or the *EXT2* gene and subsequent loss of the remaining wild-type allele in chondrocytes of the growth plate. Reduced expression of *EXT1* or *EXT2* has also been observed in sporadic osteochondromas. These genes encode enzymes that synthesize heparan sulfate glycosaminoglycans. The reduced or abnormal glycosaminoglycans may prevent normal diffusion of Indian hedgehog a local regulator of cartilage growth, thereby disrupting hedgehog signaling and chondrocyte differentiation.

MORPHOLOGY

Osteochondromas range in size from 1 to 20 cm. The cap is composed of hyaline cartilage (Fig. 19.19) covered by perichondrium. The cartilage recapitulates the growth plate and undergoes endochondral ossification, with the newly made bone forming the inner portion of the head and stalk. The cortex of the stalk merges with the cortex of the host bone resulting in continuity between the medullary cavity of the osteochondroma and the host bone.

Clinical Features. Osteochondromas usually stop growing at the time of growth plate closure and, when symptomatic, are cured by simple excision. Secondary chondrosarcoma develops only rarely, usually in tumors associated with multiple hereditary exostosis.

Chondroma

Chondromas are benign tumors of hyaline cartilage that occur in bones of endochondral origin. Tumors can arise within the medullary cavity (enchondromas) or, rarely, on the bone surface (juxtacortical chondromas). Enchondromas are usually diagnosed in individuals 20 to 50 years of age. Typically, they appear as solitary metaphyseal lesions of the tubular bones of the hands and feet. Radiographs show a circumscribed lucency with central irregular calcifications, a sclerotic rim, and an intact cortex (Fig. 19.20). *Ollier disease* and *Maffucci syndrome* are disorders characterized by the development of multiple enchondromas (enchondromatosis).

Most sporadic enchondromas of large bones are asymptomatic and are detected incidentally, but they occasionally cause painful pathologic fractures.

Pathogenesis. Heterozygous mutations in the *IDH1* and *IDH2* genes, which encode two isoforms of isocitrate dehydrogenase, have been identified in syndromic and solitary chondromas. The mutations confer a new enzymatic activity on the IDH proteins that leads to the synthesis of 2-hydroxyglutarate. As discussed in Chapter 6, this "oncometabolite" interferes with regulation of DNA methylation, an effect that likely alters the expression of a number of cancer-associated genes.

MORPHOLOGY

Chondromas are usually smaller than 3 cm, gray-blue, and translucent. They are composed of benign-appearing chondrocytes embedded in well-circumscribed nodules of hyaline cartilage (Fig. 19.21). The peripheral portion of the nodules may undergo endochondral ossification, while the center may calcify and become infarcted. Syndromic enchondromas are sometimes more cellular and display more atypia than sporadic enchondromas.

Clinical Features. The growth potential of enchondromas is limited. Treatment depends on the clinical situation and usually includes

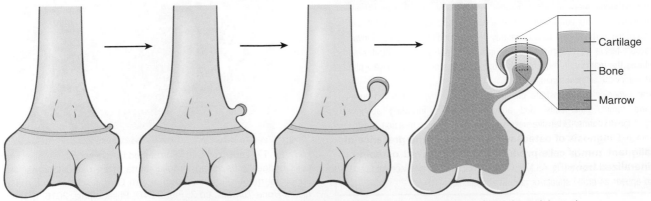

FIG. 19.18 The development of an osteochondroma, beginning with an outgrowth from the epiphyseal cartilage.

Cartilage

Bone

Marrow

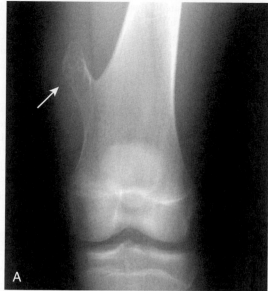

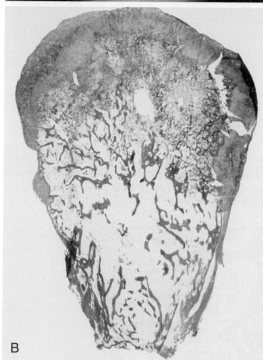

FIG. 19.19 Osteochondroma. (A) Radiograph of an osteochondroma *(arrow)* arising from the distal femur. (B) Whole mount section of narrow-pedicled osteochondroma with surface cartilage cap. (From Czerniak B: *Dorfman and Czerniak's Bone Tumors,* ed 2, Fig. 6-81D, Philadelphia, 2016, Elsevier, 2016.)

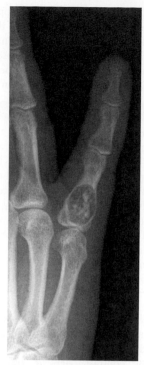

FIG. 19.20 Enchondroma of the proximal phalanx. The radiolucent nodule of cartilage with central calcification thins but does not penetrate the cortex.

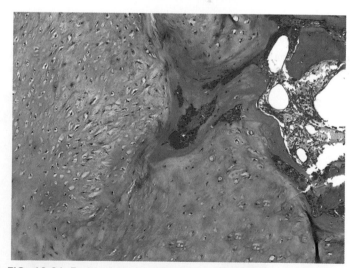

FIG. 19.21 Enchondroma composed of a nodule of hyaline cartilage encased by a thin layer of reactive bone.

observation or curettage. Solitary enchondromas rarely undergo sarcomatous transformation; by contrast, those associated with enchondromatosis do so more frequently.

Chondrosarcoma

Chondrosarcomas are malignant tumors that produce cartilage. They are the second most common malignant matrix-producing tumor of bone (after osteosarcoma). Chondrosarcomas are subclassified into *conventional* (hyaline cartilage—producing), *dedifferentiated, clear cell,* and *mesenchymal* type; approximately 90%

are of the conventional type hence our discussion will be focused on them. Patients are usually in their 40s or older, and men are affected twice as frequently as women. About 15% of conventional chondrosarcomas are secondary, arising from a preexisting enchondroma or osteochondroma. Conventional chondrosarcomas have a predilection for the axial skeleton, especially the pelvis, shoulder, and ribs. By contrast, osteosarcomas usually involve the metaphyseal region of long bones such as the femur and tibia. On imaging, the tumor may destroy the cortex and form a soft tissue mass; areas of calcified cartilage appear as flocculent densities.

Pathogenesis. Chondrosarcomas arising in multiple osteochondroma syndrome exhibit loss-of-function mutations in the *EXT1* and *EXT2* genes that regulate the synthesis of cartilaginous matrix proteins. Both chondromatosis-related and sporadic chondrosarcomas may have *IDH1* or *IDH2* mutations. Silencing of the *CDKN2A* tumor suppressor locus by DNA methylation is common in sporadic tumors.

MORPHOLOGY

Conventional chondrosarcomas are bulky tumors composed of nodules of glistening gray-white, translucent cartilage, along with gelatinous or myxoid areas (Fig. 19.22A). Focal calcifications are typically present, and central necrosis may create cystic spaces. Extracortical extension is common. Histologically, the cartilage infiltrates the marrow space and entraps normal bony trabeculae (Fig. 19.22B). Tumors vary in cellularity, cytologic atypia, and mitotic activity and are assigned a grade from 1 to 3, which correlates well with prognosis. Grade 1 tumors have low cellularity and contain neoplastic chondrocytes with plump vesicular nuclei and small nucleoli. By contrast, grade 3 chondrosarcomas are characterized by high cellularity, extreme pleomorphism with bizarre tumor giant cells, and frequent mitotic figures.

Clinical Features. Chondrosarcomas usually present as painful, progressively enlarging masses. Most conventional chondrosarcomas are grade 1 tumors, which rarely metastasize and have 5-year survival rates of 80% to 90%. By contrast, 70% of grade 3 tumors spread hematogenously (typically to the lungs) and have an overall 5-year survival of less than 50%. The treatment for conventional chondrosarcoma is wide surgical excision.

Tumors of Unknown Origin

Ewing Sarcoma

Ewing sarcoma is a malignant tumor composed of small cells and is characterized by translocations involving the *EWSR1* gene on chromosome 22. Ewing sarcoma accounts for approximately 10% of primary malignant bone tumors and follows osteosarcoma as the second most common bone sarcoma in children. Eighty percent of patients are younger than 20 years and there is a slight male predominance. Ewing sarcoma is quite uncommon: about 200 cases are diagnosed in the United States each year.

Pathogenesis. Nearly all (>90%) Ewing sarcomas contain a balanced translocation generating an in-frame fusion of the *EWSR1* gene on chromosome 22 and the *FLI1* gene on chromosome 11. This gene encodes a chimeric EWS/FLI1 protein that binds to chromatin and dysregulates transcription, leading to uncontrolled growth and abnormal differentiation through uncertain mechanisms. The cell of origin is not certain, but mesenchymal stem cells and primitive neuroectodermal cells are the most likely candidates.

MORPHOLOGY

Ewing sarcoma is usually diaphyseal and arises in the medullary cavity and invades the cortex, periosteum, and soft tissue. The periosteal reaction to the advancing tumor produces layers of reactive bone deposited with a characteristic **onion-skin appearance.** Grossly, the tumor is soft and tan-white and frequently displays areas of hemorrhage and necrosis. It is one of the small round blue cell tumors that occur in children (Chapter 4). Microscopically, there are sheets of uniform small round cells that are slightly larger and more cohesive than lymphocytes (Fig. 19.23). They have scant cytoplasm, which may appear clear because it is rich in glycogen. **Homer-Wright rosettes** (circular groupings of cells with a central fibrillary core) may be present. The tumor cells do not produce bone or cartilage.

Clinical Features. Tumors present as painful, enlarging masses that usually arise in the diaphysis of long tubular bones, but 20% are extraskeletal. The affected site is frequently tender, warm, and swollen.

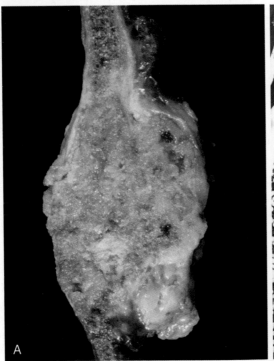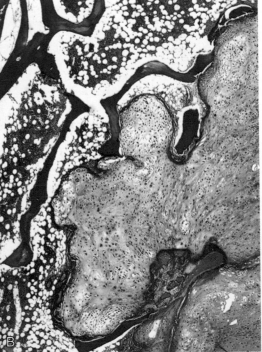

FIG. 19.22 Chondrosarcoma. (A) Nodules of hyaline cartilage permeate the medullary cavity of the sternum, grow through the cortex, and form a relatively well-circumscribed soft tissue mass in the parasternal soft tissue. (B) Chondrosarcoma permeating through preexisting trabecular bone. (From Czerniak B: *Dorfman and Czerniak's Bone Tumors,* ed 2, Figs. 7-10A, 7-14C, Philadelphia, 2016, Elsevier.)

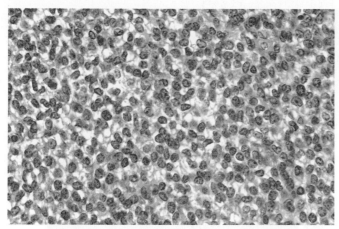

FIG. 19.23 Ewing sarcoma composed of sheets of small round cells with minimal clear cytoplasm.

Radiographs show a destructive lytic tumor with permeative margins that extend into the surrounding soft tissues. Although Ewing sarcoma is an aggressive malignancy, treatment with neoadjuvant chemotherapy followed by surgical excision with or without radiation has achieved 75% 5-year survival and 50% long-term cure rates.

Giant Cell Tumor

Giant cell tumor is characterized by the presence of multinucleate osteoclast-type giant cells, and location in epiphyses. Although giant cell tumors are benign, they can be locally aggressive. This uncommon tumor usually arises in the third through fifth decades of life.

Pathogenesis. Most of the cells within giant cell tumors are nonneoplastic osteoclasts and their precursors. The neoplastic cells are primitive osteoblast precursors that express high levels of RANKL, which promotes the proliferation of osteoclast precursors and their differentiation into mature osteoclasts. The absence of normal feedback between osteoblasts and osteoclasts results in localized, highly destructive, bone resorption.

MORPHOLOGY

Giant cell tumors typically destroy the overlying cortex, producing a bulging soft tissue mass bounded by a thin shell of reactive bone (Fig. 19.24). Grossly, they are red-brown masses that frequently undergo cystic degeneration. Microscopically, the tumor consists of numerous reactive osteoclast-type giant cells with 100 or more nuclei admixed with less conspicuous, uniform, oval mononuclear neoplastic cells (Fig. 19.25).

Clinical Features. Giant cell tumors arise in the epiphyses of long bones, most commonly the distal femur and proximal tibia. This location is distinctive, setting it apart from most other bone tumors. Their location near joints may cause arthritis-like symptoms. Occasionally, they present with pathologic fractures. These tumors are typically treated with curettage, but 40% to 60% recur locally. The RANKL inhibitor denosumab is an effective alternative to surgery in cases in which resection would be deforming or lead to loss of function. Although up to 4% of patients develop lung metastases, the clinical behavior of these foci recapitulates that of the original tumor and most patients are cured by excision of metastases.

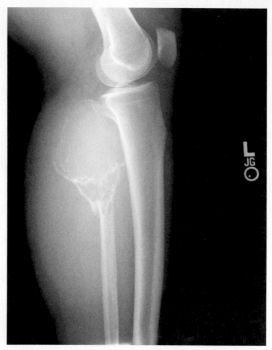

FIG. 19.24 Radiographically, giant cell tumor of the proximal fibula is predominantly lytic and expansile with destruction of the cortex. A pathologic fracture is also present.

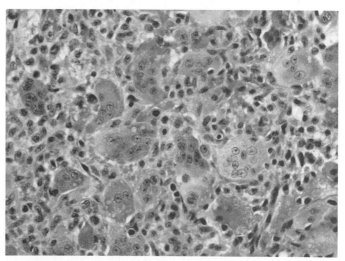

FIG. 19.25 Giant cell tumor illustrating an abundance of multinucleate giant cells with background mononuclear stromal cells.

Aneurysmal Bone Cyst

Aneurysmal bone cyst (ABC) is characterized by multiloculated blood-filled spaces. All age groups are affected, but most cases present in adolescence. It develops most frequently in the femur, tibia, and vertebral body posterior elements.

Pathogenesis. The spindle-shaped cells of ABC are of uncertain origin and frequently demonstrate rearrangements of chromosome 17p13, resulting in fusion of the coding region of the *USP6* gene to regulatory elements, most commonly of the *COL1A1* gene, leading to USP6 overexpression. The *USP6* gene encodes a deubiquitinating enzyme that upregulates the activity of the transcription factor NF-κB. This in

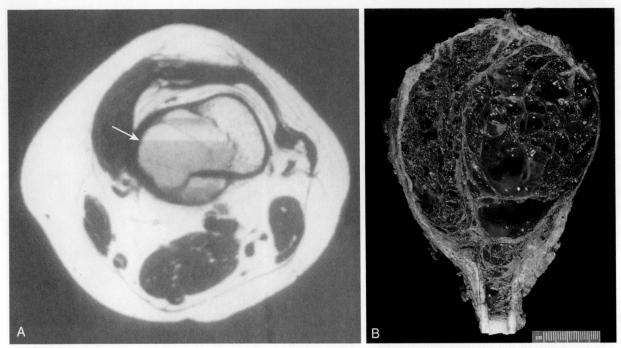

FIG. 19.26 Aneurysmal bone cyst. (A) Axial magnetic resonance image demonstrating characteristic fluid-fluid levels *(arrow)*. (B) Gross appearance of aneurysmal bone cyst. The lesion appears hemorrhagic and spongelike in this bisected portion of proximal fibula. (From Czerniak B: *Dorfman and Czerniak's Bone Tumors*, ed 2, Figs. 15-5C, 5-11B, Philadelphia, 2016, Elsevier.)

turn increases the expression of genes encoding proteins such as matrix metalloproteases that lead to cystic bone resorption.

MORPHOLOGY

Radiographically, ABC is usually an eccentric, expansile, lytic, metaphyseal lesion with well-defined margins. Computed tomography and magnetic resonance imaging may demonstrate internal septa and characteristic fluid-fluid levels (Fig. 19.26A). Grossly, it consists of multiple blood-filled cystic spaces separated by thin, tan-white septa (Fig. 19.26B). The septa lack an endothelial lining and are composed of plump uniform fibroblasts, multinucleate osteoclast-like giant cells, and reactive woven bone (Fig. 19.27).

Clinical Features. ABC presents with localized pain and swelling. Although benign, it is locally aggressive. Treatment of ABC is by curettage or excision. Recurrence occurs in 10% to 50% of cases.

Lesions Simulating Primary Neoplasms

Fibrous Cortical Defect and Nonossifying Fibroma

Fibrous cortical defects are common developmental abnormalities in which fibrous connective tissue replaces bone. These lesions are present in up to 50% of children older than 2 years of age and typically present as an incidental finding in adolescents. The vast majority arise eccentrically in the metaphysis of the distal femur and proximal tibia; almost half are bilateral or multiple. Most are less than 0.5 cm in diameter, but those that grow to 5 or 6 cm are classified as *nonossifying fibromas*. Both fibrous cortical defects and nonossifying fibromas are sharply demarcated radiolucent masses surrounded by a thin rim of sclerosis (Fig. 19.28). This appearance is sufficiently specific that biopsy is rarely necessary.

MORPHOLOGY

Nonossifying fibromas are gray to yellow-brown cellular lesions containing fibroblasts and macrophages. The cytologically bland fibroblasts are frequently arranged in a storiform (pinwheel) pattern, and the macrophages may take the form of clustered cells with foamy cytoplasm or multinucleate giant cells (Fig. 19.29). Hemosiderin is commonly present.

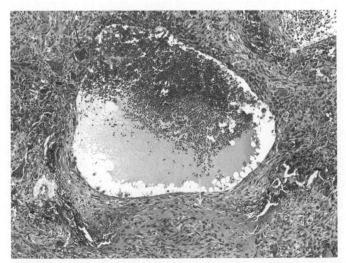

FIG. 19.27 Aneurysmal bone cyst with blood-filled cystic space surrounded by a fibrous wall containing proliferating fibroblasts, reactive woven bone *(yellow arrow)*, and osteoclast-type giant cells *(red arrows)*.

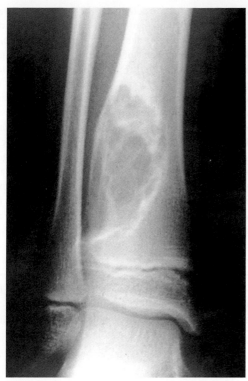

FIG. 19.28 Nonossifying fibroma of the distal tibia metaphysis producing an eccentric lobulated radiolucency surrounded by a sclerotic margin.

Clinical Features. Most small lesions resolve spontaneously within several years. The few that progressively enlarge may present with pathologic fracture and require biopsy to exclude other types of tumors. They are treated with curettage and may require bone grafting.

Fibrous Dysplasia

Fibrous dysplasia is a benign tumor that results from a localized developmental arrest; all components of normal bone are present, but they do not differentiate into mature structures. The lesions arise during skeletal development, and they may be sporadic or syndromic. They may present as follows:

- *Monostotic:* involvement of a single bone
- *Polyostotic:* involvement of multiple bones
- *Mazabraud syndrome:* fibrous dysplasia and soft tissue myxoma
- *McCune-Albright syndrome:* polyostotic fibrous dysplasia, café-au-lait skin pigmentations, and endocrine abnormalities, especially precocious puberty

Pathogenesis. All forms of fibrous dysplasia result from somatic gain-of-function mutations in *GNAS1*, a gene that is also mutated in pituitary adenomas (Chapter 18). The mutations produce a constitutively active G_s-protein that increases the cellular levels of cAMP, which promotes cellular proliferation and disrupts osteoblast differentiation. The phenotype depends on the stage of embryogenesis when the mutation is acquired and on the proportion and position of mesenchymal cells that harbor the mutation.

MORPHOLOGY

Fibrous dysplasia gives rise to intramedullary lytic lesions that may expand and cause bowing and cortical thinning. Periosteal reaction is usually absent. Lesional tissue is tan-white and gritty on gross examination and is composed of curvilinear trabeculae of woven bone without a rim of osteoblasts and surrounded by a moderately cellular fibroblastic proliferation (Fig. 19.30). Cystic degeneration, hemorrhage, and foamy macrophages are other common findings.

Clinical Features. Monostotic fibrous dysplasia often stops enlarging at the time of growth plate closure. The lesion is frequently asymptomatic, but it may cause pain and fracture. Symptomatic lesions are treated by curettage, but recurrence is common.

Polyostotic fibrous dysplasia may cause problems into adulthood. Limb girdle involvement can cause extensive deformities and fractures. Bisphosphonates can be used to reduce the severity of the bone pain. A rare complication, usually of polyostotic involvement, is malignant transformation into a sarcoma.

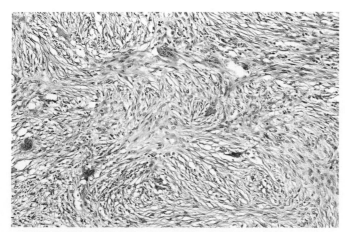

FIG. 19.29 Storiform pattern created by benign spindle cells with scattered osteoclast-type giant cells characteristic of a fibrous cortical defect.

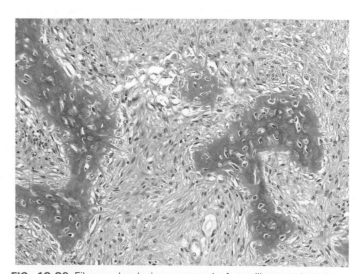

FIG. 19.30 Fibrous dysplasia composed of curvilinear trabeculae of woven bone that lack conspicuous osteoblastic rimming and arise in a background of fibrous tissue.

Metastatic Tumors

Metastatic tumors are the most common form of skeletal malignancy, greatly outnumbering primary bone cancers. The pathways of tumor spread to bone include (1) direct extension; (2) lymphatic or hematogenous dissemination; and (3) intraspinal seeding (via the Batson plexus of veins). Any cancer can spread to bone, but in adults more than 75% of skeletal metastases originate from cancers of the prostate, breast, kidney, and lung. In children, neuroblastoma, Wilms tumor, and rhabdomyosarcoma are the most common sources of metastases to bone.

Skeletal metastases are typically multifocal and involve the axial skeleton, especially the vertebral column. The radiographic appearance of metastases may be purely *lytic* (bone destroying), purely *blastic* (bone forming), or *mixed.* Some tumors like prostatic cancer typically produce osteoblastic metastases, whereas others such as renal cell carcinomas and breast cancers are most often associated with lytic lesions. Crosstalk between metastatic cancer cells and native bone cells accounts for these varied features. Tumor cells may secrete substances such as prostaglandins, cytokines, and PTH-like peptide that stimulate osteoclast activity; in turn, the resorption of bone may release matrix-bound growth factors that contribute to tumor cell growth. Sclerotic metastases may result from tumor cell secretion of WNT proteins that stimulate osteoblasts to lay down new bone.

The presence of bone metastases generally carries a poor prognosis, but metastatic breast and prostate cancers can sometimes be held in check for many years with hormone therapy. For other cancers, treatment options include systemic chemotherapy or immunotherapy, localized radiation, and bisphosphonates. Surgery may be necessary to stabilize pathologic fractures.

JOINTS

Joints allow movement while providing mechanical stability. They are classified as solid (nonsynovial) and cavitated (synovial). The solid joints, also known as *synarthroses,* provide structural stability and allow only minimal movement. They lack a joint space and include fibrous synarthroses of the cranial sutures and cartilaginous synarthroses between the sternum and the ribs and between the bones of the pelvis. Synovial joints, by contrast, have a joint space that allows a wide range of motion. Synovial membranes enclose these joints. The membranes are lined by *type A synoviocytes,* which are specialized macrophages with phagocytic activity, and *type B synoviocytes,* which are similar to fibroblasts and synthesize hyaluronic acid and various proteins. The synovial lining lacks a basement membrane, thereby allowing the efficient exchange of nutrients, wastes, and gases between blood and synovial fluid. Synovial fluid is a plasma filtrate containing hyaluronic acid produced by synovial cells that acts as a viscous lubricant and provides nutrition for the articular cartilage.

Hyaline cartilage is a unique connective tissue that serves as an elastic shock absorber and provides a wear-resistant surface. It is composed of type II collagen, proteoglycans, and chondrocytes and lacks blood and lymphatic vessels and innervation. The collagen resists tensile stresses and transmits vertical loads. The water and proteoglycans resist compression and limit friction. The chondrocytes synthesize the matrix and secrete enzymes that remodel it. These degradative enzymes are produced in inactive forms that are normally held in check by inhibitors that are also made by chondrocytes.

ARTHRITIS

Arthritis is inflammation of joints. The most common forms of arthritis are osteoarthritis and rheumatoid arthritis, which differ in their pathogenesis and clinical and pathologic manifestations (Table 19.2). Other types of arthritis are caused by immune reactions, infections, and crystal deposition.

Osteoarthritis

Osteoarthritis (OA), also called degenerative joint disease, is characterized by degeneration of cartilage that results in structural and functional failure of synovial joints. It is the most common disease of joints. Although the term osteoarthritis implies an inflammatory disease, it is primarily a degenerative disorder of articular cartilage, with inflammation acting as a secondary contributor.

In most instances, OA appears insidiously, without apparent initiating cause, as an aging phenomenon (*idiopathic* or *primary osteoarthritis*). In these cases, the disease is oligoarticular, affecting a few joints, notably weight-bearing joints. In about 5% of cases, OA appears in younger individuals with a predisposing condition such as joint deformity, previous joint injury, or an underlying systemic disease (e.g., diabetes, obesity) that places joints at risk. In these settings, the disease is called *secondary osteoarthritis.* The prevalence of OA increases exponentially beyond the age of 50; about 40% of people older than 70 are affected.

Table 19.2 Comparative Features of Osteoarthritis and Rheumatoid Arthritis

	Osteoarthritis	Rheumatoid Arthritis
Primary pathogenic abnormality	Mechanical injury to articular cartilage	Autoimmunity
Role of inflammation	May be secondary; inflammatory mediators exacerbate cartilage damage	Primary: cartilage destruction is caused by T cells and antibodies reactive with joint antigens
Joints involved	Primarily weight bearing (knees, hips)	Often begins with small joints of fingers; progression leads to involvement of multiple joints
Pathology	Cartilage degeneration and fragmentation, bone spurs, subchondral cysts; minimal inflammation	Inflammatory pannus invading and destroying cartilage; severe chronic inflammation; joint fusion (ankylosis)
Serum antibodies	None	Various, including ACPA, rheumatoid factor
Involvement of other organs	No	Yes (lungs, heart, other organs)

ACPA, Anticitrullinated peptide antibody.

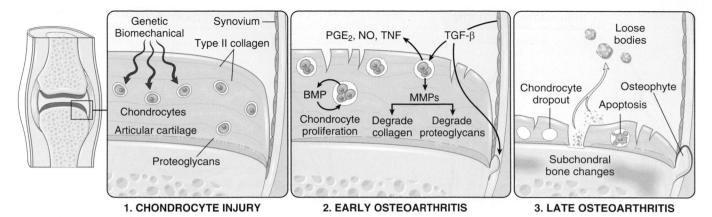

1. CHONDROCYTE INJURY   **2. EARLY OSTEOARTHRITIS**   **3. LATE OSTEOARTHRITIS**

FIG. 19.31 Schematic view of osteoarthritis (OA). OA is thought to be initiated by chondrocyte injury *(1)* in a genetically predisposed patient leading to changes in the extracellular matrix. *(2)* Although chondrocytes may proliferate and attempt to repair damaged matrix, continued degradation exceeds repair in early OA. *(3)* Late OA is evidenced by loss of both matrix and chondrocytes with subchondral bone damage. *BMP,* Bone morphogenetic protein; *MMPs,* matrix metalloproteinases; *NO,* nitric oxide; *PGE₂,* prostaglandin E₂; *TGF-β,* transforming growth factor β; *TNF,* tumor necrosis factor.

Pathogenesis. OA stems from degeneration of articular cartilage and its disordered repair. Biomechanical stress is the principal pathogenic mechanism underlying the damage, but genetic factors, including polymorphisms in genes encoding components of the matrix and signaling molecules, may predispose to chondrocyte injury and matrix alterations (Fig. 19.31). In the early stages of OA, chondrocytes proliferate, likely in response to matrix loss, and secrete matrix metalloproteinases (MMPs) that degrade the type II collagen network. Concurrently, the water content of the matrix increases and the concentration of proteoglycans decreases. The normally horizontally arranged collagen type II fibers are cleaved, yielding fissures and clefts at the articular surface (Fig. 19.32A), which becomes granular and soft. Cytokines and diffusible factors from chondrocytes, synovial cells, and macrophages recruited in response to the joint damage, particularly TGF-β (which induces the production of MMPs), IL-1, IL-6, prostaglandins, and nitric oxide, are also implicated in OA, and chronic, low-level inflammation contributes to cartilage damage and disease progression. Bone morphogenetic proteins and TGF-β appear to play a central role in the development of osteophytes, bony outgrowths at the periphery of the articular surface.

> ### MORPHOLOGY
>
> Advanced disease is characterized by chondrocyte loss, severe matrix degradation and full-thickness sloughing of portions of cartilage. The dislodged pieces of cartilage and subchondral bone tumble into the joint, forming loose bodies **(joint mice)**. The exposed subchondral bone plate becomes the new articular surface, and friction with the opposing surface burnishes the exposed bone, giving it the appearance of polished ivory **(bone eburnation)** (Fig. 19.32B). Small fractures through the articulating bone are common and the fracture gaps allow synovial fluid to be forced into the subchondral regions in a one-way, ball valve—like mechanism, leading to the formation of fibrous-walled cysts. Outgrowths **(osteophytes)** develop at the margins of the articular surface and are capped by fibrocartilage and hyaline cartilage that gradually ossify. The synovium is usually only mildly congested and fibrotic and may contain scattered chronic inflammatory cells. These morphologic alterations are quite different from those in rheumatoid arthritis (discussed later), summarized in Fig. 19.33.

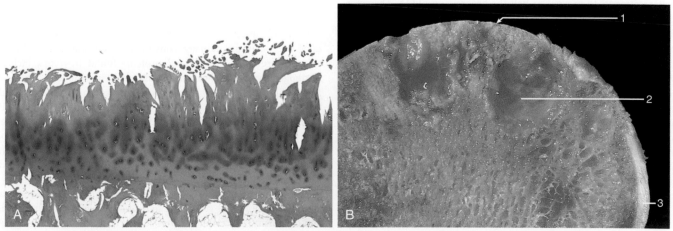

FIG. 19.32 Osteoarthritis. (A) Histologic demonstration of the characteristic fibrillation of the articular cartilage. (B) Eburnated articular surface exposing subchondral bone *(1)*, subchondral cyst *(2)*, and residual articular cartilage *(3)*.

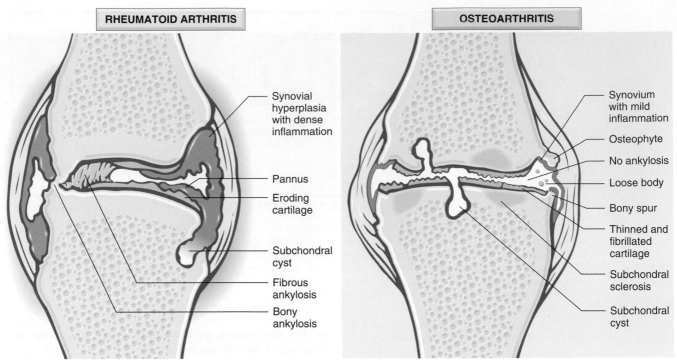

FIG. 19.33 Comparison of the morphologic features of rheumatoid arthritis and osteoarthritis.

Clinical Features. Primary OA usually presents in patients in their 50s. If a young person has significant manifestations of OA, a search for an underlying cause is warranted. Characteristic symptoms include joint pain that worsens with use, morning stiffness, crepitus, and limitation of range of movement. Impingement on spinal foramina by osteophytes results in cervical and lumbar nerve root compression and radicular pain, muscle spasms, muscle atrophy, and neurologic deficits. The joints commonly involved include the hips, knees, lower lumbar and cervical vertebrae, proximal and distal interphalangeal joints of the fingers, first carpometacarpal joints, and first tarsometatarsal joints. *Heberden nodes*, prominent osteophytes at the distal interphalangeal joints, are more common in women. With time, joint deformity may occur, but unlike in rheumatoid arthritis (discussed next) joint fusion does not take place. The level of disease severity detected radiographically does not correlate well with pain and disability. There are no treatments to prevent or halt the progression of OA. Therapies include pain management, NSAIDs to reduce inflammation, intraarticular corticosteroids, activity modification, and, for severe cases, joint replacement.

Rheumatoid Arthritis

Rheumatoid arthritis (RA) is a chronic autoimmune disorder that principally attacks the joints, producing a nonsuppurative proliferative and inflammatory synovitis. RA often progresses to the destruction of the articular cartilage and, in some cases, joint fusion (ankylosis). Extraarticular lesions may occur in the skin, heart, blood vessels, and lungs. The prevalence in the United States is 0.25% to 1%, and it is three times more common in women than in men. The peak incidence is in the third to fifth decades of life.

Pathogenesis. **The autoimmune response in RA is initiated by CD4+ helper T cells reacting against a joint antigen.** The pathologic changes are the result of inflammation caused by CD4+ T cells

and perhaps antibodies (Fig. 19.34). Numerous joint antigens have been proposed as initiators and targets of the pathologic immune response, including collagen and chemically modified peptides.

CD4+ helper T lymphocytes and other cells produce multiple cytokines that contribute to joint injury, including:
- *TNF, IL-1, and IL-6 from macrophages* recruit and activate leukocytes and other cells and stimulate the secretion of proteases that destroy hyaline cartilage. Based on the therapeutic efficacy of TNF antagonists, this cytokine is believed to be the key mediator of inflammation and joint damage.
- *IL-17 from Th17 cells* recruits neutrophils and monocytes.
- *RANKL expressed on activated T cells* stimulates osteoclasts, which cause bone resorption.

Antibodies may also contribute to joint damage. The synovium in RA often contains lymphoid follicles with germinal centers and abundant plasma cells. Many of the serum autoantibodies detected in patients are specific for *citrullinated peptides* in which arginine residues are posttranslationally converted to citrulline. The modified epitopes are present in several proteins found in joints, including fibrinogen, type II collagen, α-enolase, and vinculin. *Anticitrullinated peptide antibody* (ACPA) is a diagnostic marker that can be detected in the serum of up to 70% of RA patients. Some data suggest that ACPAs contribute to disease severity and persistence. About 80% of patients also have serum IgM or IgA autoantibodies that bind to the Fc portions of IgG. These autoantibodies are called *rheumatoid factor*; their role in disease progression is unclear, and they may also be detected in some individuals without RA.

As in other autoimmune diseases, genetic predisposition and environmental factors contribute to disease development, progression, and chronicity. It is estimated that 50% of the risk of developing RA is related to inherited genetic susceptibility. The HLA-DR4 allele is associated with ACPA-positive RA. Evidence suggests that an epitope

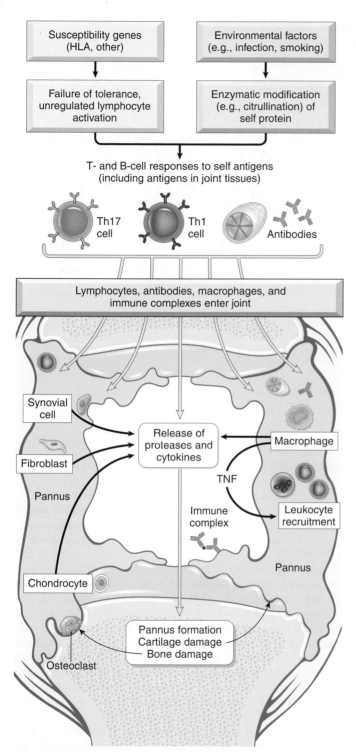

FIG. 19.34 Major processes involved in the pathogenesis of rheumatoid arthritis. *HLA*, Human leukocyte antigen; *TNF*, tumor necrosis factor.

promote citrullination of self proteins, creating new epitopes that trigger autoimmune reactions.

MORPHOLOGY

RA typically manifests as symmetric arthritis affecting the small joints of the hands and feet. The synovium becomes edematous, thickened, and hyperplastic, transforming its smooth contour to one covered by delicate and bulbous villi (Fig. 19.35A, B). The characteristic histologic features include (1) **synoviocyte hyperplasia** and proliferation; (2) **dense inflammatory infiltrates** of CD4+ helper T cells, B cells, plasma cells, and macrophages (Fig. 19.35C); (3) increased vascularity resulting from angiogenesis; (4) neutrophils and aggregates of organizing fibrin on the synovial and joint surfaces; and (5) osteoclastic activity in underlying bone, resulting in periarticular erosions and subchondral cysts. Together, these changes produce a **pannus,** a mass of edematous synovium, inflammatory cells, granulation tissue, and fibroblasts that grows over and erodes the articular cartilage. In advanced cases, the pannus can bridge the bones resulting in **fibrous ankylosis,** which may later ossify, giving rise to **bony ankylosis** (see Fig. 19.33).

Rheumatoid nodules are an infrequent manifestation of RA and typically occur in the subcutaneous tissue of the forearm, elbows, occiput, and lumbosacral area as small, firm, nontender oval masses. Microscopically, they resemble necrotizing granulomas (Fig. 19.36). Rarely, RA can involve the lungs (rheumatoid nodules, interstitial lung disease).

Clinical Features. RA can be distinguished from other forms of polyarticular inflammatory arthritis by the presence of ACPA and by characteristic radiographic findings. In about half of patients, RA begins slowly and insidiously with malaise, fatigue, and generalized musculoskeletal pain. After several weeks to months, the joints become involved. The pattern of joint involvement is generally symmetrical and the hands and feet, wrists, ankles, elbows, and knees are most commonly affected. The metacarpophalangeal and proximal interphalangeal joints are frequently involved (in contrast to OA; see earlier). While laboratory tests for ACPA and RF aid in diagnosis, about 20% of patients with RA are seronegative; in these cases, diagnosis is based on the clinical findings.

Involved joints are swollen, warm, and painful. In contrast to OA, the joints are stiff when the patient rises in the morning or following inactivity. The typical case pursues a waxing and waning course marked by progressive joint enlargement and decreased range of motion. In a minority of patients, especially those who are seronegative, the disease may stabilize or even regress.

Inflammation in the tendons, ligaments, and occasionally the adjacent skeletal muscle frequently accompanies the arthritis, leading to the characteristic ulnar deviation of the fingers and flexion-hyperextension of the fingers (producing the *swan-neck deformity* and the *boutonnière deformity*, respectively) (Fig 19.37A). Radiographic hallmarks are joint effusions, juxtaarticular osteopenia, erosion and narrowing of the joint space, and loss of articular cartilage (Fig. 19.37B).

The treatment for RA consists of corticosteroids, other immunosuppressants such as methotrexate, and, most notably, TNF antagonists. However, anti-TNF agents are not curative, and patients must be maintained on TNF antagonists to avoid disease flares. Long-term treatment with TNF antagonists predisposes individuals to infections with opportunistic organisms such as *M. tuberculosis.* Other biologic

on a citrullinated protein, vinculin, mimics an epitope on many microbes and can be presented by the class II HLA-DR4 molecule (molecular mimicry).

Many candidate environmental factors have been postulated. Insults such as infection (including periodontitis) and smoking may

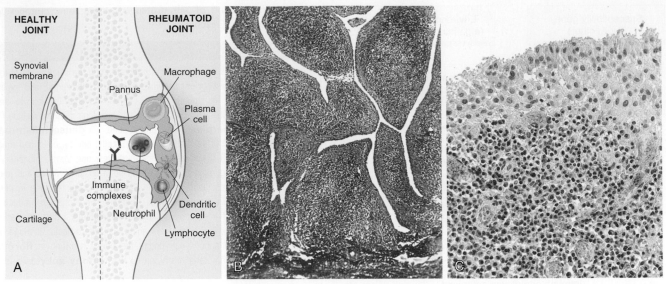

FIG. 19.35 Rheumatoid arthritis. (A) Schematic view of the joint lesion. (B) Low magnification shows marked synovial hypertrophy with formation of villi and a dense lymphocytic infiltrate. (C) At higher magnification, numerous plasma cells are seen beneath the hyperplastic synovium. (A, Modified from Feldmann M: Development of anti-TNF therapy for rheumatoid arthritis. *Nat Rev Immunol* 2:364, 2002.)

agents that interfere with T- and B-lymphocyte responses have also been approved for therapeutic use.

Juvenile Idiopathic Arthritis

Juvenile idiopathic arthritis (JIA) is a heterogeneous group of disorders of unknown cause, likely autoimmune, that present with childhood onset arthritis and usually signs of systemic inflammation. It includes several subsets that are not well defined but include systemic (polyarticular) and oligoarticular forms; they are distinctive not only in age of onset but also in clinical course.

Seronegative Spondyloarthropathies

The spondyloarthropathies are a heterogeneous group of disorders that share the following features:

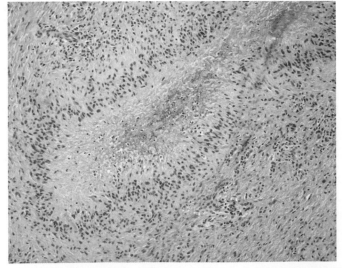

FIG. 19.36 Rheumatoid nodule composed of central necrosis rimmed by palisaded histiocytes.

- *Absence of rheumatoid factor*
- *Pathologic changes in the ligamentous attachments* rather than synovium
- *Sacroiliac and vertebral joint involvement*
- *Association with HLA-B27*
- *Bony proliferation leading to ankylosis*

The manifestations are immune mediated and are triggered by a T-cell response presumably directed against an undefined antigen, possibly infectious, that may cross-react with antigens expressed on cells of the musculoskeletal system. Two disorders in this group are described next.

Ankylosing spondylitis, the prototypical spondyloarthritis, causes destruction of articular cartilage and bony ankylosis, especially of the sacroiliac and vertebral apophyseal joints. The disease becomes symptomatic in the second and third decades of life as lower back pain and spinal immobility. Involvement of peripheral joints, such as the hips, knees, and shoulders, occurs in at least one-third of affected individuals. Approximately 90% of patients are HLA-B27 positive. The role of HLA-B27 is unknown; it is presumably related to the ability of this MHC variant to present one or more antigens that trigger the disease, but neither the antigen nor the pathogenic immune cell is known.

Reactive arthritis is defined as mono- or oligoarticular arthritis arising days to weeks after an enteric (e.g., *Shigella, Salmonella, Yersinia, Campylobacter,* and *Clostridioides difficile*) or genitourinary (e.g., *Chlamydia*) infection. A subset of patients present with a triad of symptoms: arthritis, urethritis or cervicitis, and conjunctivitis. Culture of joint fluid is negative for pathogens. Most affected individuals are young adults, and HLA-B27 positivity is common. The disease is probably caused by an autoimmune reaction initiated by the infection. Within several weeks of the initial infection, patients experience low back pain. The ankles, knees, and feet are affected most often, frequently in an asymmetric pattern. Patients with severe chronic disease have involvement of the spine that is indistinguishable from ankylosing spondylitis.

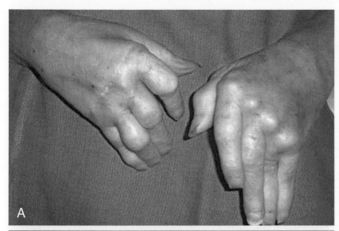

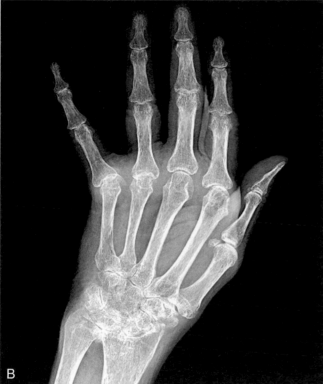

FIG. 19.37 Rheumatoid arthritis of the hand. (A) Prominent ulnar deviation of the hands and flexion-hyperextension deformities of the fingers. (B) Radiologic features include diffuse osteopenia; marked loss of the joint spaces of the carpal, metacarpal, phalangeal, and interphalangeal joints; periarticular bony erosions; and ulnar drift of the fingers. (A, From Klatt EC: *Robbins and Cotran Atlas of Pathology,* ed 4, Fig. 17.67, Philadelphia, 2021, Elsevier.)

Infectious Arthritis

Joints can become infected from hematogenous dissemination, from direct inoculation through the skin, or from contiguous spread from a soft tissue abscess or osteomyelitis. Infectious arthritis is potentially serious because it can cause rapid, permanent joint destruction.

Suppurative Arthritis

Bacteria that cause acute suppurative arthritis usually enter the joints by hematogenous spread. As with osteomyelitis, the etiologic agent depends on the anatomic location and clinical setting (e.g., trauma, intravenous drug use). *Staphylococcus aureus* is the most

common pathogen in adults and children; in neonates, group B *Streptococcus* and *Neisseria gonorrhoeae* may be responsible. Infection with gram-negative bacilli and *Pseudomonas* is generally seen in patients who are immunocompromised and in people who use intravenous drugs. Individuals with inherited deficiencies of components of the complement membrane attack complex (C5–C9) are especially susceptible to disseminated gonococcal infections and arthritis. Other predisposing conditions include immunodeficiencies (congenital and acquired), debilitating illness, joint trauma, chronic arthritis of any cause, and intravenous substance use.

The classic presentation is the sudden development of an acutely painful, warm, and swollen joint with a restricted range of motion. Fever, leukocytosis, and elevated C-reactive protein are common. The infection usually involves only a single joint, most commonly the knee, hip, shoulder, elbow, wrist, or sternoclavicular joints. The axial joints are more often involved in individuals who inject drugs. Joint aspiration is diagnostic if it yields purulent fluid in which the causative agent can be identified. Prompt recognition and effective antimicrobial therapy can prevent joint destruction.

Lyme Arthritis

Lyme arthritis is caused by the spirochete *Borrelia burgdorferi*, which is transmitted by *Ixodes* deer ticks. Lyme disease is the leading arthropod-borne disease in the United States. It is most often seen in New England, the mid-Atlantic states, and the upper Midwest, but its geographic range is widening. In its classic form, it progressively involves multiple organ systems through three clinical phases (Fig. 19.38). The initial infection of the skin, or *early localized stage,* is followed by an *early disseminated stage* involving the skin, cranial nerves, heart, and meninges. The *late disseminated* stage may be associated with chronic antibiotic-refractory disease.

Currently, arthritis occurs in less than 10% of cases because most patients are treated and cured at an earlier stage; the incidence may be higher in individuals with darker skin since the classic skin lesion, erythema migrans, is less apparent in these patients (eFig. 19.3). When untreated, approximately 60% to 80% of individuals develop a migratory arthritis (*Lyme arthritis*) lasting for weeks to months and most often affecting the knees. Spirochetes can be identified in only about 25% of arthritic joints; serologic identification of anti-*Borrelia* antibodies is diagnostic. Treatment of Lyme disease consists of antibiotics with activity against *Borrelia* and is curative in 90% of cases. In many patients with late, antibiotic-refractory arthritis, *Borrelia* cannot be detected in the joint fluid even by PCR. It has been proposed that cellular (especially Th1) and humoral responses to *Borrelia* outer surface protein A may cross-react with some unknown self antigen(s) and initiate this late, autoimmune arthritis. The chronic manifestations, in addition to joint pain, can include nonspecific symptoms (fatigue, cognitive issues), known collectively as *posttreatment Lyme disease syndrome* (PTLDS).

MORPHOLOGY

Histologically, the synovium exhibits a chronic synovitis marked by synoviocyte hyperplasia, fibrin deposition, mononuclear cell infiltrates (especially CD4+ T cells), and onion-skin thickening of arterial walls. The morphology in severe cases can resemble that of RA.

Crystal-Induced Arthritis

Articular crystal deposits are associated with a variety of joint disorders. Endogenous crystals that cause disease include monosodium

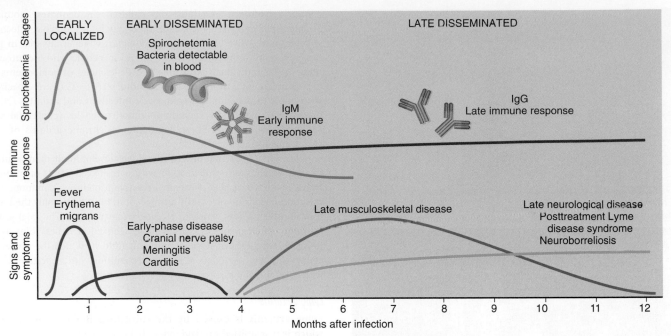

FIG. 19.38 Lyme disease progresses through three clinically recognizable phases: early localized, early disseminated, and late disseminated. Initial manifestations result directly from spirochete infection, whereas later signs and symptoms are likely immune-mediated. (Figure modified from Dr. Charles Chiu, University of California San Francisco, San Francisco, California. Used with permission.)

urate (gout), calcium pyrophosphate dehydrate (pseudogout), and basic calcium phosphate. Exogenous crystals, such as the biomaterials used in prosthetic joints, can also induce arthritis as they undergo erosion and the resultant debris accumulates with wear. All types of crystals produce disease by triggering inflammatory reactions that destroy cartilage.

Gout

Gout is marked by transient attacks of acute arthritis initiated by urate crystals deposited within and around joints. Gout, whether primary (90% of cases) or secondary to underlying disease, is characterized by abnormally high levels of uric acid in tissues and body fluids.

Pathogenesis. **Hyperuricemia (plasma urate level above 6.8 mg/dL) is necessary, but not sufficient, for the development of gout.** Elevated uric acid can result from overproduction, reduced excretion, or both. Uric acid levels are determined by several factors:

- *Synthesis.* Uric acid is the end product of purine catabolism. Increased synthesis typically reflects some abnormality in purine production. Purines are themselves the product of two interlinked pathways: the *de novo pathway*, in which purine nucleotides are synthesized from nonpurine precursors, and the *salvage pathway*, in which purine nucleotides are synthesized from free purine bases in the diet or those that are generated during the degradation of DNA and RNA.
- *Excretion.* Uric acid is filtered from the circulation by the glomerulus and virtually completely resorbed by the proximal tubule of the kidney. A small fraction of the resorbed uric acid is secreted by the distal nephron and excreted in the urine.

In primary gout, elevated uric acid most commonly results from reduced excretion, the basis of which is unknown in most patients.

Secondary gout is associated with medications or conditions that cause hyperuricemia. In a small minority of cases primary gout is caused by uric acid overproduction as a result of enzymatic defects. For example, partial deficiency of hypoxanthine guanine phosphoribosyltransferase (HGPRT) interrupts the salvage pathway, so purine metabolites cannot be recycled and are instead degraded into uric acid. Complete absence of HGPRT results not only in hyperuricemia but also neurologic manifestations *(Lesch-Nyhan syndrome)*, which dominate the clinical picture. Lesch-Nyhan syndrome is classified as a form of secondary gout. Secondary gout can also be caused by increased production (rapid lysis of tumor cells killed by chemotherapy, so-called *tumor lysis syndrome*) or decreased excretion (chronic renal disease).

The arthritis in gout is triggered by precipitation of urate crystals in the joints, stimulating the production of mediators that recruit leukocytes (Fig. 19.39). Resident macrophages in the synovium phagocytose the crystals, thereby activating a cytosolic sensor, the inflammasome (Chapter 5). The inflammasome activates caspase-1, which is involved in the production of active IL-1β. IL-1 stimulates recruitment and accumulation of neutrophils in the joint, which release other cytokines, free radicals, and proteases, as in other acute inflammatory reactions. Crystals ingested by macrophages and neutrophils also damage the membranes of phagolysosomes, leading to leakage of lysosomal enzymes. The result is an acute arthritis, which typically remits spontaneously in days to weeks. Repeated attacks of acute arthritis lead eventually to the formation of tophi, aggregates of urate crystals and inflammatory tissue, in synovial membranes and periarticular tissue. Severe damage to the cartilage develops and the function of the joints is compromised.

Only about 10% of patients with hyperuricemia develop gout. Other factors that contribute to the development of symptomatic gout include:

- *Age* of the individual and *duration* of the hyperuricemia. Gout usually appears after 20 to 30 years of hyperuricemia.

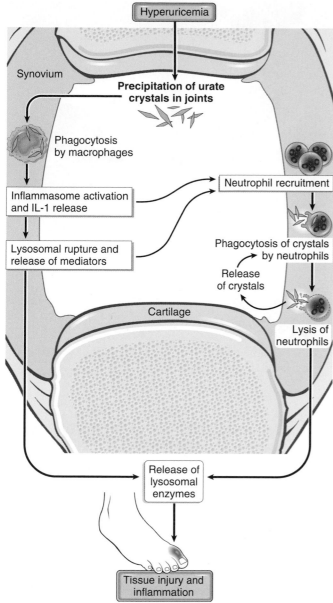

FIG. 19.39 Pathogenesis of acute gouty arthritis. Urate crystals are phagocytosed by macrophages and stimulate the production of various inflammatory mediators that elicit the inflammation characteristic of gout. Note that IL-1, one of the major proinflammatory cytokines, in turn stimulates the production of chemokines and other cytokines from a variety of tissue cells. *IL-1*, Interleukin 1.

- *Genetic predisposition.* In addition to the well-defined X-linked abnormalities of *HGPRT*, polymorphisms in genes involved with urate or ion transport and inflammation are associated with gout.
- *Alcohol* consumption
- *Obesity*
- *Drugs* (e.g., thiazides) that reduce excretion of urate

MORPHOLOGY

Acute gouty arthritis is characterized by an intense inflammatory infiltrate rich in neutrophils that permeates the synovium and synovial fluid. Urate crystals are frequently found in the cytoplasm of the neutrophils in aspirated joint fluid and are arranged in small clusters in the synovium.

They are long, slender, needle shaped, and negatively birefringent. The synovium is edematous and congested and contains neutrophils and scattered lymphocytes, plasma cells, and macrophages.

Chronic tophaceous arthritis evolves from the repetitive precipitation of urate crystals during acute attacks. The crystals encrust the articular surface and form chalky deposits in the synovium (Fig. 19.40A). The synovium becomes hyperplastic, fibrotic, and thickened by inflammatory cells and forms a pannus that destroys the underlying cartilage.

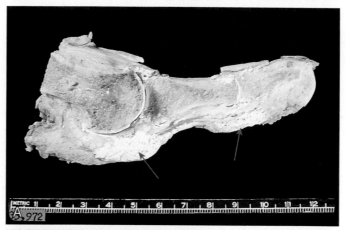

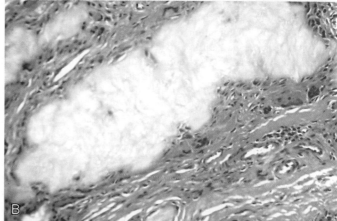

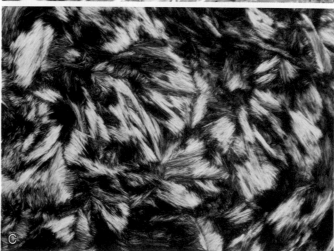

FIG. 19.40 Gout. (A) Amputated great toe with a tophi *(arrows)* involving the joint and soft tissues. (B) Gouty tophus—an aggregate of dissolved urate crystals is surrounded by reactive fibroblasts, mononuclear inflammatory cells, and giant cells. (C) Urate crystals are needle shaped and negatively birefringent under polarized light.

Tophi in the articular cartilage, ligaments, tendons, and bursae are pathognomonic of gout. They are formed by large aggregates of urate crystals surrounded by an intense foreign body giant cell reaction (Fig. 19.40B,C).

Gouty nephropathy refers to renal complications (e.g., uric acid nephrolithias [kidney stones], pyelonephritis) caused by the deposition of urate crystals or tophi in the renal medullary interstitium or tubules.

Clinical Features. Four clinical stages are recognized:

- *Asymptomatic hyperuricemia* begins around puberty in men and after menopause in women.
- *Acute arthritis* presents with sudden onset, excruciating joint pain, localized hyperemia, and warmth. Most first attacks are monoarticular and 50% occur in the metatarsophalangeal joint of the big toe. Untreated, acute gouty arthritis may last for hours to weeks but gradually resolves completely.
- *Asymptomatic intercritical period* is the symptom-free interval following resolution of acute arthritis. Without appropriate therapy, however, the attacks almost inevitably recur, become more closely spaced in time, and often become polyarticular.
- *Chronic tophaceous gout* develops on average about 10 years after the initial acute attack and is characterized by juxtaarticular bone erosion and loss of the joint space.

Treatment of gout aims at lifestyle modification (e.g., weight loss, alcohol reduction, dietary changes to reduce purine intake) and medication to reduce inflammation (e.g., NSAIDs, colchicine) and lower serum urate levels (e.g., xanthine oxidase inhibitors). Uricosuric drugs that increase renal uric acid excretion can also be used. Generally, gout does not shorten life span but can significantly affect quality of life.

Calcium Pyrophosphate Crystal Deposition Disease (Pseudogout)

Calcium pyrophosphate crystal deposition disease (CPPD), also known as *pseudogout,* usually occurs in individuals older than 50 years and becomes more common with increasing age. CPPD is divided into sporadic (idiopathic), hereditary, and secondary types. An autosomal dominant variant caused by germline mutations in the pyrophosphate transport channel results in crystal deposition and arthritis relatively early in life. Various disorders, including previous joint damage, hyperparathyroidism, hemochromatosis, hypothyroidism, and diabetes, predispose to secondary CPPD. Studies suggest that articular cartilage proteoglycans, which normally inhibit mineralization, are degraded, allowing crystallization around chondrocytes. As in gout, inflammation is caused by activation of the inflammasome in macrophages.

MORPHOLOGY

The crystals first develop in the articular cartilage, menisci, and intervertebral discs, and as the deposits enlarge they may rupture and seed the joint. The crystals form chalky, white friable deposits that are seen histologically in hematoxylin- and eosin-stained preparations as oval blue-purple aggregates (Fig. 19.41A). Crystals are rhomboid, 0.5 to 5 μm in greatest dimension (Fig. 19.41B), and positively birefringent. Inflammation is usually milder than in gout.

Clinical Features. CPPD is frequently asymptomatic. However, it may produce acute, subacute, or chronic arthritis that can be confused clinically with OA or RA. The joint involvement may last from several days to weeks and may be monoarticular or polyarticular; the knees, followed by the wrists, elbows, shoulders, and

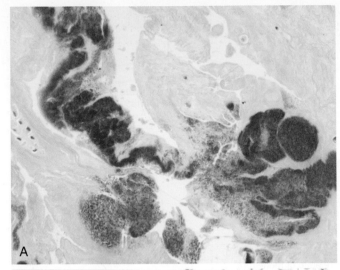

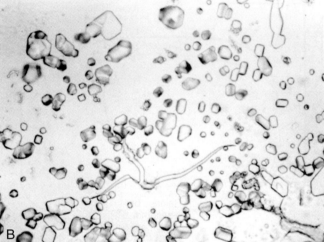

FIG. 19.41 Pseudogout. (A) Deposits are present in cartilage and consist of amorphous basophilic material. (B) Smear preparation of calcium pyrophosphate crystals.

ankles, are most commonly affected. Ultimately, approximately 50% of affected individuals experience significant joint damage. Therapy is supportive: there is no known treatment that prevents or slows crystal formation.

JOINT TUMORS AND TUMORLIKE CONDITIONS

Reactive tumorlike lesions, such as ganglions, synovial cysts, and osteochondral loose bodies, commonly involve joints and tendon sheaths. They usually result from trauma or degenerative processes and are much more common than neoplasms. Primary neoplasms are rare, usually benign, and tend to recapitulate the cells and tissue types (e.g., fat, blood vessels, fibrous tissue, and cartilage) native to joints and related structures. Synovial sarcoma, once thought to be related to or derived from the tissues of the joint, is now recognized as a sarcoma of uncertain origin and is discussed later with soft tissue tumors.

Ganglion and Synovial Cysts

A *ganglion* is a small (1–1.5 cm) cyst that is almost always located near a joint capsule or tendon sheath, often around the joints of the wrist. It appears as a firm, fluctuant, pea-sized translucent nodule. It arises as a result of cystic or myxoid degeneration of connective tissue; hence, it lacks a cellular lining and is not a true cyst. The fluid is similar to synovial fluid; however, there is no communication with the joint space. Despite the name, the lesion is unrelated to ganglia of the nervous system.

Herniation of synovium through a joint capsule or massive enlargement of a bursa may produce a *synovial cyst*. A well-recognized example is the synovial cyst that forms in the popliteal space in the setting of RA or OA *(Baker cyst)*. The synovial lining may be hyperplastic and contain inflammatory cells and fibrin.

Tenosynovial Giant Cell Tumor

Tenosynovial giant cell tumor is a benign tumor that develops in the synovial lining of joints, tendon sheaths, and bursae. It can be diffuse (previously known as *pigmented villonodular synovitis*) or localized. The localized type usually occurs as a discrete nodule attached to a tendon sheath, commonly in the hand, while the diffuse type tends to involve large joints. Both variants are most often diagnosed in patients who are in their 20s to 40s.

Pathogenesis. Both diffuse and localized tumor types harbor a reciprocal somatic chromosomal translocation, t(1;2)(p13;q37), that results in the fusion of the type VI collagen α-3 gene promoter to the *CSF1* gene, which encodes monocyte colony stimulating factor (M-CSF). Consequently, the tumor cells secrete large quantities of M-CSF, which stimulates the proliferation of macrophages in a manner similar to giant cell tumor of bone (described previously).

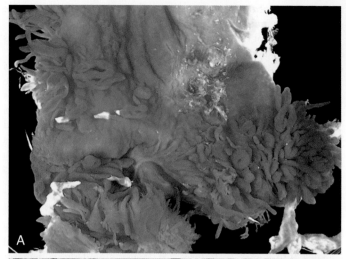

> ## MORPHOLOGY
>
> Tenosynovial giant cell tumors are red-brown to orange-yellow. In diffuse tumors, the normally smooth joint synovium is converted into a tangled mat of folds, fingerlike projections, and nodules (Fig. 19.42A). By contrast, localized (nodular) tumors are well circumscribed. The neoplastic cells, which account for only a minority of the cells in the mass, are polygonal and moderately sized and resemble synoviocytes (Fig. 19.42B). Both diffuse and localized variants may be heavily infiltrated by macrophages containing hemosiderin and foamy lipid, including some multinucleate cells.

Clinical Features. Diffuse tenosynovial giant cell tumor occurs most often in the knee (80% of cases). Affected individuals typically report pain, restricted range of motion, and recurrent swelling similar to monoarticular arthritis. Sometimes a palpable mass is present. The localized variant manifests as a solitary, slow-growing, painless mass of the hand. Some tumors erode into adjacent bones and soft tissues, thereby simulating other types of neoplasms. Surgical excision is the mainstay of treatment; recurrence is more common in the diffuse form as compared with the localized form. Clinical trials using antagonists of the M-CSF signaling pathway have yielded promising results.

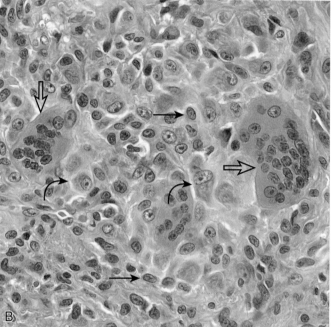

FIG. 19.42 Tenosynovial giant cell tumor. (A) Diffuse type: excised synovium with fronds and nodules. (B) Histologically, there is a mixed cell population, including epithelioid cells *(curved arrow)*, mononuclear stromal cells *(thin arrow)*, and osteoclast-like giant cells *(thick arrow)*. (B, From ExpertPath. Copyright Elsevier, 2022.)

SOFT TISSUE TUMORS

By convention, soft tissue refers to nonepithelial tissue, exclusive of the skeleton, joints, central nervous system, and hematopoietic and lymphoid tissues. With the exception of skeletal muscle neoplasms, benign soft tissue tumors are 100-fold more frequent than their malignant counterparts, the sarcomas. In the United States, the incidence of soft tissue sarcomas is approximately 12,000 per year, which is less than 1% of all cancers. Sarcomas, however, cause 2% of cancer mortality, reflecting their aggressive behavior and the lack of effective treatments. Most soft tissue tumors arise in the extremities, especially the thigh. Approximately 15% occur in children, some of whom have germline mutations that place them at increased risk.

Pathogenesis. Most sarcomas are sporadic and have no known predisposing cause. A small minority are associated with germline mutations in tumor suppressor genes that underlie various syndromes in which multiple tumors develop (e.g., neurofibromatosis 1, Gardner syndrome, Li-Fraumeni syndrome, Osler-Weber-Rendu syndrome). Others are linked to environmental exposures such as radiation, burns, or toxins.

Unlike many carcinomas and certain hematologic malignancies that arise from well-recognized precursor lesions or cells, the origin of most soft tissue sarcomas is undefined. While some sarcomas express markers of recognizable mesenchymal lineages (e.g., skeletal muscle), all are thought to arise from pluripotent mesenchymal stem cells that acquire somatic driver mutations in oncogenes and tumor suppressor genes.

The genetics of tumorigenesis is complex, but some generalizations can be made based on karyotypic abnormalities:

- *Simple karyotype* (15%—20% of sarcomas): Like many leukemias and lymphomas, sarcomas are often euploid tumors with a single or few chromosomal changes that occur early in tumorigenesis and are sufficiently specific to serve as diagnostic markers. Tumors with these features most commonly arise in younger patients and tend to have a monomorphic microscopic appearance. Examples include Ewing sarcoma, described earlier, and synovial sarcoma. In some cases, the oncogenic effect of these rearrangements is reasonably well understood. In others, the mechanisms are unknown. Oncogenic tumor-specific fusion proteins represent potential molecular targets for therapy.
- *Complex karyotype* (80%—85% of sarcomas): These tumors are aneuploid or polyploid and demonstrate multiple chromosomal gains and losses, a feature that suggests underlying genomic instability. Examples include leiomyosarcoma and undifferentiated pleomorphic sarcoma. These sarcomas are more common in adults and tend to be composed of pleomorphic tumor cells.

Classification of soft tissue tumors continues to evolve as new molecular genetic abnormalities are identified. Clinically, soft tissue tumors range from benign, self-limited lesions that require minimal treatment, to intermediate grade, locally aggressive tumors with minimal metastatic risk, to highly aggressive malignancies with significant risk of metastasis and mortality. All highly aggressive malignancies are classified as *sarcomas*, but this term is less consistently applied to locally aggressive, rarely metastasizing entities. Pathologic classification is based on the integration of morphologic (e.g., muscle differentiation), immunohistochemical, and molecular features. For most entities, tumor grade (degree of differentiation) and stage (size and depth) are important prognostic indicators.

The next section will consider representative soft tissue tumors (summarized in Table 19.3).

Table 19.3 Clinical Features of Soft Tissue Sarcomas

Category	Behavior	Tumor Type	Common Locations	Age (Years)	Morphology
Adipose	Benign	Lipoma	Superficial extremity, trunk	40—60	Mature adipose tissue
	Malignant	Well-differentiated liposarcoma	Deep extremity, retroperitoneum	50—60	Adipose tissue with scattered atypical stromal cells
		Myxoid liposarcoma	Thigh, leg	30s	Myxoid matrix, "chicken wire" vessels, round cells, lipoblasts
Fibrous	Benign	Nodular fasciitis	Arm, forearm	20—30	Spindle to stellate cells, extravasated red cells
		Deep fibromatosis	Abdominal wall	30—40	Dense collagen, long, sweeping fascicles
	Malignant	Fibrosarcoma	Deep extremities	40—60	Monomorphic spindle cells in fascicles
Skeletal muscle	Benign	Rhabdomyoma	Head and neck	0—60	Polygonal rhabdomyoblasts, "spider" cells
	Malignant	Alveolar rhabdomyosarcoma	Extremities	5—15	Uniform, round dyscohesive cells between septa
		Embryonal rhabdomyosarcoma	Genitourinary tract, head and neck	1—5	Primitive spindle cells, "strap" cells
Smooth muscle	Benign	Leiomyoma	Extremity	20s	Uniform, plump eosinophilic cells in fascicles
	Malignant	Leiomyosarcoma	Thigh, retroperitoneum	40—60	Pleomorphic eosinophilic cells
Vascular	Benign	Hemangioma	Head and neck	0—10	Circumscribed mass of capillary or venous channels
	Malignant	Angiosarcoma	Skin, deep lower extremity	50—80	Infiltrating capillary channels
Nerve sheath	Benign	Schwannoma	Head and neck	20—50	Encapsulated, fibrillar stroma, nuclear palisading
		Neurofibroma	Wide, cutaneous, subcutis	10—20+	Myxoid, ropy collagen, loose fascicles, mast cells
	Malignant	Malignant peripheral nerve sheath tumor	Extremities, shoulder girdle	20—50	Tight fascicles, atypia, mitotic activity, necrosis
Uncertain histotype	Benign	Solitary fibrous tumor	Pelvis, pleura	20—70	Branching ectatic vessels
	Malignant	Synovial sarcoma	Thigh, leg	15—40	Tight fascicles of uniform basophilic spindle cells, pseudoglandular structures
		Undifferentiated pleomorphic sarcoma	Thigh	40—70	High-grade anaplastic polygonal, round, or spindle cells, bizarre nuclei, atypical mitoses, necrosis

TUMORS OF ADIPOSE TISSUE

Lipoma

Lipoma, a benign tumor with adipocyte differentiation, is the most common soft tissue tumor in adults. Conventional lipoma is the most common subtype, from which rare variants are distinguished according to characteristic morphologic and/or genetic features. This neoplasm consisting of mature adipocytes usually arises as a well-circumscribed mass in the subcutis of the proximal extremities and trunk, typically during middle adulthood. Less commonly, lipomas are large, intramuscular, and poorly circumscribed. Most lipomas are cured by simple excision.

Liposarcoma

Liposarcoma, a malignant tumor with adipocytic differentiation, is the most common sarcoma of adulthood. They occur mainly in people in their 50s to 60s in the deep soft tissues and retroperitoneum.

The three distinct subtypes of liposarcoma (well-differentiated, myxoid, and pleomorphic) have different genetic aberrations. Well-differentiated liposarcoma harbors amplifications of chromosomal region 12q13-q15, which includes the p53 inhibitor *MDM2*. They are relatively indolent and have an excellent prognosis when complete excision is possible; however, retroperitoneal tumors frequently recur and may progress to more aggressive tumors. In myxoid liposarcoma, a fusion gene generated by a (12;16) translocation arrests adipocyte differentiation, leading to unregulated proliferation of primitive cells. They are intermediate in malignant behavior. Pleomorphic liposarcoma has a complex karyotype without reproducible genetic abnormalities. It is aggressive and frequently metastasizes.

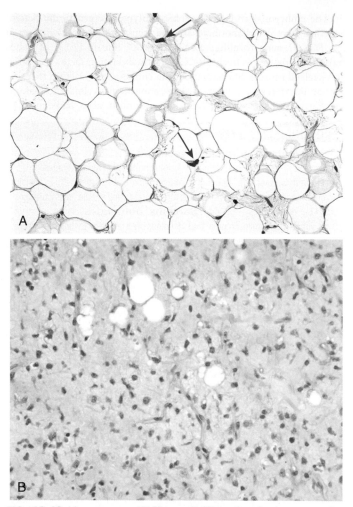

FIG. 19.43 Liposarcoma. (A) The well-differentiated subtype consists of mature adipocytes and rare, atypical stromal *(red arrows)* cells with hyperchromatic nuclei. (B) Myxoid liposarcoma with abundant ground substance and a rich capillary network in which are scattered immature adipocytes. (A from Goldblum JR, Folpe AL, Weiss SW: *Enzinger & Weiss's Soft Tissue Tumors*, ed 7, Fig. 14.12, Philadelphia, 2020, Elsevier.)

> **MORPHOLOGY**
>
> Liposarcomas are divided into three histologic subtypes:
> - *Well-differentiated liposarcoma* consists of neoplastic adipocytes with scattered atypical stromal cells (Fig. 19.43A).
> - *Myxoid liposarcoma* displays abundant basophilic extracellular matrix, arborizing capillaries, and well-spaced primitive cells reminiscent of fetal fat (Fig. 19.43B). Tumor hypercellularity is associated with a worse prognosis.
> - *Pleomorphic liposarcoma* consists of sheets of anaplastic cells, bizarre nuclei, and variable amounts of immature adipocytes (lipoblasts).

FIBROUS TUMORS

Neoplasms of fibroblasts and myofibroblasts are rare and usually benign. *Nodular fasciitis* is a self-limited fibroblastic and myofibroblastic proliferation that typically arises in the upper extremities of young adults. Though previously considered reactive, it is in fact associated with a (17;22) translocation that creates a *MYH9-USP6* fusion gene, indicating that it is a clonal, self-limited proliferation. Nodular fasciitis often spontaneously regresses and, if excised, rarely recurs. *Fibromatoses* may be superficial and follow an innocuous clinical course, or they may be deep (also called desmoid tumors); the latter are large, infiltrative masses that frequently recur but do not metastasize. Deep fibromatoses have mutations in the *CTNNB1* (β-catenin) or *APC* genes, leading to increased Wnt signaling. Most tumors are sporadic, but individuals with familial adenomatous polyposis (Gardner syndrome, Chapter 13) who have germline *APC* mutations are predisposed to deep fibromatosis.

SKELETAL MUSCLE TUMORS

In contrast to tumors of other lineages, almost all tumors showing skeletal muscle differentiation are malignant. A benign exception, *rhabdomyoma*, is frequently associated with tuberous sclerosis (Chapter 21). It may occur in the heart or in soft tissues.

Rhabdomyosarcoma

Rhabdomyosarcoma is a malignant mesenchymal tumor with skeletal muscle differentiation. Four subtypes are recognized: *alveolar* (20%), *embryonal* (50%), *pleomorphic* (20%), and *spindle cell/sclerosing* (10%). The alveolar and embryonal subtypes of rhabdomyosarcoma are the most common soft tissue sarcomas of childhood and adolescence, usually appearing before 20 years of age. Pleomorphic rhabdomyosarcoma occurs in adults and the spindle cell/sclerosing type affects all ages. Pediatric rhabdomyosarcomas often arise in the sinuses, head and neck, and genitourinary tract, locations that do not normally contain much skeletal muscle, underscoring the notion that these sarcomas arise from undifferentiated mesenchymal stem cells.

The embryonal and pleomorphic subtypes are genetically heterogeneous. Alveolar rhabdomyosarcoma frequently contains fusions of the *FOXO1* gene to either *PAX3* or *PAX7* due to (2;13) or (1;13) translocations, respectively. PAX3 is a transcription factor that initiates skeletal muscle differentiation; the chimeric PAX3-FOXO1 fusion protein interferes with differentiation, a mechanism similar to many of the transcription factor fusion proteins found in acute leukemia.

MORPHOLOGY

Grossly, **embryonal rhabdomyosarcoma** is a soft, gray, infiltrative mass. The tumor cells recapitulate skeletal muscle at various stages of differentiation and include sheets of primitive round and spindled cells in myxoid stroma. Rhabdomyoblasts with straplike cytoplasm and visible cross-striations may be present (Fig. 19.44A). **Sarcoma botryoides** is a variant of embryonal rhabdomyosarcoma that develops in the walls of hollow viscera such as the urinary bladder and vagina.

In **alveolar rhabdomyosarcoma,** fibrous septa divide the cells into clusters or aggregates reminiscent of pulmonary alveoli. The tumor cells are uniformly round with little cytoplasm and are only minimally cohesive (Fig. 19.44B).

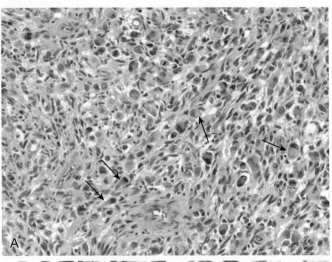

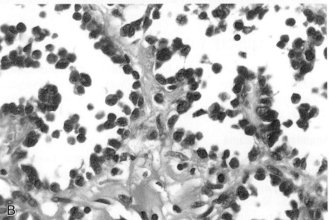

FIG. 19.44 Rhabdomyosarcoma. (A) Embryonal subtype composed of malignant cells ranging from primitive and round to densely eosinophilic with skeletal muscle differentiation *(arrows)*. (B) Alveolar rhabdomyosarcoma with numerous spaces lined by dyscohesive, uniform round tumor cells. (A, From Goldblum JR, Folpe AL, Weiss SW: *Enzinger & Weiss's Soft Tissue Tumors,* ed 7, Fig. 19.6, Philadelphia, 2020, Elsevier.)

Pleomorphic rhabdomyosarcoma is characterized by numerous large, sometimes multinucleate, bizarre eosinophilic tumor cells that may resemble those seen in other pleomorphic sarcomas. Immunohistochemical identification of muscle specific proteins such as myogenin is usually necessary to confirm rhabdomyoblastic differentiation.

Spindle cell/sclerosing rhabdomyosarcomas consist of fusiform cells with vesicular chromatin arranged in long fascicles or in a storiform pattern. Rhabdomyoblasts are occasionally present. Dense, collagenous, sclerotic stroma may be more common in adults.

Clinical Features. Rhabdomyosarcomas are aggressive neoplasms that are usually treated with surgery and chemotherapy, with or without radiation therapy. The botryoid variant of embryonal rhabdomyosarcoma has the best prognosis, whereas the pleomorphic subtype is often fatal.

SMOOTH MUSCLE TUMORS

Leiomyoma

Leiomyoma, a benign tumor of smooth muscle, arises most frequently in the uterus but can originate in any soft tissue site. Uterine leiomyomas (fibroids, Chapter 17) are common and may cause a variety of symptoms, including infertility and menorrhagia. Leiomyomas also may arise from the erector pili muscles *(pilar leiomyomas)* in the skin and rarely in the deep somatic soft tissues or gastrointestinal tract. Germline loss-of-function mutations in the fumarate hydratase *(FH)* gene are seen in an autosomal syndrome marked by the development of multiple cutaneous leiomyomas, uterine leiomyomas, and renal cell carcinoma. FH is an enzyme of the Krebs cycle, another intriguing example of the link between metabolic abnormalities and neoplasia.

Soft tissue leiomyomas are usually 1 to 2 cm in size and are composed of fascicles of densely eosinophilic spindle cells with minimal atypia and extremely rare mitotic figures. Solitary lesions are cured surgically.

Leiomyosarcoma

Leiomyosarcoma, a malignant tumor showing evidence of smooth muscle differentiation, most often develops in the deep soft tissues of the extremities and the retroperitoneum (in addition to the uterus). It accounts for 10% to 20% of soft tissue sarcomas, occurs primarily in older adults, and is more common in women than men. A particularly deadly form arises from the great vessels, often the inferior vena cava. Leiomyosarcomas have underlying defects in genomic stability leading to complex karyotypes.

MORPHOLOGY

In the deep soft tissue, leiomyosarcoma presents as a painless, firm mass. Retroperitoneal tumors may cause abdominal symptoms due to their size. They range from interweaving fascicles of eosinophilic spindle cells to sheets of pleomorphic cells. Immunohistochemical detection of smooth muscle proteins can aid in diagnosis. Mitotic activity and necrosis are common.

Clinical Features. Treatment depends on tumor size, location, and grade. Superficial leiomyosarcomas are usually small and have a good prognosis, whereas those of the retroperitoneum are difficult to control and cause death by local extension and metastatic spread, especially to the lungs.

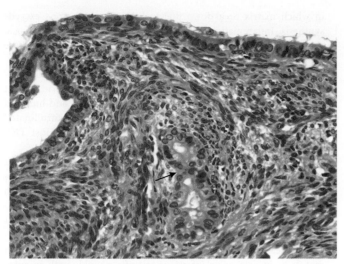

FIG. 19.45 Synovial sarcoma showing the classic biphasic spindle cell and glandlike *(arrow)* histologic appearance.

TUMORS OF UNCERTAIN ORIGIN

Although many soft tissue tumors can be assigned to recognizable histologic types, a large proportion of tumors do not recapitulate any known mesenchymal lineage. This group includes tumors with simple or complex karyotypes; an example of each is described here.

Synovial Sarcoma

Synovial sarcoma, so-named because its frequent location near joints led to the idea that it may arise from synovium, is a translocation-associated sarcoma that shows variable epithelial differentiation. Synovial sarcomas account for approximately 10% of soft tissue sarcomas. Most occur in adolescents or young adults. Individuals often present with a deep-seated, slowly growing mass of the extremities that has been present for years. Most synovial sarcomas contain a characteristic (x;18)(p11;q11) translocation that produces fusion genes composed of portions of the *SS18* gene and one of three *SSX* genes. The fusions encode chimeric proteins that interfere with normal chromatin remodeling and thereby dysregulate gene expression.

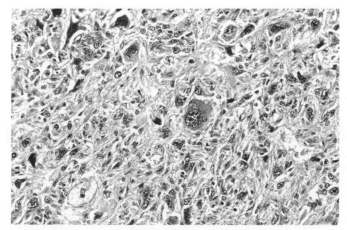

FIG. 19.46 Undifferentiated pleomorphic sarcoma showing sheets of anaplastic cells. (A, From Goldblum JR, Folpe AL, Weiss SW: *Enzinger & Weiss's Soft Tissue Tumors*, ed 7, Fig. 12.12, Philadelphia, 2020, Elsevier.)

MORPHOLOGY

Histologically, synovial sarcomas may be monophasic or biphasic. Monophasic synovial sarcoma consists of uniform spindle cells with scant cytoplasm and dense chromatin growing in short, tightly packed fascicles. The biphasic type has an additional component of glandlike structures composed of cuboidal to columnar epithelioid cells (Fig. 19.45). Immunohistochemistry is helpful in identifying these tumors, since the tumor cells, especially in the biphasic type, are positive for epithelial antigens (e.g., keratins), differentiating them from many other sarcomas.

Clinical Features. Synovial sarcomas are treated aggressively with limb-sparing surgery and frequently chemotherapy. The 5-year survival varies from 25% to 62%, related to stage and patient age. Common sites of metastases are the lung and, unusually for sarcomas, regional lymph nodes.

Undifferentiated Pleomorphic Sarcoma

Undifferentiated pleomorphic sarcoma includes malignant anaplastic mesenchymal tumors that cannot be classified into another category by morphology, immunophenotype, or genetics. Most arise in the deep soft tissues of the extremity, especially the thigh of middle-aged or older adults. These tumors are typically aneuploid with multiple structural and numerical chromosomal changes.

MORPHOLOGY

Undifferentiated pleomorphic sarcomas are usually gray-white fleshy masses that can grow quite large (10–20 cm) depending on the anatomic compartment. Necrosis and hemorrhage are common. Microscopically, they are extremely pleomorphic and are composed of sheets of large spindled to polygonal cells with hyperchromatic irregular, sometimes bizarre nuclei (Fig. 19.46). Mitotic figures, including atypical nonsymmetric forms, are abundant. By definition, the tumor cells lack differentiation along recognized lineages.

Clinical Features. Undifferentiated pleomorphic sarcomas are aggressive malignancies that are treated with surgery and adjuvant chemotherapy and/or radiation. The prognosis is generally poor. Metastases occur in 30% to 50% of cases.

■ RAPID REVIEW

Congenital Disorders of Bone and Cartilage

- Abnormalities in a single bone or a localized group of bones are called dysostoses and arise from defects in the migration and condensation of mesenchyme. They manifest as absent, supernumerary, or abnormally fused bones. Global disorganization of bone and/or cartilage are called dysplasias.
- *FGFR3* mutations are responsible for two dysplasias: achondroplasia and thanatophoric dysplasia, both of which manifest as dwarfism.
- Mutations in the genes for type I collagen underlie most types of osteogenesis imperfecta, characterized by defective bone formation and skeletal fragility.

Metabolic Disorders of Bone

- Osteopenia and osteoporosis represent histologically normal bone that is decreased in quantity. In osteoporosis, the extent of bone loss significantly increases the risk of fracture. The disease is very common, with marked morbidity and mortality from fractures. Multiple factors including peak bone mass, age, activity, genetics, nutrition, and hormonal influences contribute to its pathogenesis.
- Osteomalacia is characterized by bone that is insufficiently mineralized. In the developing skeleton, the manifestations are characterized by a condition known as rickets.
- Hyperparathyroidism arises from either autonomous or compensatory hypersecretion of PTH and can lead to osteoporosis, brown tumors, and osteitis fibrosa cystica. In higher-income countries, where early diagnosis is typical, these manifestations are rarely seen.

Bone Tumors and Tumorlike Lesions

- Primary bone tumors are classified according to the cell of origin or the matrix that they produce. The remainder are grouped according to clinicopathologic features. Most primary bone tumors are benign. Metastases, especially from lung, prostate, kidneys, and breast, are far more common than primary bone neoplasms. Major categories of primary bone tumors include:
  - Bone forming: Osteoblastoma and osteoid osteoma consist of benign osteoblasts that synthesize osteoid. Osteosarcoma is an aggressive tumor of malignant osteoblasts, predominantly occurring in adolescents.
  - Cartilage forming: Osteochondroma is an exostosis with a cartilage cap. Sporadic and syndromic forms arise from mutations in the *EXT* genes. Chondromas are benign tumors producing hyaline cartilage, usually arising in the digits. Chondrosarcomas are malignant tumors of chondroid cells that involve the axial skeleton in adults.
  - Ewing sarcoma is an aggressive, malignant, small round cell tumor associated with t(11;22).
  - Fibrous dysplasia is localized developmental arrest of bone constituents due to gain-of-function mutations in *GNAS1*.

Arthritis

- Osteoarthritis (OA, degenerative joint disease), the most common disease of the joints, is a degenerative process of articular cartilage in which matrix breakdown due to biomechanical stress exceeds synthesis. Inflammation is minimal and typically secondary. Local production of inflammatory cytokines contributes to disease progression.
- Rheumatoid arthritis (RA) is a chronic autoimmune inflammatory disease that affects mainly small joints symmetrically but can involve other joints. RA is caused by a cellular and humoral immune response against self antigens, particularly citrullinated proteins. TNF plays a central role and antagonists against TNF are of clinical benefit.
- Seronegative spondyloarthropathies are a heterogeneous group of likely autoimmune arthritides that preferentially involve the sacroiliac and vertebral joints and occur mainly in individuals with HLA-B27.
- Suppurative arthritis is caused by infection of a joint space by bacterial organisms, usually acquired hematogenously.
- Lyme disease is a systemic infection by *Borrelia burgdorferi*, which manifests, in part, as an infectious arthritis, possibly with an autoimmune component in chronic stages.
- Gout and pseudogout result from inflammatory responses triggered by precipitation of urate or calcium pyrophosphate, respectively, in joints.

Soft Tissue Tumors

- The category of soft tissue neoplasia describes tumors that arise from nonepithelial tissues exclusive of the skeleton, joints, central nervous system, and hematopoietic and lymphoid tissues. A sarcoma is a malignant mesenchymal tumor.
- Although all soft tissue tumors probably arise from pluripotent mesenchymal stem cells, rather than mature cells, they can be classified as
  - Tumors that recapitulate a mature mesenchymal tissue (e.g., fat). These can be further subdivided into benign and malignant forms.
  - Tumors composed of cells for which there is no normal counterpart (e.g., synovial sarcoma, undifferentiated pleomorphic sarcoma)
- Sarcomas with simple karyotypes demonstrate reproducible, chromosomal, and molecular abnormalities that contribute to pathogenesis and are sufficiently specific to have diagnostic use.
- Most adult sarcomas have complex karyotypes, tend to be pleomorphic, are genetically heterogeneous, and have a poor prognosis.

■ Laboratory Tests[a]

Test	Reference Values	Pathophysiology/Clinical Relevance
Anticitrullinated peptide antibodies, serum	<20 U/mL	Citrullination is a posttranslational protein modification that is associated with inflammation, particularly in synovial tissues. In rheumatoid arthritis (RA), autoantibodies are induced against a number of citrullinated antigens. These anticitrullinated peptide antibodies (ACPAs) have been identified in the synovial fluid of some patients with RA. ACPAs are found in 60%—80% of patients with RA, and ELISA-based serum tests and show specificity ranging from 85%—99%. There is also evidence that ACPAs precede the development of RA, appearing several years prior to disease presentation. Some studies suggest that levels of ACPAs correlate with disease progression and response to anti—tumor necrosis factor (TNF) antibody treatment.

Rheumatoid factor (RF), serum	<15 IU/mL	Rheumatoid factors are antibodies that react with the Fc portion of other immunoglobulin G antibodies. Despite its name, RF lacks specificity for RA and can be seen in 40%–60% of patients with Sjögren syndrome as well. RF can, however, be a prognostic indicator, as its presence correlates with increased severity of RA. RF has a sensitivity and specificity of about 70% and 85% for RA, respectively. Combination of RF and anticitrullinated peptide antibodies may have higher diagnostic yield.
Uric acid, serum	Males: <8.0 mg/dL Females: <6.1 mg/dL	Uric acid is generated by purine metabolism. Purines are synthesized by the body or are ingested, particularly in foods with abundant nucleic material (e.g., liver). About 75% of the body's uric acid is excreted in the urine. Hyperuricemia is necessary but not sufficient for development of gout. In the majority of cases of gout, the defect that causes elevation of plasma uric acid is unknown, but it most likely is due to reduced renal excretion. In a much smaller number of cases there is partial or complete absence of the enzyme hypoxanthine-guanine phosphoribosyltransferase (HGPRT), which can result in the Lesch-Nyhan syndrome. Hyperuricemia resulting in secondary gout can be seen in patients on cytotoxic drug regimens (e.g., cancer chemotherapy) and in the context of aggressive neoplasms (e.g., acute leukemia) and chronic renal failure (decreased excretion). Most patients with hyperuricemia do not develop gout.

[a]The assistance of Dr. Pankti Reid, Department of Medicine, the University of Chicago, is greatly appreciated.

References values from https://www.mayocliniclabs.com/ by permission of Mayo Foundation for Medical Education and Research. All rights reserved.

Adapted from Deyrup AT, D'Ambrosio D, Muir J, et al. Essential Laboratory Tests for Medical Education. *Acad Pathol*. 2022;9. doi: 10.1016/j.acpath.2022.100046.

Peripheral Nerves and Muscles

The peripheral nerves and skeletal muscles permit purposeful movement and provide the brain with sensory information about our surroundings. Both the anatomic distribution of lesions and their associated signs and symptoms are helpful in classifying neuromuscular diseases. The following discussion of neuromuscular disorders is organized along anatomic lines from proximal peripheral nerves to distal neuromuscular junctions and skeletal muscle.

DISORDERS OF PERIPHERAL NERVES

The two major functional elements of peripheral nerves are axonal processes and their myelin sheaths, which are made by Schwann cells. Axonal diameter and myelin thickness correlate with each other and with the conduction velocity of electrical impulses along the nerve. These characteristics distinguish different types of axons, which mediate distinct sensory inputs and motor function. Light touch, for example, is transmitted by thickly myelinated large-diameter axons with fast conduction velocities, whereas temperature sensation is transmitted by slow, lightly myelinated or unmyelinated thin axons. In the case of myelinated axons, one Schwann cell makes and maintains exactly one myelin segment, or internode, along a single axon (Fig. 20.1A). Adjacent internodes are separated by the nodes of Ranvier along which saltatory conduction occurs. Any given nerve

contains axons of different sizes and axons serving different functions. These are arranged in fascicles ensheathed by a layer of perineurial cells. Perineurial cells form a barrier between endoneurium on the inside of the fascicle and epineurium on the outside.

Patterns of Peripheral Nerve Injury

Peripheral neuropathies are often subclassified as axonal or demyelinating, even though many diseases exhibit mixed features. **Axonal neuropathies are caused by insults that directly injure the axon.** The entire distal portion of an affected axon degenerates (called *Wallerian degeneration*). Axonal degeneration is associated with secondary myelin loss (Fig. 20.1B). Regeneration takes place through axonal regrowth and subsequent remyelination of the distal axon (Fig. 20.1C). The morphologic hallmark of axonal neuropathies is a decrease in the density of axons, which in electrophysiologic studies correlates with a decrease in the signal amplitude of nerve impulses.

Demyelinating neuropathies are characterized by damage to Schwann cells or myelin and relative axonal sparing, resulting in abnormally slow nerve conduction velocity but preserved amplitude. Demyelination may occur discontinuously, affecting individual internodes along the length of an axon in a random distribution. This process is termed *segmental demyelination* (see Fig. 20.1B). Morphologically, demyelinating neuropathies show a relatively normal density of axons and features of segmental demyelination and repair. This is recognized by the presence of axons with abnormally thin myelin sheaths and short internodes (see Fig. 20.1C).

The contributions to this chapter by Dr. Peter Pytel, Department of Pathology, University of Chicago, in several previous editions of this book are gratefully acknowledged.

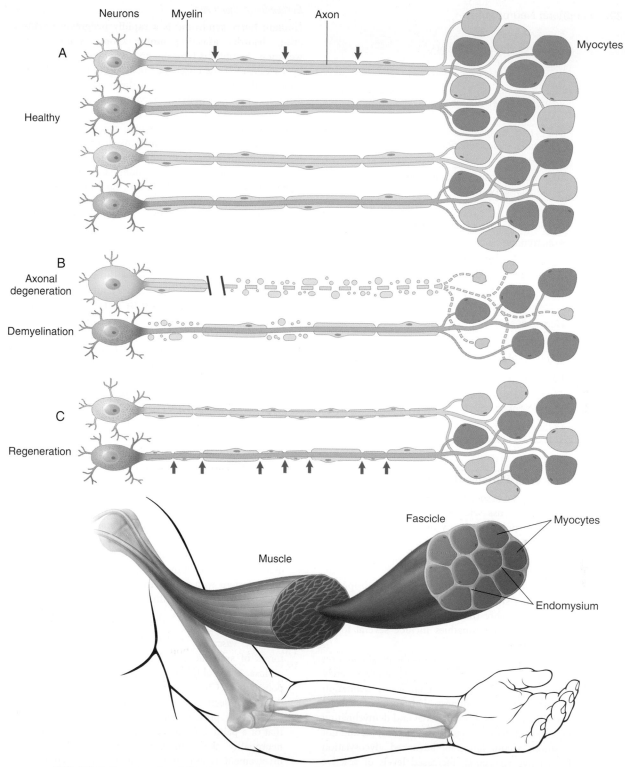

FIG. 20.1 Patterns of peripheral nerve damage. (A) In healthy motor units, type I and type II myofibers (see Table 20.2 later) are arranged in a "checkerboard" distribution. The internodes separated by nodes of Ranvier *(arrows)* along the motor axons are uniform in thickness and length. (B) Acute axonal injury *(upper axon)* results in degeneration of the distal axon and its associated myelin sheath, with atrophy of denervated myofibers. By contrast, acute demyelinating disease *(lower axon)* produces random segmental degeneration of individual myelin internodes, while sparing the axon. (C) Regeneration of axons after injury *(upper axon)* allows connections with myofibers to re-form. The regenerated axon is myelinated by Schwann cells, but the new internodes are shorter and the myelin sheaths are thinner than the original ones. Remission of demyelinating disease *(lower axon)* allows remyelination to take place, but as in regeneration of axons after injury, the new internodes are shorter and have thinner myelin sheaths than flanking healthy undamaged internodes (Nodes of Ranvier are marked by *arrows*; compare with panel A).

Table 20.1 Peripheral Neuropathies

Etiologic Category	Causative Disorders/Agents
Nutritional and metabolic	Diabetes
	Uremia
	Vitamin deficiencies—thiamine, vitamin B_6, vitamin B_{12}
Toxic	Drugs (e.g., vinblastine, vincristine, paclitaxel, cisplatin, oxaliplatin, bortezomib, colchicine, isoniazid)
	Toxins (e.g., alcohol, lead, aluminum, arsenic, mercury, acrylamide)
Vasculopathic, infiltrative	Vasculitis
	Amyloidosis, sarcoidosis, lymphoma
Inflammatory	Autoimmune diseases such as lupus, Sjögren, mixed connective tissue disorder
	Guillain-Barré syndrome
	Chronic inflammatory demyelinating polyneuropathy (CIDP)
Infections	Herpes zoster
	Leprosy
	HIV
	Lyme disease
Inherited	Charcot-Marie-Tooth neuropathy, type I, type II, and X-linked
Others	Paraneoplastic, some leukodystrophies

Disorders Associated With Peripheral Nerve Injury

Many different diseases may be associated with peripheral neuropathy (Table 20.1). We next discuss selected entities that are prototypical for a specific type of polyneuropathy or that are particularly common.

Diabetic Peripheral Neuropathy

Diabetes is the most common cause of peripheral neuropathy, usually developing with long-standing disease. Up to 80% of those who have had the disease for more than 15 years show evidence of peripheral neuropathy. Diabetic neuropathies include several forms that can occur singly or together.

- *Distal symmetric sensorimotor polyneuropathy* is the most common form of diabetic neuropathy. Sensory axons are more severely affected than motor axons, resulting in a clinical presentation dominated by paresthesias and numbness. This form of diabetic polyneuropathy exhibits features of both axonal and demyelinating injury. The pathogenesis of diabetic neuropathy is complex and not completely understood; accumulation of advanced glycosylation end products due to hyperglycemia, increased levels of reactive oxygen species, microvascular changes, and changes in axonal metabolism have all been implicated. Strict glycemic control is the best form of therapy.
- *Autonomic neuropathy* is characterized by orthostatic hypotension and changes in bowel, bladder, cardiac, and/or sexual function.
- *Lumbosacral radiculopathy* (diabetic amyotrophy) usually manifests with asymmetric pain, numbness, weakness, and muscle atrophy that typically starts in one lower extremity and may spread to the other.

Guillain-Barré Syndrome

Guillain-Barré syndrome is a rapidly progressive acute demyelinating disorder affecting motor axons, resulting in ascending weakness. Symptoms typically progress over a period of 2 weeks and by 4 weeks after the onset, vast majority of patients have reached the nadir of the disease. It is one of the most common life-threatening diseases of the peripheral nervous system. About two-thirds of Guillain-Barré syndrome cases are triggered by an infection that provokes the generation of microbe-specific T cells and antibodies, which then cross-react with antigens in the nerve sheath. Although both T cell–mediated and antibody-mediated responses are involved, the former are believed to play a dominant role. Associated infectious agents include *Campylobacter jejuni*, Epstein-Barr virus, cytomegalovirus, human immunodeficiency virus (HIV), Zika virus, and most recently SARS-CoV-2. The injury is most extensive in the nerve roots and proximal nerve segments and is associated with mononuclear cell infiltrates rich in macrophages. Treatments include plasmapheresis (to remove offending antibodies), intravenous immunoglobulin infusions (which suppress immune responses through unclear mechanisms), and supportive care, such as ventilatory support. Patients who survive the initial acute phase of the disease usually recover with time.

Chronic Inflammatory Demyelinating Polyneuropathy (CIDP)

CIDP is an inflammatory peripheral neuropathy, characterized by symmetrical mixed sensorimotor polyneuropathy that progresses for 2 months or more. Both motor and sensory abnormalities are common, such as weakness, difficulty in walking, numbness, pain, and tingling. Like Guillain-Barré syndrome, CIDP is immune mediated, but unlike Guillain-Barré syndrome it follows a chronic, relapsing-remitting, or progressive course. It occurs with increased frequency in patients with paraproteinemias, lymphoid neoplasms, and HIV infection. The peripheral nerves show segments of demyelination and remyelination.

Toxic, Vasculitic, and Inherited Forms of Peripheral Neuropathy

There are diverse other causes of peripheral neuropathy (see Table 20.1), some of which merit brief discussion.

- *Drugs* and *environmental toxins*, such as alcohol, various drugs used in cancer chemotherapy (e.g., taxanes, platinum), and arsenic, that interfere with axonal transport or cytoskeletal function produce peripheral neuropathies. The longest axons are most susceptible; hence, symptoms appear first and are most pronounced in the distal extremities.
- *Systemic vasculitis.* Peripheral nerves are damaged in different forms of systemic vasculitis (Chapter 8), including polyarteritis nodosa, cryoglobulinemia, and eosinophilic granulomatosis with polyangiitis (Churg-Strauss syndrome). Overall, peripheral nerve damage is seen in about one-third of patients with vasculitis at the time of presentation. The most common clinical picture is that of a painful asymmetric mixed sensory and motor peripheral neuropathy that randomly affects individual nerves. Patchy involvement is also apparent at the microscopic level, as single nerves may show considerable interfascicular variation in axonal damage.
- *Inherited diseases of peripheral nerves* are a heterogeneous but relatively common group of disorders. Hereditary motor and sensory neuropathies, sometimes included under the umbrella of Charcot-Marie-Tooth disease, are by far the most common inherited peripheral neuropathies, affecting up to 1 in 2500 people. They can be demyelinating or axonal. Most manifest in adulthood and follow a slowly progressive course that may mimic that of acquired

polyneuropathies. The most common causes are mutations in the genes encoding myelin-associated proteins.

- *Amyloid neuropathies are caused by deposition of amyloid fibrils in the peripheral nerves.* Light chain amyloidosis (in the setting of multiple myeloma or monoclonal gammopathy of uncertain significance) and familial transthyretin—related amyloidosis are the most common types of amyloid neuropathy. They present with progressive weakness, numbness, and neuropathic pain, with one of their characteristics being progressive autonomic manifestations, such as orthostatic hypotension, early in the course of the disease. Treatment of light chain amyloidosis includes chemotherapy to eradicate the plasma cell clones that secrete the pathogenic light chains and sometimes autologous stem cell transplantation. Liver transplantation (to eradicate the source of mutant transthyretin) has been used for the treatment of familial transthyretin related amyloidosis for 3 decades, but more recently silencing the transthyretin gene expression through gene therapy methods has become the first line of disease-modifying treatment. Several drugs that stabilize transthyretin to prevent its aggregation are also available.

Idiopathic Neuropathy

Between 30% and 40% of neuropathies are labeled idiopathic (or cryptogenic) after a workup fails to reveal a cause. Most occur in older adults (more than 55 years old) and present as slowly progressive, length-dependent, painful axonal neuropathy. Some cases of idiopathic neuropathy have been attributed to prediabetes and metabolic syndrome (a constellation of dysglycemia, hypertension, hyperlipidemia, and obesity). Treatment mainly consists of management of neuropathic pain with topical products, antiepileptics, antidepressants, and analgesics.

DISORDERS OF THE NEUROMUSCULAR JUNCTION

The neuromuscular junction is a complex, specialized structure located at the interface of motor nerve axons and skeletal muscle that serves to control muscle contraction. Here, the distal ends of peripheral motor nerves branch into small processes that terminate in bulbous synaptic boutons. Nerve impulses depolarize the presynaptic membrane, stimulating calcium influx and the release of acetylcholine into the synaptic cleft. Acetylcholine diffuses across the synaptic cleft to bind its receptor on the postsynaptic membrane, leading to depolarization of the myofiber and contraction through electromechanical coupling. Disorders of the neuromuscular junction often result in structural changes in the neuromuscular junction but may also produce functional deficits without any significant visible morphologic alterations. Considered in this section are some of the more common or pathogenically interesting disorders that disrupt the transmission of signals across the neuromuscular junction.

Myasthenia Gravis

Myasthenia gravis is an autoimmune disease with fluctuating muscle weakness that is caused by autoantibodies that target the neuromuscular junction. About 85% of patients with generalized myasthenia have autoantibodies against postsynaptic acetylcholine receptor (AChR), while most of the remaining patients have antibodies against sarcolemmal muscle-specific tyrosine kinase (MuSK). We focus here on the more common anti-AChR associated form, which has a prevalence of 150 to 200 per 1 million. There is a bimodal age distribution: early onset with a peak in the second and third decades (female predominance) and a late onset in the sixth to eighth decade (male predominance). Thymic abnormalities are common and take two forms: (1) thymic hyperplasia, actually a condition marked by the presence of reactive B-cell follicles (60% to 70% of cases); and (2) thymoma, a neoplasm of thymic epithelium (10% to 15% of cases) (Chapter 10). Both are believed to perturb tolerance to self antigens, setting the stage for the generation of anti-AChR antibodies that damage the postsynaptic membrane. AChR autoantibodies are found in 85% of patients with generalized and 50% with ocular myasthenia gravis (see below). Autoantibodies to AChR are classified as binding, blocking, or modulating. Binding antibodies cause complement activation that damages the neuromuscular junction and destroys the AChR. Blocking antibodies prevent the binding of ACh to the AChR. Modulating antibodies cross-link the receptor subunits, resulting in internalization, and are associated with myasthenia gravis due to thymoma.

Clinically, myasthenia gravis frequently manifests with *ptosis* (drooping eyelids) or *diplopia* (double vision) because of weakness in the extraocular muscles. This pattern of weakness is distinctly different from that of most primary myopathic diseases, in which there is relative sparing of facial and extraocular muscles. There are two clinical forms of myasthenia gravis: ocular and generalized. In some patients, symptoms are confined to ocular muscles, while others have both ocular and generalized weakness, including weakness of the bulbar and respiratory muscles, which may necessitate mechanical ventilation. The severity of the weakness typically fluctuates, sometimes over periods of a few minutes. Characteristically, repetitive nerve stimulation results in a decrease in the amplitude of the response. On the other hand, cholinesterase inhibitors improve strength by increasing the concentration of acetylcholine in the synaptic cleft. Effective treatments besides cholinesterase inhibitors include steroids, other immunosuppressants, complement pathway inhibitors, intravenous immunoglobulin, plasmapheresis, and, in selected patients, thymectomy. The prognosis of myasthenia gravis has significantly improved with these advancements in treatment, with most of the patients having a normal lifespan. However, about 10% of myasthenic cases are treatment refractory, and some patients still succumb to complications of the disease such as respiratory failure.

Lambert-Eaton Syndrome

Lambert-Eaton syndrome is caused by autoantibodies that inhibit the function of presynaptic calcium channels, thereby reducing the release of acetylcholine into the synaptic cleft. Patients with Lambert-Eaton syndrome experience limb and sometimes generalized muscle weakness, and there is improvement in weakness with brief muscle contraction or high-frequency repetitive nerve stimulation, which result in buildup of sufficient intracellular calcium to facilitate acetylcholine release. In about two-thirds of patients, Lambert-Eaton syndrome arises as a paraneoplastic disorder, particularly in patients with small cell lung carcinoma; in the others it is a primary autoimmune disease. Symptomatic treatment of Lambert-Eaton syndrome includes agents that block the presynaptic potassium channel, which increases the duration of action potentials in the presynaptic membrane. Unlike myasthenia gravis, cholinesterase inhibitors are not effective. Other forms of therapy include treatment of any underlying cancer and plasmapheresis or immunosuppression, which lower the concentration of the causative antibodies. The prognosis is worse than that of myasthenia gravis because of the frequent coexistence of an aggressive malignancy.

Miscellaneous Neuromuscular Junction Disorders

Several other neuromuscular junction disorders merit brief mention.

- *Congenital myasthenic syndromes* comprise a heterogeneous group of diseases that result from mutations that disrupt the function of various neuromuscular junction proteins. The causative mutations may encode presynaptic, synaptic, or postsynaptic proteins. Hence, they may present with symptoms mimicking Lambert-Eaton syndrome or myasthenia gravis. Some forms respond to treatment with acetylcholinesterase inhibitors.

- *Infections with exotoxin-producing bacteria* may be associated with defects in neural transmission and muscle contraction. *Clostridioides tetani* and *Clostridioides botulinum* both release extremely potent neurotoxins that interfere with neuromuscular transmission. Tetanus toxin blocks the action of inhibitory neurons, leading to the increased release of acetylcholine and sustained muscle contraction and spasm (tetanus). By contrast, botulinum toxin inhibits acetylcholine release, producing a flaccid paralysis. The purified toxin (Botox) is remarkably stable after injection, an attribute that has led to its widespread use as a treatment for wrinkles and a variety of other conditions associated with unwanted muscular activity (e.g., blepharospasm and strabismus).

DISORDERS OF SKELETAL MUSCLE

Patterns of Skeletal Muscle Injury and Atrophy

The principal component of the motor system is the *motor unit*, which is composed of one lower motor neuron, its neuromuscular junctions, and the skeletal muscle fibers it innervates. Skeletal muscle consists of different fiber types broadly classified as slow-twitch type I and fast-twitch type II fibers (Table 20.2). The fiber type is dependent on the innervation. All myofibers of a motor unit share the same fiber type. Normally, the fibers of different types are distributed in checkerboard patterns (see Fig. 20.1A). A number of proteins and protein complexes are crucial for the unique structure and function of skeletal muscles. These include proteins that make up the sarcomeres and the dystrophin-glycoprotein complex as well as enzymes that allow muscle

to meet its metabolic requirements. They will be discussed later when we present inherited disorders affecting muscles.

Primary muscle diseases or myopathies must be distinguished from secondary neuropathic changes caused by disorders that disrupt muscle innervation. Both are associated with altered muscle function and morphology, but each has distinctive features, illustrated in Fig. 20.2. Acquired causes of muscle injury also lead to distinctive changes. For example, prolonged disuse of muscles (e.g., due to prolonged bed rest, casting of a broken bone) may lead to focal or generalized muscle atrophy, which tends to affect type II fibers more than type I fibers. Glucocorticoid exposure, on the other hand, whether exogenous or endogenous (e.g., in Cushing syndrome), may cause preferential atrophy of proximal muscles and type II myofibers.

Inherited Disorders of Skeletal Muscle

Congenital diseases of muscle, called *muscular dystrophies* or *myopathies,* are caused by mutations in a variety of nuclear and mitochondrial genes, and present with involuntary contractions (myotonia) or weakness progressing to paralysis. In some of these disorders, the abnormalities are present almost from birth, whereas in others, the muscles are healthy at birth and the disorder develops over time. Clinically, they are heterogenous: in some, skeletal muscle is the main site of disease, while in others additional organs (e.g., the heart) are involved. Only the most common of these rare diseases are described here.

Dystrophinopathies: Duchenne and Becker Muscular Dystrophy

The most common muscular dystrophies are X-linked recessive disorders caused by mutations that disrupt the function of a large structural protein called *dystrophin* (Fig. 20.3). As a result, these diseases are referred to as *dystrophinopathies. Duchenne muscular dystrophy* (DMD) and *Becker muscular dystrophy* (BMD) are the two most important diseases in this group. DMD has an incidence of about 1 per 3500 live male births and follows an invariably fatal course. It becomes clinically evident in early childhood; most patients are wheelchair bound by the time they are teenagers and die of their disease by early adulthood. The Becker type of muscular dystrophy is less common and less severe.

Pathogenesis. **Duchenne and Becker muscular dystrophy are caused by loss-of-function mutations in the dystrophin gene on the X chromosome.** The gene encoding *dystrophin* is one of the largest human genes, spanning 2.3 million base pairs and 79 exons. Dystrophin is a key component of the dystrophin-glycoprotein complex (Fig. 20.3), consisting of dystrophin, dystroglycans, and sarcoglycans. It spans the plasma membrane and serves as a link between the cytoskeleton inside the myofiber and the basement membrane outside the cell, thereby providing mechanical stability to the myofiber and its cell membrane during muscle contraction. Defects in the complex may lead to small membrane tears that permit calcium influx, triggering events that culminate in myofiber degeneration. Duchenne muscular dystrophy is typically associated with deletions or frameshift mutations that result in total absence of dystrophin. By contrast, the mutations in Becker muscular dystrophy typically permit the synthesis of a truncated protein that retains partial function, explaining its less severe phenotype. The dystrophin-glycoprotein complex is also important for cardiac muscle function; as a result, cardiomyopathy eventually develops in many patients. Mutations affecting other components of this complex give rise to other primary muscle diseases, such as limb-girdle muscular dystrophies (described later).

Table 20.2 Muscle Fiber Types

	Type I	Type II
Action	Sustained force	Fast movement
Activity type	Aerobic exercise	Anaerobic exercise
Power produced	Low	High
Resistance to fatigue	High	Low
Lipid content	High	Low
Glycogen content	Low	High
Energy metabolism	Low glycolytic capacity, high oxidative capacity	High glycolytic capacity, low oxidative capacity
Mitochondrial density	High	Low
Myosin heavy chain gene expressed	*MYH7*	*MYH1, MYH2, MYH4*
Color	Red (high myoglobin content)	Pale red/tan (low myoglobin content)

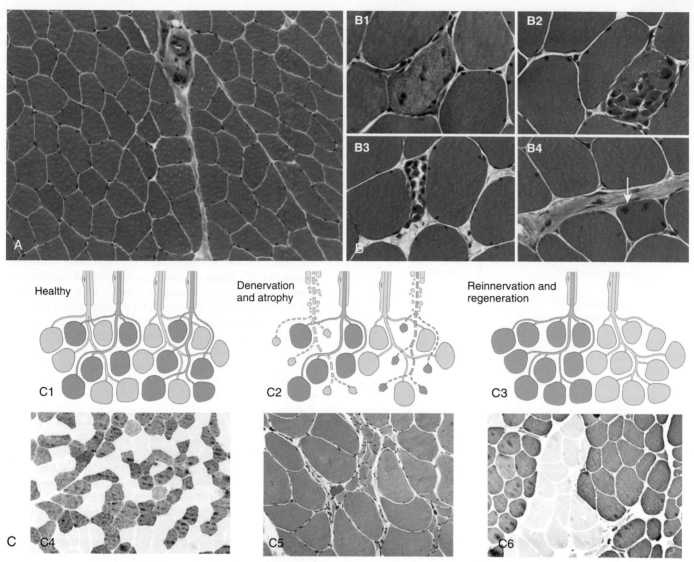

FIG. 20.2 Patterns of skeletal muscle injury. (A) Healthy skeletal muscle has relatively uniform polygonal myofibers with peripherally placed nuclei that are tightly packed together into fascicles separated by scant connective tissue. A perimysial interfascicular septum containing a blood vessel is present *(top center)*. (B) Myopathic conditions are often associated with segmental necrosis and regeneration of individual myofibers. Necrotic cells (B1–B3) are infiltrated by variable numbers of inflammatory cells. Regenerative myofibers (B4, *arrow*) are characterized by cytoplasmic basophilia and enlarged nucleoli (not visible at this power). (C) Neuropathic changes. (C1) This diagrammatic representation of four normal motor units shows a checkerboard-type admixture of light (type I) and dark (type II) stained fibers. (C2) Damage to innervating axons leads to a loss of trophic input and the atrophy of myofibers. (C3) Reinnervation of myofibers can result in a switch in fiber type and segregation of fibers of like type. As illustrated here, reinnervation is also often associated with an increase in motor unit size, with more myofibers innervated by an individual axon. (C4) Healthy muscle has a checkerboard distribution of type I *(light)* and type II *(dark)* fibers on this ATPase reaction (pH9.4), corresponding to findings in (A). (C5) Clustered flattened "angulated" atrophic fibers *(grouped atrophy)* are a typical finding associated with disrupted innervation. (C6) With ongoing denervation and reinnervation, large clusters of fibers appear that all share the same fiber type *(fiber type grouping)*.

MORPHOLOGY

The histologic alterations in skeletal muscles affected by DMD and BMD are similar, except that the changes are milder in BMD (Fig. 20.4). Immunohistochemical studies for dystrophin show absence of the normal sarcolemmal staining pattern in Duchenne muscular dystrophy and reduced staining in Becker muscular dystrophy.

The hallmarks of these as well as other muscular dystrophies are ongoing myofiber necrosis and regeneration. If degeneration outpaces repair, there is replacement of muscle tissue by fibrosis and fat. Due to ongoing repair, muscles typically show marked variation in myofiber size and abnormal internally placed nuclei. DMD and BMD also affect cardiac muscle, which shows variable degrees of myocyte hypertrophy and interstitial fibrosis.

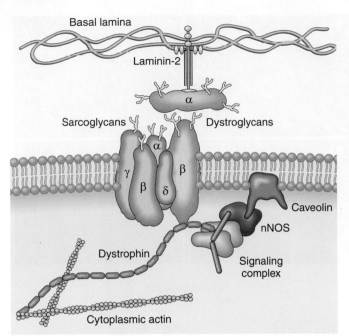

FIG. 20.3 The dystrophin-glycoprotein complex (DGC). This complex of glycoproteins serves to couple the cell membrane (the sarcolemma) to extracellular matrix proteins, such as laminin-2, and the intracellular cytoskeleton. A key set of connections is made by dystrophin, a scaffolding protein that tethers the myofibrillar cytoskeleton to transmembrane dystroglycans and sarcoglycans and binds signaling complexes, neuronal nitric oxide synthase (nNOS), and caveolin. Mutations in dystrophin are associated with X-linked Duchenne and Becker muscular dystrophies; mutations in caveolin and the sarcoglycan proteins with autosomal limb-girdle muscular dystrophies; and mutations in α2-laminin (merosin) with a form of congenital muscular dystrophy.

Clinical Features. Often the first symptoms of DMD are clumsiness and an inability to keep up with peers due to muscle weakness. The weakness typically begins in the pelvic girdle, followed by the shoulder girdle. Enlargement of the calves, termed pseudohypertrophy, is an early physical finding. The increased muscle bulk initially stems from myofiber hypertrophy, but as myofibers progressively degenerate, the muscle is increasingly replaced by adipose tissue and endomysial scar tissue. Cardiac muscle damage and fibrosis may lead to heart failure and arrhythmias, which may prove fatal. Although no structural abnormalities in the central nervous system have been described, cognitive impairment may also occur and may be severe enough to be classified as severe intellectual disability. Due to ongoing muscle degeneration, high serum creatine kinase levels are present at birth and persist through the first decade of life but then fall as muscle mass is lost with disease progression. BMD becomes symptomatic later in childhood or adolescence and progresses at a slower and more variable rate. Cardiac involvement may be the dominant clinical feature and may result in death, even in the absence of significant skeletal muscle weakness. The mean age of death for patients with Duchenne muscular dystrophy is 25 to 30 years of age, with most patients succumbing to respiratory insufficiency, pulmonary infection, or heart failure. By contrast, Becker muscular dystrophy typically presents in later childhood, adolescence, or adult life; it has slower progression; and affected individuals may have a near-normal life expectancy.

Management of patients with dystrophinopathies is challenging and currently consists primarily of supportive care. Definitive therapy would require restoration of dystrophin levels in skeletal and cardiac muscle fibers. Several genetic approaches to accomplish this are being tested. These include the administration of RNA-like molecules that alter RNA splicing and cause "skipping" of exons containing deleterious mutations, thus permitting the expression of a truncated, partially functional, dystrophin protein. This approach is clinically approved but appears to be of modest benefit. Other strategies that are still in the testing phase involves the use of drugs that promote ribosomal "read-through" of stop codons, another ploy that may enable the synthesis of some functional dystrophin protein, and delivery of dystrophin "mini-genes" using engineered viruses.

Other X-Linked and Autosomal Muscular Dystrophies

Other forms of muscular dystrophy share features with DMD and BMD but have distinct clinical, genetic, and pathologic features.

- *Myotonic dystrophy.* **Myotonia, the sustained involuntary contraction of a group of muscles, is the cardinal neuromuscular symptom in myotonic dystrophy.** Patients often report stiffness and difficulty in relaxing their grip, for example, after a handshake. Myotonic dystrophy is a trinucleotide repeat expansion disease (Chapter 4) with autosomal dominant inheritance. More than 95% of patients with myotonic dystrophy have mutations in the gene that encodes dystrophia myotonica protein kinase (DMPK). In unaffected individuals, this gene contains 5 to 37 CTG repeats, whereas affected patients usually carry 45 to several thousand. As discussed in Chapter 4, this disorder stems from a "toxic" gain of function caused by the triplet repeat expansion. Myotonic dystrophy often manifests in late childhood with gait abnormalities due to weakness of foot dorsiflexors, with subsequent progression to weakness of the intrinsic muscles of the hands and wrist extensors, atrophy of the facial muscles, and ptosis. Involvement of other organ systems results in potentially fatal cardiac arrhythmias, cataracts, early frontal balding, endocrinopathies, and testicular atrophy.

- *Limb-girdle muscular dystrophies.* **These muscular dystrophies preferentially affect the proximal musculature of the trunk and limbs.** Their genetic basis is heterogeneous. Some of the responsible mutations affect components of the dystrophin-glycoprotein complex other than dystrophin. Other mutations affect proteins involved in vesicle transport and repair of cell membranes after injury (e.g., caveolin, see Fig. 20.3), cytoskeletal proteins, or posttranslational modification of dystroglycan, a component of the dystrophin-glycoprotein complex.

- *Emery-Dreifuss muscular dystrophy* **(EMD) is a genetically heterogeneous disorder caused by mutations affecting structural proteins found in the nucleus.** An X-linked form results from mutations in the gene encoding the protein emerin, whereas an autosomal dominant form is caused by mutations in the gene encoding lamin A/C. It is hypothesized that defects in these proteins compromise the structural integrity of the nucleus in cells that are subjected to repetitive mechanical stress (e.g., cardiac and skeletal muscle). The clinical picture is characterized by progressive muscle weakness and wasting, contractures of the elbows and ankles, and cardiac disease. The cardiac involvement is severe, being associated with cardiomyopathy and arrhythmias that lead to sudden death in up to 40% of patients.

- *Facioscapulohumeral dystrophy* **is an autosomal dominant form of muscular dystrophy that is caused by genetic changes that lead to expression of DUX4, a transcription factor that is normally**

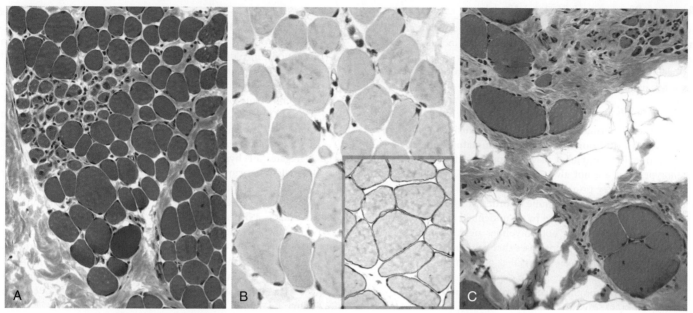

FIG. 20.4 Duchenne muscular dystrophy. Histologic images of muscle biopsy specimens from two brothers. (A—B) Specimens from a 3-year-old boy. (C) Specimen from his brother, 9 years of age. As seen in (A), at a younger age fascicular muscle architecture is maintained, but myofibers show variation in size. Additionally, there is a cluster of basophilic regenerating myofibers *(left side)* and slight endomysial fibrosis, seen as focal pink-staining connective tissue between myofibers. In (B), immunohistochemical staining shows a complete absence of membrane-associated dystrophin, seen as a brown stain in normal muscle *(inset)*. In (C), the biopsy from the older brother illustrates disease progression, which is marked by extensive variation in myofiber size, fatty replacement, and endomysial fibrosis.

repressed in mature tissues. It is thought that the disease is caused by overexpression of DUX4 target genes, many of which are involved in the normal function of skeletal muscles. Most patients become symptomatic by the age of 20 years, usually due to weakness in the facial muscles and the shoulder. The vast majority have a normal life expectancy.

Channelopathies, Metabolic Myopathies, and Mitochondrial Myopathies

Other important inherited disorders of skeletal muscle are the result of defects in ion channels (channelopathies), metabolism, and mitochondrial function.

- *Ion channel myopathies* are a group of familial disorders caused by inherited defects in ion channels that are characterized by myotonia, relapsing episodes of hypotonic paralysis associated with abnormal serum potassium levels, or both. Hypokalemic and hyperkalemic periodic paralysis both result in transient episodes of generalized muscle weakness. *Hypokalemic periodic paralysis* is more common; the paralytic attacks can last for hours to days and are precipitated by rest after exercise and high-carbohydrate meals. A mutation in a skeletal muscle calcium channel is the most common cause of hypokalemic periodic paralysis. By contrast, *hyperkalemic periodic paralysis* results from mutations in the gene encoding the skeletal muscle sodium channel, which regulates sodium entry during contraction. *Malignant hyperthermia* is a rare autosomal dominant syndrome characterized by tachycardia, tachypnea, muscle spasms, and hyperpyrexia. It is caused by mutations in the gene encoding the ryanodine receptor RYR1, a calcium efflux channel. Symptoms are triggered when patients receive halogenated anesthetic agents or succinylcholine during surgery.

Through uncertain mechanisms, exposure of the mutated receptor to the anesthetic leads to increased efflux of calcium from the sarcoplasmic reticulum, producing tetany and excessive heat production.

- *Mitochondrial myopathies* can stem from mutations in the mitochondrial or nuclear genomes since both encode proteins and RNAs that are critical for mitochondrial function. The disorders caused by mitochondrial mutations show maternal inheritance (Chapter 4). Mitochondrial myopathies usually manifest in early adulthood with proximal muscle weakness and sometimes with severe involvement of the ocular musculature *(external ophthalmoplegia)*. Some mitochondrial diseases are associated with normal muscle morphology, whereas others show aggregates of abnormal mitochondria; the latter impart a blotchy red appearance in special stains—hence the term *ragged red fibers*. On ultrastructural examination, these correspond to aggregates of mitochondria with abnormal shape and size, some containing crystalline inclusions.

- *Metabolic myopathies include several glycogen storage diseases*, the most common being McArdle disease and Pompe disease. *McArdle disease* is caused by a deficiency of myophosphorylase, which results in lack of ability of myofibers to utilize glycogen during brief, strong exercises, leading to exercise intolerance as well as exercise-induced muscle cramping and myoglobinuria. *Pompe disease* is lysosomal storage disease caused by a deficiency of acid alpha glucosidase (Chapter 4), which results in glycogen accumulation in heart, liver, and muscle (infantile type) and muscle (adult-onset type). The adult-onset type causes a proximal myopathy with predominant involvement of the respiratory muscles and diaphragm. Enzyme replacement therapy is available for the treatment of Pompe disease.

Acquired Disorders of Skeletal Muscle

A diverse group of acquired disorders may manifest with muscle weakness, muscle cramping, or muscle pain. These include inflammatory myopathies, toxic muscle injuries, postinfectious rhabdomyolysis, and muscle infarction in the setting of diabetes. In most instances, these are disorders of adults with acute or subacute onsets.

Inflammatory Myopathies

Polymyositis, dermatomyositis, and inclusion body myositis represent the traditional triad of inflammatory myopathies. This classification is a simplified view of complex diseases with variable phenotypes that are not always well delineated. The discussion that follows outlines key principles.

- *Polymyositis* is an autoimmune disorder in which CD8+ cytotoxic T lymphocytes are activated by an undefined antigen and kill muscle cells. Histologically, both myofiber necrosis and regeneration are seen (Fig. 20.5A). Many cases that were previously called polymyositis have now been reclassified as immune-mediated necrotizing myopathy (which shows sparse inflammation and some evidence of an immune mechanism), antisynthetase syndrome, or inclusion-body myositis (discussed below). Therefore, whether polymyositis is truly a distinct entity is uncertain.
- *Dermatomyositis* is the most common inflammatory myopathy in children, in whom it appears as an isolated entity. In adults, it is often a paraneoplastic disorder. In both contexts, it is believed to have an autoimmune basis. The disease is typically associated with skin manifestations such as a rash on sun-exposed skin, and may also have systemic manifestations (e.g., interstitial lung disease). There is damage to small blood vessels with secondary injury to muscles and skin. Myofiber damage is prominent in the paraseptal and perifascicular regions and may be accompanied by a mononuclear cell infiltrate (Fig. 20.5B). Anti−Mi-2 autoantibodies are highly specific for dermatomyositis, but their sensitivity is low.

- *Antisynthetase syndrome* is an autoimmune disorder associated with autoantibodies against different aminoacyl-transfer-RNAs, most common of which is anti-Jo1 antibody. It has multiple manifestations, including myositis (a polymyositis or dermatomyositis picture), fever, interstitial lung disease, and nonerosive arthritis.
- *Inclusion body myositis* is the most common inflammatory myopathy in patients older than 50 years of age. It is grouped with other forms of myositis, but it remains to be determined whether inflammation is a cause or an effect in this disorder. Its morphologic hallmark is the presence of rimmed vacuoles (Fig. 20.5C) filled with aggregates of hyperphosphorylated tau, amyloid derived from β-amyloid precursor protein, and TDP-43. These proteins are also seen in the brains of patients with neurodegenerative diseases (Chapter 21), leading some to speculate that inclusion body myositis is a degenerative disorder of aging. Other features typical of chronic inflammatory myopathies, including myopathic changes, mononuclear cell infiltrates, endomysial fibrosis, and fatty replacement, are also evident. The disease follows a chronic, progressive course and generally does not respond well to immunosuppressive agents, another feature suggesting that inflammation is a secondary event.

Toxic Myopathies

A number of toxins can cause muscle injury, which may be intrinsic (e.g., thyroxine) or extrinsic (e.g., acute alcohol intoxication, various drugs).

- *Thyrotoxic myopathy* may present as acute or chronic proximal muscle weakness and can be the first indication of thyrotoxicosis. Histologic findings include myofiber necrosis and regeneration.
- *Steroid myopathy* occurs in the setting of chronic steroid treatment or high endogenous steroid production. It is usually a proximal myopathy with a normal creatine kinase; muscle biopsy shows type 2 myofiber atrophy.

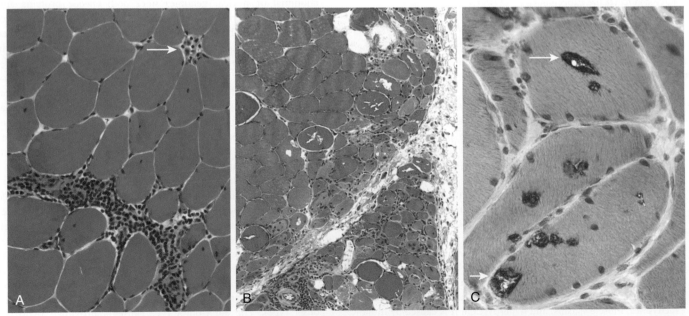

FIG. 20.5 Inflammatory myopathies. (A) Polymyositis is characterized by endomysial inflammatory infiltrates and myofiber necrosis *(arrow)*. (B) Dermatomyositis often shows prominent perifascicular and paraseptal atrophy. (C) Inclusion body myositis, showing myofibers containing rimmed vacuoles *(arrows)*. Modified Gomori trichrome stain.

- *Ethanol myopathy* occurs after an episode of binge drinking. The degree of rhabdomyolysis may be severe, sometimes leading to acute renal failure secondary to myoglobinuria. Patients usually experience acute muscle pain, which may be generalized or confined to a single muscle group. Microscopically, there is myocyte swelling, necrosis, and regeneration.

- *Drug myopathy* can be due to a variety of agents. Myopathy is the most common complication of statins (e.g., atorvastatin, simvastatin, pravastatin), occurring in approximately 1.5% of users. Two forms of statin-associated myopathy are recognized: (1) from direct toxicity of the drug and (2) an immune-mediated myopathy caused by statin-induced HMG-CoA reductase autoantibodies.

Tumors of Skeletal Muscles

Tumors showing evidence of skeletal muscle differentiation are discussed in Chapter 19 along with other tumors of soft tissues.

PERIPHERAL NERVE TUMORS

A number of different tumors arise from peripheral nerve sheaths. Such tumors may manifest as soft tissue masses, with pain or loss of function related to impingement on nerves or other surrounding structures. In most peripheral nerve tumors, the neoplastic cells show evidence of Schwann cell differentiation. These tumors usually occur in adults and include both benign and malignant variants. An important feature is their frequent association with the familial tumor syndromes neurofibromatosis type 1 (NF1) and neurofibromatosis type 2 (NF2).

Schwannomas and Neurofibromatosis Type 2

Schwannomas are benign encapsulated tumors that may occur in soft tissues, internal organs, or spinal nerve roots. The most commonly affected cranial nerve is the vestibular portion of the eighth nerve. Tumors arising in a nerve root or the vestibular nerve may be associated with symptoms related to nerve root compression, such as hearing loss in the case of vestibular schwannoma.

Most schwannomas are sporadic, but about 10% are associated with *familial neurofibromatosis type 2 (NF2)*. Patients with NF2 are at risk for developing multiple schwannomas, meningiomas, and ependymomas (Chapter 21). The presence of bilateral vestibular schwannomas is a hallmark of NF2; despite the name, neurofibromas (described later) are not found in patients with NF2.

NF2 is an autosomal dominant condition caused by loss of function mutations in the gene on chromosome 22 that encodes the protein merlin. Merlin interacts with the actin cytoskeleton and participates in several key signaling pathways that are involved in control of cell shape, cell growth, and the attachment of cells to one another (cell adhesion). Of note, merlin expression is also disrupted by somatic mutations in sporadic schwannomas.

MORPHOLOGY

Most schwannomas appear as circumscribed masses abutting an adjacent nerve. On microscopic examination, the tumors show a uniform proliferation of Schwann cells, often with an admixture of dense and loose regions referred to as Antoni A and B areas, respectively (Fig. 20.6A, B). In the dense **Antoni A** areas, bland spindle cells with buckled nuclei are arranged in intersecting fascicles. These cells often align to produce nuclear palisading, resulting in alternating bands of nuclear and anuclear areas called **Verocay bodies.** Axons are largely excluded from the tumor. In the loose, hypocellular **Antoni B** areas, the spindle cells are separated by myxoid extracellular matrix.

Neurofibromas and Neurofibromatosis Type 1

Neurofibromas are benign peripheral nerve sheath tumors. Three important subtypes are recognized:

- *Localized cutaneous neurofibromas* arise as superficial nodular or polypoid tumors. These occur either as solitary sporadic lesions or as multiple lesions in the context of neurofibromatosis 1 (NF1).
- *Plexiform neurofibromas* grow diffusely within the confines of a nerve or nerve plexus. Surgical enucleation of such lesions is therefore difficult and is often associated with lasting neurologic deficits. Plexiform neurofibromas are virtually pathognomonic for NF1

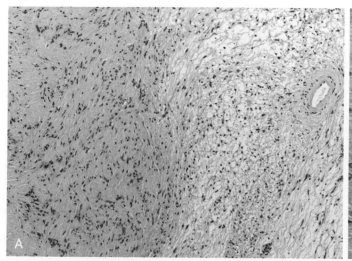
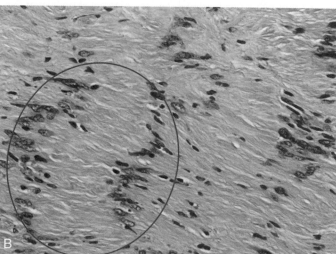

FIG. 20.6 Schwannoma and plexiform neurofibroma. (A–B) Schwannoma. As seen in (A), schwannomas often contain densely cellular Antoni A areas *(left)* and loose, hypocellular Antoni B areas *(right)*, as well as hyalinized blood vessels *(right)*. (B) Antoni A area with the nuclei of tumor cells aligned in palisading rows forming Verocay bodies (one such body is shown by the marked area).

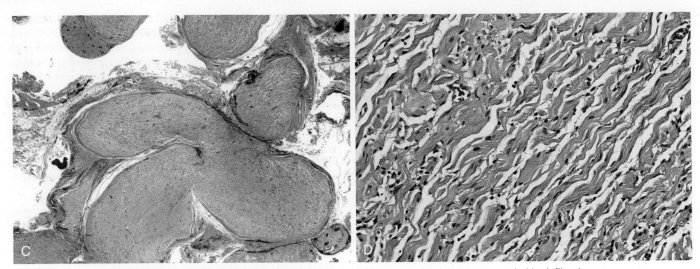

FIG. 20.6 (cont'd). (C–D) Plexiform neurofibroma. Multiple nerve fascicles are expanded by infiltrating tumor cells (C), which at higher power (D) are seen to consist of bland spindle cells admixed with wavy collagen bundles likened to carrot shavings.

(discussed below). Unlike other benign nerve sheath tumors, these tumors sometimes undergo malignant transformation.

- *Diffuse neurofibromas* are infiltrative proliferations that can take the form of large, disfiguring subcutaneous masses. These also are often associated with NF1.

NF1 is an autosomal dominant disorder caused by loss of function mutations in the gene that encodes the tumor suppressor neurofibromin, on the long arm of chromosome 17 (17q). Neurofibromin is a negative regulator of the potent oncoprotein RAS (Chapter 6). Loss of neurofibromin function and the resulting RAS hyperactivity appear to be a cardinal feature of NF1-associated tumors. In tumors arising in the setting of NF1, one *NF1* allele is lost in the germline and the other is mutated or silenced. These tumors include all three types of neurofibromas, malignant peripheral nerve sheath tumors, "optic gliomas," and other glial tumors. In addition, patients with NF1 exhibit learning disabilities, seizures, skeletal abnormalities, vascular abnormalities with arterial stenoses, pigmented nodules of the iris *(Lisch nodules)*, and pigmented skin lesions (axillary freckling and café-au-lait spots) to various degrees.

MORPHOLOGY

Unlike schwannomas, neurofibromas are not encapsulated. They may appear circumscribed, as in **localized cutaneous neurofibromas,** or may exhibit a diffusely infiltrative growth pattern. Also, in contrast to schwannomas, the neoplastic Schwann cells in neurofibroma are admixed with other cell types, including mast cells, fibroblast-like cells, and perineurial-like cells. The background stroma often contains loose wavy collagen bundles but can also be myxoid or densely fibrotic (Fig. 20.6D). **Plexiform neurofibromas** involve multiple fascicles of individual affected nerves (Fig. 20.6C). **Diffuse neurofibromas** show an extensive infiltrative pattern of growth within the dermis and subcutis of the skin.

Malignant Peripheral Nerve Sheath Tumors

Malignant peripheral nerve sheath tumors typically arise in adults and show evidence of Schwann cell derivation. In some cases they clearly originate from a peripheral nerve. They may arise from transformation of a neurofibroma, usually of the plexiform type. About one-half of such tumors arise in patients with NF1, and 3% to 10% of all patients with NF1 develop a malignant peripheral nerve sheath tumor during their lifetime. Histologically, these tumors are highly cellular and exhibit features of malignancy, including anaplasia, necrosis, infiltrative growth pattern, pleomorphism, and high proliferative activity.

Traumatic Neuroma

Traumatic neuroma is a nonneoplastic proliferation associated with transection of a peripheral nerve. Such injuries activate a regenerative program (see Fig. 20.1) characterized by sprouting and elongation of processes from the proximal axonal stump. With severe injuries that disrupt the perineurial sheath, these new processes may "miss" their target, the distal end of the transected nerve. The misguided elongating axonal processes can induce a reactive proliferation of Schwann cells, leading to the formation of a painful localized nodule consisting of a haphazard mixture of axons, Schwann cells, and connective tissue.

■ RAPID REVIEW

Peripheral Neuropathies

- Peripheral neuropathies may result in weakness and/or sensory deficits in patterns described as polyneuropathy, mononeuritis multiplex, and mononeuropathy.
- Axonal and demyelinating peripheral neuropathies can be distinguished on the basis of clinical, electromyography, and pathologic features. Some disorders are associated with a mixed pattern of injury.
- Diabetes is the most common cause of peripheral neuropathy.
- Guillain-Barré syndrome and chronic inflammatory demyelinating polyneuropathy are immune-mediated demyelinating diseases that follow acute and chronic courses, respectively.
- Metabolic diseases, drugs, toxins, connective tissue diseases, vasculitides, and infections all can result in peripheral neuropathy.
- A number of germline mutations cause peripheral neuropathy. Many of these are adult-onset diseases that may mimic the acquired ones.

Neuromuscular Junction Disorders

- Disorders of neuromuscular junctions manifest with weakness that often affects facial and extraocular muscles and may show fluctuation in severity.
- Both myasthenia gravis and Lambert-Eaton syndrome, which are the most common forms, are immune mediated, being caused by antibodies that typically target postsynaptic acetylcholine receptors and presynaptic calcium channels, respectively.
- Autoantibodies to AChR impair neuromuscular transmission by antibody- and complement-mediated damage to motor end plates.
- Myasthenia gravis is often associated with thymic hyperplasia or thymoma. Lambert-Eaton syndrome is a paraneoplastic disorder in the majority of the cases; the strongest association is with small cell lung cancer.
- Genetic defects in neuromuscular junction proteins and bacterial toxins can also cause symptomatic disturbances in neuromuscular transmission.

Disorders of Skeletal Muscle

- Skeletal muscle function can be impaired by a primary (inherited or acquired) myopathy or secondarily by disturbed muscle innervation.
- The genetic forms of myopathy fall into several fairly distinct clinical phenotypes, including muscular dystrophy, congenital myopathy, and congenital muscular dystrophy.

- Dystrophinopathies are X-linked disorders caused by mutations in the dystrophin gene and disruption of the dystrophin-glycoprotein complex. Depending on the type of mutation, the disease may be severe (Duchenne muscular dystrophy) or mild (Becker muscular dystrophy).
- Acquired myopathies have diverse causes, including inflammation and toxic exposures. Three types of inflammatory myositis are recognized, polymyositis, dermatomyositis, and inclusion body myositis, each with distinctive features.

Peripheral Nerve Sheath Tumors

- In most peripheral nerve sheath tumors, the neoplastic cells show evidence of Schwann cell differentiation.
- Peripheral nerve sheath tumors are important features of the familial tumor syndromes NF1 and NF2.
- Schwannomas are benign nerve sheath tumors. They are circumscribed tumors that abut the nerve of origin and are a feature of NF2.
- Neurofibromas may manifest as a sporadic subcutaneous nodule, as a large, poorly defined soft tissue lesion, or as a growth within a nerve. Neurofibromas are associated with NF1.
- About 50% of malignant peripheral nerve sheath tumors occur de novo in otherwise healthy persons, whereas the remainder arise from the malignant transformation of a preexisting NF1-associated neurofibroma.

The contributions to this chapter by Dr. Matthew P. Frosch, Department of Pathology, Massachusetts General Hospital, Harvard Medical School, Boston Massachusetts, and Dr. Robert Folberg in several previous editions of this book are gratefully acknowledged.

The principal focus of this chapter is on diseases of the central nervous system (CNS). At the end, we briefly describe some important disorders of the eye, which is linked anatomically and functionally to the CNS.

CENTRAL NERVOUS SYSTEM

Disorders of the CNS are some of the most serious diseases of humankind. These diseases have many unique features that reflect the highly specialized structure and functions of the CNS. The principal functional unit of the CNS is the *neuron* (gray matter). Neurons of different types and in different locations have distinct properties, including functional roles, distribution of their connections, neurotransmitters used, metabolic requirements, and levels of electrical activity at a given moment. A population of neurons may show selective vulnerability to various insults because it shares one or more of these properties. Since different regions of the brain participate in different functions, the pattern of clinical signs and symptoms that follow injury depend both on the region of brain involved and the pathologic process. Mature neurons are incapable of cell division, so destruction of even a small number of neurons essential for a specific function may cause a neurologic deficit. In addition to neurons the CNS contains other cells, such as *astrocytes* and *oligodendrocytes*, which make up the *glia* (white matter). The components of the CNS are affected by a number of unique neurologic disorders and also respond to common insults (e.g., ischemia, infection) in a manner that is distinct from other tissues.

Before delving into specific disorders, we briefly review the characteristic morphologic changes that are often seen in the CNS in the setting of injury or infection.

MORPHOLOGY

Features of Neuronal Injury. In response to injury, a number of changes occur in neurons and their processes (axons and dendrites). Within 12 hours of an irreversible hypoxic-ischemic insult, neuronal injury becomes evident on routine hematoxylin and eosin (H&E) staining (Fig. 21.1A). There is shrinkage of the cell body, pyknosis of the nucleus, disappearance of the nucleolus, loss of cytoplasmic rough endoplasmic reticulum staining (referred to as Nissl substance in neurons), and intense eosinophilia of the cytoplasm (**red neurons**). Axonal injury also leads to cell body enlargement and rounding, peripheral displacement of the nucleus, enlargement of the nucleolus, and peripheral dispersion of Nissl substance (**central chromatolysis**). In addition, acute injuries typically result in breakdown of the blood-brain barrier and variable degrees of cerebral edema (discussed later).

Many neurodegenerative diseases are associated with accumulation of abnormal proteins (e.g., amyloid plaques in Alzheimer disease) or specific **intracellular inclusions** (e.g., Lewy bodies in Parkinson disease).

Pathogenic viruses may form inclusions in infected neurons, just as in other cells, and such inclusions aid in the diagnosis. In some neurodegenerative diseases, neuronal processes become thickened and tortuous; these are termed **dystrophic neurites.**

Astrocyte Injury and Repair. Astrocytes are the principal cells responsible for repair and scar formation in the brain, a process termed **gliosis.** In response to injury, astrocytes undergo both hypertrophy and hyperplasia. The nucleus enlarges and becomes vesicular, and the nucleolus becomes prominent. The cytoplasm expands and takes on a bright pink hue, and the cell extends multiple stout, ramifying processes (**gemistocytic astrocyte;** Fig. 21.1B). In contrast to elsewhere in the body, fibroblasts do not contribute to healing after brain injury except in specific settings (e.g., penetrating brain trauma or around abscesses). In long-standing gliosis, the cytoplasm of reactive astrocytes shrinks in size, and the cellular processes become more tightly interwoven (**fibrillary astrocytes**). **Rosenthal fibers** are thick, elongated, brightly eosinophilic protein aggregates found in astrocytic processes in chronic gliosis and in some low-grade gliomas.

Oligodendrocytes, which produce myelin, exhibit a limited spectrum of specific morphologic changes in response to various injuries, such as the intranuclear viral inclusions seen in progressive multifocal leukoencephalopathy.

Microglial cells are long-lived cells derived from the embryonic yolk sac that function as the resident phagocytes of the CNS. When activated by tissue injury, infection, or trauma, they proliferate and become more prominent histologically. In areas of demyelination, organizing infarct, or hemorrhage, microglial cells resemble activated macrophages; in other settings such as infections, they develop elongated nuclei (**rod cells**). Aggregates of elongated microglial cells at sites of tissue injury are termed **microglial nodules** (Fig. 21.1C). Similar collections can be found congregating around and phagocytosing injured neurons (**neuronophagia**).

Ependymal cells line the ventricular system and the central canal of the spinal cord. Certain pathogens, particularly cytomegalovirus (CMV), can produce extensive ependymal injury, with typical viral inclusions. **Choroid plexus** is in continuity with the ependyma, and its specialized epithelial covering is responsible for the secretion of cerebrospinal fluid (CSF).

Clinical evaluation of neurologic diseases often relies on localizing signs (e.g., contralateral weakness after occlusion of a cerebral artery), which indicate the site of the abnormality, and nonlocalizing signs (e.g., altered mental status), which indicate the presence of a neurologic disorder but not its site.

EDEMA, HERNIATION, AND HYDROCEPHALUS

The brain and spinal cord are encased within the skull and spinal canal, with nerves and blood vessels passing through different foramina. Housing the delicate CNS within hard, rigid structures provides protection but leaves little room for expansion of the brain or

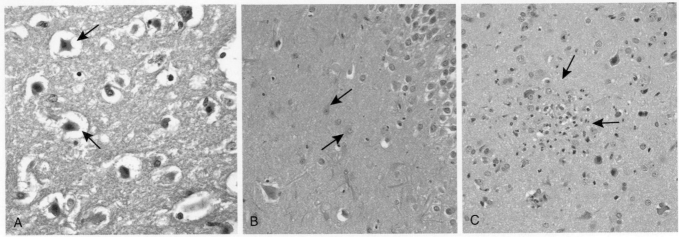

FIG. 21.1 Patterns of neuronal injury. (A) Acute hypoxic-ischemic injury in the cerebral cortex. The cell bodies are shrunken and eosinophilic ("red neurons," *arrows*), and the nuclei are pyknotic. (B) Reactive astrocytes *(arrows)*, with eosinophilic cytoplasm and multiple radiating processes. (C) Collection of microglial cells forming a poorly defined nodule *(arrow)*, a common finding in viral infections.

its surrounding fluid in disease states. As a result, virtually any expansion of skull contents brings with it an increase in intracranial pressure. Substantial increases in intracranial pressure compromise the ability of the cardiovascular system to deliver blood to the brain, resulting in decreased brain perfusion, with serious or fatal consequences. Disorders that may cause dangerous increases in intracranial contents include generalized cerebral edema, hydrocephalus, hemorrhage, ischemia, and mass lesions such as tumors.

Cerebral Edema

Cerebral edema is the accumulation of excess fluid within the brain parenchyma. There are two types, which often occur together, particularly after generalized injury.

- *Vasogenic edema* occurs when the integrity of the blood-brain barrier is disrupted, allowing fluid to shift from the vascular compartment into the extracellular spaces of the brain. Vasogenic edema can be localized (e.g., the result of increased vascular permeability due to inflammation or a tumor) or generalized.
- *Cytotoxic edema* is an increase in intracellular fluid secondary to neuronal and glial cell injury, as might follow a generalized hypoxic or ischemic insult or exposure to certain toxins.

The edematous brain is softer than normal and often appears to fill the cranial vault. In generalized edema, the gyri are flattened, the intervening sulci are narrowed, and the ventricular cavities are compressed (Fig. 21.2).

Hydrocephalus

CSF is produced by the choroid plexus within the ventricles, then circulates through the ventricular system and flows through the foramina of Luschka and Magendie into the subarachnoid space, where it is absorbed by arachnoid granulations. The balance between rates of generation and resorption regulates CSF volume.

Hydrocephalus is increase in the volume of the CSF within the ventricular system. Most often, this disorder is a consequence of impaired flow or decreased resorption of CSF. If there is a localized obstacle to CSF flow within the ventricular system, then a portion of the ventricles enlarge while the remainder do not. This pattern is referred to as *noncommunicating hydrocephalus* and is most commonly caused by

masses (e.g., tumor, hemorrhage, or infection) obstructing the foramen of Monro or compressing the cerebral aqueduct. In *communicating hydrocephalus*, the entire ventricular system is enlarged, usually secondary to reduced CSF resorption, for unknown reasons.

When hydrocephalus develops in infancy before closure of the cranial sutures, the head enlarges. Once the sutures fuse, hydrocephalus causes ventricular expansion and increased intracranial pressure, but no change in head circumference (Fig. 21.3). In contrast to these disorders, in which increased CSF volume is the primary process, a compensatory increase in CSF volume *(hydrocephalus ex vacuo)* may occur secondary to a loss of brain volume from any underlying cause (e.g., infarction, neurodegenerative disease).

Herniation

Herniation is the displacement of brain tissue past rigid dural folds (the falx and tentorium) or through openings in the skull because of increased intracranial pressure. The brain herniates when its limited capacity to accommodate the increased pressure is exceeded. Brain

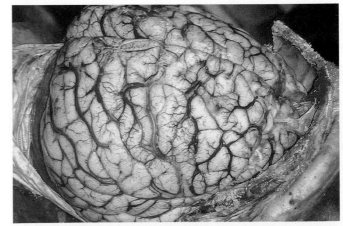

FIG. 21.2 Cerebral edema. The surfaces of the gyri are flattened as a result of compression of the expanding brain by the dura mater and inner surface of the skull. Such changes are associated with a dangerous increase in intracranial pressure.

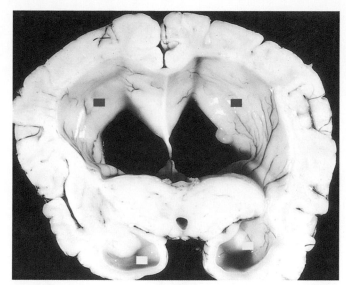

FIG. 21.3 Hydrocephalus. Dilated lateral ventricles (*red boxes*, bodies of lateral ventricles; *yellow boxes*, posterior horns of lateral ventricles) seen in a coronal section through the mid-thalamus.

herniation is most often caused by mass effects, either diffuse (generalized brain edema) or focal (tumors, abscesses, or hemorrhages). Elevated intracranial pressure may also compress the vasculature and reduce perfusion of the brain, causing ischemic injury and further exacerbating cerebral edema.

MORPHOLOGY

The brain may herniate through different openings, and if the expansion is sufficiently severe, herniation may occur simultaneously in several locations (Fig. 21.4):

- **Subfalcine (cingulate) herniation** occurs when unilateral or asymmetric expansion of a cerebral hemisphere displaces the cingulate gyrus under the edge of the falx. This may compress the anterior cerebral artery resulting in contralateral leg weakness, or aphasia if the herniation affects the dominant hemisphere.
- **Transtentorial (uncinate) herniation** occurs when the medial aspect of the temporal lobe is compressed against the free margin of the tentorium. As the temporal lobe is displaced, the third cranial nerve is compromised, resulting in pupillary dilation and impaired ocular movements on the side of the lesion ("blown pupil"). The posterior cerebral artery may also be compressed, resulting in ischemic injury to tissue supplied by that vessel, including the primary visual cortex. With further displacement of the temporal lobe, pressure on the midbrain may compress the contralateral cerebral peduncle against the tentorium, resulting in hemiparesis ipsilateral to the side of the herniation. The compression of the peduncle creates a deformation known as **Kernohan's notch.** Compression of the midbrain and the ascending reticular activating system with transtentorial herniation leads to depressed consciousness. Progression of transtentorial herniation is often accompanied by linear or flame-shaped hemorrhages in the midbrain and pons, termed **Duret hemorrhages** (Fig. 21.5). These lesions usually occur in the midline and paramedian regions and are believed to be the result of tearing of penetrating veins and arteries supplying the upper brain stem.
- **Tonsillar herniation** refers to displacement of the cerebellar tonsils through the foramen magnum. This type of herniation causes brain stem compression and compromises vital respiratory and cardiac centers in the medulla and is often rapidly fatal.

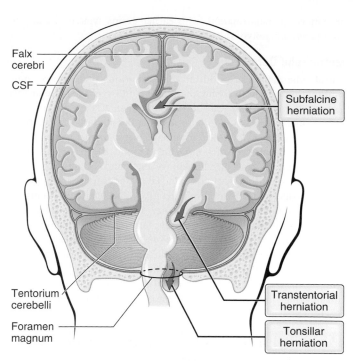

FIG. 21.4 Herniation. Displacement of brain parenchyma across fixed barriers can be subfalcine, transtentorial, or tonsillar (into the foramen magnum). *CSF,* Cerebrospinal fluid.

CONGENITAL MALFORMATIONS

The incidence of CNS malformations, giving rise to mental disability, cerebral palsy, or neural tube defects, is estimated at 1% to 2% of pregnancies. Malformations of the brain are more common in the setting of multiple anomalies. Mutations affecting genes that regulate the differentiation, maturation, or intercellular communication of neurons or glial cells can cause CNS malformation or dysfunction. Prenatal or perinatal insults, including various chemicals and infectious agents, may interfere with normal CNS development or cause tissue damage. During gestation, the timing of an injury determines

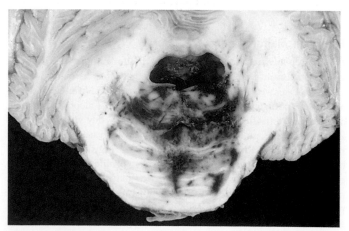

FIG. 21.5 Duret hemorrhage. As mass effect displaces the brainstem downward, there is disruption of the vessels that enter the pons along the midline, leading to hemorrhage.

the pattern of malformation, with earlier events typically leading to more severe phenotypes.

Neural Tube Defects

Neural tube defects are midline malformations that involve some combination of neural tissue, meninges, and overlying bone or soft tissue; collectively, they are the most common CNS malformations. Two distinct pathogenic mechanisms are contributory: (1) failure of neural tube closure, in which secondary mesenchymal tissue defects stem from aberrant skeletal modeling around the malformed tube (e.g., anencephaly and myelomeningocele), and (2) primary bony defects that are caused by abnormal axial mesoderm development and lead to secondary CNS abnormalities (e.g., encephalocele, meningocele, and spina bifida). Folate deficiency during the first trimester increases risk through uncertain mechanisms and represents an important opportunity for prevention, as folate supplements in women of child-bearing age reduce the incidence of neural tube defects by up to 70%. Serum α-fetoprotein (AFP) is elevated in the setting of neural tube defects; maternal screening for AFP combined with imaging studies has increased the early detection of neural tube defects.

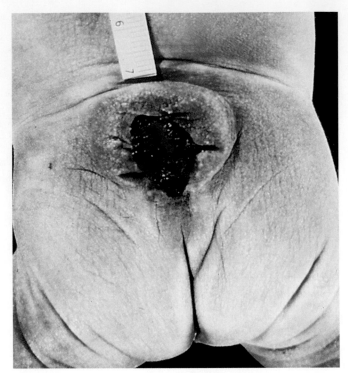

FIG. 21.6 Myelomeningocele. Both meninges and spinal cord parenchyma are included in the cystlike structure visible just above the buttocks.

MORPHOLOGY

- The most common defects involve the posterior end of the neural tube, from which the spinal cord forms. These can range from asymptomatic bony defects **(spina bifida occulta)** to **spina bifida**, a severe malformation consisting of a flat, disorganized segment of spinal cord associated with an overlying meningeal outpouching.
- **Myelomeningocele** is an extension of CNS tissue through a defect in the vertebral column that occurs most commonly in the lumbosacral region (Fig. 21.6). Patients have motor and sensory deficits in the lower extremities and problems with bowel and bladder control. The clinical problems derive from the abnormal spinal cord segment and often are compounded by infections due to defects in the thin overlying skin, which is prone to ulceration.
- **Anencephaly** is a malformation of the anterior end of the neural tube that leads to the absence of the forebrain and the top of the skull. Varying amounts of posterior fossa structures may be present.
- An **encephalocele** is a diverticulum of malformed CNS tissue extending through a defect in the cranium. It most often involves the occipital region or the posterior fossa. When it occurs anteriorly, brain tissue may extend into the sinuses.

Forebrain Malformations

Microencephaly describes the group of malformations in which the volume of brain is abnormally small; usually it is associated with a small head as well (*microcephaly*). There are a wide range of associations, including chromosome abnormalities, fetal alcohol syndrome, and in utero infection by human immunodeficiency virus (HIV) and Zika virus. The underlying mechanism is decreased generation of neurons destined for the cerebral cortex. During the early stages of brain development, as progenitor cells proliferate in the subependymal ventricular zone, the balance between cells leaving the progenitor population to form the cortex and those remaining in the proliferating pool affects the overall number of neurons and glial cells generated. If too many cells leave the progenitor pool prematurely, there is inadequate generation of mature neurons, leading to a small brain. Disruption of neuronal migration and differentiation during development can lead to abnormalities of gyration and neocortical

architecture, with neurons often ending up in the wrong location. Mutations in various genes that control migration result in a variety of malformations. A representative example is *holoprosencephaly*, characterized by disruption of normal midline patterning. Mild forms show absence of the olfactory bulbs and related structures (*arrhinencephaly*). In severe forms, the brain is not divided into hemispheres or lobes, and there may be facial midline defects such as cyclopia. The best known genetic causes involve inherited loss-of-function mutations in components of the Hedgehog signaling pathway.

Other examples include loss of gyri, which may be complete (*lissencephaly*) or partial, and increased number of irregularly formed gyri (*polymicrogyria*).

Posterior Fossa Anomalies

The most common malformations in this region of the brain result in misplacement or absence of portions of the cerebellum.

- *Arnold-Chiari malformation* (Chiari type II malformation) combines a small posterior fossa with a misshapen midline cerebellum and downward extension of the vermis through the foramen magnum; hydrocephalus and a lumbar myelomeningocele typically are also present.
- The far milder *Chiari type I malformation* has low-lying cerebellar tonsils that extend through the foramen magnum. Excess tissue in the foramen magnum results in partial obstruction of CSF flow and compression of the medulla, with symptoms of headache or cranial nerve deficits often manifesting only in adult life. Surgical intervention can alleviate the symptoms.
- *Dandy-Walker malformation* is characterized by an enlarged posterior fossa, absence of the cerebellar vermis, and a large midline cyst.

GENETIC METABOLIC DISEASES

Several genetic diseases disrupt metabolic processes in neurons and glia, resulting in progressive disorders that present early in life. These diseases can be grouped based on the cells or compartment (e.g., neurons or white matter), organelles (e.g., lysosome, peroxisome, or mitochondrion), or metabolites (e.g., sphingolipidoses, very long–chain fatty acids) that are affected. The mutations underlying these diseases typically disrupt synthetic or degradation pathways that are specific to the nervous system.

- *Neuronal storage diseases* are characterized by the accumulation of storage material within neurons, typically resulting in neuronal death. Cortical neuronal involvement leads to loss of cognitive function and also may cause seizures. Most commonly, they are autosomal recessive disorders caused by the deficiency of a specific enzyme involved in the catabolism of sphingolipids (including the gangliosides), mucopolysaccharides, or mucolipids; others appear to be caused by defects in protein or lipid trafficking within neurons. Several examples of these diseases, such as Tay-Sachs and Niemann-Pick disease and mucopolysaccharidoses (all lysosomal storage disorders) are discussed in Chapter 4.
- *Mitochondrial encephalomyopathies* are disorders of oxidative phosphorylation, often affecting multiple tissues including skeletal muscle (Chapter 20). When they involve the brain, gray matter is more severely affected than white matter due to the greater metabolic requirements of neurons. These disorders may be caused by mutations in mitochondrial or nuclear genes. They present with muscle weakness, seizures, and visual defects, alone or in combination.

CEREBROVASCULAR DISEASES

Cerebrovascular diseases are brain disorders caused by pathologic processes involving blood vessels. They are a major cause of death and morbidity in high resource parts of the world. The three main pathogenic mechanisms are (1) thrombotic occlusion, (2) embolic occlusion, and (3) vascular rupture. *Stroke* is the clinical designation applied to all these conditions when symptoms begin acutely. Thrombosis and embolism have similar consequences for the brain: loss of oxygen and metabolic substrates, resulting in infarction or ischemic injury of regions supplied by the affected vessel. Similar injury occurs globally when there is complete loss of perfusion, severe hypoxemia (e.g., hypovolemic shock), or profound hypoglycemia. Hemorrhage accompanies rupture of vessels and leads to direct tissue damage as well as secondary ischemic injury. Traumatic vascular injury is discussed separately in the context of trauma.

Hypoxia, Ischemia, and Infarction

The brain is a highly oxygen-dependent tissue that requires a continuous supply of glucose and oxygen from the blood. Although it constitutes no more than 2% of body weight, the brain receives 15% of the resting cardiac output and is responsible for 20% of total body oxygen consumption. Cerebral blood flow normally remains stable over a wide range of blood pressure and intracranial pressure because of autoregulation of vascular resistance. The brain may be deprived of oxygen by two general mechanisms:

- *Functional hypoxia,* caused by a low partial pressure of oxygen (e.g., high altitude), impaired oxygen-carrying capacity (e.g., severe anemia, carbon monoxide poisoning), or toxins that interfere with oxygen use (e.g., cyanide poisoning)
- *Ischemia,* either *transient* or *permanent,* due to tissue hypoperfusion, which can be caused by hypotension, vascular obstruction, or both

Global Cerebral Ischemia

Global cerebral hypoxia or ischemia occurs when there is a generalized reduction of cerebral perfusion (as in cardiac arrest, shock, and severe hypotension) or decreased oxygen-carrying capacity of the blood (e.g., in carbon monoxide poisoning). The clinical outcome varies with the severity and duration of the insult. When the insult is mild, there may be only transient confusion followed by complete recovery. Neurons are more susceptible to hypoxic injury than are glial cells, and the most susceptible neurons are the pyramidal cells of the hippocampus and neocortex and Purkinje cells of the cerebellum. In some cases, even mild or transient global ischemic insults may cause damage to these vulnerable areas. In severe global cerebral ischemia, widespread neuronal death occurs irrespective of regional vulnerability. Patients who survive often remain severely impaired neurologically, sometimes in a persistent vegetative state. Other patients meet the clinical criteria for so-called "brain death," in which all voluntary and reflex brain and brain stem function is absent, including respiratory drive. When patients with this form of irreversible injury are maintained on mechanical ventilation, the brain may gradually undergo autolysis.

MORPHOLOGY

In the setting of global ischemia, the brain is swollen, with wide gyri and narrowed sulci. The cut surface shows poor demarcation between gray matter and white matter. The histopathologic changes that accompany irreversible ischemic injury (infarction) are grouped into three categories. **Early changes,** occurring 12 to 24 hours after the insult, include acute neuronal cell change (red neurons) (see Fig. 21.1A) characterized initially by microvacuolation, followed by cytoplasmic eosinophilia, and later nuclear pyknosis and karyorrhexis. Similar changes occur somewhat later in astrocytes and oligodendroglia. After this, the reaction to tissue damage begins with infiltration of neutrophils. **Subacute changes,** occurring at 24 hours to 2 weeks, include necrosis of tissue, influx of macrophages, vascular proliferation, and reactive gliosis. **Repair,** seen after 2 weeks, is characterized by removal of necrotic tissue and gliosis.

Focal Cerebral Ischemia

Cerebral arterial occlusion leads first to ischemia and then to infarction in the distribution of the compromised vessel. The size, location, and shape of the infarct and the extent of tissue damage that results may be modified by collateral blood flow. Specifically, collateral flow through the circle of Willis or cortical-leptomeningeal anastomoses can limit damage in some regions. By contrast, there is little if any collateral blood flow to structures such as the thalamus, basal ganglia, and deep white matter, which are supplied by deep penetrating vessels.

Infarctions caused by emboli are more common than infarctions due to thrombosis. Cardiac mural thrombi are a frequent source of emboli; myocardial dysfunction, valvular disease, and atrial fibrillation are important predisposing factors. Thromboemboli also arise in arteries, most often from atheromatous plaques in the carotid arteries or aortic arch. Emboli of venous origin may cross over to the arterial circulation through a patent foramen ovale and lodge in the brain (paradoxical embolism; see Chapter 9); these include thromboemboli from deep leg veins and fat emboli, usually following bone trauma. The territory of the middle cerebral artery, a direct extension of the internal carotid artery, is most frequently affected by embolic occlusion. Emboli tend to lodge where vessels branch or in areas of stenosis, usually caused by atherosclerosis.

Thrombotic occlusions causing cerebral infarctions are usually superimposed on atherosclerotic plaques; common sites are the carotid bifurcation, the origin of the middle cerebral artery, and either end of the basilar artery. These occlusions may be accompanied by anterograde extension, as well as thrombus fragmentation and distal embolization. Thrombotic occlusions causing small infarcts of only a few millimeters in diameter, so-called *lacunar infarcts,* occur when small penetrating arteries get occluded due to chronic damage, usually from long-standing hypertension (discussed later).

MORPHOLOGY

Infarcts can be divided into two broad groups. **Nonhemorrhagic infarcts** result from acute vascular occlusions and may evolve into hemorrhagic infarcts when there is reperfusion of ischemic tissue, either through collaterals or after dissolution of emboli. **Hemorrhagic infarcts** usually manifest as multiple, sometimes confluent, petechial hemorrhages (Fig. 21.7A, B). The microscopic picture and evolution of hemorrhagic infarction are similar to those of nonhemorrhagic infarction, with the addition of blood extravasation and resorption. In individuals with coagulopathies, hemorrhagic infarcts may be associated with large intracerebral hematomas.

The macroscopic appearance of a nonhemorrhagic infarct evolves over time. During the first 6 hours, the tissue is unchanged in appearance, but by 48 hours, the tissue becomes pale, soft, and swollen. From days 2 to 10, the injured brain turns gelatinous and friable, and the boundary between normal and abnormal tissue becomes more distinct as edema resolves in the adjacent viable tissue. From day 10 to week 3, the tissue liquefies, eventually leaving a fluid-filled cavity, which gradually appears larger as dead tissue is resorbed (Fig. 21.7C).

Microscopically, the tissue reaction follows a characteristic sequence. After the first 12 hours, ischemic neuronal change (red neurons) (see Fig. 21.1A) and cytotoxic and vasogenic edema appear. Endothelial and glial cells, mainly astrocytes, swell, and myelinated fibers begin to disintegrate. During the first several days neutrophils infiltrate the area of injury (Fig. 21.8A), but these are replaced over the next 2 to 3 weeks by macrophages. Macrophages containing myelin or red cell breakdown products may persist in the lesion for months to years. As the process of phagocytosis and liquefaction proceeds, astrocytes at the edges of the lesion progressively enlarge, divide, and develop a prominent network of cytoplasmic extensions (gemistocytic change) (Fig. 21.8B). After several months, the striking astrocytic nuclear and cytoplasmic enlargement regresses. In the wall of the cavity, astrocyte processes form a dense feltwork of glial fibers admixed with new capillaries and a few perivascular connective tissue fibers (Fig. 21.8C).

Border zone ("watershed") infarcts occur in regions of the brain and spinal cord that lie at the most distal portions of arterial territories. They are usually seen after episodes of hypotension. In the cerebral hemispheres, the border zone between the anterior and the middle cerebral artery distributions is at greatest risk. Damage to this region produces a wedge-shaped band of necrosis over the cerebral convexity a few centimeters lateral to the interhemispheric fissure.

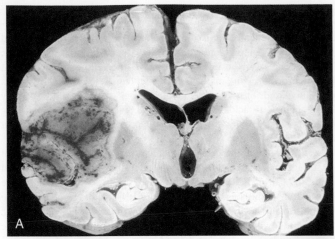

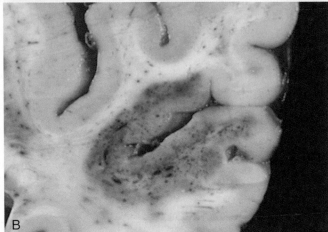

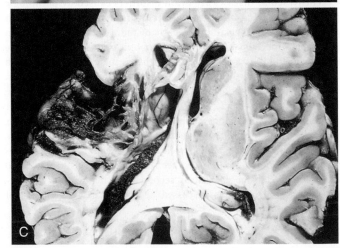

FIG. 21.7 Cerebral infarction. (A) Section of the brain showing a large, discolored, focally hemorrhagic infarct in the distribution of the left middle cerebral artery distribution. (B) An infarct with punctate hemorrhages, consistent with ischemia-reperfusion injury, is present in the temporal lobe. (C) Old cystic infarct shows destruction of cortex and surrounding gliosis.

Clinical Features. Infarcts present with combinations of localizing and nonlocalizing signs, which are usually more rapid in onset with embolic occlusions than with thromboses. Motor and/or sensory deficits (e.g., in the legs) dominate with anterior cerebral artery occlusions; aphasia, motor and/or sensory defects and hemiplegia if the middle cerebral artery in the dominant hemisphere is occluded; and visual defects with occlusion of the posterior cerebral artery.

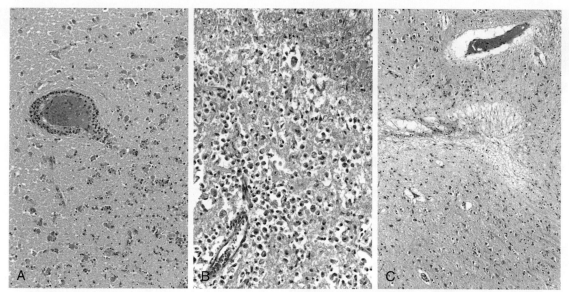

FIG. 21.8 Cerebral infarction. (A) Infiltration of a cerebral infarct by neutrophils begins at the edges of the lesion, where the vascular supply is intact. (B) By day 10, an area of infarction shows the presence of macrophages and surrounding reactive gliosis. (C) Old intracortical infarcts are seen as areas of tissue loss and residual gliosis.

Intracranial Hemorrhage

Hemorrhages within the brain are caused by (1) hypertension and other diseases leading to vascular wall injury; (2) structural lesions such as arteriovenous and cavernous malformations; (3) trauma; and (4) tumors. Hemorrhages may occur at any site within the cranium—outside the brain or within it (intraparenchymal) (Table 21.1). Hemorrhages in the epidural or subdural space are typically associated with trauma and are discussed later; by contrast, hemorrhages within the brain parenchyma and in the subarachnoid space are more commonly a manifestation of underlying cerebrovascular disease and are discussed here.

Primary Brain Parenchymal Hemorrhage

Hypertension is the most common risk factor for deep brain parenchymal hemorrhages, accounting for more than 50% of clinically significant hemorrhages and for roughly 15% of deaths among individuals with chronic hypertension. Spontaneous (nontraumatic) intraparenchymal hemorrhages are most common in mid to late adult life, with a peak incidence at about 60 years of age. Most are due to the rupture of a small intraparenchymal vessel. Intracerebral hemorrhage can be devastating when it affects large portions of the brain or extends into the ventricular system, or it can be clinically silent if it affects small regions. Hypertensive intraparenchymal hemorrhages typically occur

Table 21.1 Patterns of Hemorrhage in the Central Nervous System

Location	Etiology	Additional Features
Intraparenchymal	Trauma (contusions)	Selective involvement of the crests of gyri, where the brain is in contact with the inner surface of the skull (frontal and temporal tips, orbitofrontal surface)
	Ischemia (hemorrhagic conversion of an ischemic infarct)	Petechial hemorrhages in an area of previously ischemic brain (reperfusion injury), usually following the cortical ribbon
	Cerebral amyloid angiopathy	"Lobar" hemorrhage, involving subcortical white matter and often extending into the subarachnoid space
	Hypertension	Centered in the deep white matter, thalamus, basal ganglia, or brain stem; may extend into the ventricular system
	Tumors (primary or metastatic)	Associated with high-grade gliomas or certain types of metastatic tumors (melanoma, choriocarcinoma, renal cell carcinoma)
Subarachnoid space	Trauma	Typically associated with underlying parenchymal injury
	Vascular abnormality (arteriovenous malformation or aneurysm)	Sudden onset of severe headache, often with rapid neurologic deterioration; secondary injury may emerge and is associated with vasospasm
Epidural space	Trauma	Usually associated with skull fracture (in adults); rapidly evolving neurologic symptoms (often after a short lucid period) that require intervention
Subdural space	Trauma	May follow minor trauma; slowly evolving neurologic symptoms, often with a delay from the time of injury

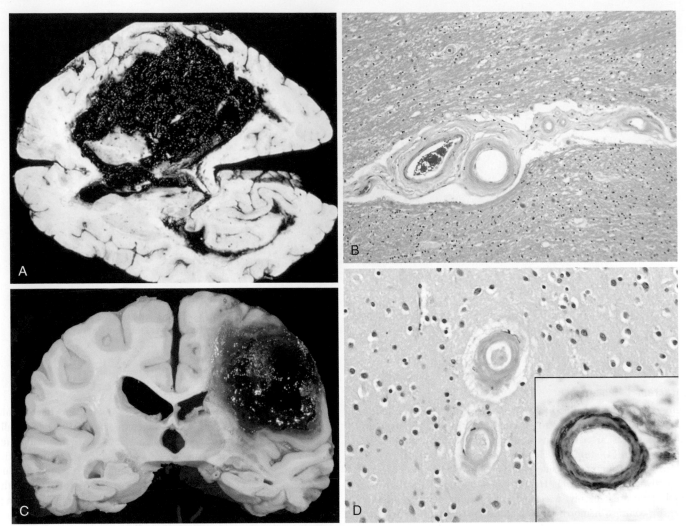

FIG. 21.9 Cerebral hemorrhage. (A) Massive hypertensive hemorrhage of the basal ganglia rupturing into a lateral ventricle. (B) Hyaline arteriolosclerosis (fibrosis and thickening of the arteriolar walls) develops in the basal ganglia and subcortical white matter of patients with long-standing hypertension; it is a risk factor for hypertensive hemorrhages as well as lacunar infarcts. (C) Large lobar hemorrhage due to cerebral amyloid angiopathy. (D) Amyloid deposition in cortical arterioles in cerebral amyloid angiopathy; *inset,* immunohistochemical staining highlights the deposited amyloid Aβ protein in the vessel wall. (C, Courtesy of Dr. Dimitri Agamanolis, http://neuropathology-web.org.)

in the basal ganglia, thalamus, pons, and cerebellum, with the location and the size of the bleed determining its clinical manifestations. If the individual survives the acute event, gradual resolution of the hematoma ensues, sometimes with considerable clinical improvement.

MORPHOLOGY

In acute intracerebral hemorrhage, extravasated blood compresses the adjacent parenchyma (Fig. 21.9A). With time, hemorrhages are converted to a cavity with a brown, discolored rim. On microscopic examination, early lesions consist of clotted blood surrounded by edematous brain tissue containing neurons and glia displaying morphologic changes typical of anoxic injury. Eventually the edema resolves, pigment- and lipid-laden macrophages appear, and a reactive astrocyte proliferation becomes visible at the periphery of the lesion. The cellular events then follow the same time course observed after cerebral infarction. Arteries may show arteriosclerosis (Fig. 21.9B).

Clinical Features. As in infarcts, the signs and symptoms of parenchymal hemorrhage are determined largely by its location. The symptoms often develop rapidly over several minutes and may continue to evolve over hours, often followed by gradual improvement. They include hemiplegia, acute-onset confusion and memory loss, and visual deficits.

Cerebral Amyloid Angiopathy

Cerebral amyloid angiopathy (CAA) is a disease in which amyloidogenic peptides, similar to those found in Alzheimer disease (discussed later), deposit in the walls of medium- and small-caliber meningeal and cortical vessels. Amyloid deposition makes vessel walls rigid and fragile, increasing the risk for hemorrhages, which differ in distribution from those associated with hypertension. CAA-associated hemorrhages often occur in the lobes of the cerebral cortex *(lobar hemorrhages)* (Fig. 21.9C, D). In addition to these symptomatic hemorrhages, CAA can also result in small (<1 mm), silent cortical hemorrhages *(microhemorrhages).*

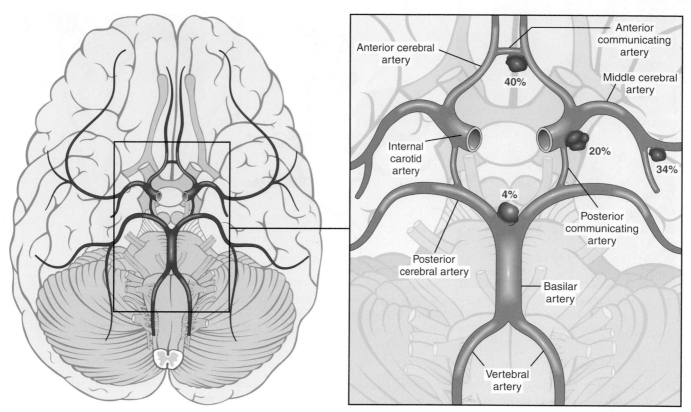

FIG. 21.10 Common sites of saccular aneurysms and the frequency of their occurrence.

Subarachnoid Hemorrhage and Saccular Aneurysms

The most frequent cause of clinically significant nontraumatic subarachnoid hemorrhage is rupture of a saccular (berry) aneurysm. Hemorrhage into the subarachnoid space may also result from vascular malformation, trauma, rupture of an intracerebral hemorrhage into the ventricular system, coagulopathies, and tumors. Epidural and subdural hemorrhages are typically secondary to trauma and are discussed later.

In about one-third of cases, rupture of a saccular aneurysm occurs because of an acute increase in intracranial pressure, such as occurs with straining at stool or sexual orgasm. Blood under arterial pressure is forced into the subarachnoid space, and the patient experiences a sudden, excruciating headache (known as a *thunderclap headache,* often described as "the worst headache I've ever had") and rapidly loses consciousness. Between 25% and 50% of affected individuals die from the first bleed, and recurrent bleeds are common in survivors. The prognosis worsens with each bleeding episode.

About 90% of saccular aneurysms occur in the anterior circulation near major arterial branch points (Fig. 21.10); multiple aneurysms exist in 20% to 30% of cases. The aneurysms are not present at birth but develop over time because of underlying defects in the vessel media. There is an increased risk for aneurysms in patients with autosomal dominant polycystic kidney disease (Chapter 12) and genetic disorders of extracellular matrix proteins (e.g., Ehler-Danlos syndrome). Overall, roughly 1.3% of aneurysms bleed per year, with the probability of rupture increasing with size. For example, aneurysms larger than 1 cm in diameter have a roughly 50% risk for bleeding per year. In the early period after a subarachnoid hemorrhage, there is an additional risk for ischemic injury from vasospasm of other vessels. Healing and the attendant meningeal fibrosis and

scarring sometimes obstruct CSF flow or disrupt CSF resorption, leading to hydrocephalus.

MORPHOLOGY

A saccular aneurysm is a thin-walled outpouching of an artery (Fig. 21.11). Beyond the neck of the aneurysm, the muscular wall and intimal elastic lamina are absent, such that the aneurysm sac is lined only by thickened hyalinized intima. The adventitia covering the sac is continuous with that of the parent artery. Rupture usually occurs at the apex of the sac, releasing blood into the subarachnoid space, the substance of the brain, or both.

Nonsaccular intracranial aneurysms may be atherosclerotic, mycotic, traumatic, and dissecting (Chapter 8). The last three types (like saccular aneurysms) are most often found in the anterior circulation, whereas atherosclerotic aneurysms are frequently fusiform and most commonly involve the basilar artery. Nonsaccular aneurysms usually manifest as cerebral infarction due to vascular occlusion instead of subarachnoid hemorrhage.

Vascular Malformations

Vascular malformations of the brain are classified into four principal types based on the nature of the abnormal vessels: arteriovenous malformations (AVMs), cavernous malformations, capillary telangiectasias, and venous angiomas. AVMs, the most common of these, affect males twice as frequently as females and most commonly manifest between 10 and 30 years of age with seizures, an intracerebral hemorrhage, or a subarachnoid hemorrhage. In the newborn period, large AVMs may lead to high-output congestive heart failure because of blood shunting from arteries to veins. The risk for bleeding makes AVM the most dangerous type of vascular malformation. Multiple

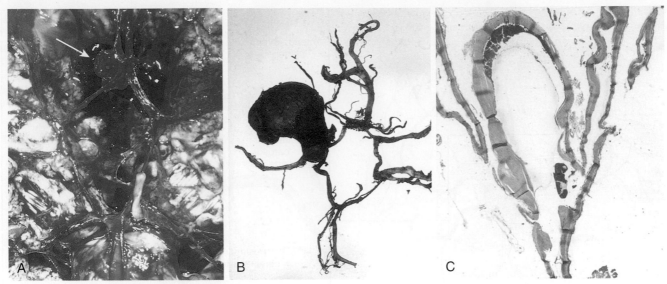

FIG. 21.11 Saccular aneurysm. (A) View of the base of the brain, dissected to show the circle of Willis with an aneurysm of the anterior cerebral artery *(arrow)*. (B) The circle of Willis is dissected to show a large aneurysm. (C) Section through a saccular aneurysm showing the hyalinized fibrous intima forming the vessel wall. Hematoxylin-eosin stain.

AVMs can be seen in the setting of hereditary hemorrhagic telangiectasia, an autosomal dominant condition often associated with mutations affecting the TGF-β pathway.

MORPHOLOGY

AVMs may involve subarachnoid vessels extending into brain parenchyma or occur exclusively within the brain. On gross inspection, they resemble a tangled network of wormlike vascular channels (Fig. 21.12). Microscopic examination shows enlarged blood vessels separated by gliotic tissue, often with evidence of previous hemorrhage.

Cavernous malformations consist of distended, loosely organized vascular channels with thin collagenized walls without intervening nervous tissue. They occur most often in the cerebellum, pons, and subcortical regions and have a low blood flow without significant arteriovenous shunting. Foci of old hemorrhage, infarction, and calcification frequently surround the abnormal vessels.

Capillary telangiectasias are microscopic foci of dilated thin-walled vascular channels separated by relatively normal brain parenchyma and occur most frequently in the pons. **Venous angiomas** (varices) consist of aggregates of ectatic venous channels. These two types of vascular malformation are unlikely to bleed or to cause symptoms, and most are incidental findings.

Other Vascular Diseases

Hypertensive Cerebrovascular Disease

Hypertension causes *hyaline arteriolar sclerosis* (Chapter 8) of the deep penetrating small arteries and arterioles that supply the basal ganglia, the hemispheric white matter, and the brain stem. Affected arteriolar walls are weakened and are vulnerable to rupture. In some instances, minute aneurysms form in vessels less than 300 μm in diameter. In addition to massive intracerebral hemorrhage (discussed earlier), several other pathologic outcomes are related to hypertension.

- *Lacunes* or *lacunar infarcts* are small cavitary infarcts, just a few millimeters in size, that are found most commonly in the deep gray matter (basal ganglia and thalamus), the internal capsule, the deep white matter, and the pons. They are caused by occlusion of a single penetrating branch of a large cerebral artery. Depending on their location, lacunes can be silent clinically or cause significant neurologic impairment.
- *Rupture of the small-caliber penetrating vessels* may occur, leading to the development of small hemorrhages. In time, these hemorrhages resorb, leaving behind a slitlike cavity *(slit hemorrhage)* surrounded by brownish discoloration.
- *Acute hypertensive encephalopathy* is most often associated with sudden sustained increases in diastolic blood pressure to greater than 130 mm Hg (so called severe, or malignant, hypertension, see Chapters 8 and 12). It is characterized by increased intracranial pressure and global cerebral dysfunction, manifesting as headaches, confusion, vomiting, convulsions, and sometimes coma. Rapid

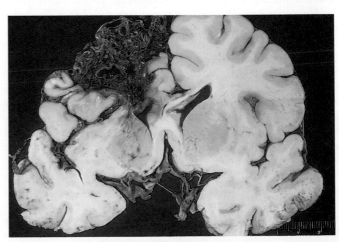

FIG. 21.12 Arteriovenous malformation.

therapeutic intervention to reduce the blood pressure is essential. Postmortem examination may show brain edema, with or without transtentorial or tonsillar herniation. Petechiae and fibrinoid necrosis of arterioles in the gray matter and white matter may be seen microscopically, as in other tissues (Chapters 8 and 12).

Vasculitis

Vasculitis in the CNS is most often the result of infections or systemic autoimmune diseases. It may impair blood flow and cause cerebral dysfunction or infarction. Infection-associated arteritis of small and large vessels was previously seen mainly in association with syphilis and tuberculosis but is now more often caused by opportunistic infections (e.g., aspergillosis, herpes zoster, or CMV) in the setting of immunocompromise. Some systemic forms of vasculitis, such as polyarteritis nodosa, may involve cerebral vessels and cause single or multiple infarcts.

Vascular Dementia

Individuals who cumulatively suffer over the course of years multiple, bilateral, gray matter (cortex, thalamus, basal ganglia) and white matter infarcts may develop a distinctive clinical syndrome characterized by dementia, gait abnormalities, and pseudobulbar signs (emotional instability), often with superimposed focal neurologic deficits. The syndrome, generally referred to as *vascular dementia,* is caused by multifocal vascular disease of several types, including (1) cerebral atherosclerosis; (2) vessel thrombosis or embolization from carotid vessels or from the heart; and (3) cerebral arteriolosclerosis from chronic hypertension. Many individuals with neurodegenerative diseases resulting in cognitive impairment or dementia also have evidence of cerebrovascular disease.

CENTRAL NERVOUS SYSTEM TRAUMA

The physical forces associated with head injury may result in skull fractures, parenchymal injury, and vascular injury; all three can coexist. The anatomic location of the lesion and the limited capacity of the brain for functional repair are major determinants of the consequences of CNS trauma. The magnitude and distribution of a traumatic brain lesion also depend on the shape of the object causing the trauma, the force of impact, and whether the head is in motion at the time of injury. A blow to the head may be penetrating or blunt; it may cause either an open or a closed injury. Injury of several cubic centimeters of brain parenchyma may be clinically silent (if in the frontal lobe), severely disabling (e.g., in the spinal cord), or fatal (e.g., in the brain stem).

Traumatic Parenchymal Injuries

When the head strikes a fixed object, brain injury may occur at the site of impact—a *coup injury*—or opposite the site of impact on the other side of the brain as the brain rebounds from the initial impact—a *contrecoup injury.* Both coup and contrecoup lesions are contusions, with comparable gross and microscopic appearances. A *contusion* is caused by rapid tissue displacement, disruption of vascular channels, and subsequent hemorrhage, tissue injury, and edema. Since they are closest to the skull, the crests of the gyri are the parts of the brain that are most susceptible to traumatic injury. Contusions are common in regions of the brain overlying rough and irregular inner skull surfaces, such as the orbitofrontal regions and the temporal lobe tips. Penetration of the brain by a projectile such as a bullet or a skull fragment from a fracture causes a laceration, with tissue tearing, vascular disruption, and hemorrhage.

MORPHOLOGY

Contusions are wedge shaped, with the widest aspect closest to the point of impact (Fig. 21.13A). Within a few hours of injury, blood extravasates throughout the involved tissue, across the width of the cerebral cortex, and into the white matter and subarachnoid spaces. Although functional effects are seen earlier, morphologic evidence of neuronal injury (i.e., nuclear pyknosis, cytoplasmic eosinophilia, cellular disintegration) takes about 24 hours to appear. The inflammatory response to the injured tissue follows its usual course, with neutrophils preceding the appearance of macrophages. In contrast with ischemic lesions, in which the superficial layer of cortex may be preserved, trauma affects the superficial layers most severely.

Old traumatic lesions characteristically appear as depressed, retracted, yellowish brown patches **(plaques jaunes)** involving the crests of gyri (Fig. 21.13B). These lesions show gliosis and residual hemosiderin-laden macrophages.

Trauma may also cause more subtle but widespread injury to axons within the brain (diffuse axonal injury), sometimes with devastating consequences. The movement of one region of brain relative to another is thought to disrupt axonal integrity and function. Angular acceleration, even in the absence of impact, may cause axonal injury as well as hemorrhage. As many as 50% of patients who develop coma shortly after trauma are believed to have white matter damage and diffuse axonal injury, which can be seen as axonal swellings that appear within hours of the injury.

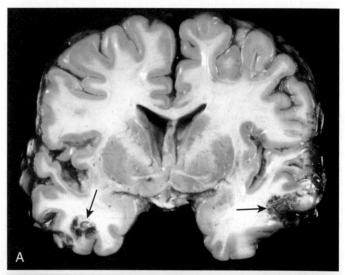

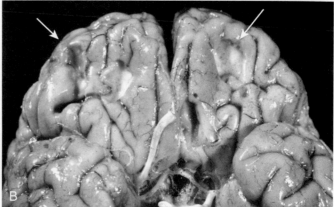

FIG. 21.13 Contusions. (A) Acute contusions are present in both temporal lobes, with areas of hemorrhage and tissue disruption *(arrows)*. (B) Remote contusions, seen as discolored yellow areas *(arrows)*, are present on the inferior frontal surface of this brain.

Concussion describes reversibly altered brain function, with or without loss of consciousness, as a result of head injury. The characteristic transient neurologic dysfunction includes loss of consciousness, temporary respiratory arrest, and loss of reflexes. Neurologic recovery is the norm, although amnesia for the event may persist. The pathogenesis of the sudden disruption of nervous activity is unknown.

Chronic Traumatic Encephalopathy

Chronic traumatic encephalopathy (CTE, previously referred to as *dementia pugilistica*) is a dementing illness that develops after repeated head trauma as may occur in football players and boxers. Affected brains are atrophic, with enlarged ventricles, and show accumulation of tau-containing neurofibrillary tangles (which are also seen in some neurodegenerative diseases, discussed later) in a characteristic pattern involving gyral depths and perivascular regions in the frontal and temporal lobe cortices. Repeated concussions predispose to the development of CTE; however, it remains uncertain what factors (e.g., the number, frequency, and/or severity of individual traumatic events, or some combination of these) determine whether encephalopathy ultimately develops.

Traumatic Vascular Injury

Vascular injury is a frequent component of CNS trauma; it results from disruption of the vessel wall and leads to hemorrhage in different anatomic sites (see Table 21.1). Depending on the affected vessel, the hemorrhage may be *epidural, subdural, subarachnoid,* or *intraparenchymal* (Fig. 21.14A), occurring alone or in combination. Subarachnoid and intraparenchymal hemorrhages were discussed earlier in the context of aneurysms and hypertension, respectively; when traumatic, they most often occur at sites of contusions and lacerations.

Epidural Hematoma

Dural vessels—especially the middle meningeal artery—are vulnerable to traumatic injury. In children and adults, tears involving dural vessels almost always stem from skull fractures. In infants, by contrast, traumatic displacement of the easily deformable skull may tear a vessel, even in the absence of a skull fracture. Once a vessel tears, blood accumulates under arterial pressure and separates the tightly applied dura away from the inner skull surface, producing a hematoma that compresses the brain surface (Fig. 21.14B; eFig. 21.1). Clinically, patients can be lucid for several hours after the traumatic event before neurologic signs appear. An epidural hematoma may expand rapidly and constitutes a neurosurgical emergency necessitating prompt drainage and repair to prevent death.

Subdural Hematoma

Rapid movement of the brain during trauma can tear the bridging veins that extend from the cerebral hemispheres through the subarachnoid and subdural space to the dural sinuses. Their disruption produces bleeding into the subdural space. Because the inner cell layer of the dura is quite thin and in very close proximity to the arachnoid layer, the blood appears to be between the dura and arachnoid, but it is actually between the two layers of the dura. In patients with brain atrophy (e.g., due to age-related changes), the bridging veins are stretched and there is additional space within which the brain can move, accounting for the higher rate of subdural hematomas in older adults, even with minor trauma. Infants are also susceptible to subdural hematomas because their bridging veins are thin walled.

Subdural hematomas typically become manifest within the first 48 hours after injury. They are most common over the lateral aspects of the cerebral hemispheres and are bilateral in about 10% of cases. Neurologic signs are attributable to the pressure exerted on the adjacent brain. Symptoms are most often nonlocalizing, taking the form of headache, confusion, and slowly progressive neurologic deterioration.

MORPHOLOGY

Acute subdural hematoma appears as a collection of freshly clotted blood apposed to the contour of the brain surface, without extension into the depths of sulci (Fig. 21.14C, eFig. 21.2). The underlying brain is flattened, and the subarachnoid space is often clear. Subdural hematomas organize by lysis of the clot (about 1 week), growth of granulation tissue from the dural surface into the hematoma (2 weeks), and fibrosis (1—3 months). Subdural hematomas commonly rebleed, presumably from the thin-walled vessels of the granulation tissue, leading to microscopic findings consistent with hemorrhages of varying ages.

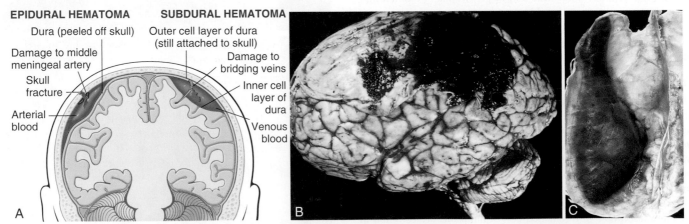

FIG. 21.14 Traumatic intracranial hemorrhages. (A) Epidural hematoma is caused by traumatic rupture of a meningeal artery, usually due to a skull fracture, leading to accumulation of arterial blood between the dura and the skull. Subdural hematoma is caused by damage to bridging veins between the brain and the superior sagittal sinus, leading to the accumulation of blood between the two layers of dura. (B) Epidural hematoma covering a portion of the dura. (C) Large organizing subdural hematoma attached to the dura. (B, Courtesy of Dr. Raymond D. Adams, Massachusetts General Hospital, Boston, Massachusetts.)

Symptomatic subdural hematomas are treated by surgical removal of the blood and associated reactive tissue.

Perinatal Brain Injury

Cerebral palsy is a term for nonprogressive neurologic motor deficits characterized by spasticity, dystonia, ataxia or athetosis, and paresis attributable to injury occurring during the prenatal and perinatal periods. There may be no associated intellectual disability. Signs and symptoms may not be apparent at birth and only declare themselves later, well after the causal event.

The two major types of injury that occur in the perinatal period are hemorrhages and infarcts. These differ from the otherwise similar lesions in adults in terms of their locations and the tissue reactions they engender. In premature infants, there is an increased risk for *intraparenchymal hemorrhage* within the germinal matrix, most often adjacent to the anterior horn of the lateral ventricle. Hemorrhages may extend into the ventricular system and from there to the subarachnoid space, sometimes causing hydrocephalus. Ischemic infarcts may occur in the supratentorial periventricular white matter *(periventricular leukomalacia),* especially in premature infants (Fig. 21.15). The residua of these infarcts are chalky yellow plaques consisting of discrete regions of white matter necrosis and dystrophic calcification. When sufficiently widespread to involve both gray matter and white matter, large cystic lesions can develop throughout the hemispheres, a condition termed *multicystic encephalopathy.*

INFECTIONS OF THE NERVOUS SYSTEM

Infections may damage the nervous system directly through injury of neurons or glia by the infectious agent, or indirectly through microbial toxins or the destructive effects of the inflammatory response. There are four principal routes by which microbes enter the nervous system:

- *Hematogenous spread* is the most common; microbes ordinarily gain access through the arterial circulation, but retrograde venous spread can occur via anastomoses between the veins of the face and the venous sinuses of the skull.
- *Direct implantation* of microorganisms is almost invariably due to open or penetrating trauma but sometimes can be associated with congenital malformations (e.g., meningomyelocele) that provide ready access for microbes.
- *Transplacental spread.* Certain perinatal infections may be acquired transplacentally or during birth and have a propensity to cause destructive brain lesions. Agents in this group include *Toxoplasma* and CMV, both of which can result in parenchymal calcifications along with tissue injury; these are discussed later.
- *Local extension* can originate from infected adjacent structures, such as air sinuses, teeth, skull, or vertebrae.
- Viruses may also be transported along the *peripheral nervous system,* as occurs with rabies and herpes zoster viruses.

In the following sections we discuss infections that are specific to the central nervous system (Table 21.2).

Meningitis

Meningitis is an inflammatory process typically induced by an infection involving the leptomeninges within the subarachnoid space; if the infection spreads into the underlying brain, it is termed meningoencephalitis. The term is also used in noninfectious settings such as *chemical meningitis,* a response to an irritant such as debris from a ruptured epidermoid cyst, and *carcinomatous meningitis,*

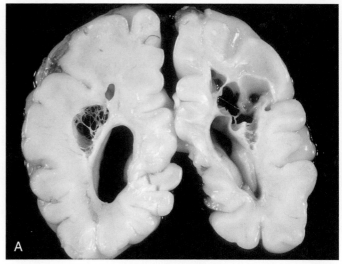

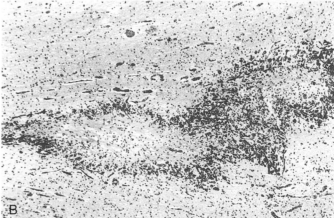

FIG. 21.15 Perinatal brain injury. (A) Chronic stage of periventricular leukomalacia. Large cystic spaces in the periventricular white matter (seen in both hemispheres of the brain) are the long-term sequelae of severe prenatal or perinatal ischemic injury. (B) Histologic section of periventricular leukomalacia shows a central focus of white matter necrosis with a peripheral rim of mineralized axonal processes.

inflammation caused by metastatic cancer cells that have spread to the subarachnoid space.

Infectious meningitis can be divided into *acute pyogenic* (usually bacterial), *aseptic* (usually viral), and *chronic* (usually tuberculous, spirochetal, or fungal) subtypes. Examination of the CSF is often useful in identifying the cause of the meningitis.

Acute Pyogenic Meningitis (Bacterial Meningitis)

The most likely causes of bacterial meningitis vary with patient age. In neonates, common organisms are *Escherichia coli* and group B streptococci. In adolescents and young adults, *Neisseria meningitidis* is the most common pathogen; in older adults, *Streptococcus pneumoniae* and *Listeria monocytogenes* are more common. Across all ages, patients typically show systemic signs of infection along with meningeal irritation and neurologic impairment, including headache, photophobia, irritability, clouding of consciousness, and neck stiffness. Lumbar puncture reveals an increased pressure; examination of the CSF shows abundant neutrophils, elevated protein, and reduced glucose. Untreated pyogenic meningitis is often fatal, but with prompt diagnosis and administration of antibiotics, most patients can be cured.

Table 21.2 Common Central Nervous System Infections

Type of Infection	Clinical Syndrome	Common Causative Organisms
Bacterial Infections		
Meningitis	Acute pyogenic meningitis	*Escherichia coli* or group B streptococci (infants)
		Neisseria meningitidis (young adults)
		Streptococcus pneumoniae or *Listeria monocytogenes* (older adults)
	Chronic meningitis	*Mycobacterium tuberculosis*
Localized infections	Abscess	Streptococci and staphylococci
	Empyema	Polymicrobial (staphylococci, anaerobic gram-negative)
Viral Infections		
Meningitis	Acute aseptic meningitis	Enteroviruses
		Measles (subacute sclerosing panencephalitis)
		Human immunodeficiency virus (HIV)
		Influenza species
		Lymphocytic choriomeningitis virus
Encephalitis	Encephalitic syndromes	Herpes simplex (HSV-1, HSV-2)
		Cytomegalovirus
		Human immunodeficiency virus
		JC polyomavirus (progressive multifocal leukoencephalopathy)
	Arthropod-borne encephalitis	West Nile virus, other arboviruses
Brain stem and spinal cord syndromes	Rhombencephalitis	Rabies
	Spinal poliomyelitis	Polio
	Encephalitis, meningitis	West Nile virus
Rickettsia, Spirochetes, and Fungi		
Meningitic syndromes	Rocky Mountain spotted fever	*Rickettsia rickettsii*
	Neurosyphilis	*Treponema pallidum*
	Lyme disease (neuroborreliosis)	*Borrelia burgdorferi*
	Fungal meningitis	*Cryptococcus neoformans*
		Candida albicans
Protozoa and Metazoa		
Meningitic syndromes	Cerebral malaria	*Plasmodium falciparum*
	Amebic encephalitis	*Naegleria* species
Localized infections	Toxoplasmosis	*Toxoplasma gondii*
	Cysticercosis	*Taenia solium*

MORPHOLOGY

In acute meningitis, an exudate is evident within the leptomeninges on the surface of the brain (Fig. 21.16). The meningeal vessels are engorged and prominent, and tracts of pus may extend along blood vessels. On microscopic examination, neutrophils may fill the entire subarachnoid space or, in less severe cases, may be confined to regions adjacent to leptomeningeal blood vessels. Particularly in untreated meningitis, gram stain reveals varying numbers of the causative organism, particularly in untreated meningitis. In fulminant meningitis, the inflammatory cells infiltrate the walls of the leptomeningeal veins and may extend focally into the substance of the brain (cerebritis); secondary vasculitis and venous thrombosis may lead to hemorrhagic cerebral infarction. Leptomeningeal fibrosis may follow pyogenic meningitis and cause hydrocephalus; it is more common as a complication of tuberculous meningitis (discussed later).

Aseptic Meningitis (Viral Meningitis)

Aseptic meningitis is a clinical term used for manifestations of meningitis, such as meningeal irritation, fever, and alterations of consciousness of relatively acute onset, in the absence of organisms detectable by bacterial culture. The disease is generally of viral etiology but may be rickettsial or autoimmune in origin (see Table 21.2). The clinical course is less fulminant than that of pyogenic meningitis, and the CSF findings also differ: in aseptic meningitis, there is a lymphocytic pleocytosis, the protein elevation is only moderate, and the glucose content is nearly always normal. The viral aseptic meningitides are usually self-limited and are treated symptomatically. The etiologic agent is identified in only a minority of cases; however, this may change through use of more sensitive and specific detection techniques (such as DNA sequencing). When pathogens are identified, enteroviruses are the most common etiology, accounting for 80% of cases.

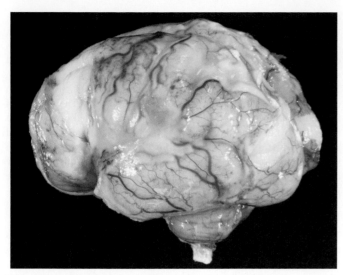

FIG. 21.16 Pyogenic meningitis. A thick layer of suppurative exudate covers the brain stem and cerebellum and thickens the leptomeninges.

Chronic Meningitis

Several pathogens, including mycobacteria, some spirochetes, and fungi, cause a chronic meningitis; infections with these organisms also may involve the brain parenchyma.

Tuberculous Meningitis. Tuberculous meningitis usually manifests with generalized signs and symptoms of headache, malaise, mental confusion, and vomiting. There is only a moderate increase in CSF cellularity, with mononuclear cells or a mixture of polymorphonuclear and mononuclear cells; the protein level is elevated, often strikingly so, and the glucose content typically is moderately reduced or normal. Infection with *Mycobacterium tuberculosis* may also result in a well-circumscribed intraparenchymal mass *(tuberculoma),* which may be associated with meningitis. Chronic tuberculous meningitis leads to arachnoid fibrosis, particularly at the base of the brain, and hydrocephalus from interference with CSF resorption.

Spirochetal Infections. *Neurosyphilis,* a tertiary stage of syphilis, occurs in about 10% of individuals with untreated *Treponema pallidum* infection. Coinfection with HIV increases the risk for developing neurosyphilis, and the disease is often more aggressive in this setting. There are several patterns of CNS involvement by syphilis, which may be present alone or in combination.

- *Meningovascular neurosyphilis* is a chronic meningitis, usually involving the base of the brain, often with an obliterative endarteritis rich in plasma cells and lymphocytes.
- *Paretic neurosyphilis* stems from parenchymal involvement by spirochetes and is associated with neuronal loss and marked proliferation of microglial cells. Clinically, this form of the disease causes an insidious progressive loss of mental and physical functions, mood alterations (including delusions of grandeur), and eventually severe dementia.
- *Tabes dorsalis* results from damage to the sensory nerves in the dorsal roots. Consequences include impaired joint position sense and ataxia; loss of pain sensation, leading to skin and joint damage *(Charcot joints);* other sensory disturbances, particularly characteristic sudden, brief, severe stabs of pain ("lightning pains"); and the absence of deep tendon reflexes.

Neuroborreliosis refers to involvement of the nervous system by the spirochete *Borrelia burgdorferi,* the causative agent of Lyme disease. Neurologic signs and symptoms are highly variable and include aseptic meningitis, facial nerve palsies, mild encephalopathy, and polyneuropathies.

Fungal Meningitis. Fungal infection of the nervous system can give rise to chronic meningitis and, as with other pathogens, can be associated with parenchymal infection. Immunocompromise increases the risk for these diseases. Several fungal pathogens cause CNS disease:

- *Cryptococcus neoformans* and *Cryptococcus gattii* both may cause meningitis and meningoencephalitis. *C. neoformans* mainly produces disease in the setting of immunocompromise, whereas *C. gattii* often causes disease in immmunocompetent individuals, usually accompanied by pulmonary involvement (Chapter 11). CNS involvement by both organisms may be fulminant and fatal in as little as 2 weeks or may be indolent, evolving over months or years. The CSF may have few cells but elevated protein. The mucoid encapsulated yeasts can be visualized on India ink preparations or detected using cryptococcal antigen tests. Extension into the brain follows vessels in the Virchow-Robin spaces. As organisms proliferate, these spaces expand, giving rise to a "soap bubble"—like appearance (eFig. 21.3).
- *Histoplasma capsulatum* commonly involves the nervous system in the setting of disseminated infection. There is an increased risk for disease in the setting of HIV infection. Histoplasmosis (like tuberculosis) typically causes a basilar meningitis, with elevated CSF protein, mildly decreased glucose, and mild lymphocytic pleocytosis. Parenchymal lesions can occur, mostly from tracking of organisms along Virchow-Robin spaces.
- *Coccidioides immitis,* a fungus endemic to desert regions of the American Southwest, most commonly causes meningitis in the setting of disseminated infection. Diagnosis can be made by examining the CSF for specific antibodies or by antigen detection. Without treatment, coccidioidal meningitis has a high fatality rate.

Parenchymal Infections

The entire spectrum of infectious pathogens (viruses to parasites) can infect the brain, often producing characteristic lesions. In general, viral infections are diffuse, bacterial infections (when not associated with meningitis) are more localized, and other organisms produce mixed patterns. In immunocompromised individuals, widespread involvement with any agent is typical.

Brain Abscesses

A brain abscess is a localized focus of necrotic brain tissue with accompanying inflammation, usually caused by a bacterial infection. Abscesses can arise by direct implantation of organisms, local extension from adjacent foci (e.g., mastoiditis, paranasal sinusitis), or hematogenous spread (usually from a primary site in the heart, lungs, or distal bones). Predisposing conditions include acute bacterial endocarditis, from which septic emboli are released that may produce multiple abscesses; cyanotic congenital heart disease, associated with a right-to-left shunt and loss of pulmonary filtration of organisms; and chronic pulmonary infections, as in bronchiectasis, which provide a source of microbes that spread hematogenously.

Abscesses are discrete destructive lesions with central liquefactive necrosis surrounded by edema (Fig. 21.17). At the outer margin of the

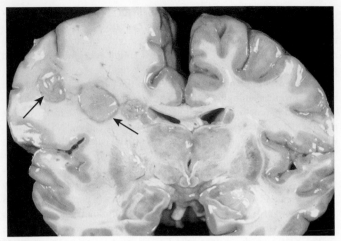

FIG. 21.17 Cerebral abscesses in the frontal lobe white matter *(arrows)*.

necrotic lesion, there is exuberant granulation tissue with neo-vascularization. The newly formed vessels are abnormally permeable, accounting for marked edema in the adjacent brain tissue. Patients often present with progressive focal neurologic deficits; signs and symptoms related to increased intracranial pressure may also develop. Typically, the CSF has a high white cell count and an increased protein concentration, but the glucose content is normal. The source of infection may be apparent or may be traced to a small (extracranial) focus that is not symptomatic. Increased intracranial pressure can lead to fatal herniation; other complications include abscess rupture with ventriculitis or meningitis, and venous sinus thrombosis. With surgery and antibiotic treatment, the otherwise high mortality rate can be reduced to less than 10%.

Viral Encephalitis

Viral encephalitis is a parenchymal infection of the brain that is almost invariably associated with meningeal inflammation *(meningoencephalitis)*. While different viruses show varying patterns of injury, the most characteristic histologic features are perivascular and parenchymal mononuclear cell infiltrates (Fig. 21.18A), microglial

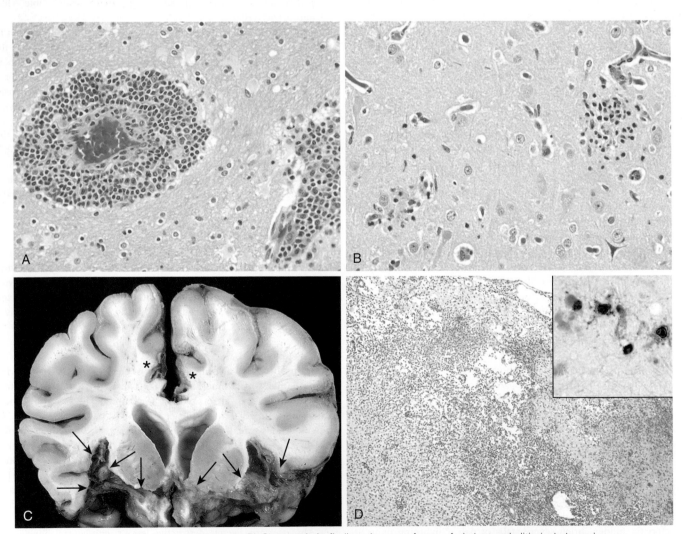

FIG. 21.18 Viral infections. (A, B) Characteristic findings in many forms of viral encephalitis include perivascular cuffs of lymphocytes (A) and microglial nodules (B). (C) Herpes encephalitis showing extensive destruction of inferior frontal and anterior temporal lobes *(arrows)* and cingulate gyri *(asterisks)*. (D) Necrotizing inflammatory process characterizes acute herpes encephalitis; nuclear viral inclusions can be highlighted by immunostaining *(inset)*. (C, Courtesy of Dr. T.W. Smith, University of Massachusetts Medical School, Worcester, Massachusetts.)

nodules (Fig. 21.18B), and neuronophagia. Certain viruses also form characteristic inclusion bodies. CSF examination helps to distinguish viral from bacterial infections of the CNS. The CSF usually shows a slightly elevated pressure and an early neutrophilic pleocytosis that rapidly converts to a lymphocytosis; the protein concentration is elevated, but glucose is normal.

The nervous system is particularly susceptible to certain viruses such as rabies virus and poliovirus. Some viruses infect specific CNS cell types, while others preferentially involve particular brain regions (e.g., medial temporal lobes, limbic system) that lie along the viral route of entry. Intrauterine viral infection following transplacental spread of rubella and CMV may cause destructive lesions, and Zika virus causes developmental abnormalities of the brain. In addition to direct infection of the nervous system, the CNS can also be injured by immune mechanisms after systemic viral infections.

Arboviruses. Arboviruses (arthropod-borne viruses) are an important cause of epidemic encephalitis, especially in tropical regions of the world, and are capable of causing serious morbidity and high mortality. Among the more commonly encountered types are Eastern and Western equine encephalitis and West Nile virus infection. Patients develop generalized neurologic symptoms, such as seizures, confusion, delirium, and stupor or coma, as well as focal signs, such as reflex asymmetry and ocular palsies.

MORPHOLOGY

Arbovirus encephalitides produce a similar histopathologic picture. Characteristically, there is a perivascular lymphocytic meningoencephalitis (sometimes with neutrophils). Multifocal gray matter and white matter necrosis is seen, often associated with neuronophagia (eFig. 21.4), the phagocytosis of neuronal debris, as well as **microglial nodules** (see Fig. 21.1C). In severe cases, there may be a necrotizing vasculitis with associated focal hemorrhages.

Herpesviruses. HSV-1 encephalitis may occur in any age group but is most common in children and young adults. It typically manifests with alterations in mood, memory, and behavior, reflecting involvement of the frontal and temporal lobes. Recurrent HSV-1 encephalitis is sometimes associated with inherited mutations that interfere with Toll-like receptor signaling (specifically that of TLR-3), which has an important role in antiviral defense.

MORPHOLOGY

Herpes encephalitis starts in and most severely affects the inferior and medial regions of the temporal lobes and the orbital gyri of the frontal lobes (Fig. 21.18C). The infection is necrotizing and often hemorrhagic in severely affected regions. Perivascular inflammatory infiltrates are usually present (Fig. 21.18D), and **large eosinophilic intranuclear viral inclusions** (Cowdry type A bodies) can be found in both neurons and glial cells.

HSV-2 also affects the nervous system. This usually takes the form of meningitis in adults, whereas disseminated severe encephalitis may occur in neonates born by vaginal delivery to women with active primary HSV genital infections.

Varicella-zoster virus (VZV) causes chickenpox during primary infection, usually without any evidence of neurologic involvement. The virus establishes latent infection in neurons of dorsal root ganglia. Reactivation in adults results in inflammation and neuronal damage in sensory ganglia. It manifests as neuropathic pain and a painful, vesicular skin eruption in the distribution of one or a few dermatomes *(shingles).* This is usually a self-limited process, but there may be a persistent pain syndrome in the affected region *(postherpetic neuralgia).* VZV also may cause a granulomatous arteritis that can lead to tissue infarcts. In patients who are immunocompromised, acute herpes zoster encephalitis can occur. Inclusion bodies can be found in glial cells and neurons.

Cytomegalovirus (CMV). CMV infects the nervous system of fetuses and individuals who are immunocompromised. All cells within the CNS (neurons, glial cells, ependyma, and endothelium) are susceptible to infection. Intrauterine infection causes periventricular necrosis, followed later by microcephaly with periventricular calcification. When adults are infected, CMV produces a subacute encephalitis, which is also often most severe in the periventricular region. Lesions can be hemorrhagic and contain cells with typical viral inclusions (eFig. 21.5).

Poliovirus. Poliovirus is an enterovirus that most often causes a subclinical or mild gastroenteritis; in a small fraction of cases, it secondarily invades the nervous system and damages motor neurons in the spinal cord and brain stem *(paralytic poliomyelitis).* The loss of motor neurons results in a flaccid paralysis with muscle wasting and hyporeflexia in the corresponding region of the body. In the acute disease, death can occur from paralysis of respiratory muscles. Long after the infection has resolved, typically 25 to 35 years after the initial illness, a poorly understood *postpolio syndrome* of progressive weakness associated with decreased muscle bulk and pain may appear. The re-emergent weakness has the same distribution as the prior polio infection. With worldwide vaccination, polio has been nearly eliminated but still persists in underresourced parts of Pakistan and Afghanistan. Additionally, in parts of the world in which endemic polio has been eliminated, such as Africa, back-mutation of the attenuated virus in oral vaccines has produced small numbers of cases of paralytic polio acquired through contaminated drinking water.

Rabies Virus. Rabies is a severe encephalitis usually transmitted to humans by the saliva of a rabid animal, including dogs, bats, or various wild mammals that are natural reservoirs. According to the WHO, about 60,000 people die of canine rabies worldwide each year. The virus enters the CNS by ascending along the peripheral nerves from the wound site, so the incubation period (usually 1 to 3 months) depends on the distance between the wound and the brain. The disease manifests initially with nonspecific symptoms of malaise, headache, and fever. As the infection advances, the patient shows extraordinary CNS excitability; the slightest touch is painful, with violent motor responses progressing to convulsions. Contracture of the pharyngeal musculature may create an aversion to swallowing even water *(hydrophobia).* Periods of mania and stupor progress to coma and eventually death in virtually all cases, typically from respiratory failure.

Human Immunodeficiency Virus. Before the availability of effective antiretroviral therapy, neuropathologic changes were demonstrated at postmortem examination in as many as 80% to 90% of AIDS cases. These changes stem from direct effects of the virus on the nervous system, opportunistic infections, and primary CNS lymphoma, most commonly an EBV-positive B-cell tumor. There has been a decrease in the frequency of these secondary effects of HIV infection due to the efficacy of multidrug antiretroviral therapy. *HIV-associated neurocognitive disorder (HAND),* a cognitive dysfunction ranging from mild to full-blown dementia, continues to be a source of morbidity, however. This syndrome is believed to stem from HIV infection of microglial cells in the brain and activation of innate immune responses. Neuronal injury likely stems from a combination of cytokine-induced inflammation and toxic effects of HIV-derived proteins.

Aseptic meningitis occurs within 1 to 2 weeks of onset of primary HIV infection in about 10% of patients; antibodies to HIV can be demonstrated, and the virus can be isolated from the CSF. The few neuropathologic studies of the early, acute phases of symptomatic or asymptomatic HIV invasion of the nervous system have shown mild lymphocytic meningitis, perivascular inflammation, and some myelin loss in the hemispheres.

When effective anti-HIV therapy is begun in the setting of established infection, there is a risk for a neurologic disorder called *immune reconstitution inflammatory syndrome (IRIS)*. Neurologic manifestations include rapidly developing cognitive impairment and cerebral edema. The pathogenesis of IRIS is unclear, but it is thought to be due to the activation of a previously suppressed inflammatory response brought about by effective treatment of HIV infection. IRIS is often associated with the presence of a mycobacterial, fungal, or viral opportunistic CNS infection, although it can also occur in the absence of any other inciting disease.

MORPHOLOGY

HIV encephalitis is a chronic inflammatory process with widely distributed **microglial nodules,** sometimes with associated foci of tissue necrosis and reactive gliosis. The microglial nodules are also found in the vicinity of small blood vessels, which show abnormally prominent endothelial cells and perivascular foamy or pigment-laden macrophages. These changes are especially prominent in the subcortical white matter, diencephalon, and brain stem. An important component of microglial nodules is macrophage-derived **multinucleate cells.** In some cases, there is also a disorder of white matter characterized by multifocal or diffuse areas of myelin loss, axonal swellings, and gliosis. HIV is present in CD4+ mononuclear and multinucleate macrophages and microglia.

Unlike HIV encephalitis, the brain lesions of IRIS may be associated with a CD8+ T-cell infiltrate, both around blood vessels and diffusely in the parenchyma, in the absence of significant HIV burden or multinucleated cells.

Polyomavirus and Progressive Multifocal Leukoencephalopathy. *Progressive multifocal leukoencephalopathy (PML)* is caused by JC virus, a polyomavirus, which preferentially infects oligodendrocytes,

resulting in demyelination as the injured cells die. Most people show serologic evidence of exposure to JC virus during childhood, and it is believed that PML results from virus reactivation, as the disease is restricted to individuals who are immunocompromised. Patients develop relentlessly progressive neurologic signs and symptoms, and imaging studies show extensive, often multifocal lesions in the hemispheric or cerebellar white matter. There is no specific treatment and the disease is usually fatal in less than a year.

MORPHOLOGY

The lesions are patchy, irregular, ill-defined areas of white matter destruction that enlarge as the disease progresses (Fig. 21.19). Each lesion is an area of demyelination, in the center of which are scattered lipid-laden macrophages and a reduced number of axons. At the edges of the lesion are greatly enlarged oligodendrocyte nuclei whose chromatin is replaced by glassy amphophilic viral inclusions. The virus also infects astrocytes, leading to bizarre giant forms with irregular, hyperchromatic, sometimes multiple nuclei that can be mistaken for a tumor.

Fungal Encephalitis

Fungal infections usually produce parenchymal granulomas or abscesses, often associated with meningitis. The most common fungal infections have the following distinctive patterns:

- *Candida albicans* usually produces multiple microabscesses, with or without granuloma formation.
- *Mucormycosis*, caused by several fungi belonging to the order *Mucorales*, typically presents as an infection of the nasal cavity or sinuses in a patient who has diabetes and ketoacidosis. It may spread to the brain through vascular invasion or by direct extension through the cribriform plate. The proclivity of *Mucor* to invade the brain directly sets it apart from other fungi, which reach the brain by hematogenous dissemination from distant sites.
- *Aspergillus fumigatus* tends to cause a distinctive pattern of widespread septic hemorrhagic infarctions because of its marked predilection for blood vessel wall invasion with subsequent thrombosis.

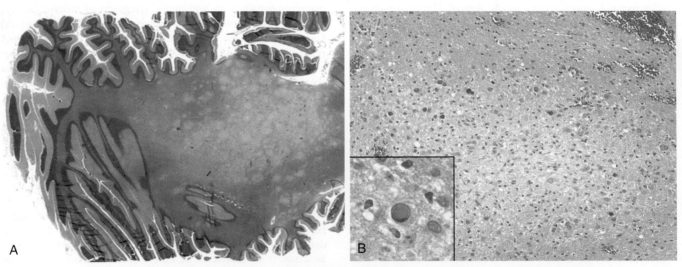

FIG. 21.19 Progressive multifocal leukoencephalopathy. (A) Section stained for myelin showing irregular, poorly defined pale areas of myelin loss, which become confluent in places. (B) Microscopically, the lesions consist of areas of demyelination. *Inset,* Enlarged oligodendrocyte nucleus containing viral inclusion characteristic of virus-infected cell.

Other Meningoencephalitides

While a wide range of other organisms can infect the nervous system and its covering, only three of the most common entities are considered here.

Cerebral Toxoplasmosis. Cerebral infection with the protozoan *Toxoplasma gondii* can occur in adults who are immunocompromised or in newborns who acquire the organism transplacentally from a mother with an active infection. The consequences include the triad of *chorioretinitis, hydrocephalus,* and *intracranial calcifications.* In adults, the clinical symptoms are subacute, evolving over weeks, and may be both localizing and diffuse. Due to inflammation and breakdown of the blood-brain barrier at sites of infection, imaging studies often show edema associated with ring-enhancing lesions.

> ### MORPHOLOGY
>
> When the infection is acquired in adults who are immunocompromised, the brain shows abscesses, frequently multiple, most often involving the cerebral cortex (near the gray-white junction) and deep gray nuclei. Acute lesions consist of central foci of necrosis surrounded by acute and chronic inflammation, macrophage infiltration, and vascular proliferation. Both free tachyzoites and encysted bradyzoites may be found at the periphery of the necrotic foci (eFig. 21.6).

Cysticercosis. Cysticercosis is the consequence of end-stage infection by the tapeworm *Taenia solium.* Ingested larvae leave the lumen of the gastrointestinal tract, where they would otherwise develop into mature tapeworms, lodge in other tissues, and encyst. Cysts can be found throughout the body and are common within the brain and subarachnoid space. Cerebral cysticercosis typically manifests as a mass lesion and can cause seizures.

The organism is found within a cyst with a smooth lining. The body wall and hooklets from mouth parts are most commonly recognized. Death of the encysted organism, as occurs after therapy, may induce an intense inflammatory reaction in the brain marked by eosinophil infiltration and gliosis, changes that may be accompanied by a worsening of symptoms.

Amebiasis. Amebic meningoencephalitis manifests with different clinical syndromes, depending on the responsible pathogen. *Naegleria fowleri,* associated with swimming in stagnant warm fresh water, causes a rapidly fatal necrotizing encephalitis. *Entameba histolytica* can spread hematogenously from the colon; cerebral amebiasis is characterized by abrupt onset of symptoms and rapid progression to death. Various species of *Acanthamoeba* cause a chronic granulomatous meningoencephalitis.

Epidural and Subdural Infections

The epidural and subdural spaces can be involved by bacterial or fungal infections, usually as a consequence of direct local spread. *Epidural abscesses* arise from an adjacent focus of infection, such as sinusitis or osteomyelitis. When abscesses occur in the spinal epidural space, they may cause spinal cord compression and constitute a neurosurgical emergency. Infections of the skull or air sinuses may also spread to the subdural space, producing *subdural empyema.* The underlying arachnoid and subarachnoid spaces are usually unaffected, but a large subdural empyema may produce a mass effect. In addition, thrombophlebitis may develop in the bridging veins that cross the subdural space, resulting in venous occlusion and infarction of the brain. Most patients are febrile, with headache and neck stiffness, and if untreated may develop focal neurologic signs referable to the site of the infection, lethargy, and coma. With treatment, including surgical drainage, resolution of the empyema occurs from the dural side; if resolution is complete, a thickened dura may be the only residual finding. With prompt treatment, complete recovery is usual.

NUTRITIONAL DISORDERS

Because of its high metabolic demands, the brain is particularly vulnerable to nutritional imbalances and alterations in the body's metabolic state. Toxic and acquired metabolic diseases, e.g., hepatic encephalopathy (Chapter 14) and alcohol poisoning (Chapter 7), are relatively common causes of neurologic illnesses. A few of the more common nutritional disorders affecting the CNS are discussed here.

Thiamine Deficiency

In addition to the systemic effects of thiamine deficiency *(beriberi)*, it can also lead to acute psychosis, abnormalities in eye movement, and ataxia, features of a syndrome termed *Wernicke encephalopathy.* Treatment with thiamine reverses these deficits, but if treatment is delayed thiamine deficiency produces a largely irreversible, profound disturbance of memory called *Korsakoff syndrome.* Because the two syndromes are closely linked, the term *Wernicke-Korsakoff syndrome* is often used. The syndrome is particularly common in the setting of chronic alcohol use disorder but also may be encountered in patients with thiamine deficiency resulting from gastric disorders, gastric bypass surgery, or persistent vomiting (e.g., hyperemesis gravidarum, bulimia nervosa).

> ### MORPHOLOGY
>
> Wernicke encephalopathy is characterized by foci of hemorrhage and necrosis in the mammillary bodies, adjacent to the ventricles, especially the third and fourth ventricles, and the hypothalamus. Resolution of the areas of necrosis produces cystic spaces associated with hemosiderin-laden macrophages. Lesions in the medial dorsal nucleus of the thalamus seem to best correlate with the memory disturbance in Korsakoff syndrome.

Vitamin B$_{12}$ Deficiency

In addition to causing anemia, deficiency of vitamin B$_{12}$ may cause diffuse demyelination and axonal loss, particularly in the white matter of the spinal cord, resulting in a syndrome called *subacute combined degeneration of the spinal cord.* Both ascending and descending tracts of the spinal cord are affected. Symptoms develop over weeks. Early clinical signs often include mild ataxia and lower-extremity numbness and tingling, which can progress to spastic weakness of the lower extremities; sometimes, complete paraplegia ensues. Prompt vitamin replacement therapy produces clinical improvement; however, if paraplegia has developed, recovery is limited.

DISEASES OF MYELIN

Within the CNS, axons are tightly ensheathed by myelin, an electrical insulator that allows rapid propagation of neural impulses. Myelin consists of multiple layers of highly specialized, closely apposed plasma membranes that are assembled by oligodendrocytes. Although myelinated axons are present in all areas of the brain, they are the dominant component in the white matter; therefore, most diseases of myelin are white matter disorders. The myelin in peripheral nerves is similar to the myelin in the CNS, but with several important differences: (1) peripheral myelin is made by Schwann cells, not oligodendrocytes; (2) each Schwann cell in a peripheral nerve provides myelin for only one internode (Chapter 20), while in the CNS, each oligodendrocyte sends out processes that create multiple internodes; and (3) the specialized proteins and lipids are different. Most diseases of CNS myelin do not involve the peripheral nerves to any significant extent, and vice versa.

In general, CNS diseases involving myelin are separated into two broad groups:

- *Demyelinating diseases* are acquired conditions characterized by damage to previously healthy myelin. The most common diseases in this group result from immune-mediated injury, such as multiple sclerosis (MS) and related disorders. Other processes that can cause demyelinating diseases include viral infection of oligodendrocytes, as in progressive multifocal leukoencephalopathy (see earlier), and injury caused by drugs and other toxic agents.
- In *leukodystrophy*, or dysmyelinating diseases, myelin is not formed properly or has abnormal turnover kinetics. Most of these are caused by mutations that disrupt the function of proteins required for the formation of normal myelin sheaths.

Multiple Sclerosis

Multiple sclerosis (MS) is an autoimmune demyelinating disorder characterized by episodes of disease activity, separated in time, that produce white matter lesions that are separated in space. It is the most common demyelinating disorder, having a prevalence of approximately 1 per 1000 individuals in the United States and Europe, and its incidence appears to be increasing. The disease may present at any age, but onset in childhood or after 50 years of age is rare. Women are affected twice as often as men.

Pathogenesis. **The lesions of MS are caused by an autoimmune response directed against components of the myelin sheath in genetically predisposed individuals.** As in other autoimmune diseases (Chapter 5), the development of MS is related to genetic susceptibility and undefined environmental triggers.

- *Genetic factors.* The incidence of MS is 15-fold higher when the disease is present in a first-degree relative and roughly 150-fold higher with an affected monozygotic twin. Only a portion of the genetic basis of the disease has been explained, and many of the identified loci are associated with other autoimmune diseases. There is a strong effect of the major histocompatibility complex; each copy of the *HLA-DRB1*1501* allele an individual inherits brings with it a roughly 3-fold increase in the risk for MS. Other genetic loci that are associated with MS include the IL-2 and IL-7 receptor genes as well as others involved in immune responses.
- *Autoimmunity.* **The disease is initiated by Th1 and Th17 T cells and B cells that react against myelin antigens and secrete cytokines.** Th1 cells secrete IFN-γ, which activates macrophages, and Th17 cells promote the recruitment of leukocytes. The demyelination is caused by activated leukocytes and their injurious products. The infiltrate in plaques and surrounding regions of the brain consists of T cells (mainly CD4+, some CD8+) and macrophages. B lymphocytes and antibodies also play an important role in the disease, as indicated by the success of B cell–depleting

therapies. An association with Epstein-Barr virus (EBV) infection has been reported, but it is not clear if or how this is related to the autoimmune response to myelin proteins.

Clinical Features. The course of MS is variable. There are three clinical types of disease.

- *Relapsing-remitting MS* is the most common form, accounting for 85% to 90% of cases. It is characterized by multiple *relapses* and episodes of *remission;* typically, recovery during remissions is not complete. Over time there is usually a gradual, often stepwise, accumulation of neurologic deficits.
- *Secondary progressive MS* has an initial relapsing-remitting phase that is followed in 10 to 20 years by progressive worsening without remissions.
- *Primary progressive MS* has progressive disability from the outset with no or minor improvements and relapses.

Clinically isolated syndrome (CIS), is a term that describes the earliest clinical manifestations of MS. Unilateral visual impairment due to involvement of the optic nerve *(optic neuritis)* is a frequent initial manifestation. However, only a minority of individuals (10% to 50%, depending on the population studied) with an episode of optic neuritis go on to develop MS (which by definition is a remitting/relapsing or progressive disorder). Involvement of the brain stem produces cranial nerve signs (ataxia, nystagmus, and internuclear ophthalmoplegia). Spinal cord lesions give rise to motor and sensory impairment of the trunk and limbs, spasticity, and loss of bladder control. Imaging studies have demonstrated that there are often more lesions in the brains of patients with MS than might be expected from the clinical examination (eFig. 21.7), and that lesions can come and go much more often than was previously suspected. Changes in cognitive function can be present but are often milder than the other deficits. In any individual patient, it is difficult to predict when the next relapse will occur; most current treatments, which are intended to control the immune response, aim at decreasing the rate and severity of relapses.

The CSF in patients with MS shows a mildly elevated protein level with an increased proportion of immunoglobulin; in one-third of cases, there is moderate pleocytosis. When the immunoglobulins are examined further, *oligoclonal bands*, each corresponding to a particular immunoglobulin, can be identified. The contribution of these antibodies to the disease process is unclear.

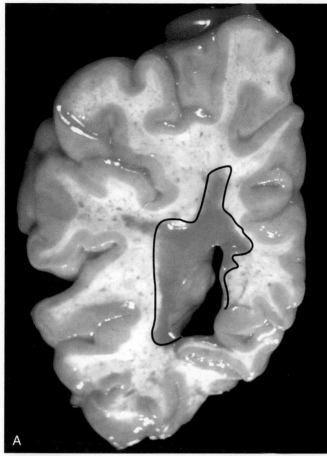

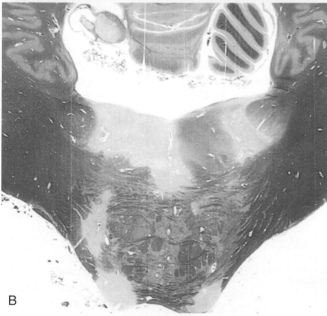

FIG. 21.20 Multiple sclerosis (MS). (A) Section of fresh brain showing a gray-brown plaque around the occipital horn of the lateral ventricle *(outlined)*. (B) Unstained regions of demyelination (MS plaques) around the fourth ventricle. Luxol fast blue—periodic acid—Schiff stain for myelin.

Other Acquired Demyelinating Diseases

Immune-mediated demyelination can occur after a number of systemic infectious illnesses, including relatively mild viral diseases.

These are not thought to be related to direct spread of the infectious agents to the nervous system. Rather, it is believed that immune cells responding to pathogen-associated antigens cross-react with myelin antigens, resulting in myelin damage.

There are two general patterns of postinfectious autoimmune reactions to myelin; unlike MS, both are associated with acute-onset monophasic illnesses. In *acute disseminated encephalomyelitis (ADEM)*, symptoms typically develop 1 or 2 weeks after an antecedent infection; in contrast with the focal findings of MS, the symptoms of ADEM are nonlocalizing (headache, lethargy, and coma). Symptoms progress rapidly, and the illness is fatal in as many as 20% of cases; in the remaining patients, there is complete recovery. *Acute necrotizing hemorrhagic encephalomyelitis* is a related disorder, which typically affects young adults and children.

Other acquired diseases of myelin include *neuromyelitis optica (NMO)*, an antibody-mediated demyelinating disease centered on the optic nerves and spinal cord, and *osmotic demyelination syndrome* caused by nonimmune damage to oligodendrocytes, typically after sudden correction of hyponatremia, that may result in a rapidly evolving quadriplegia.

As discussed earlier, *progressive multifocal leukoencephalopathy (PML)* is a demyelinating disease that occurs after reactivation of the JC virus in patients who are immunocompromised.

Leukodystrophies

Leukodystrophies are inherited dysmyelinating diseases characterized by abnormal myelin synthesis or turnover. In contrast to MS, the neurologic defects present at an early age and are progressive. Imaging studies reveal diffuse and symmetric myelin loss.

Three rare leukodystrophies merit mention:

- *Krabbe disease,* an autosomal recessive leukodystrophy resulting from a deficiency of *galactosylceramidase,* presents at between 3 to 6 months of age. Galactosylcerebroside is metabolized through an alternative pathway that generates a cytotoxic compound, galactosylsphingosine. There is loss of myelin in the brain and peripheral nerves and loss of oligodendrocytes in the CNS (eFig. 21.8). Survival beyond 2 years is rare.
- *Metachromatic leukodystrophy* is an autosomal recessive disease that results from a deficiency of the lysosomal enzyme *arylsulfatase A* that causes a buildup of sulfatides within macrophages. Sulfatides have a range of biologic actions and, when stained with certain dyes such as toluidine blue, shift the absorption spectrum of the dye, a property called metachromasia. The prognosis depends on the age at diagnosis, with earlier age of onset associated with more rapid progression.
- *Adrenoleukodystrophy* is an X-linked recessive disease associated with mutations in a member of the ATP-binding cassette transporter family of proteins (ABCD1), which is involved in the transport of molecules into the peroxisome. Very-long-chain fatty acids (VLCFAs) cannot be catabolized, resulting in elevated levels of VLCFAs in serum. Young boys present with behavioral changes and adrenal insufficiency. Death typically occurs 1 to 10 years after diagnosis.

Hematopoietic stem cell transplantation, which may allow repopulation of the CNS with enzymatically competent macrophages, has shown some benefit in Krabbe disease and metachromatic leukodystrophy.

NEURODEGENERATIVE DISEASES

Neurodegenerative diseases are characterized by the progressive loss of neurons, typically affecting groups of neurons with shared

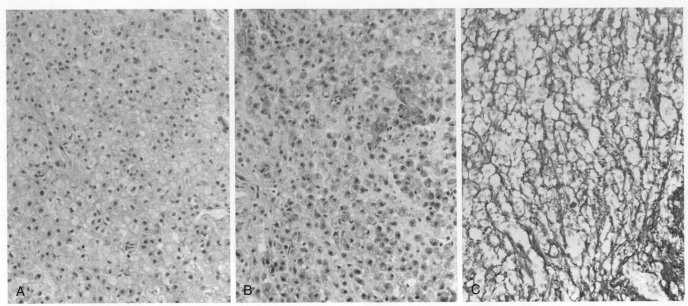

FIG. 21.21 Multiple sclerosis. (A) Active demyelinating plaques appear very cellular due to the presence of numerous lipid-laden macrophages. (B) The same lesion stained with the Luxol fast blue periodic acid–Schiff stain shows a complete absence of myelin. (C) Relative preservation of axons is seen on the neurofilament immunostain *(brown)*.

functions. Different diseases tend to affect particular neural systems and the presenting signs and symptoms reflect the site of involvement (Table 21.3):

- *Diseases that involve the hippocampus and associated cortices present with cognitive changes,* often including disturbances of memory, behavior, and language. With time these progress to dementia, as occurs with Alzheimer disease.
- *Diseases that affect the basal ganglia manifest as movement disorders;* these may be hypokinetic, as with Parkinson disease, or hyperkinetic, as with Huntington disease.
- *Diseases that affect the cerebellum or its input and output circuitry result in ataxia,* as seen in the spinocerebellar ataxias.
- *When the motor system bears the burden, weakness and difficulty with swallowing and respiration are often seen first,* as with amyotrophic lateral sclerosis.

The pathologic process that is common across most of the neurodegenerative diseases is the accumulation of protein aggregates (see Table 21.3). Protein aggregates may arise because of mutations that alter the protein's conformation or that disrupt pathways involved in protein processing or clearance. In other situations, there may be a subtle imbalance between protein synthesis and clearance (due to genetic, environmental, or unknown factors) that allows gradual accumulation of proteins. The aggregates are often resistant to degradation by normal cellular proteases, accumulate within cells or in the extracellular space, elicit an inflammatory response, and may be directly toxic to neurons. The current evidence suggests that large (i.e., microscopically visible) protein aggregates are not toxic to cells and the cellular damage may be caused by smaller (oligomeric) aggregates. However, as increasing amounts of protein are shunted into the aggregates, the normal function of the protein is reduced, and this may

Table 21.3 Features of the Major Neurodegenerative Diseases

Disease	Clinical Pattern	Protein Inclusions/Deposits
Prion disease (e.g., Creutzfeldt-Jakob disease)	Dementia	Spongiform change; PrP^{sc} protein
Alzheimer disease (AD)	Dementia	Aβ (plaques) Tau (tangles)
Frontotemporal lobar degeneration (FTLD)	Behavioral changes, language disturbance	Tau TDP43 Others (rare)
Parkinson disease (PD)	Hypokinetic movement disorder	α-synuclein
Huntington disease (HD)	Hyperkinetic movement disorder	Huntingtin (polyglutamine repeat expansions)
Spinocerebellar ataxias	Cerebellar ataxia	Various proteins (polyglutamine repeat expansions)
Amyotrophic lateral sclerosis (ALS)	Weakness with upper and lower motor neuron signs	Superoxide dismutase (SOD)1 TDP-43

also contribute to cell injury. As is evident from Table 21.3, the same proteins may be present as aggregates in multiple diseases. The intracellular protein aggregates are recognized histologically as inclusions and extracellular collections as deposits, both of which serve as diagnostic hallmarks.

Two other features are common to many neurodegenerative diseases:

- There is experimental evidence that many of the protein aggregates that accumulate in neurons in these diseases may be capable of spreading from one site in the brain to healthy neurons at another location. Thus, aggregates can seed the development of more aggregates, and the disease process can spread, like prions (described later). However, spread from an affected person to a healthy person is seen only in classic prion diseases.
- Activation of the innate immune system is a common feature of neurodegenerative diseases. Some genes that confer risk for diseases encode components of immune regulatory pathways. It is unclear if the immune system contributes to these disorders by triggering cytokine- or complement-mediated chronic inflammation or by some other mechanism.

Prion Diseases

Prion diseases are rapidly progressive neurodegenerative disorders caused by aggregation and intercellular spread of a misfolded prion protein. These include sporadic, familial, iatrogenic, and variant forms of Creutzfeldt-Jakob disease (CJD), as well as animal diseases such as scrapie in sheep and bovine spongiform encephalopathy in cattle (mad cow disease).

Pathogenesis. The causative protein, termed *prion protein (PrP),* is capable of undergoing a conformational change from its normal shape (PrP^c) to an abnormal conformation called PrP^{sc} (*sc* for *scrapie*). PrP^c is rich in α-helices, but PrP^{sc} has a high content of β-sheets, a characteristic that makes it resistant to proteolysis. When PrP^{sc} physically interacts with PrP^c molecules, it causes them to adopt the PrP^{sc} conformation (Fig. 21.22), a property that accounts for the "infectious" nature of PrP^{sc}. Over time, this self-amplifying process leads to the accumulation of pathogenic PrP^{sc} molecules in the brain. Certain mutations in the gene encoding PrP^c *(PRNP)* accelerate the rate of spontaneous conformational change; these variants are associated with early-onset familial forms of prion disease (familial Creutzfeldt-Jakob disease). PrP^c may also change its conformation spontaneously (but at an extremely low rate), accounting for sporadic cases of prion disease (sporadic Creutzfeldt-Jakob disease). Accumulation of PrP^{sc} in neural tissue seems to be the cause of cell injury, but the mechanisms underlying the cytopathic changes and eventual neuronal death are still unknown. A contributing factor may be cell death caused by misfolded prion proteins.

Creutzfeldt-Jakob Disease

Creutzfeldt-Jakob disease (CJD) is a rapidly progressive dementing illness with a typical duration of less than 1 year from first onset of subtle changes in memory and behavior to death. It is sporadic in approximately 85% of cases and has a worldwide annual incidence of about 1 per million. While commonly affecting individuals older than 70 years of age, familial forms caused by mutations in *PRNP* may present in younger individuals. In keeping with the infectious nature of PrP^{sc}, there are rare but well-established cases of iatrogenic transmission by contaminated deep implantation electrodes, administration of human growth hormone preparations, and other procedures.

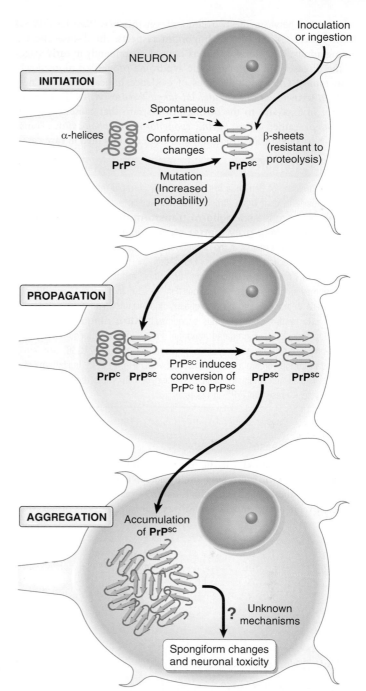

FIG. 21.22 Pathogenesis of prion disease. α-helical PrP^c may spontaneously shift to the β-sheet PrP^{sc} conformation, a change that occurs at a much higher rate in familial disease associated with PrP mutations. PrP^{sc} may also be acquired from exogenous sources, such as contaminated food, medical instrumentation, or medicines. Once present, PrP^{sc} converts additional molecules of PrP^c into PrP^{sc} through physical interaction, eventually leading to the formation of pathogenic PrP^{sc} aggregates.

Variant Creutzfeldt-Jakob Disease

Starting in 1995, cases of a CJD-like illness appeared in the United Kingdom. The neuropathologic findings and molecular features of these new cases were similar to those of CJD, suggesting a close relationship between the two illnesses, yet this new disorder differed from typical CJD in several important respects: the disease affected young adults; behavioral disorders figured prominently in early stages of the disease; and the neurologic syndrome progressed more slowly than typical CJD. Multiple lines of evidence indicate that this new disease, termed *variant Creutzfeldt-Jakob disease (vCJD)*, is a consequence of exposure to the bovine prion strain that causes the prion disease of cattle, called *bovine spongiform encephalopathy*. Transmission by blood transfusion has also been documented in rare cases.

MORPHOLOGY

The progression of dementia in CJD is usually so rapid that there is little, if any, grossly evident brain atrophy. On microscopic examination, the pathognomonic finding is a **spongiform transformation of the cerebral cortex and deep gray matter structures** (caudate, putamen); this multifocal process results in the uneven formation of small, apparently empty, microscopic vacuoles of varying sizes within the neuropil (the eosinophilic regions in gray matter that contain dendrites, axons, and synapses) and sometimes in the perikaryon of neurons (Fig. 21.23A). In advanced cases, there is severe neuronal loss, reactive gliosis, and expansion of the vacuolated areas into cystlike spaces (status spongiosus). **Kuru plaques** are extracellular deposits of aggregated abnormal PrP^sc. They are Congo red– and PAS-positive and usually occur in the cerebellum (Fig. 21.23B) and are abundant in the cerebral cortex in cases of vCJD (Fig. 21.23C). In all forms of prion disease, immunohistochemical staining demonstrates the presence of proteinase K–resistant PrP^sc in tissue.

Alzheimer Disease

Alzheimer disease (AD) is the most common cause of dementia in older adults, with increasing incidence as a function of age. The incidence is about 3% in individuals 65 to 74 years of age, 19% in those 75 to 84 years of age, and 47% in those older than 84 years of age. Most cases of AD are sporadic, but at least 5% to 10% are familial. Sporadic cases rarely present before 50 years of age, but early onset is seen with some heritable forms.

Pathogenesis. **The principal abnormality in AD is the accumulation of two proteins, Aβ and tau, in the forms of plaques and tangles, respectively, in specific brain regions; these changes result in secondary effects including neuronal dysfunction, neuronal death, and inflammatory reactions.** Plaques are deposits of aggregated Aβ peptides in the neuropil, while tangles are aggregates of the microtubule binding protein tau that develop intracellularly and then persist extracellularly after neuronal death. Both plaques and tangles appear to contribute to neural dysfunction. Deposits of Aβ and tangles begin to appear in the brain well in advance of cognitive impairment, and the presence of a large burden of plaques and tangles is strongly associated with severe cognitive dysfunction. The number of neurofibrillary tangles correlates better with the degree of dementia than does the number of neuritic plaques. The details of the interplay between the processes that lead to the accumulation of these abnormal aggregates and how the aggregates cause neuronal injury are key questions that have yet to be answered.

Role of Aβ. **Generation of a pathogenic form of Aβ, a 42-amino acid peptide, is the critical initiating event for the development of AD.** The generation of Aβ peptide may be increased by abnormal enzymatic processing or by increased production. Aβ42 is produced when the transmembrane protein amyloid precursor protein (APP) is sequentially cleaved by the enzymes β-secretase (β-amyloid–converting enzyme [BACE]) and γ-secretase (Fig. 21.24). APP can also be cleaved by α-secretase and γ-secretase, liberating a different peptide that is nonpathogenic. Mutations in *APP* or in the genes encoding two components of γ-secretase, presenilin-1 or presenilin-2, lead to familial AD characterized by an increased rate at which Aβ42 is generated. Mutations or increases in the copy number of the gene encoding APP, which is located on chromosome 21, are also associated with an elevated risk of

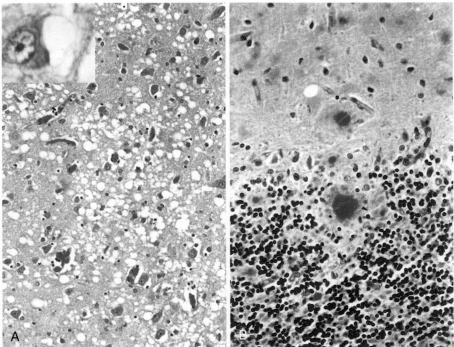

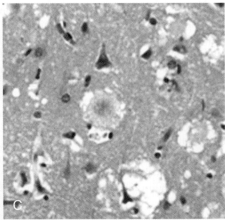

FIG. 21.23 Prion disease. (A) Spongiform change in the cerebral cortex. *Inset,* High magnification of neuron with vacuoles. (B) Cerebellar cortex showing kuru plaques (periodic acid–Schiff stain) that consist of aggregated PrP^sc. (C) Cortical kuru plaques surrounded by spongiform change in variant Creutzfeldt-Jakob disease.

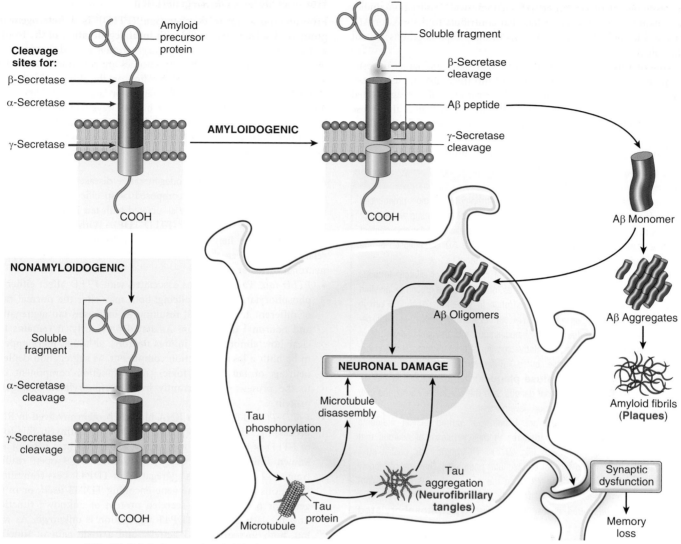

FIG. 21.24 Pathogenesis of Alzheimer disease. Amyloid precursor protein cleavage by α-secretase and γ-secretase produces a harmless soluble peptide, whereas amyloid precursor protein cleavage by β-secretase and γ-secretase releases Aβ peptides, which form pathogenic oligomers that damage neurons and larger aggregates that form characteristic extracellular plaques. The mechanism of tau hyperphosphorylation is unclear.

AD. The latter occurs in patients with trisomy 21 (Down syndrome) and individuals with interstitial duplications of the *APP* gene, presumably because the resulting increased number of *APP* gene copies leads to greater Aβ generation.

Once generated, Aβ is highly prone to aggregation; it first forms small oligomers, and these eventually propagate into large aggregates and fibrils. The large aggregates are visible as plaques, one of the pathologic hallmarks of the disease, but smaller oligomers may be the more pathogenic form. Oligomers are either formed within cells or taken up from the extracellular space. These oligomers may injure neurons by interfering with the functions of mitochondria and other organelles and by decreasing the number of synapses present and impairing the function of those that remain. Synaptic dysfunction is thought to underlie the decline in memory that is a classic feature of the disease.

Role of Tau. Because neurofibrillary tangles, the second pathologic hallmark of Alzheimer disease, contain the tau protein, there has been much interest in the role of this protein in AD. Tau is a microtubule-associated protein present in axons. In AD, tau is hyperphosphorylated, leading to loss of its ability to bind to microtubules, its normal microtubule stabilizing function, and its aggregation to form neurofibrillary tangles. The mechanism of tangle-mediated injury to neurons remains poorly understood. Two pathways have been suggested: (1) aggregates of tau elicit a stress response, which persists and eventually leads to cell death, and (2) loss of the microtubule stabilizing function of tau leads to neuronal toxicity and death.

Other Genetic Risk Factors. The genetic locus on chromosome 19 that encodes apolipoprotein E (ApoE) has a strong influence on the risk for developing AD. Three alleles of the *ApoE* gene have been identified (ε2, ε3, and ε4) based on two amino acid polymorphisms. The dosage of the ε4 allele increases the risk for AD. This ApoE isoform promotes Aβ generation and deposition and appears to exacerbate Aβ-independent, tau-mediated neurodegeneration. Overall, this locus has been estimated to convey about one-fourth of the risk for development of late-onset AD. Genome-wide association studies have identified multiple other loci that contribute to the risk for AD, but the roles of the encoded proteins in disease pathogenesis are not established.

Role of Inflammation. Both small aggregates and larger deposits of Aβ elicit an inflammatory response from microglia and astrocytes. This response probably assists in the clearance of the aggregated peptide but may also stimulate the secretion of mediators that cause damage. Additional consequences of the activation of these inflammatory cascades may include alterations in tau phosphorylation, oxidative injury to neurons, and aberrant pruning of synapses.

MORPHOLOGY

Brains involved by AD show variable cortical atrophy that is most pronounced in the frontal, temporal, and parietal lobes. The atrophy results in widening of the cerebral sulci and the loss of tissue may produce ventricular enlargement (hydrocephalus ex vacuo). At the microscopic level, AD is diagnosed by the presence of neuritic plaques and neurofibrillary tangles.

Neuritic plaques are focal, spherical collections of dilated, tortuous processes derived from dystrophic neurites, often centered around an amyloid core (Fig. 21.25A, B). Neuritic plaques range in size from 20 to 200 μm in diameter; microglial cells and reactive astrocytes are present at their periphery. Plaques can be found in the hippocampus and amygdala as well as in the neocortex, although there is relative sparing of primary motor and sensory cortices until late in the disease course. Aβ deposits that lack the surrounding neuritic reaction are called **diffuse plaques;** these are found in the superficial cerebral cortex, the basal ganglia, and the cerebellar cortex and may represent an early stage of plaque development.

Neurofibrillary tangles are bundles of paired helical filaments visible as basophilic fibrillary structures in the cytoplasm of neurons that displace or encircle the nucleus (Fig. 21.25C, D); tangles can persist after neurons die, becoming a form of extracellular pathology. They are commonly found in cortical neurons, as well as in the pyramidal cells of the hippocampus, the amygdala, the basal forebrain, and the raphe nuclei. A major component of the paired helical filaments is **hyperphosphorylated tau** (Fig. 21.25).

Other pathologic findings include **cerebral amyloid angiopathy (CAA)**, an almost invariable accompaniment of AD that can also be found in the brains of individuals without AD.

Clinical Features. The progression of AD is slow but relentless, with a symptomatic course often running more than 10 years. Initial symptoms are forgetfulness and other memory disturbances; with progression, other symptoms emerge, including language deficits and loss of mathematical skills and learned motor skills. In the final stages, affected individuals may become incontinent, mute, and unable to walk; intercurrent disease, often pneumonia, is usually the terminal event. Current clinical trials are focused on treating subjects in early, preclinical stages of the illness, using antibodies or drugs that are designed to clear Aβ from the brain or prevent alterations in tau that lead to tangle formation. An important development that is enabling early intervention trials is the identification of biomarkers of AD. It is now possible to demonstrate Aβ deposition in the brain through imaging methods, prior to the onset of symptoms. Other markers of AD include the presence of phosphorylated tau and reduced Aβ in the CSF. It is hoped that therapeutic interventions that positively impact these biomarkers will eventually prove to prevent or slow the onset or progression of AD, a hypothesis that will take many years to test rigorously.

Frontotemporal Lobar Degeneration

Frontotemporal lobar degeneration (FTLD) is a heterogeneous group of disorders associated with focal degeneration of the frontal and/or temporal lobes. The term *degeneration* is used for the pathologic changes; clinically, these syndromes are commonly referred to as *frontotemporal dementias.* Depending on the disease distribution (frontal or temporal), behavioral changes or language problems may dominate. FTLD differs from AD in two ways: (1) behavioral and language problems precede memory disturbances, and (2) the onset of symptoms occurs at younger age. These differences help in clinical discrimination between these two forms of dementia.

Pathogenesis. Like most neurodegenerative diseases, FTLD is associated with cellular inclusions composed of specific proteins; the two most common types are those associated with tau inclusions (FTLD-tau) and TDP43 inclusions (FTLD-TDP). Within each of these groups, there are heritable and sporadic forms. There is no clear relationship between the clinical subtypes of FTLD and the type of neuronal inclusion.

- *FTLD-tau.* Tau mutations associated with FTLD affect either its phosphorylation or its splicing; both may alter the normal ratio of different tau isoforms, resulting in increased tau aggregation and neuronal dysfunction. As stated previously, it remains unclear how abnormal tau injures neurons, although there appears to be both a loss-of-function component, as aggregation depletes neurons of tau, and a toxic gain-of-function component due to the presence of aberrantly hyperphosphorylated aggregated protein.

- *FTLD-TDP.* TDP43 is an RNA-binding protein involved in RNA processing. The most common genetic abnormality in this form of FTLD is a hexanucleotide repeat expansion in a gene of unknown function called *C9orf72* (chromosome 9 open reading frame #72), which causes aggregation of TDP43. Less commonly, mutations are seen in the gene encoding TDP43 itself, or in the gene for progranulin, a secreted protein of unknown function; how the latter induces TDP43 aggregation is unknown. As with tau, both loss of TDP43 activity and a toxic gain of function related to the protein aggregates may be involved in the disease. TDP43 neuronal inclusions are also found in a large proportion of cases of amyotrophic lateral sclerosis (ALS). This overlap is seen clinically, as some individuals with ALS also show evidence of FTLD.

- There are rare forms of FTLD lacking both tau- and TDP-containing inclusions. Notably, these unusual subtypes also show evidence of connections to pathways that have been implicated in FTLD-TDP.

MORPHOLOGY

The characteristic morphologic features of both types of FTLD include atrophy of frontal and temporal lobes of variable extent and severity, accompanied microscopically by neuronal loss and gliosis. In FTLD-tau, tau-containing neurofibrillary tangles are present, similar to the tangles found in AD (Fig. 21.26A). FTLD has several pathologic subtypes. In one of the subtypes called **Pick disease** the brain shows a pronounced and frequently asymmetric atrophy of the frontal and temporal lobes, with conspicuous sparing of the posterior two-thirds of the superior temporal gyrus and only rare involvement of the parietal and occipital lobes (eFig. 21.9). The atrophy can be severe, reducing gyri to a wafer-thin ("knife-edge") appearance. The neuronal loss is most severe in the outer three layers of the cortex. Some of the surviving neurons show a characteristic swelling **(Pick cells)**, and others

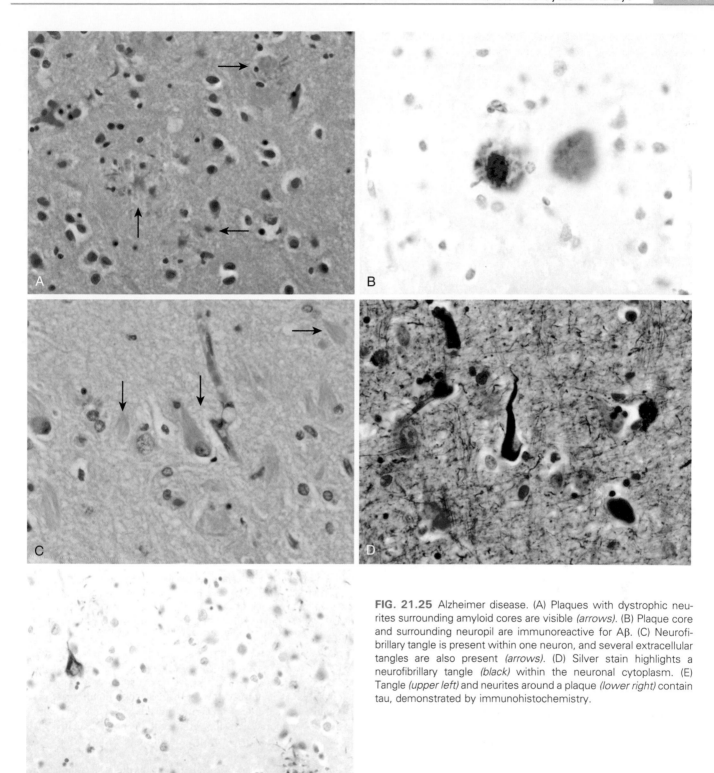

FIG. 21.25 Alzheimer disease. (A) Plaques with dystrophic neurites surrounding amyloid cores are visible *(arrows)*. (B) Plaque core and surrounding neuropil are immunoreactive for Aβ. (C) Neurofibrillary tangle is present within one neuron, and several extracellular tangles are also present *(arrows)*. (D) Silver stain highlights a neurofibrillary tangle *(black)* within the neuronal cytoplasm. (E) Tangle *(upper left)* and neurites around a plaque *(lower right)* contain tau, demonstrated by immunohistochemistry.

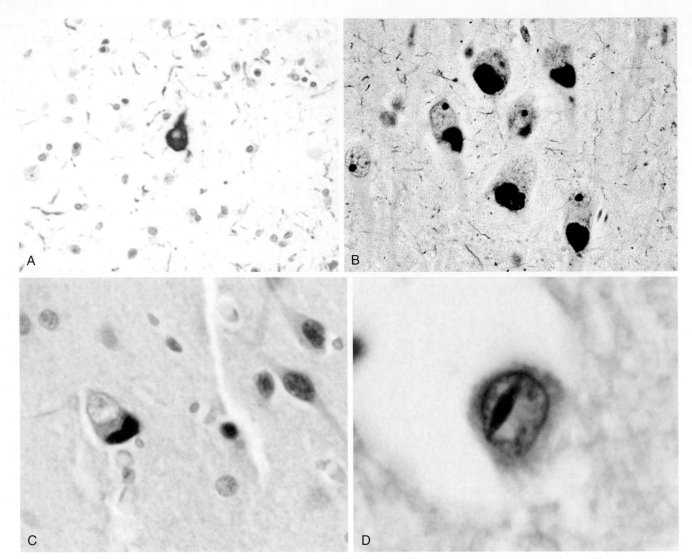

FIG. 21.26 Frontotemporal lobar degenerations (FTLDs). (A) FTLD-tau. A tangle is present along with numerous tau-containing neurites (immunohistochemical stain for tau). (B) Pick disease. Pick bodies are round, homogeneous neuronal cytoplasmic inclusions that stain intensely with silver stains. (C) FTLD-TDP. Cytoplasmic inclusions containing TDP43 are seen in association with loss of normal nuclear immunoreactivity (immunohistochemical stain for TDP43). (D) FLTD-TDP. With progranulin mutations, the TDP43—containing inclusions are commonly intranuclear.

contain **Pick bodies,** cytoplasmic, round to oval, filamentous inclusions that stain strongly with silver methods (Fig. 21.26B). In FTLD-TDP, there is loss of nuclear immunohistochemical staining for TDP43 associated with the appearance of TDP43-positive inclusions (Fig. 21.26C, D).

Parkinson Disease

Parkinson disease (PD) is a neurodegenerative disease marked by a hypokinetic movement disorder due to loss of dopaminergic neurons from the substantia nigra. Dopaminergic neurons project from the substantia nigra to the striatum and are involved in control of motor activity. *Parkinsonism* is a clinical syndrome characterized by tremor, rigidity, bradykinesia, and instability. These types of motor disturbances may be seen in a range of diseases that damage dopaminergic neurons. Parkinsonism may also be induced by drugs such as

dopamine antagonists or toxins that selectively injure these neurons. Toxins that have been implicated include chemicals found in "synthetic" heroin and pesticides. Among the neurodegenerative diseases, most cases of parkinsonism are caused by PD.

Pathogenesis. **PD is associated with protein accumulation and aggregation, mitochondrial abnormalities, and neuronal loss in the substantia nigra.** A diagnostic feature of the disease and a clue to its pathogenesis is the Lewy body, a characteristic inclusion containing α-synuclein which is normally present in neurons. α-synuclein is involved in synaptic transmission. Based on the genetics of PD, it appears that abnormal protein and organelle clearance due to defects in autophagy and lysosomal degradation have a pathogenic role. Synuclein aggregates are cleared by autophagy (Chapter 1), and several mutations associated with PD are in genes whose products (Parkin, others) appear to have roles in endosomal trafficking pathways implicated in autophagy and in mitochondrial function. While PD in most cases is sporadic, point mutations and duplications of the gene encoding α-synuclein cause autosomal dominant PD. Heterozygosity for the Gaucher disease—causing mutation in glucocerebrosidase is also a risk factor for PD (Chapter 4). Glucocerebrosidase is a lysosomal enzyme, again suggesting that abnormal turnover of cellular constituents sets the stage for the development of PD. Gain-of-function mutations in the gene encoding the kinase LRRK2 are the most common cause of autosomal dominant PD; how this abnormality leads to disease is not known.

MORPHOLOGY

A typical gross finding is **pallor of the substantia nigra** (Fig. 21.27A, B) **and locus ceruleus**. Microscopic features include loss of the pigmented, catecholaminergic neurons in these regions associated with gliosis. Remaining neurons may contain **Lewy bodies,** single or multiple cytoplasmic, eosinophilic, round to elongated inclusions (Fig. 21.27C). On ultrastructural examination, Lewy bodies consist of fine filaments composed of α-synuclein and other proteins, including neurofilaments and ubiquitin. In addition, there may be dystrophic neurites, called **Lewy neurites,** that also contain aggregated α-synuclein.

Clinical Features. PD commonly manifests as a movement disorder in the absence of a toxic exposure or other known underlying etiology. Characteristic symptoms are tremor, bradykinesia, and rigidity. Tremor is typically described as "pill-rolling" that occurs at rest. The disease usually progresses over 10 to 15 years, eventually producing severe motor slowing to the point of near immobility. Death often results from aspiration pneumonia or trauma from falls caused by postural instability.

Movement symptoms of PD initially respond to L-dihydroxy-phenylalanine (L-DOPA), but this treatment does not slow disease progression. Over time, L-DOPA becomes less effective and begins to cause problematic fluctuations in motor function. Another treatment for the motor symptoms of PD is deep brain stimulation, in which electrodes are implanted in the globus pallidus or subthalamic nucleus to modulate basal ganglia circuitry, allowing a significant reduction in L-DOPA dose in some patients.

While the movement disorder associated with loss of the nigro-striatal dopaminergic pathway is a dominant feature of PD, the disease has additional clinical and pathologic manifestations. Loss of neurons in the brain stem (in the dorsal motor nucleus of the vagus and in the reticular formation), in advance of nigral involvement, can give rise to a sleep disorder, often before motor problems arise. Dementia, typically with a mildly fluctuating course and hallucinations, emerges in many individuals with PD and is attributable to involvement of the cerebral cortex. When dementia arises within 1 year of the onset of motor symptoms, it is referred to *Lewy body dementia (LBD)*.

Atypical Parkinsonian Syndromes

These disorders have features of parkinsonism (bradykinesia and rigidity) as components of their clinical manifestations along with other symptoms and are minimally responsive to L-DOPA.

- *Progressive supranuclear palsy.* Patients develop progressive truncal rigidity, disequilibrium with frequent falls, and difficulty with voluntary eye movements. Other common symptoms include nuchal dystonia, pseudobulbar palsy, and a mild progressive dementia. The pathologic hallmark is the presence of tau-containing inclusions in neurons and glia in the brain stem and deep gray matter.
- *Corticobasilar degeneration.* This disease is most often characterized by extrapyramidal rigidity, asymmetric motor disturbances (jerking movements of limbs), and impaired higher cortical function (typically in the form of apraxia). Tau-containing inclusions are seen in the cerebral cortex.
- *Multiple system atrophy (MSA).* This sporadic disorder affects several functional systems in the brain and is marked by α-synuclein inclusions in the cytoplasm of oligodendrocytes. The clinical manifestations stem from involvement of different neural circuits: the striatonigral circuit (leading to parkinsonism), the olivopontocerebellar circuit (leading to ataxia), and the autonomic nervous system including its central elements (leading to autonomic dysfunction, with orthostatic hypotension as a prominent component). In a given individual, one of these components may predominate at the onset of the illness, but typically the other systems become affected as MSA progresses.

Huntington Disease

Huntington disease (HD) is an autosomal dominant movement disorder associated with degeneration of the striatum (caudate and putamen). The disorder is characterized by involuntary jerky movements of all parts of the body; writhing movements of the extremities

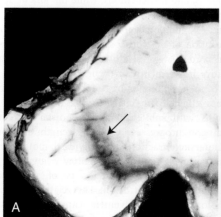
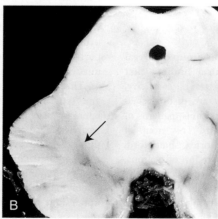
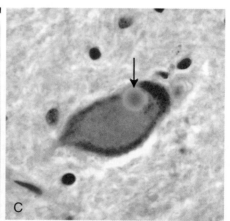

FIG. 21.27 Parkinson disease. (A) Healthy substantia nigra *(arrow)*. (B) Depigmented substantia nigra *(arrow)* in idiopathic Parkinson disease. (C) Lewy body in a neuron from the substantia nigra stains pink *(arrow)*.

are typical. The disease is relentlessly progressive, resulting in death after an average course of about 15 years. Early cognitive symptoms include forgetfulness and thought and affective disorders, and there may be a progression to severe dementia.

Pathogenesis. **HD is caused by repeat expansions of a CAG trinucleotide (encoding glutamine) in a gene that encodes the protein huntingtin.** The wild-type gene contains 11 to 34 copies of the repeat; in disease-causing alleles, the number of CAG repeats is increased, sometimes into the hundreds. There is a strong genotype-phenotype correlation, with larger numbers of repeats resulting in earlier-onset disease. Once the symptoms appear, however, the course of the illness is not affected by repeat length. Further expansions of the CAG repeats occur during spermatogenesis, so paternal transmission may be associated with earlier onset in the next generation, a phenomenon referred to as *anticipation* (Chapter 4).

HD appears to be caused by toxic gain of function related to the expanded polyglutamine tract in huntingtin, but the normal function of this protein and how the abnormal forms cause disease are unknown. The mutant protein is subject to ubiquitination and proteolysis, yielding fragments that can form large intranuclear aggregates. As in other neurodegenerative diseases, smaller aggregates of the abnormal protein fragments are suspected to be toxic. These aggregates may have a range of potentially injurious actions, including sequestration of transcription factors, disruption of protein degradation pathways, and perturbation of mitochondrial function.

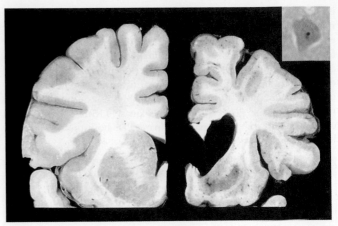

FIG. 21.28 Huntington disease. Healthy hemisphere *(left)* compared with a hemisphere with Huntington disease *(right)* showing atrophy of the striatum and ventricular dilation. *Inset,* An intranuclear inclusion in a cortical neuron is strongly immunoreactive for ubiquitin. (Gross photo courtesy of Dr. Vonsattel, Columbia University, New York, New York.)

MORPHOLOGY

On gross examination, the brain is small and shows striking atrophy of the caudate nucleus and, in some cases, to a lesser extent, the putamen (Fig. 21.28). The globus pallidus may be atrophied secondarily, and the lateral and third ventricles are dilated. Atrophy is frequently also seen in the frontal lobe, less often in the parietal lobe, and occasionally in the entire cortex.

Microscopic examination reveals severe loss of neurons from affected regions of the striatum along with gliosis. The medium-sized, spiny neurons that release the neurotransmitters γ-aminobutyric acid (GABA), enkephalin, dynorphin, and substance P are especially vulnerable, disappearing early in the disease. There is a strong correlation between the degree of degeneration in the striatum and the severity of motor symptoms; there is also an association between cortical neuronal loss and dementia. In remaining striatal neurons and in the cortex, there are intranuclear inclusions that contain aggregates of ubiquitinated huntingtin (Fig. 21.28, *inset*).

Spinocerebellar Degenerations

Spinocerebellar ataxias (SCAs) are a heterogeneous group of several dozen autosomal dominant diseases with clinical findings that include a combination of cerebellar and sensory ataxia, spasticity, and sensorimotor peripheral neuropathy. They are distinguished from one another based on different causative mutations, patterns of inheritance, age at onset, and signs and symptoms. This group of diseases affects, to a variable extent, the cerebellar cortex, spinal cord, other brain regions, and peripheral nerves. Degeneration of neurons, often without other distinctive histopathologic changes, occurs in the affected areas in association with mild gliosis. The additional clinical symptoms that accompany the ataxia can help distinguish between well-characterized subtypes. Although almost 45 distinct genetic types of SCA have been identified, there remain many cases that do not fall into one of the already characterized forms.

As with HD, several forms of SCA are caused by CAG repeat expansions encoding polyglutamine tracts in various genes. In these types of SCA, as is true for HD, neuronal intranuclear inclusions are present containing the abnormal protein, and age of onset decreases as the number of repeats increases.

Friedreich ataxia is an autosomal recessive disorder that generally manifests in the first decade of life with gait ataxia, followed by hand clumsiness and dysarthria. Most patients develop pes cavus and kyphoscoliosis, and there is a high incidence of cardiac disease and diabetes. The disease is usually caused by a GAA trinucleotide repeat expansion in the gene encoding frataxin, a protein that regulates cellular iron levels, particularly in the mitochondria. The repeat expansion results in transcriptional silencing and decreased frataxin levels, leading to mitochondrial dysfunction and oxidative damage.

Amyotrophic Lateral Sclerosis

Amyotrophic lateral sclerosis (ALS) results from the death of lower motor neurons in the spinal cord and brain stem and upper motor neurons in the cerebral cortex. The loss of lower motor neurons leads to denervation of muscles, muscular atrophy ("amyotrophy"), weakness, and fasciculations, while the loss of upper motor neurons results in paresis, hyperreflexia, and spasticity, along with a Babinski sign. An additional consequence of upper motor neuron loss is degeneration of the corticospinal tracts in the lateral portion of the spinal cord ("lateral sclerosis"). Sensation is usually unaffected, but cognitive impairment can occur.

The disease affects men slightly more frequently than women and typically becomes clinically manifest in the fifth decade or later. It usually begins with subtle asymmetric distal extremity weakness. As the disease progresses, muscle strength and bulk diminish, and involuntary contractions of individual motor units, termed *fasciculations*, occur. The disease eventually involves the respiratory muscles, leading to recurrent bouts of pulmonary infection, which is the usual cause of death. The relative degree of upper and lower motor neuron involvement can vary, although most patients exhibit both. In some cases, degeneration of the lower brain stem cranial motor nuclei occurs early and progresses rapidly, a pattern of disease referred to as *bulbar amyotrophic lateral sclerosis.* With this disease pattern, abnormalities of swallowing and speaking dominate.

Pathogenesis. While most cases are sporadic, about 10% are familial, mostly with autosomal dominant inheritance. Familial disease begins earlier in life than sporadic disease, but once symptoms appear, the clinical course is similar in both forms. Mutations in the superoxide dismutase gene, *SOD1,* on chromosome 21 were the first identified genetic cause of ALS and account for about 20% of the familial forms. These mutations are thought to generate abnormal misfolded forms of the SOD1 protein, which may trigger the unfolded protein response and cause apoptotic death of neurons.

A number of other genetic loci are associated with ALS. The most common cause of familial ALS is a hexanucleotide repeat expansion in the gene *C9orf72,* which, as mentioned earlier, is also frequently affected in frontotemporal lobar degeneration. The protein encoded by *C9orf72* associates with RNA binding proteins; notably, mutations affecting two other RNA-binding proteins may cause ALS, TDP43 (also associated with FTLD) and FUS. This convergence suggests that an abnormality of RNA processing directly or indirectly contributes to the pathogenesis of ALS, but it is uncertain how mutations in *SOD1* fit into this picture, and much remains to be discovered. As expected from the genetic overlap, there is some clinical overlap between ALS and FTLD, such as cognitive impairment.

MORPHOLOGY

The most striking gross changes are found in anterior roots of the spinal cord, which are thin and gray (Fig. 21.29A). In especially severe cases, the precentral gyrus (motor cortex) is mildly atrophic due to the death of upper motor neurons. Microscopic examination demonstrates a **reduction in the number of anterior horn cell neurons** throughout the spinal cord associated with reactive gliosis and loss of anterior root myelinated fibers (Fig. 21.29B). Similar findings are found with involvement of motor cranial nerve nuclei except those supplying the extraocular muscles, which are spared in all but a few long-term survivors. Cytoplasmic inclusions that contain TDP43 may be seen in a subset of cases. With the loss of innervation from the death of anterior horn cells, skeletal muscles show neurogenic atrophy.

Other Motor Neuron Diseases

Motor neurons are the primary target in some other diseases, similar to ALS.

- *Spinal and bulbar muscular atrophy (Kennedy disease)* is an X-linked disorder characterized by distal limb amyotrophy and bulbar signs, such as atrophy and fasciculations of the tongue and dysphagia, that are associated with degeneration of lower motor neurons in the spinal cord and brain stem. It is one of the trinucleotide expansion diseases. The expanded repeat occurs in the first exon of the androgen receptor gene on the X chromosome, impairing the function of the encoded androgen receptor; this leads to androgen insensitivity, gynecomastia, testicular atrophy, and oligospermia. Carrier females are largely unaffected. The basis for the selective motor neuron involvement is unclear, but as in other polyglutamine expansion diseases such as HD and some forms of spinocerebellar atrophy, there are intranuclear inclusions that contain the abnormal protein. Progression of the disease is slow, and most affected individuals remain ambulatory until late in the disease course. Life span is normal.

- *Spinal muscular atrophy (SMA)* includes a group of genetically linked disorders of childhood characterized by marked loss of lower motor neurons that results in progressive weakness. The disease is caused by loss-of-function mutations in the gene encoding SMN1, a protein involved in the assembly of the spliceosome. Gene therapies have been developed that produce therapeutic benefit by increasing the expression of functional SMN in motor neurons.

TUMORS

The annual incidence of CNS tumors in adults in the United States is about 24 per 100,000 individuals for intracranial tumors, about a third of which are malignant, and 1 to 2 per 100,000 individuals for intraspinal tumors. Metastases are more common than primary brain tumors. Tumors of the CNS make up a larger proportion of childhood cancers, accounting for as many of 20% of all pediatric tumors, and have replaced acute lymphoblastic leukemia as the most deadly forms of cancer in children. Childhood CNS tumors differ from those in adults in histologic subtype, mutation profile, and location. In childhood, tumors are likely to arise in the posterior fossa, whereas tumors in adults are mostly supratentorial.

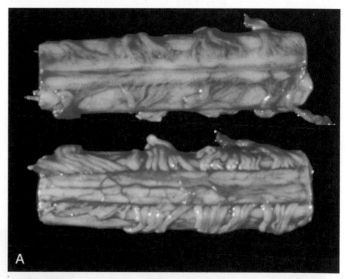
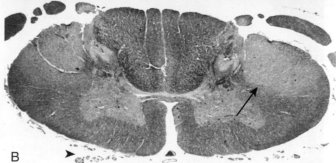

FIG. 21.29 Amyotrophic lateral sclerosis. (A) Segment of spinal cord viewed from anterior *(upper)* and posterior *(lower)* surfaces showing attenuation of anterior (motor) roots compared with posterior (sensory) roots. (B) Spinal cord showing loss of myelinated fibers (lack of stain) in corticospinal tracts (best seen on the right side of this specimen; *arrow*) as well as degeneration of anterior roots *(arrowhead).*

Tumors of the nervous system have unique characteristics that set them apart from tumors elsewhere in the body.

- CNS tumors do not have morphologically evident premalignant or in situ lesions comparable to those of carcinomas.
- Even low-grade lesions may infiltrate large regions of the brain, leading to serious clinical deficits, unresectability, and poor prognosis.
- The anatomic site of the neoplasm can influence outcome independent of tumor type and grade due to local effects (e.g., a benign meningioma may cause cardiorespiratory arrest from compression of the medulla).
- CNS tumors, even the most highly malignant gliomas, rarely spread outside of the CNS.

Gliomas

Gliomas are tumors of the brain parenchyma. The 2021 WHO classification of tumors of the central nervous system has incorporated molecular features, specifically mutations of the *IDH* gene and deletion of the chromosomal segments 1p and 19q, into the previous histology-based classification. **Based on the new classification, diffuse gliomas are grouped into adult-type and pediatric-type diffuse gliomas.** Treatment protocols and clinical trials are now based on this new WHO classification, which further segregates tumors into one of four grades according to their biologic behavior, ranging from grade 1 to grade 4. Like most cancers, lower grade brain tumors tend to progress and become more aggressive with time due to clonal evolution, a change in behavior that is often reflected in a change to a higher tumor grade.

Adult-type diffuse gliomas include three distinct types— astrocytoma, *IDH*-mutant; glioblastoma, *IDH*-wild-type; and oligodendroglioma, *IDH*-mutant and 1p/19q-codeleted. These account for most of the malignant tumors of the adult central nervous system.

Pediatric gliomas are much more heterogeneous and include both diffuse and circumscribed subtypes, with circumscribed types generally having much better prognosis. Pediatric-type diffuse gliomas are further subdivided into low-grade and high-grade; unlike adult-type, they lack *IDH* mutations and 1p/19q codeletion. This molecular distinction has prognostic implications; for instance, pediatric-type diffuse gliomas are mostly indolent compared to their adult counterparts. The discussion that follows focuses on adult-type glioma.

Astrocytoma, IDH-Mutant

IDH-mutant astrocytomas are tumors arising from astrocytes, usually in the cerebral hemispheres. They are most frequent in the fourth through the sixth decades of life. The most common presenting signs and symptoms are seizures, headaches, and focal neurologic deficits related to the anatomic site of involvement. On the basis of histologic and molecular features, they are graded as WHO grades 2 to 4. Grade 1 is not used because by convention it implies benign behavior and all diffuse gliomas are considered malignant. Molecular features are also incorporated into the grading. For instance, homozygous deletion of *CDKN2A* and/or *CDKN2B* leads to the designation of astrocytoma, *IDH*-mutant, WHO grade 4 even if the histology suggests a lower grade.

Pathogenesis. As the name implies, these tumors are characteristically associated with driver mutations of the isocitrate dehydrogenase 1 gene *IDH1*, or (less often) its homologue *IDH2* (see Chapter 6 for a discussion of these genes and their role in tumorigenesis). In addition, they frequently harbor inactivating mutations in *TP53* and *ATRX* genes.

MORPHOLOGY

Grade 2 and 3 astrocytomas are poorly defined, gray, infiltrative tumors that expand and distort the involved area of the brain without forming a discrete mass (Fig. 21.30A). Grade 4 astrocytomas diffusely infiltrate brain parenchyma without any delineated borders and, unlike *IDH*-wild-type glioblastomas, usually lack large areas of central necrosis and hemorrhage.

Microscopically, grade 2 astrocytomas are well-differentiated and characterized by a mild to moderate increase in the number of glial cell nuclei, somewhat variable nuclear pleomorphism, and an intervening network of fine, glial fibrillary acidic protein (GFAP)-positive astrocytic cell processes that give the background a fibrillary appearance (Fig. 21.30B). The transition between neoplastic and normal tissue is indistinct, and tumor cells can be seen

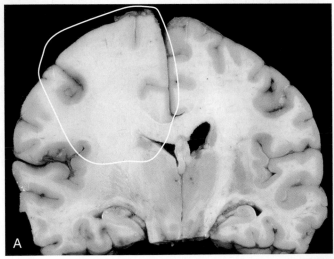
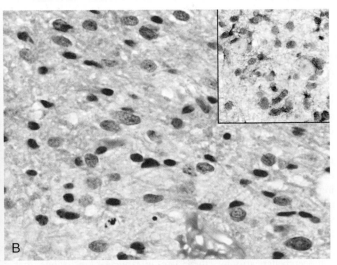

FIG. 21.30 Astrocytoma, *IDH*-mutant, grade 2. (A) On coronal section, the left frontal white matter is expanded, and there is blurring of the corticomedullary junction due to infiltrative tumor *(circled region).* (B) A histologic section of the tumor shows enlarged, irregular, large nuclei embedded within the native fibrillar matrix of the brain; the smaller round and oval nuclei are benign oligodendrocytes and reactive astrocytes, respectively. *Inset,* An immunostain for mutant IDH1 is positive in tumor cells, some of which surround unstained cortical neurons.

infiltrating healthy tissue many centimeters from the main lesion. Grade 3 astrocytomas show regions that are more densely cellular and have greater nuclear pleomorphism; mitotic figures are present. Grade 4 tumors have greater cellular crowding, cytological atypia and increased proliferative activity; additionally, they show microvascular proliferation and/or necrosis.

Clinical Features. Diffuse astrocytomas can be static for several years, but at some point they progress; the median survival is more than 5 years. Eventually, there is rapid clinical deterioration that is correlated with the appearance of high-grade histologic features and more rapid tumor growth. The median overall survival of patients with *IDH*-mutant astrocytomas is >10 years for grade 2 tumors, 5 to 10 years for grade 3 tumors, and 3 years for grade 4 tumors.

Glioblastoma, IDH-Wild-Type

Glioblastomas constitute the second type of diffuse gliomas. IDH-wild-type glioblastoma (WHO grade 4) arises from astrocytes and is the most common malignant glioma, accounting for about 50% of all primary malignant brain tumors in adults. These tumors are always considered grade 4 lesions (they do not have lower grade precursors) and have a very poor prognosis.

Pathogenesis. Glioblastomas, IDH-wild-type, harbor multiple genetic alterations that contribute to the acquisition of cancer hallmarks (Chapter 6). For example, most glioblastomas have genetic aberrations that lead to evasion of senescence (either telomerase mutations or mutations that lead to alternative lengthening of telomeres); escape from normal growth controls (biallelic deletion of *CDKN2A*, which encodes the cyclin-dependent kinase inhibitor p16); activation of growth factor signaling pathways (*EGFR* or *PDGFR* gene amplification); and resistance to apoptosis (*TP53* mutation). Another genetic alteration is methylation of the promoter of the *MGMT* gene, which

encodes a DNA repair enzyme and influences sensitivity to chemotherapeutic agents.

MORPHOLOGY

In glioblastoma, variation in the gross appearance of the tumor from region to region is characteristic. Some areas are firm and white, others are soft and yellow (due to tissue necrosis), while others show regions of cystic degeneration and hemorrhage (Fig. 21.31A, eFig. 21.10). The histologic appearance is similar to that of a grade 4 astrocytoma, with high cellularity, poorly differentiated pleomorphic cells with nuclear atypia, brisk mitotic activity, and necrosis (commonly present as serpiginous bands of necrosis with palisaded tumor cells along the border) or microvascular proliferation (Fig. 21.31B). Molecular features are also incorporated into the grading. For instance, *TERT* promoter mutation, *EGFR* gene amplification, or DNA copy number changes (+7/—10 chromosome copy-number alterations) lead to the designation of glioblastoma grade 4 even in the absence of necrosis or microvascular proliferation.

Clinical Features. Glioblastoma, IDH-wild-type, preferentially affects older patients in their 6th to 8th decades of life. Frequently affected sites include cerebral hemispheres (temporal, parietal, and frontal lobes; basal ganglia and thalamus). The tumors develop rapidly, with most patients presenting with seizures, neurocognitive impairments, nausea, vomiting, and occasionally severe pulsating headache. Rapid infiltration of the corpus callosum with subsequent growth in the contralateral hemisphere leads to a bilateral, symmetrical lesion (butterfly glioma). Imaging studies most often reveal a ring-enhancing lesion. Prognosis is very poor; even with treatment (resection, radiotherapy, and chemotherapy), the median survival is only about 15 to 18 months.

Oligodendroglioma, IDH-Mutant, and 1p/19q-Codeleted

The third major subtype of diffuse glioma is composed of cells that resemble oligodendrocytes. When corrected for tumor grade,

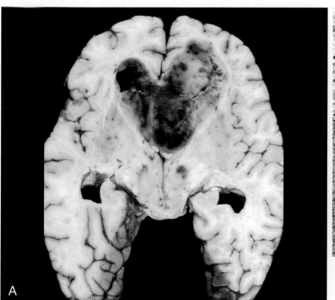

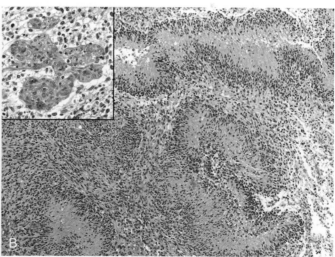

FIG. 21.31 Glioblastoma. (A) The tumor forms a necrotic, hemorrhagic, infiltrating mass. (B) Serpiginous foci of palisading necrosis (tumor nuclei lined up around the red anucleate zones of necrosis). *Inset,* Microvascular proliferation.

oligodendrogliomas (CNS WHO grade 2, 3) have the best prognosis among diffuse glial tumors; as with their astrocytic counterparts, they are now defined using morphologic and genetic features. Oligodendrogliomas account for 5% to 15% of gliomas and are most commonly detected in the fourth and fifth decades of life. Patients may have had several years of antecedent neurologic problems, often including seizures. The lesions are found mostly in the cerebral hemispheres, mainly in the frontal or temporal lobes. The combination of surgery, chemotherapy, and radiotherapy yields an average survival of 10 to 20 years for grade 2 oligodendrogliomas and 5 to 10 years for grade 3 oligodendrogliomas.

Pathogenesis. These tumors have codeletion of chromosome 1p and 19q, always in association with *IDH1* or *IDH2* mutations. Most oligodendrogliomas also have mutations in the promoter of the *TERT* gene that result in increased telomerase activity.

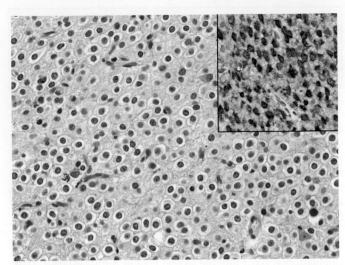

FIG. 21.32 Oligodendroglioma. Tumor cells have round nuclei, often with a clear cytoplasmic halo. Blood vessels in the background are thin and can form an interlacing pattern. *Inset,* Similar to diffuse astrocytomas, tumor cells are positive for mutant IDH1.

MORPHOLOGY

Well-differentiated oligodendrogliomas (WHO grade 2) are infiltrative tumors that form gelatinous, gray masses and may show cysts, focal hemorrhage, and calcification. On microscopic examination, the tumor is composed of sheets of regular cells with spherical nuclei containing finely granular chromatin (similar to that in normal oligodendrocytes) surrounded by a clear halo of cytoplasm giving a so-called "fried egg" appearance (Fig. 21.32). The tumor typically contains a delicate network of "chicken-wire"-like anastomosing capillaries. Calcification, present in up to 90% of these tumors, ranges in extent from microscopic foci to massive depositions. Mitotic activity is usually low. Grade 3 oligodendroglioma is a more aggressive subtype with higher cell density, nuclear anaplasia, increased mitotic activity, and often microvascular proliferation and/or necrosis.

Pilocytic Astrocytoma

Pilocytic astrocytomas are relatively benign tumors that typically affect children and young adults. They are circumscribed tumors that frequently arise in the cerebellum and present with signs and symptoms of mass effect, obstructive hydrocephalus, and increased intracranial pressure. Although most commonly located in the cerebellum, they may also involve the third ventricle, the optic pathways, the spinal cord, and occasionally the cerebral hemispheres. There is often a cyst associated with the tumor; following resection, if symptoms recur, they may be due to cyst enlargement rather than growth of the solid component. Because these tumors are well circumscribed, they are usually curable with complete resection.

A high proportion of pilocytic astrocytomas have activating mutations or translocations involving the gene encoding the serine-threonine kinase BRAF that result in activation of the mitogen-activated protein kinase (MAPK) signaling pathway. Pilocytic astrocytomas do not have mutations in *IDH1* and *IDH2*.

MORPHOLOGY

A pilocytic astrocytoma is often cystic, with a mural nodule in the wall of the cyst; if solid, it is usually well circumscribed. The tumor is composed of bipolar cells with long, thin "hairlike" processes that are GFAP-positive. **Rosenthal fibers**, eosinophilic granular bodies, and microcysts are often present, while necrosis and mitoses are rare (eFig. 21.11).

Ependymoma

Ependymomas (WHO grade 2, 3) most often arise next to the ependyma-lined ventricular system, including the central canal of the spinal cord. In the first two decades of life, they typically occur near the fourth ventricle and constitute 5% to 10% of the primary brain tumors in this age group. In adults, the spinal cord is their most common location; tumors in this site are particularly frequent in patients with neurofibromatosis type 2 (Chapter 20). Recent classification of ependymoma has incorporated histopathological features, anatomical sites (i.e., supratentorial, posterior fossa, and spinal), and molecular alterations (e.g., *ZFTA* fusion, *YAP1* fusion, *MYCN* amplification, etc.). The clinical outcome for completely resected supratentorial and spinal ependymomas is better than for those in the posterior fossa. Other ependymal tumors include subependymoma (CNS WHO grade 1) and myxopapillary ependymoma (CNS WHO grade 2).

MORPHOLOGY

In the fourth ventricle, ependymomas are typically solid or papillary masses extending from the ventricular floor (Fig. 21.33A). The tumor cells have regular, round to oval nuclei and abundant granular chromatin. Between the nuclei is a variably dense fibrillary background. Tumor cells may form round or elongated structures **(rosettes, canals)** that resemble the embryologic ependymal canal, with long, delicate processes extending into a lumen (Fig. 21.33B); more frequently present are **perivascular pseudorosettes** in which tumor cells are arranged around vessels with an intervening zone containing thin ependymal processes. Anaplastic ependymomas show increased cell density, high mitotic rates, necrosis, microvascular proliferation, and minimal ependymal differentiation.

Neuronal Tumors

Far less frequent than gliomas, tumors composed of cells with neuronal characteristics are typically lower-grade lesions that often present with

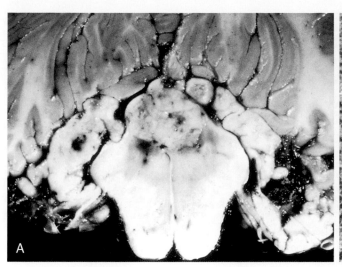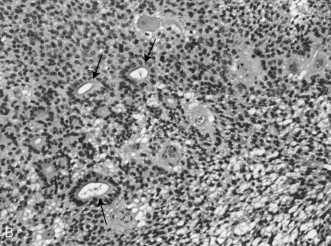

FIG. 21.33 Ependymoma. (A) Tumor of the fourth ventricle, distorting, compressing, and infiltrating surrounding structures. (B) The microscopic appearance includes both true rosettes (with a glandlike central lumen, *arrows*) and perivascular pseudorosettes (nuclear-free zone composed of fibrillary processes radiating toward a central blood vessel).

seizures, and most frequently occur in the first and second decades of life. Lesions in this group are primarily composed of cells that express neuronal markers, such as synaptophysin, neurofilament protein, and the neuronal nuclear antigen NeuN.

- *Gangliogliomas* (CNS WHO grade 1) are tumors composed of neoplastic ganglion and glial cells. Most of these tumors are slow growing and often manifest with seizures. About 20% to 50% of gangliogliomas harbor point mutations in the *BRAF* gene. They are most commonly found in the temporal lobe.
- *Dysembryoplastic neuroepithelial tumor* (CNS WHO grade 1) is a rare, low-grade tumor of children and young adults that grows slowly, often manifests as a seizure disorder, and carries a favorable prognosis after resection. It is typically located in the superficial temporal lobe and consists of small, round neuronal cells arranged in columns and around central cores of processes.

Embryonal (Primitive) Neoplasms

Some tumors of neuroectodermal origin have a primitive "small round cell" appearance that is reminiscent of progenitor cells encountered in the developing CNS. Differentiation is often limited but may progress along multiple lineages. The most common of these is the *medulloblastoma*, accounting for 20% of pediatric brain tumors.

Medulloblastoma

Medulloblastoma occurs predominantly in children and exclusively in the cerebellum. Neuronal markers are nearly always expressed, while glial markers are expressed in rare cases. It is highly malignant, and the prognosis for untreated patients is very poor; however, medulloblastoma is exquisitely radiosensitive. With total excision, chemotherapy, and irradiation, the overall 5-year survival rate may be as high as 75%.

Several molecular subtypes of medulloblastoma have been identified, including one associated with gain-of-function mutations in the sonic hedgehog (SHH) pathway, which plays an important role in normal cerebellar development and in the WNT/β-catenin signaling pathway. Notably, individuals with germline mutations in the gene *PTCH1*, which encodes a negative regulator of Hedgehog signaling, are at high risk for development of medulloblastoma and basal cell

carcinoma of the skin, a second tumor associated with unregulated Hedgehog signaling (Chapter 22). On the basis of molecular alterations (activation of WNT, activation of SHH, and mutant *TP53*), medulloblastoma has been divided into four principal groups. The molecular and histologic subtype dramatically influences prognosis, with WNT-activated medulloblastomas associated with nearly 100% survival at 5 years with standard therapeutic approaches, while most SHH-activated and *TP53*-mutant medulloblastomas have a very poor outcome.

MORPHOLOGY

In children, medulloblastomas are located in the midline of the cerebellum; lateral tumors occur more often in adults. The tumor is often well circumscribed, gray, and friable and may be seen extending to the surface of the cerebellar folia and involving the leptomeninges (Fig. 21.34A). Medulloblastomas are one of several "small blue cell" tumors of childhood. These tumors are densely cellular, with sheets of monomorphic cells (Fig. 21.34B). Individual tumor cells are small, with little cytoplasm and hyperchromatic nuclei; mitoses are abundant. Often, focal neuronal differentiation is seen in the form of rosettes, which resemble the rosettes encountered in neuroblastomas; they are characterized by primitive tumor cells surrounding central neuropil (delicate pink material formed by neuronal processes). Seeding of the cerebrospinal fluid (drop metastases) may occur.

Other Parenchymal Tumors
Primary Central Nervous System Lymphoma

Primary CNS lymphoma accounts for 2% of extranodal lymphomas and 1% of intracranial tumors. It is the most common CNS neoplasm in individuals who are immunocompromised. In populations that are not immunocompromised, the age spectrum is relatively wide, but the frequency increases after 60 years of age.

The term *primary* emphasizes the distinction between these lesions and secondary involvement of the CNS by lymphoma arising elsewhere in the body (Chapter 10). Primary brain lymphoma often demonstrates multifocal involvement of brain parenchyma and may

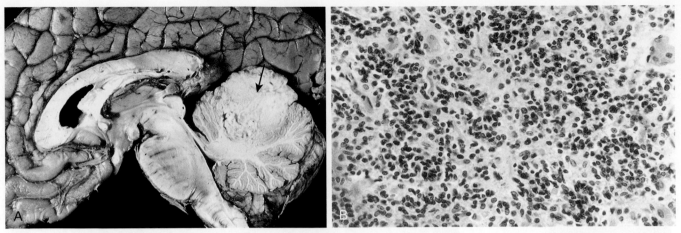

FIG. 21.34 Medulloblastoma. (A) Sagittal section of a brain showing medulloblastoma involving the superior vermis of the cerebellum *(arrow)*. (B) Microscopic appearance of medulloblastoma, showing mostly small, blue, primitive-appearing tumor cells.

also involve the eye, yet spread outside of the CNS (in lymph nodes or bone marrow) is a rare and late complication. Conversely, lymphoma arising outside the CNS rarely spreads to brain parenchyma; in this situation, secondary involvement is usually in the meninges or the CSF, where tumor is sometimes diagnosed based on the presence of malignant cells in a lumbar puncture specimen.

The vast majority of primary CNS lymphomas are diffuse large B-cell lymphomas; they are aggressive and generally have worse outcomes than diffuse large B-cell lymphomas occurring at non-CNS sites (Chapter 10). In the setting of immunocompromise, the malignant B cells are usually latently infected by Epstein-Barr virus.

MORPHOLOGY

Lesions often involve deep gray structures, as well as the white matter and the cortex. Periventricular spread is common. The tumors are relatively well defined as compared with glial neoplasms, but they are not as discrete as metastases. EBV-associated tumors often show extensive areas of necrosis. Microscopically, malignant lymphoid cells accumulate around blood vessels and infiltrate the surrounding brain parenchyma. Diagnosis of the most common subtype of primary CNS lymphoma, diffuse large B-cell lymphoma, is confirmed by immunohistochemical staining for B-cell antigens such as CD20.

Meningiomas

Meningiomas (WHO grades 1–3) are typically benign tumors that arise from the meningothelial cells of the arachnoid and are usually attached to the dura; they usually arise in adults. Meningiomas may be found along any of the external surfaces of the brain as well as within the ventricular system, where they arise from the stromal arachnoid cells of the choroid plexus. They often come to attention due to vague non-localizing symptoms, or with focal findings referable to compression of the adjacent brain. Most meningiomas are easily separable from the underlying brain, but some tumors are infiltrative, a feature associated with an increased risk for recurrence. The overall prognosis is determined by the lesion size and location, surgical accessibility, and histologic grade.

Pathogenesis. When an individual has multiple meningiomas, especially in association with eighth-nerve schwannomas or glial tumors, the diagnosis of neurofibromatosis type 2 (NF2) should be considered (Chapter 20). About half of meningiomas not associated with NF2 have somatic loss-of-function mutations in the *NF2* tumor suppressor gene. These mutations are found in all grades of meningioma, suggesting that they are involved in tumor initiation. Among sporadic tumors that lack mutations in *NF2*, several other driver mutations have been identified, including in genes that regulate the Hedgehog pathway as well as in various signaling molecules and transcription factors. The 2021 WHO classification of CNS tumors has introduced molecular biomarkers into the classification and grading of meningiomas (e.g., *BAP1* mutation in "rhabdoid" and "papillary" subtypes; *TERT* promoter mutation; and/or homozygous deletion of *CDKN2A/B* in grade 3 meningiomas).

MORPHOLOGY

Meningiomas (WHO grade 1) grow as well-defined dura-based masses that may compress the brain but do not typically invade it (Fig. 21.35A, eFig. 21.12). Extension into the overlying bone may be present. Some of the 15 histologic subtypes include **meningothelial,** named for syncytialike lobules of cells without visible cell membranes; **fibroblastic,** with elongated cells and abundant collagen deposition; **transitional,** with features of both meningothelial and fibroblastic types; **psammomatous,** with numerous psammoma bodies (Fig. 21.35B); and **secretory,** with glandlike spaces containing PAS-positive eosinophilic material.

Grade 2 meningiomas are recognized by the presence of an increased mitotic rate; unequivocal brain invasion; chordoid or clear cell subtype; or certain microscopic features, such as prominent nucleoli or foci of necrosis. These tumors demonstrate more aggressive local growth and a higher rate of recurrence and may require therapy in addition to surgery.

Grade 3 meningiomas are rare, highly aggressive tumors that resemble a high-grade sarcoma, carcinoma, or melanoma morphologically. Mitotic rates are typically much higher than in other types of meningiomas.

Metastatic Tumors and Paraneoplastic Syndromes

Metastatic lesions account for over half of intracranial tumors. The tumors that are most likely to give rise to brain metastasis are carcinomas of the lung, breast, kidney, and colon, and cutaneous melanoma, which together account for about 80% of cases. Metastases form

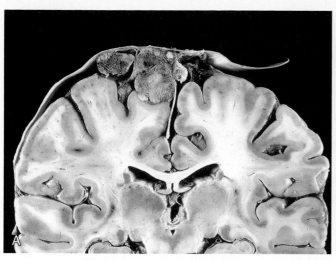
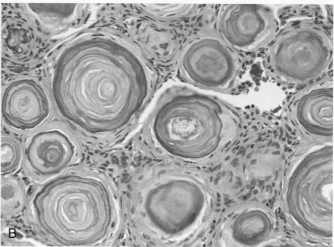

FIG. 21.35 Meningioma. (A) Parasagittal multilobular meningioma attached to the dura with compression of underlying brain. (B) Meningioma with a whorled pattern of cell growth and psammoma bodies (calcifications with concentric rings).

sharply demarcated masses, often at the gray-white matter junction, and elicit local edema and reactive gliosis.

In addition to the direct, localized CNS effects of metastases, *paraneoplastic syndromes* may involve the peripheral and central nervous systems, sometimes even preceding clinical recognition of the malignant neoplasm. Many patients with paraneoplastic syndromes have antibodies against tumor antigens. Some of the more common patterns of nervous system involvement include cerebellar degeneration (producing ataxia), limbic encephalitis (causing dementia), and sensory neuropathy.

Familial Tumor Syndromes

Several inherited syndromes caused by mutations in various tumor suppressor genes are associated with an increased risk for particular types of cancers. Those with involvement of the CNS are discussed here; familial syndromes associated with tumors of the peripheral nervous system are covered in Chapter 20.

Tuberous Sclerosis

Tuberous sclerosis is an autosomal dominant disorder characterized by the development of hamartomas and benign neoplasms involving the brain and other tissues. CNS hamartomas variously consist of glioneuronal hamartomas and subependymal hamartomas, including a form known as *subependymal giant cell astrocytoma (SEGA).* Its incidence is approximately 1 in 5,000 to 10,000 live births. Because of its proximity to the foramen of Monro, SEGA often presents acutely with obstructive hydrocephalus, which requires surgical intervention and/or therapy with an mTOR inhibitor (see later). Seizures are associated with cortical tubers and can be difficult to control with antiepileptic drugs. Extracerebral lesions include renal angiomyolipomas (Chapter 12), retinal glial hamartomas, pulmonary lymphangiomyomatosis, and cardiac rhabdomyomas (Chapter 9). Cysts may be found at various sites, including the liver, kidneys, and pancreas. Cutaneous lesions include angiofibromas, leathery thickenings in localized patches *(shagreen patches),* hypopigmented areas *(ash leaf patches),* and subungual fibromas.

Tuberous sclerosis results from disruption of either *TSC1,* which encodes hamartin, or *TSC2,* which encodes tuberin. Hamartin and tuberin form a dimeric complex that negatively regulates mTOR, a kinase that "senses" the cell's nutrient status and regulates cellular metabolism. Loss of either protein upregulates mTOR activity, which disrupts normal feedback mechanisms that restrict uptake of nutrients, leading to increased cell growth.

von Hippel–Lindau Disease

In this autosomal dominant disorder, affected individuals develop hemangioblastomas within the cerebellar hemispheres, retina, and, less commonly, the brain stem, spinal cord, and nerve roots. Patients may also have cysts involving the pancreas, liver, and kidneys and an increased propensity to develop renal cell carcinoma (Chapter 12). The disease frequency is 1 in 30,000 to 40,000. Therapy is directed at the symptomatic neoplasms, including surgical resection of cerebellar tumors and laser ablation of retinal tumors.

The affected gene, the tumor suppressor *VHL,* encodes a protein that is part of a ubiquitin-ligase complex that degrades the transcription factor hypoxia-inducible factor (HIF). Tumors arising in patients with von Hippel–Lindau disease generally have lost all VHL protein function. As a result, the tumors express high levels of HIF, which drives the expression of VEGF, various factors that promote growth, and sometimes erythropoietin; the latter effect may produce a paraneoplastic form of polycythemia.

> ### MORPHOLOGY
>
> **Hemangioblastoma,** the principal neurologic manifestation of the disease, is a highly vascular neoplasm that occurs as a mural nodule associated with a large, fluid-filled cyst. On microscopic examination, the lesion consists of numerous capillary-sized or somewhat larger thin-walled vessels separated by intervening stromal cells with a vacuolated, lightly PAS-positive, lipid-rich cytoplasm. These stromal cells express inhibin, a member of the TGF-β family, which serves as a useful diagnostic marker.

EYE

Vision is a major quality-of-life issue. Although there are conditions that are unique to the eye (e.g., cataract, glaucoma), many ocular

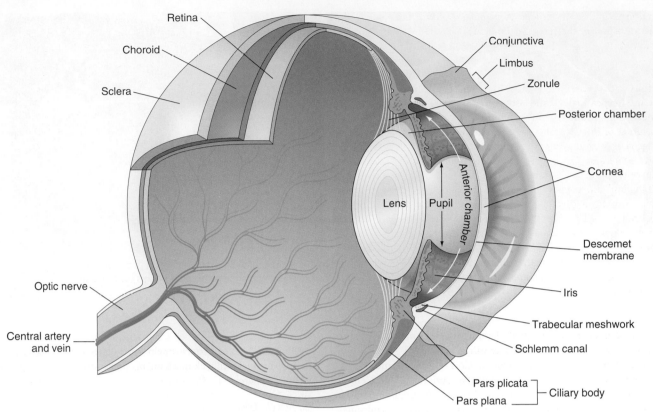

FIG. 21.36 Anatomy of the eye.

conditions share similarities with disease processes elsewhere in the body that are modified by the unique structure and function of the eye (Fig. 21.36). In recent years, the elucidation of the molecular pathogenesis of ocular disease has been translated rapidly to therapeutic applications. For instance, conditions such as corneal neovascularization, diabetic retinopathy, and certain forms of age-related neovascularization that result from pathologic angiogenesis are now successfully treated with vascular endothelial growth factor (VEGF) antagonists, saving vision in patients who even a few years ago might have been blinded.

This section of the chapter is organized on the basis of ocular anatomy and focuses on some of the most common diseases of the eye. Disorders of the eye may involve the eye itself (the globe) or the adnexa (the eyelids, orbit, conjunctiva, lacrimal glands, and optic nerve).

Conjunctiva

The conjunctiva is the mucous membrane lining the inside of the eyelids and the external surface of the eye. It consists of nonkeratinizing stratified squamous epithelium and a thin layer of underlying connective tissue.

Conjunctivitis

Bacterial and viral infections frequently cause conjunctivitis that usually heals without sequelae, but infection with the gram-negative intracellular bacterium *Chlamydia trachomatis* (*trachoma*) may produce significant conjunctival scarring. This bacterium is highly contagious, so trachoma is endemic in many lower-income countries and is the leading infectious cause of blindness worldwide. The infection initially starts with mild follicular conjunctivitis; repeated episodes lead to scarring that can invert the upper eyelids, resulting in the eyelashes turning inward (trichiasis). Repeated rubbing of the eyelashes against the eye ultimately results in corneal ulceration, scarring, and opacification.

Other Conjunctival Lesions

Actinic damage to sun-exposed regions of the conjunctiva can result in submucosal lesions called pterygium and pinguecula. Both are benign and pose no threat to vision. Biopsy may be necessary to exclude a neoplasm induced by UV radiation.

Tumors that develop in the conjunctiva include squamous cell carcinoma, which may be preceded by intraepithelial dysplastic changes, and melanocytic lesions. Conjunctival nevi are common but rarely invade the cornea and are benign. Conjunctival melanomas are unilateral, often have acquired *BRAF* mutations, and may spread to parotid or submandibular lymph nodes.

Cornea

The cornea and its overlying tear film make up the major refractive surface of the eye. The shape of the cornea has a significant influence on the refractive power of the eye, as evidenced by the success of procedures such as laser-assisted in situ keratomileusis (LASIK) to treat *myopia* (nearsightedness, when the eye is too long for its refractive power) and *hyperopia* (farsightedness, when the eye is too short).

Anteriorly, the cornea is covered by epithelium that rests on a basement membrane. The *Bowman layer,* situated just beneath the epithelial basement membrane, is acellular. The corneal stroma lacks blood vessels and lymphatics, a feature that contributes not only to the transparency of the cornea but also to the high rate of success of corneal transplantation. The corneal endothelium is derived from the neural crest and is not related to vascular endothelium. It lines the posterior aspect of the specialized basement membrane, the *Descemet membrane.*

Keratitis and Ulceration

Various pathogens—bacterial, fungal, viral (especially herpes simplex and herpes zoster), and protozoal (*Acanthamoeba*)—can cause corneal inflammation and ulceration. In all forms of keratitis, dissolution of the corneal stroma may be accelerated by activation of collagenases within corneal epithelium and stromal fibroblasts (also known as keratocytes). Exudate and cells leaking from iris and ciliary body vessels into the anterior chamber may be visible by slit-lamp examination and may accumulate in sufficient quantity to become visible even by a penlight examination *(hypopyon).* Although the associated corneal ulcer may be infectious, the hypopyon seldom contains organisms and represents a vascular response to acute inflammation. The specific forms of keratitis may have certain distinctive features. For example, chronic herpes simplex keratitis may be associated with a granulomatous reaction involving the Descemet membrane (eFig. 21.13).

Keratoconus

With an incidence of 1 in 2000, keratoconus is a fairly common disorder characterized by progressive thinning of the cornea without evidence of inflammation or vascularization. Such thinning results in a cornea that has a conical rather than spherical shape, which causes irregular astigmatism that is difficult to correct. Patients whose vision cannot be corrected with spectacles or contact lenses are candidates for corneal transplantation. Unlike many other types of degeneration, keratoconus is typically bilateral. Its development may stem from a genetic predisposition superimposed by an environmental insult, such as eye rubbing in response to atopic conditions.

MORPHOLOGY

Thinning of the cornea with breaks in the Bowman layer are the histologic hallmarks of keratoconus (Fig. 21.37). In some patients the Descemet membrane may rupture precipitously, allowing the aqueous humor in the anterior chamber to gain access to the corneal stroma. The sudden effusion of aqueous humor through a gap in the Descemet membrane—corneal **hydrops**—may cause vision to worsen suddenly. An episode of hydrops may be followed by corneal scarring that can also contribute to visual loss.

Fuchs Endothelial Dystrophy

Fuchs endothelial dystrophy, one of several dystrophies, results from loss of corneal endothelial cells, leading to edema and thickening of the stroma. It is one of the principal indications for corneal transplantation in the United States. The major clinical manifestations of Fuchs endothelial dystrophy—*stromal edema* and *bullous keratopathy*—are both related to a primary loss of endothelial cells. Early in the course of the disease, endothelial cells produce droplike deposits of abnormal basement membrane material *(guttae)* that can be visualized clinically by slit-lamp examination. With disease progression, there is a decrease in the total number of endothelial cells, and the residual cells are incapable of maintaining stromal deturgescence (relative dehydration that maintains the transparency of the cornea). Consequently, the stroma becomes edematous and thickens; it acquires a ground-glass appearance, and vision is blurred. Because of

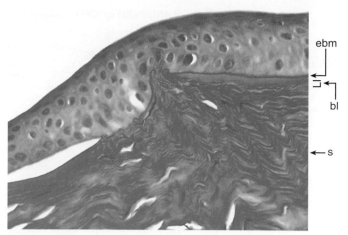

FIG. 21.37 Keratoconus. The tissue section is stained by periodic acid–Schiff to highlight the epithelial basement membrane *(ebm)*, which is intact; the Bowman layer *(bl)*, situated between the epithelial basement membrane; and the stroma *(s)*. Following the Bowman layer from the *right side* of the photomicrograph toward the *center*, there is a discontinuity, diagnostic of keratoconus.

chronic edema, the stroma may eventually become vascularized. Occasionally, the number of endothelial cells may decrease following cataract surgery even in individuals who do not have early forms of Fuchs dystrophy. This condition, known as *pseudophakic bullous keratopathy,* is also a common indication for corneal transplantation.

Anterior Segment

The anterior chamber is bounded anteriorly by the cornea, laterally by the trabecular meshwork, and posteriorly by the iris. The posterior chamber lies behind the iris and in front of the lens. *Aqueous humor,* formed by the pars plicata of the ciliary body, enters the posterior chamber, bathes the lens, and circulates through the pupil to gain access to the anterior chamber. The lens is a closed epithelial system; the basement membrane of the lens epithelium (known as the lens capsule) totally envelops the lens. Thus, the lens epithelium does not shed dead cells like the epidermis or mucosal epithelium, and, with aging, these cells accumulate in the center of the lens and become less transparent.

Cataract

Cataracts are opacities of the lens that may be congenital or acquired. Age-related cataract, which accounts for the majority of cases, typically results from opacification of the lens nucleus *(nuclear sclerosis),* presumably as a result of aging-associated cellular degeneration. Systemic diseases (e.g., galactosemia, diabetes, Wilson disease, and atopic dermatitis), drugs (especially corticosteroids), radiation, trauma, and many intraocular disorders may accelerate cataract formation. Less frequently, cataracts result from accumulation of urochrome pigment and liquefaction of the lens cortex. The technique that is most commonly used to remove opacified lenses extracts the lens contents, leaving the lens capsule intact. A prosthetic intraocular lens is then inserted into the eye.

Glaucoma

The term *glaucoma* refers to a collection of diseases in which optic neuropathy is usually associated with elevated intraocular pressure. Some individuals with normal intraocular pressure may develop characteristic optic nerve and visual field changes *(normal or*

ANTERIOR AND POSTERIOR CHAMBERS   MAJOR AQUEOUS OUTFLOW PATHWAY

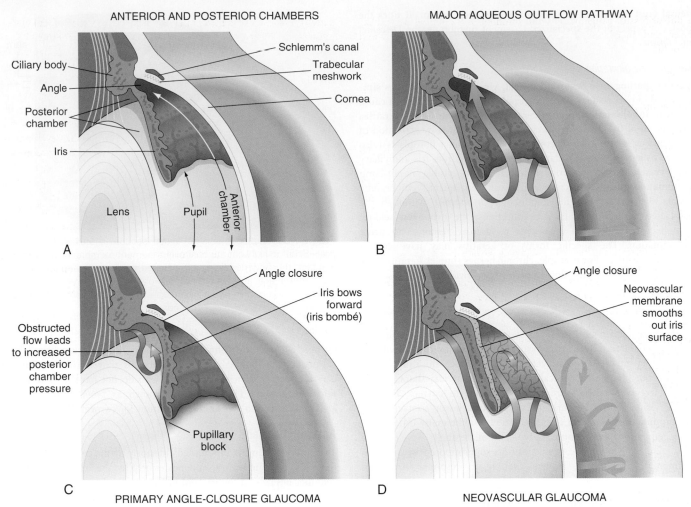

PRIMARY ANGLE-CLOSURE GLAUCOMA   NEOVASCULAR GLAUCOMA

FIG. 21.38 Glaucoma. (A) The healthy eye. Note that the surface of the iris is highly textured with crypts and folds. (B) The normal flow of aqueous humor. Aqueous humor, produced in the posterior chamber, flows through the pupil into the anterior chamber. The major pathway for the egress of aqueous humor is through the trabecular meshwork, into the Schlemm canal. (C) Primary angle-closure glaucoma. In anatomically predisposed eyes, transient apposition of the iris at the pupillary margin to the lens blocks the passage of aqueous humor from the posterior chamber to the anterior chamber. Pressure builds in the posterior chamber, bowing the iris forward (iris bombé) and occluding the trabecular meshwork. (D) Neovascular glaucoma. A neovascular membrane has grown over the surface of the iris, smoothing the iris folds and crypts. Myofibroblasts within the neovascular membrane cause the membrane to contract and to become apposed to the trabecular meshwork (peripheral anterior synechiae). Outflow of aqueous humor is blocked, and the intraocular pressure becomes elevated.

low-tension glaucoma). To understand the pathophysiology of glaucoma it is useful to consider the formation and drainage of aqueous humor (Fig. 21.38). Aqueous humor is produced in the ciliary body and passes from the posterior chamber through the pupil into the anterior chamber. Most of the aqueous humor drains through the trabecular meshwork, situated in the angle formed by the intersection between the corneal periphery and the anterior surface of the iris.

Based on the mechanism of impaired drainage, glaucoma can be classified into two major categories, which may be primary or secondary.

- *Open-angle glaucoma* is usually associated with increased intraocular pressure. It may be caused by increased production of aqueous humor or resistance to aqueous outflow in the open angle. Primary open-angle glaucoma is the most common form of glaucoma.

Secondary open-angle glaucoma may be due to deposition of particulate matter such as red cells following trauma or necrotic tumor.

- In *angle-closure glaucoma* the anterior chamber angle is narrowed or closed, physically impeding the egress of aqueous humor from the eye and resulting in increased intraocular pressure. Primary angle-closure glaucoma is most common in patients with hyperopia in which the anterior chamber is quite shallow. Secondary angle-closure glaucoma can be due to pathologic membranes that form over the iris, as in neovascular glaucoma, which is due to VEGF upregulation in the setting of chronic retinal ischemia.

Both types of glaucoma cause an optic neuropathy with visual field defects, initially affecting peripheral vision. Characteristically, there is a diffuse loss of ganglion cells and thinning of the retinal nerve fiber layer, and, in advanced cases, the optic nerve is both cupped and atrophic.

Uvea

The uvea consists of the iris, choroid, and ciliary body. The choroid is among the most richly vascularized tissues in the body.

Uveitis

Uveitis is inflammation in one or more of the tissues that compose the uvea. In clinical practice the term *uveitis* is restricted to chronic inflammatory diseases that may be either components of a systemic process or localized to the eye. Uveitis may be caused by infectious agents (e.g., *Pneumocystis jirovecii*), may be idiopathic (e.g., sarcoidosis), or may be autoimmune in origin (e.g., sympathetic ophthalmia). It may affect principally the anterior segment (e.g., in *juvenile idiopathic arthritis*) or both the anterior and posterior segments. Uveitis is frequently accompanied by retinal pathology.

Granulomatous uveitis is a common complication of sarcoidosis (Chapter 11). In the anterior segment it gives rise to an exudate that evolves into keratic precipitates. In the posterior segment, sarcoid granulomas may be seen in the choroid. Conjunctival biopsy can be used to detect granulomatous inflammation and confirm the diagnosis of ocular sarcoid.

Numerous infectious processes can affect the choroid or the retina. Inflammation in one compartment is typically associated with inflammation in the other. Retinal *toxoplasmosis* is usually accompanied by uveitis and even scleritis. Individuals with AIDS, especially if untreated, may develop cytomegalovirus retinitis and infection of the choroid by *Pneumocystis* or mycobacteria.

Sympathetic ophthalmia is an example of noninfectious uveitis limited to the eye. This condition is characterized by bilateral granulomatous inflammation typically affecting all components of the uvea. Sympathetic ophthalmia, which blinded young Louis Braille, may complicate a penetrating injury of the eye. In the injured eye, retinal antigens sequestered from the immune system may gain access to lymphatics in the conjunctiva and thus set up a delayed hypersensitivity reaction that affects not only the injured eye but also the contralateral, uninjured eye. The condition may develop from 2 weeks to many years after injury. It is characterized by diffuse granulomatous inflammation of the uvea, sometimes associated with infiltrating eosinophils. Sympathetic ophthalmia is treated with systemic immunosuppressive agents.

Neoplasms

Intraocular tumors may be primary or metastatic; the most common of these in adults is metastasis to the uvea, typically to the choroid. The occurrence of metastases to the eye is associated with an extremely short survival, and treatment of ocular metastases, usually by radiotherapy, is only palliative.

Uveal Melanoma. **Uveal melanoma is the most common primary intraocular malignancy of adults.** In the United States, these tumors account for approximately 5% of melanomas and have an age-adjusted incidence of 5 per 1 million per year. Benign uveal nevi, especially choroidal nevi, are more common, affecting about 2% of individuals.

Pathogenesis. Unlike cutaneous melanoma, the occurrence of uveal melanoma has remained stable over many years, and there is no clear link between exposure to ultraviolet light and risk. In line with this, sequencing of tumor genomes has revealed that the molecular

pathogenesis of uveal melanoma is distinct from that of cutaneous melanoma. Unlike cutaneous and conjunctival melanomas, *BRAF* mutations do not play a role in uveal melanomas. By contrast, roughly 85% of uveal melanomas harbor a gain-of-function mutation in *GNAQ* or *GNA11*, both of which encode G protein–coupled receptors that activate pathways that promote proliferation, such as the MAPK pathway (Chapter 6). Notably, uveal nevi are also associated with *GNAQ* and *GNA11* mutations, yet rarely transform to melanoma, indicating that other genetic events are required for the development of uveal melanoma. One common event is loss of chromosome 3, which leads to deletion of *BAP1*, a tumor suppressor gene that encodes a deubiquitinating enzyme. BAP1 is a component of protein complexes that place repressive marks on chromatin that lead to gene silencing; thus, uveal melanoma has joined the increasing list of cancers in which epigenetic alterations appear to have a central role in tumor pathogenesis (Chapter 6). Germline mutations in *BAP1* predispose patients to uveal melanoma and several other tumors, including malignant mesothelioma and renal cell carcinoma.

MORPHOLOGY

Histologically, uveal melanomas contain two types of cells, spindle and epithelioid, in various proportions (Fig. 21.39). **Spindle cells** are fusiform in shape, whereas **epithelioid cells** are spherical and have greater cytologic atypia. Like cutaneous melanomas, abundant tumor-infiltrating lymphocytes are seen in some cases. An unusual feature that is commonly seen is looping slitlike spaces lined by laminin that surround packets of tumor cells. These spaces (which are not blood vessels) connect to blood vessels and serve as extravascular conduits for the transport of plasma and possibly blood.

Uveal melanomas, with rare exceptions, spread by a hematogenous route. Most tumors metastasize first to the liver, a cardinal example of specific tropism of a tumor for a particular organ.

Clinical Features. Most uveal melanomas are incidental findings or present with visual symptoms related to retinal detachment or glaucoma. The prognosis of choroid and ciliary body melanomas is related to (1) size; (2) cell type (tumors containing epithelioid cells have a worse prognosis than do those containing exclusively spindle cells); (3) and proliferative index.

Uveal melanomas are treated with removal of the eye (enucleation) or radiotherapy. There seems to be no difference in survival between tumors treated with these two modalities. Radiotherapy is the preferred treatment. Melanomas situated exclusively in the iris tend to follow a relatively indolent course, whereas melanomas of the ciliary body and choroid are more aggressive.

Although the 5-year survival rate is approximately 80%, the cumulative melanoma mortality rate is 40% at 10 years, increasing 1% per year thereafter. Metastases may appear many years after treatment, typically in the liver, a remarkable example of the tendency of specific tumors to spread to particular organs. Targeted therapies such as MAPK inhibitors have shown some encouraging responses in clinical trials, but currently there is no effective treatment for metastatic uveal melanoma.

Retina

The neurosensory retina, like the optic nerve, is an embryologic derivative of the diencephalon. The retina therefore responds to injury by means of gliosis. The retinal pigment epithelium is derived

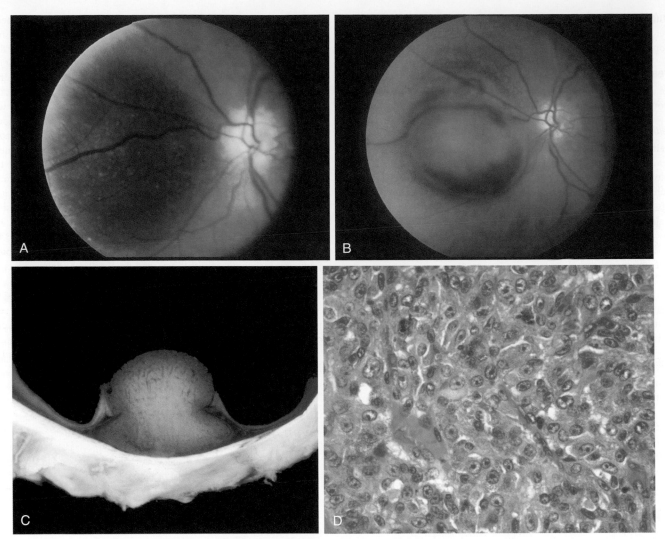

FIG. 21.39 Uveal melanoma. (A) Fundus photograph from an individual with a relatively flat pigmented lesion of the choroid near the optic disc. (B) Fundus photograph of the same individual several years later; the tumor has grown and has ruptured through the Bruch membrane. (C) Gross photograph of a choroidal melanoma that has ruptured the Bruch membrane. The overlying retina is detached. (D) Epithelioid melanoma cells. (A–C, From Folberg R: *Pathology of the Eye—An Interactive CD-ROM Program*, Philadelphia, 1996, Mosby.)

embryologically from the primary optic vesicle, an outpouching of the brain. The architecture of the retina accounts for the ophthalmoscopic appearance of a variety of ocular disorders. Exudates tend to accumulate in the outer plexiform layer of the retina, especially in the macula. With age the vitreous humor may liquefy and collapse, creating the visual sensation of "floaters." Also, with aging, the posterior face of the vitreous humor—the posterior hyaloid—may separate from the neurosensory retina (*posterior vitreous detachment*).

Retinal Detachment

Retinal detachment is separation of the neurosensory retina from the retinal pigment epithelium (RPE). There are two types, classified by etiology and on the presence or absence of a break in the retina (Fig. 21.40).

- *Rhegmatogenous retinal detachment*, the most common type of retinal detachment (Greek *rhegma* means "a break"), is associated with a full-thickness retinal defect. Retinal tears may develop after the vitreous collapses structurally, and the posterior hyaloid exerts

traction on points of strong adhesion to the retinal internal limiting membrane. Liquefied vitreous humor then seeps through the tear and gains access to the potential space between the neurosensory retina and the RPE, producing vitreous detachment. It may be complicated by *proliferative vitreoretinopathy*, the formation of epiretinal or subretinal membranes by retinal glial cells or RPE cells.

- *Nonrhegmatogenous retinal detachment* (retinal detachment without retinal break) may complicate retinal vascular disorders associated with significant exudation and any condition that damages the RPE and permits fluid to leak from the choroidal circulation under the retina. Retinal detachments associated with choroidal tumors and malignant hypertension are examples of nonrhegmatogenous retinal detachment.

Retinal Vascular Disease

Normally, the thin walls of retinal arterioles permit direct visualization of the circulating blood by ophthalmoscopy. Two systemic diseases,

RHEGMATOGENOUS
RETINAL
DETACHMENT

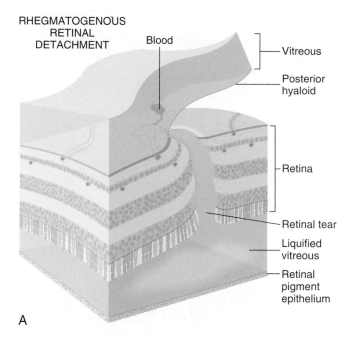

A

NONRHEGMATOGENOUS
RETINAL DETACHMENT

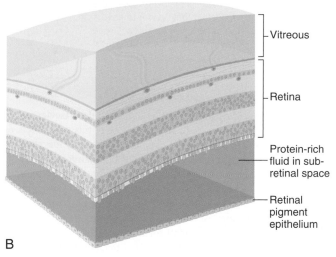

B

FIG. 21.40 Retinal detachment. (A) In rhegmatogenous retinal detachment, if the posterior hyaloid does not separate cleanly from the internal limiting membrane of the retina, the vitreous humor will exert traction on the retina, which will be torn at this point. Liquefied vitreous humor seeps through the retinal defect, and the retina is separated from the retinal pigment epithelium. (B) In nonrhegmatogenous retinal detachment the subretinal space is filled with protein-rich exudate.

hypertension and diabetes, impair the circulation and have important effects on retinal function.

Hypertension. In retinal arteriolosclerosis associated with long-standing hypertension, the thickened arteriole may compress the vein at points where the vessels cross because retinal arterioles and veins share a common adventitial sheath (Fig. 21.41A). Venous stasis distal to arteriolar-venous crossing may precipitate occlusions of the retinal vein branches. The thickened arteriolar wall changes the ophthalmic perception of circulating blood: vessels may appear narrowed, and the color of the blood column may change from bright red to copper and to silver depending on the degree of vascular wall thickness.

In severe hypertension, vessels in the retina and choroid may be damaged, producing focal choroidal infarcts. Damage to the choriocapillaris, the internal layer of the choroidal vasculature, may, in turn, damage the overlying RPE and permit exudates to accumulate in the potential space between the neurosensory retina and the RPE, producing a retinal detachment. Exudate from damaged retinal arterioles typically accumulates in the outer plexiform layer of the retina (Fig. 21.41B).

Occlusion of retinal arterioles may produce infarcts of the nerve fiber layer of the retina (axons of the retinal ganglion cell layer populate the nerve fiber layer). Axoplasmic transport in the nerve fiber layer is interrupted at the point of axonal damage, and accumulation of mitochondria at the swollen ends of damaged axons creates the histologic illusion of cells *(cytoid bodies)*. Collections of cytoid bodies populate the nerve fiber layer infarct, which is described ophthalmoscopically as a "cotton-wool spot."

Diabetes. Diabetes is the leading cause of blindness in American adults. **Ocular involvement in diabetes may take the form of retinopathy, cataract formation, or glaucoma.** Retinopathy, the most common pattern, consists of a constellation of changes that together are virtually diagnostic of diabetes. The lesion in the retina takes two forms: nonproliferative retinopathy and proliferative retinopathy.

• *Nonproliferative diabetic retinopathy* includes a spectrum of changes resulting from structural and functional abnormalities of retinal vessels, including intraretinal or preretinal hemorrhages, retinal exudates, microaneurysms, venous dilations, edema, and, most importantly, thickening of the retinal capillaries (microangiopathy). As with diabetic microangiopathy in general (Chapter 18), the basement membrane of retinal blood vessels is thickened. In addition, the number of pericytes relative to endothelial cells is diminished. Microaneurysms are discrete saccular dilations of retinal choroidal capillaries that appear through the ophthalmoscope as small red dots and are an important manifestation of diabetic microangiopathy. The retinal microcirculation in patients with diabetes may be exceptionally leaky, giving rise to macular edema, a common cause of visual loss in these patients. The vascular changes may also produce "soft" (microinfarcts) or "hard" (deposits of plasma proteins and lipids) exudates that accumulate in the outer plexiform layer, producing "cotton wool" spots that are visible with the ophthalmoscope. Although the retinal microcirculation is often hyperpermeable, it is also subject to the effects of micro-occlusion. Both vascular incompetence and vascular micro-occlusions can be visualized clinically after intravenous injection of fluorescein. Nonperfusion of the retina due to the microcirculatory changes is associated with upregulation of VEGF and intraretinal angiogenesis (located beneath the internal limiting membrane of the retina).

• *Proliferative diabetic retinopathy* is a process of neovascularization and fibrosis defined by the appearance of new vessels sprouting on the surface of either the optic nerve head or the retina (Fig. 21.42A). This lesion leads to serious consequences, including blindness, especially if it involves the macula. The term "retinal neovascularization" is used only when the newly formed vessels breach the internal limiting membrane of the retina. The web of newly formed vessels, called a neovascular membrane, is composed of angiogenic vessels with or without supportive fibrous or glial stroma (Fig. 21.42B). Neovascularization also affects the surface of the iris and may cause neovascular glaucoma. If the vitreous

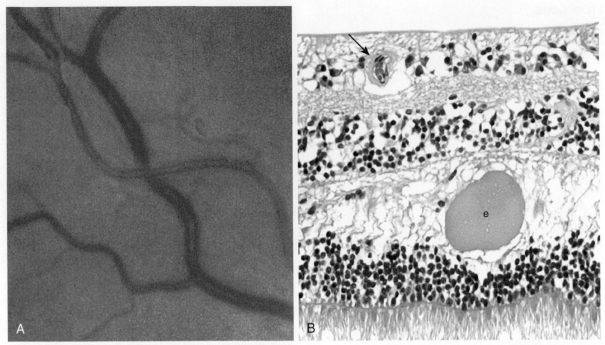

FIG. 21.41 Hypertensive retinal disease. (A) The fundus in hypertension. The diameter of the arterioles is reduced, and the color of the blood column appears to be less saturated (copper wire—like). If the wall of the vessel were thicker still, the degree of red color would diminish such that the vessels might appear to have a "silver wire" appearance. In this fundus photograph, note that the vein is compressed where the sclerotic arteriole crosses over it. (B) The wall of the retinal arteriole *(arrow)* is thick. Note the exudate *(e)* in the retinal outer plexiform layer. (A, Courtesy of Dr. Thomas A. Weingeist, Department of Ophthalmology and Visual Science, University of Iowa, Iowa City, Iowa.)

humor has not detached and the posterior hyaloid is intact, neovascular membranes extend along the potential plane between the retinal internal limiting membrane and the posterior hyaloid. If vitreous humor later separates from the internal limiting membrane of the retina (posterior vitreous detachment), there may be massive hemorrhage from the disrupted neovascular membrane. In addition, scarring associated with the organization of the retinal neovascular membrane may wrinkle the retina, disrupting the orientation of retinal photoreceptors and producing visual distortion, and may exert traction on the retina, leading to retinal detachment. Retinal neovascularization may lead to adhesions between the iris and trabecular meshwork, causing glaucoma.

The injection of VEGF inhibitors into the vitreous has been used to treat diabetic macular edema and retinal neovascularization, a successful example of how knowledge of the molecular pathogenesis of a condition may evolve into a successful therapeutic strategy.

Retinal Degenerations

***Age-Related Macular Degeneration (AMD).* AMD results from damage to the macula, which is required for central vision.** It occurs in two forms, dry and wet, that are distinguished by the presence of neoangiogenesis in the wet form and its absence in the dry form. As the name of this disorder indicates, advancing age is a risk factor. The cumulative incidence of AMD in individuals 75 years of age and older is 8%, and with increasing longevity AMD is becoming a major health problem. To understand the pathogenesis of AMD it is important to appreciate the existence of a structural and functional unit composed of the RPE, Bruch membrane (which contains the basement membrane of

the RPE), and the innermost layer of the choroidal vasculature, the choriocapillaris. Disturbance in any component of this unit affects the health of the overlying photoreceptors, producing visual loss.

- *Dry (atrophic) AMD* is characterized ophthalmoscopically by diffuse or discrete deposits in the Bruch membrane and geographic atrophy of the RPE. Loss of vision may be severe in these individuals. The oral consumption of zinc and of vitamins with antioxidant properties may slow the progression to AMD. There is currently no effective treatment for dry AMD.
- *Wet (neovascular) AMD* is characterized by choroidal neovascularization, defined by the presence of vessels that penetrate through the Bruch membrane beneath the RPE. This neovascular membrane may also penetrate the RPE and become situated directly beneath the neurosensory retina. The vessels in this membrane may leak, and the exuded blood may organize into macular scars. Occasionally, these vessels are the source of hemorrhage, leading to the localized suffusion of blood that may be mistaken clinically for an intraocular neoplasm, or give rise to diffuse vitreous hemorrhage. Currently, the mainstay of treatment for neovascular AMD is the injection of VEGF antagonists into the vitreous of the affected eye to reduce angiogenesis.

Pathogenesis. To understand the pathogenesis of AMD it is important to appreciate the existence of a structural and functional unit composed of the RPE, Bruch membrane (which contains the basement membrane of the RPE), and the innermost layer of the choroidal vasculature, the choriocapillaris. Disturbance in any component of this unit affects the health of the overlying photoreceptors, producing visual loss. Attention is now focused on the roles of several genes,

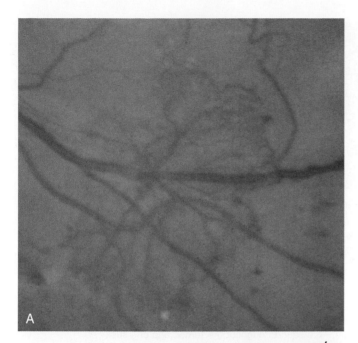

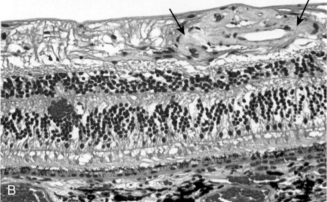

FIG. 21.42 Diabetic retinopathy. (A) Ophthalmoscopic view of retinal neovascularization creating a neovascular membrane. (B) A tangle of abnormal vessels lies just beneath the internal limiting membrane of the retina on the right half of the photomicrograph *(between arrows)*. Note the retinal hemorrhage in the outer plexiform layer in the left half.

especially *CFH* (complement factor H) and other complement regulatory genes in the pathogenesis of this condition. The complement regulatory gene variants that are associated with AMD all appear to decrease their function, implying that AMD may stem from excessive complement activity. Environmental exposures such as cigarette smoking may also increase risk of AMD, especially in genetically predisposed individuals.

Retinitis Pigmentosa. Retinitis pigmentosa is an inherited condition characterized by progressive degeneration or dysfunction of rods and cones or retinal pigment epithelium. It can cause varying degrees of visual impairment including, in some cases, total blindness. The term *retinitis* is a relic of the time when these disorders were incorrectly presumed to be inflammatory. It may occur in isolation (nonsyndromic retinitis pigmentosa, about 65% of cases) or as part of a familial syndrome such as the *Bardet-Biedl syndrome*.

Multiple mutations and patterns of inheritance have been described for nonsyndromic retinitis pigmentosa, all of which regulate the functions of either the photoreceptor cells or the RPE. Typically,

both rods and cones are lost to apoptosis, possibly as the result of accumulation of misfolded proteins. Loss of rods may lead to early night blindness and constricted visual fields. As cones are lost, central visual acuity may be affected. Clinically, retinal atrophy is accompanied by constriction of retinal vessels and optic nerve head atrophy ("waxy pallor" of the optic disc) and the accumulation of retinal pigment around blood vessels, thus accounting for the "pigmentosa" in the disease name.

Retinal Neoplasms

Retinoblastoma. Retinoblastoma is the most common primary intraocular malignancy of children. The molecular genetics of retinoblastoma are discussed in detail in Chapter 6. Although the name retinoblastoma might suggest origin from a cell that is capable of differentiation into both glial and neuronal cells, it is now clear that the cell of origin is a neuronal progenitor. Recall that in approximately 40% of cases, retinoblastoma occurs in individuals who inherit a germline mutation of one *RB* allele. Retinoblastoma arises when a second, somatic mutation occurs in the retinal progenitor and *RB* gene function is lost. In sporadic cases, both *RB* alleles are lost by somatic mutations. Retinoblastomas arising in those with germline mutations are often bilateral. In addition, they may be associated with pineoblastoma ("trilateral" retinoblastoma), which has a very poor prognosis.

MORPHOLOGY

The pathology of hereditary and sporadic retinoblastoma is identical. The tumors are often nodular masses, usually in the posterior retina and sometimes with satellite seedings. They may contain both undifferentiated and differentiated elements. The former appear as collections of small, round cells with hyperchromatic nuclei resembling retinoblasts, placing the tumors in the "small round blue cells" group of tumors. In well-differentiated tumors there are **Flexner-Wintersteiner rosettes** and fleurettes reflecting photoreceptor differentiation, consisting of clusters of cuboidal or short columnar cells around a central lumen. Viable tumor cells are found encircling blood vessels with zones of necrosis typically found in relatively avascular areas, illustrating the dependence of retinoblastoma on its blood supply (Fig. 21.43). Focal zones of dystrophic calcification are characteristic.

Retinoblastoma tends to spread to the brain, skull, and bone marrow and seldom disseminates to the lungs. Prognosis is adversely affected by extraocular extension and invasion along the optic nerve and by choroidal invasion. In an effort to preserve vision and eradicate the tumor, many ophthalmic oncologists now attempt to reduce tumor burden by administration of chemotherapy, including selective delivery of the drug to the eye through the ophthalmic artery; after chemoreduction, tumors may be obliterated by laser treatment or cryopexy.

Optic Nerve

As a sensory tract of the central nervous system, the optic nerve is surrounded by meninges, and cerebrospinal fluid circulates around the nerve. The pathology of the optic nerve is similar to the pathology of the brain. For example, the most common primary neoplasms of the optic nerve are gliomas (typically pilocytic astrocytoma in young individuals and diffuse glioma in older adults) and optic nerve sheath meningioma.

Papilledema

Papilledema refers to bilateral swelling of the optic nerve head as a result of elevated intracranial pressure. Edema of the head of the

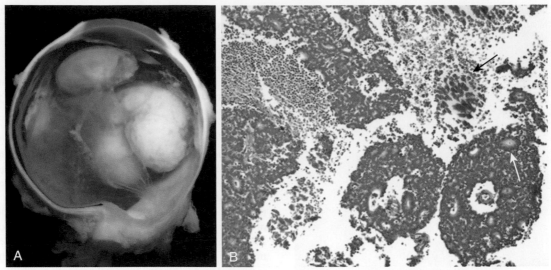

FIG. 21.43 Retinoblastoma. (A) Gross photograph of retinoblastoma. (B) Tumor cells appear viable when in proximity to blood vessels, but necrosis is seen as the distance from the vessel increases. Dystrophic calcification *(black arrow)* is present in the zones of tumor necrosis. Flexner-Wintersteiner rosettes—arrangements of a single layer of tumor cells around an apparent "lumen"—are seen throughout the tumor, and one such rosette is indicated by the *white arrow.*

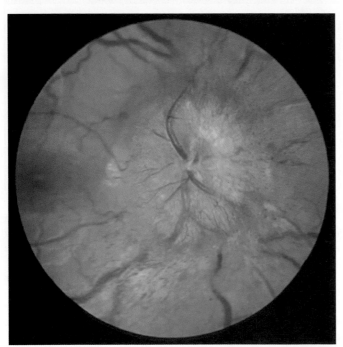

FIG. 21.44 Papilledema. In papilledema secondary to increased intracranial pressure, the optic nerve is typically swollen and hyperemic. (Courtesy Dr. Sohan S. Hayreh, Department of Ophthalmology and Visual Science, University of Iowa, Iowa City, Iowa.)

optic nerve may also develop as a consequence of compression of the nerve (as in a primary neoplasm of the optic nerve when swelling of the nerve head produces unilateral disc edema). The increase in pressure encircling the nerve contributes to venous stasis and interferes with axoplasmic transport, leading to nerve head swelling. Typically, acute papilledema from increased intracranial pressure is not associated with visual loss. Ophthalmoscopically, the optic nerve head is swollen and hyperemic (Fig. 21.44). It may remain congested for a prolonged period of time.

Optic Neuritis and Neuropathy

Many unrelated conditions have historically been grouped under the heading of optic neuritis, but in common clinical usage the term *optic neuritis* is used to describe a loss of vision secondary to demyelinization of the optic nerve. One of the most important causes of optic neuritis is multiple sclerosis (discussed earlier). Indeed, optic neuritis may be the first manifestation of this disease. Individuals with a single episode of optic nerve demyelination may recover vision and remain disease free.

Nonischemic forms of *optic neuropathy* may be inherited or secondary to nutritional deficiencies or toxins such as methanol. Individuals may experience severe visual compromise.

■ RAPID REVIEW

Central Nervous System

Edema, Herniation, and Hydrocephalus

- Cerebral edema is the accumulation of excess fluid within the brain parenchyma. Hydrocephalus is an increase in CSF volume within the ventricular system.
- Increases in brain volume (as a result of increased CSF volume, edema, hemorrhage, or tumor) raise the pressure inside the fixed capacity of the skull, which can damage the brain by decreasing perfusion or by displacing tissue across dural partitions inside the skull or through openings in the skull (herniations).

Congenital Malformations

- Malformations of the brain can occur because of genetic factors or external insults.
- Various malformations stem from failure of neural tube closure (spina bifida, myelomeningocele), improper formation of neural

structures, altered neuronal migration (e.g., microencephaly), and abnormal cerebellar development (e.g., Arnold-Chiari malformation).

Genetic Metabolic Diseases

- Inherited systemic diseases that affect neurons or white matter include neuronal storage diseases (e.g., Tay-Sachs, Niemann-Pick diseases) and disorders caused by mitochondrial abnormalities.

Cerebrovascular Diseases

- Stroke is the clinical term for acute-onset neurologic deficits resulting from hemorrhagic or obstructive vascular lesions.
- Cerebral infarction follows loss of blood supply and can be widespread or focal, or affect regions with the least robust vascular supply ("watershed" infarcts).
- Focal cerebral infarcts are most commonly embolic; with subsequent dissolution of the embolus and reperfusion, a nonhemorrhagic infarct can become hemorrhagic.
- Primary intraparenchymal hemorrhages typically are due to either hypertension (most commonly in white matter, deep gray matter, or posterior fossa contents) or cerebral amyloid angiopathy (cerebral cortex).
- Spontaneous subarachnoid hemorrhage usually is caused by a structural vascular abnormality, such as an aneurysm or arteriovenous malformation.

Central Nervous System Trauma

- Physical injury to the brain can occur when the inside of the skull comes into forceful contact with the brain.
- In blunt trauma, there may be brain injury both at the original point of contact (coup injury) and on the opposite side of the brain (contrecoup injury) owing to impacts with the skull.
- Rapid displacement of the head and brain can tear axons (diffuse axonal injury), often causing severe, irreversible neurologic deficits.
- Traumatic tearing of blood vessels, depending on the location, leads to epidural, subdural, or intraparenchymal hematoma as well as subarachnoid hemorrhage.
- Perinatal brain injury may cause (1) hemorrhage, often in the region of the germinal matrix with the risk for extension into the ventricular system, and (2) ischemic infarcts, leading to periventricular leukomalacia.

Infections of the Nervous System

- Different pathogens use distinct routes to reach the brain, and they cause different patterns of disease.
- Bacterial infections may cause meningitis, cerebral abscesses, or a chronic meningoencephalitis.
- Viral infections can cause meningitis or meningoencephalitis.
- Fungi and protozoan parasites cause diverse lesions.

Acquired Metabolic and Toxic Diseases

- Nutritional disorders: Thiamine deficiency causes focal hemorrhage and necrosis (Wernicke-Korsakoff syndrome); vitamin B_{12} deficiency causes subacute combined degeneration of the spinal cord.
- Metabolic disorders: Hypoglycemia causes neuronal injury, hyperglycemia causes stupor and coma, and elevated ammonia in liver disease affects astrocytes (hepatic encephalopathy).
- Toxic disorders: Metals (e.g., lead), industrial chemicals, and environmental pollutants (e.g., carbon monoxide) cause injury to different structures, and ethanol can cause brain swelling and cerebellar abnormalities.

Diseases of Myelin

- Multiple sclerosis, an autoimmune demyelinating disease, is the most common disorder of myelin, affecting young adults. It often pursues a relapsing-remitting course, with eventual progressive accumulation of neurologic deficits.
- Other, less common forms of immune-mediated demyelination often follow infections and are more acute illnesses.
- Leukodystrophies are genetic disorders in which myelin production or turnover is abnormal.

Neurodegenerative Diseases

- Neurodegenerative diseases cause symptoms that depend on the pattern of brain involvement. Cortical disease usually manifests as cognitive change, alterations in personality, and memory disturbances; basal ganglia disorders usually manifest as movement disorders.
- Many of the neurodegenerative diseases are associated with various protein aggregates, which serve as pathologic hallmarks. Familial forms of these diseases are associated with mutations in the genes encoding these proteins or controlling their metabolism.
- Prion diseases are caused by an altered form of a normal cellular protein, PrP. They can be sporadic, transmitted, or inherited.
- Among dementias, Alzheimer disease (with plaques of Aβ and tangles of tau) is the most common; other predominantly dementing diseases include the various forms of FTLDs (both forms with tau-containing lesions and with other types of inclusions) and dementia with Lewy bodies (with α-synuclein containing lesions).
- Among the hypokinetic movement disorders, Parkinson disease is the most common, with α-synuclein containing inclusions.
- Amyotrophic lateral sclerosis (ALS) is the most common form of motor neuron disease, with diverse genetic causes as well as sporadic forms.

Tumors of the Central Nervous System

- Primary tumors of the CNS most often arise from the cells of the coverings (meningiomas) or the brain parenchyma (gliomas, neuronal tumors, choroid plexus tumors).
- Even low-grade or benign tumors can have poor clinical outcomes, depending on where they occur in the brain.
- Distinct types of tumors affect specific brain regions (e.g., cerebellum for medulloblastoma) and specific age populations (medulloblastoma and pilocytic astrocytomas in pediatric age groups, and glioblastoma and lymphoma in older patients).
- Glial tumors are broadly classified into astrocytoma, glioblastoma, oligodendroglioma, and ependymoma. Increasing tumor malignancy is associated with anaplasia, increased cell density, necrosis, and mitotic activity.

Eye

Conjunctiva

- Conjunctivitis is caused by a variety of bacterial and viral infections and is usually self-limited. Trachoma, caused by *Chlamydia trachomatis*, common in lower-income countries, is often a chronic infection that may distort the eyelids and result in corneal scarring and blindness.

Cornea

- Inflammations of the cornea may be accompanied by a noninfectious exudative process in the anterior chamber that may organize to distort anterior segment anatomy and contribute to secondary glaucoma and to cataract.
- Keratoconus is an example of a condition that distorts the contour of the cornea and alters its refractive surface, producing an irregular form of astigmatism.

Anterior Segment

- Cataracts are opacities of the lens that may be congenital or acquired.
- The term glaucoma describes a group of conditions characterized by optic neuropathy with distinctive changes in the visual field and the size and shape of the optic nerve cup, usually the result of elevation in intraocular pressure.
- Glaucoma may be the result of increased production of aqueous humor or its defective outflow and is classified into open-angle and angle-closure types.

Uvea

- Uveitis is restricted to a diverse group of chronic diseases that may be either components of a systemic process or localized to the eye.

- Sarcoid is an example of a systemic condition that may produce granulomatous uveitis, and sympathetic ophthalmia may produce bilateral granulomatous inflammation as a possible consequence of penetrating injury to one eye.
- The most common intraocular tumor of adults is metastasis to the eye.
- The most common primary intraocular tumor of adults is uveal melanoma. The genetics of uveal melanoma is different from that of cutaneous melanoma. Uveal melanoma disseminates hematogenously and the first metastases are typically in the liver.

Retina

- Retinal detachment, a separation of the neurosensory retina from the RPE, may be the consequence of a break in the retina (rhegmatogenous retinal detachment) or may develop without a retinal break because of pathology within or beneath the retina (nonrhegmatogenous retinal detachment).
- Several major causes of blindness result from pathologic intraocular angiogenesis, including proliferative diabetic retinopathy and exudative (wet) age-related macular degeneration. VEGF antagonists may prevent visual loss in many of these conditions. Hypertension also causes vascular lesions in the retina.
- Retinoblastoma is the most common primary intraocular tumor of children.

Optic Nerve

- Bilateral swelling of the optic nerve head known as papilledema may develop as a consequence of elevated cerebrospinal fluid pressure and stasis of axoplasmic transport within the optic nerve. Unilateral disc edema can result from compression by a local tumor.
- Optic neuropathy may be inherited (as in Leber hereditary optic neuropathy) or may result from acquired conditions, amongst which multiple sclerosis is an important cause.

OUTLINE

Skin disorders are common and diverse, ranging from irritating itching to life-threatening melanoma. Many of these conditions are confined to the skin, but others are manifestations of multiorgan diseases, such as systemic lupus erythematosus or neurofibromatosis. In such instances, pathologic changes involving the skin often offer the first clue to the underlying diagnosis.

As the largest interface between the body and the external environment, the skin is the site of important immunologic responses. It is constantly exposed to microbial and nonmicrobial antigens from the environment that are captured and processed by epidermal Langerhans cells and dermal dendritic cells, which transport their antigenic cargo to regional lymph nodes and initiate immune responses. The squamous cells *(keratinocytes)* that make up the epidermis help maintain skin homeostasis by providing a physical barrier to environmental insults and by secreting cytokines that influence both the epidermal and dermal microenvironments. The underlying dermis contains resident populations of CD4+ helper and CD8+ cytotoxic T lymphocytes, regulatory T cells (Tregs), and occasional B cells. The epidermis normally contain a population of γδ T cells, while the dermis contains perivascular mast cells and scattered macrophages, all components of the innate immune system. Responses involving these immune cells and locally released cytokines account for the morphologic patterns and clinical expressions of inflammatory and infectious skin disorders.

This chapter focuses on common and pathogenically illustrative skin diseases. In considering these diseases, it is important to appreciate that the practice of dermatopathology relies on close interactions with clinicians, particularly dermatologists, as the clinical history, gross appearance, and distribution of lesions are often as important as the microscopic findings in arriving at a specific diagnosis. Diseases of the skin can be confusing for the student, in part because dermatologists and dermatopathologists communicate using a "skin-specific" lexicon that one must become familiar with in order to understand these diseases. The most important of these terms and definitions are listed in Table 22.1.

ACUTE INFLAMMATORY DERMATOSES

Thousands of inflammatory dermatoses exist, challenging the diagnostic acumen of even experienced clinicians. In general, acute lesions, defined as days to several weeks in duration, are characterized by inflammation, edema, and variable epidermal, vascular, or subcutaneous injury. Acute dermatoses are often marked by infiltrates consisting of mononuclear cells rather than neutrophils, unlike acute inflammatory disorders at most other sites. Some acute lesions may persist, transitioning to a chronic phase, while others are self-limited.

Urticaria

Urticaria ("hives") is a common disorder mediated by localized mast cell degranulation, which leads to dermal microvascular hyperpermeability. The resulting erythematous, edematous, and pruritic plaques are termed *wheals.*

Pathogenesis. In most cases, urticaria stems from an immediate (type 1) hypersensitivity reaction (Chapter 5), in which environmental antigens trigger mast cell degranulation by binding to immunoglobulin E (IgE) antibodies attached to the mast cell surface through the

The contributions to this chapter by Dr. Alexander J. Lazar, Department of Pathology, MD Anderson Cancer Center, Houston, Texas, in several previous editions of this book are gratefully acknowledged.

Table 22.1 Nomenclature of Skin Lesions

Macroscopic Lesions	Definition
Excoriation	Traumatic lesion breaking the epidermis and causing a raw linear area (i.e., deep scratch); often self-inflicted
Lichenification	Thickened, rough skin (similar to lichen on a rock); usually the result of repeated rubbing
Macule, patch	Circumscribed, flat lesion distinguished from surrounding skin by color. Macules are 5 mm in diameter or less, while patches are greater than 5 mm in size.
Papule, nodule	Elevated dome-shaped or flat-topped lesion. Papules are 5 mm in diameter or less, while nodules are greater than 5 mm in size.
Plaque	Elevated flat-topped lesion, usually greater than 5 mm in diameter (may be formed by coalescence of papules)
Pustule	Discrete, pus-filled, raised lesion
Scale	Dry, horny, platelike excrescence; the result of thickening of the cornified layer
Vesicle, bulla, blister	Fluid-filled raised lesion 5 mm or less in diameter (vesicle) or greater than 5 mm in diameter (bulla). Blister is the common term for both lesions.
Wheal	Itchy, transient, elevated lesion with variable blanching and erythema formed as the result of dermal edema

Microscopic Lesions	Definition
Acanthosis	Diffuse epidermal hyperplasia
Dyskeratosis	Abnormal, premature keratinization within cells below the stratum granulosum
Hyperkeratosis	Thickening of the stratum corneum, often associated with a qualitative abnormality of keratin
Papillomatosis	Surface elevation caused by hyperplasia and enlargement of contiguous dermal papillae
Parakeratosis	Retention of nuclei in the stratum corneum of squamous epithelium. On mucous membranes, parakeratosis is normal.
Spongiosis	Intercellular edema of the epidermis

IgE-specific Fc receptor. Responsible antigens may come from a variety of sources, including viruses, pollens, foods, drugs, and insect venoms. IgE-independent urticaria may also result from exposure to substances that directly incite mast cell degranulation, such as opiates and certain antibiotics. In the vast majority of cases, no cause is discovered, even with extensive investigation.

MORPHOLOGY

The histologic features of urticaria are subtle. There is usually a sparse superficial perivenular infiltrate of mononuclear cells, rare neutrophils, and sometimes eosinophils. Superficial dermal edema causes splaying of collagen bundles, making them more widely spaced than normal. Mast cells, which reside around superficial dermal venules, may be difficult to appreciate with routine hematoxylin-eosin (H&E) stains but are readily visualized using Giemsa stains.

Clinical Features. Urticaria most commonly affects individuals between 20 and 40 years of age. Individual lesions usually develop and fade within hours, but episodes may persist for days or even months. Lesions range from small, pruritic papules to large, edematous, erythematous plaques. They may be localized to a particular part of the body or generalized. In a specific type of urticaria termed *pressure urticaria*, lesions are found only in areas exposed to pressure (such as the feet or buttocks). Although not life threatening, severe pruritus may compromise quality of life. Most cases respond to antihistamines, but severe, refractory disease may require treatment with leukotriene antagonists, monoclonal antibodies that block the action of IgE, or immunosuppressive drugs.

Eczematous Dermatitis

Eczema (literally, "to boil") is a clinical term that embraces a number of conditions with varied underlying etiologies. New lesions take the form of erythematous papules, often with overlying vesicles, which ooze and become crusted. Pruritus is characteristic. With persistence, lesions coalesce into raised, scaling plaques. The nature and degree of these changes vary among the clinical subtypes, which include the following:

- *Atopic dermatitis* is an immune response to environmental antigens that appears to stem from defects in epidermal barrier function that increase the permeability of the skin to antigens.
- *Allergic contact dermatitis* stems from topical exposure to an allergen and is caused by delayed hypersensitivity reactions.
- *Drug-related eczematous dermatitis* is caused by a hypersensitivity reaction to drugs.
- *Photoeczematous dermatitis* is an abnormal reaction to UV or visible light.
- *Primary irritant dermatitis* results from exposure to substances that chemically, physically, or mechanically damage the skin.

While the barrier defect that underlies atopic dermatitis stems from a genetic predisposition and can persist for years or decades, other forms of eczematous dermatitis resolve completely when the offending stimulus is removed or exposure is limited, stressing the importance of investigating the underlying cause. Only the most common forms, atopic dermatitis and contact dermatitis, are considered here.

Atopic dermatitis most often presents during childhood and is common, affecting 5% to 20% of children worldwide. It is associated with elevated levels of IgE and is part of the so-called *atopic triad*, which also includes asthma and food allergies. Affected individuals often have a family history of atopy and frequently carry genetic variants that disrupt the function of filaggrin, a structural protein that is essential for the creation of the epidermal barrier.

Allergic contact dermatitis (also called *contact sensitivity*) is triggered by exposure to an environmental agent that chemically reacts with self proteins, creating neoantigens that are recognized by the T-cell arm of the adaptive immune system. A classic example is *urushiol*, a reactive substance found in poison ivy, oak, and sumac. The self proteins modified by the agent are processed by epidermal and dermal dendritic cells, which migrate to draining lymph nodes and present the antigen to naïve T cells. This sensitization event leads to acquisition of immunologic memory; on reexposure to the antigen, the activated memory CD4+ T lymphocytes migrate to the affected skin sites. There they release cytokines that recruit

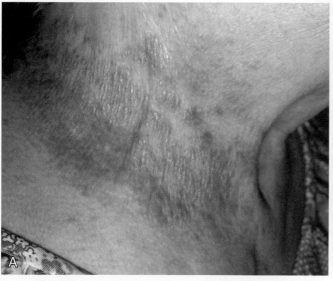

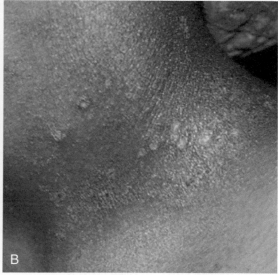

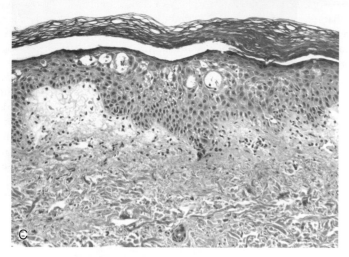

FIG. 22.1 Eczematous dermatitis. (A) Patterned erythema and scale stemming from a nickel-induced contact dermatitis produced by a necklace in an individual with lighter skin. (B) By contrast, eczematous dermatitis can appear hyperpigmented in individuals with darker skin, as in this case of atopic dermatitis. In other cases, postinflammatory hypopigmentation may be seen in darker skin types (not shown). (C) Microscopically, there is an accumulation of fluid (spongiosis) between epidermal cells, which may progress to blister formation. (B, Reprinted with permission from Cutis. 2019;104:164–168. ©2019, Frontline Medical Communications Inc.)

additional inflammatory cells and also mediate epidermal damage, as in any delayed-type hypersensitivity reaction (Chapter 5).

MORPHOLOGY

As the name implies, skin involvement in contact dermatitis is limited to sites of direct contact with the triggering agent (Fig. 22.1A), whereas in other forms of eczema, lesions may be widely distributed (Fig. 22.1B). Grossly, lesions may appear erythematous or hyper- or hypopigmented, depending on skin type. Acute lesions are pruritic, edematous, oozing plaques, often containing vesicles and bullae. With persistent antigen exposure, the epidermis may become scaly (hyperkeratotic) and thickened (acanthotic). Some changes are produced or exacerbated by scratching of the lesion (see lichen simplex chronicus, discussed later).

Histologically, **spongiosis** (epidermal edema) characterizes all forms of acute eczematous dermatitis—hence the synonym **spongiotic dermatitis**. Edema fluid seeps into the epidermis, where it splays apart keratinocytes (Fig. 22.1C). Intercellular bridges are stretched and become more prominent and easier to visualize. This change is accompanied by a superficial perivascular lymphocytic infiltrate, edema of dermal papillae, and mast cell degranulation. Eosinophils may be present and are especially prominent in spongiotic eruptions provoked by drugs, but in general the histologic features are similar regardless of cause, emphasizing the need for careful clinical correlation.

Clinical Features. Treatment of allergic contact dermatitis involves eliminating exposure to the causative allergen and topical treatment with antiinflammatory agents. Atopic dermatitis often remits spontaneously in adults, but can sometimes be chronic and severe. Treatment options range from topical antiinflammatory agents and antihistamines (to control pruritus) to systemic therapy with antibodies that block IL-4 and IL-13, cytokines with important roles in Th2 immune responses.

Erythema Multiforme

Erythema multiforme is characterized by epithelial injury mediated by skin-homing CD8+ cytotoxic T lymphocytes. It is an uncommon, usually self-limited disorder that appears to be a hypersensitivity response to certain infections and drugs. Antecedent infections include those caused by herpes simplex, mycoplasma, and some fungi, while implicated drugs include sulfonamides, penicillin, salicylates, hydantoins, and antimalarials. The T-cell attack is focused on the basal cells of cutaneous and mucosal epithelia, presumably due to recognition of still unknown antigens. Certain human leukocyte antigen (HLA) haplotypes are associated with the disease.

Affected individuals present with a wide array of lesions, which may include macules, papules, vesicles, and bullae (hence the term multiforme). Well-developed lesions have a characteristic "**targetoid**" appearance (Fig. 22.2A), which may be less apparent in darker skin types (Fig. 22.2B). Early lesions show a superficial perivascular lymphocytic infiltrate associated with dermal edema and margination of lymphocytes along the dermoepidermal junction in intimate association with apoptotic keratinocytes (Fig. 22.2C). With time, discrete, confluent zones of basal epidermal necrosis appear, leading to blister formation.

Clinical Features. The most common precipitant of erythema multiforme is recent herpes simplex virus infection, usually a week or so before the appearance of the characteristic skin eruptions. Erythema multiforme has a broad range of severity. The forms associated with infection (e.g., herpesvirus) are less severe.

CHRONIC INFLAMMATORY DERMATOSES

Chronic inflammatory dermatoses are persistent skin conditions that exhibit their most characteristic features over many months to years, although they may begin with an acute stage. The skin surface in some chronic inflammatory dermatoses is roughened as a result of excessive or abnormal scale formation and shedding *(desquamation)*.

Psoriasis

Psoriasis is a common chronic inflammatory dermatosis, affecting 1% to 2% of individuals residing in the United States. Epidemiologic studies have shown that patients with psoriasis are at increased risk for death from cardiovascular disease, possibly because psoriasis creates a chronic inflammatory state.

Pathogenesis. **Psoriasis is a T cell—mediated inflammatory disease, presumed to be autoimmune in origin,** although the initiating antigens are not defined. Both genetic (HLA types and other susceptibility loci) and environmental factors contribute to the risk. It is unclear whether the inciting antigens are self antigens, environmental antigens, or some combination of the two. Sensitized populations of T cells home to the skin, mainly CD4+ Th1 and Th17 cells, and accumulate in the epidermis. These cells secrete cytokines and growth factors that induce keratinocyte hyperproliferation, resulting in the characteristic lesions. Psoriatic lesions can be elicited in susceptible individuals by local trauma *(Koebner phenomenon)*, which may induce a local inflammatory response that promotes lesion development. Genome-wide association studies have linked an increased risk for psoriasis to polymorphisms in HLA loci and genes encoding proteins that are involved in adaptive immunity, TNF signaling, and skin barrier function. Several loci are also associated with the development of psoriatic arthritis, a more severe complication of this disease that is seen in up to 10% of patients.

In light skin types, the typical lesion is a well-demarcated **pink to salmon-colored plaque covered by loosely adherent silver-white scale** (Fig. 22.3A). In patients with darker skin types, plaques range from **salmon colored to hyperpigmented and demonstrate gray scale** (Fig. 22.3B). There is marked epidermal thickening **(acanthosis),** with regular downward elongation of the rete ridges (Fig. 22.3C). The pattern of this downward growth has been likened to "**test tubes in a rack.**" Increased epidermal cell

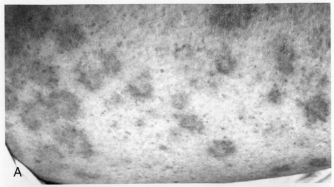

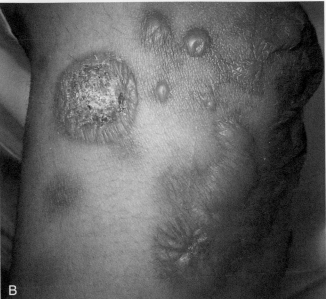

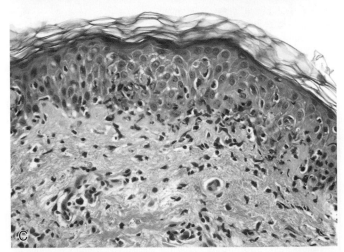

FIG. 22.2 Erythema multiforme. (A) On more lightly pigmented skin, well-demarcated, erythematous targetoid plaques are the hallmark of erythema multiforme. (B) On more darkly pigmented skin, the lesions may appear to be hyperpigmented and to have gray-silver central areas. (C) Early lesions show lymphocytes along the dermoepidermal junction (interface dermatitis) associated with scattered apoptotic keratinocytes, marked by dark shrunken nuclei and eosinophilic cytoplasm. (B, From *Immunity and Immunologic Oral Lesions*, in *Oral Pathology for the Dental Hygienists, with General Pathology Introductions,* Peters SM and Ibsen OAC, eds., Elsevier, 2023.)

turnover and lack of maturation results in **loss of the stratum granulosum** and **extensive parakeratotic scale**. Also seen is thinning of the epidermal cell layer overlying the tips of dermal papillae and dilated and tortuous blood vessels within the papillae. These vessels bleed when the scale is removed, giving rise to multiple punctate bleeding points **(Auspitz sign)**. Neutrophils form small aggregates within both the spongiotic superficial epidermis **(spongiform pustule of Kogoj)** and the parakeratotic stratum corneum **(Munro microabscesses)**. Similar changes can be seen in superficial fungal infections, which must be excluded with appropriate special stains.

Clinical Features. Psoriasis most frequently affects the skin of the elbows, knees, posterior scalp, lumbosacral areas, intergluteal cleft, glans penis, and vulva. Nail changes on the fingers and toes occur in 30% of cases. In most cases psoriasis is mild and limited in distribution, but in others it is widespread and severe. Treatment is aimed at preventing the release or actions of inflammatory mediators. Mild disease is treated topically with ointments containing corticosteroids or other immunomodulatory agents, whereas more severe disease is treated with phototherapy (which has immunosuppressive effects) and immunosuppressive agents that block TNF function or Th17 immune responses.

Lichen Planus

"Pruritic, purple, polygonal, planar papules, and plaques" are the tongue-twisting *P*s that describe this disorder of skin and squamous mucosa. The lesions may result from a CD8+ T cell—mediated cytotoxic response to unknown antigens expressed by basal keratinocytes or deposited at the dermoepidermal junction.

MORPHOLOGY

Cutaneous lesions of lichen planus consist of **pruritic, violaceous, flat-topped papules** that may coalesce focally to form plaques (Fig. 22.4A). These papules are highlighted by white dots or lines termed **Wickham striae**. Hyperpigmentation may result from melanin loss into the dermis from damaged keratinocytes. Microscopically, lichen planus is a prototypical **interface dermatitis,** so called because the inflammation and damage are concentrated at the interface of the squamous epithelium and papillary dermis. There is a dense, continuous infiltrate of lymphocytes along the dermoepidermal junction (Fig. 22.4B). The lymphocytes are intimately associated with basal keratinocytes, which often atrophy or become necrotic. Perhaps as a response to damage, the basal cells take on the appearance of the more mature cells of the stratum spinosum ("squamatization"). This pattern of inflammation causes the dermoepidermal interface to assume an angulated, zigzag contour **(saw-toothing)**. Anucleate, necrotic basal cells are seen in the inflamed papillary dermis and are referred to as colloid bodies or **Civatte bodies**. Although these changes bear some similarities to those in erythema multiforme (another type of interface dermatitis discussed earlier), lichen planus shows well-developed changes of chronicity, including epidermal hyperplasia, hypergranulosis, and hyperkeratosis.

Clinical Features. Lichen planus is an uncommon disorder that usually presents in middle-aged adults. The cutaneous lesions are multiple and usually symmetrically distributed, particularly on the extremities, and often occur around the wrists and elbows and on the vulva and glans penis. Approximately 70% of cases also involve the oral mucosa, where the lesions manifest as white papules with a reticulate or netlike appearance. The cutaneous lesions of lichen planus usually resolve spontaneously within 1 to 2 years, but the oral lesions may persist and be of sufficient severity to interfere with food intake.

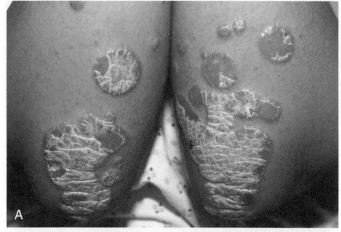
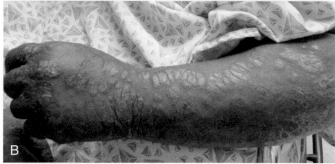
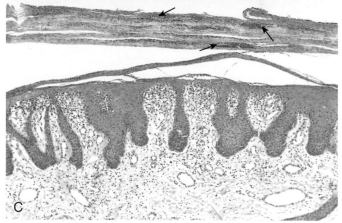

FIG. 22.3 Chronic psoriasis. (A) Erythematous psoriatic plaques covered by silvery-white scale in an individual with lighter skin. (B) In patients with darker skin, plaques range from salmon colored to hyperpigmented and typically demonstrate gray scale. (C) Microscopic examination shows marked epidermal hyperplasia, downward extension of rete ridges (psoriasiform hyperplasia), and prominent parakeratotic scale with infiltrating neutrophils *(Munro microabscesses, arrows)*. (B, Courtesy of Dr. Sarah Wolfe, Department of Dermatology, Duke University Medical Center, Durham, North Carolina.)

Lichen Simplex Chronicus

Lichen simplex chronicus manifests as roughening of the skin, which takes on an appearance reminiscent of lichen on a tree. This change is a response to local repetitive trauma, usually from rubbing or scratching. Nodular forms exist that are referred to as *prurigo nodularis*. The pathogenesis of lichen simplex chronicus is not understood, but the trauma induces epithelial hyperplasia and eventual dermal scarring.

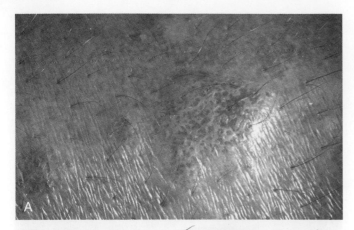

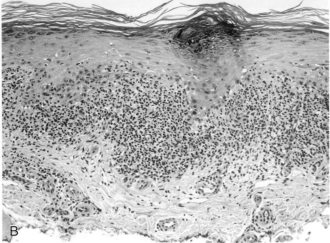

FIG. 22.4 Lichen planus. (A) Flat-topped pink-purple polygonal papules with white lacelike markings referred to as *Wickham striae*. (B) Microscopic examination shows a bandlike infiltrate of lymphocytes along the dermoepidermal junction, hyperkeratosis, hypergranulosis, and pointed rete ridges ("sawtoothing"), which results from chronic injury of the basal cell layer.

MORPHOLOGY

Lichen simplex chronicus is characterized by **acanthosis, hyperkeratosis,** and **hypergranulosis.** Also seen are elongation of the rete ridges, fibrosis of the papillary dermis, and a dermal chronic inflammatory infiltrate (Fig. 22.5). Of interest, these lesions are similar in appearance to normal volar (palms and soles) skin, in which skin thickening serves as an adaptation to repetitive mechanical stress.

Clinical Features. The lesions are often raised, erythematous, or hyperpigmented scaly plaques and may be mistaken for keratinocytic neoplasms. Lichen simplex chronicus may be superimposed on and mask another (often pruritic) dermatosis. It is therefore important to rule out an underlying cause while recognizing that the lesion may be entirely related to trauma.

INFECTIOUS DERMATOSES

Bacterial Infections

Numerous bacterial infections occur in the skin. These range from superficial infections known as *impetigo* to deeper dermal abscesses

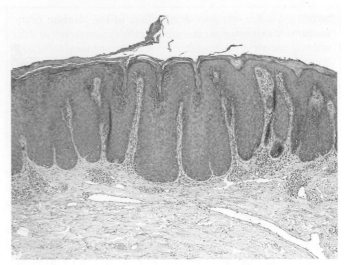

FIG. 22.5 Lichen simplex chronicus. Note the distinctive acanthosis, hyperkeratosis, and hypergranulosis. Superficial dermal fibrosis and vascular ectasia, both common features, also are present.

caused by bacteria such as Pseudomonas aeruginosa that infect puncture wounds. The pathogenesis is similar to that for microbial infections elsewhere. Only impetigo is discussed here.

MORPHOLOGY

Impetigo is characterized by an accumulation of neutrophils beneath the stratum corneum that often produces a subcorneal pustule. Nonspecific reactive epidermal alterations and superficial dermal inflammation accompany these findings. Bacterial cocci in the superficial epidermis can be demonstrated by gram stain.

Clinical Features. Impetigo, one of the most common bacterial infections of the skin, is seen primarily in children. The causative organism, usually *Staphylococcus aureus* or less commonly *Streptococcus pyogenes*, is typically acquired through direct contact with a source. Impetigo often begins as a single small macule, usually on the extremities or the face near the nose or the mouth, which rapidly evolves into a larger circular plaque (Fig. 22.6), often with a honey-colored crust of dried serum. Individuals who are colonized by *S. aureus* or *S. pyogenes* (usually nasal or anal) are more likely to be affected. A

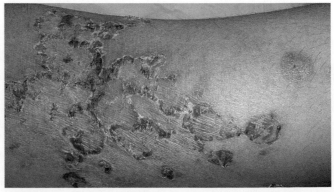

FIG. 22.6 Impetigo. A child's arm involved by a superficial bacterial infection showing the characteristic erythematous scab-like lesions crusted with dried serum. (Courtesy of Dr. Angela Wyatt, Bellaire, Texas.)

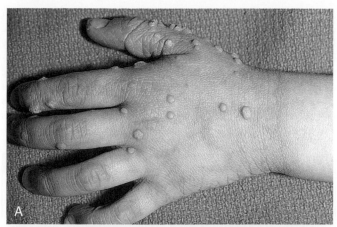

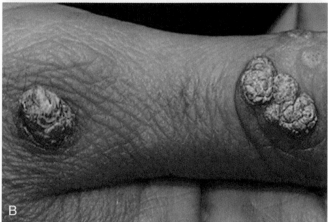

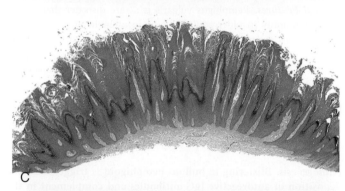

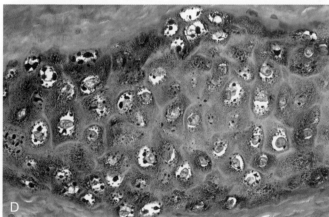

less common bullous form of childhood impetigo may mimic an autoimmune blistering disorder.

Fungal Infections

Fungal infections are varied, ranging from superficial infections with *Tinea* or *Candida* spp. to life-threatening *Aspergillus* spp. infections in individuals who are immunocompromised. Fungal infections can be superficial (stratum corneum, hair, and nails), deep (dermis or subcutis), or systemic, the last type arising through hematogenous spread, often in a patient who is immunocompromised.

MORPHOLOGY

The histologic appearance varies depending on the organism and the host response. Superficial infections are typically associated with a neutrophilic infiltrate in the epidermis. Deep fungal infections produce greater tissue damage and tend to elicit a granulomatous response. *Aspergillus* is often angioinvasive. Periodic acid–Schiff (PAS) and Gomori methenamine silver stains are helpful in identifying the fungal organisms.

Clinical Features. Superficial infections usually produce erythematous to brown-gray macules, depending on the patient's skin type, with superficial scale, and may be pruritic. Superficial fungal infections sometimes have an annular appearance. However, they may also induce lesions that mimic psoriasiform or eczematous dermatoses, so it is important to consider the possibility of fungal infection when these conditions are in the differential diagnosis. Deeper infections such as those seen with *Aspergillus* spp. can appear as erythematous, violaceous, or hyperpigmented nodules or plaques. Such lesions are sometimes associated with local hemorrhage or ulceration.

Verrucae (Warts)

Verrucae are proliferative lesions of squamous epithelial cells that are caused by human papillomavirus (HPV). They are most common in children and adolescents but may be encountered in any age group. HPV infection usually stems from direct contact with an infected individual. Verrucae are generally self-limited, most often regressing spontaneously within 6 months to 2 years.

Pathogenesis. While some members of the HPV family are associated with preneoplastic and invasive cancers of the oropharynx and anogenital region (Chapters 6, 13, 16, and 17), cutaneous warts are mainly caused by low-risk HPV subtypes that lack transforming potential. Like high-risk HPV, low-risk viruses express viral E6 and E7 oncoproteins that lead to dysregulated epidermal cell growth and increased survival. Structural variation in E6 and E7 proteins that affect their interactions with host proteins explains why low-risk viruses cause warts instead of cancer. Because the growth of warts is normally halted by the immune response, immunodeficiency is associated with larger, more numerous verrucae.

MORPHOLOGY

Warts are differentiated on the basis of their gross appearance and location and are generally caused by distinct HPV subtypes. **Verruca vulgaris** (Fig. 22.7A), the most common type, may occur anywhere but is found most

FIG. 22.7 Verruca vulgaris. (A) Multiple warts, with characteristic rough, pebblelike surfaces. (B) On more darkly pigmented skin, warts often appear to be hyperpigmented. (C) Microscopically, common warts contain zones of papillary epidermal proliferation that often radiate symmetrically like the points of a crown. (D) At higher power, pallor or halos around nuclei, prominent keratohyalin granules, and related cytopathic changes are seen. (B, From Plastic Surgery Key, https://plasticsurgerykey.com/27-viral-diseases-of-skin-and-mucosa/.)

frequently on the hands, particularly on the dorsal surfaces and periungual areas. On lighter skin, it appears as a gray-white to gray-brown, flat to convex, 0.1- to 1-cm papule with a rough, pebblelike surface, whereas on darker skin it may appear to be hyperpigmented (Fig. 22.7B). **Verruca plana** (flat wart) is common on the face or dorsal surfaces of the hands, where they appear as flat, smooth, tan or dark brown macules. **Verruca plantaris** and **verruca palmaris** occur on the soles and palms, respectively. These rough, scaly lesions can reach 1 to 2 cm in diameter and may coalesce to form a surface that can be confused with ordinary calluses. **Condyloma acuminatum** (genital wart) occurs on the penis, female genitalia, urethra, and perianal areas (Chapters 16 and 17). Histologic features common to verrucae include epidermal hyperplasia (so-called **verrucous** or **papillomatous epidermal hyperplasia**) (Fig. 22.7C) and cytoplasmic vacuolization **(koilocytosis),** which preferentially involves the more superficial epidermal layers, producing halos of pallor surrounding the nuclei of infected cells. Lesional cells also contain prominent keratohyalin granules and eosinophilic cytoplasmic protein aggregates as a result of impaired squamous maturation (Fig. 22.7D).

BLISTERING (BULLOUS) DISORDERS

Although vesicles and bullae (blisters) occur as secondary phenomena in several unrelated conditions (e.g., herpesvirus infection, spongiotic dermatitis), there is a group of disorders in which blisters are the primary and most distinctive feature. Blistering in these diseases tends to occur at specific levels within the skin, a morphologic distinction that is critical for diagnosis (Fig. 22.8).

Pemphigus Vulgaris and Pemphigus Foliaceus

Pemphigus is an uncommon autoimmune blistering disorder resulting from loss of normal intercellular attachments within the epidermis and the squamous mucosal epithelium. There are three major variants:
- Pemphigus vulgaris (the most common type)
- Pemphigus foliaceus
- Paraneoplastic pemphigus

The last entity is associated with internal malignancy and is not discussed here.

Pathogenesis. **Pemphigus vulgaris and pemphigus foliaceus are autoimmune diseases caused by antibody-mediated (type II) hypersensitivity reactions** (Chapter 5). The pathogenic antibodies are IgG autoantibodies that bind to intercellular desmosomal proteins (desmoglein types 1 and 3) found in the skin and mucous membranes

(eFig. 22.1). The antibodies disrupt the intercellular adhesive function of desmosomes and may activate intercellular proteases as well. The location of the blisters within the epidermis is determined in part by the distribution of desmoglein proteins and the specificity of the autoantibodies, but other unknown factors also appear to influence the clinical phenotypes. By direct immunofluorescence, lesions show a characteristic *fishnetlike pattern* of intercellular IgG deposits (Fig. 22.9). As with many other autoimmune diseases, pemphigus is associated with particular HLA alleles.

MORPHOLOGY

The common histologic denominator in all forms of pemphigus is **acantholysis,** the loss of the intercellular adhesive junctions that normally cement neighboring squamous epithelial cells together. **Pemphigus vulgaris,** caused by antibodies to DSG1 and DSG3, involves both mucosa and skin, especially on the scalp, face, axillae, groin, trunk, and points of pressure. The lesions consist of superficial flaccid vesicles and bullae that rupture easily, leaving deep and often extensive erosions covered with a serum crust (Fig. 22.10A). In pemphigus vulgaris, acantholysis selectively involves the layer of cells immediately above the basal cell layer, giving rise to a suprabasal acantholytic blister (Fig. 22.10B). **Pemphigus foliaceus,** caused by antibodies to DSG1 alone, is a rare, milder form of pemphigus. It results in bullae that are mainly confined to the skin, with only infrequent involvement of mucous membranes. The blisters in this disorder are superficial, and erythema and crusting of ruptured blisters are more limited (Fig. 22.11A). In pemphigus foliaceus, acantholysis selectively involves the superficial epidermis at the level of the stratum granulosum, resulting in subcorneal blisters (Fig. 22.11B).

Clinical Features. Pemphigus vulgaris is a rare disorder that occurs most commonly in older adults and more often in women than in men. Lesions are painful, particularly when ruptured, and frequently develop secondary infections. Most affected patients have oropharyngeal involvement at some point in their course. The mainstay of treatment is immunosuppressive therapy, sometimes for life.

Bullous Pemphigoid

Bullous pemphigoid is another distinctive acquired blistering disorder with an autoimmune basis.

Pathogenesis. **Blistering in bullous pemphigoid is triggered by the deposition of autoreactive IgG antibodies and complement in the epidermal basement membrane** (Fig. 22.12A). Bullous pemphigoid is caused by autoantibodies that bind to proteins that are required for

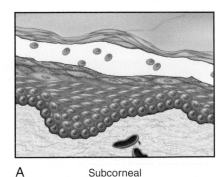 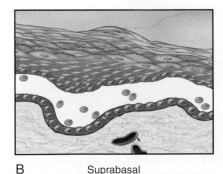 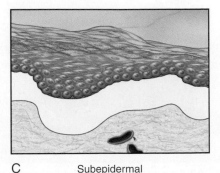

A   Subcorneal   B   Suprabasal   C   Subepidermal

FIG. 22.8 Levels of blister formation. (A) Subcorneal (as in pemphigus foliaceus). (B) Suprabasal (as in pemphigus vulgaris). (C) Subepidermal (as in bullous pemphigoid or dermatitis herpetiformis).

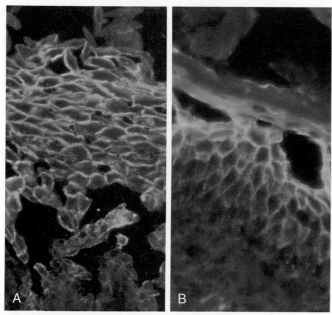

FIG. 22.9 Direct immunofluorescence findings in pemphigus. (A) Pemphigus vulgaris. Note the uniform deposition of immunoglobulin *(green)* along keratinocyte cell membranes in a characteristic "fishnet" pattern. (B) Pemphigus foliaceus. Immunoglobulin deposits are confined to superficial layers of the epidermis.

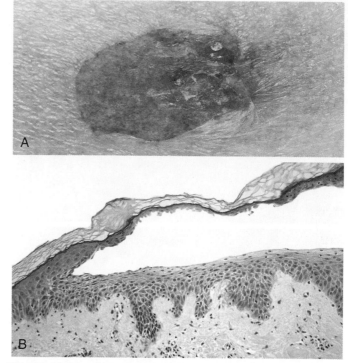

FIG. 22.11 Pemphigus foliaceus. (A) A typical blister, which is more superficial than those seen in pemphigus vulgaris. (B) Microscopic appearance of a characteristic subcorneal blister.

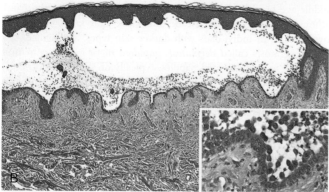

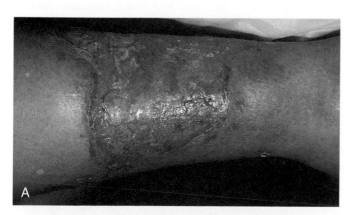

FIG. 22.10 Pemphigus vulgaris. (A) An erosion on the leg arising from coalescence of a group of "unroofed" blisters. (B) Suprabasal intraepidermal blister in which rounded, dissociated (acantholytic) keratinocytes are plentiful *(inset)*.

adherence of basal keratinocytes to the basement membrane (see eFig. 22.1). Most antibody deposition occurs in a continuous linear pattern at the dermoepidermal junction (Fig. 22.12A), where specialized structures called hemidesmosomes link basal keratinocytes to the underlying basement membrane. The so-called bullous pemphigoid antigens (BPAGs) are components of hemidesmosomes. Antibodies against one such component called BPAG2 (type XVII collagen) are proven to cause blistering (Fig. 22.12B). Binding of pathogenic antibodies also leads to the recruitment of neutrophils and eosinophils (Fig. 22.12C). Bullous pemphigoid and pemphigus vulgaris are thus caused by similar pathogenic mechanisms but differ in their clinical presentation and course due to differences in the location of the target antigen (hemidesmosomes in bullous pemphigoid, desmosomes in pemphigus).

MORPHOLOGY

Bullous pemphigoid is associated with tense **subepidermal bullae** filled with clear fluid (Fig. 22.12B). The overlying epidermis characteristically lacks acantholysis. Early lesions show variable numbers of eosinophils at the dermoepidermal junction, occasional neutrophils, superficial dermal edema, and basal cell layer vacuolization. The vacuolated basal cell layer eventually gives rise to a fluid-filled blister (Fig. 22.12C). The blister roof consists of full-thickness epidermis with intact intercellular junctions, a key distinction from the blisters seen in pemphigus.

Clinical Features. The lesions of bullous pemphigoid do not rupture as readily as in pemphigus and, if uncomplicated by infection, heal without scarring. Pruritus is a prominent feature. The disease tends to follow a remitting and relapsing course and responds to topical or systemic immunosuppressive agents. Gestational pemphigoid (also

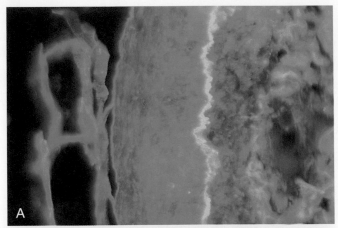

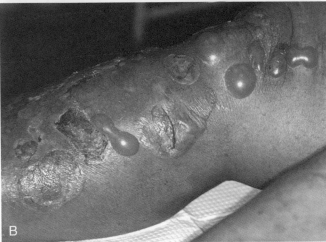

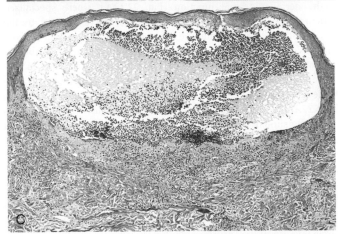

FIG. 22.12 Bullous pemphigoid. (A) Deposition of IgG antibody (detected by direct immunofluorescence) in the subepidermal basement membrane (epidermis is on the left side of the fluorescent band). (B) Gross appearance of characteristic tense, fluid-filled blisters. (C) Subepidermal vesicle with an eosinophil-rich inflammatory infiltrate. (C, Courtesy of Dr. Victor G. Prieto, Houston, Texas.)

known as *herpes gestationis*, a misnomer since there is no viral etiology) is a clinically distinct subtype that appears suddenly during the second or third trimester of pregnancy. Gestational pemphigoid typically resolves after childbirth but may recur with subsequent pregnancies.

Dermatitis Herpetiformis

Dermatitis herpetiformis is an autoimmune blistering disorder associated with gluten sensitivity that is characterized by extremely pruritic, grouped vesicles and papules. The disease predominantly affects males, often in the third and fourth decades of life. Up to 80% of cases are associated with celiac disease, but only a small fraction of patients with celiac disease develop dermatitis herpetiformis. Like celiac disease, dermatitis herpetiformis responds to a gluten-free diet.

Pathogenesis. **In dermatitis herpetiformis, genetically predisposed individuals develop IgA antibodies to dietary gliadin (derived from the wheat protein gluten) as well as IgA autoantibodies that cross-react with endomysium and tissue transglutaminases, including epidermal transglutaminase expressed by keratinocytes** (Chapter 13). By direct immunofluorescence, the skin shows discontinuous, granular deposits of IgA selectively localized in the tips of dermal papillae (Fig. 22.13A) due to binding of the IgA antibodies to fibrils that connect hemidesmosomes to the dermis (see eFig. 22.1). The resultant injury and inflammation produce a subepidermal blister.

MORPHOLOGY

The vesicles and erosions of dermatitis herpetiformis are bilateral, symmetric, and grouped, erythematous or hyperpigmented, and preferentially involve the extensor surfaces, elbows, knees, upper back, and buttocks (Fig. 22.13B, C). Depending on the skin color of the patient, the lesions may be erythematous or hyperpigmented, neutrophils accumulate selectively at the tips of dermal papillae, forming small **microabscesses** (Fig. 22.13D). The basal cells overlying these microabscesses show vacuolization and eventually dissociate from the basement membrane, allowing **subepidermal blisters** to form.

TUMORS OF THE SKIN

Benign and Premalignant Epithelial Lesions

Benign epithelial neoplasms are common and arise from stem-like cells residing in the epidermis and hair follicles. These tumors grow to a limited size and generally do not undergo malignant transformation.

Seborrheic Keratosis

This common pigmented epidermal tumor occurs most frequently in middle-age or older individuals. It preferentially involves the trunk, although the extremities, head, and neck may also be sites of involvement. In individuals with darker skin types, a variant of seborrheic keratosis called *dermatosis papulosa nigra* manifests as multiple small hyperpigmented papules, typically on the face and neck.

Seborrheic keratoses are caused by acquired activating mutations in growth factor signaling pathways. A significant fraction of these tumors harbor activating mutations in fibroblast growth factor receptor 3 (FGFR3), which possesses a tyrosine kinase activity that stimulates RAS and the PI3K/AKT pathway, while others have activating mutations in downstream pathway components such as RAS and PI3K. Except for cosmetic concerns, seborrheic keratoses and dermatosis papulosa nigra are usually of little clinical importance. However, in rare patients hundreds of seborrheic keratoses appear suddenly as a paraneoplastic syndrome *(sign of Leser-Trelat)*. Patients with this presentation may harbor internal malignancies, most commonly gastrointestinal tract carcinomas,

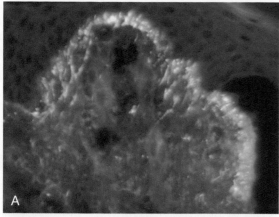

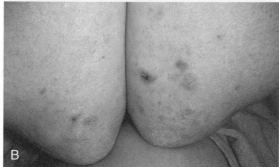

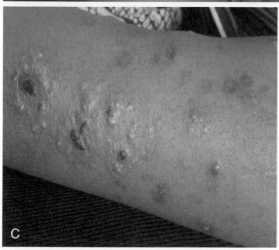

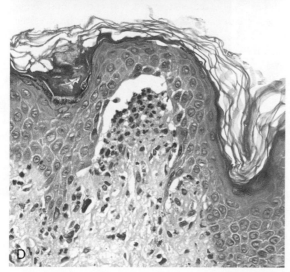

which produce growth factors that stimulate the proliferation of seborrheic keratoses.

> ## MORPHOLOGY
>
> Seborrheic keratoses are **exophytic, coinlike plaques** that vary in diameter from millimeters to centimeters and have a **"stuck-on"** appearance (Fig. 22.14, *inset*). They are tan to dark brown and have a velvety- to granular-appearing surface. Occasionally, their dark or irregular color is suggestive of melanoma, leading to biopsy for further evaluation.
>
> Microscopically, seborrheic keratoses are composed of monotonous sheets of small cells that resemble the basal cells of the normal epidermis (see Fig. 22.14). Variable melanin pigmentation is present within these basaloid cells, accounting for the brown coloration seen grossly. Hyperkeratosis occurs at the surface, and the presence of small keratin-filled cysts **(horn cysts)** and infolding of surface keratinocytes into the main tumor mass **(pseudo-horn cysts)** are characteristic features. Dermatosis papulosa nigra shows similar features.

Actinic Keratosis

Actinic keratosis is a premalignant lesion caused by UV-induced DNA damage that is associated with mutations in *TP53* and other genes that are frequently mutated in squamous cell carcinoma of the skin. Because such lesions are usually the result of chronic exposure to sunlight and are associated with hyperkeratosis, they are called *actinic* (sun-related). The rate of progression to squamous cell carcinoma is small, varying from 0.1% to 2.6% per year. Most regress or remain stable.

> ## MORPHOLOGY
>
> Actinic keratoses are usually less than 1 cm in diameter, tan-brown or red, and rough to the touch (Fig. 22.15A). Microscopically, lower portions of the epidermis show **cytologic atypia,** often associated with hyperplasia of basal cells (Fig. 22.15B) or with atrophy and diffuse thinning of the epidermal surface. The dermis contains thickened, blue-gray elastic fibers (solar elastosis), the result of chronic sun damage. The stratum corneum is thickened and shows abnormal retention of nuclei (parakeratosis). Uncommonly, full-thickness epidermal atypia is seen; such lesions are considered squamous cell carcinoma in situ (Fig. 22.15C).

Clinical Features. Actinic keratoses are very common in fair-skinned individuals and increase in incidence with age and sun exposure. As would be expected, there is a predilection for sun-exposed skin on the face, arms, and dorsum of the hands. Despite the low risk for malignant progression, actinic keratoses are often treated, either to prevent progression or for cosmetic reasons. Local eradication with

FIG. 22.13 Dermatitis herpetiformis. (A) Characteristic selective deposition of IgA autoantibody at the tips of the dermal papillae. (B) Lesions consist of intact and eroded (usually scratched) erythematous (B) or hyperpigmented (C) blisters, often grouped (seen here on elbows and arms). (D) Blisters associated with basal cell layer injury, initially caused by accumulation of neutrophils (microabscesses) at the tips of the dermal papillae. (A, Courtesy of Dr. Victor G. Prieto, Houston, Texas; C, From Dermatitis herpetiformis—Machona MS, Gupta M, Mudenda V, Ngalamika O. Dermatitis herpetiformis in an African woman. *Pan Afr Med J.* 2018 Jun 12;30:119. doi: 10.11604/pamj.2018.30.119.14012. PMID: 30364361; PMCID: PMC6195247.)

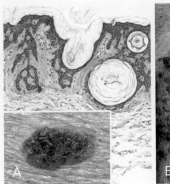

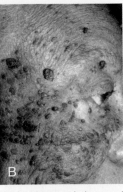

FIG. 22.14 Seborrheic keratosis. (A) A characteristic roughened, brown, waxy lesion that appears to be "stuck on" the skin *(inset)*. Microscopic examination shows an orderly proliferation of uniform, basaloid keratinocytes that tend to form keratin microcysts (horn cysts). (B) In individuals with darker skin, the lesions are often hyperpigmented and may cluster on the face and neck (dermatosis papulosa nigra). (B, From *Andrews' Diseases of the Skin*, 13e, Elsevier, 2020, Fig. 29.7.)

cryotherapy (superficial freezing) or topical agents is effective and safe.

Malignant Epidermal Tumors

Squamous Cell Carcinoma

Squamous cell carcinoma is a common tumor that typically arises on sun-exposed sites in older adults with lighter skin types. These tumors have a higher incidence in men than in women.

Pathogenesis. **Cutaneous squamous cell carcinoma is mainly caused by UV light exposure, which leads to widespread DNA damage and extremely high mutational loads** (Chapter 6). Patients with the rare disorder *xeroderma pigmentosum,* which disrupts repair of UV-induced DNA damage, are at exceptionally high risk. *TP53* mutations are common, as are activating mutations in *RAS* and loss-of-function mutations in genes encoding Notch receptors, which

transmit signals that regulate the orderly differentiation of normal squamous epithelia.

Immunosuppression, particularly in organ transplant recipients, is associated with an increased incidence of cutaneous squamous cell carcinomas, indicating that immune surveillance likely has an important role in limiting the development of this tumor. Other predisposing factors include oncogenic human papilloma viruses (in genital skin), industrial carcinogens (tars and oils), chronic non-healing ulcers, old burn scars, ingestion of arsenicals, and ionizing radiation.

MORPHOLOGY

Squamous cell carcinomas in situ appear as sharply defined **hyperkera-totic plaques or nodules** that range from erythematous to skin colored; some lesions appear to arise in association with prior actinic keratoses. Microscopically, squamous cell carcinoma in situ is characterized by highly atypical cells at all levels of the epidermis, with nuclear crowding and disorganization. More advanced, invasive squamous cell carcinomas are nodular, often scaly lesions that may ulcerate (Fig. 22.16A). Such tumors show variable degrees of differentiation, ranging from tumors with cells arranged in orderly lobules that exhibit extensive keratinization to neoplasms consisting of highly anaplastic cells with foci of necrosis and only abortive, single-cell keratinization (dyskeratosis) (Fig. 22.16B).

Clinical Features. Invasive squamous cell carcinomas of the skin are often discovered while they are small and easily resected. Approximately 4% will have metastasized to regional lymph nodes at diagnosis. The likelihood of metastasis is related to the thickness of the lesion, degree of invasion into the subcutis, and location, with higher risk being associated with lesions near the ear or the lips. Tumors arising from actinic keratoses may be locally aggressive but generally metastasize only after long periods of time, while those arising in burn scars, ulcers, and nonsun-exposed skin often behave more aggressively. Likely because of their high mutational burden, metastatic cutaneous squamous cell carcinomas are highly responsive to immune checkpoint inhibitor therapy, offering hope to the unusual patient who develops metastatic disease.

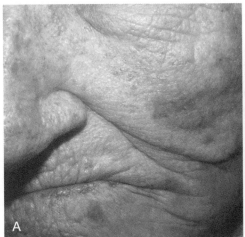

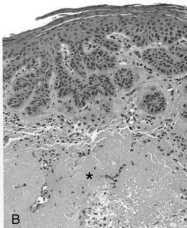

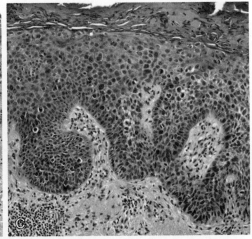

FIG. 22.15 Actinic keratosis. (A) Red, rough (sandpaper-like) lesions owing to excessive scale are present on the cheek and nose. (B) Basal cell layer atypia (dysplasia) with epithelial buds associated with marked hyperkeratosis, parakeratosis, and dermal solar elastosis *(asterisk)*. (C) Squamous cell carcinoma in situ lesion showing full-thickness epithelial atypia.

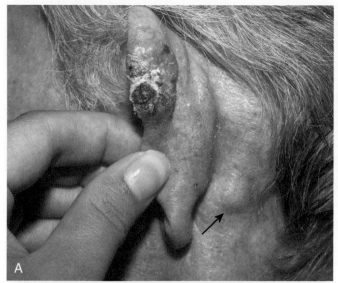

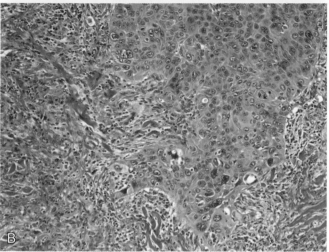

FIG. 22.16 Invasive squamous cell carcinoma. (A) A nodular, hyperkeratotic lesion occurring on the ear, associated with metastasis to a prominent postauricular lymph node *(arrow)*. (B) Tumor invades the dermal soft tissue as irregular projections of atypical squamous cells exhibiting acantholysis.

Basal Cell Carcinoma

Basal cell carcinoma is a common, slow-growing cancer that rarely metastasizes. It tends to occur at sites of chronic sun exposure and in individuals with lighter skin types.

Pathogenesis. **The molecular hallmark of basal cell carcinoma is loss-of-function mutations in *PTCH1*, a tumor suppressor gene that negatively regulates Hedgehog signaling; hence, tumors exhibit constitutive Hedgehog pathway activation.** Excessive activation of Hedgehog in turn activates a host of downstream genes implicated in cell growth and survival and other phenotypes linked to malignant transformation. In sporadic basal cell carcinoma, *PTCH1* mutations bear the telltale signs of UV light–induced DNA damage. The central role of increased Hedgehog signaling in basal cell carcinoma is emphasized by *Gorlin syndrome,* an autosomal dominant disorder caused by inherited defects in *PTCH1* that is associated with familial basal cell carcinoma as well as increased risk of odontogenic keratocystic tumors (Chapter 13) and medulloblastoma (Chapter 21).

The Hedgehog pathway is an important regulator of embryonic development, and patients with Gorlin syndrome also often have subtle developmental anomalies. Acquired mutations in *TP53* caused by UV light–induced damage are common in both familial and sporadic tumors.

MORPHOLOGY

Basal cell carcinomas manifest as a raised nodule or papule with irregular or rolled edges, sometimes ulcerated, often with prominent, dilated subepidermal blood vessels **(telangiectasia)** (Fig. 22.17A). While typically erythematous in individuals with lighter skin, some tumors, particularly those in individuals with darker skin, contain melanin pigment and can have an appearance similar to melanocytic nevi or melanomas (Fig. 22.17B). Microscopically, the tumor cells resemble the normal epidermal basal cell layer or germinative elements of hair follicles. Because they only arise from the epidermis or the follicular epithelium, they are not encountered on mucosal surfaces. Two common patterns are seen: **multifocal superficial growths** originating from the epidermis, and **nodular lesions,** which grow downward into the dermis as cords and islands of variably basophilic cells with hyperchromatic nuclei embedded in a fibrotic or mucinous stromal matrix (Fig. 22.17C). Tumor cell nuclei align (palisade) in the outermost layer the tumor cell nests, which tend to artifactually separate from the underlying stroma in tissue sections, creating a characteristic cleft (Fig. 22.17D).

Clinical Features. It is estimated that more than 1 million basal cell carcinomas are treated in the United States annually. By far the most important risk factor is cumulative sun exposure. Basal cell carcinoma is more common in warm southern regions of the United States, and its incidence is 40-fold higher in sunny climates near the equator, such as Australia, than it is in Northern European locales. Individual tumors are usually cured by local excision, but approximately 40% of patients develop another basal cell carcinoma within 5 years. Advanced lesions may ulcerate and extensive local invasion of bone or facial sinuses may occur if the tumor is neglected. Metastasis is rare. Hedgehog pathway inhibitors are used to treat locally advanced or metastatic tumors.

Melanocytic Proliferations

Melanocytic Nevi

Strictly speaking, the term *nevus* denotes any congenital lesion of the skin. *Melanocytic nevus,* however, refers to a benign congenital or acquired neoplasm of melanocytes. Melanocytic nevi are more common in individuals with lighter skin types.

Pathogenesis. **Melanocytic nevi are benign neoplasms caused by somatic gain-of-function mutations in *BRAF* or *RAS*.** Nevi are derived from melanocytes, pigment-producing cells with dendritic projections that are normally interspersed among basal keratinocytes. As previously discussed, *BRAF* encodes a serine/threonine kinase that lies downstream of RAS in the extracellular regulated kinase (ERK) pathway (Chapter 6). Experimental evidence suggests that unrestricted BRAF/RAS signaling initially induces melanocytic proliferation followed by senescence. How these opposing effects are coordinated is unclear, but it is believed that the "brake" on proliferation provided by senescence explains why very few nevi transform into malignant melanomas. Indeed, the growth and migration of nevus cells from the dermoepidermal junction into the underlying dermis is accompanied by morphologic changes that are consistent with cellular senescence (Fig. 22.18). Superficial nevus cells are larger and tend to produce

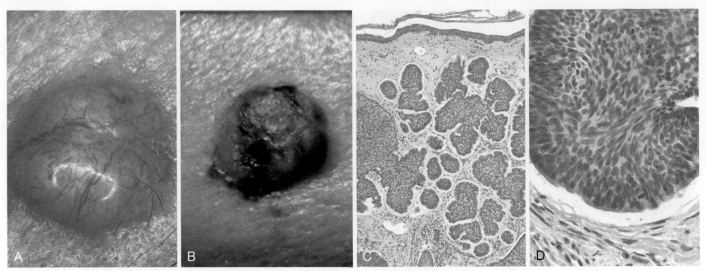

FIG. 22.17 Basal cell carcinoma. (A) On lightly pigmented skin, the lesion typically appears as smooth-surfaced, pearly papule with telangiectatic vessels. (B) On darker skin, the lesion often appears hyperpigmented. (C) Tumor is composed of nests of basaloid cells infiltrating a fibrotic stroma. (D) Tumor cells with scant cytoplasm and small hyperchromatic nuclei that palisade on the outside of the nest. The cleft between the tumor cells and the stroma is a highly characteristic artifact of sectioning. (B, Reproduced with permission from ©DermNet NZ www.dermnetnz.org 2022.)

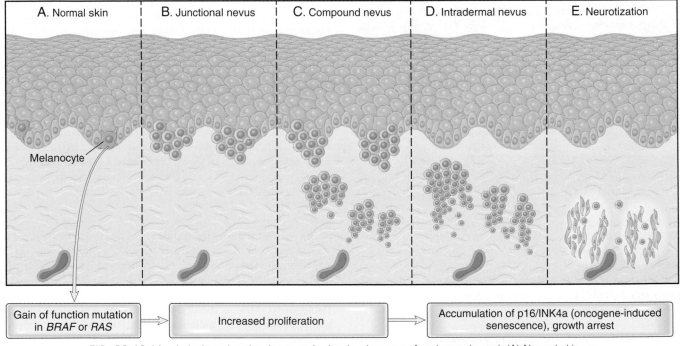

FIG. 22.18 Morphologic and molecular steps in the development of melanocytic nevi. (A) Normal skin uninvolved by nevi shows only scattered melanocytes. (B) An activating mutation in *BRAF* or *RAS* drives proliferation of junctional melanocytes, leading to the formation of a nevus. (C) Over time, nests of melanocytes may penetrate into the dermis, producing a compound nevus. (D, E). Subsequent accumulation of the tumor suppressor molecule p16 (also known as INK4a) appears to induce senescence, leading to permanent growth arrest and "maturation" of intradermal nevoid cells, a process referred to as "neurotization."

melanin pigment and grow in nests; deeper nevus cells are smaller, produce little or no pigment, and grow in cords or single cells. The deepest nevus cells have fusiform contours and grow in fascicles. This sequence of morphologic changes is of diagnostic importance, since they are absent in melanomas.

MORPHOLOGY

Common melanocytic nevi are tan-to-brown, uniformly pigmented, small papules (5 mm or less across) with well-defined, rounded borders (Fig. 22.19A). Early lesions are composed of cells with round, uniform nuclei, inconspicuous nucleoli, and little or no mitotic activity that grow in "nests" along the dermoepidermal

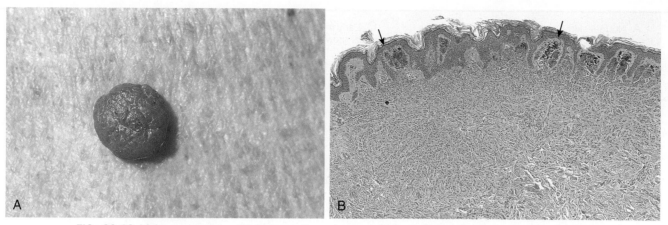

FIG. 22.19 Melanocytic nevus. (A) Melanocytic nevi are relatively small, symmetric, and uniformly pigmented. (B) A compound nevus composed of nests of heavily pigmented superficial melanocytes *(arrows)* and dermal melanocytes with little or no pigment.

junction. Such early-stage lesions are called **junctional nevi** (see Fig. 22.18). Eventually, most junctional nevi grow into the underlying dermis as nests or cords of cells **(compound nevi),** and in older lesions the epidermal nests may be lost entirely, creating **intradermal nevi** (Fig. 22.19B).

Clinical Features. There are numerous types of melanocytic nevi with varied appearances. Although these lesions are usually of only cosmetic concern, they may cause irritation or mimic melanoma, requiring their surgical removal. Compound and intradermal nevi are often more elevated than junctional nevi.

Dysplastic Nevi

Dysplastic nevi are most common in individuals with lighter skin types and may be sporadic or familial. The latter are important clinically because they identify individuals who have an increased risk of developing melanoma. As with conventional melanocytic nevi, activating *RAS* or *BRAF* mutations are commonly found in dysplastic nevi and are believed to have a pathogenic role.

Clinical Features. Unlike ordinary nevi, dysplastic nevi have a tendency to occur on body surfaces not exposed to the sun as well as on sun-exposed sites. *Familial dysplastic nevus syndrome* is strongly associated with melanoma, as the lifetime risk for the development of melanoma in affected individuals is close to 100%. In sporadic cases, only individuals with 10 or more dysplastic nevi appear to be at an increased risk for melanoma. Transformation of dysplastic nevi to melanoma has been documented, both clinically and histologically. However, such cases are the exception, as most melanomas appear to arise *de novo* and not from a preexisting nevus. Thus, the likelihood that any particular nevus, dysplastic or otherwise, will develop into melanoma is low, and these lesions are best viewed as markers of melanoma risk.

Melanoma

Melanoma is less common but much more deadly than basal or squamous cell carcinoma. The reported incidence of melanoma has increased dramatically over the past several decades, partly because of increasing exposure of at-risk individuals to UV light and partly because

MORPHOLOGY

Dysplastic nevi are larger than most acquired nevi (often more than 5 mm across) and may number in the hundreds (Fig. 22.20A). They are flat macules to slightly raised plaques, with a "pebbly" surface. They usually have variable pigmentation (variegation) and irregular borders (Fig. 22.20A, *inset*).

Microscopically, dysplastic nevi are mostly compound nevi that exhibit both architectural and cytologic evidence of abnormal growth. Nevus cell nests within the epidermis may be enlarged and exhibit abnormal fusion or coalescence with adjacent nests (bridging). As part of this process, single nevus cells begin to replace the normal basal cell layer along the dermoepidermal junction, producing so-called "**lentiginous hyperplasia**." Cytologic atypia consisting of irregular, often angulated, nuclear contours and hyperchromasia is frequently observed. Associated alterations also occur in the superficial dermis. These consist of a sparse lymphocytic infiltrate, release of melanin pigment that is phagocytosed by dermal macrophages (melanin incontinence), and linear fibrosis surrounding epidermal nests of melanocytes (Fig. 22.20B). These dermal changes are elements of the host response to these lesions.

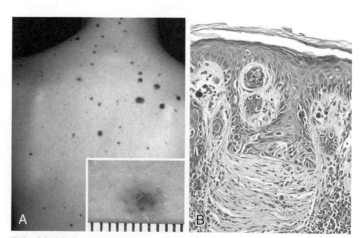

FIG. 22.20 Dysplastic nevus. (A) Numerous irregular nevi on the back of a patient with dysplastic nevus syndrome. The lesions are usually greater than 5 mm in diameter and have irregular borders and variable pigmentation *(inset).* (B) A characteristic feature is the presence of parallel bands of fibrosis in the superficial dermis.

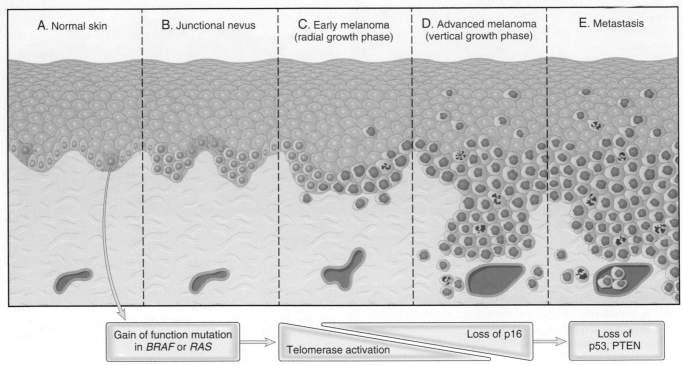

FIG. 22.21 Morphologic and molecular steps in the development of melanoma. (A) Normal skin shows only scattered melanocytes. (B) An activating mutation in *BRAF* or *RAS* drives proliferation of junctional melanocytes, a lesion that may take the form of a nevus. (C) Additional mutations, particularly mutations that activate telomerase expression, lead to transformation and development of early melanoma, which spreads laterally (radial growth phase). (D) Additional events such as the loss of the tumor suppressor p16 produces more invasive growth (vertical growth phase). (E) Metastatic spread is associated with acquisition of mutations that lead to loss of function of the tumor suppressors PTEN and p53.

of increased detection of early lesions due to vigorous surveillance. Today, as a result of increased public awareness of the earliest signs of skin melanomas, most melanomas are cured surgically.

***Pathogenesis.* As with other cutaneous malignancies, melanoma is mainly caused by UV light—induced DNA damage that leads to the stepwise acquisition of driver mutations.** The incidence is highest in sun-exposed skin and in geographic locales such as Australia, where sun exposure is high and much of the population is fair skinned. Intense intermittent sun exposure at an early age appears to convey the highest risk. Hereditary predisposition also plays a role in an estimated 5% to 10% of cases, as already discussed under familial dysplastic nevus syndrome. For example, germline mutations in the *CDKN2A* locus are found in as many as 40% of the rare individuals who suffer from familial melanoma. This complex locus encodes two tumor suppressors: p16, a cyclin-dependent kinase inhibitor that regulates the G_1-S transition of the cell cycle by maintaining the retinoblastoma tumor suppressor protein in its active state; and p14, which augments the activity of the p53 tumor suppressor by preventing its degradation (Chapter 6).

Key phases of melanoma development are marked by radial and vertical growth. The earliest recognizable phase of melanoma development is proposed to consist of lateral expansion of melanocytes along the dermoepidermal junction (lentiginous hyperplasia and junctional nevus; Fig. 22.21A—C). This then progresses to early melanoma, which is marked by a *radial growth phase* within the epidermis, often for a prolonged period (Fig. 22.21D). During this stage, melanoma cells do not have the capacity to invade and

metastasize. With time, a *vertical growth phase* supervenes, in which the tumor grows downward into the deeper dermal layers as an expansile mass lacking cellular maturation (Fig. 22.21E). This event is often heralded by the development of a nodule in a previously flat lesion and correlates with the emergence of metastatic potential.

DNA sequencing of familial and sporadic cases, including cases that appear to have arisen from benign nevi, has provided important insights into the molecular pathogenesis of melanoma (see Fig. 22.21). The initiating event appears to be an activating mutation in *BRAF* or (less commonly) *RAS*. In the vast majority of cases, this produces only a benign nevus unless other mutations are superimposed. Sequencing of nevi with "atypical" morphologic features suggestive of melanoma as well as melanomas in the radial phase of growth has shown that they commonly harbor mutations that activate the expression of telomerase, which is proposed to break senescence (the usual fate of benign nevi). With additional mutations or epigenetic aberrations that lead to loss of *CDNK2A* and its encoded tumor suppressor p16, the tumor shifts to the invasive vertical phase of growth. Throughout this cutaneous phase of tumor evolution, exposure to UV light adds to the mutational burden and increases the chances of tumor progression. Finally, with additional mutations in tumor suppressor genes such as *TP53* and *PTEN*, the tumor acquires the capacity for metastasis. This phase is marked by the appearance of aneuploidy and genomic copy number alterations, which add to the genetic heterogeneity of the evolving tumor.

By contrast, the less common melanomas that arise in non—sun-exposed acral and mucosal sites follow different molecular courses. One common initiating event in these tumors is a gain-of-function mutation in the KIT receptor tyrosine kinase gene. Similarly, melanomas arising in the uvea of the eye also have a distinct set of driver gene mutations, most notably mutually exclusive mutations that activate the GTP-binding proteins GNAQ or GNA11.

Melanomas that develop in sun-exposed sites have a high burden of mutations induced by UV light, some of which create neoantigens. It follows that for melanoma to develop, tumor cells must acquire the ability to either suppress or evade the host immune response. **The importance of immune evasion has been proven by the response of many advanced melanomas to immune checkpoint inhibitors, agents that unleash muzzled melanoma-specific T cells, allowing them to attack the tumor** (described later).

MORPHOLOGY

Unlike benign nevi, melanomas often exhibit **striking variations in pigmentation,** including shades of black, brown, red, dark blue, and gray (Fig. 22.22A). The **borders are irregular** and often "notched." Microscopically, malignant cells grow as poorly formed nests or as individual cells at all levels of the epidermis (pagetoid spread) and in expansile dermal nodules; these constitute the radial and vertical growth phases, respectively (Fig. 22.22B, C). Of note, superficial spreading melanomas are often associated with a brisk lymphocytic infiltrate (Fig. 22.22B), a feature that may reflect a host response to tumor-specific antigens. **Increasing thickness strongly correlates with worse biologic behavior.** By recording and using these and other variables in aggregate, accurate prognostication is possible.

Individual melanoma cells are usually considerably larger than nevus cells. Typically they have large nuclei with irregular contours, chromatin that is characteristically clumped at the periphery of the nuclear membrane, and prominent "cherry red" eosinophilic nucleoli (Fig. 22.22D). Immunohistochemical stains can be helpful in identifying metastatic deposits (Fig. 22.22D, *inset*).

Clinical Features. Although most of these lesions arise in the skin, they may also occur in the oral and anogenital mucosal surfaces, the esophagus, the meninges, and the eye. The incidence of cutaneous melanoma is inversely related to the extent of skin pigmentation.

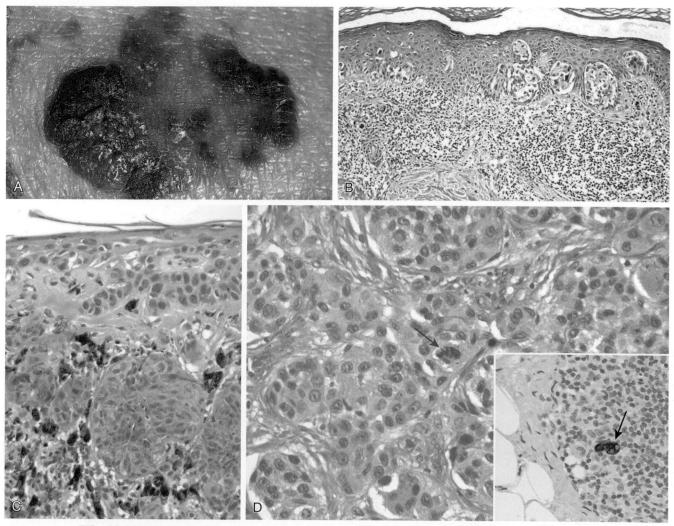

FIG. 22.22 Melanoma. (A) Lesions tend to be larger than nevi, with irregular contours and variable pigmentation. Macular areas indicate superficial (radial) growth, while elevated areas indicate dermal invasion (vertical growth). (B) Radial growth phase, with spread of nested and single melanoma cells within the epidermis. (C) Vertical growth phase, with nodular aggregates of infiltrating tumor cells within the dermis. (D) Melanoma cells with hyperchromatic irregular nuclei of varying size that have prominent nucleoli. An atypical mitotic figure is present in the center of the field *(red arrow).* The *inset* shows a sentinel lymph node containing a tiny cluster of metastatic melanoma *(arrow),* detected by staining for the melanocytic marker HMB-45.

While melanoma is more common in individuals of lighter skin types, melanoma does arise in individuals with darker skin types, most commonly on the sole (so-called acral melanoma), palm, or nail bed.

Cutaneous melanoma is usually asymptomatic; occasionally, pruritus is an early manifestation. The most important clinical sign is a change in the color or size of a pigmented lesion. The main clinical warning signs are as follows:

1. Rapid enlargement of a preexisting nevus
2. Itching or pain in a lesion
3. Development of a new pigmented lesion during adult life
4. Irregularity of the borders of a pigmented lesion
5. Variegation of color within a pigmented lesion

These principles are expressed in the so-called "ABCs" of melanoma: *a*symmetry, *b*order, *c*olor, *d*iameter, and *e*volution (change of an existing nevus). It is vital to recognize melanomas and intervene as rapidly as possible. The vast majority of superficial lesions are curable surgically, while metastatic melanoma often proves to be fatal.

The probability of metastasis is predicted by measuring the depth of invasion in millimeters of the vertical growth phase nodule from the top of the granular cell layer of the overlying epidermis (termed the *Breslow thickness*). Risk of metastasis is also increased in tumors with a high mitotic rate and in those that fail to induce a local immune response. When metastases occur, they may involve not only regional lymph nodes but also the liver, lungs, brain, and virtually any other site. Sentinel lymph node biopsy (of the first draining node[s] of a primary melanoma) at the time of surgery provides additional information on biologic aggressiveness.

Agents that selectively inhibit BRAF and KIT have produced dramatic responses in patients with metastatic tumors with *BRAF* and *KIT* mutations, respectively, although many tumors eventually recur due to the development of drug resistance. More recently, immune checkpoint inhibitors that augment host antitumor cytotoxic T-cell responses (Chapter 6) have been shown to be effective at stabilizing metastatic disease and in some instances causing remarkable tumor regression and even clinical remissions. Current treatment of advanced disease involves the use of combinations of different checkpoint inhibitors and targeted therapies such as BRAF inhibitors.

■ RAPID REVIEW

Inflammatory Dermatoses

- Many specific inflammatory dermatoses exist that are variously mediated by IgE antibodies *(urticaria),* antigen-specific T cells (*eczema, erythema multiforme,* and *psoriasis*), or trauma (lichen simplex chronicus).
- Underlying genetic susceptibility plays a role in atopic dermatitis and psoriasis.
- These disorders can be grouped based on patterns of inflammation (e.g., interface dermatitis in lichen planus and erythema multiforme).
- Clinical correlation is essential to diagnose specific skin diseases, since many have overlapping, nonspecific histologic features.

Blistering Disorders

- Blistering disorders are classified based on the level of the epidermis that is affected.

- These disorders are often caused by autoantibodies specific for epithelial or basement membrane proteins that lead to unmooring of keratinocytes (acantholysis).
- *Pemphigus* is associated with IgG autoantibodies to various intercellular desmogleins (part of the desmosome), resulting in bullae that are either subcorneal (pemphigus foliaceus) or suprabasal (pemphigus vulgaris).
- *Bullous pemphigoid* is associated with IgG autoantibodies to basement membrane proteins (part of the hemidesmosome) and produces a subepidermal blister.
- *Dermatitis herpetiformis* is associated with IgA autoantibodies to transglutaminase (as in celiac disease) and is characterized by subepidermal blisters.

Benign and Premalignant Epithelial Lesions

- *Seborrheic keratosis:* Round, flat plaques made up of proliferating monotonous epidermal basal cells, which sometimes contain melanin. Hyperkeratosis and keratin-filled cysts are characteristic.
- *Actinic keratosis:* Present on sun-exposed skin, these lesions show cytologic atypia in lower parts of the epidermis and infrequently progress to carcinoma in situ.
- Although both these lesions are associated with oncogenic mutations, malignant transformation is exceedingly rare in seborrheic keratoses and occurs in only a small subset of actinic keratoses.

Malignant Epidermal Tumors

- The incidence of both basal cell carcinoma and squamous cell carcinoma is strongly correlated with increasing lifetime sun exposure.
- Risk factors for cutaneous squamous cell carcinoma include fair skin, UV light exposure, oncogenic human papillomavirus, exposure to carcinogenic chemicals, chronic skin inflammation and scarring, and immunosuppression.
- Cutaneous squamous cell carcinoma has the potential for metastasis but is usually recognized and excised before it does so.
- Basal cell carcinoma, the most common malignancy worldwide, is a locally aggressive tumor associated with mutations in the Hedgehog pathway. Metastasis is very rare.

Melanocytic Lesions, Benign and Malignant

- Most *melanocytic nevi* have activating mutations in *BRAF* or less often *RAS,* but the vast majority do not undergo malignant transformation.
- Most sporadic *dysplastic nevi* are best regarded as markers of melanoma risk rather than premalignant lesions. They are characterized by architectural disorder and cytologic atypia.
- *Melanoma* is a highly aggressive malignancy; tumors only a few millimeters in thickness can give rise to deadly metastases.
- In most cases, melanoma progresses from an intraepithelial (in situ) to an invasive (dermal) form. Characteristics of the dermal tumor such as depth of invasion and mitotic activity correlate with survival.
- Melanoma occurring in sun-exposed skin is often associated with activating mutations in the BRAF serine-threonine kinase and is responsive to treatment with BRAF inhibitors and immune checkpoint inhibitors. As in other malignant tumors, melanomas develop by accumulation of mutations in several oncogenes (*BRAF* and *RAS*) and tumor suppressor genes (p16, *TP53,* and *PTEN*).

■ Laboratory Tests[a]

Test	Reference Values	Pathophysiology/Clinical Relevance
BP180 (BPAG2), BP230 (BPAG1) antibodies, serum	<20 RU/mL	BPAG1 and BPAG2 are molecules in the hemidesmosomes that anchor the basal epithelial cells to the basal lamina. They are the antigenic targets in bullous pemphigoid. Although BPAG1 and BPAG2 antibodies are present in most patients with bullous pemphigoid, a negative test does not exclude the disease. If clinical suspicion is high but the test is negative, a cutaneous immunofluorescent test is recommended. Antibody titer correlates with disease severity in some patients.
Deamidated gliadin IgG and IgA antibody, serum	Negative: <20.0 U Weak positive: 20.0–30.0 U Positive: >30.0 U	A test for tissue transglutaminase IgA antibody (see below) is the first line serologic test for patients with celiac disease and dermatitis herpetiformis. However, approximately 2% of patients with celiac disease (and a low fraction of those with dermatitis herpetiformis) are IgA deficient. In this setting, an alternative test for deamidated gliadin IgG antibody is used to identify patients with celiac disease and dermatitis herpetiformis. The sensitivity of this test is reduced if patients are on a gluten-free diet prior to testing.
Desmoglein 1/3 IgG antibodies, serum	<20 RU/mL	Desmoglein 1 (DSG1) and desmoglein 3 (DSG3) are adhesion molecules on cell surface desmosomes. DSG1 is distributed from the stratum corneum to the basement membrane, whereas DSG3 is limited to the lower portion of the epidermis. Autoantibodies to these proteins are seen in pemphigus foliaceus (DSG1) and pemphigus vulgaris (DSG3 and DSG1); they disrupt intercellular adhesions, leading to blistering.
Endomysial antibody, IgA, serum	Negative	IgA autoantibodies to the endomysium (connective tissue surrounding muscle cells) are elevated in 70% to 80% of patients with celiac disease or dermatitis herpetiformis. By comparison, antitissue transglutaminase (TTG) autoantibodies have a sensitivity and specificity of 90% to 98% and 95% to 97%, respectively; therefore, antiendomysial antibody testing is not a first-line test. It also is not useful in patients with IgA deficiency. Titer generally correlates with disease severity and declines with strict adherence to a gluten-free diet.
Tissue transglutaminase (TTG) IgA antibody, serum	<4.0 U/mL (negative) 4.0–10.0 U/mL (weak positive) >10.0 U/mL (positive)	TTG deamidates gliadin, which binds with increased affinity to HLA-DQ2 and DQ8 molecules on antigen presenting cells, leading to a CD4+ T-cell response. Enzyme-linked immunoabsorbant assay (ELISA) for IgA antiTTG autoantibodies is a sensitive and specific test for dermatitis herpetiformis (DH). Since it assesses the presence of IgA antibodies, it is negative in patients with IgA deficiency (about 2% of patients with celiac disease; less commonly in patients with DH). The test may be negative when patients are on a gluten-free diet and is useful in monitoring adherence to a gluten-free diet.

[a]The review of this table by Dr. Angad Chada, Department of Medicine, University of Chicago, is gratefully acknowledged.

References values from https://www.mayocliniclabs.com/ by permission of Mayo Foundation for Medical Education and Research. All rights reserved.

Adapted from Deyrup AT, D'Ambrosio D, Muir J, et al. Essential Laboratory Tests for Medical Education. *Acad Pathol.* 2022;9. doi: 10.1016/j.acpath.2022.100046.

INDEX

Pages followed by *b*, *t*, *f*, or *e* refer to boxes, tables, figures or online-only content, respectively.

A

AA protein, in amyloidosis, 178
AAA. *See* Abdominal aortic aneurysm
Aβ protein, in Alzheimer disease, 750–751, 751f
ABC. *See* Aneurysmal bone cyst
Abdominal aortic aneurysm (AAA)
　clinical consequences, 290
　inflammatory, 290b
　mycotic, 289–290
　risk for rupture of, 290
Abetalipoproteinemia, 509
ABL gene, 197
ABL proto-oncoprotein, 202
Abrasion, defined, 252b
Abscesses
　in acute pyelonephritis, 465b, 466f
　brain, 741–742, 742f
　"cold", 33
　crypt, 517b–518b
　defined, 40–41
　epidural, 745
　lung, 427, 427b
　ring, 332b
　stellate, 597b
Acantholysis, in pemphigus, 782b
Acanthosis, definition of, 776t
Acetaldehyde
　in alcohol metabolism, 246
　in ethanol metabolism, 246
Acetaminophen
　adverse reactions to, 249
　hepatotoxicity of, 546
　overdose of, 535, 536f
Achalasia, of esophagus, 490
Achondroplasia, 683
Acid aerosols, health effects of, 239t
Acinar cell injury, 574
Acinar cells, of pancreas, 572
Acinus, of lung, 404
Acquired immunodeficiency syndrome (AIDS),
　170–177
　central nervous system disease in, 176
　characteristics of, 170–177
　clinical features of, 175–177
　　effects of antiretroviral drug therapy,
　　176–177
　　opportunistic infections, 175–176
　　tumors, 176
　epidemiology of, 170–171
　morphology of, 177b
　pathogenesis of, 170
　transmission of, 170–171
　tuberculosis in patients with, 432–433
Acromegaly, 640
Actinic keratosis, 785–786
　clinical features of, 785–786
　morphology of, 785b, 786f
Activated partial thromboplastin time (aPTT),
　390t

Activation-induced cytosine deaminase (AID),
　220
Acute chest syndrome, in sickle cell anemia, 351
Acute coronary syndrome, 316, 317f
Acute kidney injury, causes of, 467
Acute lymphoblastic leukemia (ALL), 365–368
　clinical features of, 367–368
　flow cytometry results for, 367f
　genetics of, 366b–367b
　immunophenotyping of, 366b–367b
　morphology of, 366f, 366b–367b
　pathogenesis of, 365–367
Acute myeloid leukemia (AML)
　bone marrow aspirate of, 381f
　clinical features of, 367–368
　epigenetic alterations in, 365–366
　flow cytometry results for, 367f
　morphology of, 366b–367b
Acute-phase response, in inflammation, 46
Acute postinfectious glomerulonephritis, 454t,
　460–461
　clinical features of, 461
　morphology of, 460f, 460b
　pathogenesis of, 460
Acute respiratory distress syndrome (ARDS), 75,
　401–402
　alveoli in, 402f
　from burns, 253
　clinical features of, 402, 402.e1f
　DAD in, 403f
　inflammatory reaction in, 26t
　morphology of, 402b, 403f
　pathogenesis of, 401–402
Acute tubular injury (ATI), 467–469
　causes of, 467–469
　clinical features of, 469
　ischemic, 467
　morphology of, 469f, 469b
　nephrotoxic, 467
　pathogenesis of, 467–469, 468f
AD. *See* Alzheimer disease
ADA. *See* American Diabetes Association
ADAMTS13 activity, plasma, 390t
Adaptations
　cellular, 2
　pathologic, 17
　physiologic, 17
　to stress, 17–20
　　atrophy, 19
　　hyperplasia, 18–19
　　hypertrophy, 16f, 17–18
　　metaplasia, 19–20
Addison disease, 670–671
Adenocarcinoma in situ (AIS), of lung, 440b,
　440.e1f
Adenocarcinomas
　of appendix, 528
　of bladder, 591
　of cervix, 608

Adenocarcinomas (*Continued*)
　colon, 524–527
　　clinical features of, 525–527, 527f
　　epidemiology of, 524
　　morphology of, 525b, 526f–527f
　　pathogenesis of, 524–525, 526f
　colorectal, 521–523
　designation as, 188
　esophageal
　　clinical features of, 495
　　incidence of, 493–494
　　morphology of, 494f, 494b
　　pathogenesis of, 494
　　risk for development of, 493–494
　of fallopian tube, 614
　of female breast, 625
　gastric, 500–502
　　clinical features of, 501–502
　　epidemiology of, 501
　　morphology of, 501b, 502f
　　pathogenesis of, 501
　infiltrating ductal of pancreas of, 578
　poorly differentiated, 526–527, 527f
　of prostate, 588, 589f
　well-differentiated, 527f
Adenomas
　of appendix, 528
　classification of, 522b–523b
　colonic, 521–523
　colorectal, 521–523
　corticotroph, 640
　hepatocellular, 561, 562f
　lactotroph, 639–640
　morphology of, 522f, 522b, 523f, 523b
　parathyroid, 653b–654b
　pituitary, 638
　　abnormalities associated with, 639
　　classification of, 638, 639t
　　familial, 639
　　functioning or nonfunctioning, 638
　　monomorphism of, 639b, 640f
　　morphology of, 639b, 640f
　　nonfunctioning, 638, 641
　pleomorphic, 188, 488–489
　　defined, 488
　　incidence of, 488–489
　　morphology of, 488b, 489f
　somatotroph, 640
　of thyroid, 647–648
　thyrotroph, 641
Adenomatous polyposis coli (*APC*) gene, 208,
　209f, 523
Adenomyosis, 609
Adenosine deaminase (ADA), mutations in, 166
Adipocytes, 268
Adiponectin
　cancer and, 268
　metabolic effects of, 268
Adipose tissue, 268